Pharmaceutical Biotechnology

Daan J. A. Crommelin • Robert D. Sindelar
Bernd Meibohm
Editors

Pharmaceutical Biotechnology

Fundamentals and Applications

Fifth Edition

Springer

Editors
Daan J. A. Crommelin
Utrecht University
Utrecht
The Netherlands

Bernd Meibohm
College of Pharmacy
University of Tennessee
Health Science Center
Memphis, TN
USA

Robert D. Sindelar
Faculty of Pharmaceutical Sciences and The Centre for Health Evaluation & Outcomes Sciences (CHEOS)
The University of British Columbia (UBC)
Vancouver, BC
Canada

ISBN 978-3-030-00709-6 ISBN 978-3-030-00710-2 (eBook)
https://doi.org/10.1007/978-3-030-00710-2

This Springer imprint is published by the registered company Springer Nature Switzerland AG
The registered company address is: Gewerbestrasse 11, 6330 Cham, Switzerland

Contents

Preface

Over the past 30 years, the share of biotechnologically derived drug products in the arsenal of medicinal products has been growing steadily. These drug products include proteins, such as monoclonal antibodies, antibody fragments, endogenous or modified hormones, and growth factors, as well as antisense oligonucleotides, RNA, DNA preparations for gene therapy, and stem cell therapies. In 2017, 12 out of the 46 approved marketing authorizations for new molecular entities by the US Food and Drug Administration (FDA) were biotech products, mainly from the monoclonal antibody family (Mullard 2018). Drug products such as epoetin-α (Epogen®, Eprex®, Procrit®), interferon-α (Intron®A, Roferon®A) and interferon-β (Avonex®, Rebif®, Betaseron®), anti-TNF-α agents, etanercept (Enbrel®), infliximab (Remicade®), adalimumab (Humira®), bevacizumab (Avastin®), and trastuzumab (Herceptin®) are all examples of highly successful biotech drugs that have revolutionized the pharmacotherapy of previously unmet medical needs. And, last but not least, biotech drugs also have a major socioeconomic impact. In 2017, 7 of the 10 top selling drugs in the world were biotechnologically derived drug products, with sales varying between 5–16 billion US dollars, totaling 75 billion dollars. The revenues of biotechnology-based medication are annually growing at a 10% pace and will reach 300 billion US dollars in 2021, i.e., one third of the total global revenues for brand medicines in that year (IFPIA 2017).

The techniques of biotechnology are a driving force of modern drug discovery as well. Due to the rapid growth in the importance of biopharmaceuticals and the techniques of biotechnologies to modern medicine and the life sciences, the field of pharmaceutical biotechnology has become an increasingly important component in the education of today's and tomorrow's pharmacists and pharmaceutical scientists. We believe that there is a critical need for an introductory textbook on Pharmaceutical Biotechnology that provides well-integrated, detailed coverage of both the relevant science and clinical application of pharmaceuticals derived by biotechnology.

Previous editions of the textbook *Pharmaceutical Biotechnology: Fundamentals and Applications* have provided a well-balanced framework for education in various aspects of pharmaceutical biotechnology, including production, dosage forms, administration, economic and regulatory aspects, and therapeutic applications. Rapid growth and advances in the field of pharmaceutical biotechnology, however, made it necessary to revise this textbook in order to provide up-to-date information and introduce readers to the cutting-edge knowledge and technology of this field.

This fifth edition of the textbook *Pharmaceutical Biotechnology: Fundamentals and Applications* builds on the successful concept used in the preceding editions and further expands its availability as electronic versions of the full book as well as individual chapters are readily available and downloadable through online platforms.

The textbook is structured into two sections. An initial basic science and general features section comprises the first 17 chapters introducing the reader to key concepts at the foundation of the technology relevant for protein therapeutics, including molecular biology, production and analytical procedures, formulation development, pharmacokinetics and pharmacodynamics, immunogenicity, and chapters dealing with regulatory, economic, and pharmacy practice considerations and with evolving new technologies and applications. The second section (Chaps. 18–27) discusses the various therapeutic classes of protein biologics and nucleotide- and cell-based therapeutics.

All chapters of the previous edition were revised; some were completely overhauled and two added ("Analytical Toolbox" and "Therapeutic Proteins in Evidence-Based Practice"). The section on monoclonal antibodies is differentiated into a section on general considerations for this important class of biologics and sections focused on their application in oncology, transplantation, and inflammation in order to allow for a comprehensive discussion of the substantial number of approved antibody drugs (see above).

In accordance with previous editions, the new edition of *Pharmaceutical Biotechnology: Fundamentals and Applications* will have as a primary target students in undergraduate and professional pharmacy programs as well as graduate students in the pharmaceutical sciences. Additional important audiences are pharmaceutical scientists in industry and academia, particularly those that have not received formal training in pharmaceutical biotechnology and are inexperienced in this field.

We are convinced that this fifth edition of *Pharmaceutical Biotechnology: Fundamentals and Applications* makes an important contribution to the education of pharmaceutical scientists, pharmacists, and other healthcare professionals as well as serving as a ready resource on biotechnology. By increasing the knowledge and expertise in the development, application, and therapeutic use of "biotech" drugs, we hope to help facilitate a widespread, rational, and safe application of this important and rapidly evolving class of therapeutics.

Utrecht, The Netherlands — Daan J. A. Crommelin
Vancouver, BC, Canada — Robert D. Sindelar
Memphis, TN, USA — Bernd Meibohm

March 2019

REFERENCES

IFPIA (2017) The pharmaceutical industry and global health: facts and figures 2017. https://www.ifpma.org/wp-content/uploads/2017/02/IFPMA-Facts-And-Figures-2017.pdf

Mullard A (2018) FDA drug approvals 2017. Nat Rev Drug Discov 17:81–85

Abbreviations

α2-PI	α2-Plasmin inhibitor
γ-RV	Gamma retrovirus
μg	Micrograms
3D	Three-dimensional
4-OHT	4-hydroxytamoxifen
5-FC	5-Fluorocytosine
5-FU	5-Fluorouridine
AAV	Adeno associated virus
AAV2	AAV serotype 2
Ad	Adenovirus
ADA	Adenosine deaminase deficiency
ADA	Anti-drug antibodies
ADA	Adenosine deaminase
ADCC	Antibody-dependent cellular cytotoxicity
ADME	Absorption, distribution, metabolism, elimination
ADRs	Adverse drug reactions
AEX	Anion exchange
AF4	Asymmetrical flow field-flow fractionation
AHFS	American Hospital Formulary Service
AI	Artificial Intelligence
AIDS	Acquired immunodeficiency syndrome
aie	After initial entry into vial
ALL	Acute lymphoblastic leukaemia
AMD	Age related macular degeneration
APC	Activated protein C
APC	Antigen-presenting cell
APE1	Apurinic/apyrimidinic endonucleases from human
API	Active pharmaceutical ingredient
ART	Assisted reproductive technologies
ASO	Antisense oligonucleotide
ATF	Alternating tangential flow
ATMPs	Advanced therapy medicinal products
AUC	Area under the curve/analytical ultracentrifugation
BCA	Bicinchoninic Acid
BCG	Bacillus Calmette-Guérin
BCGF	B-cell growth factor
BCR	B-cell receptor
BDD-FVIII	B-domain deleted factor VIII
BFU	Bone marrow erythroid progenitor cells
BHK	Baby hamster kidney
BM	Bone marrow
BMP	Bone morphogenetic protein
BPCI	Biologics Price Competition and Innovation
BRMs	Biological (immune) response modifiers

BSA	Bovine serum albumin
BSE	Bovine spongiform encephalopathy
BSE/TSE	Bovine/transmittable spongiform encephalopathy, mad cow disease
BSI	British standards institution
CAPEX	Capital expenditures
CAR	Chimeric antigen receptor
CAR	Coxsackievirus and adenovirus receptors
Cas	CRISPR-associated proteins
Cas9	CRISPR-associated protein 9
CAT	Committee for advanced therapies
CBA	Cost-benefit analysis
CBER	Center for Biologics Evaluation and Research
CD	Circular dichroism spectroscopy
CD	Cluster of differentiation
CD	Crohn's disease
CD	Cytosine deaminase
cDNA	Copy or Complementary DNA
CDR	Complementarity-determining region
CE SDS	Capillary electrophoresis sodium dodecyl sulfate
CEA	Carcinoembryonic antigen
CEA	Cost-effectiveness analysis
CEX	Cation exchange
CF	Cystic fibrosis
CFR	Code of Federal Regulations
CFTR	Cystic fibrosis transmembrane conductance regulator
CG	Chorionic gonadotropin
CGH	Comparative genomic hybridization
cGMP	Current Good Manufacturing Practice
CHMP	Committee for Medicinal Products for Human Use
CHO cells	Chinese hamster ovary cells
CHO	Chinese hamster ovary
CIP	Clean-in-place
CK	Chemokines
CLL	Chronic lymphocytic leukemia
CM	Capacitance manometer
CMA	Cost-minimization analysis
CMA	Critical material attribute
CMC	Chemical, manufacturing and controls
CMS	US Centers for Medicare & Medicaid Services
CMV	Cytomegalovirus
COI	Cost of illness
COPD	Chronic obstructive pulmonary disease
COS	Controlled ovarian stimulation
CpG	Cytosine-phosphodiester-guanine
CPG2	Carboxypeptidase G2
CPP	Cell-penetrating peptide
CPP	Critical process parameters
CQA	Critical quality attribute
CRISPR	Cluster regularly interspaced short palindrome repeat
CSF	Cerebrospinal fluid
CSF-1R	Colony-stimulating factor 1 receptor
CT	Cholera toxin
CTI	Computed tomography imaging
CTL	Cytotoxic T lymphocyte
CTP	Carboxy terminal peptide

CUA	Cost-utility analysis
CXC	Chemokine (of the CXC chemokine family)
CZE	Capillary zone electrophoresis
DC	Dendritic cell
DCC	Dual-chamber cartridge
DC-Chol	3-β[N(NV,NV-dimethylaminoethane)-carbamoyl] cholesterol
DHHS	Department of Health and Human Services
DLBCL	Diffuse large B-cell lymphoma
DLS	Dynamic light scattering
DM	Diabetes mellitus
DMARD	Disease-modifying anti-rheumatic drugs
DMD	Duchenne's muscular dystrophy
DMSO	Dimethyl sulfoxide
DNA	Deoxyribonucleic acid
DNase I	Deoxyribonuclease I
DO	Dissolved oxygen
DOPE	Dioleoylphosphatidylethanolamine
DOTMA	2, 3-Dioleyloxypropyl-1-trimethyl ammonium bromide
Dox	Doxycycline
DP	Drug product
DS	Drug substance
DSB	Double-strand break
DSC	Differential scanning calorimeter
DSP	Downstream processing
dsRNA	Double-stranded RNA
E. coli	*Escherichia coli*
EC	European commission
EDF	Eosinophil differentiation factor
EDSS	Expanded disability status scale
EDTA	Ethylene diaminetetraacetic acid
EGF	Epidermal growth factor
EGFRvIII	Epidermal growth factor receptor variant III
EI	Electrospray ionization mass spec
ELISA	Enzyme-linked immunosorbent assay
ELSI	Ethical, legal, and societal issues
EMA	European Medicines Agency
EMBL	European Molecular Biology Laboratory
ENV	Envelope
Eo-CFC	Eosinophil-leukocyte Colony Forming Cell
EPAR	European Public Assessment Report
EPO	Erythropoietin
ESC	Embryonic stem cell
ESCF	Epidemiologic Study of Cystic Fibrosis
EU	European Union
EUTCD	European tissues and cells directive
FACS	Fluorescence-activated cell sorting
F-actin	Filamentous actin
FBS	Fetal bovine serum
Fc	Immunoglobulin constant region
FcRn	Neonatal Fc receptor
FCS	Fetal calf serum
FDA	Food and Drug Administration
FDC	Food, Drug, and Cosmetic
FE	Foregut endoderm
FEV_1	Mean forced expiratory volume in 1 s

FFF	Field-flow fractionation
FGF	Fibroblast growth factor
FGF2	Fibroblast growth factor-2
FIH	First in human
FISH	Fluorescence in situ hybridization
FMEA	Failure mode and effects analysis
FSC	Forward scatter
FSH	Follicle-stimulating hormone
FTET	Frozen-thawed embryo transfer
FTIR	Fourier- transform infrared spectroscopy
FVC	Forced vital capacity
FVIII, FIX etc	Factor VIII, factor IX etc
GAD	Glutamic acid decarboxylase
GAG	Group-specific antigen
GalNAc	N-acetylgalactosamine
GCP	Good clinical practice
G-CSF	Granulocyte colony-stimulating factor
GDP	Good distribution practice
GFP	Green fluorescent protein
GI	Gastrointestinal track
Gla	γ-Carboxyglutamic acid
GlcNAc	*N*-acetylglucosamine
GLP	Glucagon-1-like peptide
GLP	Good laboratory practice
GM-CSF	Granulocyte-macrophage colony-stimulating factor
GMO	Genetically modified organism
GMP	Good manufacturing practice
GSD II	Glycogen storage disease II
GSK-3β	Glycogen synthase kinase-3β
GST	Glutathione S-transferase
GTAC	Gene Therapy Advisory Committee
GTMP	Gene therapy medicinal product
GvHD	Graft versus host disease
GWAS	Genome-wide association studies
HAMA	Human antibodies to murine antibodies
HBsAg	Hepatitis B surface antigen
HBV	Hepatitis B virus
HCA	Human Cell Atlas
hCG	Human chorionic gonadotropin
HCP	Health care provider
HCT/P	Human cells, tissues, and cellular and tissue-based products
HCV	Hepatitis C virus
HDR	Homology-directed repair
HEK	Human embryonic kidney
HEK293	Human embryonic kidney cells 293
HER	Electronic health records
hESC	Human embryonic stem cell
HF	Hollow fiber
HGF	Hepatocyte growth factor
hGH	Recombinant human growth hormone
HGI	Human Genome Initiative
HGNC	Human genome nomenclature committee
HGP	Human Genome Project
Hib	Haemophilus influenzae type B

HIC	Hydrophobic interaction chromatography
HIV	Human immunodeficiency virus
HLA	Human leukocyte antigen
HMDB	Human Metabolome Database
HMP	Human Microbiome Project
HPLC	High-performance liquid chromatography
HPP	Human Proteome Project
HPV	Herpes virus
HPV	Human papilloma virus
HP-β-CD	2-Hydroxypropyl-beta-cyclodextrin
HSA	Human serum albumin
HSC	Hematopoietic stem cell
HSV	Herpes simplex Type-I
HSV-TK	Herpes simplex I virus thymidine kinase
HTS	High-throughput screening
HuBMAP	Human BioMolecular Atlas Program
HUPO	Human Proteome Organization
IBC	Institutional Biosafety Committees
IBD	Inflammatory bowel disease
ICH	International Conference on harmonisation
ICSI	Intracytoplasmic sperm injection
IEC	Ion-exchange chromatography
IEF	Isoelectric focusing
IFN	Interferon
IL	Interleukin
IL-6	Interleukin-6
IM	Intramuscular
IND	Investigational New Drug
INN	International Nonproprietary Name
IP	Intraperitoneal
iPSC	Induced pluripotent stem cell
IRB	Institutional Review Board
ITRs	Inverted terminal repeats
IU	International Units
IV	Intravenous
IVF	In vitro fertilization
JAK-STAT	Janus activated kinase, signal transducer and activator of transcription
J-Code	US reimbursement-related codes
kDa	Kilo dalton
kGy	Kilo gray
LAL	Limulus amebocyte lysis
LC	Liquid chromatography
LC/MS/MS	Liquid chromatography tandem mass spectrometry
LDL	Low-density lipoprotein
LH	Luteinizing hormone
LHRH	Luteinizing hormone-releasing hormone
LIF	Leukemia inhibitory factor
LLO	Listeriolysin O
LNA	Locked nucleic acid
LNGFR	Low affinity nerve growth factor receptor
LO	Light obscuration
LPLD	Familial lipoprotein lipase deficiency
LPS	Lipopolysaccharide

LT-α	Lymphotoxin alpha
LTRs	Long terminal repeats
LV	Lentivirus
LyE	Lethal lysis *gene E*
M cell	Microfold cell
MA(A)	Marketing authorization (application)
Mab	Monoclonal antibody
mAb	Monoclonal antibody
MACI	Matrix-assisted chondrocyte implantation
MACS	Magnetic-activated cell sorting
MALDI	Matrix-assisted laser desorption/ionization mass spec
MBP	Maltose-binding protein
MCB	Master cell bank
MCS	Multiple cloning site
M-CSF	Macrophage colony-stimulating facto
MDCK	Madin-Darby canine kidney
MDR	Multidrug resistance
MDS	Myelodysplastic syndromes
MDSCs	Myeloid derived suppressor cells
MGDF	Megakaryocyte growth and development factor
MHC	Major histocompatibility complex
MHCI	Major histocompatibility complex class I
MHCII	Major histocompatibility complex class II
MiRNA	Micro RNA
MIU	Million international units
mL	Milliliter
MMAD	Mass median aerodynamic diameter
MMR	Measles-mumps-rubella
MoA	Mode of action
MRI	Magnetic resonance imaging
mRNA	Messenger RNA
MS	Mass spectrometry
MSC	Mesenchymal stromal cell
MxA protein	Myxovirus resistance protein 1
NA	Not applicable
NCA	National competent authority
NCATS	US National Center for Advancing Translational Sciences
NCBI	National Center for Biotechnology Information
nc-RNA	Non-coding RNA
NDA	New Drug Application
NET	Neutrophil extracellular trap
NGF	Nerve growth factor
NGS	Next-generation genome sequencing
NHEJ	Non-homologous end-joining
NIH	National Institute of Health
NK	Natural killer
NMR	Nuclear magnetic resonance spectroscopy
NOR	Normal operating range
NS	Normal saline
NSCLC	Non-small-cell lung cancer
NTA	Nanoparticle tracking analysis
OAS	Oligoadenylate synthetase
OBA	Office of Biotechnology Activities
OBRR	Office of Blood Research and Review

OCTGT	Office of Cellular, Tissue and Gene Therapies
OHRP	Office for Human Research Protections
OOPD	Office of Orphan Products Development
OPEX	Operating expenditures
ORFs	Open reading frames
ORi	Origin of replication
OTAT	Office of Tissues and Advanced Therapies
OVRR	Office of Vaccines Research and Review
P4 Medicine	Preventative, predictive, personalized and participatory Medicine
PAI-1	Plasminogen activator inhibitor-1
PAM	Protospacer adjacent motif
PAMP	Pathogen-associated molecular pattern
PAP	Prostatic acid phosphatase
PAR	Proven acceptable range
PAS	Publicly available specification
PBM	Pharmacy benefits management
PBMCs	Peripheral blood mononuclear cells
PCR	Polymerase chain reaction
PCSK9	Proprotein convertase subtilisin/kinesin type 9
PD	Pharmacodynamics
PDA	Parenteral drug association
PEC	Pancreatic endotherm cell
PEG	Polyethylene glycol
PEI	Polyethyleneimine
PEI-β-CyD	Cyclodextrin-PEI-based polymer
PF	Posterior foregut
PFS	Prefilled syringe
pg	Picogram
PhRMA	Pharmaceutical Research and Manufacturers of America
PHS	Public Health Service
pI	Isoelectric point
PIC	Polyion complex
PK	Pharmacokinetics
PK/PD	Pharmacokinetic/pharmacodynamics
PLGA	Polylactic acid–polyglycolic acid
PLL	Poly (L-lysine)
PNA	Peptide nucleic acid
POL	Polymerase
polyA	Polyadenylation
poly-IC	Polyinosinic and polycytidylic acid
poly-ICLC	Polylysine-complexed poly-IC
PRCA	Pure red cell aplasia
PRR	Pathogen recognition receptor
PS	Phosphorothioate
PSMA	Prostate-specific membrane antigen
PTM	Post-translational modification
QA	Quality assurance
QALY	Quality-adjusted life-year
Qbd	Quality by design
QC	Quality control
QCM	Quartz crystal microbalance
QP	Qualified person
q-PCR	Quantitative PCR
R&D	Research & development

RAC	Recombinant DNA Advisory Committee
RCA	Replication-competent adenovirus
RCL	Replication-competent lentiviruses
rDNA	Recombinant DNA
REMS	Risk evaluation and mitigation strategies
RES	Reticuloendothelial system
RGD	Arginine-glycine-aspartic acid
rhIFNα-2b	Recombinant human interferon α-2b
rhIFNβ	Recombinant human interferon β
RISC	RNA-induced silencing complex
RLD	Reference Listed Drug
RNA	Ribonucleic acid
RNAi	RNA interference
RNP	Ribonucleoprotein
RPE	Retinal pigmented epithelial cells
RP-HPLC	Reversed-phase high-performance liquid chromatography
RSV	Respiratory syncytial virus
RSV	Rous sarcoma virus
RT	Reverse transcriptase
RT	Room temperature
RT-PCR	Reverse transcriptase polymerase chain reaction
RV	Retrovirus
SARS	Severe acute respiratory syndrome
SBGN	Systems Biology Graphical Notation
SBWFI	Sterile bacterial water for injection
SC	Subcutaneous
SCC	Single-chamber cartridge
SCF	Stem cell factor
SCID	Severe combined immunodeficiency
SCNT	Somatic cell nuclear transfer
SCPF	Stem cell proliferation factor
SCTMP	Somatic cell therapy medicinal product
SD	Standard deviation
SDF	Stromal cell-derived factor
SDF-1	Stromal cell-derived factor-1
SDR	Specificity determining residues
SDS-PAGE	Sodium dodecyl sulfate polyacrylamide gel electrophoresis
SDV	Single-dose vials
SEC	Size exclusion chromatography
SELEX	Systematic evolution of ligands by exponential enrichment
SERCA2a	Sarcoendoplasmic reticulum calcium-ATPase 2a
SIP	Steam-in-place
siRNA	Small interfering RNA
SIV	Simian immunodeficiency virus
SLE	Systemic lupus erythematosus
SLP	Synthetic long peptide
SLS	Static light scattering
SMase	Sphingomyelin phosphodiesterase
SNPs	Single-nucleotide polymorphisms
SOCS	Suppressors of cytokine signaling family
SPR	Surface plasmon resonance
SSC	Side scatter
ssRNA	Single-stranded RNA
STR	Short tandem repeat

SUB	Single-use bioreactor
SUF	Single-use fermentor
SV40	Simian viral 40
SWFI	Sterile water for injection
TALEN	Transcription activator-like effector nucleases
TALEs	TAL effectors
Tc	Collapse temperature
TCGA	The Cancer Genome Atlas
TCGF	T-cell growth factor
TCR	T-cell receptor
Te	Eutectic temperature
TEP	Tissue engineered product
Tet	Tetracycline
TetR	Tetracycline repressor
TF	Tissue factor
TFF	Tangential flow filtration
Tfh	Follicular helper cell
Tg	Glass transition temperature of (freeze-)dried product
Tg′	Glass transition temperature of frozen liquid
TGF	Transforming growth factor
TGF-β	Transforming growth factor beta
Th1	T-helper 1
Th2	T-helper 2
TIL	Tumor infiltration lymphocyte
TK	Thymidine kinase
TLR	Toll-like receptor
TNF	Tumor necrosis factors
TO%	Total relative uptake
t-PA	Tissue-type plasminogen activator
TPMT	Thiopurine methyltransferase
TPO	Thrombopoietin
TPP	Therapeutic protein product
TRE	Tetracycline response element
Treg	Regulatory T cell
TRF	T-cell replacement factor
tRNA	Transfer RNA
TSE	Transmissible spongiform encephalopathies
TSH	Thyroid-stimulating hormone
tTA	Chimeric tetracycline transactivator protein
TTR	Transthyretin
UF/DF	Ultrafiltration/diafiltration
UFH	Unfractionated heparin
UK	United Kingdom
UPDRS	Unified Parkinson's Disease Rating Scale
UPLC	Ultra performance liquid chromatography
US/USA	United States of America
USP	Upstream processing
UTR	Untranslated regions
UV	Ultraviolet
VEGF	Vascular endothelial growth factor
VLP	Virus-like particle
VLS	Vascular leak syndrome
VSV-G	Vesicular stomatitis virus-G
VWF	von Willebrand factor

WCB	Working cell bank
WGS	Whole-genome sequencing
WHO	World Health Organization
WT1	Wilms tumor protein 1
XNA	Xeno nucleic acids
ZFN	Zinc-finger nucleases
ZNF	Zinc finger nucleases

Contributors

David P. Allen Lilly Research Laboratories, Bioproduct Research and Development, Eli Lilly and Company, Indianapolis, IN, USA

Rita R. Alloway Division of Nephrology, Department of Internal Medicine, University of Cincinnati, Cincinnati, OH, USA

C. Andrew Boswell Preclinical and Translational Pharmacokinetics, Genentech Inc., South San Francisco, CA, USA

Jürgen Barth Justus-Liebig-Universität, Medizinische Klinik IV, Universitätsklinik, Giessen, Germany

John M. Beals Lilly Research Laboratories, Biotechnology Discovery Research, Eli Lilly and Company, Indianapolis, IN, USA

Ingrid Beierle Germantown, TN, USA

Erik Oude Blenke Department of Pharmaceutics, Utrecht Institute for Pharmaceutical Sciences, Utrecht University, Utrecht, The Netherlands

D. Bruce Baldwin Lilly Research Laboratories, Technical Services and Manufacturing Sciences, Eli Lilly and Company, Indianapolis, IN, USA

Amit Kumar Chaudhary Department of Pharmaceutical Sciences, College of Pharmacy, University of Nebraska Medical Center, Omaha, NE, USA

Shan Chung Bioanalytical Sciences, Genentech Inc., South San Francisco, CA, USA

Emile van Corven Bioceros, Utrecht, The Netherlands

Daan J. A. Crommelin Department of Pharmaceutics, Utrecht Institute for Pharmaceutical Sciences, Utrecht University, Utrecht, The Netherlands

Le N. Dao Clinical Pharmacology, Genentech Inc., South San Francisco, CA, USA

Michael R. DeFelippis Lilly Research Laboratories, Bioproduct Research and Development, Eli Lilly and Company, Indianapolis, IN, USA

Rong Deng Clinical Pharmacology, Genentech Inc., South San Francisco, CA, USA

Amit Garg Clinical Pharmacology, Genentech Inc., South San Francisco, CA, USA

Ashish Garg Lilly Research Laboratories, Bioproduct Research and Development, Eli Lilly and Company, Indianapolis, IN, USA

Sandhya Girish Clinical Pharmacology, Genentech Inc., South San Francisco, CA, USA

Andrea Hawe Coriolis Pharma, Martinsried, Germany

Karin H. Hoogendoorn Leiden University Medical Center, Hospital Pharmacy, Interdivisional GMP Facility, Leiden, The Netherlands

Wim Jiskoot Division of BioTherapeutics, Leiden Academic Centre for Drug Research (LACDR), Leiden University, Leiden, The Netherlands

Gideon F. A. Kersten Institute for Translational Vaccinology, Bilthoven, The Netherlands

Grzegorz Kijanka Division of BioTherapeutics, Leiden Academic Centre for Drug Research (LACDR), Leiden University, Leiden, The Netherlands

Atanas Koulov Analytical Development and Quality Control, Drug Product Services, Lonza AG, Basel, Switzerland

Michael Laird Division of Medical Affairs, Department of Bioprocess Development, Genentech Inc., South San Francisco, CA, USA

Robert A. Lazarus Department of Early Discovery Biochemistry, Genentech Inc., South San Francisco, CA, USA

Renato de Leeuw DeLeeuw Consultancy, Heesch, The Netherlands

Chunze Li Clinical Pharmacology, Genentech Inc., South San Francisco, CA, USA

Barbara Lippe Endocrine Care, Genentech Inc., South San Francisco, CA, USA

Alfred Luitjens Batavia Biosciences, Leiden, The Netherlands

Ram I. Mahato Department of Pharmaceutical Sciences, College of Pharmacy, University of Nebraska Medical Center, Omaha, NE, USA

Enrico Mastrobattista Department of Pharmaceutics, Utrecht University, Utrecht, The Netherlands

James P. McCormack Faculty of Pharmaceutical Sciences, University of British Columbia, Vancouver, BC, Canada

Holly B. Meadows Department of Pharmacy, Medical University of South Carolina, Charleston, SC, USA

Bernd Meibohm Department of Pharmaceutical Sciences, University of Tennessee Health Science Center, College of Pharmacy, Memphis, TN, USA

Alexander B. Meijer Department of Pharmaceutical Sciences, Utrecht Institute for Pharmaceutical Sciences, Utrecht University, Utrecht, The Netherlands

Koen Mertens Department of Pharmaceutical Sciences, Utrecht Institute for Pharmaceutical Sciences, Utrecht University, Utrecht, The Netherlands

Ronald S. Oosting Division of Pharmacology, Utrecht Institute for Pharmaceutical Sciences, Utrecht University, Utrecht, The Netherlands

Chad D. Paavola Lilly Research Laboratories, Biotechnology Discovery Research, Eli Lilly and Company, Indianapolis, IN, USA

Amit S. Patel Department of Pharmacy, University of Mississippi, Oxford, MS, USA

Department of Pharmacy, Medical Marketing Economics, LLC, Oxford, MS, USA

Juan Jose Pérez-Ruixo Department of Clinical Pharmacology, Janssen Research & Development, Beerse, Belgium

Sidney Pestka† PBL Interferon Source, Piscataway, NJ USA

Nicole A. Pilch Department of Pharmacy Practice and Outcomes Sciences, Medical University of South Carolina, Charleston, SC, USA

Wendy S. Putnam Clinical Pharmacology, Genentech Inc., South San Francisco, CA, USA

Theo Rispens Department of Immunopathology, Sanquin, Amsterdam, The Netherlands

Jean-Charles Ryff Biotechnology Research and Innovation Network, Basel, Switzerland

Tom Sam GlobalPharmCMC, Heesch, The Netherlands

Raymond M. Schiffelers Laboratory Clinical Chemistry & Haematology, University Medical Center Utrecht, Utrecht, The Netherlands

Vinod P. Shah VPS Consulting, LLC, North Potomac, MD, USA

Amarnath Sharma Clinical Pharmacology and Pharmacometrics, Janssen Research and Development, Spring House, PA, USA

Kartick P. Shirur Medical Marketing Economics, LLC, Oxford, MS, USA

Robert D. Sindelar Faculty of Pharmaceutical Sciences and The Centre for Health Evaluation & Outcomes Sciences (CHEOS), The University of British Columbia (UBC), Vancouver, BC, Canada

Global Drug Commercialization Centre (GDCC)-China and GDCC-worldwide, Chengdu, China

Bram Slütter Division of BioTherapeutics, Leiden Academic Centre for Drug Research (LACDR), Leiden University, Leiden, The Netherlands

Meina T. Tang Clinical Pharmacology, Genentech Inc., South San Francisco, CA, USA

Jeffrey S. Wagener† Department of Pediatrics, University of Colorado School of Medicine, Aurora, CO, USA

Hao Wu WuXi Biologics, a WuXi AppTec Affiliate, Shanghai, China

Yan Xu Clinical Pharmacology and Pharmacometrics, Janssen Research and Development, Spring House, PA, USA

Honghui Zhou Clinical Pharmacology and Pharmacometrics, Janssen Research and Development, Spring House, PA, USA

About the Editors

Daan J. A. Crommelin is Professor Emeritus, Department of Pharmaceutical Sciences, Utrecht Institute for Pharmaceutical Sciences at Utrecht University, Utrecht, the Netherlands, and Adjunct Professor in the Department of Pharmaceutics and Pharmaceutical Chemistry at the University of Utah, Salt Lake City, UT, USA.

Robert D. Sindelar is Professor and former Dean of the Faculty of Pharmaceutical Sciences and the Centre for Health Evaluation & Outcomes Sciences (CHEOS) at the University of British Columbia (UBC), Vancouver, BC, Canada, and President of Global Drug Commercialization Centre (GDCC)-China and GDCC-worldwide, Chengdu, China.

Bernd Meibohm is Professor of Pharmaceutical Sciences and Associate Dean for Research and Graduate Programs at the University of Tennessee Health Science Center, Memphis, TN, USA.

1

Molecular Biotechnology: From DNA Sequence to Therapeutic Protein

Ronald S. Oosting

INTRODUCTION

Proteins are already used for more than 100 years to treat or prevent diseases in humans. It started in the early 1890s with "serum therapy" for the treatment of diphtheria and tetanus by Emile von Behring and others. The antiserum was obtained from immunized rabbits and horses. Behring received the Nobel Prize for Medicine in 1901 for this pioneering work on passive immunization. A next big step in the development of therapeutic proteins was the use of purified insulin isolated from pig or cow pancreas for the treatment of diabetes type I in the early 1920s by Banting and Best (in 1923 Banting received the Nobel Prize for this work). Soon after the discovery of insulin, the pharmaceutical company Eli Lilly started large-scale production of the pancreatic extracts for the treatment of diabetes. Within 3 years after the start of the experiments by Banting, already enough animal-derived insulin was produced to supply the entire North American continent. Compare this to the present average time-to-market of a new drug (from discovery to approval) of 13.5 years (Paul et al. 2010). Note: Both the European Medicines Agency (EMA) and the US Food and Drug Administration (FDA) have accelerated approval procedures to speed up the market introduction of new drugs with "meaningful advantages" over the available therapies.

Thanks to advances in biotechnology (e.g., recombinant DNA technology, hybridoma technology), we have moved almost entirely away from animal-derived proteins to proteins with the complete human amino acid sequence.

Such therapeutic human proteins are less likely to cause side effects and to elicit immune responses. Banting and Best were very lucky. They had no idea about possible sequence or structural differences between human and porcine/bovine insulin. Nowadays, we know that porcine insulin differs only by one amino acid from the human sequence and bovine insulin differs by three amino acids (see Fig. 1.1). Thanks to this high degree of sequence conservation, porcine/bovine insulin can be used to treat human patients. In 1982, human insulin became the first recombinant human protein approved for sale in the USA (also produced by Eli Lilly) (cf. Chap. 16). Since then a large number of biopharmaceuticals have been developed. There are now several hundreds of human proteins marketed for a wide range of therapeutic areas.

PHARMACEUTICAL BIOTECHNOLOGY, WHY THIS BOOK, WHY THIS CHAPTER?

In this book we define pharmaceutical biotechnology as all technologies needed to produce biopharmaceuticals (other than (non-genetically modified) animal- or human blood-derived medicines). Attention is paid both to these technologies and the products thereof. Biotechnology makes use of findings from various research areas, such as molecular biology, biochemistry, cell biology, genetics, bioinformatics, microbiology, bioprocess engineering, and separation technologies. Progress in these fields has been and will remain a major driver for the development of new biopharmaceuticals. Biopharmaceuticals form a fast-growing segment in the world of medicines opening new therapeutic options for patients with severe diseases. This success is also reflected by the fast growth in global sales.

Until now biopharmaceuticals are primarily proteins, but therapeutic DNA or RNA based molecules (think about gene therapy products, DNA vaccines, and RNA interference-based products; Chaps. 14, 15, and 16, respectively) may soon become part of our therapeutic arsenal.

Therapeutic proteins differ in many aspects from classical, small molecule drugs. They differ in size, composition, production, purification, contaminations, side

R. S. Oosting (✉)
Division of Pharmacology, Utrecht Institute for Pharmaceutical Sciences, Utrecht University, Utrecht, The Netherlands
e-mail: r.s.oosting@uu.nl

D. J. A. Crommelin et al. (eds.), *Pharmaceutical Biotechnology*, https://doi.org/10.1007/978-3-030-00710-2_1

a

```
                 signal peptide                          beta chain
human     MALWMRLLPLLALLALWGPDPAAAFVNQHLCGSHLVEALYLVCGERGFFYTPKTRREAED
porcine   MALWTRLLPLLALLALWAPAPAQAFVNQHLCGSHLVEALYLVCGERGFFYTPKARREAEN
bovine    MALWTRLAPLLALLALWAPAPARAFVNQHLCGSHLVEALYLVCGERGFFYTPKARREVEG
          **** ** *********.* ** ****************************:***.*
                                         alpha chain
human     LQVGQVELGGGPGAGSLQPLALEGSLQKRGIVEQCCTSICSLYQLENYCN
porcine   PQAGAVELGGGLG--GLQALALEGPPQKRGIVEQCCTSICSLYQLENYCN
bovine    PQVGALELAGGPG-----AGGLEGPPQKRGIVEQCCASVCSLYQLENYCN
           *.* :**.** *       .***  **********:*:***********
```

b

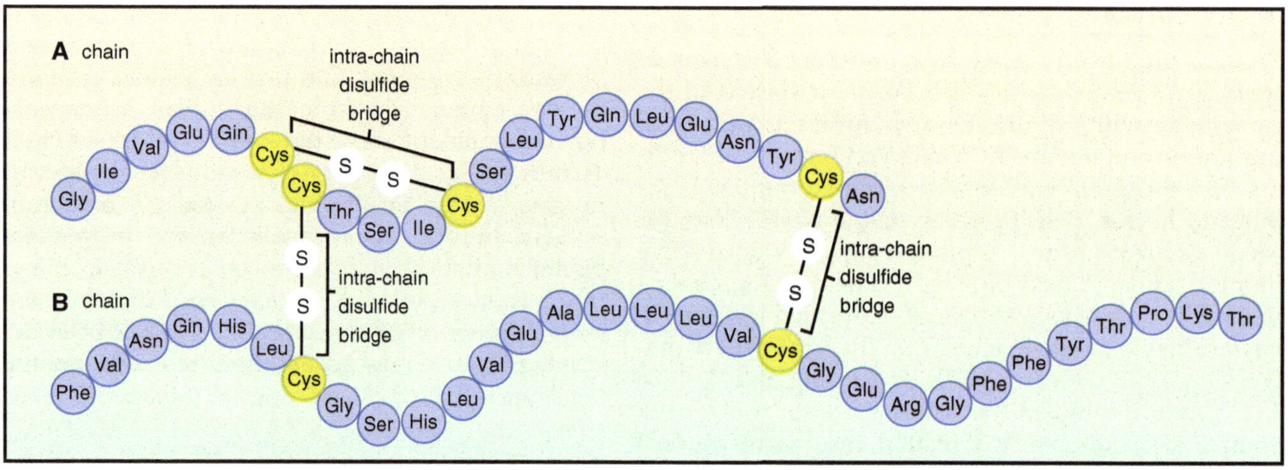

Figure 1.1 ■ (**a**) Multiple alignment (http://www.ebi.ac.uk/Tools/msa/clustalw2) of the amino acid sequences of human, porcine, and bovine preproinsulin. (*): identical residue. (**b**) Schematic drawing of the structure of insulin. The alpha and beta chain are linked by two disulfide bridges. Both the one-letter and three-letter codes for the amino acids are used in this figure: alanine (Ala, A), arginine (Arg, R), asparagine (Asn, N), aspartic acid (Asp, D), cysteine (Cys, C), glutamic acid (Glu, E), glutamine (Gln, Q), glycine (Gly, H), histidine (His, H), isoleucine (Ile, I), leucine (Leu, L), lysine (Lys, K), methionine (Met, M), phenylalanine (Phe, F), proline (Pro, P), serine Sser, S), threonine (Thr, T), tryptophan (Trp,W), tyrosine (Tyr, Y), and valine (Val, V) (**b** is taken from Wikipedia)

effects, stability, formulation, regulatory aspects, etc. These fundamental differences justify paying attention to therapeutic proteins as a family of medicines. These general aspects are discussed in the first 17 chapters of this book. After those general topics, the different families of biopharmaceuticals are dealt with in detail. This first chapter should be seen as a chapter where many of the basic elements of the selection, design, and production of biopharmaceuticals are touched upon. For in detail information the reader is referred to relevant literature and other chapters in this book.

ECONOMICS AND USE

Newly introduced biopharmaceuticals are very expensive. This is partly due to the high development costs (Paul et al. 2010), combined with high -initial- production costs and, for many therapeutic proteins, a relatively low number of patients. In addition, the relatively high price of (bio)pharmaceuticals is also due to too many failures during the drug discovery and development process. The few products that actually reach the market have to compensate for all the expenses made for failed products. For a monoclonal antibody, the probability to proceed from the preclinical discovery stage into the market is around 17% (for small molecule drugs the probability of success is even lower, ~7%). Economic aspects of biopharmaceuticals are discussed in Chap. 11.

As mentioned above, the number of patients for many marketed therapeutic proteins is relatively small. This has several reasons. The high price of therapeutic proteins makes that they are used primarily for the treatment of the relative severe cases. The specificity of many therapeutic proteins makes that they are only effective in subgroups of patients (personalized medicine). This is in particular true for the monoclonal antibodies used to treat cancer patients. For instance, the antibody trastuzumab (Herceptin®) is only approved for breast cancer patients with high expression levels of the HER2 receptor on the tumor cells (±20% of breast cancer cases). Other examples from the cancer field are the monoclonal antibodies cetuximab and panitumumab for the treatment of metastatic colorectal cancer. Both antibodies target the epidermal growth factor (EGF) receptor. Successful treatment of a patient with one of these monoclonal antibodies depends on (1) the presence of the EGF receptor on the tumor and (2) the absence of mutations in signaling proteins downstream of the EGF receptor (KRAS and BRAF). Mutations in downstream signaling proteins cause the tumor to grow independently from the EGF receptor and make the tumor nonresponsive to the antagonistic monoclonal antibodies.

Some diseases are very rare and thus the number of patients is very small. Most of these rare diseases are due to a genetic defect. Examples are cystic fibrosis (CF) and glycogen storage disease II (GSD II). CF is most common in Caucasians. In Europe 1:2000–3000 babies are affected annually. GSD II is even rarer. It affects 1:140,000 newborns. The effects of GSD II can be reduced by giving the patients recombinant myozyme. It is clear that developing a drug for such a small patient population is commercially not very interesting. To booster drug development for the rare diseases (known as orphan drugs and orphan diseases) specific legislation exists in the USA, Europe and Japan. These programs are very successful. It is expected that the orphan drug (both biopharmaceuticals and small molecule drugs) market will almost double between 2016 and 2022 ($209 bn in 2022, EvaluatePharma 2017).

FROM AN IN SILICO DNA SEQUENCE TO A THERAPEUTIC PROTEIN

We will discuss now the steps and methods needed to select, design, and produce a recombinant therapeutic protein (see also Fig. 1.2). We will not discuss in detail the underlying biological mechanisms. The reader is referred to Box 1.1, for a short description of the central dogma of molecular biology, which describes the flow of information from DNA via RNA into a protein.

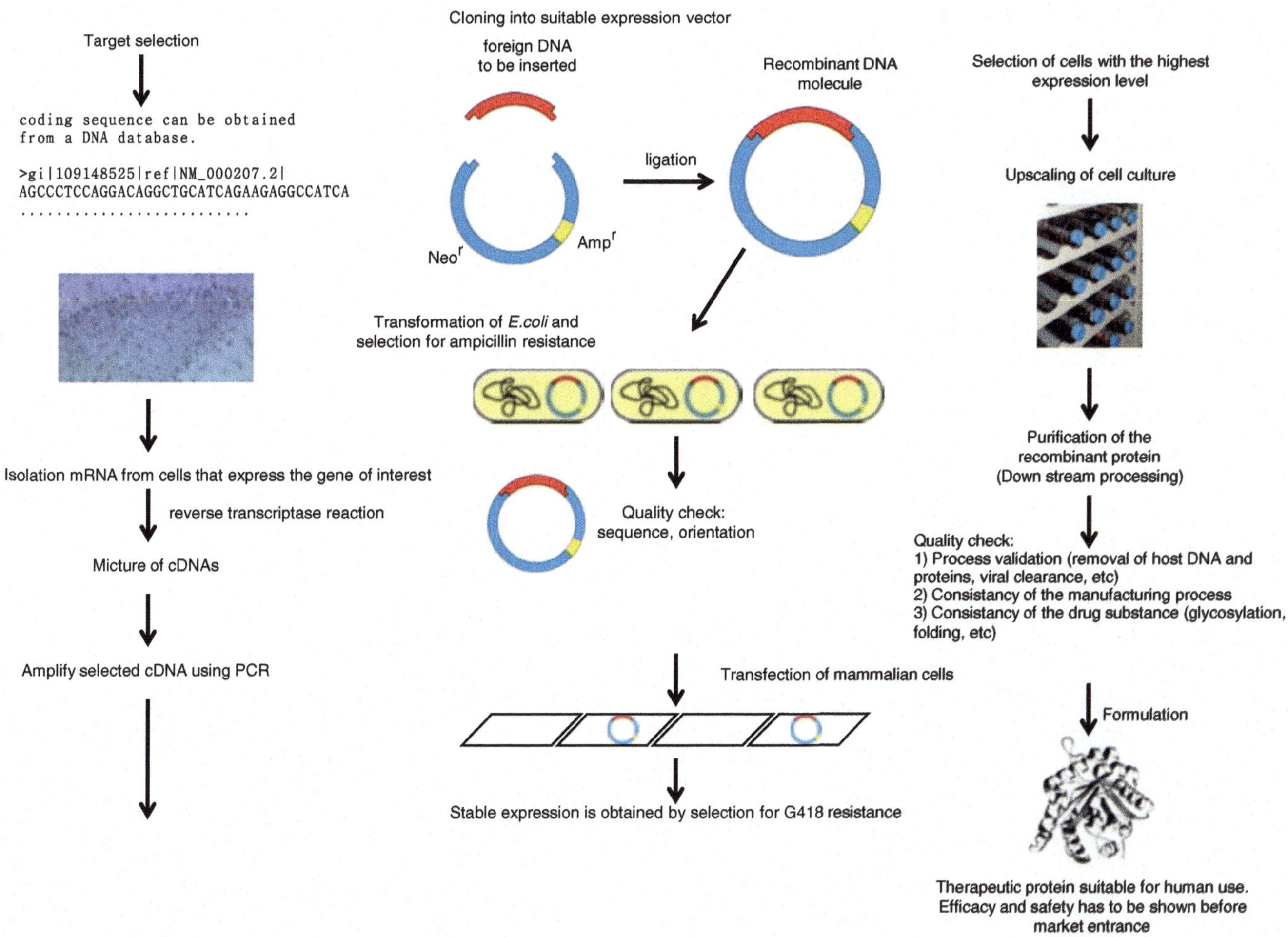

Figure 1.2 ■ Schematic representation of all the steps required to produce a therapeutic protein. *cDNA* copy DNA, *PCR* polymerase chain reaction

a

```
>gi|109148525|ref|NM_000207.2| Homo sapiens insulin (INS), transcript
variant 1, mRNA
5'AGCCCTCCAGGACAGGCTGCATCAGAAGAGGCCATCAAGCAGATCACTGTCCTTCTGCCATGGCCCTGT
GGATGCGCCTCCTGCCCCTGCTGGCGCTGCTGGCCCTCTGGGGACCTGACCCAGCCGCAGCCTTTGTGAAC
CAACACCTGTGCGGCTCACACCTGGTGGAAGCTCTCTACCTAGTGTGCGGGGAACGAGGCTTCTTCTACAC
ACCCAAGACCCGCCGGGAGGCAGAGGACCTGCAGGTGGGGCAGGTGGAGCTGGGCGGGGGCCCTGGTGCAG
GCAGCCTGCAGCCCTTGGCCCTGGAGGGGTCCCTGCAGAAGCGTGGCATTGTGGAACAATGCTGTACCAGC
ATCTGCTCCCTCTACCAGCTGGAGAACTACTGCAACTAGACGCAGCCCGCAGGCAGCCCCACACCCGCCGC
CTCCTGCACCGAGAGAGATGGAATAAAGCCCTTGAACCAGCAAAA 3'
```

b

```
>gi|4557671|ref|NP_000198.1| insulin preproprotein [Homo sapiens]
(NH2)MALWMRLLPLLALLALWGPDPAAAFVNQHLCGSHLVEALYLVCGERGFFYTPKTRREAEDLQVGQV
ELGGGPGAGSLQPLALEGSLQKRGIVEQCCTSICSLYQLENYCN-(COOH)
```

Figure 1.3 ■ DNA sequences are always written from the 5′ → 3′ direction and proteins sequences from the amino-terminal to the carboxy-terminal. (**a**) nucleotide code, (**b**) amino acid code, see legend to Fig. 1.1

■ Selection of a Therapeutic Protein

The selection of what protein should be developed for a treatment of a particular disease is often challenging, with lots of uncertainties. This is why most big pharmaceutical companies only become interested in a certain product when there is some clinical evidence that the new product actually works and that it is safe. This business model gives opportunities for startup biotech companies and venture capitalists to engage in this important early development process.

Sometimes the choice for a certain protein as a therapeutic drug is very simple. Think, for instance, about replacement of endogenous proteins such as insulin and erythropoietin for the treatment of diabetes type I and anemia, respectively. For many other diseases it is much more difficult to identify an effective therapeutic protein or target. For instance, an antibody directed against a growth factor receptor on a tumor cell may look promising based on *in vitro* and animal research but may be largely ineffective in human cancer patients.

It is beyond the scope of this chapter to go further into the topic of therapeutic protein and target discovery. For further information the reader is referred to the large number of scientific papers on this topic, as can be searched using PubMed (http://www.ncbi.nlm.nih.gov/pubmed).

In the rest of this chapter, we will mainly focus on a typical example of the steps in the molecular cloning process and production of a therapeutic protein. At the end of this chapter, we will briefly discuss the cloning and large-scale production of monoclonal antibodies (see also Chap. 8).

Molecular cloning is defined as the assembly of recombinant DNA molecules (most often from two different organisms) and their replication within host cells.

■ DNA Sequence

The DNA, mRNA, and amino acid sequence of every protein in the human genome can be obtained from publicly available gene and protein databases, such as those present at the National Center for Biotechnology Information (NCBI) in the USA and the European Molecular Biology Laboratory (EMBL). Their websites are http://www.ncbi.nlm.nih.gov/ and http://www.ebi.ac.uk, respectively.

DNA sequences in these databases are always given from the 5′ end to the 3′ end and protein sequences from the amino- to the carboxy-terminal end (see Fig. 1.3). These databases also contain information about the gene (e.g., exons, introns, and regulatory sequences. See Box 1.1 for explanations of these terms) and protein structure (domains, specific sites, posttranslation modifications, etc.). The presence or absence of certain posttranslational modifications determines what expression hosts (e.g., *Escherichia coli* (*E. coli*), yeast, or a mammalian cell line) may be used (see below).

■ Selection of Expression Host

Recombinant proteins can be produced in *E. coli*, yeast, plants (e.g., rice and tomato), mammalian cells, and even by transgenic animals. All these expression hosts have different pros and cons (see Chap. 4 for more details).

Most marketed therapeutic proteins are produced in cultured mammalian cells. In particular Chinese hamster ovary (CHO) cells are used (more than 70% of marketed proteins are produced in CHO cells). On first sight, mammalian cells are not a logical choice. They are much more difficult to culture than, for instance, bacteria or yeast. On average, mammalian cells divide only once every 24 h, while cell division in *E. coli* takes ~30 min and in yeast ~1 h. In addition, mammalian cells need expensive growth media and in many cases bovine (fetal) serum as a source of growth factors (see Table 1.1 for a comparison of the various expression systems). Since the outbreak of the bovine or transmissible spongiform encephalopathy epidemic (BSE/TSE, better known as mad cow disease) in cattle in the United Kingdom, the use of bovine serum for the production of therapeutic proteins is considered a safety risk by the

	Prokaryotes *E. coli*	Yeast *Pichia pastoris Saccharomyces cerevisiae*	Mammalian cells (e.g., CHO or HEK293 cells)
+	Easy manipulation Rapid growth Large-scale fermentation Simple media High yield	Grows relatively rapidly Large-scale fermentation Performs some posttranslational modifications	May grow in suspension, perform all required posttranslational modifications
–	Proteins may not fold correctly or may even aggregate (inclusion bodies) Almost no posttranslational modifications	Posttranslational modifications may differ from humans (especially glycosylation)	Slow growth Expensive media Difficult to scale up Dependence on serum (BSE)

Table 1.1 ■ Pros and cons of different expression hosts

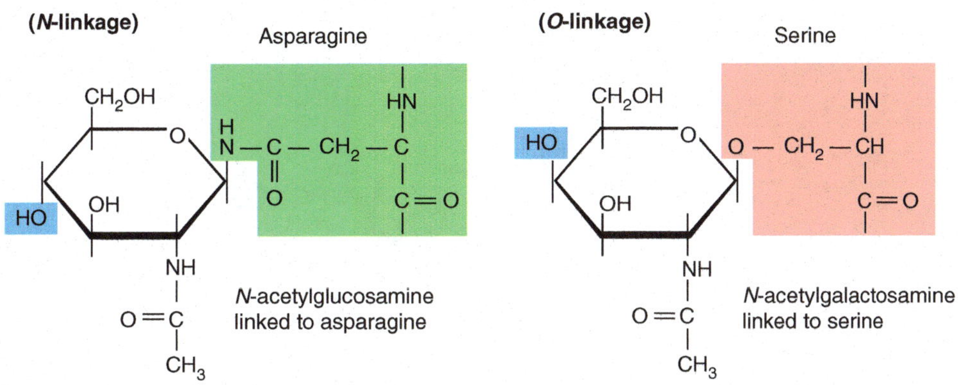

Figure 1.4 ■ Glycosylation takes place either at the nitrogen atom in the side chain of asparagine (N-linked) or at the oxygen atom in the side chain of serine or threonine. Glycosylation of asparagine takes place only when this residue is part of an Asn-X-Ser or Ans-X-Thr (X can be any residue except proline). Not all potential sites are glycosylated. Which sites become glycosylated depends also on the protein structure and on the cell type in which the protein is expressed

regulatory authorities (such as the EMA in Europe and the FDA in the USA). To minimize the risk of transmitting TSE via a medicinal product, bovine serum has to be obtained from animals in countries with the lowest possible TSE risk, e.g., the USA, Australia, and New Zealand. Because of the inherent risk of using animal-derived products, serum-free culture media containing recombinant growth factors, are increasingly used.

The main reason why mammalian cells are used as production platform for therapeutic proteins is that in these cells posttranslational modification (PTM) of the synthesized proteins resembles most closely the human situation. An important PTM is the formation of disulfide bonds between two cysteine moieties. Disulfide bonds are crucial for stabilizing the tertiary structure of a protein. Wild type *E.coli* is only able to produce disulfide bonds in the periplasm, the space between the inner cytoplasmic membrane and the bacterial outer membrane. Cytosolic expression of recombinant protein in *E.coli* is needed for high level expression and proper folding. By knocking out two major reducing enzymes: thioredoxin reductase and glutathione reductase, *E.coli* strains have been produced that are able to express disulfide bonds. Unfortunately, the yield of recombinant disulfide bonded proteins by such strains are usually low. However, new developments in this area are very promising (e.g., co-expression of the disulfide bonded protein with sulfhydryl oxidase and disulfide bond isomerase, see Gaciarz et al. 2017) and may ultimately result in an *E.coli*-based expression system suited for high level expression of therapeutic proteins with disulfide bonds.

Another important PTM of therapeutic proteins is glycosylation. Around 70% of all marketed therapeutic proteins, including monoclonal antibodies, are glycosylated. Glycosylation is the covalent attachment of oligosaccharides to either asparagine (N-linked) or serine/threonine (O-linked) (see Fig. 1.4). The oligosaccharide moiety of a therapeutic protein affects many of its pharmacological properties, including stability, solubility, bioavailability, in vivo activity, pharmacokinetics, and immunogenicity. Glycosylation differs between species, between different cell types within a species, and even between batches of in cell culture produced therapeutic proteins. N-linked glycosylation is found in all eukaryotes (and also in some bacteria, but not in wildtype *E. coli*; see Nothaft and Szymanski 2010) and takes place in the lumen of the endoplasmatic reticulum and the Golgi system (see Fig. 1.5). All N-linked oligosaccharides have a common pentasaccharide core containing three mannose and two

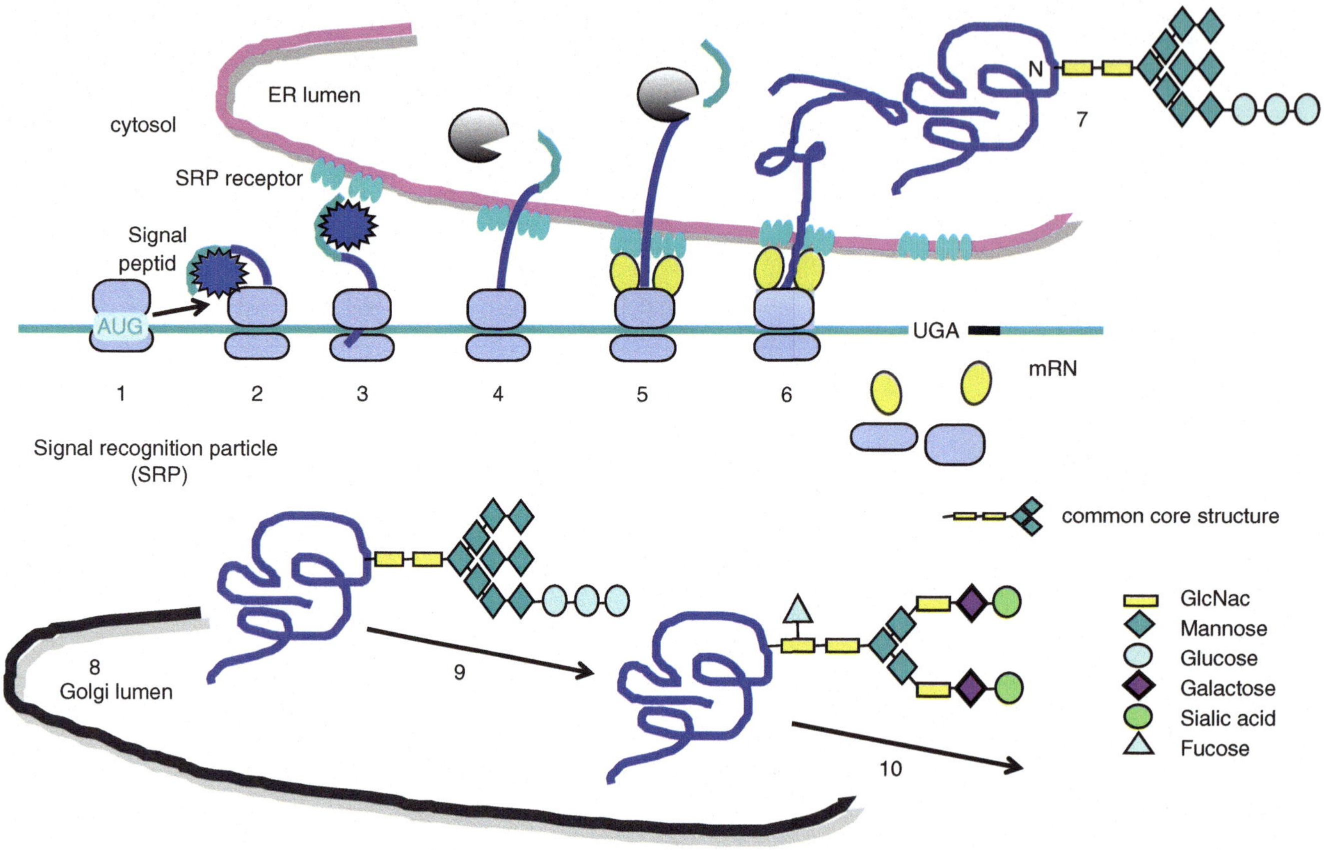

Figure 1.5 Schematic drawing of the N-linked glycosylation process as it occurs in the endoplasmic reticulum (ER) and Golgi system of an eukaryotic cell. (*1*) The ribozyme binds to the mRNA and translation starts at the AUG. The first ~20 amino acids form the signal peptide. (*2*) The signal recognition particle (SRP) binds the signal peptide. (*3*) Next, the SRP docks with the SRP receptor to the cytosolic side of the ER membrane. (*4*) The SRP is released and (*5*) the ribosomes dock onto the ER membrane. (*6*) Translation continues until the protein is complete. (*7*) A large oligosaccharide (activated by coupling to dolichol phosphate) is transferred to the specific asparagine (N) residue of the growing polypeptide chain. (*8*) Proteins in the lumen of the ER are transported to the Golgi system. (*9*) The outer carbohydrate residues are removed by glycosidases. Next, glycosyltransferases add different carbohydrates to the core structure. The complex type carbohydrate structure shown is just an example out of many possible varieties. The exact structure of the oligosaccharide attached to the peptide chain differs between cell types and even between different batches of in cell culture-produced therapeutic proteins. (*10*) Finally, secretory vesicles containing the glycoproteins are budded from the Golgi. After fusion of these vesicles with the plasma membrane, their content is released into the extracellular space

N-acetylglucosamine (GlcNAc) residues. Additional sugars are attached to this core. These maturation reactions take place in the Golgi system and differ between expression hosts. In yeast, the mature glycoproteins are rich in mannose, while in mammalian cells much more complex oligosaccharide structures are possible. To make yeast more suitable for expressing human glycosylated proteins, yeast strains with humanized glycosylation pathways have been developed. Unfortunately, the protein yields with these strains were too low and the level of glycosylation too heterogenous (see also Wells and Robinson 2017). O-linked glycosylation takes place solely in the Golgi system.

■ CopyDNA

The next step is to obtain the actual DNA that codes for the protein. This DNA is obtained by reverse-transcribing the mRNA sequence into copyDNA (cDNA). To explain this process, it is important to discuss first the structure of a mammalian gene and mRNA.

Most mammalian genes contain fragments of coding DNA (exons) interspersed by stretches of DNA that do not contain protein-coding information (introns). Messenger RNA synthesis starts with the making of a large primary transcript. Then, the introns are removed via a regulated process, called splicing. The mature mRNA contains only the exon sequences. Most mammalian mRNAs contain also a so-called poly-A "tail," a string of 100–300 adenosine nucleotides. These adenines are coupled to the mRNA molecule in a process called polyadenylation. Polyadenylation is initiated by binding of a specific set of proteins at the polyadenylation site at the end of the mRNA. The poly-A tail is important for transport of the mRNA from the nucleus into the cytosol, for translation, and it protects the mRNA from degradation.

Box 1.1 ■ The Central Dogma of Molecular Biology

The central dogma of molecular biology was first stated by Francis Crick in 1958 and deals with the information flow in biological systems and can best be summarized as "DNA makes RNA makes protein" (this quote is from Marshall Nirenberg who received the Nobel Prize in 1968 for deciphering the genetic code). The basis of the information flow from DNA via RNA into a protein is pairing of complementary bases; thus, adenine (A) forms a base pair with thymidine (T) in DNA or uracil in RNA and guanine (G) forms a base pair with cytosine (C).

To make a protein, the information contained in a gene is first transferred into a RNA molecule. RNA polymerases and transcription factors (these proteins bind to regulatory sequences on the DNA, such as promoters and enhancers) are needed for this process. In eukaryotic cells, genes are built of exons and introns. Intron sequences (the term intron is derived from intragenic region) are removed from the primary transcript by a highly regulated process which is called splicing. The remaining mRNA is built solely of exon sequences and contains the coding sequence or sense sequence. In eukaryotic cells, transcription and splicing take place in the nucleus.

The next step is translation of the mRNA molecule into a protein. This process starts by binding of the mRNA to a ribosome. The mRNA is read by the ribosome as a string of adjacent 3-nucleotide-long sequences, called codons. Complexes of specific proteins (initiation and elongation factors) bring aminoacylated transfer RNAs (tRNAs) into the ribosome-mRNA complex. Each tRNAs (via its anticodon sequence) base pairs with its specific codon in the mRNA, thereby adding the correct amino acid in the sequence encoded by the gene. There are 64 possible codon sequences. Sixty-one of those encode for the 20 possible amino acids. This means that the genetic code is redundant (see Table 1.2).

Translation starts at the start codon AUG, which codes for methionine and ends at one of the three possible stop codons: UAA, UGA, or UAG. The nascent polypeptide chain is then released from the ribosome as a mature protein. In some cases the new polypeptide chain requires additional processing to make a mature protein.

		2nd		Base			
		U	C	A	G		
	U	Phe	Ser	Tyr	Cys	U	
		Phe	Ser	Tyr	Cys	C	
		Leu	Ser	Stop	Stop	A	
1		Leu	Ser	Stop	Trp	G	3
s	C	Leu	Pro	His	Arg	U	R
t		Leu	Pro	His	Arg	C	D
		Leu	Pro	Gln	Arg	A	
b		Leu	Pro	Gln	Arg	G	B
a	A	Ile	Thr	Asn	Ser	U	A
s		Ile	Thr	Asn	Ser	C	S
e		Ile	Thr	Lys	Arg	A	E
		Met	Thr	Lys	Arg	G	
	G	Val	Ala	Asp	Gly	U	
		Val	Ala	Asp	Gly	C	
		Val	Ala	Glu	Gly	A	
		Val	Ala	Glu	Gly	G	

Table 1.2 ■ The genetic code

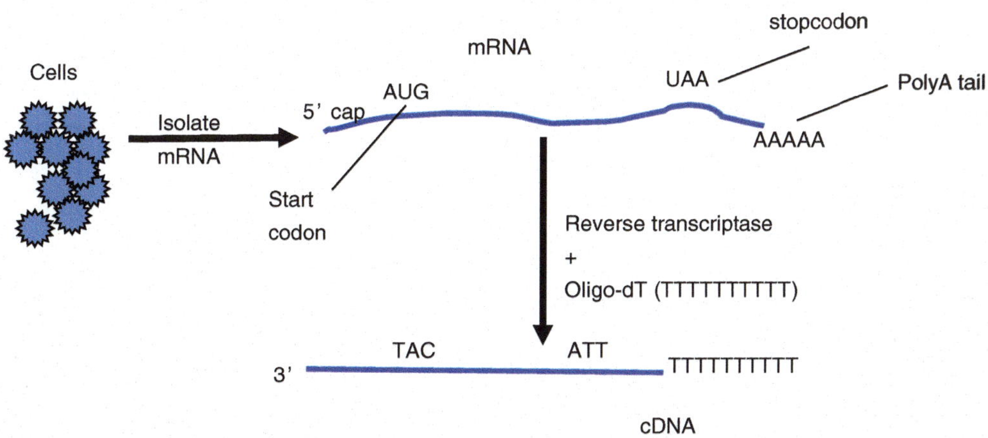

Figure 1.6 ■ Reverse transcriptase reaction

An essential tool in cDNA formation is reverse transcriptase (RT). This enzyme was originally isolated from retroviruses. These viruses contain an RNA genome. After infecting a host cell, their RNA genome is reverse-transcribed first into DNA. The finding that RNA can be reverse-transcribed into DNA by RT is an important exception of the central dogma of molecular biology (as discussed in Box 1.1).

To obtain the coding DNA of the protein, one starts by isolating (m)RNA from cells/tissue that expresses the protein. Next, the mRNA is reverse-transcribed into copyDNA (cDNA) (see Fig. 1.6). The RT reaction is performed in the presence of an oligo-dT (a single-stranded oligonucleotide containing ~20 thymidines). The oligo-dT binds to the poly-A tail and reverse transcriptase couples deoxyribonucleotides complementary to the mRNA template, to the 3′end of the growing cDNA. In this way a so-called library of cDNAs is obtained, representing all the mRNAs expressed in the starting cells or tissue.

The next step is to amplify specifically the cDNA for the protein of interest using the polymerase chain reaction (PCR, see Fig. 1.7). A PCR reaction uses a (c) DNA template, a forward primer, a reverse primer, deoxyribonucleotides (dATP, dCTP, dGTP, and dTTP), Mg^{2+}, and a thermostable DNA polymerase. DNA polymerase adds free nucleotides only to the 3′ end of the newly forming strand. This results in elongation of the new strand in a 5′→3′ direction. DNA polymerase can add a nucleotide only to a preexisting 3′-OH end, and therefore it needs a primer at which it can add the first nucleotide. PCR primers are single-stranded oligonucleotides around 20 to 30 nucleotides long, flanking opposite ends of the target DNA (see Fig. 1.8). The PCR is usually carried out for 30 cycles. Each cycle consists of three stages: a denaturing stage at ~94 °C (the double-stranded DNA is converted into single-stranded DNA), a primer annealing stage at ~60 °C (the optimal anneal temperature depends on sequences of the primers and template), and an extension stage at 72 °C. Theoretically, the amount of DNA should double during each cycle. A 30-cycle-long PCR should therefore result in a 2^{30}-fold (~10^9) increase in the amount of DNA. In practice this is never reached. In particular at later cycles, the efficiency of the PCR reaction reduces.

PCR makes use of a thermostable DNA polymerase. These polymerases were obtained from Archaea living in hot springs such as those occurring in Yellowstone National Park (see Fig. 1.9) and at the ocean bottom. DNA polymerases make mistakes. When the aim is to clone and express a PCR product, a thermostable DNA polymerase should be used with 3′→5′ exonuclease "proofreading activity." Innovations in this area still continue. The reader is referred to websites of companies, such as NEB, Roche, Invitrogen and others, to look for the latest additions to the PCR toolbox.

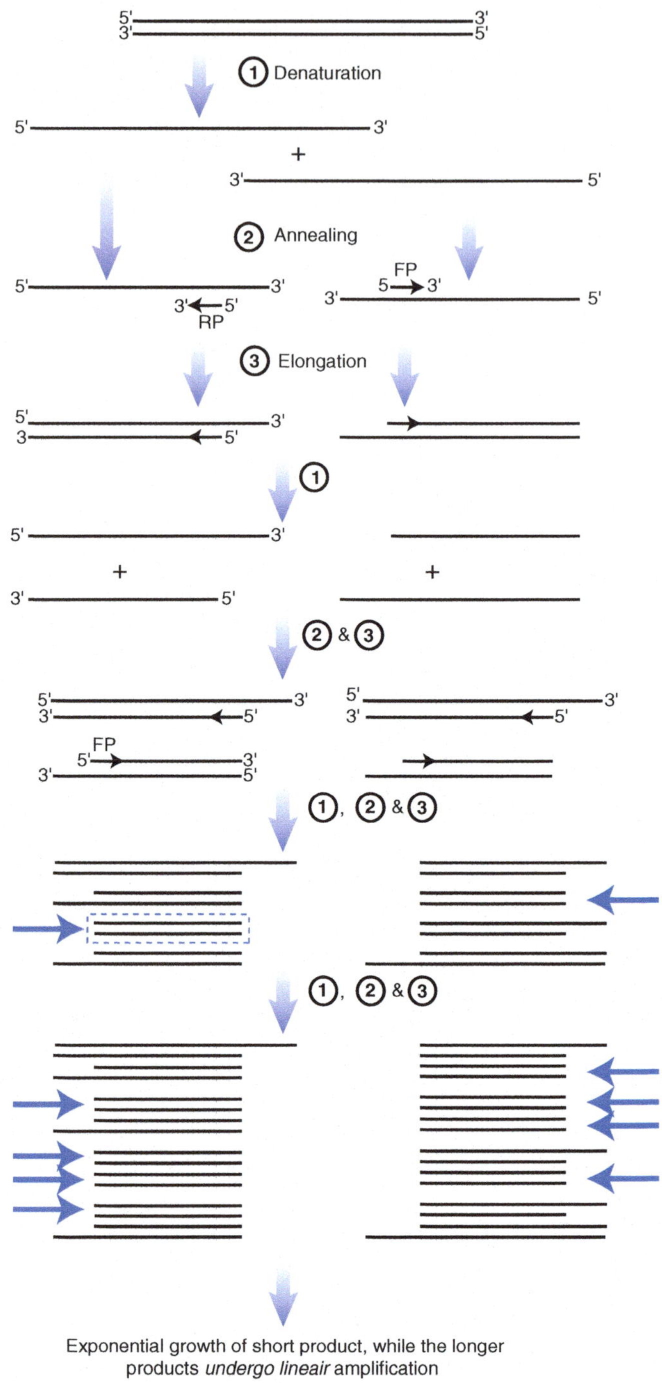

Figure 1.7 ■ The PCR process. (*1*) DNA is denatured at 94–96 °C. (2) The temperature is lowered to ±60 °C. At this temperature the primers bind (anneal) to their target sequence in the DNA. (*3*) Next, the temperature is raised to 72 °C, the optimal temperature for Taq polymerase. Four cycles are shown here. A typical PCR reaction runs for 30 cycles. The *arrows* point to the desired PCR product

■ Cloning PCR Products into an Expression Vector

There are several ways to clone a PCR product. One of the easiest ways is known as TA cloning (see Fig. 1.10). TA cloning makes use of the property of Taq polymerase to add a single adenosine to the 3′end of a PCR product. Such a PCR product can subsequently be ligated (using DNA ligase, see Molecular Biology toolbox) into a plasmid with a 5′ thymidine overhang (see Box 1.2 for a general description of expression plasmids). PCR products obtained with a DNA polymerase with proofreading activity have a blunt end, and thus they do not contain the 3′ A overhang. However, such PCR fragments can easily be A-tailed by incubating for a short period with Taq polymerase and dATP. Blunt PCR products can also directly be cloned into a linearized plasmid with 2 blunt ends. However, the efficiency of blunt-end PCR cloning is much lower than

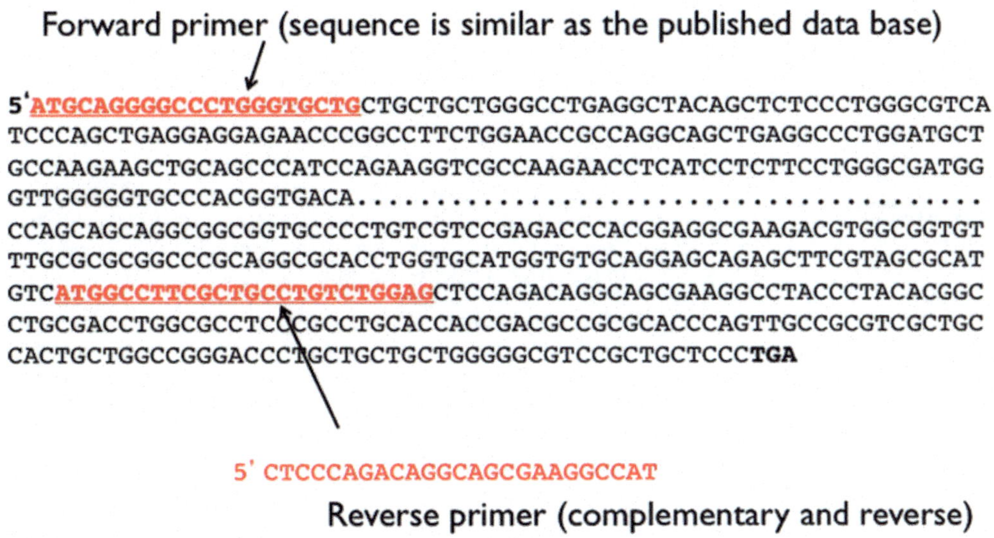

Figure 1.8 ■ PCR primer design

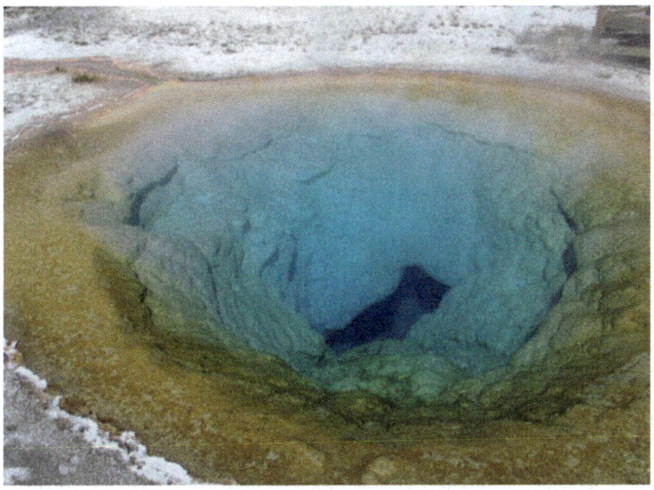

Figure 1.9 ■ A hot spring in Yellowstone National Park. In hot springs like this one, Archaea, the bacterial source of thermostable polymerases, live

that of TA cloning. A disadvantage of TA and blunt-end cloning is that directional cloning is not possible, so the PCR fragment can be cloned either in the sense or antisense direction (see Fig. 1.10). PCR products can also be cloned by adding unique recognition sites of restriction enzymes to both ends of the PCR product. This can be done by incorporating these sites at the 5′end of the PCR primers. Although this strategy looks very straightforward, it is also not very efficient.

After ligation, the plasmid is introduced into *E. coli* by a process called transformation. There are several ways to transform *E. coli*. Most used are the calcium chloride method (better known as heat shock) and electroporation (the bacteria are exposed to a very high electric pulse). Whatever the transformation method, channels in the membrane are opened through which the plasmid can enter the cell. Next, the bacteria are plated onto an agar plate with an antibiotic. Only bacteria that have taken up the plasmid with an antibiotic-resistant gene and thus produce a protein that degrades the antibiotic will survive. After an overnight incubation at 37 °C, the agar plate will contain a number of clones. The bacteria in each colony are the descendants of one bacterium. Subsequently, aliquots of a number of these colonies are grown overnight in liquid medium at 37 °C. From these cultures, plasmids can be isolated (this is known as a miniprep). The next steps will be to determine whether the obtained plasmid preparations contain an insert, and if so, to determine what the orientation is of the insert relative to the promoter that will drive the recombinant protein expression. The orientation can, for instance, be determined by cutting the obtained plasmids with a restriction enzyme that cuts only once somewhere in the plasmid and with another enzyme that cuts once somewhere in the insert. On the basis of the obtained fragment sizes (determined via agarose gel electrophoresis using appropriate molecular weight standards), the orientation of the insert in the plasmid can be determined (see Fig. 1.10).

As already discussed above, DNA polymerases make mistakes, and therefore, it is crucial to determine the nucleotide sequence of the cloned PCR fragment. DNA sequencing is a very important method in biotechnology (the developments in high-throughput sequencing have enabled the sequencing of many different genomes, including that of humans) and is therefore further explained in Box 1.3.

■ Transfection of Host Cells and Recombinant Protein Production

Introducing DNA into a mammalian cell is called transfection (and as already mentioned above, transformation in *E. coli*). There are several methods to introduce DNA into a mammalian cell line. Most often,

Box 1.2 ■ Plasmids and enzyme toolbox

Schematic drawing of an expression plasmid for a mammalian cell line

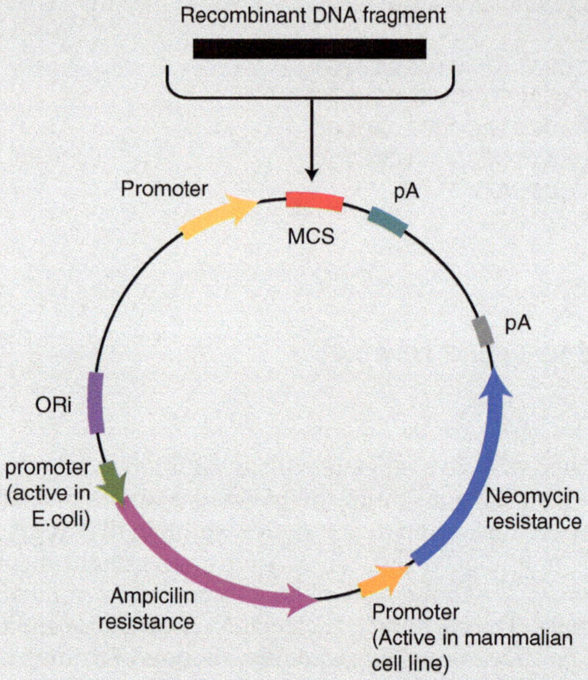

Plasmids are self-replicating circular extrachromosomal DNA molecules. The plasmids used nowadays in biotechnology are constructed partly from naturally occurring plasmids and partly from synthetic DNA. The figure above shows a schematic representation of a plasmid suitable for driving protein expression in a mammalian cell. The most important features of this plasmid are:

1. An origin of replication (ORi). The ori allows plasmids to replicate separately from the host cell's chromosome.
2. A multiple cloning site (MCS). The MCS contains recognition sites for a number of restriction enzymes. The presence of the MCS in plasmids makes it relatively easy to transfer a DNA fragment from one plasmid into another.
3. Antibiotic-resistant genes. All plasmids contain a gene that makes the recipient E. coli resistant to an antibiotic, in this case resistant to ampicillin. Other antibiotic-resistant genes that are often used confer resistance to tetracycline and Zeocin®. The expression plasmid contains also the neomycin resistance gene. This selection marker enables selection of those mammalian cells that have integrated the plasmid DNA in their chromosome. The protein product of the neomycin resistance gene inactivates the toxin Geneticin®.
4. Promoter to drive gene expression. Many expression vectors for mammalian cells contain the cytomegalovirus (CMV) promoter, which is taken from the cytomegaloma virus and is constitutively active. To drive recombinant protein expression in other expression hosts, other plasmids with other promoter sequences have to be used.
5. Poly (A) recognition site. This site becomes part of the newly produced mRNA and binds a protein complex that adds subsequently a poly (A) tail to the 3′ end of the mRNA. Expression vectors that are used to drive protein expression in E. coli do not contain a poly(A) recognition site.

Enzyme Toolbox

DNA polymerase produces a polynucleotide sequence against a nucleotide template strand using base pairing interactions (G against C and A against T). It adds nucleotides to a free 3′OH, and thus it acts in a 5′ → 3′ direction. Some polymerases have also 3′ → 5′ exonuclease activity (see below), which mediates proofreading.

Reverse transcriptase (RT) is a special kind of DNA polymerase, since it requires an RNA template instead of a DNA template.*Restriction enzymes* are endonucleases that bind specific recognition sites on DNA and cut both strands. Restriction enzymes can either cut both DNA strands at the same location (blunt end) or they can cut at different sites on each strand, generating a single-stranded end (better known as a sticky end).

Examples:

HindIII	5′A^{a}AGCTT 3′TTCGA^{a}A	XhoI	5′C^{a}TCGAG 3′GAGCT^{a}C
KpnI	5′GGTAC^{a}C 3′C^{a}CATGG	EcoRV	5′GAT^{a}ATC 3′CTA^{a}TAG
NotI	5′GC^{a}GGCCGC 3′CGCCGG^{a}CG	PacI	5′TTAAT^{a}TAA 3′AAT^{a}TAATT

^{a}Location where the enzyme cuts

DNA ligase joints two DNA fragments. It links covalently the 3′-OH of one strand with the 5′-PO_4 of the other DNA strand. The linkage of two DNA molecules with complementary sticky ends by ligase is much more efficient than blunt-end ligation.

Alkaline phosphatase. A ligation reaction of a blunt-end DNA fragment into a plasmid also with blunt ends will result primarily in empty plasmids, being the result of self-ligation. Treatment of a plasmid with blunt ends with alkaline phosphatase, which removes the 5′PO_4 groups, prevents self-ligation.

Exonucleases remove nucleotides one at a time from the end (exo) of a DNA molecule. They act, depending on the type of enzyme, either in a 5′ → 3′ or 3 → 5′ direction and on single- or double-stranded DNA. Some polymerases have also exonuclease activity (required for proofreading). Exonucleases are used, for instance, to generate blunt ends on a DNA molecule with either a 3′ or 5′ extension.

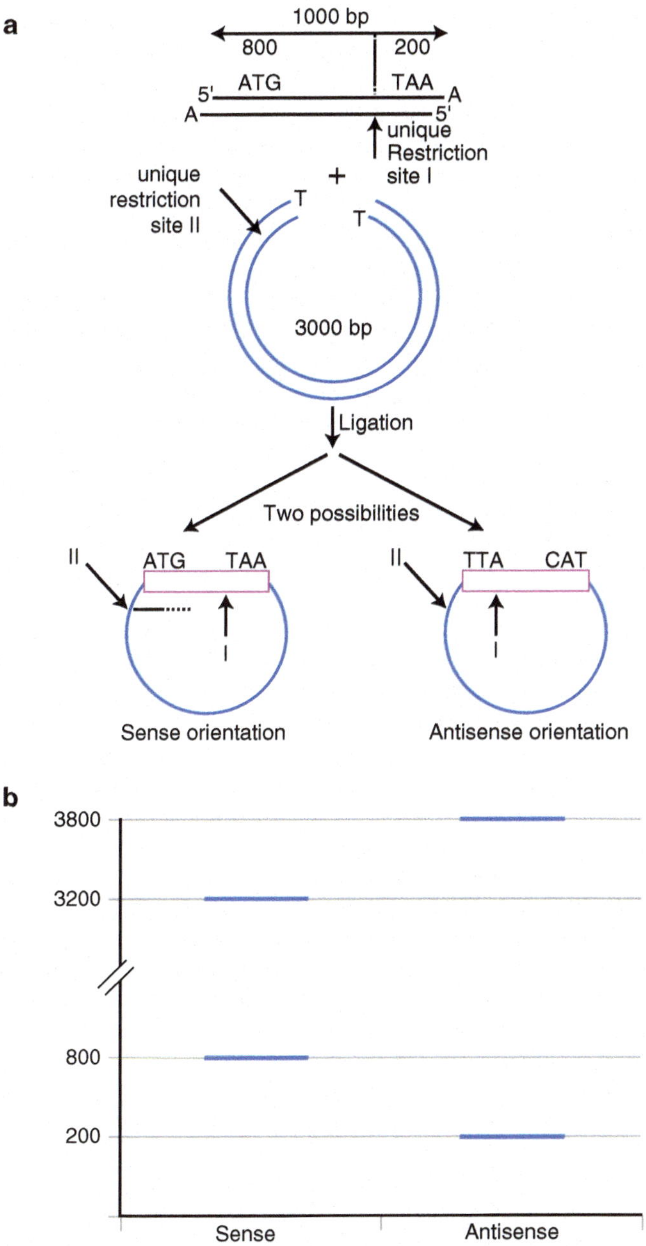

Figure 1.10 ■ Cloning of a PCR product via TA cloning (**a**). This cloning strategy makes use of the property of Taq polymerase to add an extra A to the 3′ end of the PCR product. To determine the orientation of the insert, the plasmid is cut by enzymes I and II (enzyme I cuts in the insert and enzyme II cuts in the plasmid). On the basis of the obtained fragment size (as determined by agarose electrophoresis), the orientation of the insert can be deduced (**b**)

the plasmid DNA is complexed to cationic lipids (such as Lipofectamine) or polymers (such as polyethyleneimines or PEI) and then pipetted to the cells. Next, the positively charged aggregates bind to the negatively charged cell membrane and are subsequently endocytosized (see Fig. 1.11). Then, the plasmid DNA has to escape from the endosome and has to find its way into the nucleus where mRNA synthesis can take place. This is actually achieved during cell division when the nuclear membrane is absent. Another way to introduce DNA into the cytosol is through electroporation. During electroporation, an electric pulse is applied

Box 1.3 ■ DNA Sequencing

Technical breakthroughs in DNA sequencing, the determination of the nucleotide sequence, permit the sequencing of entire genomes, including the human genome. It all started with the sequencing in 1977 of the 5386-nucleotide-long single-stranded genome of the bacteriophage φX174.

Chain-Termination Method and High-Throughput Sequencing

The most frequently used method for DNA sequencing is the chain-termination method, also known as the dideoxynucleotide method, as developed by Frederick Sanger in the 1970s.

The method starts by creating millions of copies of the DNA to be sequenced. This can be done by isolating plasmids with the DNA inserted from bacterial cultures or by PCR. Next, the obtained double-stranded DNA molecules are denatured, and the reverse strand of one of the two original DNA strands is synthesized using DNA polymerase, a DNA primer complementary to a sequence upstream of the sequence to be determined, normal deoxynucleotidetriphosphates (dNTPs), and dideoxyNTPs (ddNTPs) that terminate DNA strand elongation. The four different ddNTPs (ddATP, ddGTP, ddCTP, or ddTTP) miss the 3'OH group required for the formation of a phosphodiester bond between two nucleotides and are each labeled with a different fluorescent dye, each emits light at different wavelengths. This reaction results in different reverse strand DNA molecules extended to different lengths. Following denaturation and removal of the free nucleotides, primers, and the enzyme, the resulting DNA molecules are separated on the basis of their molecular weight with a resolution of just one nucleotide (corresponding to the point of termination). The presence of the fluorescent label attached to the terminating ddNTPs makes a sequentially read out in the order created by the separation process possible. See also the figures below. The separation of the DNA molecules is nowadays carried out by capillary electrophoresis. The available capillary sequencing systems are able to run in parallel 96 or 384 samples with a length of 600 to 1000 nucleotides. With the more common 96 capillary systems, it is possible to obtain around 6 million bases (Mb) of sequence per day.

Next-Generation Sequencing

The capillary sequencing systems are still used, but are more and more replaced by alternative systems with a much higher output and at the same time a strong reduction in the costs. The fastest machine available today (2018) is the HiSeqX ten from Illumina. It is capable of sequencing 0.6 Terabase (0.6 × 10^{12} base)/day.

The description of these really high-throughput systems is beyond the purpose of this book. An excellent review about this topic is written by Reuter et al. (2015).

(continued)

Box 1.3 ■ (continued)

Schematic representation of the DNA sequencing process

a DNA synthesis in the presence of dNTPs and fluorescently labeled ddNTPs (T,C,A,or G)

Target sequence
3' ---GGGTCCAGTGGCAGAGGATTCCGCC
5' ---CCCAGG →

primer extension
---CCCAGGT
---CCCAGGTC
---CCCAGGTCA
---CCCAGGTCAC
---CCCAGGTCACC
---CCCAGGTCACCG

b Separation of the synthesized DNA molecules by capillary electrophoresis and read out of fluorescence

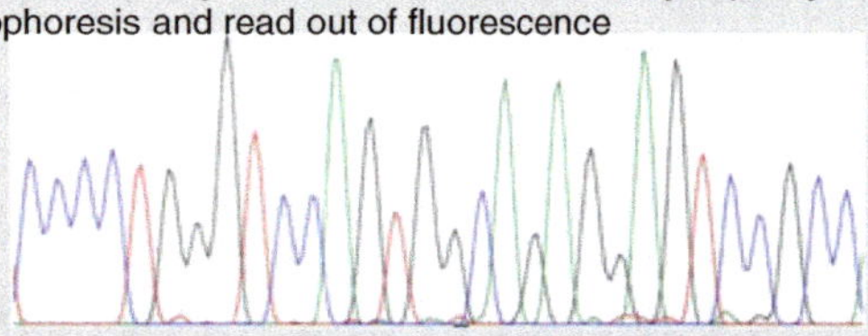

Schematic representation of the DNA sequencing process

to the cells, which results in the formation of small pores in the plasma membrane. Through these pores the plasmid DNA can enter the cells.

Transfection leads to transient expression of the introduced gene. The introduced plasmids are rapidly diluted as a consequence of cell division or even degraded. However, it is possible to stably transfect cells leading to long expression periods. Then, the plasmid DNA has to integrate into the chromosomal DNA of the host cell. To accomplish this, a selection gene is normally included into the expression vector, which gives the transfected cells a selectable growth advantage. Only those cells that have integrated the selection marker (and most likely, but not necessary, also the gene of interest) into their genome will survive. Most expression plasmids for mammalian cells contain as selection marker the neomycin resistance gene (Neo^r). This gene codes for a protein that neutralizes the toxic drug Geneticin, also known as G418. The entire selection process takes around 2 weeks and results in a tissue culture dish with several colonies. Each colony contains the descendants of 1 stably transfected cell. Then, the cells from individual colonies have to be isolated and further expanded. The next step will be to quantify the recombinant protein production of the obtained cell cultures and to select those with the highest yields.

Transfection of mammalian cells is a very inefficient process (compared to transformation of *E. coli*) and needs relatively large amounts of plasmid DNA. Integration of the transfected plasmid DNA into the genome is a very rare event. As a typical example, starting with 10^7 mammalian cells, one obtains usually not more than 10^2 stably expressing clones.

■ Cell Culture

A big challenge is to scale up cell cultures from lab scale (e.g., a 75 cm^2 tissue culture bottle) to a large-scale production platform (like a bioreactor). Mammalian cells are relatively weak and may easily become damaged by stirring or pumping liquid in or out a fermenter (shear stress). In this respect, *E. coli* is much sturdy, and thus this bacterium can therefore be grown in much larger fermenters.

A particular problem is the large-scale culturing of adherent (versus suspended) mammalian cells. One way to grow adherent cells in large amounts is on the surface of small beads. After a while the surface of the beads will be completely covered (confluent) with cells, and then, it is necessary to detach the cells from the beads and to redivide the cells over more (empty) beads and to transfer them to a bioreactor compatible with higher working volumes. To loosen the cells from the beads, usually the protease trypsin is used. It is very important that the trypsinization process is well timed: if it is too short, many cells are still on the beads, and if it is too long, the cells will lose their integrity and will not survive this treatment.

Some companies have tackled the scale-up problem by "simply" culturing and expanding their adherent cells in increasing amounts of roller bottles. These bottles revolve slowly (between 5 and 60 revolutions per hour), which bathes the cells that are attached to the inner surface with medium (see Fig. 1.12). See Chap. 4 for more in-depth information in this book. For in depth knowledge of recombinant protein production in CHO cells, the reader in referred to the reviews by Kim et al. (2012) and Kunert and Reinhart (2016).

■ Purification; Downstream Processing

Recombinant proteins are usually purified from cell culture supernatants or cell extracts by filtration and conventional column chromatography, including affinity chromatography (see Chap. 4).

The aim of the downstream processing (DSP) is to purify the therapeutic protein from (potential) endogenous and extraneous contaminants, such as host cell proteins, DNA, and viruses.

It is important to mention here that slight changes in the purification process of a therapeutic protein may affect its activity and the amount and nature of the co-purified impurities. This is one of the main reasons (in addition to differences in expression host and culture conditions) why follow-on products (after expiration of the patent) made by a different company will never be identical to the original preparation and that is why they are not considered a true generic product (see also Chap. 12). A generic drug must contain the same active ingredient as the original drug, and in the case of a therapeutic protein, this is almost impossible and that is why the term "biosimilar" was invented.

Although not often used for the production of therapeutic proteins, recombinant protein purification

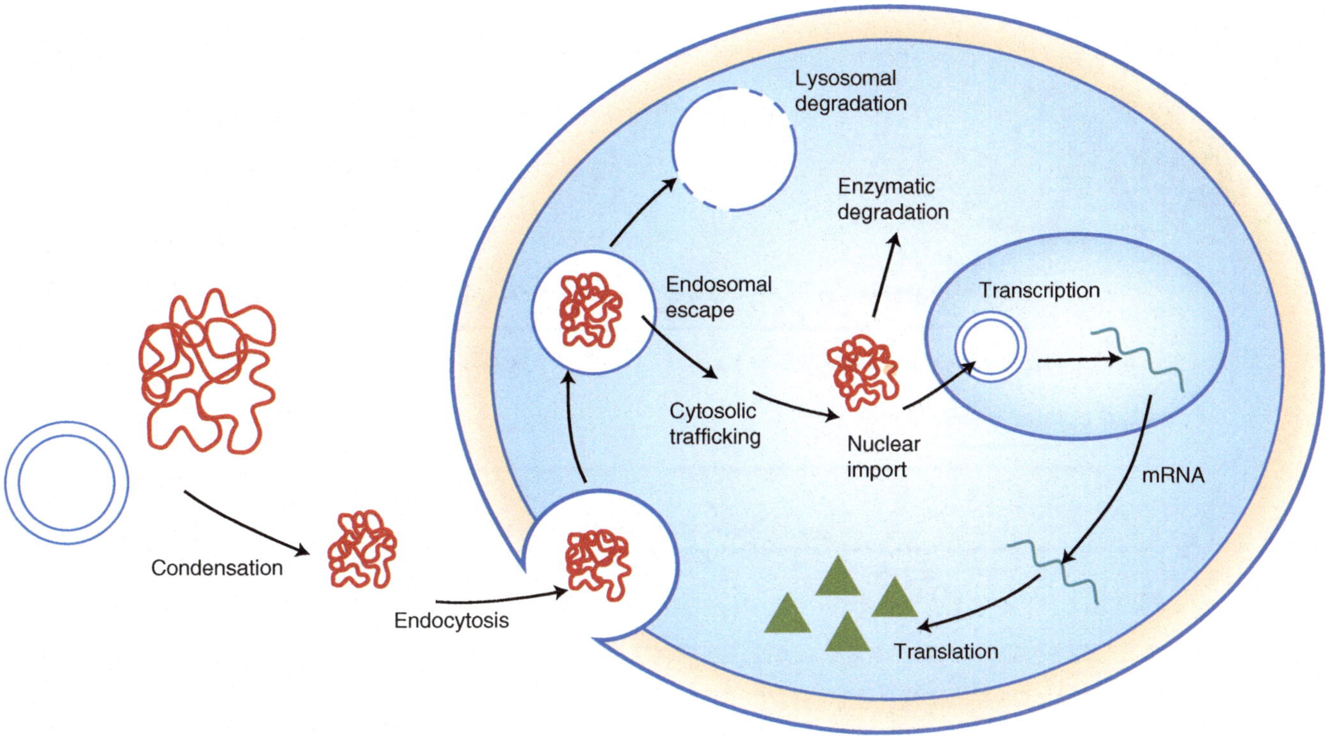

Figure 1.11 ■ Carrier-mediated transfection of mammalian cells

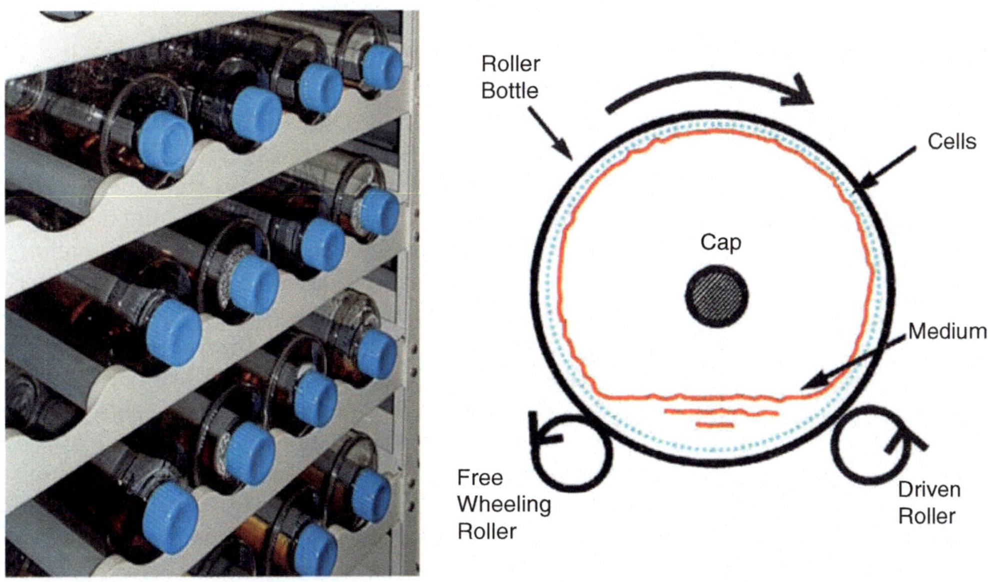

Figure 1.12 ■ Cell culturing in roller bottles

may be simplified by linking it with an affinity tag, such as the his-tag (6 histidines). His-tagged proteins have a high affinity for Ni^{2+}-containing resins. There are two ways to add the 6 histidine residues. The DNA encoding the protein may be inserted into a plasmid encoding already a his-tag. Another possibility is to perform a PCR reaction with a regular primer and a primer with at its 5′end 6 histidine codons (CAT or CAC) (see Fig. 1.13). To enable easy removal of the his-tag from the recombinant protein, the tag may be followed by a suitable amino acid sequence that is recognized by an endopeptidase.

In *E. coli*, recombinant proteins are often produced as a fusion protein with another protein such as thioredoxin, maltose-binding protein (MBP), and glutathione S-transferase (GST). These fusion partners may improve the proper folding and solubility of the recombinant protein and act as affinity tags for purification. For a review on recombinant protein expression in E.coli see Rosno and Ceccarelli (2014).

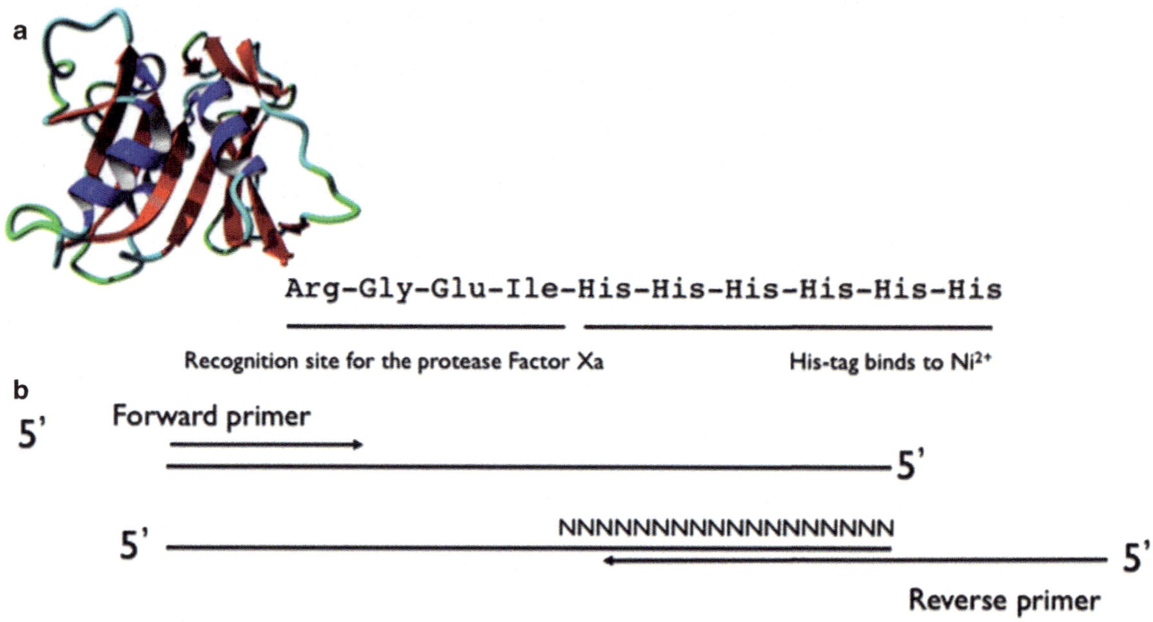

XXX XXX XXX XXX XXX XXX ILE GLU GLY ARG HIS HIS HIS HIS HIS HIS **stop**

5'NNN NNN NNN NNN NNN NNN ATT GAA GGA CGT CAT CAT CAT CAT CAT CAT TAA

REVERSE PRIMER:

5" TTA ATG ATG ATG ATG ATG ATG ACG TCC TTC AAT NNN NNN NNN NNN NNN NNN

Figure 1.13 ■ (**a**) Schematic drawing of a his-tagged fusion protein. (**b**) Design of the primers needed to generate a his-tag at the carboxy-terminal end of a protein

MONOCLONAL ANTIBODIES

So far, we discussed the selection, design, and production of a protein starting from a DNA sequence in a genomic database. There is no database available of the entire repertoire of human antibodies. Potentially there are millions of different antibodies possible, and our knowledge about antibody-antigen interactions is not large enough to design a specific antibody from scratch.

Many marketed therapeutic proteins are monoclonal antibodies (cf. Chaps. 8, 23, 25, and 26). We will focus here on the molecular biological aspects of the design and production of (humanized) monoclonal antibodies in cell culture (primarily CHO cells are used). For a description of the structural elements of monoclonal antibodies, we refer to Chap. 8, Figs. 8.1 and 8.2.

The classic way to make a monoclonal antibody starts by immunizing a laboratory animal with a purified human protein against which the antibody should be directed (see Fig. 1.14). In most cases, mice are used. The immunization process (a number of injections with the antigens and an adjuvant) will take several weeks. Then the spleens of these mice are removed and lymphocytes are isolated. Subsequently, the lymphocytes are fused with a myeloma cell using polyethylene glycol (PEG). The resulting hybridoma cell inherited from the lymphocytes the ability to produce antibodies and from the myeloma cell line the ability to divide indefinitely. To select hybridoma cells from the excess of non-fused lymphocytes and myeloma cells, the cells are grown in HAT selection medium. This culture medium contains hypoxanthine, aminopterin, and thymidine. The myeloma cell lines used for the production of monoclonal antibodies contain an inactive hypoxanthine-guanine phosphoribosyltransferase (HGPRT), an enzyme necessary for the salvage synthesis of nucleic acids. The lack of HGPRT activity is not a problem for the myeloma cells because they can still synthesize purines de novo. By exposing the myeloma cells to the drug aminopterin also de novo synthesis of purines is blocked and these cells will not survive anymore. Selection against the unfused lymphocytes is not necessary, since these cells, like most primary cells, do not survive for a long time in cell culture. After PEG treatment, the cells are diluted and divided over several dishes. After approximately 2 weeks, individual clones are visible. Each clone contains the descendants of one hybridoma cell and will produce one particular type of antibody (that is why they are called monoclonal antibodies). The next step is to isolate hybridoma cells from individual clones and grow them in separate wells of a 96-well plate. The hybridomas secrete antibodies into the culture medium. Using a suitable test (e.g., an ELISA), the obtained culture media can be screened for antibody

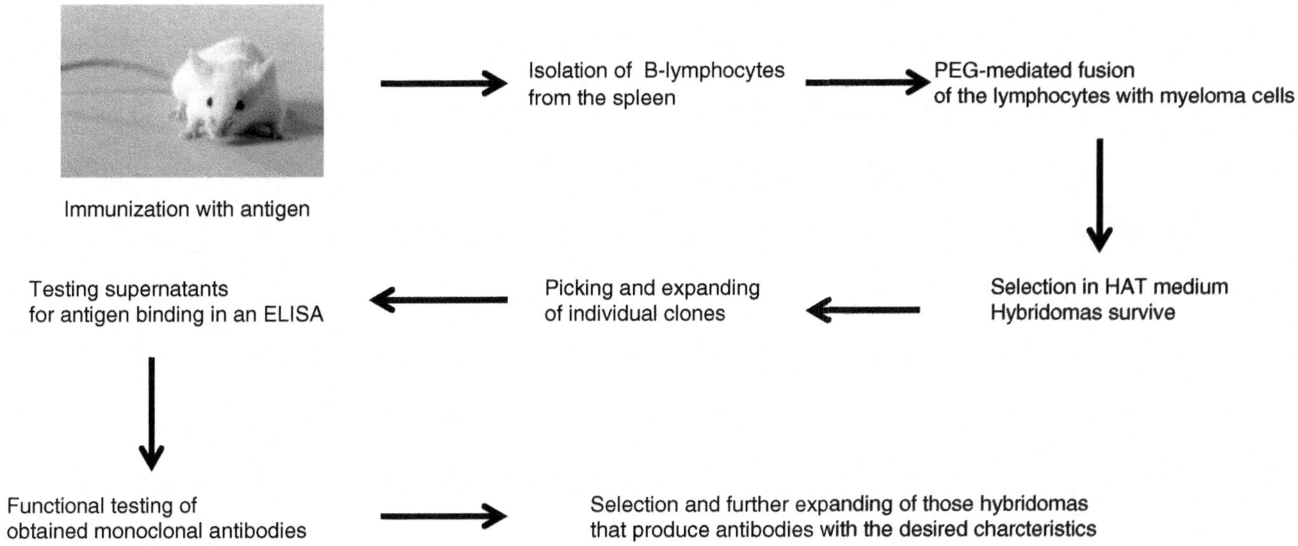

Figure 1.14 ■ The making of a mouse monoclonal antibody

binding to the antigen. The obtained antibodies can then be further characterized using other tests. In this way a mouse monoclonal antibody is generated.

These mouse monoclonal antibodies cannot be used directly for the treatment of human patients. The amino acid sequence of a mouse antibody is too different from the sequence of an antibody in humans and thus will elicit an immune response. To make a mouse antibody less immunogenic, the main part of its sequence must be replaced by the corresponding human sequence. Initially, human-mouse chimeric antibodies were made. These antibodies consisted of the constant regions of the human heavy and light chain and the variable regions of the mouse antibody. Later, so-called humanized antibodies were generated by grafting only the complementarity-determining regions (CDRs), which are responsible for the antigen-binding properties, of the selected mouse antibody onto a human framework of the variable light (V_L) and heavy (V_H) domains. The humanized antibodies are much less immunogenic than the previously used chimeric antibodies. To even further reduce immunogenicity, specificity determining residues (SDR) grafting is used (Kashmiri et al. 2005). SDR stands for 'specificity determining residues'. From the analysis of the 3-D structure of antibodies, it appeared that only ~30% of the amino acid residues present in the CDRs are critical for antigen binding. These residues, which form the SDR, are thought to be unique for a given antibody.

Humanization of a mouse antibody is a difficult and tricky process. It results usually in a reduction of the affinity of the antibody for its antigen. One of the challenges is the selection of the most appropriate human antibody framework. This framework determines basically the structure of the antibody and thus the orientation of the antigen recognition domains in space. Sometimes it is necessary to change some of the residues in the human antibody framework to restore antigen binding. To further enhance the affinity of the humanized antibody for its antigen, mutations within the CDR/SDR sequences are introduced. How this in vitro affinity maturation is done is beyond the scope of this chapter.

So far the generation of a humanized antibody has been described in a rather abstract way. How is it done in practice? First, the nucleotide sequence of each of the V_L and V_H regions is deduced (contains either the murine CDRs or SDRs). Next, the entire sequence is divided over four or more alternating oligonucleotides with overlapping flanks (see Fig. 1.15). These relatively long oligonucleotides are made synthetically. The reason why the entire sequence is divided over four nucleotides instead of over two or even one is that there is a limitation to the length of an oligonucleotide that can be synthesized reliably (a less than 100% yield of each coupling step (nucleotides are added one at the time) and the occurrence of side reactions make that oligonucleotides hardly exceed 200 nucleotide residues).

To the four oligonucleotides, a heat-stable DNA polymerase and the 4 deoxyribonucleotides (dATP, dCTP, dGTP, and dTTP) are added, and the mixture is incubated at an appropriate temperature. Then, 2 primers, complementary to both ends of the fragment, are added, which enable the amplification of the entire sequence. The strategy to fuse overlapping oligonucleotides by PCR is called PCR sewing.

Finally, the PCR product encoding the humanized V_L and V_H region is cloned into an expression vectors carrying the respective constant regions and a signal peptide. The signal peptide is required for glycosylation. Subsequently, the expression constructs will

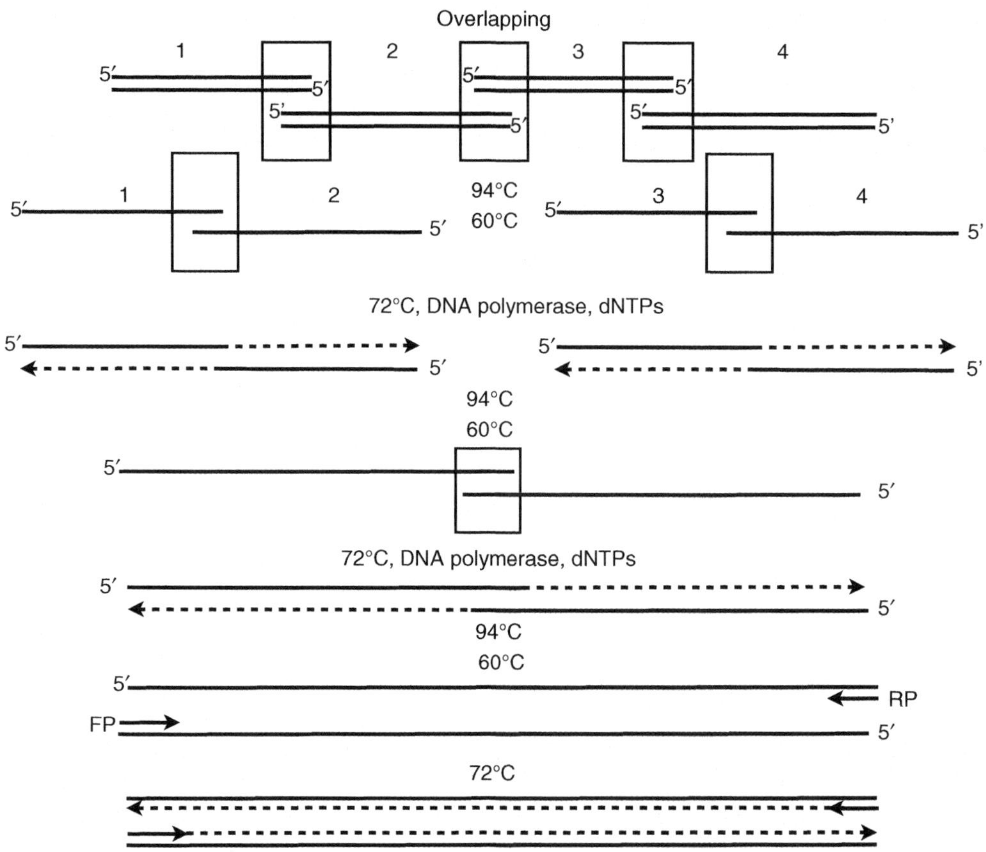

Figure 1.15 ■ The making of a sequence containing the humanized V_L or V_H region of an antibody by PCR sewing. Both the V_L and V_H regions contain three highly variable loops (known as complementarity-determining regions 1, 2, and 3). The V_L and V_H regions are approximately 110 amino acids in size. Four alternating oligonucleotides with overlapping flanks are incubated together with a DNA polymerase and deoxynucleotides. DNA polymerase fills in the gaps. The sequences of these oligonucleotides are based upon the original mouse CDR/SDR sequences inserted into a human V_L or V_H framework. Next, the entire sequence is PCR amplified using end primers (*FP* forward primer, *RP* reverse primer). The resulting PCR fragments will be around 330 base pair in size

be used to stably transfect CHO cells. The obtained clones will be tested for antibody production, and clones with the highest antibody production capacity will be selected for further use.

YIELDS

To give an idea about the production capacity needed to produce a monoclonal antibody, we will do now some calculations. The annual amount needed for the most successful therapeutic monoclonal antibodies is around 1000 kg. In cell culture, titers of up to 10 g/L are reached (in fed-batch cultures) and the yield of the DSP is around 80%. Thus, to produce 1000 kg monoclonal antibody, one needs at least 100,000 L of cell culture supernatant. In Chap. 4 more details can be found.

CONCLUSION

Thanks to advances in many different areas, including molecular biology, bioinformatics, and bioprocess engineering, we have moved from an animal-/human-derived therapeutic protein product towards in vitro-produced therapeutic proteins with the fully human sequence and structure. Importantly, we have now access to potentially unlimited amounts of high-quality therapeutic proteins. Of course, there will always be a risk for (viral) contaminations in the in vitro-produced therapeutic protein preparation, but this risk is much smaller than when the protein has to be isolated from a human source (examples from the past include the transmission of hepatitis B and C and human immunodeficiency virus (HIV) via blood-derived products and the transmission of Creutzfeldt-Jakob disease from human growth hormone preparations from human pituitaries).

As basic knowledge in molecular biology and engineering keeps on growing, the efficiency of the cloning and production process will increase in parallel.

SELF-ASSESSMENT QUESTIONS

■ Questions

1. A researcher wanted to clone and subsequently express the human histone H4 protein in *E. coli*.

   She obtained the sequence below from the NCBI, as shown below. The start and stop codons are underlined.

   >gi|29553982|ref|NM_003548.2| Homo sapiens histone cluster 2, H4a (HIST2H4A), mRNA

   AGAAGCTGTCTATCGGGCTCCAGCGGTC ATGTCCGGCAGAGGAAAGGGCGGAAAA GGCTTAGGCAAAGGG

GGCGCTAAGCGCCACCGCAAGGTCTTGA GAGACAACATTCAGGGCATCACCAAGCC TGCCATTCGGCGTC

TAGCTCGGCGTGGCGGCGTTAAGCGGAT CTCTGGCCTCATTTACGAGGAGACCCGCGG TGTGCTGAAGGT

GTTCCTGGAGAATGTGATTCGGGACG CAGTCACCTACACCGAGCACGCCAAGCGCA AGACCGTCACAGCC

ATGGATGTGGTGTACGCGCTC AAGCGCCAGGGGCGCACCCTGTACGGC TTCGGAGGCTAGGCCGCCGCTC

CAGCTTTGCACGTTTCGATCCCAAAGG CCCTTTTTAGGGCCGACCA.

(i) Is *E. coli* a suitable expression host for the H4 protein?

(ii) Design primers for the amplification of the coding sequence of the H4 protein by PCR.

(iii) To ease purification the researcher decided to add an affinity tag (Trp-Ser-His-Pro-Gln-Phe-Glu-Lys) to the carboxy-terminal end of the H4 protein. PCR was used to clone this tag in frame with the H4 protein. What was the sequence of the primers she probably used?

To answer this question, make use of the table below.

		2nd		Base			
		U	C	A	G		
	U	Phe	Ser	Tyr	Cys	U	
		Phe	Ser	Tyr	Cys	C	
		Leu	Ser	Stop	Stop	A	
1		Leu	Ser	Stop	Trp	G	3
s	C	Leu	Pro	His	Arg	U	r
t		Leu	Pro	His	Arg	C	d
		Leu	Pro	Gln	Arg	A	
b		Leu	Pro	Gln	Arg	G	b
a	A	Ile	Thr	Asn	Ser	U	a
s		Ile	Thr	Asn	Ser	C	s
e		Ile	Thr	Lys	Arg	A	e
		Met	Thr	Lys	Arg	G	
	G	Val	Ala	Asp	Gly	U	
		Val	Ala	Asp	Gly	C	
		Val	Ala	Glu	Gly	A	
		Val	Ala	Glu	Gly	G	

(iv) And finally, she decided to optimize the codon usage for expression in *E. coli*. What is coding optimalization? What is its purpose?

(v) Design a strategy/method to optimize the codon usage of the H4 protein.

(vi) The human H4 mRNA differs from most other human mRNAs by lacking a poly-A tail (instead the H4 mRNA is protected by a palindromic termination element), and thus the cDNA encoding this protein cannot be obtained by a reverse transcriptase reaction using an oligo-dT as primer. Describe a method to obtain the H4 cDNA.

2. Ampicillin, G418, and HAT medium are used to select for transformed *E. coli*, transfected mammalian cells, and hybridomas, respectively. Describe shortly the mechanism underlying the three mentioned selection strategies.
3. *E. coli* does not take up plasmid DNA spontaneously. However, the so-called chemical competent *E. coli* is able to take up plasmids following a heat shock (30 s 42 °C, followed by an immediate transfer to 0 °C). These competent bacteria can be obtained by extensive washing with a 100 mM $CaCl_2$ solution.

Transformation of competent *E. coli* of good quality results in $\pm 10^8$ colonies/µg of supercoiled plasmid DNA. The bacteria in each colony are the descendants of one bacterium that had initially taken up one plasmid molecule.

Calculate the transformation efficiency defined as the number of plasmids taken up by the competent bacteria divided by the total number of plasmids added. Make the calculation for a plasmid of 3333 base pairs (the MW of a nucleotide is 300 g/mol and the Avogadro constant is 6×10^{23} molecules/mol).

Answers

1. (i) Information about the protein structure can be obtained from http://www.expasy.org/. The H4 protein does not contain disulfide bridges and is unglycosylated. It is therefore likely that *E. coli* is able to produce a correctly folded H4 protein. (ii) PCR primers are usually around 18–20 nucleotides long. The sequences of the forward and reverse primer are *ATG* TCC GGC AGA GGA AAG (identical to the published sequence) and *CTA* GCC TCC GAA GCC GTA (complementary and reverse), respectively. (iii) The forward primer will be as above. At the 5′ end of the reverse primer, additional sequences must be added. First, the DNA sequence encoding the affinity tag Trp-Ser-His-Pro-Gln-Phe-Glu-Lys must be determined using the codon usage table: TCG CAC CCA CAG TTC GAA AAG. It is important to place the tag in front of the stop codon (TAG). The sequence of the reverse primer will then be 5′-CTA CTT TTC GAA CTG TGG GTG CGA CCA GCC TCC GAA GCC GTA CAG-3′. (iv) For most amino acids more than one codon exists (see the codon usage table).

Differences in preferences for one of the several codons that encode the same amino acid exist between organisms. In particular in fast-growing organisms, such as *E. coli*, the optimal codons reflect the composition of their transfer RNA (tRNA) pool. By changing the native codons into those codons preferred by *E. coli*, the level of heterologous protein expression may increase. Alternatively, and much easier, one could use as expression host an *E. coli* with plasmids encoding extra copies of rare tRNAs. (v) The H4 protein is 103 amino acids long. The easiest way to change the sequence at many places along the entire length of the coding sequence/mRNA is by designing four overlapping oligonucleotides. Next, the four overlapping oligonucleotides must be "sewed" together by a DNA polymerase in the presence of dNTPs. Finally, by the addition of two flanking primers, the entire, now optimized, sequence can be amplified. (vi) An oligo-dT will not bind to the mRNA of H4, and therefore one has to use a H4-specific primer. One could use for instance the reverse primer as designed by question 1.ii.

2. (a) *Selection of transformed bacteria using ampicillin.* The antibiotic ampicillin is an inhibitor of transpeptidase. This enzyme is required for the making of the bacterial cell wall. The ampicillin resistance gene encodes for the enzyme beta-lactamase, which degrades ampicillin. (b) *Selection of stably transfected mammalian cells using G418.* Most expression plasmids for mammalian cells contain as selection marker the neomycin resistance gene (Neo^r). This gene codes for a protein that neutralizes the toxic drug Geneticin, also known as G418. G418 blocks protein synthesis both in prokaryotic and eukaryotic cells. Only cells that have incorporated the plasmid with the Neo^r gene into their chromosomal DNA will survive. (c) *Selection of hybridomas using HAT medium.* HAT medium contains hypoxanthine, aminopterin, and thymidine. The myeloma cell lines used for the production of monoclonal antibodies contain an inactive hypoxanthine-guanine phosphoribosyltransferase (HGPRT), an enzyme necessary for the salvage synthesis of nucleic acids. The lack of HGPRT activity is not a problem for the myeloma cells because they can still synthesize purines de novo. By exposing the myeloma cells to the drug aminopterin also de novo synthesis of purines is blocked and these cells will not survive anymore. Selection against the unfused lymphocytes is not necessary, since these cells, like most primary cells, do not survive for a long time in cell culture.
3. First, calculate the molecular weight of the plasmid: $3333 \times 2 \times 300 = 2 \times 10^6$ g/mol. → 2×10^6 g plasmid $= 6 \times 10^{23}$ molecules. → 1 g plasmid $= 3 \times 10^{17}$ molecules. →1 μg (1×10^{-6} g) $= 3 \times 10^{11}$ molecules. 1 μg gram plasmid results in 10^8 colonies. Thus, only one in 3000 plasmids is taken up by the bacteria.

SUGGESTED READING

Brekke OH, Sandlie I (2003) Therapeutic antibodies for human diseases at the dawn of the twenty-first century. Nat Rev Drug Discov 2(1):52–62

EvaluatePharma® World Preview 2017 (2017) Outlook to 2022. http://info.evaluategroup.com/rs/607-YGS-364/images/WP17.pdf. Accessed 3 Apr 2018.

GAciarz A, Khatri NK, Velez-Superbie ML, Saaranen MJ, Uchida Y, Keshavarz-Moore E, Ruddock LW (2017) Efficient soluble expression of disulfide bonded proteins in the cytoplasm of Escherichia coli in fed batch fermentations on chemically defined minimal media. Microbio Cell Fact 16:108

Kashmiri SV, De Pascalis R, Gonzales NR, Schlom J (2005) SDR grafting-a new approach to antibody humanization. Methods 36(1):2–34

Kim JY, kim Y-G, Lee GM (2012) CHO cells in biotechnology for production of recombinant proteins: current state and further potential. Appl Microbiol Biotechnol 93:917–930

Kircher M, Kelso J (2010) High-throughput DNA sequencing-concepts and limitations. Bioessays 32(6):524–536

Kunert R, Reinhart D (2016) Advances in recombinant antibody manufacturing. Appl Microbiol Biotechnol 100:3451–3461

Leader B, Baca QJ, Golan DE (2008) Protein therapeutics: a summary and pharmacological classification. Nat Rev Drug Discov 7(1):21–39

Lodish H, Berk A, Kaiser CA, Krieger M, Scott MP (2007) Molecular cell biology, 6th edn. WH. Freeman & CO, New York

Nothaft H, Szymanski CM (2010) Protein glycosylation in bacteria: sweeter than ever. Nat Rev Microbiol 8(11):765–778

Paul SM, Mytelka DS, Dunwiddie CT, Persinger CC, Munos BH, Lindborg SR, Schacht AL (2010) How to improve R&D productivity: the pharmaceutical industry's grand challenge. Nat Rev Drug Discov 9(3):203–214

Rosano GL, Ceccarelli EA (2014) Recombinant protein expression in Escherichia coli: advances and challenges. Front Microbiol 5(172):1–17

Strohl WR, Knight DM (2009) Discovery and development of biopharmaceuticals: current issues. Curr Opin Biotechnol 20(6):668–672

Wells EA, Robinson AS (2017) Cellular engineering fro therapeutic protein production: product quality, host modification, and process improvement. Biotechnol J 12:16001015, 1–16001015,12

2

Biophysical and Biochemical Characteristics of Therapeutic Proteins

Wim Jiskoot and Daan J. A. Crommelin

INTRODUCTION

For a recombinant human protein to become a therapeutic product, its biophysical and biochemical characteristics must be well understood. These properties serve as a basis for understanding the behavior of the protein under various circumstances, e.g., for establishing the range of conditions to properly purify the protein and to stabilize it during production, storage and shipping.

PROTEIN STRUCTURE

Primary Structure

Most proteins which are developed for therapy perform specific functions by interacting with other small and large molecules, e.g., cell-surface receptors (mostly proteins), nucleic acids, carbohydrates, and lipids. The functional properties of proteins are derived from their folding into distinct three-dimensional structures. Each protein fold is based on its specific polypeptide sequence in which different natural amino acids are connected through peptide bonds in a specific way. This alignment of the 20 amino acid residues, called a primary sequence, has in general all the information necessary for folding into a distinct tertiary structure comprising different secondary structures such as α-helices and β-sheets (see below). Because the 20 amino acids possess different side chains, polypeptides with widely diverse properties are obtained.

All of the natural amino acids consist of a C_α carbon to which an amino group, a carboxyl group, a hydrogen, and a side chain are covalently attached. All natural amino acids, except glycine (having a proton as the side chain), are chiral and have an L-configuration (Fig. 2.1). In a polypeptide these amino acids are joined by condensation to yield peptide bonds consisting of the C_α-carboxyl group of an amino acid joined with the C_α-amino group of the next amino acid (Fig. 2.2).

The condensation gives an amide (NH) group at the N-terminal side of C_α and a carbonyl (C=O) group at the C-terminal side. These groups, as well as the side chains, play important roles in protein folding. Owing to their ability to form hydrogen bonds, they make major energetic contributions to the formation of two important secondary structures, α-helix and β-sheet. The peptide bonds between various amino acid residues are very much equivalent, however, so that they do not determine which part of a sequence should form an α-helix or β-sheet. Sequence-dependent secondary structure formation is determined by the side chains.

The 20 natural amino acids commonly found in proteins are shown in Fig. 2.3. They are described by their full names and three- and one-letter codes. Their side chains are structurally different in such a way that at physiological pH values, aspartic and glutamic acid are negatively charged and lysine and arginine are positively charged. At pH 7.4, a minor fraction of the histidine side chains is positively charged (pKa = 6). Tyrosine and cysteine are protonated and uncharged at physiological pHs, but become negatively charged above pH 10 and 8, respectively.

This text is a revised and abbreviated version of the chapter by Tsutomu Arakawa and John S. Pilo in the fourth, previous edition of this book. The discussion of techniques to physicochemically characterize protein structures was taken out and forms now a separate chapter, Chap. 3.

W. Jiskoot (✉)
Division of BioTherapeutics, Leiden Academic Centre for Drug Research (LACDR), Leiden University, Leiden, The Netherlands
e-mail: w.jiskoot@lacdr.leidenuniv.nl

D. J. A. Crommelin
Department of Pharmaceutics, Utrecht Institute for Pharmaceutical Sciences, Utrecht University, Utrecht, The Netherlands
e-mail: d.j.a.crommelin@uu.nl

D. J. A. Crommelin et al. (eds.), *Pharmaceutical Biotechnology*, https://doi.org/10.1007/978-3-030-00710-2_2

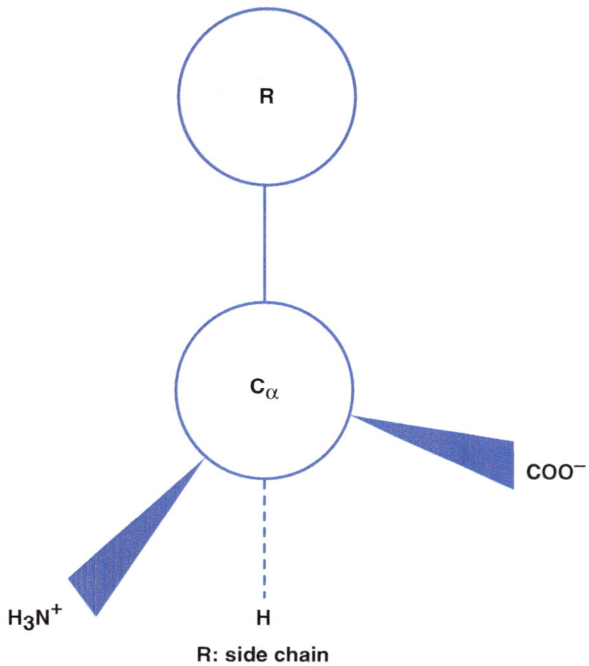

Figure 2.1 ■ Structure of L-amino acids

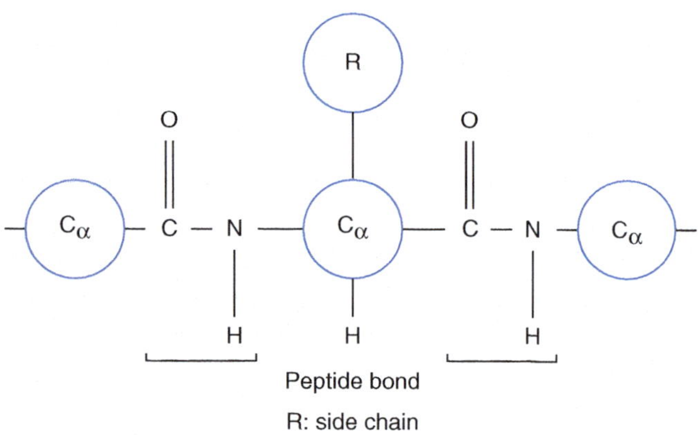

Figure 2.2 ■ Schematical structure of two sequential peptide bonds

Polar amino acids consist of serine, threonine, asparagine, and glutamine, as well as cysteine, while nonpolar amino acids consist of alanine, valine, phenylalanine, proline, methionine, leucine, and isoleucine. Glycine behaves neutrally while cystine, the oxidized form of two cysteines (i.e., a Cys-Cys, or disulfide bridge), is characterized as hydrophobic. Although tyrosine and tryptophan often enter into polar interactions, they are better characterized as nonpolar, or hydrophobic, as described later.

These 20 amino acids are incorporated into a unique sequence based on the genetic code, as the example in Fig. 2.4 shows. This is an amino acid sequence of human granulocyte-colony-stimulating factor (G-CSF), which selectively regulates proliferation and maturation of neutrophils. Although several properties of this protein depend on the location of each amino acid and hence the location of each side chain in the three-dimensional structure, some properties can be estimated simply from the amino acid composition, as shown in Table 2.1.

Using the pK_a values of these side chains, one amino terminus and one carboxyl terminus, one can calculate total charges (positive plus negative charges) and net charges (positive minus negative charges) of a protein as a function of pH, i.e., a titration curve. Since cysteine can be oxidized to form a disulfide bond or can be in a free form, accurate calculation above pH 8 requires knowledge of the status of cysteinyl residues in the protein. The titration curve thus obtained is only an approximation, since some charged residues may be buried and the effective pKa values depend on the local environment of each residue. Nevertheless, the calculated titration curve gives a first approximation of the overall charged state of a protein at a given pH and hence its solubility (Cf. Fig. 5.5, Chap. 5). Other molecular parameters, such as isoelectric point (pI, where the net charge of a protein becomes zero), molecular weight, extinction coefficient, partial specific volume, and hydrophobicity, can also be estimated from the amino acid composition, as shown in Table 2.1.

The primary structure of a protein, i.e., the sequence of the 20 amino acids, can lead to the three-dimensional structure because the various amino acids have diverse physicochemical properties. As an example, Fig. 2.5 shows a cartoon of the three-dimensional structure of filgrastim (recombinant human G-CSF). Each type of amino acid has the tendency to be more preferentially incorporated into certain secondary structures. The frequencies with which each amino acid is found in α-helix, β-sheet, and β-turn, secondary structures that are discussed later in this chapter, can be calculated as an average over a number of proteins whose three-dimensional structures have been solved. These frequencies are listed in Table 2.2. The β-turn has a distinct configuration consisting of four sequential amino acids and there is a strong preference for specific amino acids in these four positions. For example, asparagine has an overall high frequency of occurrence in a β-turn and is most frequently observed in the first and third position of a β-turn. This characteristic of asparagine is consistent with its side chain being a potential site of N-linked glycosylation (see below). Furthermore, effects of glycosylation on the biological and physicochemical properties of proteins are extremely important. However, their contribution to structure is not readily predictable.

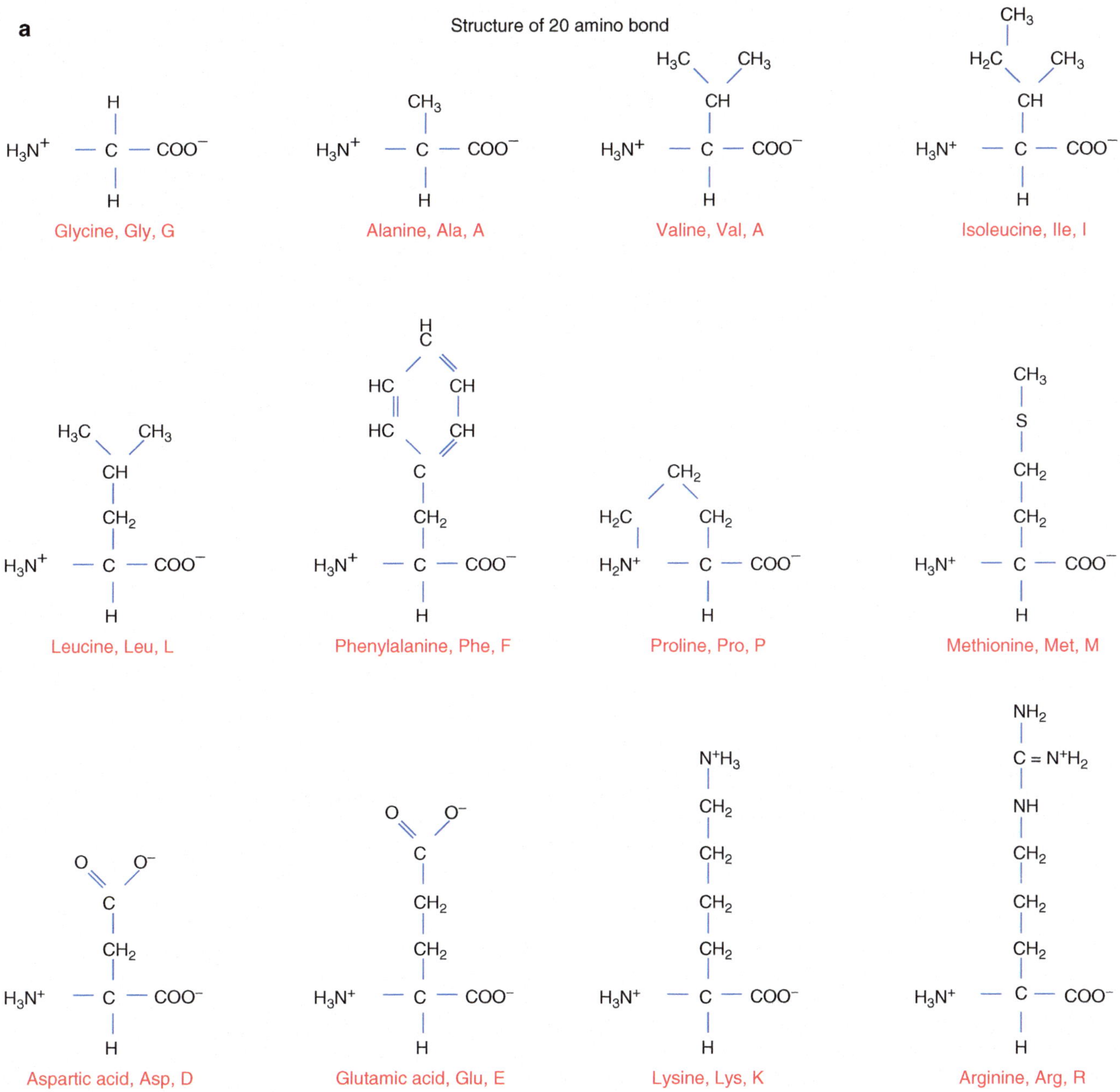

Figure 2.3 ■ **a**, **b** Chemical structure of the 20 natural amino acids, which are the building blocks commonly found in proteins

Another property of amino acids, which impacts protein folding, is the hydrophobicity of their side chains. Although nonpolar amino acids are basically hydrophobic, it is important to know how hydrophobic they are. This property has been determined by measuring the partition coefficient or solubility of amino acids in water and organic solvents and normalizing such parameters relative to glycine. Relative to the side chain of glycine, a single hydrogen, such normalization shows how strongly the side chains of nonpolar amino acids prefer the organic phase to the aqueous phase. A representation of such measurements is shown in Table 2.3. The values indicate that the free energy increases as the side chain of tryptophan and tyrosine are transferred from an organic solvent to water and that such transfer is thermodynamically unfavorable. Although it is unclear how comparable the hydrophobic property is between an organic solvent and the interior of protein molecules, the hydrophobic side chains favor clustering together, resulting

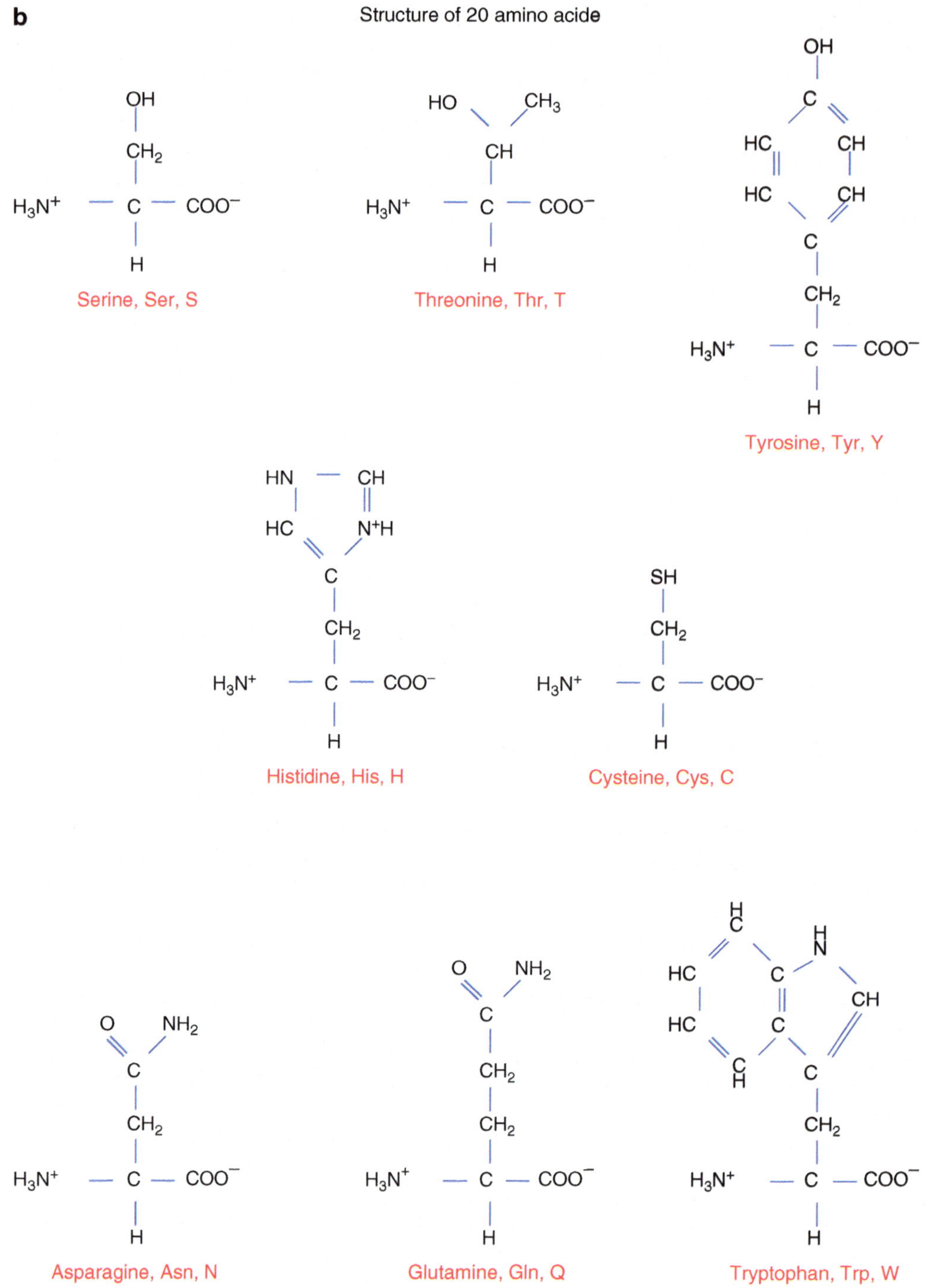

Figure 2.3 ■ (continued)

TPLGPASSLPQSFLLKCLEQVRKIQGDGAALQEKLCATYK 40
LCHPEELVLLGHSLGIPWAPLSSCPSQALQLAGCLSQLHS 80
GLFLYQGLLQALEGISPELGPTLDTLQLDVADFATTIWQQ 120
MEELGMAPALQPTQGAMPAFASAFQRRAGGVLVASHLQSF 160
LEVSYRVLRHLAQP

Figure 2.4 ■ Amino acid sequence of human granulocyte-colony-stimulating factor

Parameter		Value	
Molecular weight		18,673	
Total number of amino acids		174	
1 μg		53.5 pmol	
Molar extinction coefficient		15,820	
1 A (280)		1.18 mg/mL	
Isoelectric point		5.86	
Charge at pH 7		−3.39	
Amino acid	**Number**	**% By weight**	**% By frequency**
A Ala	19	7.23	10.92
C Cys	5	2.76	2.87
D Asp	4	2.47	2.30
E Glu	9	6.22	5.17
F Phe	6	4.73	3.45
G Gly	14	4.28	8.05
H His	5	3.67	2.87
1 Me	4	2.42	2.30
K Lys	4	2.75	2.30
L Leu	33	20.00	18.97
M Met	3	2.11	1.72
N Asn	0	0.00	0.00
P Pro	13	6.76	7.47
Q Gln	17	11.66	9.77
R Arg	5	4.18	2.87
S Ser	14	6.53	8.05
T Thr	7	3.79	4.02
V Val	7	3.71	4.02
W Trp	2	1.99	1.15
Y Tyr	3	2.62	1.72

Table 2.1 ■ Amino acid composition and physicochemical parameters of granulocyte-colony-stimulating factor

in a core structure with properties similar to those of an organic solvent. These hydrophobic characteristics of nonpolar amino acids and hydrophilic characteristics of polar amino acids generate a partition of amino acyl residues into a hydrophobic core and a hydrophilic surface, which contributes to the conformational stability of folded proteins.

■ Secondary Structure

Immediately evident in the primary structure of a protein is that each amino acid is linked by a peptide bond (Fig. 2.2). The amide, NH, is a hydrogen donor and the carbonyl, C=O, is a hydrogen acceptor, and they can form a stable hydrogen bond when they are positioned in an appropriate configuration of the polypeptide chain. Such structures of the polypeptide chain are called secondary structure. Two main structures, α-helix and β-sheet, accommodate such stable hydrogen bonds. Besides α-helices and β-sheets, loops and turns are common secondary structures found in proteins.

α-Helix

The α-helix is a right-handed helix that makes one turn per 3.6 residues. The overall length of α-helices can vary widely. Figure 2.6 shows an example of a short α-helix. In this case, the C=O group of residue 1 forms a hydrogen bond with the NH group of residue 5 and the C=O group of residue 2 forms a hydrogen bond with the NH group of residue 6. All the hydrogen bonds are aligned along the helical axis. Since peptide NH and C=O groups both have electric dipole moments pointing in the same direction, they will add to a substantial dipole moment throughout the entire α-helix, with the negative partial charge at the C-terminal side and the positive partial charge at the N-terminal side.

The side chains project outward from the α-helix. This projection means that all the side chains surround the outer surface of an α-helix and interact both with each other and with side chains of other regions within the protein that come in contact with these side chains. These interactions, so-called long-range interactions, can stabilize the α-helical structure and help it to act as a folding unit. Often an α-helix serves as a building block for the three-dimensional structure of globular proteins by bringing hydrophobic side chains to one side of a helix and hydrophilic side chains to the opposite side of the same helix. Distribution of side chains along the α-helical axis can be viewed using the helical wheel. Since one turn in an α-helix is 3.6 residues long, each residue can be plotted every 360°/3.6 = 100° around a circle (viewed from the top of the α-helix), as shown in Fig. 2.7. Such a plot shows the projection of the position of the residues onto a plane perpendicular to the helical axis. One of the helices in erythropoietin is shown in Fig. 2.7, using an open circle for hydrophobic side chains and an open rectangle for hydrophilic side chains. It becomes immediately obvious that one side of the α-helix is highly hydrophobic, suggesting that this side forms an internal core, while the other side is relatively hydrophilic and is hence most likely exposed to the surface. Since many biologically important proteins function by interacting with other macromolecules, the information obtained from the helical wheel is extremely useful. For example, mutations of amino acids in the solvent-exposed side may lead to identification of regions responsible for biological activity, while mutations in the internal core may lead to altered protein stability.

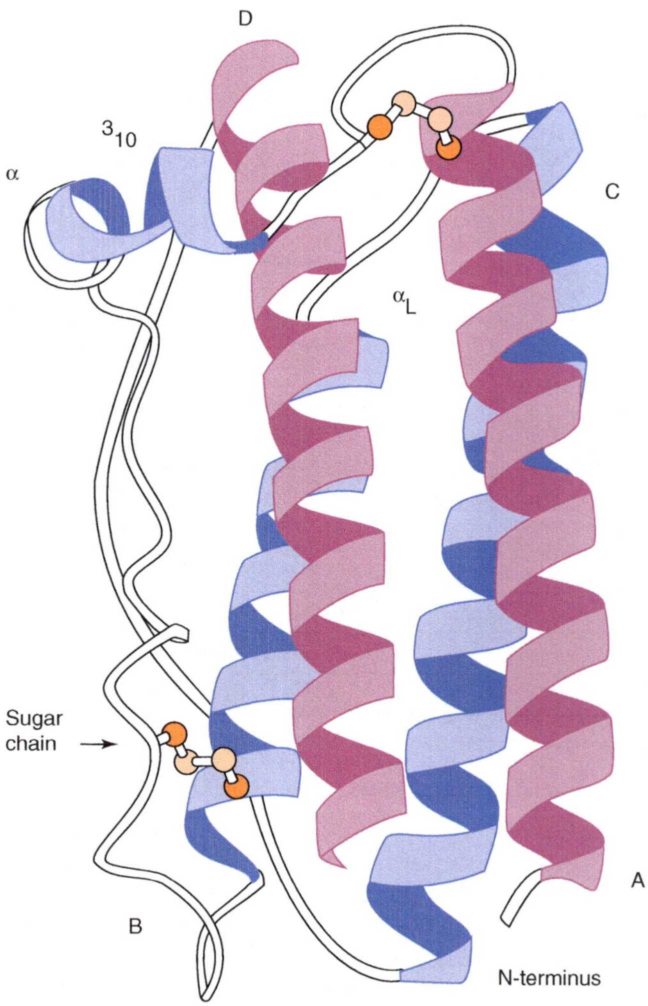

Figure 2.5 ■ Schematic illustration of the three-dimensional structure of filgrastim (recombinant human G-CSF). Filgrastim is a 175-amino acid protein. Its four antiparallel alpha helices (*A*, *B*, *C*, and *D*) and short 3-to-10 type helix (3_{10}) form a helical bundle. The two biologically active sites (α and α_L) are remote from modifications at the N-terminus of the α-helix and the sugar chain attached to loops *C–D*. Note: filgrastim is not glycosylated; the sugar chain is included to illustrate its location in endogenous G-CSF

β-*Sheet*

The second major secondary structural element found in proteins is the β-sheet. In contrast to the α-helix, which is built up from a continuous region with a peptide hydrogen bond linking every fourth amino acid, the β-sheet comprises peptide hydrogen bonds between different regions of the polypeptide that may be far apart in sequence. β-strands can interact with each other in one of the two ways shown in Fig. 2.8, i.e., either parallel or antiparallel. In a parallel β-sheet, each strand is oriented in the same direction with peptide hydrogen bonds formed between the strands, while in antiparallel β-sheets, the polypeptide sequences are oriented in the opposite direction. In both structures, the C=O and NH groups project into opposite sides of the polypeptide chain, and hence, a β-strand can interact from either side of that particular chain to form peptide hydrogen bonds with adjacent strands. Thus, more than two β-strands

α-Helix		β-Sheet		β-Turn		β-Turn position 1		β-Turn position 2		β-Turn position 3		β-Turn position 4	
Glu	1.51	Val	1.70	Asn	1.56	Asn	0.161	Pro	0.301	Asn	0.191	Trp	0.167
Met	1.45	Lie	1.60	Gly	1.56	Cys	0.149	Ser	0.139	Gly	0.190	Gly	0.152
Ala	1.42	Tyr	1.47	Pro	1.52	Asp	0.147	Lys	0.115	Asp	0.179	Cys	0.128
Leu	1.21	Phe	1.38	Asp	1.46	His	0.140	Asp	0.110	Ser	0.125	Tyr	0.125
Lys	1.16	Trp	1.37	Ser	1.43	Ser	0.120	Thr	0.108	Cys	0.117	Ser	0.106
Phe	1.13	Leu	1.30	Cys	1.19	Pro	0.102	Arg	0.106	Tyr	0.114	Gln	0.098
Gln	1.11	Cys	1.19	Tyr	1.14	Gly	0.102	Gln	0.098	Arg	0.099	Lys	0.095
Trp	1.08	Thr	1.19	Lys	1.01	Thr	0.086	Gly	0.085	His	0.093	Asn	0.091
Ile	1.08	Gln	1.10	Gln	0.98	Tyr	0.082	Asn	0.083	Glu	0.077	Arg	0.085
Val	1.06	Met	1.05	Thr	0.96	Trp	0.077	Met	0.082	Lys	0.072	Asp	0.081
Asp	1.01	Arg	0.93	Trp	0.96	Gln	0.074	Ala	0.076	Tyr	0.065	Thr	0.079
His	1.00	Asn	0.89	Arg	0.95	Arg	0.070	Tyr	0.065	Phe	0.065	Leu	0.070
Arg	0.98	His	0.87	His	0.95	Met	0.068	Glu	0.060	Trp	0.064	Pro	0.068
Thr	0.83	Ala	0.83	Glu	0.74	Val	0.062	Cys	0.053	Gln	0.037	Phe	0.065
Ser	0.77	Ser	0.75	Ala	0.66	Leu	0.061	Val	0.048	Leu	0.036	Glu	0.064
Cys	0.70	Gly	0.75	Met	0.60	Ala	0.060	His	0.047	Ala	0.035	Ala	0.058
Tyr	0.69	Lys	0.74	Phe	0.60	Phe	0.059	Phe	0.041	Pro	0.034	Ile	0.056
Asn	0.67	Pro	0.55	Leu	0.59	Glu	0.056	Ile	0.034	Val	0.028	Met	0.055
Pro	0.57	Asp	0.54	Val	0.50	Lys	0.055	Leu	0.025	Met	0.014	His	0.054
Gly	0.57	Glu	0.37	Ile	0.47	Ile	0.043	Trp	0.013	Ile	0.013	Val	0.053

Taken and edited from Chou PY, Fasman GD (1978) Empirical predictions of protein conformation. Ann Rev Biochem 47: 251–276 with permission from Annual Reviews, Inc.

Table 2.2 ■ Frequency of occurrence of 20 amino acids in α-helix, β-sheet, and β-turn

Amino acid side chain	Cal/mol
Tryptophan	3400
Norleucine	2600
Phenylalanine	2500
Tyrosine	2300
Dihydroxyphenylalanine	1800
Leucine	1800
Valine	1500
Methionine	1300
Histidine	500
Alanine	500
Threonine	400
Serine	–300

Taken from Nozaki Y, Tanford C (1971) The solubility of amino acids and two glycine peptides in aqueous ethanol and dioxane solutions. Establishment of a hydrophobicity scale. J Biol Chem 246:2211–2217 with permission from American Society of Biological Chemists

Table 2.3 ■ Hydrophobicity scale: transfer free energies of amino acid side chains from organic solvent to water

can contact each other either in a parallel or in an antiparallel manner, or even in combination. Such clustering can result in all the β-strands lying in a plane as a sheet. The β-strands which are at the edges of the sheet may have unpaired alternating C = O and NH groups.

Side chains project perpendicularly to this plane in opposite directions and can interact with other side chains within the same β-sheet or with other regions of the molecule, or may be exposed to the solvent.

However, in almost all known protein structures, β-strands are right-handed twisted. This way, the β-strands adapt into widely different conformations. Depending on how they are twisted, all the side chains in the same strand or in different strands do not necessarily project in the same direction.

Loops and Turns

Loops and turns serve to connect other secondary structure elements, such as α-helices and β-strands. They are comprised of an amino acid sequence which is usually hydrophilic and exposed to the solvent.

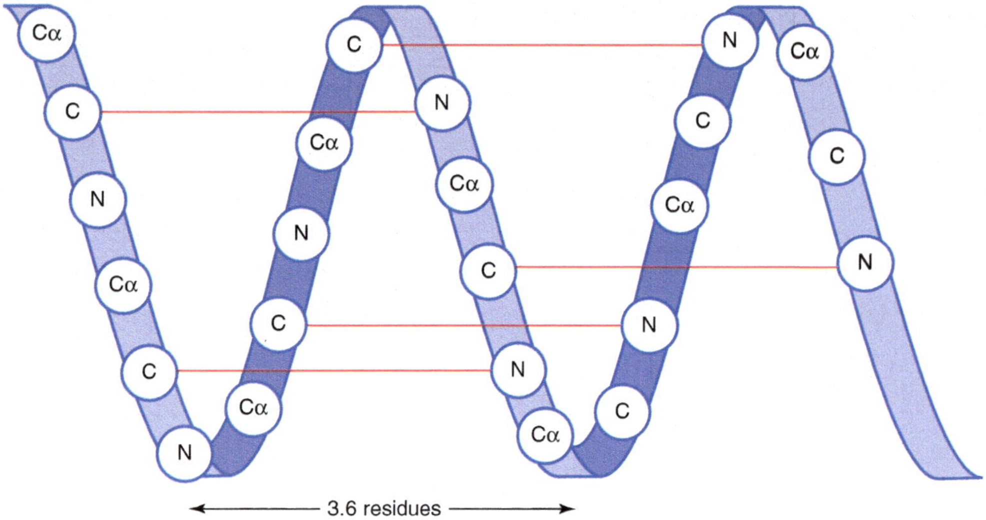

Figure 2.6 ■ Schematic illustration of the structure of an α-helix

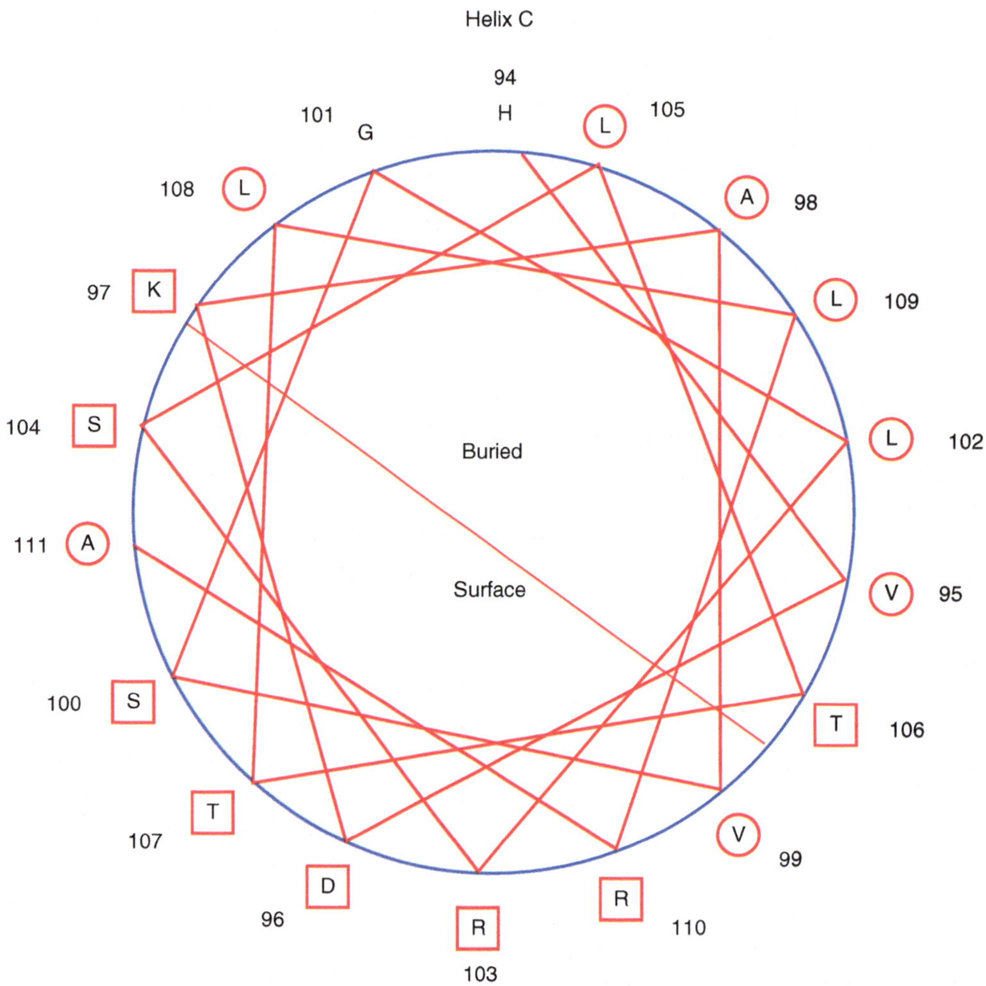

Figure 2.7 ■ Helical wheel analysis of erythropoietin sequence, from His94 to Ala111, with amino acid residues indicated in one-letter code; open circle = hydrophobic side chain, open rectangle = hydrophilic side chains) (Elliott S, personal communication, 1990)

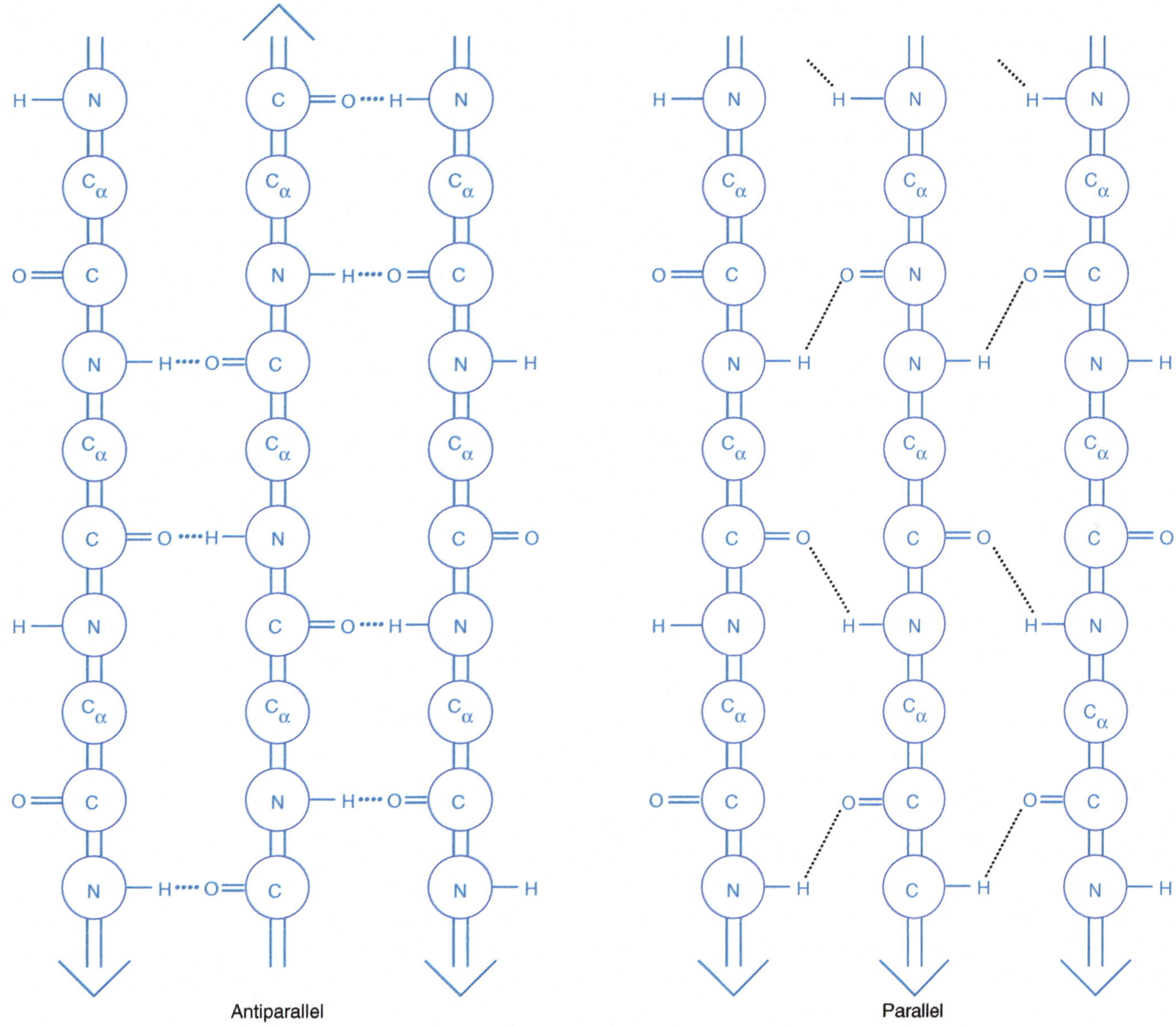

Figure 2.8 ■ Schematic illustration of the structure of an antiparallel (*left side*) and a parallel (*right side*) β-sheet. *Arrow* indicates the direction of amino acid sequence from the N-terminus to C-terminus

These regions consist of β-turns (reverse turns), short hairpin loops, and long loops. Loops and turns usually cause a change in direction of the polypeptide chain, allowing it to fold back to create a compact three-dimensional structure. Turns are short, typically consisting of four amino acid residues, and are stabilized by hydrogen bonds. Loops can be longer and are typically unstructured. Many hairpin loops are formed to connect two antiparallel β-strands.

The amino acid sequences which form β-turns are relatively easy to predict, since turns must be present periodically to fold a linear sequence into a globular structure. Amino acids found most frequently in the β-turn are usually not found in α-helical or β-sheet structures. Thus, proline and glycine represent the least-observed amino acids in these typical secondary structures. However, proline has an extremely high frequency of occurrence at the second position in the β-turn, while glycine has a high preference at the third and fourth position of a β-turn.

Although loops are not as predictable as β-turns, amino acids with high frequency for β-turns also can form a long loop. Loops are an important secondary structure, since they form a highly solvent-exposed region of the protein molecules and allow the protein to fold onto itself.

Tertiary Structure and Quaternary Structure

The spatial arrangement of the various secondary structures in a protein results in its three-dimensional structure. Many proteins fold into a fairly compact, globular structure. Larger proteins usually are folded into several structural domains. Examples are immunoglobulins and Factor VIII.

The folding of a protein molecule into a distinct three-dimensional structure determines its function. Enzyme activity requires the exact coordination of catalytically important residues in the three-dimensional space. Binding of antibodies to antigens and binding of growth factors and cytokines to their receptors all require a distinct, specific surface for high-affinity binding. These interactions do not occur if the tertiary structures of antibodies, growth factors, and cytokines are altered.

A unique tertiary structure of a protein can often result in the assembly of the protein into a distinct quaternary structure consisting of a fixed stoichiometry of protein chains within the complex. Assembly can occur between identical or between different polypeptide chains. Each molecule in the complex is called a subunit. For instance, actin and tubulin self-associate into F-actin and microtubule; hemoglobin is a tetramer consisting of two α- and two β-subunits; among the cytokines and growth factors, interferon-γ is a homodimer, while platelet-derived growth factor is a homodimer of either A or B chains or a heterodimer of the A and B chain. The formation of a quaternary structure occurs via non-covalent interactions and may be stabilized through disulfide bonds between the subunits, such as in the case of the two heavy chains and two light chains of immunoglobulins.

Forces

Interactions occurring between chemical groups in proteins are responsible for formation of their specific secondary, tertiary, and quaternary structures. Either repulsive or attractive interactions can occur between different groups. Repulsive interactions consist of steric hindrance and electrostatic effects. Like charges repel each other and bulky side chains, although they do not repel each other, cannot occupy the same space. Folding is also against the natural tendency to move toward randomness, i.e., increasing entropy. Folding leads to a fixed position of each atom and hence a decrease in entropy. For folding to occur, this decrease in entropy, as well as the repulsive interactions, must be overcome by attractive interactions, i.e., hydrophobic interactions, hydrogen bonds, electrostatic attraction, and van der Waals interactions. Hydration of proteins, discussed in the next section, also plays an important role in protein folding.

These interactions are all relatively weak and can be easily broken and formed. Hence, each folded protein structure arises from a fine balance between these repulsive and attractive interactions. The stability of the folded structure is a fundamental concern in developing protein therapeutics.

Hydrophobic Interactions

The hydrophobic interaction reflects a summation of the van der Waals attractive forces among nonpolar groups in the protein interior, which change the surrounding water structure necessary to accommodate these groups if they become exposed. The transfer of nonpolar groups from the interior to the surface requires a large decrease in entropy, so that hydrophobic interactions are essentially entropically driven. The resulting large positive free energy change prevents the transfer of nonpolar groups from the largely sheltered interior to the more solvent-exposed exterior of the protein molecule. Thus, nonpolar groups preferentially reside in the protein interior, while the more polar groups are exposed to the surface and surrounding environment. The partitioning of different amino acyl residues between the inside and outside of a protein correlates well with the hydration energy of their side chains, that is, their relative affinity for water.

Hydrogen Bonds

The hydrogen bond is ionic in character since it depends strongly on the sharing of a proton between two electronegative atoms (generally oxygen and nitrogen atoms). Hydrogen bonds may form either between a protein atom and a water molecule or exclusively as protein intramolecular hydrogen bonds. Intramolecular interactions can have significantly more favorable free energies (because of entropic considerations) than intermolecular hydrogen bonds, so the contribution of all hydrogen bonds in the protein molecule to the stability of protein structures can be substantial. In addition, when the hydrogen bonds occur in the interior of protein molecules, the bonds become stronger due to the hydrophobic environment.

Electrostatic Interactions

Electrostatic interactions occur between any two charged groups. According to Coulomb's law, if the charges are of the same sign, the interaction is repulsive with an increase in energy, but if they are opposite in sign, it is attractive, with a lowering of energy. Electrostatic interactions are strongly dependent upon distance, according to Coulomb's law, and inversely related to the dielectric constant of the medium. Electrostatic interactions are much stronger in the interior of the protein molecule because of a lower dielectric constant. The numerous charged groups present on protein molecules can provide overall stability by the electrostatic attraction of opposite charges, for example, between negatively charged carboxyl groups and positively charged amino groups. However, the net effects of all possible pairs of charged groups must be considered. Thus, the free energy derived from electrostatic interactions is actually a property of the whole structure, not just of any single amino acid residue or cluster.

Van der Waals Interactions

Weak van der Waals interactions exist between atoms (except the bare proton), whether they are polar or nonpolar. They arise from net attractive interactions between permanent dipoles and/or induced (temporary and fluctuating) dipoles. However, when two atoms approach each other too closely, the repulsion between their electron clouds becomes strong and counterbalances the attractive forces.

■ Hydration

Water molecules are bound to proteins internally and externally. Some water molecules occasionally occupy small internal cavities in the protein structure and are hydrogen bonded to peptide bonds and side chains of the protein and often to a prosthetic group, or cofactor, within the protein. The protein surface is large and consists of a mosaic of polar and nonpolar amino acids, and it binds a large number of water molecules, from the surrounding environment, i.e., it is hydrated. As described in the previous section, water molecules trapped in the interior of protein molecules are bound more tightly to hydrogen-bonding donors and acceptors because of a lower dielectric constant.

Solvent around the protein surface clearly has a general role in hydrating peptide and side chains but might be expected to be rather mobile and nonspecific in its interactions. Well-ordered water molecules can make significant contributions to protein stability. One water molecule can hydrogen bond to two groups distant in the primary structure on a protein molecule, acting as a bridge between these groups. Such a water molecule may be highly restricted in motion and can contribute to the stability, at least locally, of the protein, since such tight binding may exist only when these groups assume the proper configuration to accommodate a water molecule that is present only in the native state of the protein. Such hydration can also decrease the flexibility of the groups involved.

There is also evidence for solvation over hydrophobic groups on the protein surface. So-called hydrophobic hydration occurs because of the unfavorable nature of the interaction between water molecules and hydrophobic surfaces, resulting in the clustering of water molecules. Since this clustering is energetically unfavorable, such hydrophobic hydration does not contribute to the protein stability. However, this hydrophobic hydration facilitates hydrophobic interaction. This unfavorable hydration is diminished as the various hydrophobic groups come in contact either intramolecularly or intermolecularly, leading to the folding of intrachain structures or to protein-protein interactions.

Both the loosely and strongly bound water molecules can have an important impact, not only on protein stability but also on protein function. For example, certain enzymes function in nonaqueous solvent provided that a small amount of water, just enough to cover the protein surface, is present. Bound water can modulate the dynamics of surface groups, and such dynamics may be critical for enzyme function. Dried enzymes are, in general, inactive and become active after they absorb 0.2 g water per g protein. This amount of water is only sufficient to cover surface polar groups, yet may give sufficient flexibility for function.

Evidence that water bound to protein molecules has a different property from bulk water can be demonstrated by the presence of non-freezable water. Thus, when a protein solution is cooled below −40 °C, a fraction of water, ~0.3 g water/g protein, does not freeze and can be detected by high-resolution nuclear magnetic resonance (NMR). Several other techniques also detect a similar amount of bound water. This unfreezable water reflects the unique property of bound water that prevents it from adopting an ice structure.

Proteins are dissolved under physiological conditions or in test tubes in aqueous solutions containing not only water but also other solution components, e.g., salts, metals, amino acids, sugars, and many other minor components (cf. Chap. 5). These components also interact with the protein surface and affect protein folding and stability. For examples, sugars and amino acids are known to enhance folding and stability of the proteins, as described later.

■ Post-translational Modifications

In eukaryotic cells the amino acid sequence of a protein is synthesized in the ribosomes. Subsequently, so-called post-translational modification processes in the endoplasmatic reticulum and the Golgi body of the cell may change the 'amino-acid-only' structure. For instance, sugar groups (glycosylation), phosphate groups (phosphorylation), sulfate groups (sulfation) can be enzymatically attached to the primary amino acid structure of the protein. Disulfide bridge formation is a post-translational modification as well. For therapeutic proteins that undergo post-translational modifications, glycosylation and disulfide bridging are the most relevant ones. An important family of glycosylated and disulfide bridges-carrying molecules is the monoclonal antibody family (Cf. Chap. 8). Other examples of highly glycosylated proteins (also called glycoproteins) are follicle stimulating hormone (Chap. 19), erythopoeitin (Chap. 24) and Factor VIII (Chap. 21). On the other hand, proteins such as insulins, human growth hormone and interferon alfa lack sugar chains. But, all those proteins contain disulfide bonds.

Protein disulfide bonds are essential for the proper folding, functioning and stability of proteins. Oxidative enzymatic steps in the endoplasmatic reticulum lead to cystine bridge formation. When a protein product goes through red-ox cycling, disulfide bonds may open up and form again. Then, disulfide bond shuffling may result in improper protein structures and covalent aggregates.

Glycosylation is a process where many different enzymes generate often complex sugar structures. During glycosylation various sugars can be attached via glycosidic linkages in chains of different lengths and complexity. An important prerequisite for glycosylation is that the protein has sites for N-linked (via asparagine) or O-linked (usually via serine or threonine) glycosylation. Some sugar chains are unbranched, others are branched chains. Common units found in sugar chains of glycoproteins are mannose, galactose, xylose, sialic acid (derivatives of N-acetylneuraminic acid, negatively charged) and N-acetylgalactosamine, N-acetylglucosamine. Figure 2.9 shows examples of glycosylation patterns found for the monoclonal antibody rituximab.

Glycosylation plays a prominent role in the folding process of proteins and their stability, e.g., against aggregation. Moreover, therapeutic activity may be affected as, e.g., with monoclonal antibodies, where the antibody dependent cellular cytotoxicity (ADCC) depends on the glycosylation pattern. Finally, glycosylation, in particular the presence of sialic acid affects PK profiles. High sialic acids densities cause prolonged circulation times (cf. Fig. 19.3).

Standard prokaryotic cells such as *E. coli* don't perform glycosylation reactions. That may be different for engineered prokaryotes (cf. Chap. 4). Proteins expressed in eukaryotic cells can attach sugar chains to their primary structure. They undergo varying degrees of glycosylation depending on the host cell used and cell culture conditions. Moreover, downstream processing conditions may affect (and are sometimes exploited to adjust) the glycosylation profile of the final

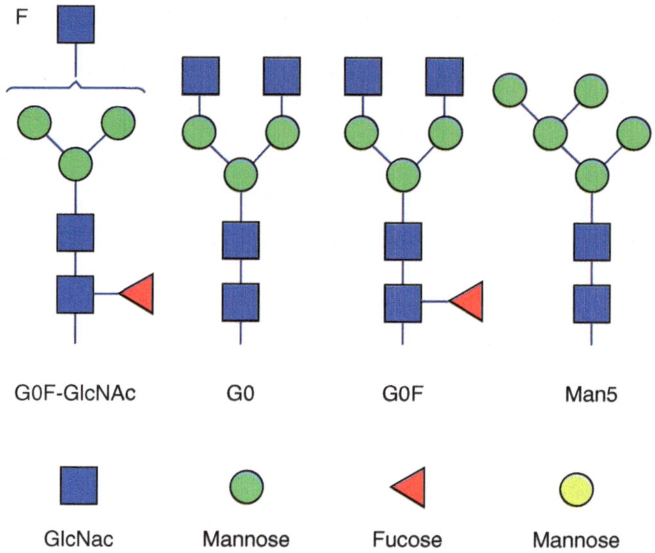

Figure 2.9 ■ Glycosylation pattern of the monoclonal antibody rituximab (Rituxan®/Mabthera®). From: Schiestl et al. (2011) Acceptable changes in quality attributes of glycosylated biopharmaceuticals. Nature Biotechnology 29: 310–312

drug substance. Mammalian cells have an advantage over yeast or plant production cells. Their sugar chain composition closest resembles the 'natural' one. The sugar chains produced in yeast are rich in mannose; their sialic acid content is low. This will increase the clearance rate of these glycoproteins upon injection. Plant derived glycoproteins are rich in fucose and xylose levels. Those structures are believed to increase immunogenicity. As with yeast-derived glycoproteins, they have a relatively low sialic acid content, which affects the pharmacokinetic profile, i.e., accelerated clearance from the blood.

It is important to realize that, unlike the synthesis of a protein's unique primary structure, post-translational modifications result in multiple chemical species, i.e., they introduce heterogeneity in the chemical structure of a protein. For instance, glycosylation variants within one batch of a glycoprotein (e.g., follicle stimulating hormone, FSH, monoclonal antibodies, cf. Fig. 2.9), yield a mixture of various molecular species within one product. This heterogeneity complicates protein characterization but can be identified by analytical techniques such as isoelectric focusing and mass spectrometry (see Chap. 3).

PROTEIN FOLDING

Proteins become functional only when they assume a distinct tertiary structure. Many physiologically and therapeutically important proteins present their surface for recognition by interacting with molecules such as substrates, receptors, signaling proteins, and cell-surface adhesion macromolecules. Upon biosynthesis in vivo, proteins fold in a spatially organized environment that is comprised of ribosomes, ribosome-associated enzymes, chaperones and a highly concentrated macromolecule solution (200–400 mg/mL). The nascent peptide chain often may fold co-translationally. The interplay of codon usage and tRNA abundance plays an important role in introducing appropriate translation pauses in order to regulate the in vivo speed of protein synthesis to achieve correct folding.

The majority of the current therapeutic proteins require several post-translational modifications, such as disulfide formation and glycosylation, in order to be functional (see above). This is why mammalian cell line expression platforms such as CHO and HEK293 are best suited for expression of proteins that require post-translational modifications for their activity. Several *E. coli* strains have been engineered to translocate recombinant protein to the periplasmic space around the *E. coli* cell membrane, which harbors enzymes that can introduce or break disulfide bonds. However, when recombinant proteins are produced in *E. coli*, they often form inclusion bodies into which they are deposited as insoluble proteins. Therefore, an in vitro process is required to refold insoluble recombinant proteins into their native, physiologically active state. This is usually accomplished by solubilizing the insoluble proteins with detergents or denaturants, followed by the purification and removal of these reagents concurrent with refolding the proteins (see Chap. 4).

Unfolded states of proteins are usually highly stable and soluble in the presence of denaturing agents. Once the proteins are folded correctly, they are also relatively stable. During the transition from the unfolded form to the native state, the protein must go through a multitude of other transition states in which it is not fully folded, and denaturants or solubilizing agents are at low concentrations or even absent.

The refolding of proteins can be achieved in various ways. The dilution of proteins at high denaturant concentration into aqueous buffer will decrease both denaturant and protein concentration simultaneously. The addition of an aqueous buffer to a protein-denaturant solution also causes a decrease in concentrations of both denaturant and protein. The difference in these procedures is that, in the first case, both denaturant and protein concentrations are the lowest at the beginning of dilution and gradually increase as the process continues. In the second case, both denaturant and protein concentrations are highest at the beginning of dilution and gradually decrease as the dilution proceeds. Dialysis or the diafiltration of protein in the denaturant against an aqueous buffer resembles the second case, since the denaturant concentration decreases as the procedure continues. In this case, however, the protein concentration remains practically unchanged. Refolding can also be achieved by first binding the protein in denaturants to a solid phase, i.e., to a column matrix, and then equilibrating it with an aqueous buffer. In this case, protein concentrations are not well defined. Each procedure has advantages and disadvantages and may be applicable to one protein, but not to another.

If proteins in the native state have disulfide bonds, cysteines must be correctly oxidized. Such oxidation may be done in various ways, e.g., air oxidation, glutathione-catalyzed disulfide exchange, or mixed-disulfide formation followed by reduction and oxidation or by disulfide reshuffling.

Protein folding has been a topic of intensive research since Anfinsen's demonstration that ribonuclease can be refolded from the fully reduced and denatured state in in vitro experiments. This folding can be achieved only if the amino acid sequence itself contains all information necessary for folding into the native structure. This is the case, at least partially, for many proteins. However, a lot of other proteins do not refold in a simple one-step process. Rather, they refold via various intermediates which are relatively compact and possess varying degrees of secondary structures, but which lack a rigid tertiary structure. Intrachain interactions of these preformed secondary structures eventually lead to the native state. However, the absence of a rigid structure in these preformed secondary structures can also expose a cluster of hydrophobic groups to those of other polypeptide chains, rather than to their own polypeptide segments, resulting in intermolecular aggregation. High efficiency in the recovery of native protein depends to a large extent on how this aggregation of intermediate forms is minimized. The use of chaperones or polyethylene glycol has been found quite effective for this purpose. The former are proteins, which aid in the proper folding of other proteins by stabilizing intermediates in the folding process and the latter serves to solvate the protein during folding and diminishes interchain aggregation events.

Protein folding is often facilitated by cosolvents, such as polyethylene glycol or glycerol. As described above, proteins are functional and highly hydrated in aqueous solutions. True physiological solutions, however, contain not only water but also various ions and low- and high-molecular-weight solutes, often at very high concentrations. These ions and other solutes play a critical role in maintaining the functional structure of the proteins. When isolated from their natural environment, the protein molecules may lose these stabilizing factors and hence must be stabilized by certain compounds, often at high concentrations. These solutes are also used in vitro to assist in protein folding and to help stabilize proteins during large-scale purification and production as well as for long-term storage. These solutes encompass sugars, amino acids, inorganic and organic salts, and polyols. They may not strongly bind to proteins, but instead typically interact weakly with the protein surface to provide significant stabilizing energy without interfering with their functional structure.

SELF-ASSESSMENT QUESTIONS

Questions

1. What is the net charge of granulocyte-colony-stimulating factor at pH 2.0, assuming that all the carboxyl groups are protonated?
2. Based on the above calculation, do you expect the protein to unfold at pH 2.0?
3. Are hydrophilic and hydrophobic amino acids ad random distributed in an alfa-helix primary sequence of a folded protein?
4. (A) What are the different types of forces that stabilize the secondary, tertiary and, eventually, quaternary structure of a protein? (B) Why are solutes changing these folded structures?

Answers

1. Based on the assumption that glutamyl and aspartyl residues are uncharged at this pH, all the charges come from protonated histidyl, lysyl, arginyl residues, and the amino terminus, i.e., 5 His + 4 Lys + 5 Arg + N-terminal = +15.
2. Whether a protein unfolds or remains folded depends on the balance between the stabilizing and destabilizing forces. At pH 2.0, extensive positive charges destabilize the protein, but whether such destabilization is sufficient or insufficient to unfold the protein depends on how stable the protein is in the native state. The charged state alone cannot predict whether a protein will unfold.
3. An α-helix serves as a building block for the three-dimensional structure of globular proteins by bringing hydrophobic side chains to one side of a helix and hydrophilic side chains to the opposite side of the same helix.
4. (A) These forces are covalent forces (disulfide bonds), hydrophobic interactions, hydrogen bonds, electrostatic interactions, van der Waals interactions and hydration forces. (B) These components interact with the protein surface and affect protein folding and stability. For example, sugars and amino acids are known to enhance folding and stability of the proteins, as described below. Another example is buffers that change the pH and by that the charge on the proteins and by that electrostatic intereactions, or (high) concentrations of surfactants that denature (unfold) proteins.

FURTHER READING

Buxbaum E (2015) Fundamentals of protein structure and function, 2nd edn. Springer, New York

Creighton TE (ed) (1989) Protein structure: a practical approach. IRL Press, Oxford

Gregory RB (ed) (1994) Protein-solvent interactions. Marcel Dekker, New York

Schulz GE, Schirmer RH (eds) (1979) Principles of protein structure. Springer, New York

Shirley BA (ed) (1995) Protein stability and folding. Humana Press, Totowa

Whitford D (2005) Proteins: structure and function. Wiley, Hoboken, NJ

3 Protein Stability and Characterization

Atanas Koulov

INTRODUCTION

One of the main tasks in the development of protein therapeutics is the detailed characterization of the recombinant protein—drug candidate. Gaining intimate knowledge of the molecular characteristics of the protein is required for understanding and controlling the manufacturing process, and also the stability of the molecule. The latter is critical for developing a stable and fit-for-purpose drug product, as well as defining an appropriate control strategy for monitoring the stability during long-term storage.

ANALYTICAL TOOLBOX: GENERAL OVERVIEW

The large diversity of possible protein modifications necessitates the use of a broad array of analytical approaches. Naturally, the largest share of analytical methods comes from well-established and traditional technologies of separation science, such as chromatography and electrophoresis. Over the last couple of decades, mass spectrometry approaches have also gained vast popularity, largely owed to the very rapid development of the technology in this field. Unlike traditionally used separation technology approaches, mass spectrometry allows for elucidating the structure of protein modifications and in turn monitoring specific molecular modifications (e.g. oxidation at a specific amino acid residue), as opposed to measuring global (population) changes in the protein structure.

■ Chromatography

Chromatography techniques are extensively used in biotechnology, not only in protein purification procedures (see Chap. 4) but also in assessing the integrity of the product. Routine procedures are highly automated so that comparisons of similar samples can be made. An analytical chromatographic system consists of an autosampler, which will take a known amount (usually a known volume) of material for analysis and automatically places it in the solution stream (mobile phase) headed toward a separation column used to fractionate the sample. Another part of this system is a pump module, which provides a reproducible flow rate. In addition, the pumping system can provide a gradient, which changes the properties of the mobile phase such as pH, ionic strength, and polarity. A detection system (or possibly multiple detectors in series) is located at the outlet of the column. This measures the relative amount of protein exiting the column. Coupled to the detector is a data acquisition system. This takes the signal from the detector and integrates it into a value related to the amount of material (see Fig. 3.1). When the protein solution emerges from the column, the signal begins to increase, and as the protein passes through the detector, the signal subsequently decreases. The area under the peak of the signal is proportional to the amount of material that has passed through the detector. By analyzing known amounts of protein, a peak area versus amount of protein plot can be generated and this may be used to estimate the amount of this protein in the sample under other circumstances. Another benefit of this integrated chromatography system is that low levels of components which appear over time can be estimated relative to the major, desired protein being analyzed. This is a particularly useful function when the long-term stability of the product is under evaluation.

During the more than 100 years of history of chromatography, a large variety of separation modes has been developed and many of these are actively used today for characterization of proteins. Proteins and peptides can be chromatographically separated based on their polarity (reversed-phase chromatography, hydrophobic interaction chromatography, hydrophilic interaction chromatography), charge distribution (ion exchange chromatography), size (size exclusion chromatography), etc. In addition, mixed-mode chromatography (using

A. Koulov (✉)
Analytical Development and Quality Control, Drug Product Services, Lonza AG, Basel, Switzerland
e-mail: atanas.koulov@lonza.com

D. J. A. Crommelin et al. (eds.), *Pharmaceutical Biotechnology*, https://doi.org/10.1007/978-3-030-00710-2_3

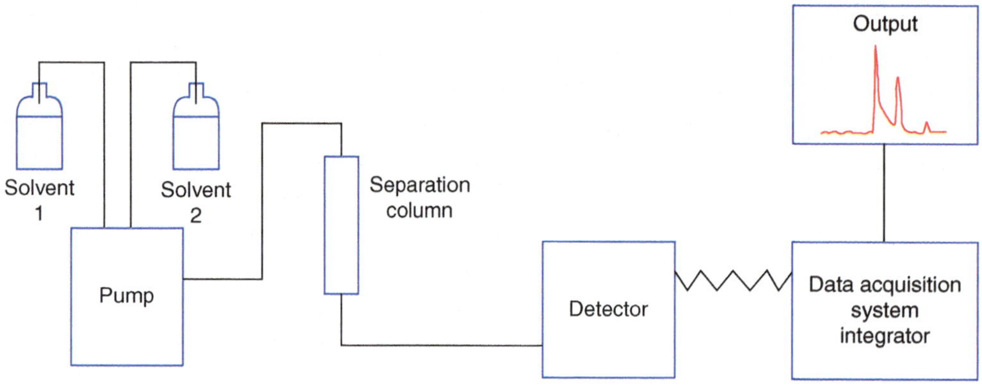

Figure 3.1 ■ *Components* of a typical chromatography station. The pump combines solvents one and two in appropriate ratios to generate a pH, salt concentration, and/or hydrophobic gradient. Proteins that are fractioned on the column pass through a detector, which measures their occurrence. Information from the detector is used to generate chromatograms and estimate the relative amount of each component

columns with both hydrophobic and charged groups, i.e., a combination of ion-exchange and hydrophobic interaction chromatography) and two-dimensional chromatographic approaches (using a sequential combination of separation modes e.g. reversed phase and ion exchange chromatography) are regularly used when characterizing proteins and peptides.

■ Electrophoresis

Generally speaking, the family of electrophoretic techniques separates proteins in an electrical field, based on their charge-to-mass ratio. The charge of the protein depends on the presence of acidic and basic amino acids (cf. Chap. 2) and can be controlled by the pH of the solution in which the protein is separated. The farther away the pH of the solution is from the pI value of the protein, that is, the pH at which it has a net charge of zero, the greater is the net charge and hence the greater is its charge to mass ratio. Alternatively, additives, such as sodium dodecyl sulphate (SDS), may impart an overwhelming negative charge to the protein molecules. This phenomenon forms the basis of the SDS-PAGE (sodium dodecyl sulphate polyacrylamide gel electrophoresis) technique that is/was extensively used to determine the molecular weight of proteins (see section "Polyacrylamide Gel Electrophoresis ((SDS)-PAGE)" and section "Capillary Electrophoresis Sodium Dodecyl Sulfate (CE-SDS)").

Throughout the twentieth century, gel electrophoresis was one of the main methods of choice for characterization of proteins. Since the advent of capillary electrophoresis in the 1980s, significant improvements were achieved in the electrophoretic separation of proteins. Today, capillary electrophoresis is the main electrophoretic method used in the biopharmaceutical analytics.

■ Mass Spectrometry

Mass spectrometry (MS) is a technique in which ions of the various species present in the sample are generated using different ionization techniques and where their molecular masses are measured with high accuracy. This technique is one of the most impactful analytical methods in the current biopharmaceutical analytical practice. While this method was used in the past to analyze small, relatively volatile molecules, the molecular weights of highly charged proteins with masses of over 100 kDa can now be accurately determined. Together with the rapid development of informatics and MS analytical instrumentation incorporating different ionization and detection modes, a large number of different variants of MS have been developed and are currently in use.

One of the main advantages of MS is its ability to determine molecular masses with unparalleled accuracy. This attribute has enabled measuring posttranslational modifications with mass differences of only 1 Da and specific modifications that arise during stability studies. For example, an increase in mass of 16 Da suggests that an oxygen atom has been added to the protein as happens when a methionyl residue is oxidized to a methionyl sulfoxide residue. The molecular mass of peptides obtained after proteolytic digestion and separation by high performance liquid chromatography (HPLC) indicates from which region of the primary structure they are derived. Such an HPLC chromatogram is called a "peptide map." An example is shown in Fig. 3.2. This is obtained by digesting a protein with pepsin and by subsequently separating the digested peptides by reverse HPLC. This highly characteristic pattern for a protein is called a "protein fingerprint." Peaks are identified by elution times on HPLC. If peptides have molecular masses differing from those expected from the primary sequence, the nature of the modification to that peptide can be implicated. Moreover, molecular mass estimates can be made for peptides obtained from unfractionated proteolytic digests. Molecular masses that differ from expected values indicate that a part of the protein molecule has been altered, e.g. that a different glycosylation pattern occurs, that a different or degraded amino acid has been found, or that the protein under investigation still contains contaminants.

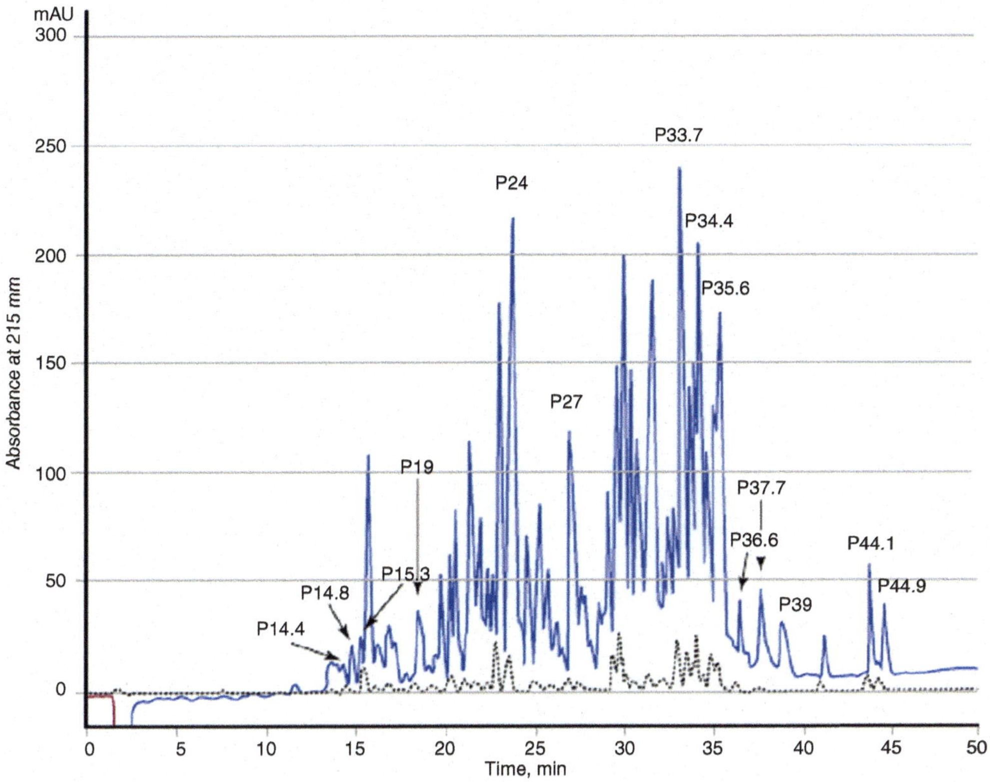

Figure 3.2 ■ Peptide map of a pepsin digest of recombinant human β-secretase. Each peptide is labeled by elution time in HPLC

Another way of using mass spectrometry as an analytical tool is in the sequencing of peptides. A recurring structure, the peptide bond, in peptides tends to yield fragments of the mature peptide, which differ stepwise by an amino acyl residue. The difference in mass between two fragments indicates the amino acid removed from one fragment to generate the other. Except for leucine and isoleucine, each amino acid has a different mass and hence a sequence can be read from the mass spectrometer. Stepwise removal can occur from either the amino terminus or carboxy terminus. In addition, subsequent fragmentation of the individual peptides (MS^2) yields a highly regular fragmentation pattern, which enables sequencing of the parent peptide.

By changing three basic components of the mass spectrometer, i.e. the ion source, the analyzer, and the detector, different types of measurement may be undertaken. Typical ion sources that volatilize proteins are electrospray ionization, fast atom bombardment, and liquid secondary ionization. Common analyzers include quadrupole, magnetic sector, and time-of-flight, electrostatic sector, quadripole ion trap and ion cyclotron resonance instruments. The function of the analyzer is to separate the ionized biomolecules based on their mass-to-charge ratio. The detector measures a current whenever impinged upon by charged particles. Electrospray ionization (El) and matrix-assisted laser desorption (MALDI) are two sources that can generate high-molecular-weight volatile proteins. In the former method, droplets are generated by spraying or nebulizing the protein solution into the source of the mass spectrometer. As the solvent evaporates, the protein remains behind in the gas phase and passes through the analyzer to the detector. In MALDI, proteins are mixed with a matrix, which vaporizes when exposed to laser light, thus carrying the protein into the gas phase. An example of MALDI-mass analysis is shown in Fig. 3.3, indicating the singly charged ion (116, 118 Da) and the doubly charged ion (58,036.2) for a purified protein. Since proteins may carry multiple charges, a number of components are observed representing mass-to-charge forms, each differing from the next by one charge. By imputing various charges to the mass-to-charge values, a molecular mass of the protein can be estimated. The latter step is empirical since only the mass-to-charge ratio is detected and not the net charge for that particular particle.

■ Spectroscopic and Other Techniques for Studying Higher Order Structure

A variety of spectroscopic techniques have found broad use for studying protein structure. These techniques differ significantly by the information content provided and by the amount of expert knowledge required for operation and data interpretation. As a rule: the higher the information content (spatial resolution of the structure) provided by a given method, the more laborious, complex to operate and interpret the data obtained it is.

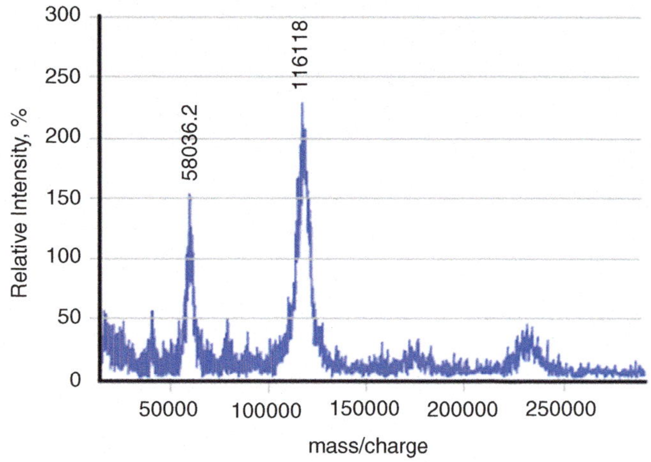

Figure 3.3 ■ MALDI-mass analysis of a purified recombinant human β-secretase. Numbers correspond to the singly charged and doubly charged ions

Circular Dichroism (CD) is a method that utilizes the property of proteins as chiral molecules to differently absorb the right- and left-handed polarized light across the UV and visible parts of the spectrum. CD is used extensively for probing the secondary and tertiary structure of proteins.

Fourier Transformed Infrared Spectroscopy (FTIR) is used to measure the absorption of infrared (IR) light by proteins due to vibrational transitions of various functional groups. In this technique, the absorption of IR light over a broad wavelength range is measured simultaneously, using a device called interferometer. Different factors (such as hydrogen bonding, redox state, bond angles and conformation) can influence the absorption of the vibrating group, which is why FTIR spectroscopy is widely used to probe a protein structure. The repeat units in proteins give rise to several characteristic absorption bands, of which the Amide I (1700–1600 cm^{-1}) bands are perhaps the most useful, due to their sensitivity to the protein secondary structure.

Fluorescence is another widely used spectroscopic technique to study protein conformation, its secondary, tertiary and quaternary structure. In this technique, the fluorescence of the two main fluorophores (Tyr and Trp) present in proteins is used. Trp fluorescence is of particular interest due to the peculiar properties of this fluorophore. One of the two overlapping transitions in Trp is highly sensitive to hydrogen bonding of the indole's –NH group, which in practical terms gives rise to a high sensitivity of the Trp fluorescence spectrum to exposure to water. This property of Trp fluorescence is used to indirectly measure the protein structure as a function of Trp exposure to the aqueous environment.

Some mass spectrometry techniques have been developed with the specific goal to study the higher order protein structure. The most prominent example is Hydrogen-Deuterium exchange MS (HDX-MS). In this technique the different exchange rates of the amide hydrogens over the peptide backbone of the protein are measured using a highly specialized LC-MS system after exposing the protein to deuterium (D_2O) for a brief period of time, followed by quenching of the exchange and a rapid peptide mapping measurement (enzymatically digesting the protein into peptide fragments and measuring the deuteration levels of the individual peptides). Kinetic experiments allow measuring the rates of deuteration of the different peptides, which largely depend on the local structural environment—the level of exposure to the aqueous environment, as well as the conformational flexibility of the given peptide. The results from HDX-MS experiments are visualized using protein maps indicating the rates of exchange in the different protein regions. These maps are extremely useful in understanding the protein dynamics, flexibility and accessibility.

Ion mobility MS (IMS-MS) is another MS technique to study the higher order structure of a protein. Briefly, this technique measures the differential mobility of different protein species in the gas phase in an electric field. This method is mostly used to measure the aggregation state of protein mixtures.

Nuclear Magnetic Resonance (NMR) is a technique that has made major contributions to elucidate the 3D structure of proteins and is becoming more and more popular with the concomitant development of the analytical instrumentation. Very briefly, this technique measures the magnetic properties of atomic nuclei (more specifically the interaction of the magnetic moment of an atomic nucleus with an external magnetic field) which strongly depends of their local environment. Thus, when employing various experimental strategies including 2-D (two dimensional) NMR approaches (also including measurements of different nuclei) in principle allows the determination of the 3D (three dimensional) structure of a protein at atomic resolution. One advantage that NMR has over other high-resolution techniques such as X-ray diffraction, see below) is that one can directly observe protein dynamics in kinetic experiments in solution.

X-ray diffraction is still considered the ultimate technique for studying the structure of proteins. This technique uses the phenomenon of diffraction of a monochromatic X-ray beam by protein crystals. In a protein crystallography experiment the diffraction pattern of the protein crystal is captured from many different orientations of the crystal. From the diffraction patterns obtained (intensity and location of the resulting spots) the positions of the atoms in the molecule can be determined which in turn allows for a calculation of a molecular model of the protein in crystal form, often at atomic resolution.

In the next sections of this chapter, the wide-ranging arsenal of analytical methods to separate and characterize various protein structural modifications is presented in the specific context of these protein modifications. More precisely, applicable analytical techniques are discussed in the context of specific protein attribute(s) altered by a given modification. For example, analytical methods to characterize protein charge heterogeneity are discussed in the context of the modifications which introduce change in protein charge, etc.

PROTEIN STABILITY: WHAT CAN GO WRONG AND HOW TO MEASURE IT?

All levels of structural organization of proteins (See Chap. 2) are susceptible to damage as a consequence of physical or chemical stress (Table 3.1). Different modifications of the protein structure may be manifested as changes in various attributes (properties) of the protein. This is why assessing the stability of protein therapeutics is a complex and multifaceted task. In the following sections of this chapter the most common structural modifications of proteins are presented together with the typical analytical approaches currently applied to measure these modifications.

■ Protein Modifications Introducing Changes in Charge Heterogeneity

Deamidation and Isomerization

Some of the most common and most significant modifications in terms of impact on the properties of protein biopharmaceuticals are the deamidation of asparagine (Asn) and isomerization of aspartate (Asp). The mechanism of deamidation involves the formation of a cyclic imide intermediate (succinimide), which in turn hydrolyzes spontaneously to a mixture of isoaspartic/aspartic acid at an approximate ratio of 3:1. This reaction may be accompanied by further racemization of the

Protein modification	Typical causes and important factors	Physical property affected	Method of analysis
Oxidation Cys Disulfide Intrachain Interchain Met, Trp, Tyr	Light, metal ions, peroxides	Hydrophobicity	RP-HPLC, HIC and mass spectrometry
Fragmentation	pH, sequence (nearest AA neighbor)	Size	Size-exclusion chromatography, SDS-PAGE
N to O migration Ser, Thr		Hydrophobicity	RP-HPLC inactive in Edman reaction
α-Carboxy to β-carboxy migration Asp, Asn		Hydrophobicity	RP-HPLC inactive in Edman reaction
Deamidation Asn, Gln	pH, sequence (nearest AA neighbor), HOS	Charge	Ion-exchange chromatography
Acylation α-Amino group, ε-amino group		Charge	Ion-exchange chromatography mass spectrometry
Esterification/carboxylation Glu, Asp, C-terminal		Charge	Ion-exchange chromatography mass spectrometry
Secondary structure changes		Hydrophobicity	RP-HPLC
		Size	Size-exclusion chromatography
		Sec/tert structure	CD
		Sec/tert structure	FTIR
Aggregation		Sec/tert structure	Fluorescence Light scattering
			Analytical ultracentrifugation, AF4

Table 3.1 ■ Common protein modifications and corresponding methods of analysis

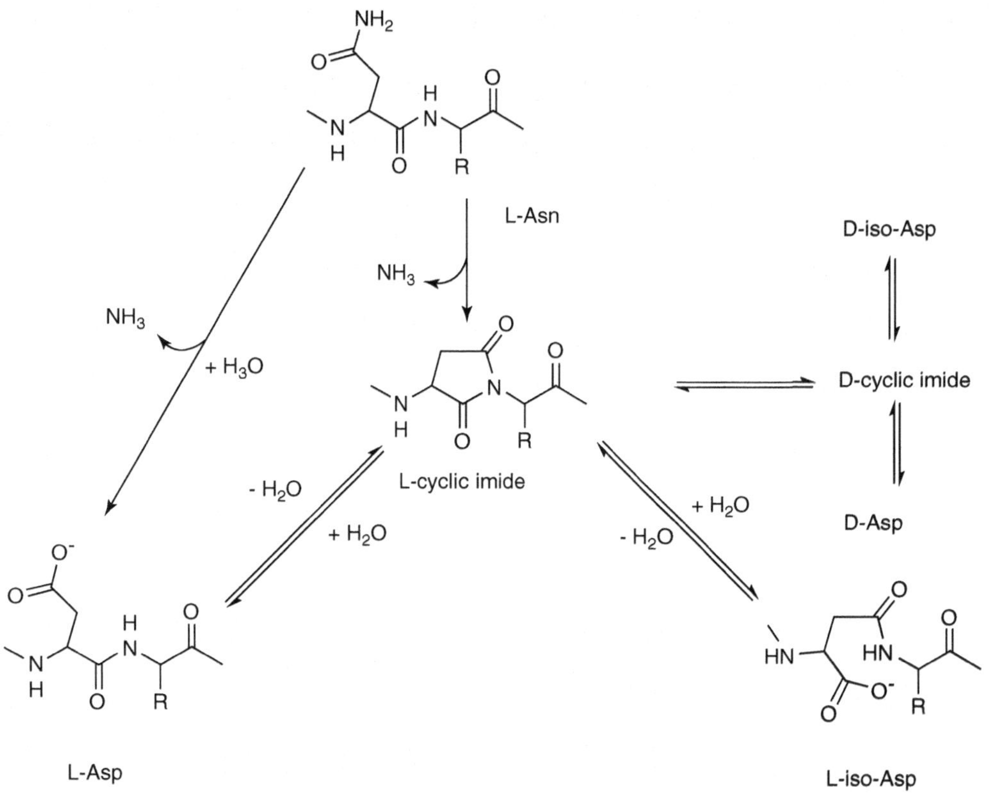

Figure 3.4 ■ Deamidation, isomerization and succinimide formation

isoaspartyl and aspartyl residues via the succinimide intermediate (See Fig. 3.4). Typically, the succinimide intermediate is short-lived at neutral pH, but in some cases may be stabilized.

Isomerization of Asp to isoAsp and deamidation of Asn occur frequently in biotherapeutics. In some cases, these modifications may be benign, but in others they may result in severe consequences for the product, for example in cases when the complementarity-determining regions (CDR) regions of MABs are affected. The biological activity of these molecules may be altered. The most important factors that influence deamidation and isomerization rates are temperature, pH, local protein structure and flanking aminoacyl residues. All chemical reactions mentioned above either result in changes in the charge of the affected protein (deamidation and succinimide formation), or in changes of the surface charge distribution (isomerization). Whereas deamidation results in an increase of acidic species, succinimide formation contributes to an increase of basic variants of the protein.

In should be noted that deamidation can also occur in glutamine (Gln) residues. However, the rates of Gln deamidation are much slower than Asn deamidation rates.

Pyro-Glu Formation

Another common modification that results in a change in the protein charge heterogeneity is the formation of pyroglutamate (pyro-Glu). Cyclization of the N-terminal glutamate (Glu) to pyroGlu (see Fig. 3.5) may occur either enzymatically or spontaneously. PyroGlu formation typically results in protein species with a higher pI than the main isoform.

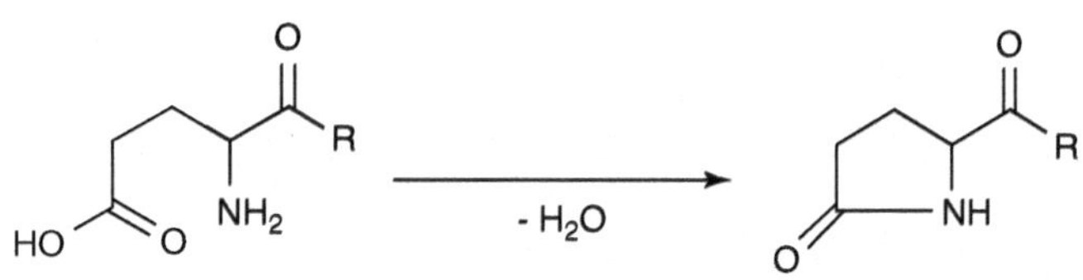

Figure 3.5 ■ Pyro-Glu formation

Glycation

Glycation of proteins is the addition of reducing sugars (e.g. glucose or lactose) to the primary amine of lysine residues. It typically occurs during manufacturing in glucose-containing culture media. The glycation of proteins results in the increase of acidic protein variants.

Additional Modifications Inducing Changes in Protein Charge Heterogeneity

All protein charge modifications mentioned above occur as a result of chemical instability of proteins, i.e. under various types of physico-chemical stress: extreme pH, high temperature, etc. Other modifications that may result in the formation of protein

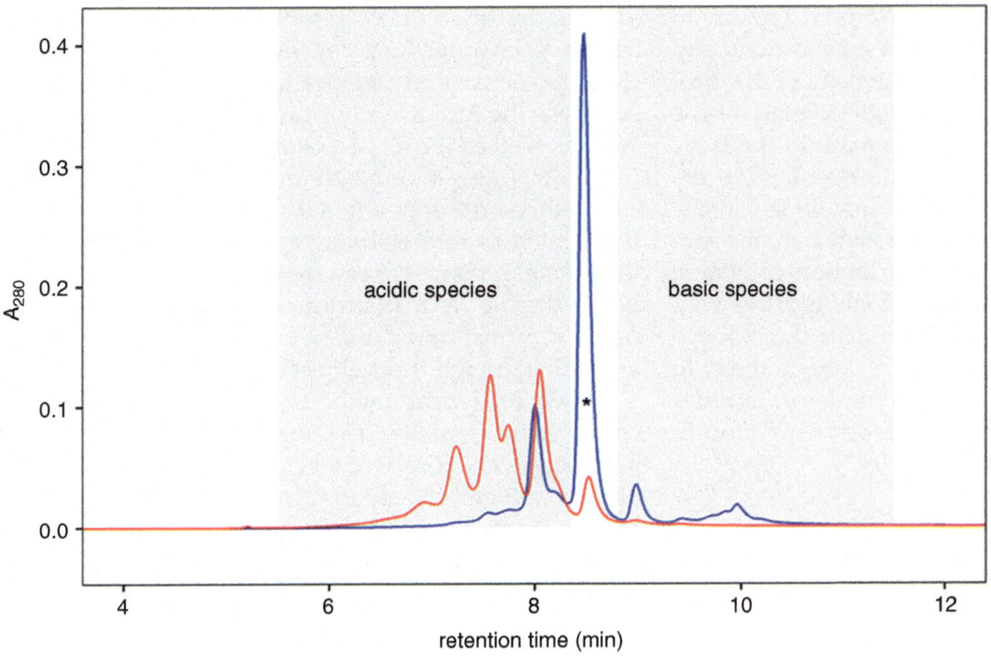

Figure 3.6 ■ Charge heterogeneity profile of a MAB using Cationic Exchange Chromatography: control (blue line) and stressed (red line) acidic species formed during incubation at 40 °C and pH 4.5. The main peak is indicated by a star

charge variants occur as a result of enzymatic reactions—typically during the fermentation process while manufacturing biopharmaceuticals. Such modifications are, for example, the formation of C-terminal Lys variants and the sialylation of proteins.

■ Measuring Changes in Protein Charge Heterogeneity

A number of different protein modifications occurring either during long term storage or during fermentation (upstream processing) may result in changes of the protein charge heterogeneity profile (e.g. deamidation, isomerization, glycation, etc.—see previous section). Because these modifications commonly occur simultaneously, in practice the resulting charge heterogeneity patterns of proteins are often relatively complex. Thus, characterization of the various species underlying the complex protein charge heterogeneity may require the application of different analytical approaches.

There are two main groups of techniques commonly used to measure changes in the charge profile distribution of protein therapeutics: electrophoretic techniques (IEF/icIEF, CZE) and chromatographic techniques (IEC), see below.

Ion-Exchange Chromatography (IEC)

A group of methods that has traditionally been applied for assessment of charge heterogeneity and still finds a very broad use in this context is the group of analytical ion exchange chromatographic techniques (IEC or IEX). The commercial availability of a variety of stationary phases (chromatographic columns) for separation of charge variants using HPLC provides a choice of separation modes (anionic or cationic, strong or weak) and the opportunity for a very good separation and fractionation of variants that are difficult to separate by other techniques.

This technique takes advantage of the electric charge properties of proteins. Some of the amino acyl residues are negatively charged and others are positively charged. The net charge of the protein can be modulated by the pH of its environment relative to the pI value of the protein. At a pH value lower than the pI, the protein has a net positive charge, whereas at a pH value greater than the pI, the protein has a net negative charge. IEC utilizes various resins (chromatographic stationary phases), containing functional groups with either positive or negative charges (anion- or cation-exchange chromatography, correspondingly), depending on the pI of the separated protein. Positively charged proteins bind to negatively charged matrices and negatively charged proteins bind to positively charged matrices. Proteins bound to the chromatographic column are displaced (eluted) from the resin either by increasing the salt concentration of the mobile phase (screening the protein-column charge-charge interactions), or changing the pH of the mobile phase (effectively changing the charge of the protein). Proteins or protein variants with different net charges are separated from one another during elution with the change in the gradient (salt or pH). The choice of the charged resin and elution conditions are dependent upon the protein of interest.

Figure 3.6 shows an example separation of a monoclonal antibody using cationic exchange chromatography (CEX). Acidic isoforms elute before (left side of the chromatogram) and basic isoforms after (right side of the chromatogram) the main isoform. Upon exposure to low pH and elevated temperature stress conditions, significant changes in the charge heterogeneity of this protein can be observed. One finds a large decrease of the main isoform, accompanied by a decrease in the basic and increase in the acidic charge isoforms. Due to the complexity of the possible reactions mentioned in the previous section, it is difficult to assess what are the specific changes underlying the re-distribution of charge variants using this chromatogram alone. For this purpose, typically, it is necessary to fractionate the individual peaks (or groups of peaks) and subject them to further analyses (typically mass spectrometry) in order to establish unequivocally the specific sequence modifications (see section "Mass spectrometry").

Isoelectric Focusing (IEF/cIEF)

Another family of analytical methods to separate proteins based on their electric charge properties is isoelectric focusing (IEF). Isoelectric focusing techniques rely on separating proteins based on their isoelectric point (pI). In a first run, a pH gradient is established within a polyacrylamide gel (or a capillary in cIEF) using a mixture of small-molecular-weight ampholytes with varying pI values. After introduction of the protein sample and application of an electric field, all proteins or protein species/variants migrate within the pH gradient to the pH where their corresponding net charge is zero (their apparent pI). This technique is very useful for separating protein charge variants, such as deamidated or glycated species, from the native protein.

Isoelectric focusing (IEF), or its capillary configuration: Imaged Capillary Isoelectric Focusing (icIEF), has the advantages that it can be applied to a broad variety of molecules and that it typically requires minimal method development efforts. icIEF has found particularly broad use in the biotech industry as a "platform" or "generic" charge heterogeneity assessment method due to its relative ease of use, minimal sample requirements and its broad applicability.

Capillary Zone Electrophoresis (CZE)

Another method which has gained an increased presence over the last decades is Capillary Zone Electrophoresis (CZE). Rather than separating the proteins in a matrix, as in polyacrylamide gel electrophoresis through which the proteins migrate, in CZE the proteins are free in solution in an electric field within the confines of a capillary tube with a diameter of 25–50 μm. After passing through the capillary tube, proteins encounter an UV absorbance or fluorescence detector which can be used to quantify the proteins. The movement of one protein relative to another is a function of the molecular mass and the net charge on the protein. The latter can be influenced by pH and analytes in the solution. Typically, various additives or capillary coatings (e.g. epsilon amino caproic acid (EACA), or triethylenetetramine (TETA)) are used to suppress the interaction of proteins with the capillary wall, as well as the electro-osmotic flow.

CZE offers several advantages over other analytical methods described here to assess charge heterogeneity, such as the relatively easy implementation and low development efforts required. This makes CZE very suitable as a platform method. In addition, it offers a robust and rapid separation, which makes it amenable to high throughput applications.

All analytical methods for measuring protein charge heterogeneity described in this chapter have advantages and disadvantages. The specific application of a given method depends on the given protein or protein mixture measured (e.g. the column, selection of method conditions,) and on the type of modification of the protein structure. Surface modifications for example, are easily detected by IEC, whereas modifications buried within the structure of the protein may be detected better by IEF and CZE. Additional considerations for method selection depend on the specific purpose of the analyses. In cases where the characterization goal is to simply measure the changes under given stress condition, an IEF or a CZE measurement may be sufficient. However, one disadvantage of these electrophoretic methods is the inability for direct fractionation of molecular variants and online coupling (hyphenation) to mass spectrometry for measurements of changes in the primary sequence. Thus, if the goal of the investigation is to understand the chemical nature of these changes and additional measurements (e.g. MS) may be required, IEC may be preferred. In practice, often a combined approach is used—e.g. electrophoretic methods may be used to measure charge heterogeneity routinely, while complementary IEC methods are used for fractionation of specific variants when needed.

■ Protein Modifications Introducing Changes in Size

Proteins can undergo a number of changes that affect their size. These changes may be either covalent modifications such as fragmentation of the polypeptide chain and intermolecular disulfide scrambling, or non-covalent modifications such as protein aggregation and particle formation. Often, such changes dramatically affect protein biopharmaceuticals' potency and safety profiles.

Protein Fragmentation

Despite the fact the peptide bond as such is remarkably stable, fragmentation of the polypeptide backbone of recombinant proteins is a commonly observed modification. The reason for this apparent contradiction is that often, the adjacent amino acid side-chains

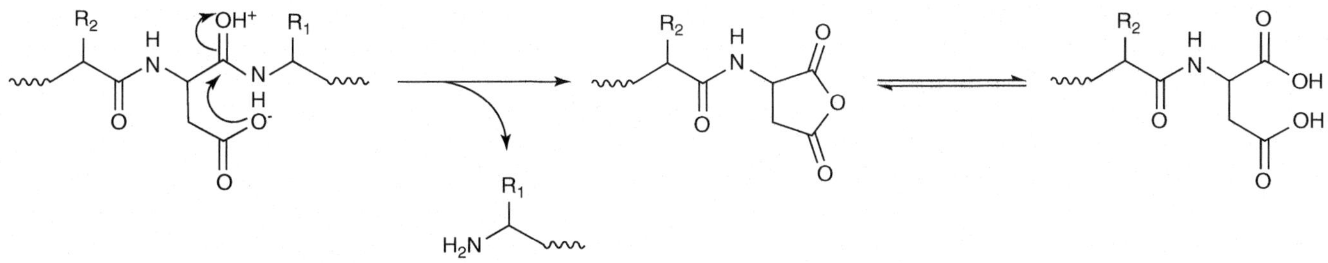

Figure 3.7 ■ Fragmentation of a polypeptide chain at an "Asp-X" site

or local structure flexibility may contribute significantly to rendering a site susceptible to fragmentation. Neighboring amino acid side chains (most commonly Asp, Ser/Thr, Cys/Cys-Cys, Asn) may result in fragmentation which may occur via distinct mechanisms (see details below). In addition, flexible regions, such as disordered loops or the IgG hinge regions, for example, may be particularly prone to fragmentation. Various additional factors and conditions (such as pH, temperature, the presence of radicals) may contribute to increased fragmentation of the polypeptide chain of a protein as well. One of the most common examples of polypeptide chain fragmentation in recombinant proteins is fragmentation at an Asp-X site, where X is any amino acid residue (shown in Fig. 3.7). In this example, at low pH a nucleophilic attack of the ionized side-chain carboxylate of the Asp on the protonated carbonyl carbon of the peptide bond takes place, followed by release of the C-terminal peptide, cyclization and a further hydrolysis of the unstable aspartic anhydride to an Asp residue.

There are many other reported mechanisms of fragmentation of the polypeptide chain, which involve various amino acid residues. Depending on the specific mechanism, various factors affect the rate of fragmentation. In the example above, low pH and small amino acid residues at position X favor the fragmentation reaction. Typically, the structural context (three-dimensional structure of the protein) also influences fragmentation with more disordered regions being more susceptible.

Protein Aggregation

The term "protein aggregation" refers to the process of agglomeration of two or more protein molecules, but it is typically distinct from functional protein-protein binding or quaternary structure formation. This term is too general for practical use, as it encompasses a vast diversity of different molecular phenomena. Protein aggregates can be reversible or irreversible, soluble or insoluble, covalent or non-covalent, etc. Furthermore, protein aggregates are typically present as a continuum of species spanning an enormous size range: from a few nm to >100 μm. Despite various attempts to categorize protein aggregation in a systematic fashion, to date there is still no sufficient clarity and agreement on nomenclature.

Protein aggregation may take place as a result of a variety of phenomena, such as local unfolding or perturbation of the protein secondary, tertiary or quaternary structure. This general mechanism is typically evoked in cases when the system (e.g. protein solution) receives an excess of energy, such as during thermal stress. The physical stability of a protein is expressed as the difference in free energy, ΔG_U, between the native and denatured states. Thus, protein molecules are in equilibrium between the above two states. As long as this unfolding is reversible and ΔG_U is positive, it does not matter how small the ΔG_U is. In many cases, this reversibility does not hold. This is often seen when ΔG_U is decreased by heating. Most proteins denature (i.e., unfold) upon heating and subsequent aggregation of the denatured molecules results in irreversible denaturation. Thus, reversible unfolding is made irreversible by aggregation:

$$\text{Native state} \overset{\Delta G_U}{\Leftrightarrow} \text{Denatured state} \overset{k}{\Rightarrow} \text{Aggregated state}$$

Therefore, any stress that decreases ΔG_U and increases k will cause the accumulation of irreversibly inactivated forms of the protein. Such stresses may include chemical modifications as described above. Protein aggregation may occur as a result of oxidative processes such as disulfide scrambling or the chosen physical conditions, such as pH, ionic strength, protein concentration, and temperature. Development of a suitable formulation that prolongs the shelf life of a recombinant protein is essential when it is to be used as a human therapeutic (cf. Chap. 5).

Despite the variety of molecular mechanisms via which protein aggregation may ensue, the final outcome is the generation of protein species larger than the original molecule. Thus, all techniques for measuring protein aggregation are size-based.

■ Measuring Changes in Protein Size

Similar to all other analytical techniques, the size-based protein characterization methods each have their advantages and disadvantages. Thus, some find more extensive use in characterizing small protein fragments and others in measuring large molecular weight species and proteinaceous particles. Because of the huge diversity of protein aggregation mechanisms and products, naturally there is a large array of analytical techniques, which have been developed to study specifically protein aggregation and assess its various aspects. Some techniques are suitable for measuring and characterizing small aggregates (oligomers), whereas others are useful for measuring exclusively high-molecular weight species (protein particles). Some techniques are specifically utilized to evaluate covalent aggregates, whereas others are used for non-covalent aggregates. However, in reality nearly all of the common size-based protein characterization analytical techniques find dual use—for assessment of fragmentation and aggregation alike. This section will present only the most commonly used techniques, without delving into details and discussing the highly specialized technologies with very limited, niche use.

Size-Exclusion Chromatography

As the name implies, this technique separates proteins based on their size or molecular weight or shape. The matrix consists of very fine beads containing cavities and pores accessible to molecules of a certain size or smaller, but inaccessible to larger molecules. The principle of this technique is the distribution of molecules between the volume of solution within the beads and the volume of solution surrounding the beads (cf. Fig. 4.6). Small molecules have access to a larger volume than large molecules. As the solution flows through the column, molecules can diffuse back and forth, depending upon their size, in and out of the pores of the beads. Smaller molecules can reside within the pores for a finite period whereas larger molecules, unable to enter these spaces, continue along in the fluid stream. Intermediate-sized molecules spend an intermediate amount of time within the pores. They can be fractionated from large molecules that cannot access the matrix space at all and from small molecules that have free access to this volume and spend most of the time within the beads.

Size-exclusion chromatography can be used to estimate the mass of proteins by calibrating the column with a series of globular proteins of known mass. However, the separation depends on molecular shape (conformation) as well as mass and highly elongated proteins—proteins containing flexible, disordered regions—and glycoproteins will often appear to have masses as much as two to three times the true value. Other proteins may interact weakly with the column matrix and be retarded, thereby appearing to have a smaller mass. Size-exclusion chromatography can be used to measure both protein fragmentation and protein aggregation, with the latter being more the common application. Sedimentation (ultracentrifugation), light scattering or MS methods are preferred for accurate mass measurement.

Polyacrylamide Gel Electrophoresis ((SDS)-PAGE)

One of the earliest methods for analysis of proteins is polyacrylamide gel electrophoresis (PAGE). Polyacrylamide gels are used as a sieve. By adjusting the concentration of acrylamide that is used in these gels, one can control the migration rate of material within the gel. The more acrylamide, the more hindrance for the protein to migrate in an electrical field. The polyacrylamide gel provides not only a separation matrix, but also a matrix to hold the proteins in place until they can be detected with suitable reagents.

The direction and speed of migration of the protein in a gel depend on the pH of the gel. If the pH of the gel is above its pI value, then the protein is negatively charged and hence migrates toward the positive electrode. The higher the pH of the gel, the faster the migration. This type of electrophoresis is called native gel electrophoresis.

The addition of a detergent, sodium dodecyl sulfate (SDS), to the electrophoretic separation system allows for the separation to take place primarily as a function of the size of the protein. Dodecyl sulfate ions form complexes with proteins, resulting in an unfolding of the proteins, and the amount of detergent that is complexed is proportional to the mass of the protein. The larger the protein, the more detergent that is complexed. Dodecyl sulfate is a negatively charged ion. When proteins are in a solution of SDS, the net effect is that the own charge of the protein is overwhelmed by that of the dodecyl sulfate complexed with it, so that the proteins take on a net negative charge proportional to their mass. Polyacrylamide gel electrophoresis in the presence of sodium dodecyl sulfate is commonly known as SDS-PAGE. All the proteins take on a net negative charge, with larger proteins binding more SDS but with the charge to mass ratio being fairly constant among the proteins. Since all proteins have essentially the same charge to mass ratio, how can separation occur? This is done by controlling the concentration of acrylamide in the path of proteins migrating in an electrical field. The greater the acrylamide concentration, the more difficult it is for large protein molecules to migrate relative to smaller protein molecules. This is sometimes thought of as a sieving effect, since the greater the acrylamide concentration, the smaller the pore size within the polyacrylamide gel. Indeed, if the acrylamide concentration is sufficiently high, some high-molecular-weight proteins may not migrate at all within the gel. Since in SDS-PAGE the proteins are denatured, their hydrodynamic size, and hence the degree of retardation by the sieving effects, is directly related to their mass. Proteins containing disulfide bonds will have a much more compact structure and higher mobility for their mass unless the disulfides are reduced prior to electrophoresis.

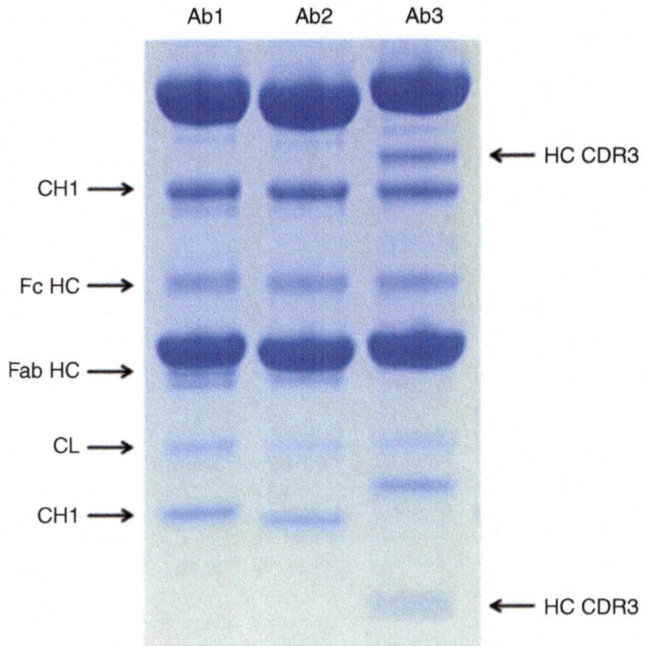

Figure 3.8 ■ Fragmentation of three (Ab1, Ab2 and Ab3) monoclonal antibodies monitored using SDS-PAGE (*taken from Vlasak et al., MAbs (2011) 3:3, 253–263*); CH1—heavy chain constant domain 1, Fc HC—heavy chain Fc domain, Fab HC—heavy chain Fab domain, CL—light chain constant domain, HC—heavy chain, CDR3—complementarity-determining region 3

An example of SDS-PAGE is shown in Fig. 3.8. Here, SDS-PAGE is used to monitor the polypeptide chains of three different monoclonal antibodies and their various fragmentation products.

As described above, native gel electrophoresis and SDS-PAGE are quite different in terms of the mechanism of protein separation. In native gel electrophoresis, the proteins are in the native state and migrate on their own charges. Thus, this electrophoresis can be used to characterize proteins in the native state. In SDS-PAGE, proteins are unfolded and migrate based on their molecular mass.

Detection of Proteins Within Polyacrylamide Gels

Although the polyacrylamide gels provide a flexible support for the proteins, with time the proteins will diffuse and spread within the gel. Consequently, the usual practice is to fix the proteins using fixing solutions (rendering the proteins insoluble) or trap them at the location where they migrated to.

There are many methods for staining proteins in gels, but the two most common and well-studied methods are either staining with a dye called Coomassie blue or by a method using silver. The latter method is used if a very low limit of detection needs to be achieved. The principle of developing the Coomassie blue stain is the hydrophobic interaction of a dye with the protein. Thus, the gel takes on a color wherever a protein is located. Using standard amounts of proteins, the amount of protein or contaminant may be estimated. Quantification using the silver staining method is more complex.

Blotting Techniques

Blotting methods form an important niche in the analytical toolbox of biotech products. Typically, they are used to detect very low levels of unique molecules in a milieu of proteins, nucleic acids, and other cellular components. For example, they can be used to detect components from the host cells used for the production of recombinant proteins (cf. Chap. 4). When blotting, biomolecules are transferred to a synthetic membrane ("blotting"), and this membrane is then probed with specific reagents to detect the molecule of interest. Membranes used in protein blots are made of a variety of materials including nitrocellulose, nylon, and polyvinylidene difluoride (PVDF), all of which avidly bind protein.

Liquid samples can be analyzed by methods called dot blots or slot blots. A solution containing the biomolecule of interest is filtered through a membrane, which captures the biomolecule. Often, the sample is subjected to some type of fractionation, such as polyacrylamide gel electrophoresis, prior to the blotting step. An early technique, Southern blotting, named after the discoverer, E.M. Southern, is used to detect DNA fragments. When this procedure was adapted to RNA fragments and to proteins, other compass coordinates were chosen as labels for these procedures, i.e., northern blots for RNA and western blots for proteins. Western blots involve the use of labeled antibodies to detect specific proteins.

Following polyacrylamide gel electrophoresis, the transfer of proteins from the gel to the membrane can be accomplished in a number of ways. Originally, blotting was achieved by capillary action. The transfer of proteins to the membrane can occur under the influence of an electric field, as well. The electric field is applied perpendicularly to the original field used in separation so that the maximum distance the protein needs to migrate is only the thickness of the gel, and hence, the transfer of proteins can occur very rapidly. This latter method is called electroblotting.

Once the transfer has occurred, the next step is to identify the presence of the desired protein. In addition to various colorimetric staining methods, the blots can be probed with reagents specific for certain proteins, as for example, antibodies to a protein of interest. This technique is called immunoblotting. In the biotechnology field, immunoblotting is used as an identity test for the product of interest. An antibody that recognizes the desired protein is used in this instance. Secondly,

1. Antibodies are labeled with radioactive markers such as ^{125}I
2. Antibodies are linked to an enzyme such as horseradish peroxidase (HRP) or alkaline phosphatase (AP). On incubation with substrate, an insoluble colored product is formed at the location of the antibody. Alternatively, the location of the antibody can be detected using a substrate which yields a chemiluminescent product, an image of which is made on photographic film
3. Antibody is labeled with biotin. Streptavidin or avidin is added to strongly bind to the biotin. Each streptavidin molecule has four binding sites. The remaining binding sites can combine with other biotin molecules which are covalently linked to HRP or to AP

Table 3.2 ■ Detection methods used in blotting techniques (further explained in the text below)

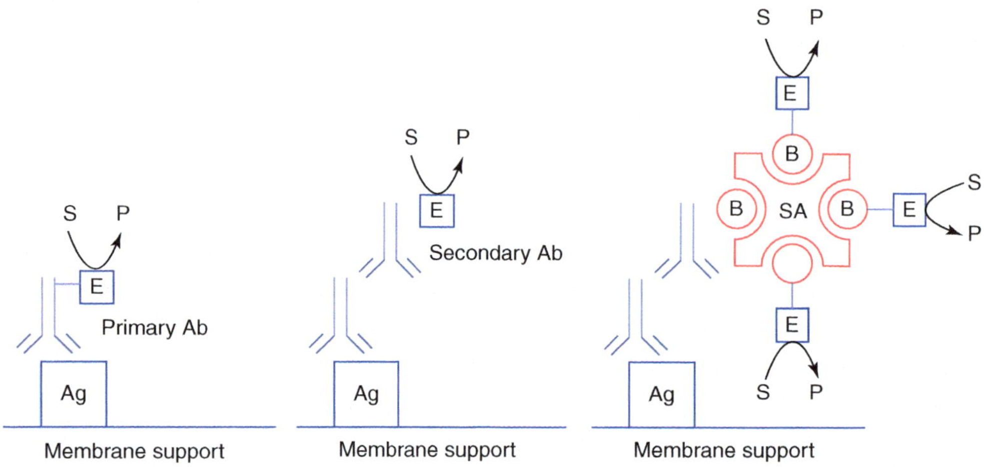

Figure 3.9 ■ Common immunoblotting detection systems used to detect antigens (protein of interest). Ag, on membranes. Abbreviations used: *Ab* antibody, *E* enzyme, such as horseradish peroxidase or alkaline phosphatase, *S* substrate, *P* product, either colored and insoluble or chemiluminescent, *B* biotin, *SA* streptavidin

immunoblotting is sometimes used to show the absence of host proteins. In this instance, the antibodies are raised against proteins of the organism in which the recombinant protein has been expressed. This latter method can attest to the purity of the desired protein.

The antibody reacts with a specific protein on the membrane only at the location of that protein because of its specific interaction with its antigen. When immunoblotting techniques are used, methods are still needed to recognize the location of the interaction of the antibody with its specific protein. A number of procedures can be used to detect this complex (see Table 3.2).

The antibody itself can be labeled with a radioactive marker such as ^{125}I and placed in direct contact with X-ray film. After exposure of the membrane to the film for a suitable period, the film is developed and a photographic negative is made of the location of radioactivity on the membrane. Alternatively, the antibody can be linked to an enzyme that, upon the addition of appropriate reagents, catalyzes a color or light reaction at the site of the antibody. These procedures entail purification of the antibody and specifically label it. More often, "secondary" antibodies are used. The primary antibody is the one that recognizes the protein of interest. The secondary antibody is then an antibody that specifically recognizes the primary antibody. Quite commonly, the primary antibody is raised in rabbits. The secondary antibody may then be an antibody raised in another animal, such as a goat, which recognizes rabbit antibodies. Since this secondary antibody recognizes rabbit antibodies in general, it can be used as a generic reagent to detect rabbit antibodies in a number of different proteins of interest that have been raised in rabbits. Thus, the primary antibody specifically recognizes and complexes a unique protein, and the secondary antibody, suitably labeled, is used for detection (see also section "ELISA" and Fig. 3.9).

The secondary antibody can be labeled with a radioactive or enzymatic marker group and used to detect several different primary antibodies. Thus, rather than purifying a number of different primary antibodies, only one secondary antibody needs to be purified and labeled for recognition of all primary antibodies. Because of their wide use, many common secondary antibodies are commercially available in kits containing the detection system and follow routine, straightforward procedures.

In addition to antibodies raised against the amino acyl constituents of proteins, specific antibodies can be used which recognize unique posttranslational components in proteins, such as phosphotyrosyl residues, which are important during signal transduction, and carbohydrate moieties of glycoproteins.

Figure 3.9 illustrates the above mentioned detection methods that can be used on immunoblots. The primary antibody, or if convenient, the secondary antibody, can have an appropriate label for detection. They may be labeled with a radioactive tag as mentioned previously. Secondly, these antibodies can be coupled with an enzyme such as horseradish peroxidase (HRP) or alkaline phosphatase (AP). Substrate is added and is converted to an insoluble, colored product at the site of the protein-primary antibody-secondary antibody-HRP product. An alternative substrate can be used which yields a chemiluminescent product. A chemical reaction leads to the production of light that can detected by photographic or X-ray film. The chromogenic and chemiluminescent detection systems have comparable sensitivities to radioactive methods. The former detection methods are displacing the latter method, since problems associated with handling radioactive material and radioactive waste solutions are eliminated.

As illustrated in Fig. 3.9, streptavidin, or alternatively avidin, and biotin can play an important role in detecting proteins on immunoblots. This is because biotin forms very tight complexes with streptavidin and avidin. Secondly, these proteins are multimeric and contain four binding sites for biotin. When biotin is covalently linked to proteins such as antibodies and enzymes, streptavidin binds to the covalently bound biotin, thus recognizing the site on the membrane where the protein of interest is located.

Capillary Electrophoresis Sodium Dodecyl Sulfate (CE-SDS)

Today, the traditional slab gel SDS-PAGE is increasingly being replaced by capillary electrophoresis sodium dodecyl sulfate (CE-SDS) due to the improved convenience and possibilities for automation, superior separation and reproducibility of this newer technique. In CE-SDS the separation is carried out in a capillary in the presence of a sieving matrix. Whereas the basic electrophoretic separation principle of CE-SDS is the same as the one of SDS-PAGE, there are also some significant differences. Unlike SDS-PAGE, where only cross-linked polyacrylamide is used as a sieving matrix, in CE-SDS a variety of linear or slightly branched polymers may be used for the same purpose (e.g. linear polyacrylamide, polyethylene oxide, polyethylene glycol, dextran, pullulan). This contributes to the method's flexibility. Another aspect where CE-SDS differs is the detection mode. In this technique, the laborious step of post-separation staining of the SDS-PAGE gels is eliminated and replaced by online UV or highly sensitive fluorescence detection. The elimination of the staining/destaining step as well as the need for scanning of the gels in CE-SDS (online detection generates quantitative electropherograms), together with the CE instrument design contributes to faster and more reproducible analysis, as well as amenability to automation. Altogether, CE-SDS is considered a superior method, demonstrating better accuracy, linearity and precision than SDS-PAGE, which is why the latter has been effectively replaced by CE-SDS in the current pharmaceutical analytical practice.

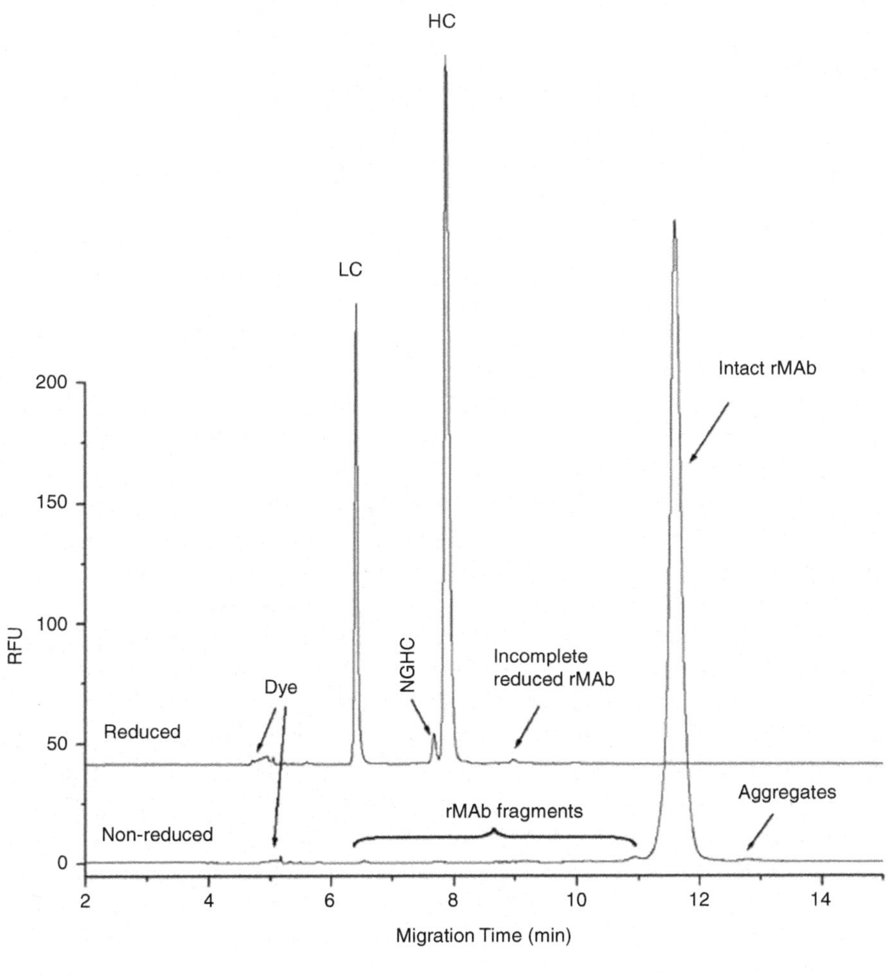

Figure 3.10 CE-SDS reduced and non-reduced separations of a monoclonal antibody, showing the intact MAB, the heavy (HC) and light chains (LC) as well as various fragments, non-glycosylated form and incompletely reduced recombinant rMAB. Taken from Salas-Solano and Felten (2008)

Figure 3.10 shows an example of reduced and non-reduced CE-SDS separations of a monoclonal antibody.

An interesting new trend in the CE instrument development that has emerged recently—the development of new systems based on a microchip technology—has promised to revolutionize these analyses even further. These new chip- or cartridge-based configurations of CE-SDS (also IEF) enable the fully automatic separation of a larger number of samples and improve the ease of use even further. They achieve even faster and higher throughput separations, while maintaining the advantages of CE-SDS over SDS-PAGE.

Asymmetric Field Flow Field Fractionation

Protein aggregation is a process that can produce species spanning a vast size-range, stretching from a few nanometers (oligomeric species) to hundreds of micrometers (visible particles). Measuring the various species across this continuum is impossible using one single technique. Whereas the methods described above (section "Electrophoresis") are limited by the corresponding separation matrices (columns, gels) and can measure protein aggregates up to a certain range (depending on the protein size typically large oligomeric species), for quantifying larger protein species the application of other techniques is required. One of the best techniques for measuring high order protein aggregates is Asymmetric Field Flow Fractionation (AF4). Although this technique was discovered in the 1960s and its application for separation of proteins developed in the 1980s, it has only gained popularity in the last decade.

AF4 is based on the migration of analytes in a mobile phase flowing through a channel with a semi-permeable bottom wall. During the separation, as the analytes advance through the channel they are subjected to an asymmetric field, generated by the application of a flow perpendicular to the sample flow. This leads to the differential migration of the analytes—smaller species eluting faster due to their faster lateral diffusion and larger species eluting slower. Thus, a separation of aggregates of various sizes is achieved without using a stationary phase. The lack of a stationary phase is an advantage as it eliminates the filter effect of columns, column frits and gels, which often leads to exclusion of the large aggregate/particle species from separation altogether. A second advantage is its very wide size range of separation—it can separate aggregates ranging from several nanometers to hundreds of nanometers and even micrometers.

Techniques for Measuring Sub-Visible Particles

Protein aggregate species of tens of nanometers and larger are commonly termed "sub-viosible particles" (SvP). Because the sub-visible particles are a critical quality attribute of protein therapeutics (cf. Chap. 7), their accurate and precise measurements are of high importance for the development of biotherapeutics. Due to the broad size-range span of these species, the simultaneous application of several techniques is required in order to measure all applicable species (See Table 3.3).

The traditional and "gold standard" method for measuring particles in the micrometer size-range is Light Obscuration (LO). This method uses a flow cell through which the sample is led. A Laser illuminates the flow cell. A particle passing with the liquid flow casts a shadow over the photodiode detector, which is registered and quantified via the resulting current drop.

A newer technique is Flow Imaging Microscopy (FIM). In this technique, instead of photodiode detector, a high-speed camera is used to capture the images of all individual particles imaged via a microscope. This invention allows for studying the morphology of the particles detected and potentially provides the option to draw conclusions about their composition and origin.

Other methods for particle characterization include some newly emerged techniques, such as Resonance Mass Measurement (RMM) or Nano Tracking Analysis (NTA). Both of these techniques allow measuring the concentrations of sub-micrometer particles, which is their major application. Nanotracking Analysis uses single particle tracking to calculate the diffusion coefficient of each individual particle and in turn—its size. The concentrations of particles in solution are then inferred from the small subset measured. Due to the unique capability of this technique to measure particles >30 nm it finds extensive use in vaccine development and recombinant virus characterization. RMM also offers some unique features, namely the ability to distinguish between particles with different densities. The latter is very useful in discriminating proteinaceous particles from silicone oil droplets (often present in biopharmaceutical drug products in pre-filled syringes or cartridges), for example.

The availability of the various SvP methods allows for coverage of the entire particle size-range. However, as with all analytical methodologies, an important consideration when using different SvP characterization methods in parallel is to recognize the specific advantages and shortcomings that apply to each of them.

	Method principle and data analysis	Size (μm)												Optimal sample concentration (part./ mL)
		0.03	0.05	0.20	0.30	0.50	0.60	0.80	1.00	2.00	5.00	10.00	25.00	
NTA	***Tracking of Brownian motion of individual particles:*** Hypothetical hard spheres that diffuse at the same speed of the tracked particles are assumed. The hydrodynamic diameter is obtained according to the 2D-modified Stokes-Einstein equation. For count determinations the averaged particle abundance (average number of particles per frame) is divided by the estimated volume of the sample chamber.	■	■	■	■	■	■	■						$3x10^8$-$1x10^9$ ~20-70 centers per frame
RMM	***Changes in frequency due to added mass:*** Shifts in frequency with respect to sensor baseline resonance are convert ed into buoyant mass using the sensor-specific sensitivity. Sensitivity is obtained using size standards as calibrators. Knowing the fluid's and particle's density, buoyant mass is converted into dry mass. Assuming a sphere shape, particle diameter is calculated. Concentration is obtained relating the number of events (particles) registered with the volume of sample dispensed			■	■	■	■	■	■	■				< $8x10^6$
EZS	***Changes in resistance due to volume displacement:*** The impedance pulses generated as particles are pumped through an orifice in a glass tube are individually analyzed by the instrument electronic components. As the electrical current is constrained in the aperture orifice each pulse is directly proportional to the volume that the particle displaced and its size. Concentration is obtained relating the number of events (particles) registered with the volume of sample dispensed						■	■	■	■	■	■	■	~ $2x10^5$ Coincidence <5%
FIM	***Image analysis of single particles:*** Digital images of the particles in the sample are captured and analyzed by the instrument software. Following background comparison, intensity values are assigned to each activated pixel. Adjoining pixels below 96% of the maximum brightness is grouped as particles. Internal algorithms are used to generate morphological descriptors per each particle. Concentration is obtained relating the number of events (particles) registered with the volume of sample dispensed.								■	■	■	■	■	< $9x10^4$
LO	***Drop in current due to light obscuration:*** A calibration curve size vs. voltage is defined using calibration size standards. Particle size is obtained by direct interpolation in the calibration curve of the voltage recorded when a particle blocks the sensor. Concentration is obtained relating the number of events (particles) registered with the volume of sample dispensed.									■	■	■	■	< $1.8x10^4$

Reproduced with modifications from Ríos Quiroz et al. (2016)
NTA nano tracking analysis, *RMM* resonance mass measurement, *EZS* electrical zone sensing, *FIM* flow imaging microscopy, *LO* light obscuration

Table 3.3 ■ Analytical techniques commonly used for measuring and characterizing sub-visible particles

Protein Modifications Introducing Changes in Hydrophobicity

Protein Oxidation

Oxidation is a common degradative pathway for proteins. It often has profound effects on their physicochemical properties. Such major property changes may in turn result in alteration of the biological functions of the affected protein, such as loss of binding, reduction of enzymatic activity, unexpectedly rapid clearance. Thus, monitoring protein oxidation is very critical for the successful development of biopharmaceuticals.

Protein oxidation may occur during all stages of protein manufacturing, processing and storage, whenever the proteins may be exposed to oxidative agents. The latter may include peroxides, transition metal ions, exposure to light, etc.

Whereas theoretically all amino acids can be oxidized, in practice the most commonly oxidized amino acid residues are Trp, Met, Tyr, His, Phe and Cys.

Tryptophan residues are particularly susceptible to oxidation due to the relatively high reactivity of the aromatic indole with reactive oxygen species. Tryptophan oxidation typically requires some level of exposure of the Trp residues, which a commonly buried in the three-dimensional structure of proteins. However, when oxidized, tryptophan residues may convert to a large variety of products (see Figs. 3.11 and 3.12), all of which with properties very different from the original Trp. The most common pathway for Trp oxidation includes the formation of N-formylkinurenine.

Another commonly oxidized amino acid is methionine. The sulfur atom in the Met residue can accept either one or two oxygen atoms leading to the formation of sulfoxide or sulfone, correspondingly (see Fig. 3.12). Due to the typically high surface exposure of Met, this modification is relatively common.

Measuring Changes in Protein Hydrophobicity

Most oxidative modifications of proteins result in some changes of the polarity of the affected residues. In the Met and Trp oxidation examples shown here, the resulting products differ from the original residues by their relative hydrophobicity. Thus, protein oxidation is commonly detected and quantified with analytical methods utilizing polarity-based separation. The most common technique using this separation principle is reversed-phase chromatography.

Reversed-Phase High-Performance Liquid Chromatography

Reversed-phase high-performance liquid chromatography (RP-HPLC) takes advantage of the hydrophobic properties of proteins. The functional groups on the column matrix may contain from one to up to 18 carbon atoms in a hydrocarbon chain. The longer this chain, the more hydrophobic is the matrix. The hydrophobic patches of proteins interact with the hydrophobic chromatographic matrix. Proteins are then eluted from the matrix by increasing the hydrophobic nature of the solvent passing through the column. Acetonitrile is a solvent commonly used, although other organic solvents such as ethanol also may be employed. The solvent is made acidic by the addition of trifluoroacetic acid, since proteins have increased solubility at pH values further removed from their pI. A gradient with increasing concentration of hydrophobic solvent is passed through the column. Different proteins have different hydrophobicities and are eluted from the column depending on the "hydrophobic potential" of the solvent.

This technique can be very powerful. It may detect the addition of a single oxygen atom to the protein, as is the case when a methionyl residue is oxidized or when the hydrolysis of an amide moiety on a glutamyl or asparaginyl residue occurs. Disulfide bond formation or shuffling also changes the hydrophobic characteristic of the protein. Hence, RP-HPLC can be used not only to assess the homogeneity of the protein but also to follow degradation pathways occurring during long-term storage.

RP-HPLC does not always provide sufficient resolution for separation of oxidized species of an intact protein, particularly when larger and more complex proteins are analyzed (such as monoclonal antibodies). In such cases various methods can be applied to solve this problem. For example, the intact protein can be digested into subdomains, such as the Fab and Fc fragments in the case of a MAB, or even smaller fragments (cf. Chap. 8). This latter approach typically employs more frequently-cutting enzymes, such as trypsin, or Lys-C, in order to generate a large number of small peptide fragments, which can be better separated on a RP-HPLC from their oxidized isoforms (see Fig. 3.13).

Such RP-HPLC separations of proteolytic digests of recombinant proteins typically yield complex and unique separation patterns ("peptide maps"), which are often used as a method to identify a protein. Several different proteases, such as trypsin, chymotrypsin, and other endoproteinases, are used for these identity tests (see below under section "Mass Spectrometry").

Hydrophobic Interaction Chromatography

A companion to RP-HPLC is hydrophobic interaction chromatography (HIC). In principle, this latter method is normal-phase chromatography, i.e., here an aqueous solvent system rather than an organic one is used to fractionate proteins. The hydrophobic characteristics of the solution are modulated by inorganic salt concentrations. Ammonium sulfate and sodium chloride are often used,

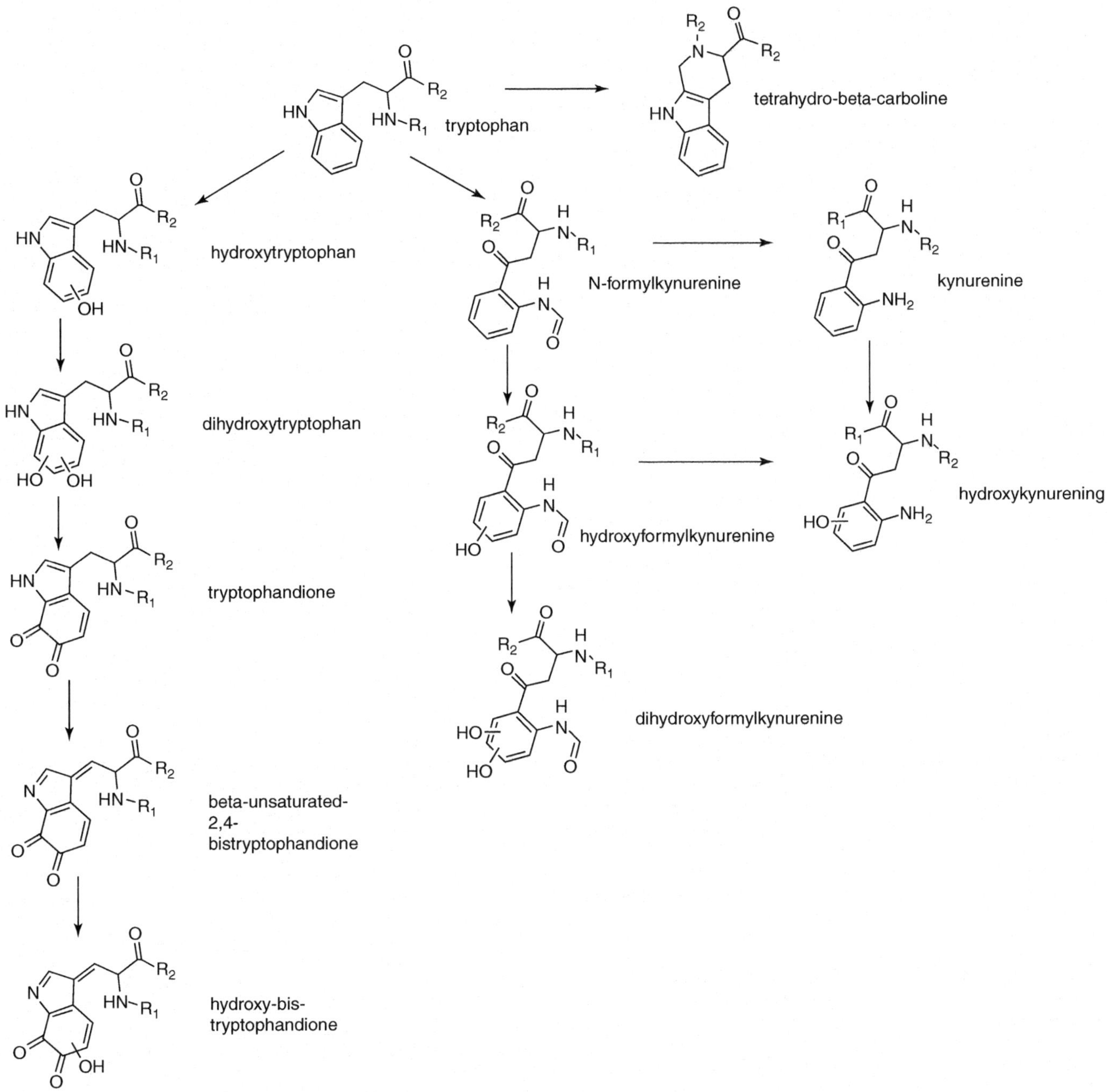

Figure 3.11 ■ Possible oxidation products of tryptophan

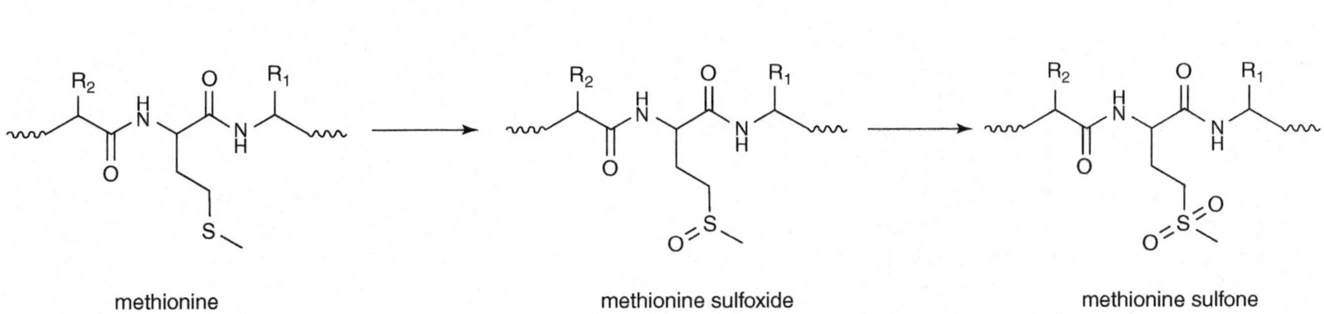

Figure 3.12 ■ Oxidation of a methionine-containing peptide

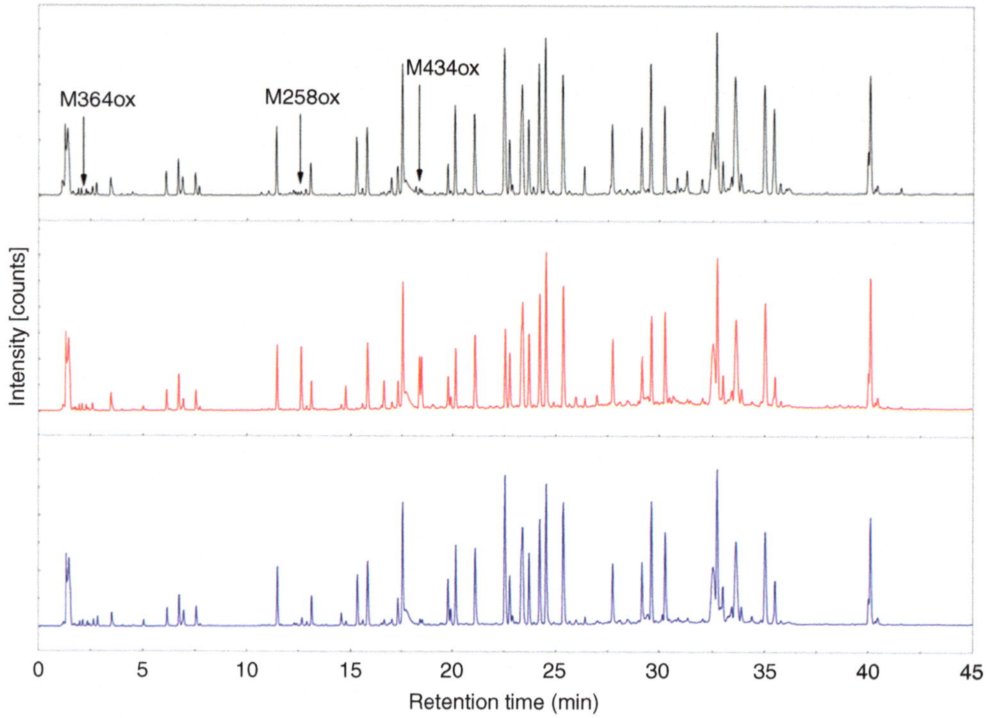

Figure 3.13 ■ A RP-HPLC peptide map of a MAB showing the oxidation of individual methionine residues (indicated by arrows). Top trace shows the peptide map of a non-oxidized protein sample, middle trace—sample oxidized using H_2O_2 and bottom—sample to which H_2O_2 and an antioxidant have been added

since these compounds are highly soluble in water. In the presence of high salt concentrations (up to several molar), proteins are attracted to hydrophobic surfaces on the matrix of resins used in this technique. As the salt concentration decreases, proteins have less affinity for the matrix and eventually elute from the column. This method lacks the resolving power of RP-HPLC, but is gentler, since low pH values or organic solvents as used in RP-HPLC can be detrimental to some proteins.

■ Two-Dimensional (Hyphenated) Techniques

Some analytical techniques can be combined (hyphenated) to achieve additional functionality. Two prominent examples are discussed below.

2-Dimensional Gel Electrophoresis and Differential Gel Electrophoresis

Isoelectric focusing and SDS-PAGE can be combined into a procedure called 2-D gel electrophoresis. Briefly, proteins are first fractionated by isoelectric focusing based upon their pI values. They are then subjected to SDS-PAGE run perpendicular to the first dimension and fractionated based on the molecular weights of the proteins. These separations produce a gel on which each protein appears as a separate spot, corresponding to a specific molecular weight and pI value combination. This setup allows for separating very complex protein mixtures (e.g. extracted from cells or tissues) and is commonly used in the proteomic field (cf. Chap. 9). Another situation where 2D Gel Electrophoresis is regularly applied concerns profiling of host cell proteins.

Another 2-dimensional gel technique is Differential Gel Electrophoresis (DIGE). This technique is essentially 2D Gel Electrophoresis where 2 or 3 different samples are separated simultaneously. The proteins in the samples are labeled with differently colored fluorescent dyes (typically Cy2, Cy3 and Cy5, which are charge- and mass- matched). The proteins co-migrate on the gel and are typically detected simultaneously using a multi-channel scanner or a camera. The overlay of the different channels allows for identifying/visualization of individual proteins being over- or underrepresented in the different samples, which is otherwise very difficult to find out with complex protein mixtures.

2-Dimensional Chromatography

One important strategy for improving the selectivity (specificity) of chromatographic separations is the coupling of two or more columns—for example, an ion exchange column, directly followed by a reversed phase column. This strategy allows for the separation of highly complex analyte mixtures, such as the mixtures of peptides generated during shotgun proteomic experiments. In these experiments multiprotein (up to thousands of proteins) mixtures are digested using a protease (typically trypsin) to produce an even richer mixture of peptides. These peptide mixtures are separated on a 2D chromatographic system in order to reduce the complexity and are commonly analyzed using an MS as a detector. MS/MS fragmentation of the individual peptides allows for the sequencing and identification of each peptide and correspondingly—protein, thus permitting the semi-quantitative analysis of the original protein mixtures. Such approaches are very commonly used in host cell protein (HCP) profiling, and biomarker research.

MODIFICATIONS TO THE HIGHER ORDER STRUCTURE OF PROTEINS

All levels of protein structural organization can be altered as a consequence of physical or chemical stress. These alterations can be manifested in a large diversity of protein modifications, each changing the physicochemical and biological properties of the protein. See Table 3.1.

In addition to covalent modifications (modifications to the primary structure/amino-acid sequence) described in earlier sections, the higher order structure of proteins can undergo changes as well. Such changes can be relatively minor, such as alterations of the quaternary structure (subunit configuration) of a protein complex due to an incorrect disulfide bridge, or more substantial like perturbation of the tertiary structure of a given domain. Some of these possible modifications are described in the following section.

■ Measuring Changes in Higher Order Structure of Proteins

A large number of analytical techniques can be used to measure the structural organization of proteins. However, all these methods differ significantly from each other by the level of information content they provide and the ease of use. Typically, the most accessible and easy to use methods provide a relatively low information content, whereas higher resolution methods (providing specific information about the structure of separate domains and even functional groups and atoms) require highly specialized and expensive equipment and dedicated, highly trained specialized personnel.

Lower Resolution Techniques: CD, FTIR, Fluorescence

Most of the spectroscopic techniques used for characterization of the higher order protein structure (See section "Spectroscopic and Other Techniques for Studying Higher Order Structure") are relatively easy to use, although interpretation of the experimental results typically requires expert knowledge. Very often in biotech development spectroscopic measurements such as CD, FTIR or fluorescence spectroscopy are applied in order to compare protein therapeutic products from different manufacturing batches (typically after changes introduced into the manufacturing process), asking the specific question whether significant differences (alterations of the secondary or tertiary structure) are present between the different batches. In these, so called "comparability studies" (cf. Chap. 12) the first goal is to identify if such changes are present at all. To answer this question, it is sufficient to overlay the CD, FTIR or fluorescence spectra from the different batches and look for any differences. However, one common downside of CD, FTIR and fluorescence spectroscopy is the fact that if differences are seen, it is difficult to judge to which region of the molecule these differences are related. The reason for this is that all of the above-mentioned techniques provide a summary/population information for all of the spectroscopically active functional groups in the molecule (chromophores in the case of CD, fluorophores in the case of fluorescence and amide absorption bands in case of FTIR) and do not provide specific spacial information for individual groups. This means that using the results from such experiments one cannot pinpoint where exactly in the structure of the molecule the detected changes are located. To answer that question, additional analytical work employing higher resolution techniques (see below) is required.

One additional complication resulting from the fact that the methods mentioned above measure the overall molecular population present in the test solution is the fact that the limit of detection (LOD) of specific structural changes is relatively high. More specifically, if a given structural modification has occurred only within a small portion of the overall population (for example, let us say in only 5% of the molecules), this change is unlikely to give sufficiently strong spectral signals to modify the overall (summary) spectrum collected in the experiment. Thus, the techniques described above are typically useful for the detection of gross modifications of the secondary, tertiary (CD, FTIR and fluorescence) and quaternary (fluorescence) structure.

Higher Resolution Techniques

In contrast to the spectroscopic methods described in the previous section, some techniques are capable of providing specific spatial information for specific domains, functional groups or even individual atoms in proteins. The degree of structural detail available varies from method to method and typically, the higher the information content (structural details) —the more complex and specialized the method.

An increasingly popular technique for higher order structures (HOS) determination is HDX-MS (see section "Spectroscopic and Other Techniques for Studying Higher Order Structure"). This method typically provides much higher spatial resolution than the spectroscopic techniques mentioned above, although not as high as X-ray crystallography or NMR (see below). What is typically achieved using HDX-MS is at peptide–level information, allowing to map individual sub-domains according to their mobility and solvent accessibility. These maps (using 3D molecular models) can be extremely useful in understanding structural alterations limited to small regions of the protein. Compared to the higher resolution methods described below, HDX-MS is more accessible (both in terms of instrumentation and also expertise) and it is not limited by the protein size, crystallographic properties or required sample amounts, which are some of the downsides for NMR and X-ray crystallography.

X-ray crystallography is the ultimate spatial resolution method. Using this technique, it is quite common to determine protein structures at an atomic resolution. This technique is indispensable in research focused on enzymes or specific protein binding sites. A number of X-ray crystallographic structure analyses of Ab-Ag complexes, for example, or drug-target molecule complexes have been very illuminating and were critical with respect to advancing drug discovery. In drug development this technique typically does not find as broad use, due to the huge efforts required. Despite advances in this field, including the use of robotics and machine learning approaches, it is not uncommon to take year(s) for solving a given structure, not to mention the fact that solving some structures is currently impossible due to the fact that some proteins are exceedingly difficult to crystalize.

Another very high resolution technique is NMR (See section "Spectroscopic and Other Techniques for Studying Higher Order Structure"). One very significant advantage that this method offers is the fact that experiments can be carried out in solution, meaning that often important aspects of the protein dynamics can be interrogated, a feature not available with other high resolution techniques. Until recently, major limitations of this technique came from the need to label the proteins prior to analyses using stable isotopes and also the size limit to the proteins analyzed. More recent advances in the protein NMR field led to the possibility to obtain 2D ^{13}C NMR methyl fingerprint data for structural mapping of an intact MAB at natural isotopic abundance (Arbogast et al. 2015) which significantly ameliorated the shortcomings mentioned above.

One technique which has undergone a development boom in the twenty-first century is Cryo Electron Microscopy (CryoEM). This technique also allows looking at native structures and complexes in some cases to near-atomic resolution. The huge impact of this technique on biological research and studies of protein complexes was recognized in 2017, when the co-discoverers of the method received the Nobel Prize for Chemistry (Henderson 2018).

BIOLOGICAL ACTIVITY (POTENCY) ASSAYS/ BIOASSAYS

■ Binding Assays (ELISA), Surface Plasmon Resonance (SPR)

Immunoassays

Enzyme-linked immunosorbent assay (ELISA) provides a means to quantitatively measure extremely small amounts of proteins. This procedure utilizes the fact that plastic surfaces are able to adsorb low but detectable amounts of proteins. Typically, antibodies against a certain protein of interest are allowed to adsorb to the surface of microtitration plates. Each plate may contain up to 96 or 384 wells so that multiple samples can be assayed. After incubating the antibodies in the wells of the plate for a specific period, excess antibody is removed and residual protein binding sites on the plastic are blocked by incubation with an inert protein. Several microtitration plates can be prepared at one time since the antibodies coating the plates retain their binding capacity for an extended period. During the ELISA, the sample solution containing the protein of interest is incubated in the wells and the protein (Ag) is captured by the antibodies coating the well surface. Excess sample is removed and other antibodies which now have an enzyme (E) linked to them are added to react with the bound antigen.

The format described above is called a sandwich assay since the antigen (protein of interest) is located between the antibody on the titer well surface and the antibody containing the linked enzyme. Figure 3.14 illustrates a number of formats that can be used in an ELISA. A suitable substrate is added and the enzyme linked to the antibody-antigen-antibody well complex converts this compound to a colored product. The amount of product obtained is proportional to the enzyme adsorbed in the well of the plate. A standard curve can be prepared if known concentrations of antigen (protein of interest) are tested in this system and the amount of antigen in unknown samples can be estimated from this standard curve. A number of enzymes can be used in ELISAs. However, the most common ones are horseradish peroxidase and alkaline phosphatase. A variety of substrates for each enzyme is available; they yield colored products catalyzed by the antibody-linked enzyme. Absorbance of the colored product solutions is measured on plate readers, instruments that rapidly measure the absorbance in all 96 wells of the microtitration plate. Data processing can be automated for rapid throughput of information. Note that detection approaches partly parallel those discussed in the section on "Blotting." The above ELISA format (sandwich assay) is only one of many different ELISA set ups. For example, the microtitration wells may be coated directly with the antigen

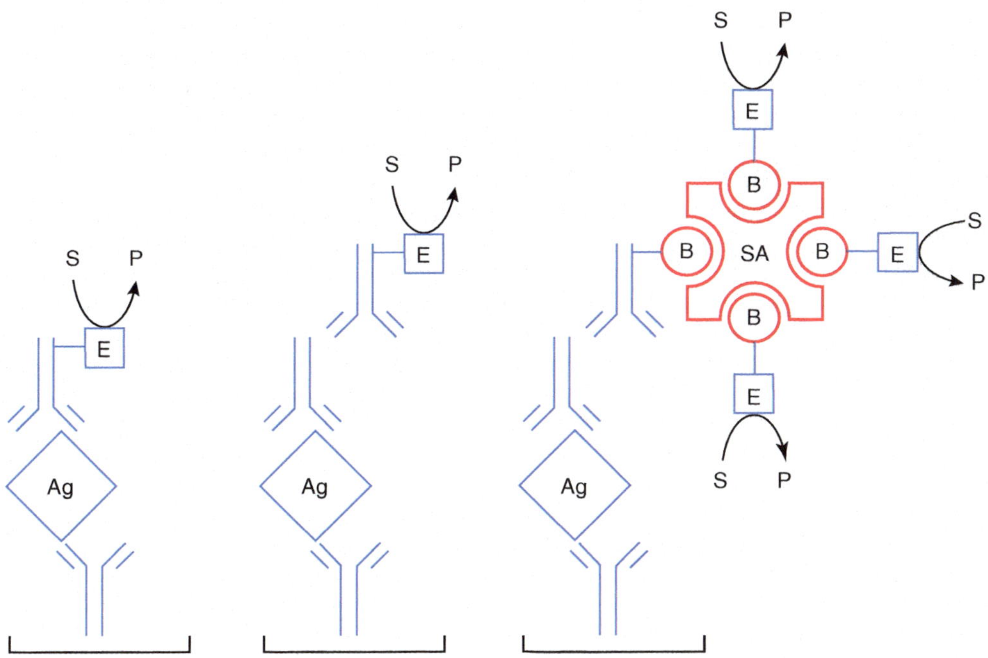

Figure 3.14 ■ Examples of several formats for ELISA in which the specific antibody is adsorbed to the surface of a microtitration plate. See Fig. 3.9 for abbreviations used. The antibody is represented by the Y-type structure. The product *P* is colored and the amount generated is measured with a spectrometer or plate reader

rather than having a specific antibody attached to the surface. The concentration of antigen is established by comparison with known quantities of antigen (protein of interest) used to coat individual wells.

Another approach is to use—this time subsequent to the binding of the antigen (protein of interest) either directly to the surface or to an antibody on the surface—an antibody specific to the antibody binding the protein antigen, that is, a secondary antibody (see section "Blotting Techniques"; Fig. 3.9). This latter, secondary, antibody contains the linked enzyme used for detection. As already discussed in the section on "Blotting," the advantage of this approach is that such antibodies can be obtained in high purity and with the desired enzyme linked to them from commercial sources. Thus, a single source of enzyme-linked antibody can be used in assays for different protein antigens. Should a sandwich assay be used, then antibodies from different species need to be used for each side of the sandwich. A possible scenario is that rabbit antibodies are used to coat the microtitration wells; mouse antibodies, possibly a monoclonal antibody, are used to complex with the antigen; and then, a goat anti-mouse immunoglobulin containing linked HRP or AP is used for detection purposes.

As with immunoblots discussed above, streptavidin or avidin can be used in these assays if biotin is covalently linked to the antibodies and enzymes.

SPR-Based Binding Assays

Surface plasmon resonance techniques are based on the excitation of free electrons (called surface plasmons when excited) by polarized light from a metal film at an interface with a medium having a different refractive index. Binding of molecules to this interfacial layer results in shifts in their reflection curves. Since the refractive index changes are linearly proportional to the number of molecules bound, this technique can be used to calculate a number of binding parameters such as the equilibrium association constant (K_A), equilibrium dissociation constant (K_D), as well as the concentration of a protein in solution. In practice, these measurements are carried out using commercially available SPR chips, which are typically covalently derivatized with antibodies or antigens to which the protein of interest can bind. The solution with the protein of interest flows over the chip at a defined rate and from the SPR signals the characteristics mentioned above can be calculated.

Today, both ELISA- and SPR- based binding assays are extensively used in the development of biopharmaceuticals. Although neither method has undergone fundamental changes over the last decade or so, one recent improvement which has been broadly implemented is the automation of these assays. Since these techniques typically require a significant hands-on time for analysis, recent advances as the introduction of robotic systems have increased the throughput significantly.

■ Cell-Based Activity Assays

Paramount to the development of a protein therapeutic is to have an assay that identifies its biological function. Chromatographic and electrophoretic methodologies can address the purity of a biotherapeutic and be useful in investigating stability parameters. However, it is also essential to ascertain whether the therapeutic protein has adequate bioactivity. Typically, bioassays (potency assays) are carried out in vitro by monitoring the biological response in cells when the therapeutic protein is added to the system. These biological responces need to reflect the mode of action (MoA) of the therapeutic. There is a wide and ever-increasing variety of cell-based assays.

Common cell-based bioassays are:

(a) Cell proliferation/anti-proliferation assays in which the proliferation (or reduction of proliferation) of the cells in culture is measured as a response to the drug,
(b) Cytotoxicity assays in which cell death occurring as a response to the drug is measured,
(c) Adhesion assays in which the influence of the drug on the adhesion properties of the cells are measured,
(d) Kinase receptor activation assays in which the phosphorylation of a tyrosine kinase as a response to the drug as a ligand is measured by capture-ELISA after cell lysis,
(e) Cellular response to the biopharmaceutical is often monitored via the activation of a specific cellular signaling cascade,
(f) Antibody-Dependent Cell-mediated Cytotoxicity (ADCC) assays are assays in which cell lysis by immune system effector cells upon their activation by a therapeutic antibody bound to a receptor of the target cell is measured,
(g) Complement-Dependent Cytotoxicity (CDC) assays are assays in which the lysis of the target cell by components of the complement system are measured after complement activation by the therapeutic antibody bound to a cellular receptor,
(h) Cytokine release assays measure the release of cytokines by the target cell as a response to the protein therapeutic.

An interesting new approach to cell-based potency assays is the use of reporter genes. In the reporter gene assays the activation of a gene regulatory element (as a response to a signaling cascade activation) is monitored using a common reporter gene, for example luciferase. The assay readout is the expression of the reporter gene as response to the drug. The advantage of this approach is the potential for using it as a generic (platform) approach to a number of different bioassays, thus simplifying the bioassay development, cell banking, etc.

CONCLUDING REMARKS

With the ever-increasing application and variety of human recombinant proteins as therapeutics, the need for characterization of their structure, function, and purity has also increased. Naturally, the analytical technology has also undergone a rapid evolution. Today, a large array of techniques is used to characterize the primary, secondary, tertiary and quaternary structure of proteins and to determine the quality, purity, and stability of the recombinant drug product.

The information provided in this chapter offers only a general guidance on the process and tools for analytical characterization of various protein modifications. In reality, this process is rarely straightforward and is often convoluted by a number of factors. For example, a lot of different protein modifications occur simultaneously, thus inducing simultaneous changes in a number of molecular attributes. Often the results of these simultaneous changes may be masked. For example, it is possible that no changes in the IEX charge heterogeneity profile of a protein molecule are detected when simultaneous succinimide formation (inducing the formation of more basic species) and deamidation (inducing the formation of acidic species) occur, in spite of a significant redistribution of various charged species.

Many protein modifications result in changes in more than one molecular attribute. Thus, more than one analytical technique should be used to characterize these modifications. For example, pyro-Glu formation may be measured using either charge based techniques (e.g. IEX) or techniques measuring changes in polarity (e.g. RP-HPLC). Moreover, the extent to which the molecular properties of a protein are modified as a result of a given modification, depends on the structural context in which this modification occurs (overall molecular charge, hydrophobicity, size, etc.). For example, clipping of a small fragment of a very large protein may not be easy to detect using size-exclusion chromatography, due to the resolution limits of this technique.

Because of the complexity of the interplay between various potential protein modifications, the definition of the characterization and quality control strategies is an important intellectual challenge for the analytical experts in the therapeutic protein development teams, and critical for the success of every development program.

SELF-ASSESSMENT QUESTIONS

Questions

1. What are the most common chemical modifications resulting in changes in protein charge heterogeneity?
2. What are the three most common techniques for measuring charge heterogeneity of proteins?
3. What is the transfer of proteins to a membrane such as nitrocellulose or PDVF called?
4. What are the two most commonly oxidized amino acids in protein biotherapeutics? How can one

detect these oxidized amino acids in molecular structure?
5. In a 2-dimensional electrophoresis analysis of a protein mixture the first method of separation is an IEF run, followed by a SDS-PAGE run in a perpendicular direction to the first run? If one runs the SDS-PAGE analysis first, followed by the IEF run, would one get a similar result?
6. List three techniques for separating proteins based on molecular size.
7. Which technique provides the ultimate (atomic) resolution of the structure of a protein?
8. What are limitations of an ELISA when analyzing a protein product?

Answers

1. Deamidation and isomerization.
2. Ion exchange chromatography, Isoelectric focusing, capillary zone electrophoresis.
3. This method is called blotting. If an electric current is used, then the method is called electroblotting.
4. Methionine and tryptophan. MS, RP-HPLC and HIC are preferred analytical techniques to detect oxidation of proteins.
5. No. In the SDS-PAGE analysis the protein is denatured (unfolds) and SDS interacts with the protein giving it a uniform negative charge that masks the amino acids charges in the protein. The pI of the protein(s) cannot be determined in a subsequent IEF run.
6. Size-exclusion chromatography, SDS-PAGE, Asymmetric Field Flow Field Fractionation (AFFF).
7. X-ray crystallography.
8. The ELISA (sandwich assay set up) may measure degradation products and/or product-related variants with similar affinity to intact molecules.

Acknowledgements This chapter is a re-work of part (including a number of figures) of the chapter *"Biophysical and Biochemical Analysis of Recombinant Proteins"*, by Tsutomu Arakawa and John Philo, which appeared in the previous editions of this book—cf. fourth edition, 2013. Despite the significant changes made to the original chapter, it still contains fragments of the excellent original text by Arakawa and Philo.

The author thanks Abbas Razvi and Marigone Lenjani for providing chromatograms and electropherograms shown in this chapter.

FURTHER READING

Arbogast LW, Brinson RG, Marino JP (2015) Mapping monoclonal antibody structure by 2D 13C NMR at natural abundance. Anal Chem 87(7):3556–3561

Berkowitz SA, Engen JR, Mazzeo JR, Jones GB (2012) Analytical tools for characterizing biopharmaceuticals and the implications for biosimilars. Nat Rev Drug Discov 11(7):527–540

Butler JE (ed) (1991) Immunochemistry of solid-phase immunoassay. CRC Press, Boca Raton

Cavanagh J, Fairbrother WJ, Skelton NJ (2007) Protein NMR spectroscopy: principles and practice book, 2nd edn. Academic Press, San Diego

Chirino AJ, Mire-Sluis A (2004) Characterizing biological products and assessing comparability following manufacturing changes. Nat Biotechnol 22(11):1383–1391

Coligan J, Dunn B, Ploegh H, Speicher D, Wingfield P (eds) (1995) Current protocols in protein science. Wiley, New York

Crabb JW (ed) (1995) Techniques in protein chemistry VI. Academic, San Diego

Domon B, Aebersold R (2006) Mass spectrometry and protein analysis. Science 312(5771):212–217

Du Y, Walsh A, Ehrick R, Xu W, May K, Liu H (2012) Chromatographic analysis of the acidic and basic species of recombinant monoclonal antibodies. MAbs 4(5):578–585

Dunbar BS (1994) Protein blotting: a practical approach. Oxford University Press, New York

Fekete S, Guillarme D, Sandra P, Sandra K (2016) Chromatographic, electrophoretic, and mass spectrometric methods for the analytical characterization of protein biopharmaceuticals. Anal Chem 88(1):480–507

Folzer E, Diepold C, Bomans K, Finkler C, Schmidt R, Bulau P, Huwyler J, Mahler H-C, Koulov AV (2015) Selective oxidation of methionine and tryptophan residues in a therapeutic IgG1 molecule. J Pharm Sci 104:2824–2831

Gahoual R, Beck A, Leize-Wagner E, François YN (2016) Cutting-edge capillary electrophoresis characterization of monoclonal antibodies and related products. J Chromatogr B Analyt Technol Biomed Life Sci 1032:61–78

Hames BD, Rickwood D (eds) (1990) Gel electrophoresis of proteins: a practical approach, 2nd edn. IRL Press, New York

Henderson R (2018) From electron crystallography to single particle Cryo EM (Nobel lecture). Angew Chem Int Ed Engl 57(34):10804–10825

Jiskoot W, Crommelin DJA (eds) (2005) Methods for structural analysis of protein pharmaceuticals. AAPS Press, Arlington

Kahle J, Wätzig H (2018) Determination of protein charge variants with (imaged) capillary isoelectric focusing and capillary zone electrophoresis. Electrophoresis 39(20):2492–2511

Kaltashov IA, Bobst CE, Abzalimov RR, Wang G, Baykal B, Wang S (2012) Advances and challenges in analytical characterization of biotechnology products: mass spectrometry-based approaches to study properties and behavior of protein therapeutics. Biotechnol Adv 30(1):210–222

Liu H, Gaza-Bulseco G, Faldu D, Chumsae C, Sun J (2008) Heterogeneity of monoclonal antibodies. J Pharm Sci 97(7):2426–2447

McEwen CN, Larsen BS (eds) (1998) Mass spectrometry of biological materials, 2nd edn. Dekker, New York

Moritz B, Schnaible V, Kiessig S, Heyne A, Wild M, Finkler C, Christians S, Mueller K, Zhang L, Furuya K, Hassel M, Hamm M, Rustandi R, He Y, Solano OS, Whitmore C, Park SA, Hansen D, Santos M, Lies M (2015) Evaluation of capillary zone electrophoresis for charge heterogeneity testing of monoclonal antibodies. J Chromatogr B Analyt Technol Biomed Life Sci 983-984:101–110

Müllertz A, Perrie Y, Rades T (eds) (2016) Analytical techniques in the pharmaceutical sciences. Springer, New York

Pace CN, Grimsley GR, Scholtz JM, Shaw KL (2014) Protein stability. In: eLS. Wiley, Chichester

Parr MK, Montacir O, Montacir H (2016) Physicochemical characterization of biopharmaceuticals. J Pharm Biomed Anal 130:366–389

Ponniah G, Nowak C, Neill A, Liu H (2017) Characterization of charge variants of a monoclonal antibody using weak anion exchange chromatography at subunit levels. Anal Biochem 520:49–57

Rathore D, Faustino A, Schiel J, Pang E, Boyne M, Rogstad S (2018) The role of mass spectrometry in the characterization of biologic protein products. Expert Rev Proteomics 15(5):431–449

Ríos Quiroz A, Lamerz J, Da Cunha T, Boillon A, Adler M, Finkler C, Huwyler J, Schmidt R, Mahler H-M, Koulov AV (2016) Factors governing the precision of subvisible particle measurement methods—a case study with a low-concentration therapeutic protein product in a prefilled syringe. Pharm Res 33:450–461

Salas-Solano O, Felten O (2008) Capillary electrophoresis methods for pharmaceutical analysis. Sep Sci Technol 9:401

Shirley BA (ed) (1995) Protein stability and folding. Humana Press, Totowa

Strege MA, Lagu AL (eds) (2004) Capillary electrophoresis of proteins and peptides. Humana Press, Totowa

Thorpe R, Wadhwa M, Mire-Sluis A (1997) The use of bioassays for the characterisation and control of biological therapeutic products produced by biotechnology. Dev Biol Stand 91:79–88

Vlasak J, Ionescu R (2011) Fragmentation of monoclonal antibodies. MAbs 63:253–263

Vlasak J, Ionescu R (2008) Heterogeneity of monoclonal antibodies revealed by charge-sensitive methods. Curr Pharm Biotechnol 9:468–481

Wei H, Mo J, Tao L, Russell RJ, Tymiak AA, Chen G, Iacob RE, Engen JR (2014) Hydrogen/deuterium exchange mass spectrometry for probing higher order structure of protein therapeutics: methodology and applications. Drug Discov Today 19(1):95–102

Wild D (ed) (2013) The immunoassay handbook theory and applications of ligand binding, ELISA and related techniques, 4th edn. Elsevier, New York

4 Production and Purification of Recombinant Proteins

Alfred Luitjens and Emile van Corven

INTRODUCTION

The growing therapeutic use of proteins increases the need for practical and economical processing techniques. As a result, biotechnological production methods have advanced significantly over the past three decades. Also, single-use production technology that has the potential to mitigate many of the economical and quality issues arising from manufacturing has evolved rapidly (Hodge 2004; Luitjens et al. 2012).

When producing proteins for therapeutic use, a number of issues must be considered related to the manufacturing, purification, and characterization of the products. Biotechnological products for therapeutic use have to meet strict specifications especially when used via the parenteral route. The regulatory agencies both in Europe (EMA: European Medicines Agency) and in the United States of America (FDA: Food and Drug Administration) play a pivotal role in providing legal requirements and guidelines (www.ICH.org, www.FDA.gov).

In this chapter the focus is on the technical aspects of production (upstream processing) and purification (downstream processing) of recombinant therapeutic proteins. However, a majority of the techniques discussed can also be applied to vaccines and viral vector production. For further details, the reader is referred to the literature mentioned.

A. Luitjens
Batavia Biosciences, Leiden, The Netherlands
e-mail: a.luitjens@bataviabiosciences.com

E. van Corven (✉)
Bioceros, Utrecht, The Netherlands
e-mail: e.vancorven@bioceros.com

UPSTREAM PROCESSING

Expression Systems

General Considerations

Expression systems for proteins of therapeutic interest include both pro- and eukaryotic cells (bacteria, yeast, fungi, plants, insect cells, mammalian cells) and transgenic animals. The choice of a particular system will be determined to a large extent by the nature and origin of the desired protein, the intended use of the product, the amount needed, and the cost.

In principle, any protein can be produced using genetically engineered organisms, but not every type of protein can be produced by every type of cell. In most cases, the protein is foreign to the host cells that have to produce it, and although the translation of the genetic code can be performed by the cells, the post-translation modifications of the protein might be different compared to the native product.

About 5% of the mammalian proteome is thought to comprise enzymes performing over 200 types of posttranslation modifications of proteins (Walsh 2006). These modifications are species and/or cell-type specific. The metabolic pathways that lead to these modifications are genetically determined by the host cell. Thus, even if the cells can produce the desired post-translation modification, such as glycosylation, still the resulting glycosylation pattern might be different from that of the native protein. Correct N-linked glycosylation of therapeutically relevant proteins is important for full biological activity, immunogenicity, stability, targeting, and pharmacokinetics. Prokaryotic cells, such as bacteria, are sometimes capable of producing N-linked glycoproteins. However, the observed N-linked structures differ from the structures found in eukaryotes (Dell et al. 2011). Yeast cells are able to produce recombinant proteins such as albumin, and has been engineered to produce glycoproteins with human-like glycan structures including terminal sialylation (reviewed by Celik and Calik 2012).

D. J. A. Crommelin et al. (eds.), *Pharmaceutical Biotechnology*, https://doi.org/10.1007/978-3-030-00710-2_4

Still, most products on the market and currently in development use cell types that are, if possible, closely related to the original protein-producing cell type. Therefore, for human-derived proteins, typically mammalian cells are chosen for production as prokaryotic cells are less effective in producing post-translational modifications. Those are often essential when it comes to complex protein structures such as monoclonal antibodies. However, driven by the increasing demand for inexpensive products, especially for costly antibody therapies, two trends opened new opportunities to produce antibody fragments in *E. coli*; (i) generation of improved engineered *E. coli* strains and (ii) new knowledge in using biologically functional antibody fragments. Based on this, two *E. coli* derived antibody fragments (Ranibizumab and Certolizumab pegol) have been approved by the regulatory bodies. It is expected that in the near future more antibody fragments will be launched. Therefore, although still to be further developed, bacteria and yeast may keep on playing a role as future production systems given their ease and low cost of large-scale manufacturing.

Generalized features of proteins expressed in different biological systems are listed in Table 4.1 (see also Walter et al. 1992; Yao et al. 2015). However, it should be kept in mind that there are exceptions to this table for specific product/expression systems.

Transgenic Animals

Foreign genes can be introduced into animals like mice, rabbits, pigs, sheep, goats, and cows through nuclear transfer and cloning techniques. Using milk-specific promoters, the desired protein can be expressed in the milk of the female offspring. During lactation the milk is collected, the milk fats are removed, and the skimmed milk is used as the starting material for the purification of the protein.

The advantage of this technology is the relatively cheap method to produce the desired proteins in vast quantities when using larger animals such as cows. Disadvantages are the long lead time to generate a herd of transgenic animals and concerns about the health of the animal, food safety and ethics (see: report Bundesministerium für Gesundheit, Familie und Jugend, Sektion IV http://www.science-art.at/uploads/media/report_transgenic_animals_02.pdf). Some proteins expressed in the mammary gland leak back into the circulation and cause serious negative health effects. An example is the expression of erythropoietin in cows. Although the protein was well expressed in the milk, it caused severe health effects and these experiments were stopped.

The purification strategies and purity requirements for proteins from milk can be different from those derived from bacterial or mammalian cell systems. Often the transgenic milk containing the recombinant protein also contains significant amounts of the nonrecombinant counterpart. To separate these closely related proteins poses a purification challenge. The "contaminants" in proteins for oral use expressed in milk that is otherwise consumed by humans are known to be safe for consumption.

The transgenic animal technology for the production of pharmaceutical proteins has progressed within the last few years. The FDA and EMA approved recombinant antithrombin III (ATryn®, GTC Biotherapeutics) produced in the milk of transgenic goats, as well as recombinant human C1 esterase inhibitor (Ruconest®,

Protein feature	Prokaryotic bacteria	Eukaryotic yeast	Eukaryotic mammalian cells	Eukaryotic plant cells	Transgenic animals
Concentration	High	High	High	Low	Medium-High
Molecular weight	Low	High	High	High	High
S-S bridges	Limitation	No limitation	No limitation	No limitation	No limitation
Secretion	No	Yes/no	Yes	Yes/no	Yes
Aggregation state	Inclusion body	Singular, native	Singular, native	Singular, native	Singular, native
Folding	Risk of misfolding	Correct folding	Correct folding	Correct folding	Correct folding
Glycosylation (human-like)	Limited	Limited	Possible	Limited	Possible
Contamination risk	Possible (endotoxin)	Low	Possible (virus, prion, oncogenic DNA)	Low	Very possible (virus, prion, endotoxin)
Cost to manufacture	Low	Low	High	High[a]	Medium-high

[a]Due to current limited scalability (Shukla et al. 2017)

Table 4.1 ■ Generalized features of proteins of different biological origin

Pharming Group N.V.) produced in the milk of transgenic rabbits. More details about this technology are presented in Chap. 9.

Plants

Therapeutic proteins can also be expressed in plants and plant cell cultures (see also Chap. 1). For instance, human albumin has been expressed in potatoes and tobacco. Whether these production vehicles are economically feasible has yet to be established. The lack of genetic stability of plants was sometimes a drawback. Stable expression of proteins in edible seeds has been obtained. For instance, rice and barley can be harvested and easily kept for a prolonged period of time as raw material sources. Especially for oral therapeutics or vaccines, this might be the ideal solution to produce large amounts of cheap therapeutics, because the "contaminants" are known to be safe for consumption. However, challenges are the presence of high endotoxin levels, a relatively low expression level of the product, and secretion of proteases limiting the shelf life of plant extracts (Shukla et al. 2017). A better understanding of the plant molecular biology together with more sophisticated genetic engineering techniques and strategies to increase yields and optimized glycan structures resulted in an increase in the number of products in development including late-stage clinical trials (reviewed by Orzaez et al. 2009, and Peters and Stoger 2011). Biosafety concerns (such as pollen contamination and immunogenicity of plant-specific glycans) and costly downstream extraction and purification requirements, however, have hampered moving therapeutic protein production in plants from the laboratory to industrial size application (Yao et al. 2015).

More details about the use of plant systems for the production of pharmaceutical proteins are presented in Chap. 9.

Cultivation Systems

The remainder of this chapter will focus on mammalian cell-based expression systems. Non-mammalian expression systems will only briefly be discussed.

General

Cells can be cultivated in vessels containing an appropriate liquid growth medium in which the cells are either immobilized and grow as a monolayer, attached to microcarriers, in suspension, or entrapped in matrices. The culture method will determine the scale of the separation and purification methods. Production-scale cultivation is commonly performed in fermentors, used for bacterial and fungal cells, or bioreactors, used for mammalian and insect cells. Bioreactor systems can be classified into four different types:

- Stirred tank (Fig. 4.1a)
- Airlift (Fig. 4.1b)
- Fixed bed (Fig. 4.1c)
- Membrane bioreactors (Fig. 4.1d)

Because of its reliability and experience with the design and scaling up potential, the stirred tank is still the most commonly used bioreactor. This type of bioreactor is not only used for suspension cells like CHO, HEK293, and PER.C6® cells, it is also used for production of adherent cells like Vero and MDCK cells. In the latter case the production is performed on microcarriers (Van Wezel et al. 1985).

Bioreactor Processes

The kinetics of cell growth and product formation will not only dictate the type of bioreactor used but also how the growth process is performed. Three types of bioreactor processes are commonly employed and discussed below:

- Batch

  In a batch process, the bioreactor is filled with the entire volume of medium needed during the cell growth and/or production phase. No additional supplements are added to increase the cell growth or production during the process. Waste products, such as lactate and ammonium, and the product itself accumulate in the bioreactor. The product is harvested at the end of the process. Maximum cell density and product yields will be lower compared to a fed-batch process.
- Fed-batch

  In a fed-batch process, a substrate is supplemented to the bioreactor. The substrate consists of the growth-limiting nutrients that are needed during the cell growth phase and/or during the production phase of the process. Like the batch process, waste products accumulate in the bioreactor. The product is harvested at the end of the process. With the fed-batch process, higher cell densities and product yields can be reached compared to the batch process due to the extension of production time that can be achieved compared to a batch process. The substrate used is highly concentrated and can be added to the bioreactor at certain points in time or as a continuous feed. The fed-batch mode is currently widely used for the production of proteins. The process is well understood and characterized.
- Perfusion

  In a perfusion process, the media and waste products are continuously exchanged and the product is harvested throughout the culture period. A membrane device is used to retain the cells in the bioreactor, and waste medium is removed from the bioreactor by this device (Fig. 4.2). To keep the medium level constant in the bioreactor, fresh

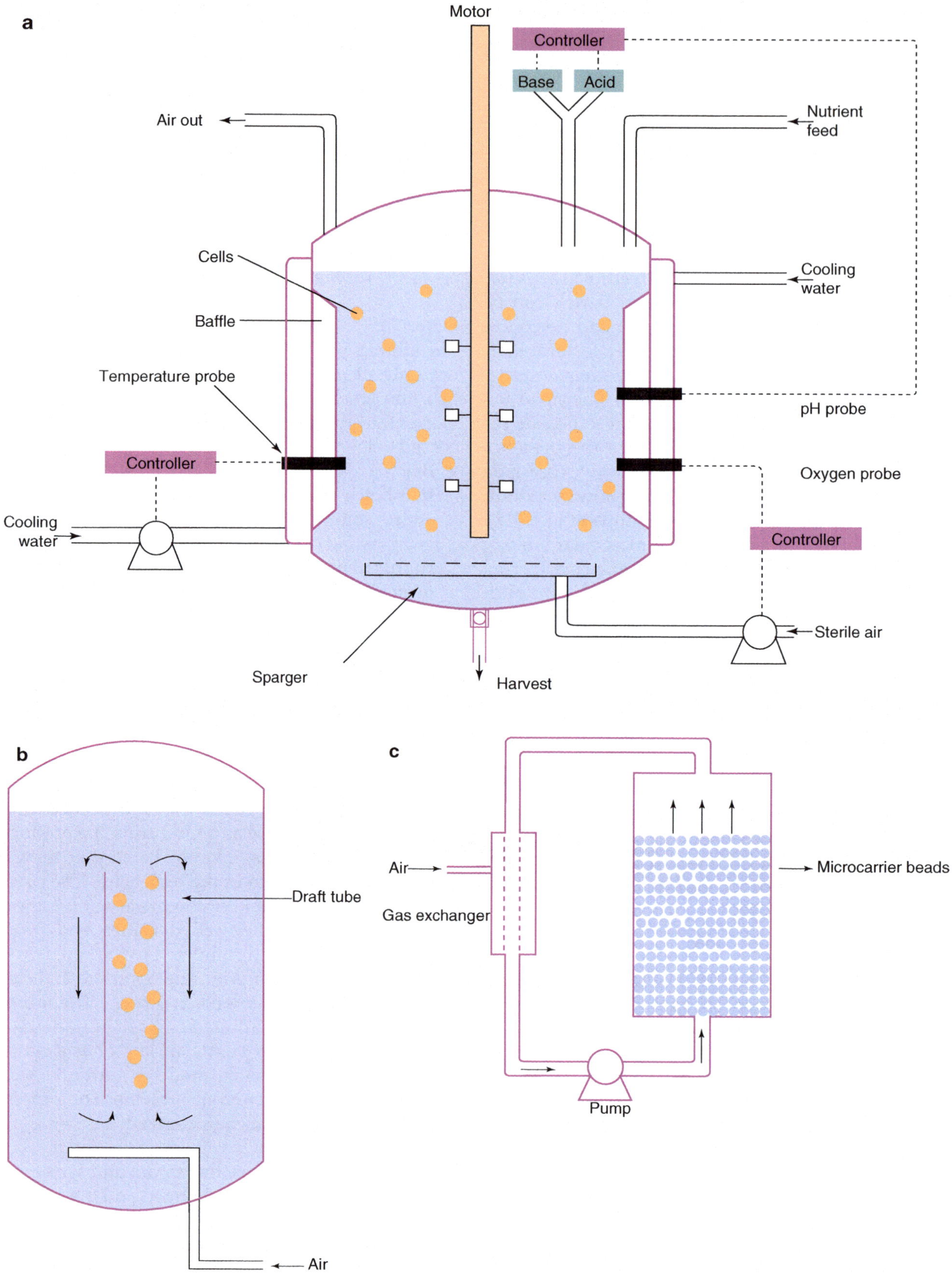

Figure 4.1 ■ (**a**) Schematic representation of stirred-tank bioreactor. (**b**) Schematic representation of airlift bioreactor. (**c**) Schematic representation of fixed-bed stirred-tank bioreactor. (**d**) Schematic representation of hollow fiber perfusion bioreactor. All schematics are adapted from Klegerman and Groves (1992)

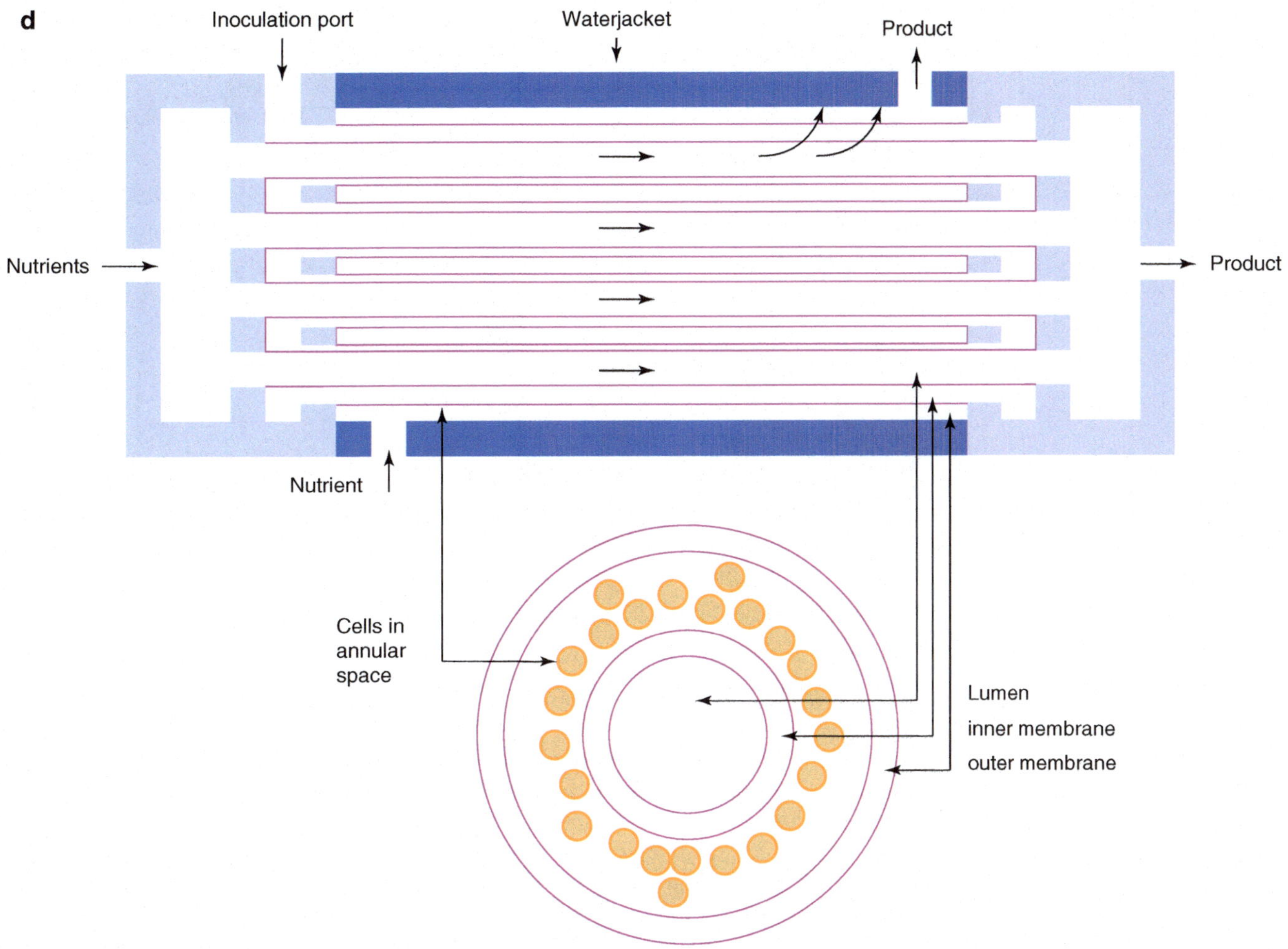

Figure 4.1 ■ (continued)

medium is supplemented to the bioreactor. By operating in perfusion mode, the level of waste products will be kept constant and one generates a stable environment for the cells to grow or to produce (see below). With the perfusion process, much higher cell densities can be reached and therefore higher productivity (Compton and Jensen 2007).

In all these three protocols, the cells go through four distinctive phases:

1. Lag phase
   In this phase the cells are adapting to the conditions in the bioreactor and do not yet grow.
2. Exponential growth phase
   During this phase, cells grow in a more or less constant doubling time for a fixed period. However under the right process conditions mammalian cell doubling time is dependent on the cell type used, and will usually vary between 20 and 40 h. Plotting the natural logarithm of cell concentration against time produces a straight line. Therefore, the exponential growth phase is also called the log phase. The growth phase will be affected by growth conditions such as temperature, pH, oxygen pressure, and external forces like stirring and baffles that are inserted into the bioreactor. Furthermore, the growth rate is affected by the supply of sufficient nutrients, buildup of waste products, etc.
3. Stationary phase
   In the stationary phase, the growth rate of the cells slows down since nutrients are depleted and/or build up of toxic waste products like lactate and ammonium. In this phase, constant cell concentrations are found because a balance between cell growth and cell death has been reached.

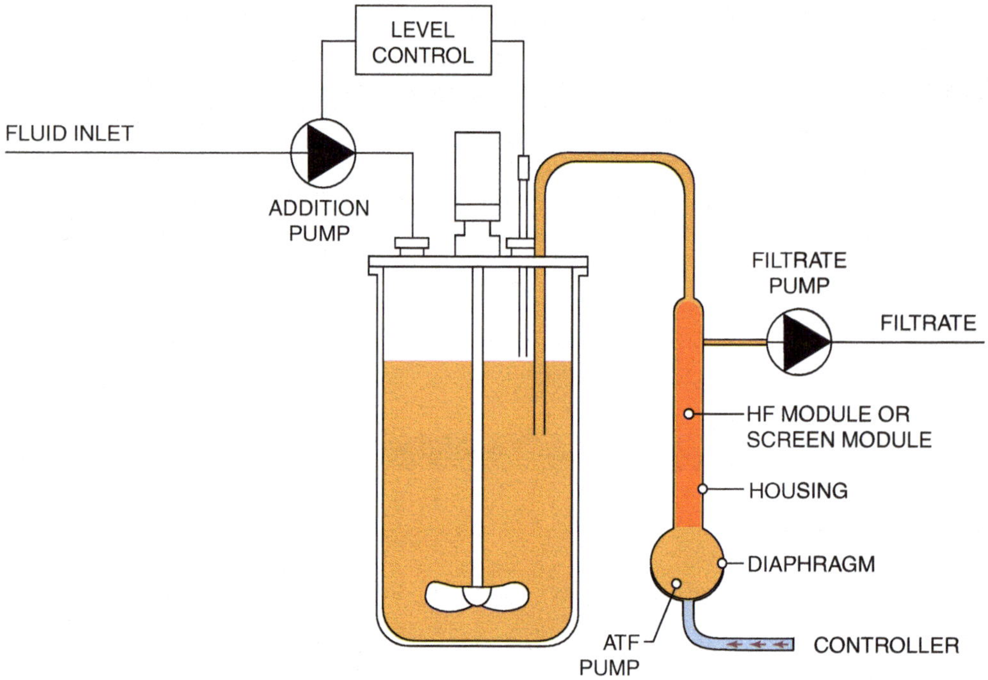

Figure 4.2 ■ Schematic representation of perfusion device coupled to a stirred-tank bioreactor. *ATF* alternating tangential flow

4. Death phase
   Cells die due to depletion of nutrients and/or presence of high concentrations of toxic products such as lactate and ammonium.

Examples of animal cells that are commonly used to produce recombinant proteins of clinical interest are Chinese Hamster Ovary cells (CHO), immortalized human embryonic retinal cells (PER.C6® cells), baby hamster kidney cells (BHK), lymphoblastoid tumor cells (interferon production), melanoma cells (plasminogen activator), and hybridized tumor cells (monoclonal antibodies).

The cell culture has to be free from undesired microorganisms that may destroy the cell culture or present hazards to the patient by producing endotoxins. Therefore, strict measures are required for both the production procedures and materials used (WHO 2010; Berthold and Walter 1994) to prevent a possible contamination with extraneous agents such as viruses, bacteria, and mycoplasma. Furthermore, strict measures are needed, especially with regard to the raw materials used, to prevent contaminations with transmissible spongiform encephalopathies (TSEs).

■ Cultivation Medium

In order to achieve optimal growth of cells and optimal production of recombinant proteins, it is of great importance not only that conditions such as stirring, pH, oxygen pressure, and temperature are chosen and controlled appropriately but also that a cell growth and protein production medium with the proper nutrients are provided for each stage of the production process.

The media used for mammalian cell culture are complex and consist of a mixture of diverse components, such as sugars, amino acids, electrolytes, vitamins, fetal calf serum (caveat, see below), and/or a mixture of peptones, growth factors, hormones, and other proteins (see Table 4.2). Many of these ingredients are pre-blended either as concentrate or as homogeneous mixtures of powders. To prepare the final medium, components are dissolved in purified water before sterilization. The preferred method for sterilization is heat (≥15 min at 121 °C). However most components used in cell culture medium can not be sterilized by heat, therefore filtration is used. Then, the medium is filtrated through 0.1 μm (to prevent mycoplasma and bacterial contamination) or 0.2 μm filters (to prevent bacterial contamination). Some supplements, especially fetal bovine serum, contribute considerably to the presence of contaminating proteins and may seriously complicate purification procedures. Moreover, the composition of serum is variable. It depends on the individual animal, season of the year, processing differences between suppliers, etc. The use of serum may introduce adventitious material such as viruses, mycoplasma, bacteria, and fungi into the culture system (Berthold and Walter 1994). Furthermore, the possible presence of prions that can cause transmissible spongiform encephalitis almost precludes the use of materials from animal origin. However, if use of this material is inevitable, one must follow the

Type of nutrient	Example(s)
Sugars	Glucose, lactose, sucrose, maltose, dextrins
Fat	Fatty acids, triglycerides
Water (high quality, sterilized)	Water for injection
Amino acids	Glutamine
Electrolytes	Calcium, sodium, potassium, phosphate
Vitamins	Ascorbic acid, -tocopherol, thiamine, riboflavine, folic acid, pyridoxin
Serum (fetal calf serum, 'synthetic' serum)	Albumin, transferrin
Trace minerals	Iron, manganese, copper, cobalt, zinc
Hormones	Growth factors

Table 4.2 ■ Major components of growth media for mammalian cell structures

relevant guidelines in which selective sourcing of the material is the key measure to safety (EMA 2011). A measure to prevent the contaminations mentioned above is gamma irradiation of the fetal bovine serum at 25 kGy and use sourcing from countries that have a TSE/BSE free status (Australia, New Zealand, Tasmania, USA, etc.). Many of these potential problems when using serum in cell culture media led to the development of chemically defined medium, free from animal components and material derived from animal components. These medium formulations were not only developed by the suppliers. There is the trend that the key players in the biotech industry develop their own chemically defined medium for their specific production platforms. The advantage of this is that manufacturers are less dependent on medium suppliers, and have full knowledge on the composition of the medium used for their products. The chemically defined media have been shown to give satisfactory results in large-scale production settings for monoclonal antibody processes. However, hydrolysates from non-animal origin, such as yeast and plant sources, are more and more used for optimal cell growth and product secretion (reviewed by Shukla and Thömmes 2010).

DOWNSTREAM PROCESSING

Introduction

Recovering a biological reagent from a cell culture supernatant is one of the critical parts of the manufacturing procedure for biotech products, and purification costs typically outweigh those of the upstream part of the production process. For the production of monoclonal antibodies, protein A resin and virus removal by filtration can account for a significant part, e.g., 40%, of the cost (Gottschalk 2006, Sinclair et al. 2016).

In the 1980s and early 1990s, the protein of interest was produced in bioreactors at low concentrations (e.g., 10–200 mg/L). At the most concentrations up to 500–800 mg/L could be reached (Berthold and Walter 1994). Developments in cell culture technology through application of genetics, proteomics, medium compositions and increased understanding of bioreactor technology resulted in product titers well above 1 g/L. Product titers above 20 g/L are also reported (Monteclaro 2010). These high product titers pose a challenge to the downstream processing unit operations (Shukla and Thömmes 2010).

With the low-yield processes, a concentration step is often required to reduce handling volumes for further purification. Usually, the product subsequently undergoes a series of purification steps (Fig. 4.3). The first step in a purification process is to remove cells and cell debris from the process fluids ('clarification'). This process step is normally performed using centrifugation and/or depth filters. Depth filters are often used in combination with filter aid/diatomaceous earth. Often the clarification step is regarded as a part of the upstream process. Therefore, the first actual step in the purification process is a capture step. Subsequent steps remove the residual bulk contaminants, and a final step removes trace contaminants and sometimes variant forms of the molecule. Alternatively, the reverse strategy, where the main contaminants are captured and the product is purified in subsequent steps, might result in a more economic process, especially if the product is not excreted from the cells. In the case where the product is excreted into the cell culture medium, the product will generally not represent more than 1–5% of total cellular protein, and a specific binding of the cellular proteins in a product-specific capture step will have a high impact on the efficiency of that step. If the bulk of the con-

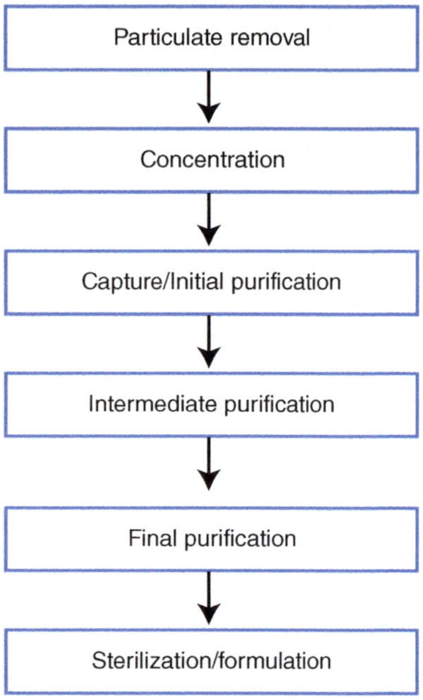

Figure 4.3 ■ Basic operations required for the purification of a biopharmaceutical macromolecule. For monoclonal antibody processes the concentration occurs within the capture step. Final purification is often called "polishing"

taminants can be removed first, the specific capture step will be more efficient and smaller in size and therefore more economic. Subsequent unit operation steps (e.g., chromatography columns) can be used for further purification.

After purification, additional steps are performed to bring the desired product into a formulation buffer in which the product is stabilized and can be stored for the desired time until further process steps are performed. Before storage of the final bulk drug substance, the product will be subjected to a bioburden reduction step. Normally this will be performed by a 0.2 μm filtration step. Formulation aspects will be dealt with in Chap. 5).

When designing an upstream and purification protocol, the possibility for scaling up should be considered carefully. A process that has been designed for small quantities is most often not suitable for large quantities for technical, economic, and safety reasons. Developing a process to purify the desired product is also called the downstream process (DSP). Two stages can be defined: *design* and *scale-up*.

As mentioned above, separating the impurities from the product protein requires a series of purification steps (*process design*), each removing some of the impurities and bringing the product closer to its final specification. In general, the starting feedstock contains cell debris and/or whole-cell particulate material that must be removed. Defining the major contaminants in the starting material is helpful in the downstream process design. This includes detailed information on the source of the material (e.g., bacterial or mammalian cell culture) and major contaminants that are used or produced in the upstream process (e.g., albumin, serum, or product analogs). Moreover, the physico-chemical characteristics of the product versus the known contaminants (stability, isoelectric point, molecular weight, hydrophobicity, density, specific binding properties) largely determine the process design. Processes used for production of therapeutics in humans should be safe, reproducible, robust, and produced at the desired cost of goods. The DSP steps may expose the protein molecules to high physical stress (e.g., high temperatures and extreme pH) which can alter the protein properties possibly leading to loss in efficacy. Any substance that is used by injection must be sterile. Furthermore, the endotoxin concentration must be below a certain level depending on the product. Limits are stated in compound specific compendial monographs (e.g., European Pharmacopoeia: <0.2 endotoxin units per kg body mass for intrathecal application). Aseptic techniques have to be used wherever possible and necessitate procedures throughout with clean air and microbial control of all materials and equipment used. During validation of the purification process, one must also demonstrate that potential viral contaminants are inactivated and removed (Walter et al. 1992). The purification matrices should be at least sanitizable or, if possible, steam-sterilizable. For depyrogenation, the purification material must withstand either extended dry heat at ≥180 °C or treatment with 1–2 M sodium hydroxide. If any material in contact with the product inadvertently releases compounds, these leachables must be analyzed and their removal by subsequent purification steps must be demonstrated during process validation, or it must be demonstrated that the leachables are below a toxic level. The increased use of plastic film-based single-use production technology (e.g. sterile single-use bioreactor bags, bags to store liquids and filter housings) has made these aspects more significant in the last decade. Suppliers have reacted by providing a significant body of information regarding leachables and biocompatibility for typical solutions used during processing. The problem of leachables is especially hampering the use of affinity chromatography (see below) in the production of pharmaceuticals for human use, in which the removal of any leached ligands well below a toxic level has to be demonstrated. Because leached affinity ligands will bind to the product, the removal might be cumbersome.

Scale-up is the term used to describe a number of processes employed in converting a laboratory procedure into an economical, industrial process. During the scale-up phase, the process moves from the laboratory to the pilot plant and finally to the production plant. The objective of scale-up is to reproducibly produce a product of high quality at a competitive price. Since the costs of downstream processing can be as high as 50–80% of the total cost of the final drug product, practical and economical ways of purifying the product should be used. Superior protein purification methods hold the key to a strong market position (Wheelwright 1993).

Basic operations required for a downstream purification process used for macromolecules from biological sources are shown in Fig. 4.3.

As mentioned before, the design of downstream processing is highly product dependent. Each product requires a specific multistage purification procedure. The basic scheme as represented in Fig. 4.3 becomes complex. Two typical examples of a process flow for downstream processing are shown in Fig. 4.4. These schemes represent the processing of a monoclonal antibody (about 150 kDa) and another glycosylated protein (recombinant interferon; about 28 kDa) produced in mammalian cells. The aims of the individual unit operations are described in the figure as well.

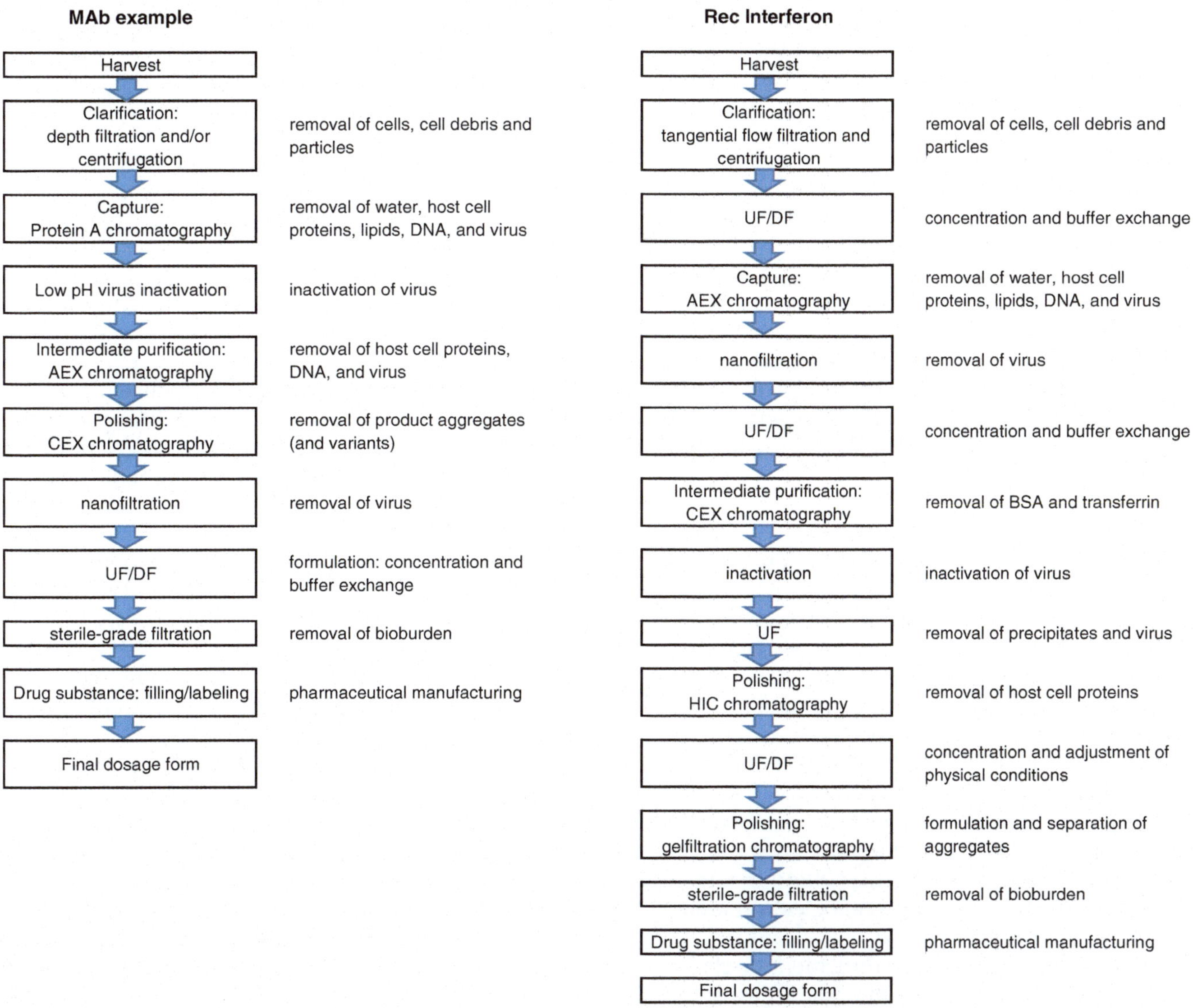

Figure 4.4 ■ Downstream processing of a monoclonal antibody (MAb) and a glycosylated recombinant interferon, describing the purpose of the inclusion of the individual unit operations. (*F* filtration, *TFF* tangential flow filtration, *UF* ultrafiltration, *DF* diafiltration, *A* adsorption; Rec Interferon adapted from Berthold and Walter 1994). For MAbs, the sequence of anion exchange chromatography (AEX), cationic exchange chromatography (CEX), and nanofiltration steps can change. Also, instead of ion exchange ligands, hydrophobic interaction chromatography (HIC) or mixed mode ligands are used (Shukla et al. 2017)

Separation technique	Mode/principle	Separation based on
Filtration	Microfiltration	Size
	Ultrafiltration	Size
	Nanofiltration	Size
	Dialysis	Size
	Charged membranes	Charge
	Depth filtration	Size
Centrifugation	Isopycnic banding	Density
	Non-equilibrium setting	Density
Extraction	Fluid extraction	Solubility
	Liquid/liquid extraction	Partition, change in solubility
Precipitation	Fractional precipitation	Change in solubility
Chromatography	Ion exchange	Charge
	Gel filtration	Size
	Affinity	Specific ligand-substrate interaction
	Hydrophobic interaction	Hydrophobicity
	Adsorption	Covalent/non-covalent binding

Table 4.3 ■ Frequently used separation processes and their physical basis

A number of purification methods are available to separate proteins on the basis of a wide variety of different physico-chemical criteria such as size, charge, hydrophobicity, and solubility (Table 4.3). Detailed information about some separation and purification methods commonly used in purification schemes is provided below.

■ Centrifugation

Recombinant protein products in a cell harvest must be separated from suspended particulate material, including whole cells, lysed cell material, and fragments of broken cells generated when cell breakage has been necessary to release intracellular products. Most downstream processing flow sheets will, therefore, include at least one unit operation for the removal ("clarification") of particulates. Most frequently used methods are centrifugation and filtration techniques. However, the expense and effectiveness of such methods is highly dependent on the physical nature of the particulate material, of the product and the scale of the unit operation. Various clarification technologies are summarized in Turner et al. (2017).

Besides the use of centrifugation for clarification also subcellular particles and organnelles, suspended in a viscous liquid (for example the particles produced when cells are disrupted by mechanical procedures) can be separated by centrifugation. However, subcellular particles and organelles are difficult to separate either by using one fixed centrifugation step (or by filtration), but they can be isolated efficiently by centrifugation at different speeds. For instance, nuclei can be obtained by centrifugation at 400 × *g* for 20 min, while plasma membrane vesicles are pelleted at higher centrifugation rates and longer centrifugation times (fractional centrifugation). In many cases, however, total biomass can easily be separated from the medium and classified by a simple centrifugation step (e.g., a continuous disc-stack centrifuge). Buoyant density centrifugation can be useful for separation of particles as well. This technique uses a viscous fluid with a continuous gradient of density in a centrifuge tube. Particles and molecules of various densities within the density range in the tube will cease to move when the isopycnic region has been reached. Both techniques of continuous (fluid densities within a range) and discontinuous (blocks of fluid with different density) density gradient centrifugation are used in buoyant density centrifugation on a laboratory scale. However, for application on an industrial scale, continuous centrifuges (e.g. tubular bowl centrifuges) are only used for discontinuous buoyant density centrifugation of protein products. This type of industrial centrifuge is mainly applied to recover precipitated proteins or contaminants.

■ Filtration

Filtration is often applied at various stages during downstream processing. The most successful set ups being normal flow depth filtration, membrane filtration and tangential flow filtration (TFF, also referred to as "cross flow"). Separation is achieved based on particle size differences. Below the main types of filtration are described.

Depth Filtration

Depth filters are often applied in the clarification of cell harvest to remove cells and cell debris. Depth filters consist of a complex porous matrix of materials, often including charged components and filter aids such as diatomaceous earth, enabling cellular debris and other contaminants to be retained at both the surface and internal layers of the depth filter (Turner et al. 2017). Issues at large manufacturing scale are usually the large membrane area needed to prevent clogging/fouling, and the large hold up volumes. For large harvest volumes depth filters are also used in combination with centrifugation.

Membrane Filtration

Depth filters retain contaminants within the filter structure, while membrane filters have defined pore size ranges (e.g., in the micrometer or nanometer range) that trap supra-pore size particles on the membrane surface while allowing passage of smaller particles. The main membrane filters are either used in a dead-end mode in which the retained particles collect on the surface of the filter media as a stable filter cake that grows in thickness and increases flow resistance, or in a tangential flow mode in which the high shear across the membrane surface limits fouling, gel layer formation and concentration polarization. Important applications of membrane filters within pharmaceutical processes are described below.

Tangential Flow Filtration

Tangential flow filtration (TFF) is often used for the concentration and buffer exchange of purified product and used sometimes within clarification processes. Depending upon the molecules/particles to be separated or concentrated, ultrafilter or micro membranes are used. Mixtures of molecules of highly different molecular dimensions are separated by passage of a dispersion under pressure across a membrane with a defined pore size. In general, ultrafiltration achieves little purification of protein product from other molecules with a comparable size, because of the relatively large pore size distribution of the membranes. As mentioned, this technique is widely used to concentrate macromolecules, and also to change the aqueous phase (e.g. re buffer components) in which the particles are dispersed or in which molecules are dissolved (diafiltration) to one required for the subsequent purification steps.

Sterilizing-Grade Filtration

Bioburden reduction filters are an essential part of most pharmaceutical processes. These dead-end filters consist of a membrane with an average pore size of 0.1 or 0.2 μm and a narrow size distribution). They are very effective in the removal of (possible) bioburden, and as such used at various steps in the purification process, e.g. at hold steps, and at the final steps to produce drug substance or drug product.

Virus Filtration

As mentioned later in this chapter, removal of potential contaminating viruses is essential in a pharmaceutical process. Nanofiltration is an elegant and effective technique and the validation aspects of this technology are well described (PDA technical report 41 2005). Filtration through 15 nm pore membranes can remove even the smallest non-enveloped viruses such as bovine parvovirus (Maerz et al. 1996). Nanofilters are a major contributor to the costs of the downstream process.

Charged Membranes

A type of membrane that is increasingly used within the biopharmaceutical industry is the charged membrane (Zhou and Tressel 2006; Etzel and Arunkumar 2017). As for ion exchange chromatography (see below), negatively (sulphonic, S) or positively (quaternary ammonium, Q) charged ligands are attached to the multilayer membranes, enabling the removal of residual impurities such as host cell DNA, viruses or host cell proteins from the recombinant protein product. In contrast to ion exchange chromatography, the open structure of the charged membranes enables relatively high diffusion rates of product/contaminants, thus a fast process step. A downside is the lower capacity. Charged membranes are often used in a flow-through mode in e.g. monoclonal antibody production processes, as such replacing the Q-based chromatography columns.

■ Extraction

Extraction, including liquid-liquid extraction, is a technique often used in the chemical industry, but rarely used for biopharmaceuticals. Liquid-liquid extraction basically separates molecules on solute affinity due to differences in the molecule's physical-chemical properties in a mixture of two immiscible phases (reviewed by Dos Santos et al. 2018). Traditionally the phases consist of an aqueous and an organic phase. Upon phase separation, the target molecules are extracted to one of the two phases allowing its concentration and sometimes purification. Due to the possible impact of organic solvents on the structure and biological activity of biopharmaceuticals as well as the environmental impact, this traditional extraction method is rarely used.

To overcome the main concerns, aqueous two phase systems are developed. The compounds enabling separation of biopharmaceuticals encompass polymers, salts, surfactants, amino acids and ionic liquids. Compared to chromatography the operational costs of the two phase systems are relatively low, scale up is straightforward and the technique can be easily integrated in the early steps of a downstream process. However, two phase systems are rarely applied in biopharmaceutical processes due to in general relatively low recovery values and limited purification abilities (reviewed by Dos Santos et al. 2018). A better understanding of the partitioning processes may reduce these limitations in the future.

Precipitation

The solubility of a particular protein depends on the physicochemical environment, for example, pH, ionic species, and ionic strength of the solution (see also Chap. 5). A slow continuous increase of the ionic strength (of a protein mixture) will selectively drive proteins out of solution. This phenomenon is known as "salting out." A wide variety of agents, with different "salting-out" potencies are available. Chaotropic series with increasing "salting-out" effects of negatively (1) and positively (2) charged molecules are given below:

1. SCN^-, I^-, CLO_4^-, NO_3^-, Br^-, Cl^-, CH_3COO^-, PO_4^{3-}, SO_4^{2-}
2. Ba^{2+}, Ca^{2+}, Mg^{2+}, Li^+, Cs^+, Na^+, K^+, Rb^+, NH_4^+

Ammonium sulfate is highly soluble in cold aqueous solutions and is frequently used in "salting-out" purification.

Another method to precipitate proteins is to use water-miscible organic solvents (change in the dielectric constant). Examples of precipitating agents are polyethylene glycol and trichloroacetic acid. Under certain conditions, chitosan and nonionic polyoxyethylene detergents also induce precipitation (Cartwright 1987; Homma et al. 1993; Terstappen et al. 1993). Cationic detergents have been used to selectively precipitate DNA.

Precipitation is a scalable, simple, and relatively economical procedure for the recovery of a product from a dilute feedstock. It has been used for the isolation of proteins from culture supernatants. Unfortunately, with most bulk precipitation methods, the gain in purity is generally limited and product recovery can be low. Moreover, extraneous components are introduced which must be eliminated later. Finally, large quantities of precipitates may be difficult to handle. Despite these limitations, recovery by precipitation has been used with considerable success for some products.

Chromatography

In preparative chromatography systems, molecular species are primarily separated based on differences in distribution between two phases: one is the stationary phase (mostly a solid phase) and the other moves. This mobile phase may be liquid or gaseous (see also Chap. 3). Nowadays, almost all stationary phases (fine particles providing a large surface area) are packed into a column. The mobile phase is passed through by pumps. Downstream protein purification protocols usually have at least two to three chromatography steps. Chromatographic methods used in purification procedures of biotech products are listed in Table 4.3 and are briefly discussed in the following sections.

Chromatographic Stationary Phases

Chromatographic procedures often represent the rate-limiting step in the overall downstream processing. An important primary factor governing the rate of operation is the mass transport into the pores of conventional packing materials. Adsorbents employed include inorganic materials such as silica gels, glass beads, hydroxyapatite, various metal oxides (alumina), and organic polymers (cross-linked dextrans, cellulose, agarose). Separation occurs by differential interaction of sample components with the chromatographic medium. Ionic groups such as amines and carboxylic acids, dipolar groups such as carbonyl functional groups, and hydrogen bond-donating and bond-accepting groups control the interaction of the sample components with the stationary phase, and these functional groups slow down the elution rate if interaction occurs.

Chromatographic stationary phases for use on a large scale are evolving over time. An approach to the problems associated with mass transport in conventional systems is to use chromatographic particles that contain some large "through pores" in addition to conventional pores (see Fig. 4.5). These flow-through or "perfusion chromatography" media enable faster convective mass transport into particles and allow operation at much higher speeds without loss in resolution or binding capacity (Afeyan et al. 1989; Fulton 1994).

The ideal stationary phase for protein separation should possess a number of characteristics, among which are high mechanical strength, high porosity, no nonspecific interaction between protein and the support phase, high capacity and mass transfer rate, biocompatibility, and high stability of the matrix in a variety of solvents. The latter is especially true for columns used for the production of pharmaceuticals that need to be cleaned, depyrogenized, disinfected, and sterilized at regular intervals.

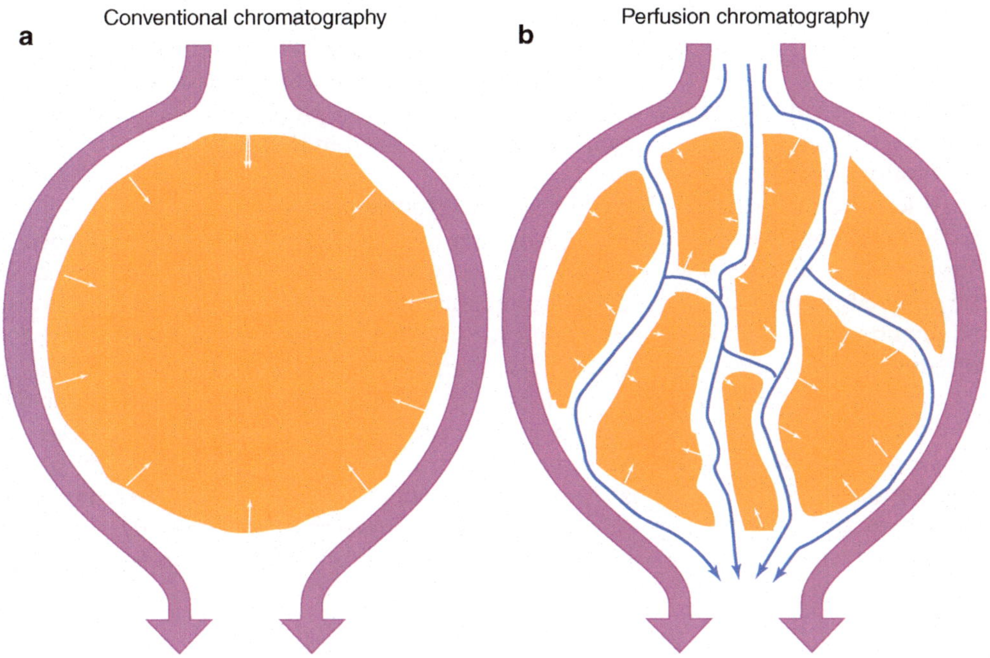

Figure 4.5 ■ The structure of conventional chromatographic particles (**a**) and the perfusion of flow through chromatographic particles (**b**) (adapted from Fulton 1994)

In production environments, chromatography columns which operate at relatively low back pressure are often used. These can be made of stainless steel. But the low back pressure allows the introduction of disposable (plastic) columns in a GMP manufacturing environment. Unlike conventional stainless steel, plastic columns are less sensitive to e.g. salt corrosion. A disadvantage can be leaching of plastic components into the product stream. Disposable plastic columns permit the efficient separation of proteins in a single batch, making this an attractive unit operation in a manufacturing process. A new development is the use of chromatography equipment with fully disposable flow paths that resists almost all chemicals used in protein purification including disinfection and sterilization media.

Adsorption Chromatography

In adsorption chromatography (also called "normal phase" chromatography), the stationary phase is more polar than the mobile phase. The protein of interest selectively binds to a static matrix under one condition and is released under a different condition. Adsorption chromatography methods enable high ratios of product load to stationary phase volume. Therefore, this principle is economically scalable.

Ion-Exchange Chromatography

Ion-exchange chromatography can be a powerful step early in a purification scheme. It can be easily scaled up. Ion-exchange chromatography can be used in a negative mode, i.e., the product flows through the column under conditions that favor the adsorption of contaminants to the matrix, while the protein of interest does not bind (Tennikova and Svec 1993). The type of the column needed is determined by the properties of the proteins to be purified (e.g., isoelectric point and charge density). Anion exchangers bind negatively charged molecules and cation exchangers bind positively charged molecules. In salt-gradient ion-exchange chromatography, the salt concentration in the perfusing elution buffer is increased continuously or in steps. The stronger the binding of an individual protein to the ion exchanger, the later it will appear in the elution buffer. Likewise, in pH-gradient chromatography, the pH is changed continuously or in steps. Here, the protein binds at one pH and is released at a different pH. As a result of the heterogeneity in glycosylation (e.g., a varying number of sialic acid moieties), glycosylated proteins may elute over a relatively broad pH range (up to 2 pH units).

In order to simplify purification, a specific amino acid tail can be added to the protein at the gene level to create a "purification handle". For example, a short tail consisting of arginine residues allows a protein to bind to a cation exchanger under conditions where almost no other cell proteins bind. However, this technique is useful for laboratory-scale isolation of the product and generally not at production scale due to regulatory problems related to the removal of the arginine or other specific tags from the protein.

(Immuno)Affinity Chromatography

Affinity Chromatography

Affinity chromatography is based on highly specific interactions between an immobilized ligand and the protein of interest. Affinity chromatography is a very powerful method for the purification of proteins. Under physiological conditions, the protein binds to the ligand. Extensive washing of this matrix will remove contaminants, and the purified protein can be recovered by the addition of ligands competing for the stationary phase binding sites or by changes in physical conditions (such as low or high pH of the eluent) that greatly reduce the affinity. Examples of affinity chromatography include the purification of glycoproteins, that bind to immobilized lectins, and the purification of serine proteases with lysine binding sites, that bind to immobilized lysine. In these cases, a soluble ligand (sugar or lysine, respectively) can be used to elute the required product under relatively mild conditions. Another example is the use of the affinity of protein A and protein G for antibodies. Protein A and protein G have a high affinity for the Fc portions of many immunoglobulins from various animals. Protein A and G matrices can be commercially obtained with a high degree of purity. Protein A resins are often used in the capture of biotherapeutic monoclonal antibodies at large scale, and these resins are also one of the most expensive parts of the production process. In the last decade the amino acid composition has been modified to generate Protein A ligands that are more resistant to hydroxide, allowing better cleaning of the resin. Also, the coupling chemistry has been improved to allow re-use of the resin for over a hundred cycles, and by that reducing the cost of goods.

For the purification of, e.g., hormones or growth factors, the receptors or short peptide sequence that mimic the binding site of the receptor molecule can be used as affinity ligands. Some proteins show highly selective affinity for certain dyes commercially available as immobilized ligands on purification matrices. When considering the selection of these ligands for pharmaceutical production, one must realize that some of these dyes are carcinogenic and that a fraction may leach out during the process.

An interesting approach to optimize purification is the use of a gene that codes not only for the desired protein but also for an additional sequence that facilitates recovery by affinity chromatography. At a later stage the additional sequence is removed by a specific cleavage reaction. As mentioned before, this is a complex process that needs additional purification steps.

In general, the use of affinity chromatography in the production process for therapeutics may lead to complications during validation of the removal of free ligands or protein extensions. Consequently, except for monoclonal antibodies where affinity chromatography is part of the purification platform at large scale, this technology is rarely used in the industry.

Immunoaffinity Chromatography

The specific binding of antibodies to their epitopes is used in immunoaffinity chromatography (reviewed by Abi-Ghanem and Berghman 2012). This technique can be applied for purification of either the antigen or the antibody. The antibody can be covalently coupled to the stationary phase and act as the "receptor" for the antigen to be purified. Alternatively, the antigen, or parts thereof, can be attached to the stationary phase for the purification of the antibody. Advantages of immunoaffinity chromatography are its high specificity and the combination of concentration and purification in one step.

A disadvantage associated with immunoaffinity methods is the sometimes very strong antibody-antigen binding. This requires harsh conditions during elution of the ligand. Under such conditions, sensitive ligands could be harmed (e.g., by denaturation of the protein to be purified). This can be alleviated by the selection of antibodies and environmental conditions with high specificity and sufficient affinity to induce an antibody-ligand interaction, while the antigen can be released under mild conditions. Another concern is disruption of the covalent bond linking the "receptor" to the matrix. This would result in elution of the entire complex. Therefore, in practice, a further purification step after affinity chromatography as well as an appropriate detection assay (e.g., Enzyme-Linked Immuno Sorbent Assay, ELISA) is almost always necessary. On the other hand, improved coupling chemistry that is less susceptible to hydrolysis has been developed to prevent leaching.

Scale-up of immunoaffinity chromatography is often hampered by the relatively large quantity of the specific "receptor" (either the antigen or the antibody) that is required and the lack of commercially available, ready-to-use matrices. The use of immunoaffinity in pharmaceutical processes will have major regulatory consequences since the immunoaffinity ligand used will be considered by the regulatory bodies as a "second product", thus will be subjected to the nearly the same regulatory scrutiny as the drug substance. Moreover, immunoaffinity ligands can have a significant effect on the final costs of goods.

Examples of proteins of potential therapeutic value that have been purified using immunoaffinity chromatography are interferons, urokinase, epoetin, interleukin-2, human factor VIII and X, and recombinant tissue plasminogen activator.

Hydrophobic Interaction Chromatography

Under physiological conditions, most hydrophobic amino acid residues are located inside the protein core, and only a small fraction of hydrophobic amino acids is exposed on the "surface" of a protein. Their exposure is suppressed because of the presence of hydrophilic amino acids that attract large clusters of water molecules and form a "shield." High salt concentrations reduce the hydration of a protein, and the surface-exposed hydrophobic amino acid residues become more accessible. Hydrophobic interaction chromatography (HIC) is based on non-covalent and non-electrostatic interactions between proteins and the stationary phase. HIC is a mild technique, usually yielding high recoveries of proteins that are not damaged, are folded correctly, and are separated from contaminants that are structurally related. HIC is ideally placed in the purification scheme after ion-exchange chromatography, where the protein usually is released in high ionic strength elution media (reviewed by Chen et al. 2015).

Gel-Permeation Chromatography

Gel-permeation or size-exclusion chromatography, also known as gel filtration, separates molecules according to their shape and size (see Fig. 4.6). Inert gels with narrow pore-size distributions in the size range of proteins are available. These gels are packed into a column. The protein mixture is loaded on top of the column and the proteins diffuse into the gel. The smaller the protein, the more volume it will have available in which to disperse. Molecules that are larger than the largest pores are not able to penetrate the gel beads and will therefore stay in the void volume of the column. When a continuous flow of buffer passes through the column, the larger proteins will elute first and the smallest molecules last. Gel-permeation chromatography is a good alternative to membrane diafiltration for buffer exchange at almost any purification stage, and it is often used in laboratory design. At production scale, the use of this technique is usually limited, because it is a slow process and only relatively small sample volumes can be loaded on a large column (up to one-third of the column volume in the case of "buffer exchange"). It is therefore best avoided or used late in the purification process when the protein is available in a highly concentrated form. Gel filtration is sometimes used as the final step in the purification to bring proteins in the appropriate buffer used in the final formulation. In this application, its use has little if no effect on the product purity characteristics.

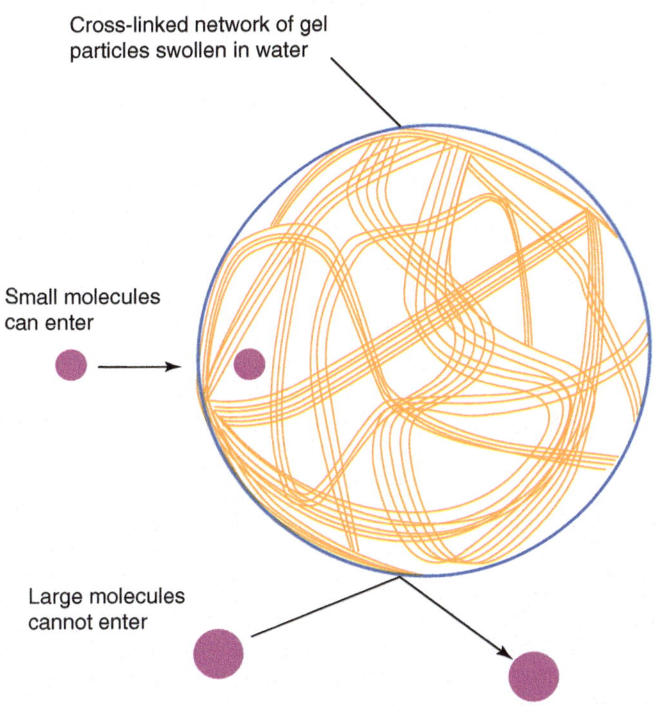

Figure 4.6 ■ Schematic representation of gel filtration (Adapted from James 1992)

Expanded Beds

As mentioned before, purification schemes are based on multistep protocols. This not only adds greatly to the overall production costs but also can result in significant loss of product. Therefore, there still is an interest in the development of new methods for simplifying the purification process. Adsorption techniques are popular methods for the recovery of proteins, and the conventional operating format for preparative separations is a packed column (or fixed bed) of adsorbent. Particulate material, however, can be trapped near the bed, which results in an increase in the pressure drop across the bed and eventually in clogging of the column. This can be avoided by the use of pre-column filters (e.g., 0.2 μm pore size) to save the column integrity. Another solution to this problem may be the use of expanded beds (Chase and Draeger 1993; Fulton 1994), also called fluidized beds (see Fig. 4.7). In principle, the use of expanded beds enables clarification, concentration, and purification to be achieved in a single step. The concept is to employ a particulate solid-phase adsorbent in an open bed with upward liquid flow. The hydrodynamic drag around the particles tends to lift them upwards, which is counteracted by gravity because of a density difference between the particles and the liquid phase. The particles remain suspended if particle diameter, particle density, liquid viscosity, and liquid density are properly balanced by choosing the correct flow rate. The expanded bed allows particulates (e.g., cells and cell debris) to pass through, whereas molecules in solution are selectively retained (e.g., by the use of ion-exchange or affinity adsorbents) on the adsorbent particles. Feedstocks can be applied

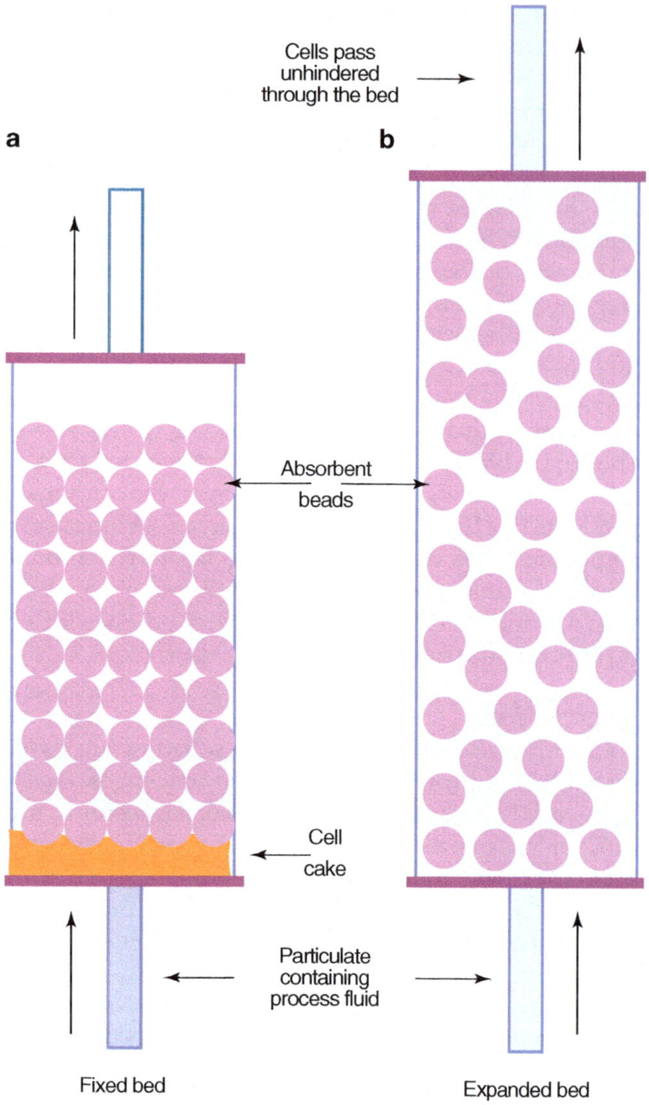

Figure 4.7 ■ Comparison between (**a**) a packed bed and (**b**) an expanded bed (adapted from Chase and Draeger 1993)

to the bed without prior removal of particulate material by centrifugation or filtration, thus reducing process time and costs. Fluidized beds have been used previously for the industrial-scale recovery of antibiotics such as streptomycin and novobiocin (Fulton 1994; Chase 1994). Stable, expanded beds can be obtained using simple equipment adapted from that used for conventional, packed bed adsorption and chromatography processes. Ion-exchange adsorbents are likely to be chosen for such separations.

SINGLE-USE SYSTEMS

In the last decade the development of single-use production systems has been boosting. This is reflected by the growing number of single-use systems available for mammalian cell culture and microbial cultures (see below). Single-Use systems are currently not only developed for culturing, but also for downstream unit operations such as the filtration (depth, membrane) and chromatography steps. It is currently possible to produce proteins with only single-use systems.

Single-use bioreactors for mammalian cell culture and protein production applications are characterized by a low power input, low mixing capabilities, limited oxygen transfer, restrictive exhaust capacity and limited foam management. Therefore, transferring these single-use bioreactors into single-use fermentors that can be used for microbial production is a challenge. The present generation of single-use fermentors is only used in the production of the least challenging five percent of microbial fermentations (Jones 2015).

Single-use bioreactors are used for the manufacturing of products in development and on the market. Shire (Dublin, Ireland) was the first company that used single-use bioreactors up to 2000 L for the manufacturing of one of its products. The advantages of the single-use technology are:

- Cost-effective manufacturing technology
  By introducing single-use systems, the design is such that all items not directly related to the process can be removed from the culture system, such as clean-in-place (CIP) and steam-in-place (SIP) systems that are critical within a stainless steel plant. Furthermore, a reduction in capital costs (CAPEX) is achieved by introducing single-use systems. In a case study that compares the costs for a single-use versus multi-use stainless steel 2 × 1000 L new facility, the single-use facility reduces CAPEX significantly, while operating costs (OPEX) are increased. Overall these studies show that investing in a flexible single-use facility is beneficial compared to a fixed stainless steel facility (Eibl and Eibl 2011; Goldstein and Molina 2016). It must be noted that investment decisions on new production facilities must be taken before the product is licensed by regulatory bodies.
- Increases the number of GMP batches
  By introducing single-use systems, it is possible to increase the number of GMP batches that can be produced within a manufacturing campaign since cleaning and sterilization of the equipment is not needed anymore. The turnover time needed from batch to batch is shortened.
- Provides flexibility in GMP facility design
  When stainless steel systems are used, changes to the equipment might have an impact on the design of the stainless steel tanks, piping, etc. These equipment changes will influence the overall validation status of the facility. By using single-use systems,

equipment changes can easily be incorporated as the setup of the single-use process is flexible. As with the stainless steel systems, in case a change will influence the validated process, the validated status of the process must be reconsidered and a revalidation might be needed.

- Speeds up implementation and time to market
  Due to the great flexibility of the single-use systems, the speed of product to market is less influenced by process changes that might be introduced during the different development stages of the production process than 'traditional' stainless steel equipment. However, the process needs to be validated before market introduction. When changes are introduced after process validation, a revalidation might be needed. Here again, there is no difference in this respect to the traditional stainless steel setup.
- Reduces water and wastewater costs
  Since the systems are single-use, there will be a great reduction in the total costs for cleaning. Not only through a reduction in water consumption but also a reduction in the number of hours needed to clean systems and to set them up for the next batch of product.
- Reduces validation costs
  No annual validation costs for cleaning and sterilization are needed anymore when single-use systems are used.

A disadvantage of the single-use system is that the operational expenses will increase and storage facilities for single-use bags and tubing are needed. Moreover, the dependence of the company on one supplier of single-use systems is a factor to consider. Finally, leachables and extractables from the single use plastics may end up in your product, causing potential safety and efficacy issues.

The advantages of the stainless steel bioreactors are obvious as this traditional technology is well understood and controlled, although the stainless steel pathway had and still has major disadvantages such as expensive and inflexible design, installation and maintenance costs combined with significant expenditures of time in facilities and equipment qualification and validation efforts. For very large volume products stainless steel is still the most economically viable option due to limited scalability of current single-use bioreactors (i.e., 2000 L max).

CONTAMINANTS

Parenteral product purity mostly is ≥99% (Berthold and Walter 1994; ICH 1999a). Purification processes should yield potent proteins with well-defined characteristics for human use from which "all" contaminants have been removed to a major extent. The purity of the drug protein in the final product largely depends upon the applied purification technology.

Origin	Contaminant
Host-related	Viruses
	Bacteria (mycoplasma)
	Host-derived proteins and DNA
	Endotoxins (from gram-negative bacterial hosts)
Product-related	Glycosylation variants
	Amino acid substitution and deletion
	Denatured protein (loss of secondary, tertiary, quaternary structure)
	Oxidized variants
	Conformational isomers
	Dimers and aggregates
	Disulfide pairing variants
	Succinimide formation
	(De)amidated species
	Protein fragments
Process-related	Viruses
	Bacteria
	Cell culture medium components
	Purification reagents
	Metals
	Column materials/leachables
	Leachables from single-use system (tubes, bags, etc.)

Table 4.4 ■ Potential contaminants/variants in recombinant protein products derived from bacterial and mammalian hosts

Table 4.4 lists potential contaminants and product variants that may be present in recombinant protein products from bacterial and mammalian sources. These contaminants can be host-related, process-related and product-related. In the following sections, special attention is paid to the detection and elimination of contamination by viruses, bacteria, cellular DNA, and undesired proteins.

■ Viruses

Endogenous and adventitious viruses, which require the presence of living cells to propagate, are potential contaminants of animal cell cultures and, therefore, of the final drug product. If present, their concentration in the purified product will be very low and it will be difficult to detect them. Viruses such as retrovirus can be visualized by (nonsensitive) electron microscopy. For retroviruses, a highly sensitive RT-PCR (reverse-transcriptase polymerase chain reaction) assay is available, but for other viruses, a sensitive in vitro assay might be lacking. The risks of some viruses (e.g., hepatitis virus) are known (Walter et al. 1991; Marcus-Sekura 1991), but there are other viruses whose risks cannot be properly judged because of lack of solid

Category	Types	Example
Inactivation	Heat treatment	Pasteurization
	pH extremes	Low pH
	Radiation	UV-light
	Dehydration	Lyophilization
	Cross linking agents, denaturating or disrupting agents	β-propiolactone, formaldehyde, NaOH, organic solvents (e.g., chloroform), detergents (e.g., Na-cholate)
	Neutralization	Specific, neutralizing antibodies
Removal	Chromatography	Ion-exchange, immuno-affinity chromatography
	Filtration	Nanofiltration, Q-charged membranes
	Precipitation	Cyroprecipitation

Table 4.5 ■ Methods for reducing or inactivating viral contaminants

experimental data. Some virus infections, such as parvovirus, can have long latent periods before their clinical effects show up. Long-term effects of introducing viruses into a patient treated with a recombinant protein should not be overlooked. Therefore, it is required that products used parenterally are free from viruses. The specific virus testing regime required will depend on the cell type used for production (Löwer 1990; Minor 1994).

Viruses can be introduced by nutrients, by an infected production cell line, or they are introduced (by human handling) during the production process. The most frequent source of virus introduction is animal serum. In addition, animal serum can introduce other unwanted agents such as bacteria, mycoplasmas, prions, fungi, and endotoxins. Appropriate screening of cell banks and growth medium constituents for viruses and other adventitious agents should be strictly regulated and supervised (Walter et al. 1991; FDA 1993; ICH 1999b; WHO 2010). Validated, orthogonal methods (cf Chap. 5) to inactivate and remove possible viral contaminants during the production process are mandatory for licensing of therapeutics derived from mammalian cells or transgenic animals (EMA 1996; ICH 1999b). Viruses can be inactivated by physical and chemical treatment of the product. Heat, irradiation, sonication, extreme pH, detergents, solvents, and certain disinfectants can inactivate viruses. These procedures can be harmful to the product as well and should therefore be carefully evaluated and validated (Walter et al. 1992; ICH 1999b). As mentioned in the filtration section removal of viruses by nanofiltration is an elegant and effective technique and the validation aspects of this technology are well described (PDA technical report 41 2005). A significant log reduction of even the smallest non-evelopped viruses such as bovine parvovirus can be obtained by filtration through 15 nm membranes (Maerz et al. 1996). Another common, although less robust, method to remove viruses in antibody processes is by ion-exchange chromatography and Q-charged membranes (Zhou and Tressel 2006). A number of methods for removing or inactivating viral contaminants are mentioned in Table 4.5.

In general, a protein production process should contain two or more orthogonal virus reduction steps. As mentioned, virus validation studies need to be performed on the developed production process and they should show sufficient removal or inactivation of spiked model viruses before the start of clinical studies. The choice of viruses to be spiked depends upon the production cell line, the ease of growing model viruses to high titers, and should include various types of virus (large vs small, enveloped vs non-enveloped, DNA vs. RNA). These types of studies are performed in specialized laboratories.

■ Bacteria

Bacterial contamination may be a problem for cells in culture or during pharmaceutical purification. Usually the size of bacteria allows simple filtration over 0.2 μm (or smaller) filters for adequate removal. Special attention is given to potential contaminations with mycoplasma, a genus of bacteria having no cell wall around their cell membrane. Some mycoplasma species are pathogenic to humans, and hundreds of mycoplasma species infect animals (Larsen and Hwang 2010). Testing for mycoplasma is a regulatory requirement for human biopharmaceuticals.

In order to further prevent bacterial contamination during production, the raw materials used have to be sterilized, preferably at 121 °C or higher, and the products are manufactured under strict aseptic conditions wherever possible. Production most often takes place in so-called clean rooms in which the chance of environmental contamination is reduced through careful control of the environment, for example, filtration of air. Additionally, antibiotic agents can be added to the culture media in some cases but have to be removed further downstream in the purification process. However, the use of beta-lactam antibiotics such as penicillin is strictly prohibited due to oversensitivity of some individuals to these compounds. Because of the persistence of antibiotic residues, which are difficult to eliminate from the product, appropriately designed manufacturing plants and extensive quality control systems for added reagents (medium, serum, enzymes, etc.) permitting antibiotic-free operation are preferable.

Pyrogens

Pyrogens are compounds that induce fever. Humans are sensitive to pyrogen contamination at very low concentrations (picograms per mL). Exogenous pyrogens (pyrogens introduced into the body, not generated by the body itself) can be derived from bacterial, viral, or fungal sources. Bacterial pyrogens are mainly endotoxins shed from gram-negative bacteria. They are lipopolysaccharides, and Fig. 4.8 shows the basic structure. The conserved structure in the full array of thousands of different endotoxins is the lipid-A moiety. Another general property shared by endotoxins is their high, negative electrical charge. Their tendency to aggregate and to form large units with M_W of 10^4 to over 10^6 Daltons in water, and their tendency to adsorb to surfaces indicate that these compounds are amphipathic in nature. Sensitive tests to detect and quantify pyrogens are commercially available.

They are stable under standard autoclaving conditions but break down when heated in the dry state. For this reason equipment and container are treated at temperatures above 160 °C for prolonged periods (e.g., 30 min dry heat at 250 °C). Removal is complicated because pyrogens vary in size and chemical composition. Pyrogen removal of recombinant products derived from bacterial sources should be an integral part of the preparation process. Ion exchange chromatographic procedures (utilizing its negative charge) can effectively reduce endotoxin levels in solution.

Excipients used in the protein formulation should be essentially endotoxin-free. For solutions "water for injection" (compendial standards) is (freshly) distilled or produced by reverse osmosis. The aggregated endotoxins cannot pass through the reverse osmosis membrane. Removal of endotoxins immediately before filling the final container can be accomplished by using activated charcoal or other materials with large surfaces offering hydrophobic interactions. Endotoxins can also be inactivated on utensil surfaces by oxidation (e.g., peroxide) or dry heating (e.g., 30 min dry heat at 250 °C).

Cellular DNA

The application of continuous mammalian cell lines for the production of recombinant proteins might result in the presence of oncogene-bearing DNA fragments in the final protein product (Walter and Werner 1993; Löwer 1990). A stringent purification protocol that is capable of reducing the DNA content and fragment size to a safe level is therefore necessary (Berthold and Walter 1994; WHO 2010; ICH 2017). A number of approaches are available to validate that the purification process removes cellular DNA and RNA. One such approach involves incubating the cell line with radiolabeled nucleotides and determining radioactivity in the purified product obtained through the purification protocol. Other methods are dye-binding fluorescence-enhancement assays for nucleotides and PCR-based methods. If the presence of nucleic acids persists at significant levels in a final preparation, then additional steps must be introduced in the purification process. The question about a safe level of nucleic acids

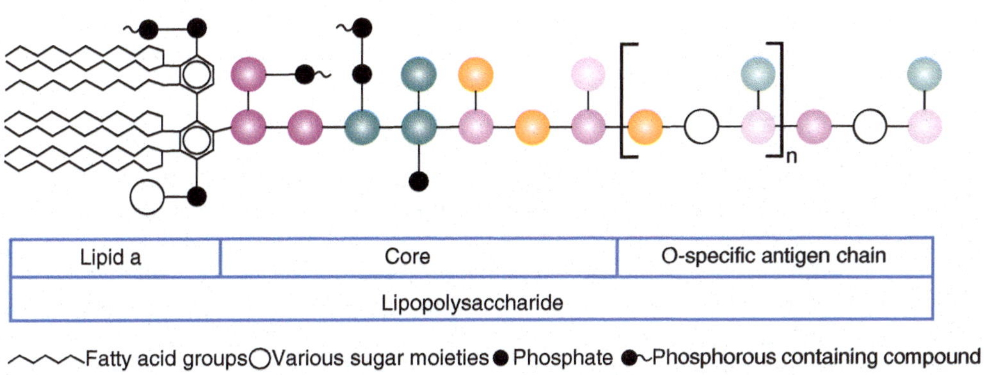

Figure 4.8 ■ Generalized structure of endotoxins. Most properties of endotoxins are accounted for by the active, insoluble "lipid A" fraction being solubilized by the various sugar moieties (circles with different colors). Although the general structure is similar, individual endotoxins vary according to their source and are characterized by the O-specific antigenic chain (adapted from Groves 1988)

in biotech products is difficult to answer. Transfection with so-called naked DNA is very difficult and a high concentration of DNA is needed. Nevertheless, it is agreed for safety reasons that final product contamination by nucleic acids should not exceed 100 pg or 10 ng per dose depending on the type of cells used to produce the pharmaceutical (WHO 2010; European Pharmacopoeia 2011).

■ Protein Contaminants and Product Variants

As mentioned before, minor amounts of host-, process-, and product-related protein contaminants will likely be present in biotech products. These types of contaminants are a potential health hazard because, if present, they may be recognized as antigens by the patient receiving the recombinant protein product. On repeated use the patient may show an immune reaction caused by the contaminant, while the protein of interest is performing its beneficial function. In such cases the immunogenicity may be misinterpreted as being due to the recombinant protein itself. Therefore, one must be very cautious in interpreting safety data of a given recombinant therapeutic protein. Some contaminants may also affect efficacy of the product, for example if they bind to an epitope important for the product to exert its function. Hence, careful control is needed.

Generally, the sources of host- and process-related protein contaminants are the cell culture medium used and the host proteins of the cells. Among the host-derived contaminants, the host species' version of the recombinant protein could be present (WHO 2010). As these proteins are similar in structure, it is possible that undesired proteins are co-purified with the desired product. For example, urokinase is known to be present in many continuous cell lines. The synthesis of highly active biological molecules such as cytokines by hybridoma cells might be another concern (FDA 1990). Depending upon their nature and concentration, these cytokines might enhance the antigenicity of the product.

"Known" or expected contaminants should be monitored at the successive stages in a purification process by suitable in-process controls, e.g., sensitive immunoassay(s). Tracing of the many "unknown" cell-derived proteins is more difficult. When developing a purification process, other less-specific analytical techniques such as SDS-PAGE (sodium dodecyl sulfate–polyacrylamide gel electrophoresis) are usually used in combination with various staining techniques.

Product-related contaminants may pose a safety issue for patients. These contaminants can, for example, be aggregated, deamidated or oxidized forms of the product. And, importantly, one has to keep in mind that recombinant proteins produced in cells are inherently variable, for example at the level of glycosylation. Such molecules are generally considered product variants. Some of these contaminants/variants are described in the following paragraphs.

N- and C-Terminal Heterogeneity

A major problem connected with the production of biotech products is the problem associated with the amino (NH2)-terminus of the protein, e.g., in E. coli systems, where protein synthesis always starts with methylmethionine. Obviously, it has been of great interest to develop methods that generate proteins with an NH2-terminus as found in the authentic protein. When the proteins are not produced in the correct way, the final product may contain several methionyl variants of the protein in question or even contain proteins lacking one or more residues from the amino terminus. This is called the amino-terminal heterogeneity. This heterogeneity can also occur with recombinant proteins (e.g., α-interferon) susceptible to proteases that are either secreted by the host or introduced by serum-containing media. These proteases can clip off amino acids from the C-terminal and/or N-terminal of the desired product (amino- and/or carboxy-terminal heterogeneity). Amino- and/or carboxy-terminal heterogeneity is not desirable since it may cause difficulties in purification and characterization of the proteins. In case of the presence of an additional methionine at the N-terminal end of the protein, its secondary and tertiary structure can be altered. This could affect the biological activity and stability and may make it immunogenic. Moreover, N-terminal methionine and/or internal methionine is sensitive to oxidation (Sharma 1990).

C-terminal lysine clipping is often observed in monoclonal antibodies produced in mammalian cells. This does not have to be an issue, since the C-terminal lysine is clipped off rapidly in the blood upon injection in humans. The glutamine on the N-terminus of monoclonal antibodies can be converted in pyro-glutamate, increasing the acidity of the antibody. These types of posttranslational modifications should be controlled within a certain range to ensure a robust production process.

Conformational Changes/Chemical Modifications

Although mammalian cells are able to produce proteins structurally equal to endogenous proteins, some caution is needed. Transcripts containing the full-length coding sequence could result in conformational isomers of the protein because of unexpected secondary structures that affect translational fidelity (Sharma 1990). Another factor to be taken into account is the possible existence of equilibria between the desired form and other forms such as dimers. The correct folding of proteins after biosynthesis is important because it determines the specific activity of the protein). Therefore, it is important to determine if all molecules of a given recombinant protein secreted by a mammalian expression system are folded in their native conformation.. Apart from conformational changes, proteins can undergo chemical alterations, such as proteolysis, deamidation, and hydroxyl and sulfhydryl oxidations during the purification process (cf. Chaps. 2 and 3) These alterations can result in (partial) denaturation of the protein. Vice versa, denaturation of the protein may cause chemical modifications as well (e.g., as a result of exposure of sensitive groups).

Glycosylation (also cf. Chap. 2)

Many therapeutic proteins produced by recombinant DNA technology are glycoproteins of which the majority are monoclonal antibodies. The presence and nature of oligosaccharide side chains in proteins affect a number of important characteristics, such as the proteins' serum half-life, solubility, and stability, and sometimes even the pharmacological function (Cumming 1991). Darbepoetin, a second-generation, genetically modified erythropoietin, has a carbohydrate content of 80% compared to 40% for the native molecule, which increases the in vivo half-life after intravenous administration from 8 h for erythropoietin to 25 h for darbepoetin (Sinclair and Elliott 2005). Antibody-dependent cell cytotoxicity (ADCC) is dependent on the degree of fucosylation of the antibody product (Hossler et al. 2009; reviewed by Krasnova and Wong 2016). As a result, the therapeutic profile may be "glycosylation" dependent. As mentioned previously, protein glycosylation is not determined by the DNA sequence. It is an enzymatic modification of the protein after translation and depends on the metabolic state of the cell (Hossler et al. 2009). Although mammalian cells are very well able to glycosylate proteins, it is hard to fully control glycosylation. Carbohydrate heterogeneity can occur through the size of the chain, type of oligosaccharide, and sequence of the carbohydrates. This has been demonstrated for a number of recombinant products including monoclonal antibodies, interleukin-4, chorionic gonadotropin, erythropoietin, and tissue plasminogen activator. Carbohydrate structure and composition in recombinant proteins may differ from their native counterparts, because the enzymes required for synthesis and processing vary among different expression systems, e.g. glycoproteins from insect cells are frequently smaller than the same glycoproteins expressed in mammalian cells or even from one mammalian system to another.

Proteolytic Processing

Proteases play an important role in processing, maturation, modification, or isolation of recombinant proteins. Proteases from mammalian cells are involved in secreting proteins into the cultivation medium e.g. by cleaving of a signal peptide. Proteases are released if cells die and undergo lysis during production in the bioreactor and at harvest. It is therefore important to control growth and harvest conditions in order to minimize this effect. Another source of proteolytic attack is found in the components of the medium in which the cells are grown. For example, serum contains a number of proteases and protease zymogens that may affect the secreted recombinant protein. If present in small amounts and if the nature of the proteolytic attack on the desired protein is identified, appropriate protease inhibitors to control proteolysis could be used. It is advised to document the integrity of the recombinant protein after each purification step.

Proteins become much more susceptible to proteases at elevated temperatures. Purification strategies should be designed to carry out all the steps at 2–8 °C (Sharma, 1990) if proteolytic degradation occurs. Alternatively, Ca^{2+} complexing agents (e.g., citrate) can be added as many proteases depend on Ca^{2+} for their activity. From a manufacturing perspective, however, cooling large-scale downstream process unit operations, although not impossible, is a complicating and expensive factor.

BACTERIA: PROTEIN INCLUSION BODY FORMATION

In bacteria soluble proteins can form dense, finely granular inclusions within the cytoplasm. These "inclusion bodies" often occur in bacterial cells that overproduce proteins by plasmid expression. The protein inclusions appear in electron micrographs as large, dense bodies often spanning the entire diameter of the cell. Protein inclusions are probably formed by a buildup of amorphous protein aggregates held together by covalent and non-covalent bonds. The inability to measure inclusion body proteins directly may lead to the inaccurate assessment of recovery and yield and may cause problems if protein solubility is essential for efficient, large-scale purification (Berthold and Walter 1994). Several schemes for recovery of proteins from inclusion bodies have been described. The recovery of proteins from inclusion bodies requires cell breakage and inclusion body recovery. Dissolution of inclusion proteins is the next step in the purification scheme and typically takes place in extremely dilute solutions, thus increasing the volumes of the unit operations during the manufacturing phases. This can make process control more difficult if, for example, low temperatures are required during these steps. Generally, inclusion proteins dissolve in denaturing agents such as sodium dodecyl sulfate (SDS), urea, or guanidine hydrochloride. Because bacterial systems generally are incapable of forming disulfide bonds, a protein containing these bonds has to be refolded under oxidizing conditions to restore these bonds and to generate the biologically active protein. This so-called renaturation step is increasingly difficult if more S-S bridges are present in the molecule and the yield of renatured product could be as low as only a few percent. Once the protein is solubilized, conventional chromatographic separations can be used for further purification of the protein.

Aggregate formation at first sight may seem undesirable, but there may also be advantages as long as the protein of interest will unfold and refold properly. Inclusion body proteins can easily be recovered to yield proteins with >50% purity, a substantial improvement over the purity of soluble proteins (sometimes below 1% of the total cell protein). Furthermore, the aggregated forms of the proteins are more resistant to proteolysis, because most molecules of an aggregated form are not accessible to proteolytic enzymes. Thus the high yield and relatively cheap production using a bacterial system can offset a low-yield renaturation process. For a non-glycosylated, simple protein molecule, this production system is still used.

QUALITY BY DESIGN

The current expectations of regulatory agencies, particularly in implementing the twenty-first century's risk-based GMPs, is to employ the principles of risk analysis, design space (see below), control strategy and Quality by Design (QbD). Implementing QbD should result in a manufacturing process that consistently delivers a high quality product. Furthermore, it ensures that the critical sources of variability are identified and controlled through appropriate control strategies. A detailed end-to-end assessment of the product, its manufacturing process and raw materials will result in the definition of:

1. Critical quality attributes (CQAs)
   The definition of a CQA according to ICH Q8 (R2), 2009 is as follows: "a physical, chemical, biological, or microbiological property or characteristic that should be within an appropriate limit, range, or distribution to ensure the desired product quality". The CQAs of biologics are basically assessed by measuring their impact on safety and efficacy.
2. Critical process parameters (CPPs)
   CPPs are according to ICH Q8(R2) (2009) "process parameters whose variability has an impact on a critical quality attributes". They are identified by sound scientific judgement and based on prior knowledge, development, scale-up and manufacturing experience. CPPs should be controlled and monitored to confirm that the product quality is comparable to or better than historical data from development and manufacturing. Quality attributes that should be considered in defining CPPs are for example purity, qualitative and quantitative impurities, microbial quality, biological activity and content.
3. Critical material attributes (CMAs)
   CMAs are materials used in the process that affect the quality attributes. They are judged as described above for the CPPs. CMAs should be controlled and monitored by validated incoming goods assays.
4. Control strategy
   The control strategy for the product is defined by controlling CPPs and the CMAs. Based on the risks related to the CPPs/CMAs an appropriate control strategy should be designed. A proper control strategy will decrease the probability/likelihood of out of range CQA and increase the detectability of CPP/CMA failure. During the lifecycle of the product the control strategy should be adjusted based on new knowledge. The control strategy will be assessed by means of a risk assessment (e.g., failure mode effects analysis, FMEA).

Above mentioned analysis must be performed during various stages of process development. However, the starting point for a QbD excercise is to study the (potential) CQAs that are defined in early stage discovery. The analysis should continue during early and late development and commercial scale manufacturing. Prior knowledge, analytical development, comparability studies, and (non-) clinical study results contribute to the understanding of CQAs. By performing this analysis during various stages, the QbD principles will be continuously updated as they are based on increased know-how during product development and commercial scale manufacturing.

Although not obligatory, the authorities encourage to implement a design space in the processes. ICH Q8 defines the design space of a process as follows: "the multidimensional combination and interaction of input variables (e.g., material attributes) and process parameters that have been demonstrated to provide assurance of quality. Working within the design space is not considered as a change. Movement out of the design space is considered to be a change and would normally initiate a regulatory postapproval change process. The design space is proposed by the manufacturer. The advantage of the design space that it is usually broader than the operating ranges".

Based on these assessments the CPPs and CMAs are specified for:

(a) Normal operating ranges (NOR)
   A process range that is representative of historical variability in the manufacturing process

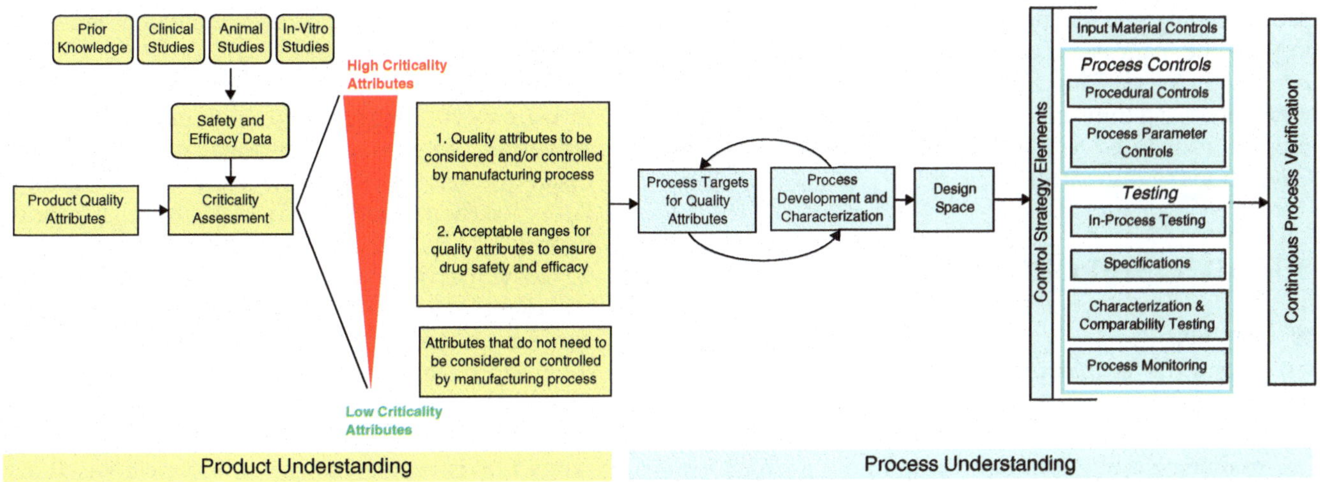

Figure 4.9 ■ The overall approach for A-Mab product realization illustrates a sequence of activities that starts with the design of the molecule and spans the development process ultimately resulting in the final process and control strategy used for commercial scale manufacturing (adapted from Berridge et al. 2009)

(b) Acceptable operating ranges
A range that is specified in the manufacturing batch record

(c) Proven acceptable range (PAR)
A characterized range of the process which will result in producing a product meeting the relevant quality criteria.

Company representatives of the Biotechnology Industry were brought together in 2008 helping to advance the principles which are contained in ICH Q8 (R2), Q9 and Q10, focusing on the principles of Quality by Design. The outcome of this collaboration resulted in a unique document: "A-Mab: A case study in BioProcess Development" (Berridge et al. 2009). The case study is a must read for people involved in the biotechnology industry. Figure 4.9 shows the overall approach for A-Mab product realization.

COMMERCIAL-SCALE MANUFACTURING AND INNOVATION

A major part of the recombinant proteins on the market consist of monoclonal antibodies produced in mammalian cells. Pharmaceutical production processes have been set up since the early 1980s of the twentieth century. These processes essentially consist of production in stirred tanks bioreactors, clarification using centrifugation, and membrane technology, followed by protein A capture, low-pH virus inactivation, cation-exchange and anion-exchange chromatography (or an alternative chromatographic ligand), virus filtration, and UF/DF for product formulation (Shukla and Thömmes 2010). Such platform processes run consistently at very large scale (e.g. multiple 10,000 L bioreactors and higher volumes). Product recovery is generally very high (>70%). Since product titers in the bioreactors have increased to a level where further increases have no or a minimal effect on the cost of goods, the focus of process development in companies having these large-scale manufacturing plants working at full capacity is shifting to understanding the process fundamentals of the current platform (Kelley 2009). However, it is also anticipated that the monoclonal antibody demands for some disease indications may decrease due to the introduction of more efficacious products such as antibody-drug conjugates (e.g. Adcetris®, Seattle Genetics) and increased competition with biosimilar products (e.g., Celltrion's Remsina®/Infectra® as biosimilar of the Johnson & Johnson blockbuster Remicade®), and the introduction of new products with (much) smaller market sizes, including those used in personalized medicines approaches. A lower demand together with the increase in recombinant protein titers and yields will lead to a decrease in bioreactor size, an increase in the need for flexible facilities, and faster turnaround times leading to a growth in the use of disposables and other innovative technologies as discussed above (Shukla and Thömmes 2010). Such innovative technologies and capabilities encompass process intensification, in which production is intensified by using highly concentrated product and reactants, and in which process steps are combined into single units. Innovation is also seen in the introduction of continuous processing strategies in the pharmaceutical industry, as well as steps towards fully automated facilities, enabling a fast response to capacity demands at lower costs and higher quality. Facilities will become modular and mobile, allowing standardized "plug and play" manufacturing systems to be configured, assembled and relocated quickly. A further introduction of process analytical technology (PAT) is expected, allowing in-line process monitoring and real time drug product release. This includes development of software enabling multivariate data analysis, predictive models and closed feedback control loops (BioPhorum Operations Group 2017).

SELF-ASSESSMENT QUESTIONS

Questions

1. Name the four expression systems mentioned in this chapter?
2. What is the main reason to use eukaryotic mammalian cells as expression system?
3. What are the main reasons for manufacturing companies to change from stainless steel system to single-use systems?
4. Which bioreactor processes are generally used for production of biopharmaceuticals?
5. Membrane filters are frequently used within the purification process of biotech products. Name four different membrane filter types.
6. Compared to other chromatographic methods, what is in general the most significant advantage and disadvantage of affinity purification chromatography?
7. Name at least six different product-related variants.
8. What is the difference between a NOR and PAR? Which of these two parameters gives most flexibility in a process?
9. What are the major safety concerns in the purification of cell-expressed proteins?
10. Glycosylation may affect several properties of the protein. Mention at least three possible effects in case of changing a glycosylation pattern.
11. What is in general the expectation of the size of future GMP manufacturing facilities? What is the reasoning behind this?

Answers

1. Prokaryotic bacteria, eukaryotic yeast, eukaryotic mammalian cells, and eukaryotic plant cells.
2. For biopharmaceutical products used in human health care the glycosylation process is the most important reason. The glycosylation pattern should be human-like which is possible with the eukaryotic mammalian cell system.
3. The main reasons are the speed to market, possibility to increase the number of batches produced per year in a manufacturing facility, providing flexibility in facility design, reduction of water consumption and reduced validation costs.
4. The main bioreactor processes are batch, fed-batch and perfusion.
5. Sterilizing-grade filters, tangential flow filters, virus removal filters, charged filters.
6. Advantage: high degree of purity can be obtained; disadvantage: usually very costly, and extra regulatory burden due to characterization of affinity ligand.
7. Glycosylations variants, amino acid substitution and deletion, denatured protein, oxidized variants, conformational isomers, dimers and aggregates, disulfide paring variants, succinimide formation, (de)amidated variants, protein fragments.
8. The Normal Operating Range (NOR) is a process range that is representative of historical variability in the manufacturing process, while a Proven Acceptable Range (PAR) is a characterized range of the process which will result in producing a product meeting the relevant quality criteria. The PAR gives most flexibility since it allows operation beyond the NOR.
9. Removal of viruses, bacteria, protein contaminants and cellular DNA.
10. Solubility, pKa, charge, stability and biological activity.
11. GMP manufacturing facilities will become smaller, modular and mobile. Rationale: manufacturing volumes will become smaller due to process intensification and the generation of products with a smaller market capture.

REFERENCES

Abi-Ghanem DA, Berghman LR (2012) Immunoaffinity chromatography: a review. http://cdn.intechopen.com/pdfs-wm/33050.pdf

Afeyan N, Gordon N, Mazsaroff I, Varady L, Fulton S, Yang Y, Regnier F (1989) Flow-through particles of the high-performance liquid chromatographic separation of biomolecules, perfusion chromatography. J Chromatogr 519:1–29

Berridge J, Seamon K, Venugopal S (2009) A-Mab: a case study in BioProcess development, version 2.1, 30th October 2009. http://c.ymcdn.com/sites/www.casss.org/resource/resmgr/imported/A-Mab_Case_Study_Version_2-1.pdf

Berthold W, Walter J (1994) Protein purification: aspects of processes for pharmaceutical products. Biologicals 22:135–150

BioPhorum Operations Group (2017) Biomanufacturing technology roadmap. www.biophorum.com/wp-content/uploads/2017/07/SupplyPartMgmnt.pdf

Cartwright T (1987) Isolation and purification of products from animal cells. Trends Biotechnol 5:25–30

Celik E, Calik P (2012) Production of recombinant proteins by yeast cells. Biotechnol Adv 30(5):1108–1118

Chase H, Draeger N (1993) Affinity purification of proteins using expanded beds. J Chromatogr 597:129–145
Chase HA (1994) Purification of proteins by adsorption chromatography in expanded beds. Trends Biotechnol 12:296–303
Chen T, Zhang K, Gruenhagen J, Medley CD (2015) Hydrophobic interaction chromatography for antibody drug conjugate drug distribution analysis. american pharmaceutical review. www.americanpharmaceuticalreview.com/Featured-Articles/177927
Compton B, Jensen J (2007) Use of perfusion technology on the Rise – New modes are beginning to gain ground on Fed-Batch strategy. Genet Eng Biotechnol News 27:48
Council of Europe (2011) Cell substrates for the production of vaccines for human use. In: European Pharmacopoeia, 7th edn. Council of Europe, Strasbourg
Cumming DA (1991) Glycosylation of recombinant protein therapeutics: Control and functional implications. Glycobiology 1:115–130
Dell A, Galadari A, Sastre F, Hitchen P (2011) Similarities and differences in the glycosylation mechanisms in prokaryotes and eukaryotes. Int J Microbiol 2010:148178
Dos Santos NV, De Carvalho Santos-Ebinuma V, Pessoa A Jr, Brandao Pereira JF (2018) Liquid-liquid extraction of biopharmaceuticals from fermented broth: trends and future prospects. J Chem Technol Biotechnol 93(7):1845–1863
Eibl R, Eibl D (eds) (2011) Single-use technology in biopharmaceuticalmanufacture. Wiley, Hoboken
EMA (2011) Note for guidance on minimising the risk of transmitting animal spongiform encephalopathy agents via human and veterinary medicinal products (EMA/410/01 rev.3)
Etzel MR, Arunkumar A (2017) Charged ultrafiltration and microfiltration membranes for antibody purification. In: Gottschalk U (ed) Process scale purification of antibodies. Wiley, Hoboken. https://doi.org/10.1002/9781119126942.ch12
European Agency for the Evaluation of Medicinal Products (EMA) (1996) Note for guidance for virus validation studies: design, contribution and interpretation of studies validating the inactivation and removal of viruses (CPMP/BWP/268/95)
FDA, Center for Biologics Evaluation and Research (1990) Cytokine and growth factor pre-pivotal trial information package with special emphasis on products identified for consideration under 21 CFR 312 Subpart E. FDA, Bethesda
FDA, Office of Biologicals Research and Review (1993) Points to consider in the characterization of cell lines used to produce biologicals. FDA, Rockville Pike
Fulton SP (1994) Large scale processing of macromolecules. Curr Opin Biotechnol 5:201–205
Goldstein A, Molina O (2016) Implementation strategies and challenges: single use technologies. PepTalk Presentation
Gottschalk U (2006) The renaissance of protein purification. BioPharm Int 19:S8–S9
Groves MJ (1988) Parenteral technology manual: an introduction to formulation and production aspects of parenteral products. Interpharm Press, Buffalo Grove
Hodge G (2004) Disposable components enable a new approach to biopharmaceutical manufacturing. BioPharm Int 15:38–49
Homma T, Fuji M, Mori J, Kawakami T, Kuroda K, Taniguchi M (1993) Production of cellobiose by enzymatic hydrolysis: removal of ß-glucosidase from cellulase by affinity precipitation using chitosan. Biotechnol Bioeng 41:405–410
Hossler P, Khattak SF, Li ZJ (2009) Optimal and consistent protein glycosylation in mammalian cell culture. Glycobiology 19:936–949
ICH (International Conference on Harmonization) Topic Q6B (1999a) Specifications: test procedures and acceptance criteria for biotechnology/biological products.
ICH (International Conference on Harmonization) Topic Q5A (1999b) Viral safety evaluation of biotechnology products derived from cell lines of human or animal origin
ICH (International Conference on Harmonization) Topic Q8 (R2) (2009) Pharmaceutical development.
ICH (International Conference on Harmonization) (2017) Guideline M7 on assessment and control of DNA reactive (mutagenic) impurities in pharmaceuticals to limit potential carcinogenic risk
James AM (1992) Introduction fundamental techniques. In: James AM (ed) Analysis of amino acids and nucleic acids. Butterworth-Heinemann, Oxford, pp 1–28
Jones N (2015) Single-Use Processing for Microbial Fermentations. BioProcess Int 13:56–62
Kelley B (2009) Industrialization of mAb production technology. MAbs 1:443–452
Klegerman ME, Groves MJ (1992) Pharmaceutical biotechnology. Interpharm Press, Buffalo Grove
Krasnova L, Wong CH (2016) Understanding the chemistry and biology of glycosylation with glycan synthesis. Annu Rev Biochem 85:599–630
Larsen B, Hwang J (2010) Mycoplasma, ureaplasma, and adverse pregnancy outcomes: a fresh look. Infect Dis Obstet Gynecol 2010:1–7
Löwer J (1990) Risk of tumor induction in vivo by residual cellular DNA: quantitative considerations. J Med Virol 31:50–53
Luitjens A, Lewis J, Pralong A (2012) Single-use biotechnologies and modular manufacturing environments invite paradigm shifts in bioprocess development and biopharmaceutical manufacturing. In: Subramanian G (ed) Biopharmaceutical production technology, vol 1&2. Wiley-VCH Verlag GmbH & Co. KGaA, Weinheim, pp 817–857
Maerz H, Hahn SO, Maassen A, Meisel H, Roggenbuck D, Sato T, Tanzmann H, Emmrich F, Marx U (1996) Improved removal of viruslike particles from purified monoclonal antibody IgM preparation via virus filtration. Nat Biotechnol 14:651–652
Marcus-Sekura CJ (1991) Validation and removal of human retroviruses. Center for Biologics Evaluation and Research, FDA, Bethesda
Minor PD (1994) Ensuring safety and consistency in cell culture production processes: viral screening and inactivation. Trends Biotechnol 12:257–261

Monteclaro F (2010) Protein expression systems, ringing in the new. Innov Pharm Technol 12:45–49

Orzaez D, Granell A, Blazquez MA (2009) Manufacturing antibodies in the plant cell. Biotechnol J 4:1712–1724

PDA (2005) PDA technical report no. 41: virus filtration. PDA J Pharm Sci Technol 59(S-2):1–42

Peters J, Stoger E (2011) Transgenic crops for the production of recombinant vaccines and anti-microbial antibodies. Hum Vaccin 7:367–374

Sharma SK (1990) Key issues in the purification and characterization of recombinant proteins for therapeutic use. Adv Drug Deliv Rev 4:87–111

Shukla AA, Thömmes J (2010) Recent advances in large-scale production of monoclonal antibodies and related proteins. Trends Biotechnol 28:253–261

Shukla AA, Wolfe LS, Mostafa SS, Norman C (2017) Evolving trends in mAb production processes. Bioeng Transl Med 2:58–69

Sinclair A, Brower M, Lopes AG, Pollard D, Abe Y (2016) Standardized economic cost modeling for next-generation MAb production. BioProcess Int 14:14–23

Sinclair AM, Elliott S (2005) Glycoengineering: the effect of glycosylation on the properties of therapeutic proteins. J Pharm Sci 94:1626–1635

Tennikova T, Svec F (1993) High performance membrane chromatography: highly efficient separation method for proteins in ion-exchange, hydrophobic interaction and reversed phase modes. J Chromatogr 646:279–288

Terstappen G, Ramelmeier R, Kula M (1993) Protein partitioning in detergent-based aqueous two-phase systems. J Biotechnol 28:263–275

Turner R, Joseph A, Titchener-Hooker N, Bender J (2017) Manufacturing of proteins and antibodies: chapter downstream processing technologies, harvest operations. In: Advances biochemical engineering/biotechnology. Springer, Berlin

Van Wezel AL, Van der Velden-de Groot CA, De Haan HH, Van den Heuvel N, Schasfoort R (1985) Large scale animal cell cultivation for production of cellular biologicals. Dev Biol Stand 60:229–236

Walsh C (2006) Posttranslational modification of proteins: expanding nature's inventory, vol xxi. Roberts and Co. Publishers, Englewood, p 490

Walter J, Werner RG (1993) Regulatory requirements and economic aspects in downstream processing of biotechnically engineered proteins for parenteral application as pharmaceuticals. In: Kroner KH, Papamichael N, Schütte H (eds) Downstream processing, recovery and purification of proteins, a handbook of principles and practice. Carl Hauser Verlag, Muenchen

Walter J, Werz W, McGoff P, Werner RG, Berthold W (1991) Virus removal/inactivation in downstream processing. In: Spier RE, Griffiths JB, MacDonald C (eds) Animal cell technology: development, processes and products. Butterworth-Heinemann Ltd. Linacre House, Oxford, pp 624–634

Walter K, Werz W, Berthold W (1992) Virus removal and inactivation, concept and data for process validation of downstream processing. Biotech Forum Eur 9:560–564

Wheelwright SM (1993) Designing downstream processing for large scale protein purification. Biotechnology 5:789–793

WHO (World Health Organization) (2010) Recommendations for the evaluation of animal cell cultures as substrates for the manufacture of biological medicinal products and for the characterization of cell banks. Technical report series, proposed replacement of 878, annex 1. WHO, Geneva

Yao J, Weng Y, Dickey A, Tressel KY (2015) Plants as factories for human pharmaceuticals: applications and challenges. Int J Mol Sci 16:28549–28565

Zhou JX, Tressel T (2006) Basic concepts in Q membrane chromatography for large scale antibody production. Biotechnol Prog 22:341–349

5 Formulation of Biologics Including Biopharmaceutical Considerations

Daan J. A. Crommelin, Andrea Hawe, and Wim Jiskoot

INTRODUCTION

This chapter provides an introduction to the process of formulating biologics. In this formulation process, a drug *substance* (DS), also called active pharmaceutical ingredient (API), is turned into a drug *product* that can be administered to the patient. It addresses questions regarding the tests to be run, e.g., to characterize the DS and to ensure its stability, and the chotice of excipients and delivery system. It also discusses biopharmaceutical issues such as the route and rate of administration.

The text concentrates on formulating proteins used in therapy, but the same principles also apply to other biologics, such as vaccines and oligonucleotide based products as discussed in Chaps. 14 and 15 of this book.

Formulating a protein is not a one-step, routine process with fixed strategies. Several different, sometimes overlapping, phases can be recognized during the product development process, as depicted in Fig. 5.1. In the formulation development process one starts with preformulation activities and ends up –after months/years of running tests– with late-stage fine tuning of the selected, optimized product composition-dosage form. Therefore, the formulation used in the preclinical and clinical development phases may change according to the insights gained up to that moment: from 'initial formulation' to 'commercial drug product'.

POINTS TO CONSIDER IN THE PROCESS OF FORMULATING A THERAPEUTIC PROTEIN

■ Protein Structure and Protein Stability

Table 5.1 lists 'points to consider' when formulating a protein. An early and deep understanding of the structural properties of the protein at hand such as primary structure, higher-order structures, molecular weight, isoelectric point, post-translational modifications, hydrophobicity, and its physical (unfolding and aggregation) and chemical stability (cf. Table 5.2) as function of its direct environment (e.g., pH, ionic strength) will speed up the formulation process. This basic information helps to design a product that is stable not only on the shelf, but also under real-life conditions, e.g., during transportation, compounding (e.g., dilution in an intravenous infusion bag) and administration (Jiskoot et al., 2017; Nejadnik et al., 2018). Table 5.3 (adapted from Hawe et al., 2012) shows various stress factors a product can encounter.

D. J. A. Crommelin (✉)
Department of Pharmaceutical, Utrecht Institute for Pharmaceutical Sciences, Utrecht University, Utrecht, The Netherlands
e-mail: d.j.a.crommelin@uu.nl

A. Hawe
Coriolis Pharma, Martinsried, Germany
e-mail: Andrea.Hawe@coriolis-pharma.com

W. Jiskoot
Division of BioTherapeutics, Leiden Academic Centre for Drug Research (LACDR), Leiden University, Leiden, The Netherlands
e-mail: w.jiskoot@lacdr.leidenuniv.nl

D. J. A. Crommelin et al. (eds.), *Pharmaceutical Biotechnology*, https://doi.org/10.1007/978-3-030-00710-2_5

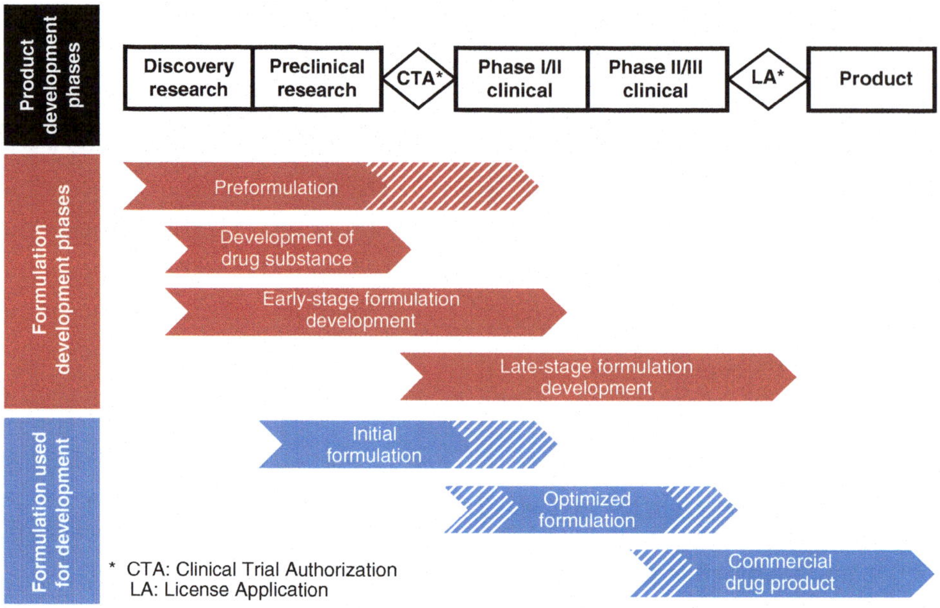

Figure 5.1 ■ Diagram of a formulation development process. Modified from Chang and Hershenson (2002)

Factor	Description/attributes/examples
API or drug substance	Type of protein, physico-chemical properties, e.g., molecular weight, pI, hydrophobicity, solubility, post-translational modifications, pegylation, physical and chemical stability and concentration, available amount, purity
Clinical factors	Patient population (e.g., age and concomitant medication), self-administration versus administration by professional, compatibility with infusion solution, indication (e.g., one-time application or chronical application)
Route of administration	Subcutaneous, intravenous injection or infusion, intramuscular, intravitreal, intra-articular, intradermal, pulmonal
Dosage form	Single- or multi-dose, prefilled syringe, dual chamber cartridge, pen cartridge; liquid, lyophilizate, frozen liquid, API concentration, injection volume, injection rate, controlled delivery/release
Primary packaging material	Glass, polymers, rubber, silicone oil, metals, leachables (anti-oxidants, plasticizers, etc.)
Excipients	Pharmaceutical quality, safety record (for intended administration route and dose), manufacturer, tested for critical impurities, stability
Analytical methods	Characterization of API, stability-indicating assays, quality control assays

Adapted from Weinbuch et al. (2018)
API active pharmaceutical ingredient

Table 5.1 ■ Points for consideration in the formulation process of pharmaceutical proteins

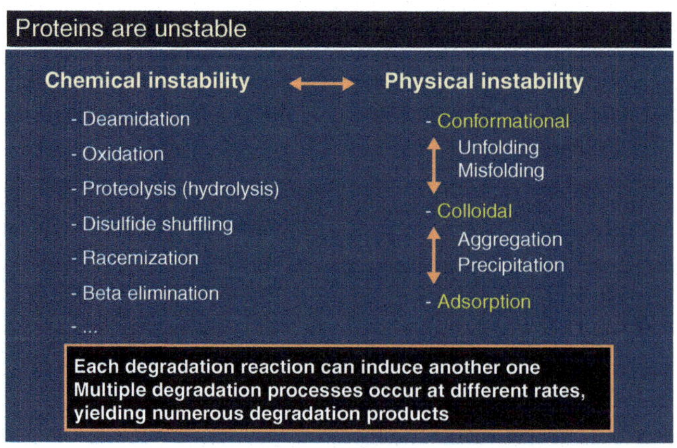

Table 5.2 ■ Chemical and physical reactions jeopardizing protein stability (cf. Table 3.1)

Stress factor	When encountered/examples
Elevated temperature, temperature excursions	Production (upstream and downstream processing); improper shipment; storage or handling deviations
Freezing, freeze-thawing	Storage of frozen (bulk) material; accidental freezing during storage or shipment; lyophilization
Mechanical stress	Production (e.g., pumping, stirring, filtration)
Light	Production; shipment; storage; handling
Oxidative stress	Production (exposure to oxygen); exposure to peroxide or metal ion impurities in excipients; shipment (cavitation)
pH changes	Production (downstream processing); freezing; formulation; dilution in infusion liquids; administration
Interfaces	Air-water interface; filters; primary packaging material; infusion bags and administration lines; particulate impurities
X-ray	Air freight transportation

Adapted from Hawe et al. (2012)

Table 5.3 ■ Stress factors a therapeutic protein may encounter

Box 1: Orthogonal vs Complementary Analytical Techniques

Orthogonal analytical techniques are combinations of techniques that monitor the same (similar) properties of a protein (in its formulation) with a different measurement principle (cf. Table 5.4).

For example,

- Size-exclusion chromatography (SEC), asymmetrical flow field flow fractionation (AF4) and analytical ultracentrifugation (AUC)
- Near-UV circular dichroism (CD) and intrinsic fluorescence spectroscopy
- Far-UV circular dichroism (CD) and Fourier transform infrared (FTIR) spectroscopy
- Light obscuration (LO), flow-Imaging microscopy and electric zone sensing

Complementary analytical techniques are techniques that measure different properties of a protein (in its formulation) with a different measurement principle (cf. Table 5.4).

For example when monitoring aggregation of the protein,

- Size-exclusion chromatography (SEC) for oligomers and dynamic light scattering for nanometer size aggregates
- Analytical ultracentrifugation (AUC) for oligomers and nanoparticle tracking analysis (NTA) for nanometer size aggregates,
- Light obscuration or flow imaging microscopy for micrometer size aggregates, visual inspection for larger, visible particles
- Techniques for sizing (see above) and methods for conformational analysis (CD, FTIR, fluorescence spectroscopy)
- Techniques for size (e.g., SEC), charge (e.g., ion-exchange chromatography) and hydrophobicity (RP-HPLC)

■ Analytical Toolbox

The need for an 'analytical toolbox' with stability-indicating orthogonal and complementary analytical techniques (see Box 1) to characterize a protein in various stages of formulation development in as much detail as possible is evident. Table 5.4 (adapted from Hawe et al., 2012) lists selected analytical methodologies that are being used to monitor protein stability.

These analytical techniques will provide the necessary data and guide the formulator through the subsequent stages of the development process ending up with the marketed drug product. More information about protein (in)stability and analytical methodology can be found in Chap. 3 of this book and in articles/books by Manning et al. (1989, 2010), Jiskoot and Crommelin (2005); Kamerzell et al. (2011); Zölls et al. (2012); Hawe et al. (2012); Weinbuch et al. (2018).

■ Physical and Chemical Stability

Already in an early stage, data on physical stability (colloidal and conformational stability) and on chemical stability of the API and formulations are collected. Monitoring and controlling aggregate formation is particularly important, because protein aggregates are

Type of degradation product	Examples of analytical techniques
Soluble aggregates (dimers, trimers, oligomers) and fragments	Size-exclusion HPLC/UPLC, AF4, analytical ultracentrifugation, SDS-PAGE, CE-SDS
Nanometer-sized aggregates	Dynamic light scattering; nanoparticle tracking analysis; AF4; Taylor dispersion analysis; turbidimetry/nephelometry; static light scattering
Micrometer-sized aggregates	Light obscuration; light microscopy; flow imaging microscopy; coulter counter; fluorescence microscopy; turbidimetry/nephelometry; Raman microscopy
Visible particles	Visual inspection; (semi-)automated visual inspection
Conformational changes	Circular dichroism, infrared, intrinsic fluorescence, extrinsic fluorescence spectroscopy and secondary-derivative UV spectroscopy
Chemical changes	Reversed-phase HPLC/UPLC; (HPLC-)mass spectrometry; ion-exchange chromatography; (capillary) isoelectric focusing

AF4 asymmetrical flow field-flow fractionation, *CE-SDS* capillary electrophoresis sodium dodecyl sulfate, *HPLC* high performance liquid chromatography, *UPLC* ultra performance liquid chromatography
Adapted from Hawe et al. (2012)

Table 5.4 ■ Examples of protein degradation products and techniques to analyze them

Type of stress	Examples of stress conditions	Anticipated instability types
Temperature	Real time (2–8 °C; up to several years) Accelerated (e.g., 25 °C, 40 °C, up to several months)	Aggregation, conformational changes, chemical changes
Mechanical	Shaking (50–500 rpm, hours-days) Stirring, 50–500 rpm, hours-days) Freeze-thawing, (1–5 cycles, from 25 °C to −20 °C or −80 °C)	Aggregation, adsorption, conformational changes
Oxidation	H_2O_2 (1–5%, 1–2 days)	Chemical changes, aggregation, conformational changes
Humidity*	0–100% relative humidity	Aggregation, conformational changes, chemical changes

* Specifically for lyophilized products. Adapted from Weinbuch et al. (2018)

Table 5.5 ■ Examples of accelerated stability and forced degradation studies

readily formed under a variety of conditions and have been associated with enhanced risk of immunogenicity of therapeutic proteins (cf. Chap. 7). It should be emphasized that aggregation of proteins can happen at concentrations much below their solubility and at temperatures far below their denaturation temperature. Proteins in solution have an increased tendency to aggregate upon mechanical stress and interaction with interfaces. Therefore, protein stability should not only be studied under quiescent conditions, but tests should be performed on protein stability in tubes, pipes, columns and pumps, during handling and the fill-finish process to ensure stability during manufacturing.

For shelf life assessment of the drug product typically 'real time'data at 2–8 °C is collected in combination with data from forced degradation studies. These include collecting stability information under stress conditions such as exposure to elevated temperatures e.g., 25 °C and 40 °C, to mechanical stress (cavitation, shear, interfacial effects) or to light. This information is used to assess the overall robustness of a formulation during manufacturing. The ICH (International Conference on Harmonization) guideline Q5C provides global information about accelerated stability testing of biological products but does not outline exact conditions for forced degradation studies, except light stress. Table 5.5 lists a typical set of stress test conditions that are used in practice. With respect to temperature stress, one should realize that protein degradation typically does not follow Arrhenius kinetics; this is due to the complexity of the different degradation reactions that may run parallel to each other (Manning et al., 2010). Therefore, accelerated degradation studies at elevated temperatures can never replace real-time experiments (Hawe et al., 2012). Typically, a shelf life of at least 18–24 months for the drug product in its final primary packaging container (e.g., vial, syringe, cartridge pen, autoinjector) is desired. Various strategies are available to increase a protein's shelf life to or beyond the preferred 24 months range. These follow later in this chapter.

Primary Packaging

The vast majority of therapeutic proteins is parenterally administered by injection. Various primary packaging materials are available to the formulator, such as vials, cartridges and syringes (see Fig. 5.2 and Sacha et al. 2010; Sacha et al. 2015). The choice of the primary packaging material depends on a number of factors. For chronic therapy, the subcutaneous route of administration is often preferred as the patient can self-administer the drug. Convenience of use then excludes vial containers. One can choose among pen injectors and prefilled syringes (cf. Fig. 5.2). Pen injectors are cartridge-based syringes for multidose administration. They are typically used when frequent subcutaneous injections of variable doses of the drug are required, such as with insulin. The patient has to insert the needle her/himself. Prefilled syringes for subcutaneous administration are gaining increased popularity, especially in combination with an autoinjector to facilitate controlled and reproducible self-administration.

Typically, vials and the barrel of pre-filled syringes consist of glass. Glass has the advantage of transparency, which allows visual inspection of the injected solution. Pre-filled glass syringes are coated with silicone oil that acts as a lubricant to help moving the plunger. Fully polymer-based syringes start to offer an alternative option. A disadvantage of pre-filled glass syringes is that a small fraction of the silicone oil coating can be released in the solution in the form of (subvisible) oil droplets. Proteins can adsorb to these silicone oil droplets, which potentially leads to aggregation. Adding non-ionic surfactants to the formulation can prevent protein adsorption and aggregation. Furthermore, in the manufacturing process of glass syringes tungsten, which has been associated with protein aggregate formation as well, may end up in the product.

On storage of glass vials and syringes, the glass surface can release (heavy) metal ions; organic compounds may leach out of the polymer-based materials as used in vial stoppers, syringe plungers and barrels of polymer-based syringes. The formulator should collect information on these leachables and take proper action when necessary, such as changing packaging material or its vendor, add coatings or adjust formulation characteristics such as the pH.

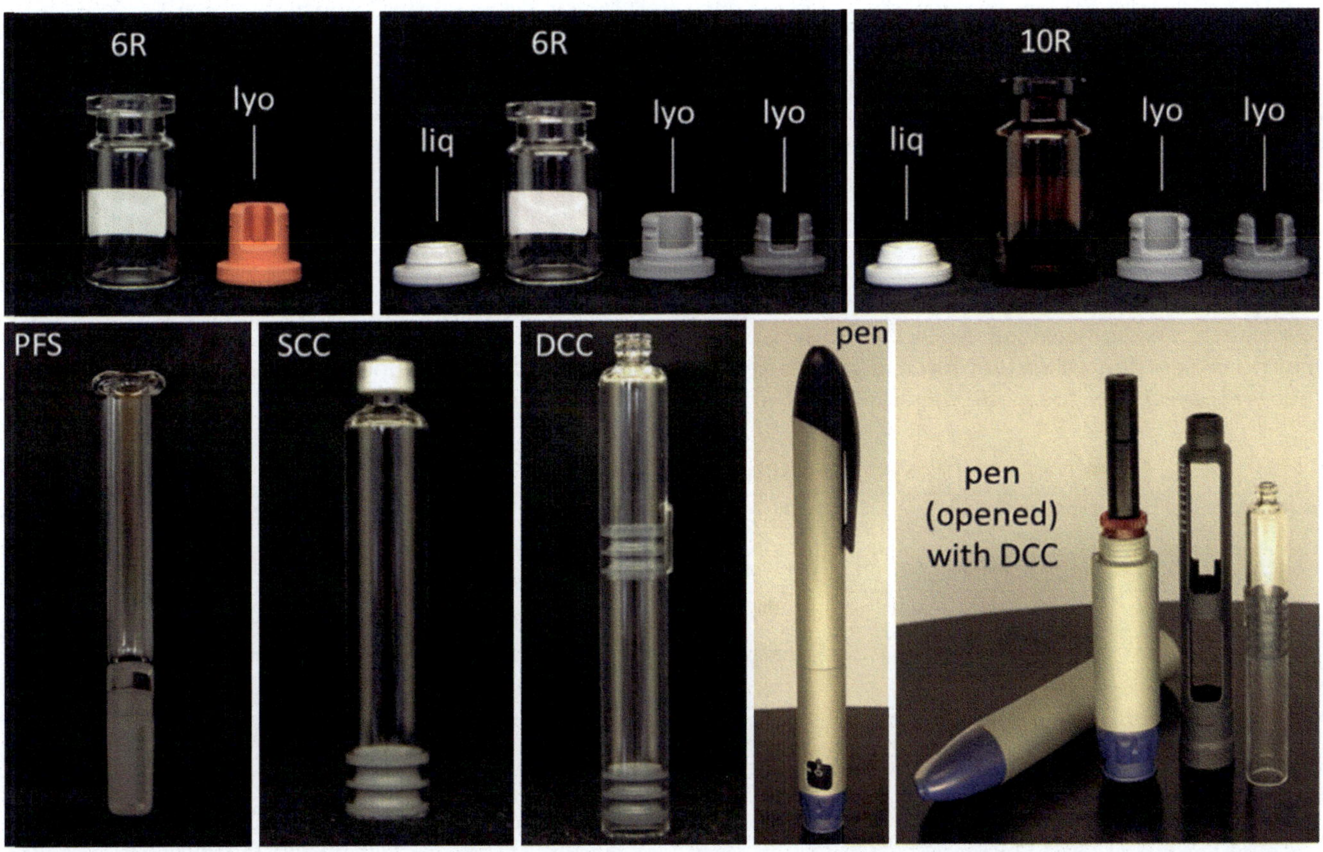

Figure 5.2 ■ Examples of primary packaging materials and a pen device (pen): 6-ml (6R) vials and 10-ml (10R) vial with corresponding stoppers for liquid (liq) and lyophilized (lyo) formulations; (empty) pre-filled syringe (PFS), single-chamber cartridge (SCC) and dual-chamber cartridge (DCC). Scaling of the pictures is not identical. Photos taken by Matthias Wurm

Higher gauge (G) –i.e., thinner– needles are preferred by patients as the pain sensation during injection decreases with a decreasing needle diameter. However, these narrow needles will negatively affect the 'syringeability': the force required to inject a certain volume at a certain rate through a needle with a certain length. The narrower the needle, the more force is needed. The same occurs when increasing the viscosity of the protein solution as is seen with highly (>50 mg/ml) concentrated monoclonal antibody solutions for subcutaneous injection.

Formulation Development of Marketed Products

A marketed drug product may undergo changes in its formulation and the way it is used. For instance, the company may introduce a new type of primary packaging material, a change in route of administration, a change in master cell bank, or new column material in the purification process. Such changes may affect protein structure and its stability profile and thereby the safety and efficacy profile of the product. Chapter 7 (immunogenicity) mentions an example of a formulation change of an epoetin product that caused a dramatic increase in the incidence of anti-drug antibody induced pure red cell aplasia, a serious adverse effect. Dependent on the proposed change, regulatory bodies may request new data to exclude changes in structure and shelf life of the new product and ensure that protein efficacy and safety have not changed. These comparability studies may include clinical studies, if analytical, preclinical and pharmacokinetic studies are considered insufficient to prove the claim of 'comparability' (cf. Chap. 12, biosimilars).

Excipients

In a protein formulation one finds, apart from the API, a number of excipients that are selected to serve different purposes. This selection process should be carried out with great care to ensure therapeutically effective and safe products. The nature of the protein (e.g., stability) and its therapeutic use (e.g., multiple injection systems for chronic use) can make these formulations complex in terms of excipient profile and manufacturing (freeze-drying, aseptic preparation). Table 5.1 mentions clinical factors, route of administration and dosage form as points to consider when designing the formulation. For example, the choice of an intravenously administered product (hospital setting) versus a subcutaneously administered product (self-administration) impacts the selection of excipients.

Both the choice of the excipient and its concentration are important. For instance, low concentrations of polysorbates may stabilize the protein (see below), while higher concentrations may cause denaturation. On the other hand, too low concentrations of polysorbates may result in particle formation during storage caused by polysorbate degradation when the cleaved fatty acids (from the polysorbate) are no longer solubilized by the remaining polysorbate; moreover, polysorbate degradation may lead to a surfactant concentration that is insufficient to stabilize the protein.

Table 5.6 lists components commonly found in presently marketed formulations. Clearly, an excipient can have different functions. For instance, sugars may be added for achieving isotonicity, as conformation stabilizer in liquid products, and as bulking agent and lyoprotectant in freeze-dried products. Kamerzell et al. (2011) discuss in detail the role of different classes of excipients in protein formulations and their mechanism of action.

In the following sections the reasons for including excipients from this list to protein products are discussed in more detail.

Solubility Enhancement

Approaches to enhance protein solubility include the selection of the proper pH (see below) and ionic strength conditions. Addition of amino acids, such as

Excipient class	Function	Examples
Buffers	pH control, tonicity	Histidine, phosphate, acetate, citrate, succinate
Salts	Tonicity, stabilization, viscosity reduction	Sodium chloride
Sugars[a], polyols	Tonicity, stabilization, cryoprotection, lyoprotection[b], bulking agent[b], reconstitution improvement[b]	Sucrose, trehalose, mannitol, sorbitol
Surfactants	Adsorption prevention, solubilization, stabilization, reconstitution improvement[b]	Polysorbate 20, polysorbate 80, poloxamer 188
Amino acids	Stabilization, viscosity reduction, tonicity, pH control, bulking agent[b]	Arginine, glycine, histidine, lysine, proline
Anti-oxidants	Oxidation prevention	Methionine, sodium edetate
Preservatives[c]	Bacterial growth prevention	m-cresol, benzyl alcohol, phenol

Adapted from Weinbuch et al. (2018)
[a]Only non-reducing sugars
[b]For freeze-dried products
[c]Multi-dose containers

Table 5.6 Common excipients in protein drug products

arginine, or surfactants can also help to increase the solubility. The mechanism of action of these solubility enhancers depends on the type of enhancer and the protein involved and is not always fully understood. As an example, Fig. 5.3 shows the dramatic effect of the arginine concentration on the apparent solubility of tissue plasminogen activator (alteplase).

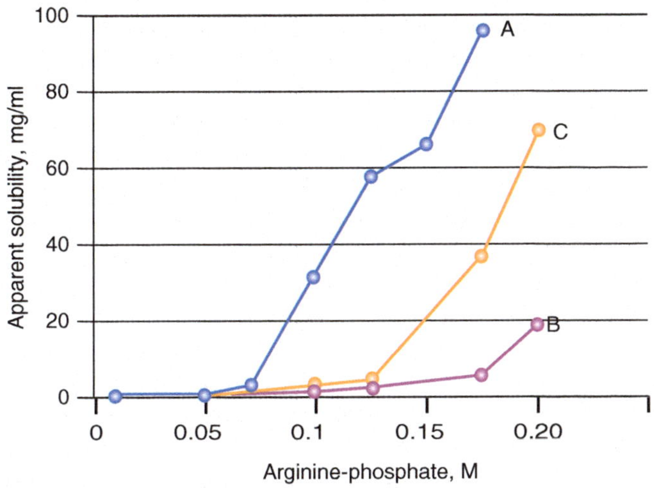

Figure 5.3 ■ Effect of arginine concentration on the apparent solubility of (A) type I and (B) type II alteplase, and (C) a 50:50 mixture thereof at pH 7.2 and 25 °C (From Nguyen and Ward 1993)

Protection Against Adsorption, Interfacial Stress and Aggregation in the Bulk Solution

Most proteins are prone to adsorb to interfaces. Upon adsorption, proteins tend to expose hydrophobic sites, normally present in the core of the native protein structure when an interface is present. Examples of interfaces are the formulation liquid–air interface, the liquid–container wall interface, or interfaces formed between the liquid and utensils used to administer the drug (e.g., infusion bags and lines, syringes, needles). Importantly, adsorbed, partially unfolded protein molecules not only present a loss of API but also may form aggregates, leave the surface, return to the aqueous phase, and form larger aggregates. Figure 5.4 (adapted from Sediq et al. 2016) shows a schematic representation of this mechanism of aggregation at a solid surface. A similar situation may occur at gas-liquid interfaces. For some proteins the reconstitution protocol for the freeze-dried cake explicitly stipulates to swirl the vial instead of shaking it to avoid protein exposure to large liquid-air interfaces.

Many protein formulations include a surfactant to reduce protein adsorption. Surfactants readily adsorb to hydrophobic interfaces with their own hydrophobic groups and render this interface hydrophilic by exposing their hydrophilic groups to the aqueous phase. Protein accumulation at the interface is suppressed and thereby aggregate formation. The most commonly used surfactants for parenteral use are poly-

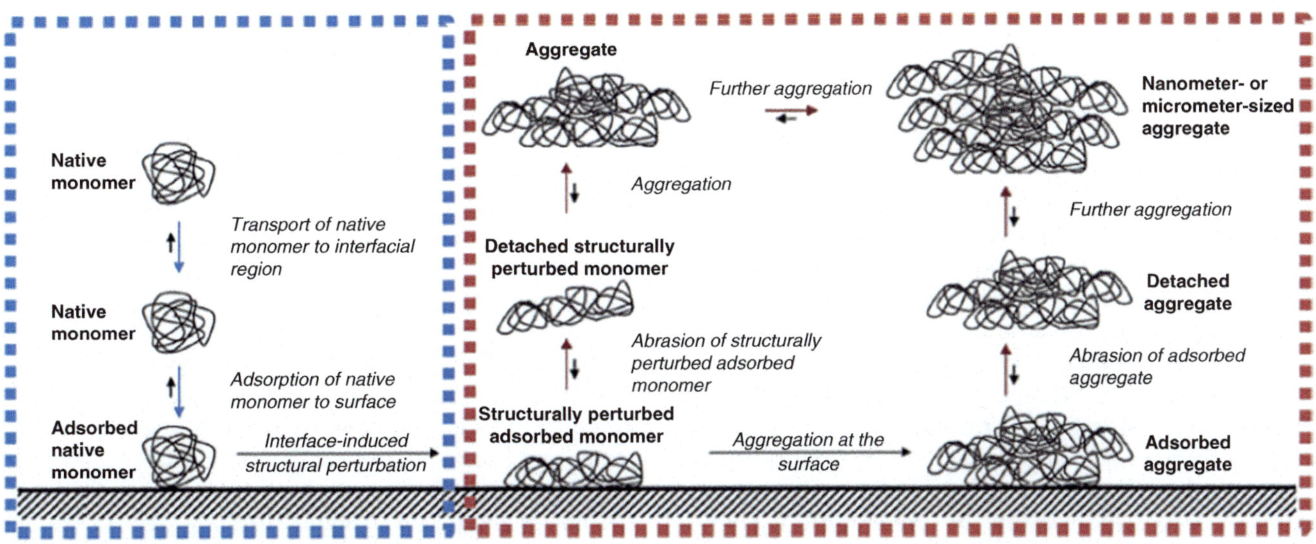

Figure 5.4 ■ Schematic representation of the suggested mechanism of stirring-induced protein aggregation. The left part (framed in blue) depicts the process of protein adsorption onto solid surfaces with potential perturbation of the native structure of the protein on adsorption. This process is followed by aggregation at the surface and in the bulk (framed in red). Contact sliding results in abrasion of the adsorbed protein layer, leading to renewal of the surface for adsorption of a fresh protein layer. Addition of surfactants, such as polysorbate 20, and avoidance of contact stirring will inhibit the steps shown as blue and red arrows, respectively. Adapted from Sediq et al. (2016)

sorbate 20 and 80. Poloxamer 188 is also used and is gaining importance because of issues with polysorbate degradation (Martos et al., 2017). Furthermore, 2-hydroxypropyl-beta-cyclodextrin can prevent adsorption and is accepted as an excipient for parenteral use as well. Human serum albumin prevents adsorption, but is nowadays rarely used because of potential infectious content and interference with analytical characterization of the API.

Apart from interface-induced aggregation, aggregates may be formed in the bulk of a solution because of colloidal and/or conformational instability (Chi et al. 2003). Sugars, selection of a proper pH value and buffer components may mitigate the tendency to this bulk aggregation.

Glucose may perfectly act as a conformational stabilizer, but will induce chemical instability through the Maillard reaction. Primary amino groups of the proteins react with the reducing sugar, resulting in brownish/yellow solutions. Sucrose should not be used below pH 6 because of hydrolysis, leading to formation of fructose and glucose, both being reducing sugars. Polyols such as mannitol and sorbitol may be used as well, also at low pH.

These excipients (sugars and polyhydric alcohols) may not be inert; they may influence protein stability. For example, sugars and polyhydric alcohols can stabilize the protein structure through the principle of "preferential exclusion" (Arakawa et al. 1991). They enhance the interaction of the solvent with the protein and are themselves excluded from the protein surface layer; the protein is preferentially hydrated. This results in an increased conformational stability of the protein.

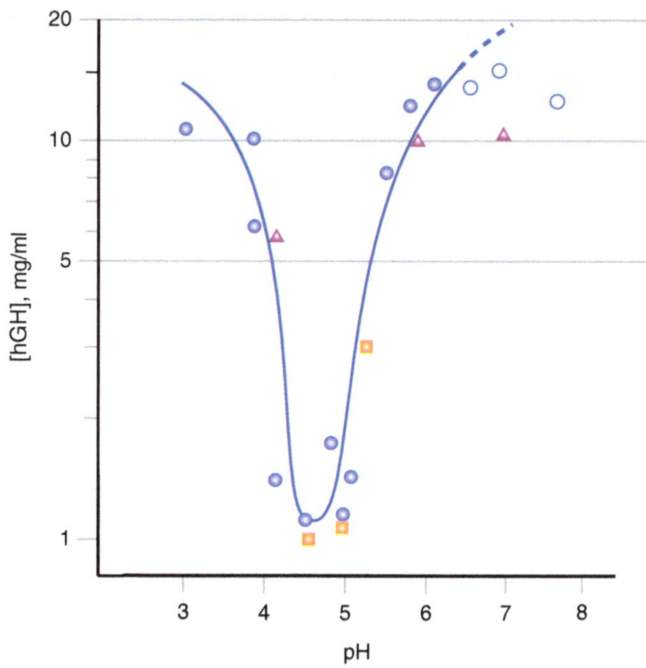

Figure 5.5 ■ A plot of the solubility of various forms of hGH as a function of pH. Samples of hGH were either recombinant hGH (circles), Met-hGH (triangles), or pituitary hGH (squares). Solubility was determined by dialyzing an approximately 11 mg/ml solution of each protein into an appropriate buffer for each pH. Buffers were citrate, pH 3–7, and borate, pH 8–9, all at 10 mM buffer concentrations. Concentrations of hGH were measured by UV absorbance as well as by RP-HPLC, relative to an external standard. The closed symbols indicate that precipitate was present in the dialysis tube after equilibration, whereas open symbols mean that no solid material was present, and thus the solubility is at least this amount (From Pearlman and Bewley 1993)

Buffer Selection

Buffer selection is an important part of the formulation process, because of the pH dependence of protein solubility, as illustrated in Fig. 5.5. Moreover, both the pH and the buffer species itself can have profound effects on the physical (aggregation) and chemical stability of proteins (Zbacnik et al. 2017) (cf. Fig. 5.6). Buffer systems regularly encountered in protein formulations are phosphate, citrate, histidine, succinate, glutamate and acetate. Highly concentrated protein solutions (protein concentration >50 mg/ml) may not need a buffer as they have sufficient intrinsic buffer capacity (Bahrenburg et al., 2015). Even short, temporary pH changes can cause protein aggregation. These conditions can occur, for example, during elution of a monoclonal antibody from a protein A column at low pH (see Chap. 4) or during the freezing step in a freeze-drying process, when one of the buffer components is crystallizing and the other is not. For instance, in a sodium phosphate buffer, Na_2HPO_4 crystallizes faster than NaH_2PO_4. This causes a pronounced drop in pH during the freezing step (see below). In the presence of high concentrations of a sugar, which is typically added as lyo- and cryoprotectant during lyophilization, the effect of pH changes is less pronounced. Other buffer components do not crystallize but form amorphous systems, and then pH changes are negligible.

Protection Against Oxidation

Methionine, cysteine, tryptophan, tyrosine, and histidine are amino acid residues that are readily oxidized (see Chap. 3). As these amino acid residues occur in almost all proteins, oxidative degradation is a regular threat to the stability of proteins. The sensitivity of an amino acid residue towards oxidation depends on its position within the protein, as this determines its accessibility for oxidative reagents. Replacement of oxygen by inert gases (e.g., argon) in the vials or minimizing the headspace, such as in pre-filled syringes, helps reducing oxidative stress. Moreover, one may consider the addition of antioxidants, such as methionine, which competes with methionine residues for oxidation. Interestingly, some antioxidants can accelerate protein

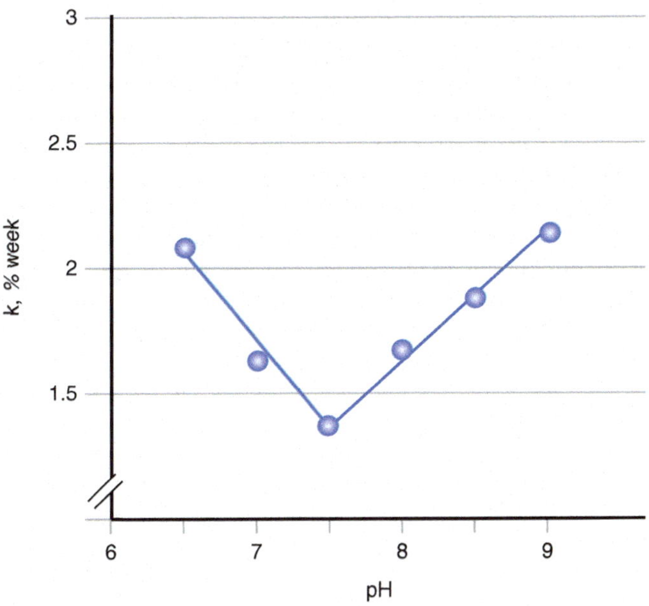

Figure 5.6 ■ pH stability profile (at 25 °C) of monomeric recombinant α1-antitrypsin (rAAT) by size exclusion-HPLC assay, k degradation rate constant. Monomeric rAAT decreased rapidly in concentration both under acidic and basic conditions. Optimal stability occurred at pH 7.5 (Adjusted from Vemuri et al. 1993)

oxidation (Vemuri et al. 1993). Ascorbic acid, for example, can act as an oxidant in the presence of trace amounts of heavy metals which may be present as impurities. To reduce the catalytic activity of heavy metals, one may consider introducing chelators such as EDTA (ethylenediaminetetraacetic acid) (Kamerzell et al. 2011).

Preservation

Proteins may be marketed in containers designed for multiple injections. After administering the first dose, contamination with microorganisms may occur. Therefore, formulations in multi-dose containers must contain a preservative. Common antimicrobial agents include phenol, meta-cresol, benzyl alcohol, and chlorobutanol (Kamerzell et al., 2011). These preservative molecules can interact with the protein, which may compromise both the activity of the protein and the effectivity of the preservative. An example is the well-established interaction between insulin and phenols (Chap. 18). A caveat is the incompatibility of polysorbates and m-cresol, which may lead to precipitation.

Tonicity Adjustment

For proteins the regular rules apply for adjusting the tonicity of parenteral products. Formulation excipients, such as buffers and amino acids, contribute to the tonicity. Disaccharides, polyols and sodium chloride are commonly added to reach isotonicity.

Protection Against Freezing and Drying

Cryoprotectants are excipients that protect a protein during freezing or in the frozen state (mainly sugars: sucrose, trehalose and sugar alcohols: mannitol, sorbitol). This is relevant for the development of frozen liquid formulations. The key stabilizing mechanisms is 'preferential exclusion'. As explained above, these additives ('water structure promoters') enhance the interaction of the solvent (water) with the protein and are themselves excluded from the protein surface layer; the protein is preferentially hydrated.

Lyoprotectants protect the protein in the lyophilized state (e.g., sugars). The key mechanisms of protection described for lyoprotectants are (cf. Mensink et al. 2017): (1) the 'water replacement theory': replacement of water as stabilizing agent by forming hydrogen bonds with the protein and (2) the 'vitrification theory': formation of a glassy amorphous matrix keeping protein molecules separated from each other.

When stored in the presence of reducing sugars, such as glucose and lactose, the Maillard reaction (see above) may occur also in the dried state and the cake color turns yellow brown. Therefore, reducing sugars should not be used as lyoprotectant and non-reducing sugars such as sucrose (above pH 6) or trehalose are preferred.

■ Freeze-Drying of Proteins

The abundant presence of water in liquid protein formulations promotes chemical and physical degradation processes. This explains why proteins in solution often do not meet the preferred stability requirements for industrially produced pharmaceutical products (shelf life >2 years), even when kept permanently under refrigerator conditions (cold chain).

Freeze-drying may provide the required stability (Constantino and Pikal 2004). During freeze-drying water is removed through sublimation. The freeze-drying process consists of three steps: (1) freezing (if required, this includes an annealing step), (2) primary drying, and (3) secondary drying. Figure 5.7 shows what happens with chamber pressure and temperature over time during these stages.

Although aimed to improve protein stability, freeze-drying may cause irreversible damage to the protein. This is particularly true when applying improper lyophilization process conditions (see below) and/or selecting improper excipients (see above). Table 5.6 lists excipients typically encountered in successfully freeze-dried protein products.

Freezing

In the freezing step (see Fig. 5.7) the temperature of the solution (typically in vials) is lowered. Ice crystal formation does not start right at the thermodynamic or equilibrium freezing point, but supercooling occurs. That means that ice crystallization often only occurs when reaching temperatures of −15 °C or lower. During ice crystallization the temperature temporarily rises in the vial, because of the generation of crystallization heat. During the cooling stage, concentration of the protein and excipients occurs because of the growing ice crystal mass at the expense of the liquid aqueous phase. This can cause precipitation of one or more of the excipients, which may result in pH shifts (see above and Fig. 5.8) and ionic strength changes. It may also induce protein denaturation. Cooling of the vials is done through lowering the shelf temperature. Selecting the proper cooling scheme for the shelf –and consequently the vials– is important, as it dictates the degree of supercooling and ice crystal size. Small crystals form during fast cooling; large crystals form at lower cooling rates. Small ice crystals are required for porous cakes and fast sublimation rates (Pikal 1990).

Ice nucleation is a random and stochastic approach, which may lead to inhomogeneity in pore size and cake structure. Controlled nucleation can be applied to assure freezing at a defined temperature. This results in reduced primary drying times and shorter reconstitution times of highly concentrated lyophilized protein formulations (Geidobler and Winter 2013).

When choosing the freezing temperature it is important to assure that the product is fully frozen. Crystallizing compounds (e.g. NaCl, mannitol) need to be cooled below the eutectic temperature (Te) and compounds forming amorphous structures (e.g. sugars) below the glass transition temperature of the maximally freeze-concentrated solution (Tg′). In the amorphous phase the viscosity changes dramatically in the

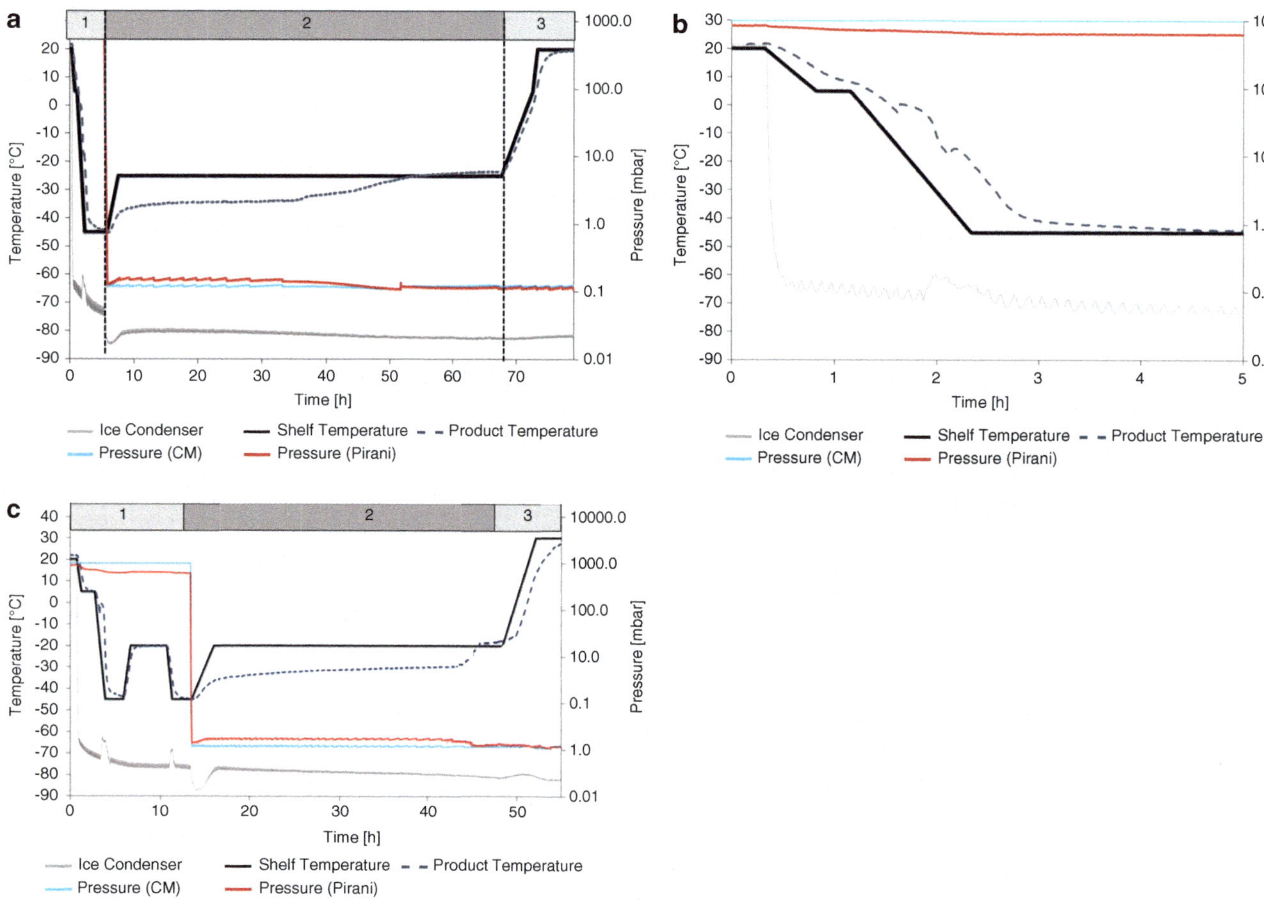

Figure 5.7 ■ **(a)** Example of freeze-drying showing shelf temperature, product temperature, pressure (by Pirani and CM and ice condenser temperature. 1 = freezing stage, 2 = primary drying stage, 3 = secondary drying stage. See the text for explanation of CM and Pirani measurement. **(b)** Zoom in on the freezing stage. **(c)** Similar to **(a)**, but now with annealing step in the freezing stage (temperature rise form −45 °C tot −20 °C and drop again to −45 °C)

temperature range around Tg′: A "rubbery" state exists above and a glass state below the Tg′.

Lyophilized formulations can be either amorphous (e.g. sugar-based) or (partially) crystalline (e.g. mannitol-based). To assure that bulking agents such as mannitol crystallize, an annealing step can be included to promote crystallization during freezing: The frozen mass is then kept at a temperature above the Tg′ for some time and then refrozen, before moving towards primary drying. At the start of the primary drying stage, no "free and fluid" water should be present in the vials. Minus forty to minus fifty degrees Celsius is a typical freezing temperature range where sublimation is initiated through chamber pressure reduction.

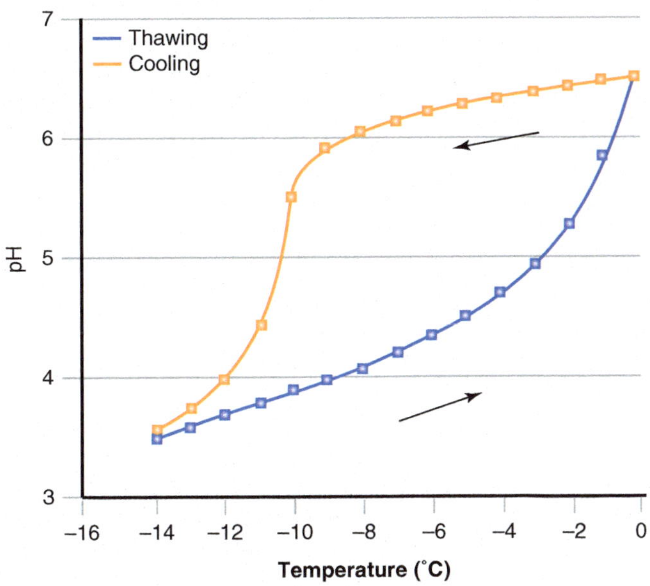

Figure 5.8 ■ The effect of freezing-thawing on the pH of a citric acid–disodium phosphate buffer system (Cited in Pikal 1990)

Primary Drying

In the primary drying stage (see Fig. 5.7), sublimation of the water mass in the vial starts by lowering the pressure. The water vapor condenses on a condenser, with a (substantially) lower temperature than the shelf with the vials (typically −80 °C). Sublimation costs energy (about 2500 kJ/g ice). The supply of heat from the shelf to the vial prevents the vial temperature to drop. Thus, the shelf is heated during this stage.

The pressure (vacuum) and the heat supply rate control the resulting product temperature. It is important to keep the product temperature below the Tg′ (e.g., determined by differential scanning calorimetry (DSC)) or the collapse temperature (Tc) (e.g., determined by freeze-drying microscopy). At and above the collapse temperature the material softens and cannot support its own structure anymore (see below). Collapse causes a strong reduction in sublimation rate and poor cake formation, resulting in non-elegant cake appearance and long reconstitution times. Although cake appearance is negatively affected, collapse may result in products with acceptable protein stability (Schersch et al. 2010). An example of a DSC scan providing information on the Tg′ is presented in Fig. 5.9.

Heat reaches the vial through (1) direct shelf–vial contact (conductance), (2) radiation, and (3) gas conduction (Fig. 5.10). Gas conduction depends on the pressure: if one selects relatively high gas pressures, heat transport increases because of a high conductivity. However, it reduces mass transfer, because of a low driving force: the pressure between equilibrium vapor

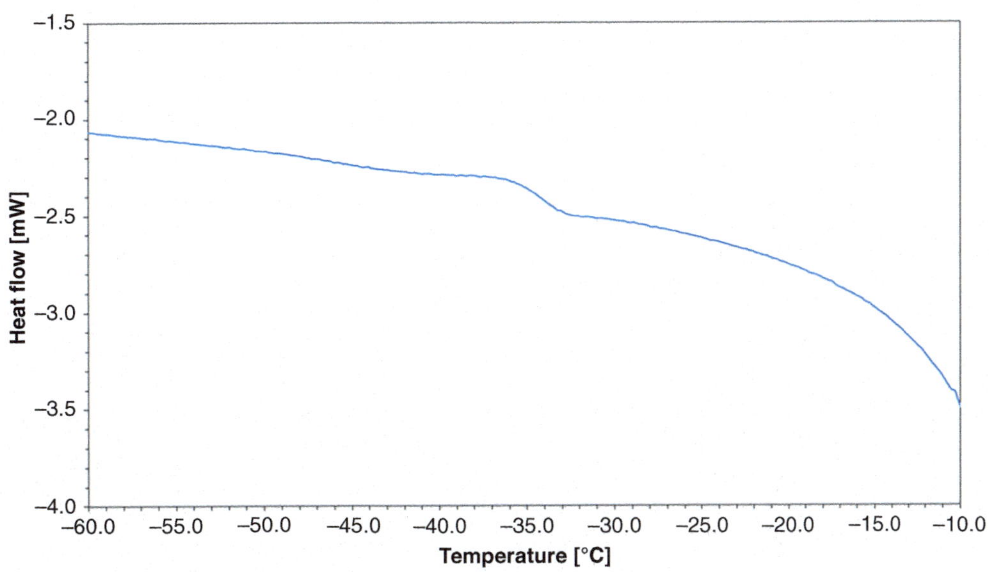

Figure 5.9 ■ Differential Scanning Calorimetry trace of a 5% sucrose solution with a Tg about −35 °C

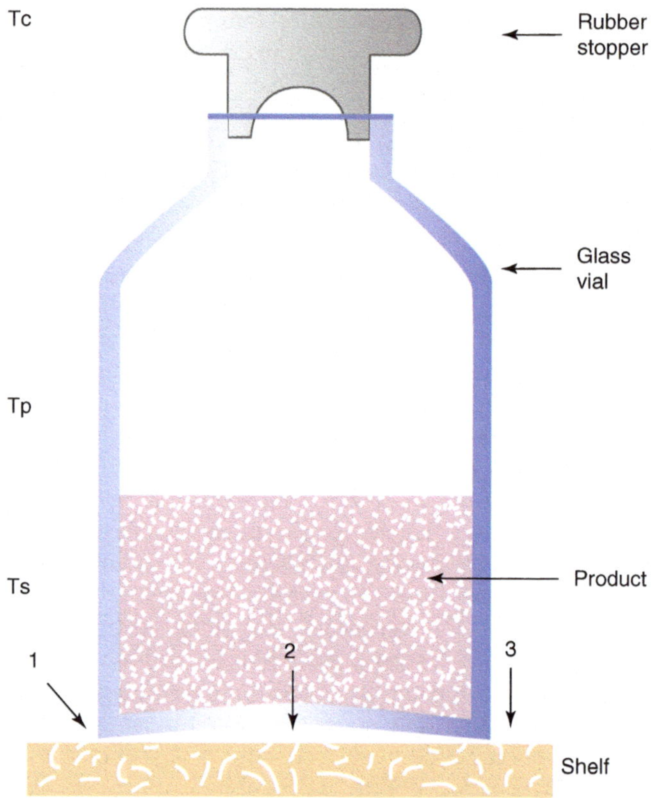

Figure 5.10 ■ Heat transfer mechanisms during the freeze-drying process: (1) Direct conduction via shelf and glass at points of actual contact. (2) Gas conduction: contribution heat transfer via conduction through gas between shelf and vial bottom. (3) Radiation heat transfer. Ts shelf temperature, Tp temperature sublimating product, Tc temperature condensor. Ts > Tp > Tc

pressures at the interface between the frozen mass/dried cake and the chamber pressure (Pikal 1990). During the primary drying stage, one transfers heat from the shelf through the vial bottom and the frozen mass to the interface frozen mass/dry powder, to keep the sublimation process going.

During this drying stage the product temperature should never reach Te or Tg′/Tc, as the cake may collapse. Typically a safety margin of 2–5 °C is used. For highly concentrated protein formulations Tc is typically higher than Tg′, and the products can be dried at product temperatures above Tg′ (below Tc) without resulting in collapse. Therefore, knowledge of Te and Tg′ is of great importance to develop a rationally designed freeze-drying protocol.

Heat transfer resistance decreases during the drying process by the reduction of the transport distance as the interface retreats. With the mass transfer resistance (transport of water vapor), however, the opposite occurs. Mass transfer resistance increases during the drying process, as the dry cake becomes thicker. Therefore, parameters such as chamber pressure and shelf temperature are not necessarily constant during the primary drying process. They should be carefully chosen and adjusted as the drying process proceeds.

When all frozen or "unbound" water (i.e., not bound to protein or excipients) has been removed, the primary drying step has finished (Fig. 5.7). The primary drying process can be monitored by following individual vials (e.g., product temperature of individual vials) or batch methods e.g., comparative pressure measurements, manometric temperature measurement/pressure rise test, mass spectrometry to monitor gas composition in the chamber or tunable diode laser absorption spectroscopy to provide information on the sublimation rate.

The end of the primary drying stage can be measured by thermocouples within the product vials: the end of primary drying is reached when product temperature and shelf temperature become equal, or when the partial water pressure drops (Pikal 1990).

Comparative pressure measurement with a Pirani gauge and a capacitance manometer (CM) is another approach next to thermocouples to detect the end of primary drying. This is based on the gas composition dependent reading of a Pirani gauge, whereas a capacitance manometer reading is not influenced by the gas composition. Consequently, the Pirani gauge (which is typically calibrated under nitrogen or air) shows higher pressure values than the CM in the presence of water vapor in the chamber, i.e., as long as primary drying is progressing. The end of primary drying, i.e., when sublimation of "unbound" water has finished, is indicated when the pressure measured by the Pirani gauge and the CM show the same signal.

Secondary Drying

In the secondary drying stage, the temperature is slowly increased to remove "bound" water; the chamber pressure is still kept low. The temperature should stay all the time below the collapse/eutectic temperature, which continues to rise as the residual water content drops. Typically, the secondary drying step ends when the product has been kept at 20–40 °C for several hours. The residual water content of the product (e.g., determined by a Karl Fischer assay) is a critical, end point-indicating parameter. Values as low as 1% residual water in the cake have been recommended; however, this needs to be evaluated on a product specific basis and certain products may require higher or lower residual moisture contents to result in a stable product. Figure 5.11 (Pristoupil 1985; Pikal 1990) exemplifies the decreasing stability of freeze-dried hemoglobin with increasing residual water content.

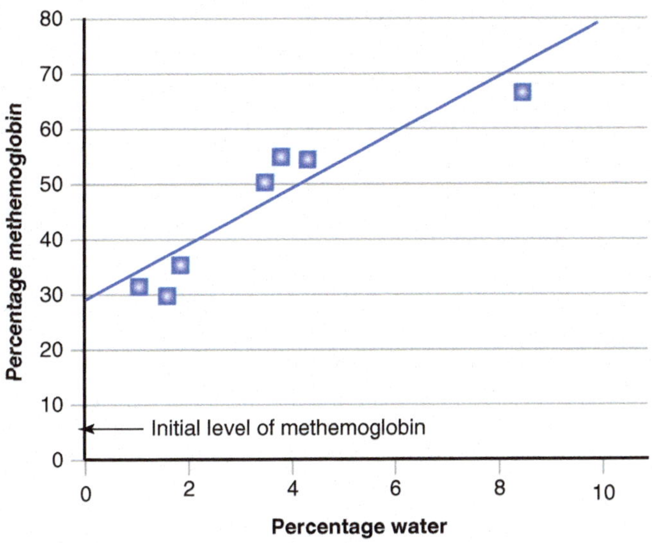

Figure 5.11 ■ The effect of residual moisture on the stability of freeze-dried hemoglobin (–6%) formulated with 0.2 M sucrose; decomposition to methemoglobin during storage at 23 °C for 4 years (From Pikal 1990). Data reported by Pritoupil et al. (1985)

HANDLING OF PHARMACEUTICAL PROTEINS POST-PRODUCTION

In the formulation process, the manufacturer will expose the protein product under development to a number of stress factors as mentioned in Table 5.3. The composition of the final formulation of the protein product will reflect the outcome of those (laboratory) stress experiments in combination with real-time stability testing: optimum formulation conditions for chemical and physical stability of the protein will be chosen. In spite of all these efforts, pharmaceutical proteins remain sensitive to 'real life' handling and may readily show degradation reactions that obviously affect both efficacy and safety. Therefore, the manufacturer—together with the regulatory authorities—creates a package insert text that points out to health care professionals and patients the conditions that should be maintained for the product, e.g., storage temperature window, avoidance of shaking/shear, exposure to light. As an example, the package insert of trastuzumab states: 'Swirl the vial gently to aid reconstitution. Trastuzumab may be sensitive to shear-induced stress, e.g., agitation or rapid expulsion from a syringe. DO NOT SHAKE' (FDA web site).

Surprisingly, little information is available on the actual storage and administration practices for pharmaceutical proteins in hospitals. Anecdotal information of exposing protein solutions to high shear conditions (shaking, use of pneumatic tube transport) and the use of incorrect administration techniques can be found in the literature. This is also true for the patient's home setting. However, recently, real data became available of a group of rheumatoid arthritis patients of whom only a small minority stored their protein product (anti-TNF-alpha therapy) in the prescribed temperature window, i.e. 2–8 °C. Both freezing and storing above 25 °C occurred (Vlieland et al., 2016). The consequences of this behavior for the stability of this protein, in particular aggregate formation, may be an increased chance of formation of anti-drug antibodies (Jiskoot et al., 2017; Vlieland et al., 2018). Considering the clinical importance of these medicines and the high prices paid, it is time to teach health care professionals and patients the importance of' 'Good Handling Practices for Biologicals' (Nejadnik et al., 2018).

DELIVERY OF PROTEINS: ROUTES OF ADMINISTRATION

■ The Parenteral Route of Administration

Parenteral administration is here defined as administration via those routes where a needle is used, including intravenous (IV), intramuscular (IM), subcutaneous (SC), intracutaneous, intraperitoneal (IP) and intravitreal injections. Chapter 6 provides more information on the pharmacokinetic behavior of recombinant proteins. It suffices here to state that the blood half-life of biotech products can vary over a wide range. For example, the blood circulation half-life of tissue plasminogen activator is a few minutes, whereas monoclonal antibodies have half-lives of a few days to weeks.

A simple way to expand the mean residence time for short half-life proteins is to switch from IV to IM or SC administration. One should realize that by doing that, changes in disposition may occur with a significant impact on the bioavailability (slower uptake in the blood compartment and lower extent of absorption) and therapeutic performance of the biologic. For instance, the extent of absorption of SC administered protein injections (compared to IV administration) may be as low as 30% (Richter et al., 2012; Kinnunen and Mrsny, 2014). This change in disposition is caused by various factors such as: (1) the prolonged residence time at the IM or SC site of injection compared to IV administration, differences in protein environment upon injection and enhanced exposure to degradation reactions (peptidases), and (2) differences in disposition.

Regarding point 1: For instance, diabetics can become "insulin resistant" through high tissue peptidase activity (Maberly et al. 1982). Other factors that can contribute to absorption variation are differences in level of activity of the muscle at the injection site and also massage and heat at the injection site. The state of the tissue, for instance, the occurrence of pathological conditions, may be important as well.

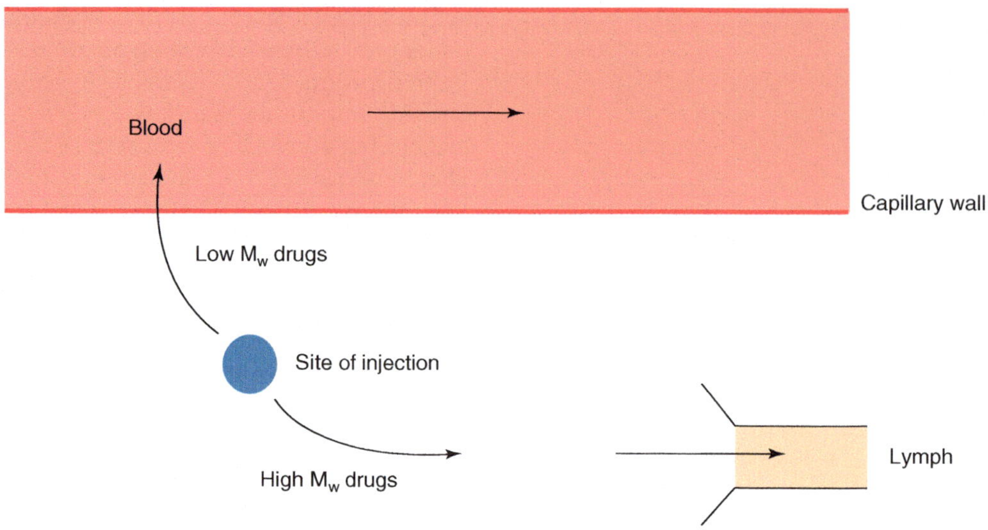

Figure 5.12 ■ Routes of uptake of SC- or IM-injected drugs

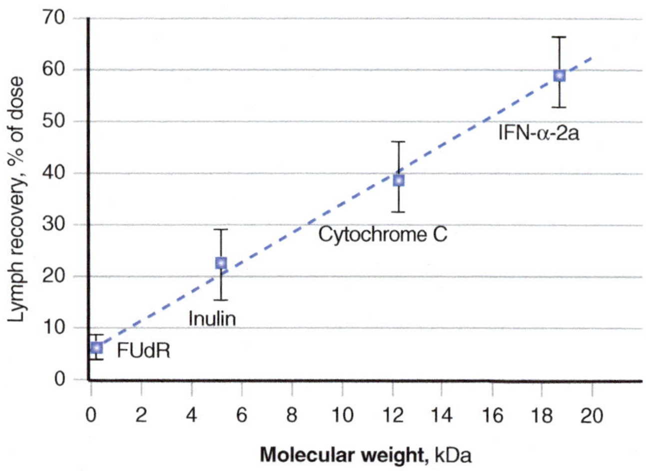

Figure 5.13 ■ Correlation between the molecular weight and the cumulative recovery of rIFN alpha-2a (Mw 19 kDa), cytochrome c (Mw 12.3 kDa), insulin (Mw 5.2 kDa), and FUdR, 5-fluorodeoxyuridine, (Mw 256.2 Da) in the efferent lymph from the right popliteal lymph node following SC administration into the lower part of the right hind leg of sheep. Each point and bar shows the mean and standard deviation of three experiments performed in separate sheep. The line drawn is the best fit by linear regression analysis calculated with the four mean values. The points have a correlation coefficient r of 0.998 ($p < 0.01$) (From Supersaxo et al. 1990)

Regarding point 2: Upon administration, the protein may reach the blood through the lymphatics or enter the blood circulation through the capillary wall at the site of injection (Figs. 5.12 and 5.13). The fraction of the administered dose taking this lymphatic route depends on the molecular weight of the protein (Supersaxo et al. 1990). Lymphatic transport takes time (hours), and uptake in the blood circulation is highly dependent on the injection site. On its way to the blood, the lymph passes through draining lymph nodes. There, contact is possible between lymph contents and cells of the immune system, such as macrophages and B and T lymphocytes residing in the lymph nodes.

■ Other Routes of Administration

For several reasons, e.g., ease of administration, patient friendliness and cost, alternative administration routes to the parenteral route would be welcome for the successful systemic delivery of recombinant proteins. This is particularly true for the oral route. Nature, unfortunately, does not allow us to use the oral route of administration for therapeutic proteins if a high (or at least constant) bioavailability is required. The two main reasons (A and B) for this failure of uptake are: (A) protein degradation in the GI (gastrointestinal track) and (B) poor permeability of the wall of the GI tract in case of a passive transport process.

Regarding point A: Protein degradation. The human body has developed a very efficient system to break down proteins in our food to amino acids or di- or tripeptides. These building stones for body proteins are actively absorbed for use in newly formed proteins. The stomach secretes pepsins, a family of aspartic proteases. They are particularly active between pH 3 and 5 and lose activity at higher pH values. Pepsins are endopeptidases capable of cleaving peptide bonds distant from the ends of the peptide chain. They preferentially cleave peptide bonds between two hydrophobic amino acids. Other endopeptidases are active in the gastrointestinal tract at neutral pH values, e.g., trypsin, chymotrypsin, and elastase. They have different, complementary peptide bond cleavage characteristics. Exopeptidases, proteases degrading peptide chains from their C- or N-terminus, are present as well. In the intestinal epithelium, brush border and cytoplasmic proteases of the enterocytes continue to cut proteins into fragments down to amino acids, di- and tripeptides.

Regarding point B: Permeability. High-molecular-weight molecules with a hydrophilic 'coat' such as therapeutic proteins do not readily penetrate the intact and mature epithelial barrier of the intestinal lumen. Active transport of intact proteins over the GI-epithelium has not been described. This leaves diffusion to and partitioning into the enterocyte membrane as the sole pathway for mass transfer. Diffusion coefficients and partition coefficients are low for intact therapeutic proteins leading to very low extent of uptake. Some oral vaccines, however, are available on the market, as discussed in Chap. 14. For those products only a (small) fraction of the antigen has to reach its target site to illicit an immune response.

Some proteins are administered locally for local therapy. For instance, ranibizumab (Fab fragment), aflibercept (a recombinant fusion protein consisting of vascular endothelial growth factor (VEGF)-binding portions from the extracellular domains of human VEGF receptors 1 and 2, which are fused to the Fc portion of human IgG1) and bevacizumab are proteins to block neovascularization in the retina. When injected in the vitreous cavity of the eye, they interact with vascular endothelial growth factor (VEGF) and slow down wet, age-related macular degeneration. Another example of administering a biologic near its site of action is dornase alfa (Pulmozyme). It is taken via inhalation to break down DNA in sputum of cystic fibrosis patients (cf. Chap. 22).

Apart from the oral route, the eye and lungs (as mentioned above when discussing local therapy), the nose, rectum, oral cavity (buccal absorption) and skin have been studied as potential sites of application. Table 5.7 lists the potential pros and cons for the different relevant routes. Moeller and Jorgensen (2009) and Jorgensen and Nielsen (2009) describe "the state of the art" in more detail. The nasal, buccal, rectal, and transdermal routes all are of little clinical relevance if systemic action is required. In general, bioavailability is too low and varies too much. The pulmonary route may be the exception to this rule.

FDA approved the first pulmonary insulin formulation (Exubera®) in January 2006. However, the supplier took it off the market in 2008 because of poor market penetration. Inhalation technology plays a critical role when considering the prospects of the pulmonary route for the systemic delivery of therapeutic proteins. Dry powder inhalers and nebulizers are the delivery systems considered and tested. The fraction of protein that is ultimately absorbed depends on (1) the

Route of administration
Oral
+ Easy to access, proven track record with "conventional" medicines, sustained/controlled release possible
– Negligible bioavailability for proteins
Nasal
+ Easily accessible, fast uptake, proven track record with a number of "conventional" medicines, probably lower proteolytic activity than in the GI tract, avoidance of first pass effect, spatial containment of absorption enhancers is possible
– Reproducibility (in particular under pathological conditions), safety (e.g., ciliary movement), negligible bioavailability for proteins
Pulmonary
+ Relatively easy to access, fast uptake, proven track record with "conventional" medicines, substantial –in the 10% range- fractions of insulin are absorbed, lower proteolytic activity than in the GI tract, avoidance of hepatic first pass effect
– Reproducibility (in particular under pathological conditions, smokers/nonsmokers), safety (e.g., immunogenicity), presence of macrophages in the lung with high affinity for particulates
Rectal
+ Easily accessible, partial avoidance of hepatic first pass, probably lower proteolytic activity than in the upper parts of the GI tract, spatial containment of absorption enhancers is possible, proven track record with a number of "conventional" drugs
– Negligible bioavailability for proteins
Buccal
+ Easily accessible, avoidance of hepatic first pass, probably lower proteolytic activity than in the lower parts of the GI tract, spatial containment of absorption enhancers is possible, option to remove formulation if necessary
– Negligible bioavailability of proteins, no proven track record yet
Transdermal
+ Easily accessible, avoidance of hepatic first pass effect, removal of formulation if necessary is possible, spatial containment of absorption enhancers, proven track record with "conventional" medicines, sustained/controlled release possible
– Negligible bioavailability of proteins
Intravitreal
+ Direct access to vitreous, delivery close to the target site
– Not suitable for systemic effects

+ Relative advantage, – Relative disadvantage

Table 5.7 ■ Alternative routes of administration to the IV, IM and SC route for biopharmaceuticals

fraction of the inhaled/nebulized dose that is actually leaving the device, (2) the fraction that is actually deposited in the lung, and (3) the fraction that is being absorbed, i.e., total relative uptake (TO%) = % uptake from device × % deposited in the lungs × % actually absorbed from the lungs. For insulin, TO% is estimated to be about 10% (Patton et al. 2004). The fraction of insulin that is absorbed from the lung is about 20%. The reproducibility of the blood glucose response to inhaled insulin was equivalent to SC-injected insulin. These figures demonstrate that insulin absorption via the lung may be a promising route, but the fraction that reaches the blood circulation is small and commercial success failed to materialize until now.

DELIVERY OF PROTEINS BY THE PARENTERAL ROUTE: APPROACHES FOR RATE-CONTROLLED DELIVERY

Presently used therapeutic proteins widely differ in their pharmacokinetic characteristics (see Chap. 6). If they are recombinant counterparts of endogenous agents such as insulin, tissue plasminogen activator, growth hormone, epoetin, interleukins, or factor VIII, it is important to realize why, when, and where –by which cells– they are secreted. Cells can communicate with each other through the endocrine, paracrine and/or autocrine pathway leading to secretion of mediator molecules (Table 5.8).

The presence of these mediators may activate a complex cascade of events that needs to be carefully controlled. Therefore, key issues for their therapeutic success are (1) access to target cells, (2) retention at the target site, and (3) proper timing of delivery.

In particular, for paracrine- and autocrine-acting proteins, such as tumor necrosis factor and interleukin-2 severe side effects were reported upon parenteral (IV or SC) administration. The occurrence of these side effects limits the therapeutic potential of these compounds. Therefore, the delivery of these proteins at the proper site, rate, and dose is crucial for their therapeutic success.

Endocrine hormones
A hormone secreted by a distant cell to regulate cell functions distributed widely through the body. The bloodstream plays an important role in the transport process
Paracrine-acting mediators
The mediator is secreted by a cell to influence surrounding cells, short-range influence
Autocrine-acting mediators
The agent is secreted by a cell and affects the cell by which it is generated, (very) short-range influence

Table 5.8 ■ Communication between cells: chemical messengers

Various technologies similar to those used for "small, low molecular weight" medicines may achieve rate control. E.g., for insulin one can choose from a spectrum of options (see Chap. 18). Moreover, continuous/"smart" infusion systems are on the market for insulin, see below.

■ Mechanical Pumps

In general, proteins are parenterally administered as an aqueous solution. Only recombinant vaccines and a number of insulin formulations are (colloidal) dispersions. For continuous and controlled administration of these solutions pump systems are used: continuous infusion. These pumps typically deliver the protein formulation via the intravenous route. However, patients may receive subcutaneously up to 25 ml over prolonged periods (up to 1 h) with a pump system (20% immune globulin solution; Hizentra, 2017). Table 5.9 lists some of the technologically feasible options. They are briefly touched upon below.

Pumps can be chosen in various sizes/prices, being portable or not, for inside/outside the body, with/without sophisticated rate control software. A pump system needs constant attention as it may fail because of power failure (batteries serve as backup power supply), problems with the syringe, accidental needle withdrawal, leakage of the catheter, and problems at the injection or implantation site. Moreover, long-term protein drug stability may become a problem. The protein should be stable at 37 °C or ambient temperature (for internal/implanted and external devices, respectively) between two refills.

Controlled administration of a drug does not necessarily imply a constant input rate. Pulsatile or variable-rate delivery is the desired mode of input for a number of proteins. For these biologics pumps should provide options for a flexible input rate. Insulin is a prime example of a therapeutic protein, where there is a need to adjust the input rate to the needs of the body. Today by far most experience has been gained with pump systems with adjustable input rates in an ambulatory setting with this protein drug. Even with high-tech pump systems,

• Continuous infusion with pumps. Input: Preset with limited variability. E.g. elastomer or spring driven pumps
• Continuous infusion with pumps. Input: Variable, controlled by health care professional or patient. E.g. mechanically/electronically driven (smart) pumps
• Rate control through implants. Input: limited control. E.g. biodegradable, polymer based microspheres
• Rate control through a closed-loop approach/feedback system. E.g. biosensor-pump combination

Table 5.9 ■ Controlled release and input systems for parenteral delivery

the patient still has to collect data to adjust the pump rate. This implies invasive sampling of body fluids on a regular basis, followed by calculations and setting of the required input rate. Progress made on developing the concept of closed-loop systems integrating these three actions: monitoring, calculating and choosing the rate of administration, i.e. a "natural" biofeedback system, is discussed under 'Biosensor-Pump Combinations'.

Biodegradable Microspheres

Polylactic acid–polyglycolic acid (PLGA)-based delivery systems are being used extensively for the delivery of therapeutic peptides, in particular for luteinizing hormone-releasing hormone (LHRH) agonists, such as leuprolide in the therapy of prostate cancer. The first LHRH agonist-controlled release formulations were implants, rods containing leuprolide with dosing intervals of 1–3 months. Later, microspheres loaded with leuprolide entered the market with dosing intervals up to 6 months. Considerations to design these controlled release systems are (1) the drug has to be highly potent (only a small dose is required over the dosing interval) and stable in the dosage form until release, (2) a sustained presence in the body is required, and (3) no adverse reactions at the injection site should occur. Only two such microsphere products for sustained delivery of therapeutic proteins instead of peptides made it to the market. Nutropin Depot® released recombinant human growth hormone over prolonged periods (monthly injection). Introduced in 1999, it was taken off the market in 2004 because of low perceived added therapeutic value, manufacturing problems and costs. A glucagon-like protein-1 (GLP-1, 39 amino acids) slow release formulation (Bydureon™) based on PLGA microspheres for once a week administration to type II diabetics was released in 2012.

Biosensor-Pump Combinations

If input rate control is desired to stabilize a certain body function, then this function or a suitable biomarker should be monitored. An algorithm converts this data into a drug-input rate and corresponding pump settings. If there is a known relationship between plasma level of the biomarker and pharmacological effect, these systems contain (Fig. 5.14):

1. A biosensor, measuring the (plasma) level of the biomarker
2. An algorithm, to calculate the required input rate for the delivery system
3. A pump system, able to administer the drug at the required rate over prolonged periods

The concept of a fully integrated closed-loop delivery of proteins still has to overcome a number of conceptual and practical hurdles. A simple relationship between plasma level and therapeutic effect does not always exist (see Chap. 6). There are many exceptions known to this rule; for instance, "hit and run" drugs can have long-lasting pharmacological effects after only a short exposure time. Also, drug effect–blood level relationships may be time dependent, as in the case of downregulation of relevant receptors on prolonged stimulation. Finally, if circadian rhythms exist, these will be responsible for variable PK/PD (pharmacokinetic/pharmacodynamic) relationships as well.

If PK/PD relationships can be established, as with insulin in selected groups of diabetics, then integrated

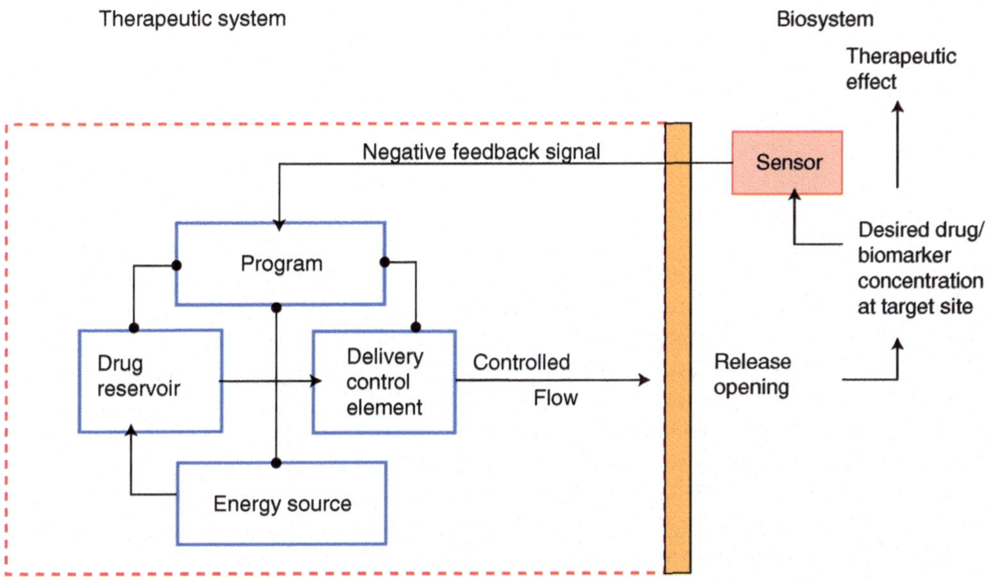

Figure 5.14 ■ Therapeutic system with closed control loop (From Heilmann 1984). (1) A biosensor, measuring the plasma level of the protein. (2) An algorithm, to calculate the required input rate for the delivery system. (3) A pump system, able to administer the drug at the required rate over prolonged periods

biosensor–pump combinations are available that almost act as biofeedback systems (Schaepelynck et al. 2011; Hovorka 2011). In 2016, FDA approved an integrated diabetes management system: insulin pump, continuous glucose monitoring biosensor, and diabetes therapy management software (Runge and Brown, 2016). The biosensor measures interstitial fluid glucose levels every 5 min and sends the outcome (wireless) to a therapy management algorithm. This software program adjusts the insulin pump settings to deliver an appropriate dose of insulin for basal glucose levels. However, the patient still has to inject a bolus before meals. Biosensor stability, robustness, absence of histological reactions and handling postprandial highs are still challenges in the design of fully integrated closed loop systems for chronic use. Trevitt et al. (2016) describe the state of the art in this fast-moving field.

DELIVERY OF PROTEINS BY THE PARENTERAL ROUTE: HALF-LIFE EXTENSION BY MODIFICATION OF THE API

Chemical modifications can change protein characteristics. For example, insulin half-life can be prolonged by exploiting the long circulation time of serum albumin and its high binding affinity for fatty acids such as myristic acid. In insulin detemir (Levemir®) lysine replaces the C-terminal threonine of insulin and myristic acid is chemically coupled through this lysine. After subcutaneous injection the myristic acid–insulin combination reaches the blood circulation and binds to albumin. Thereby the half-life of insulin is prolonged from less than 10 min to over 5 h. A similar approach is used with glucagon-1-like peptide (GLP-1 (7–37)) for the treatment of diabetes. Conjugating myristic acid to GLP-1 (amino acids 7–37) (liraglutide marketed as Victoza®) increases the plasma half-life from 2 min to over 10 h.

Another chemical modification approach that has been very successful in prolonging plasma circulation times and dosing intervals is the covalent attachment of polyoxyethylene glycol (PEG) to proteins. Figure 5.15 shows an example of this approach. Commercially highly successful examples that were developed later are PEGylated interferon alfa-2a and -2b and PEGylated hG-CSF (human granulocyte colony stimulating factor, filgrastim; see Chaps. 24 and 27). Furthermore, genetic modification of APIs has been successful in a number of cases. For example, fusion proteins with human serum albumin or Fc-parts (e.g., etanercept, aflibercept) from monoclonal antibodies are strategies to prolong the half-life. Both serum albumin and antibodies are physiological molecules with a long plasma half-life (see e.g. Chap. 8). With epoetins another approach was followed. Darbepoetin alfa (Aranesp) is a hyperglycosylated form of epoetin. It has the same mechanism of action but has a three-fold longer half-life compared to epoetin.

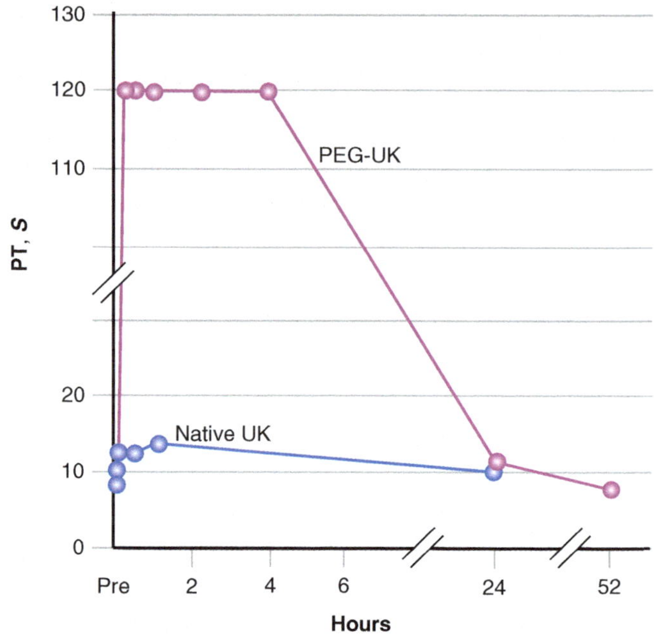

Figure 5.15 ■ Influence of chemical grafting of polyethylene glycol (PEG) on the ability of urokinase (UK) to affect the prothrombin time in seconds (PT) in vivo in beagles as function of time after a single administration (through Tomlinson 1987)

CONCLUDING REMARKS

In order to formulate a protein API successfully and turn it into a medicinal product that can be administered to a patient, the first requirement is an in depth understanding of the chemical and physical characteristics of the molecule in question, including its stability under the preferred storage conditions. A set of stability-indicating, complementary and orthogonal analytical techniques (see Box 1) should be available to help in successfully selecting the route of administration, the proper excipients, the packaging material for a stable product (freeze-dried or not).

In spite of considerable efforts made over almost 100 years, the parenteral route is the only one that allows us to administer protein-based medicines for systemic delivery to the patient. All other routes of administration failed so far.

SELF-ASSESSMENT QUESTIONS

Questions

1. A protein, which is poorly water soluble around its pI (pH 7.4), has to be formulated for subcutaneous administration. What conditions would one select to produce a water-soluble, injectable solution?
2. Why are many proteins to be used in the clinic formulated in freeze-dried form? Why is, as a rule, the presence of a lyoprotectant required? Why is it

important to know the glass transition temperature or eutectic temperature of the system?

3. Why should glucose be avoided as an excipient in protein formulations?
4. Why has oral delivery of therapeutic proteins failed so far?
5. What is the impact on the pharmacokinetics when changing from the IV to the SC route of administration of a therapeutic protein?
6. A company decides to explore the possibility to develop a biofeedback system for a therapeutic protein. What information should be available for estimating the chances for success?
7. What is the function of a preservative? For which type of protein formulations are they required? Example? Potential disadvantage?
8. Why do many protein formulations contain a surfactant? Example? Potential disadvantage?

Answers

1. Both solubility and stability should be considered. As both the aqueous solubility and the stability will be pH dependent, information on the solubility and stability as function of pH should be collected. The pH should be controlled by using a buffer. If needed, other excipients can be added to improve both the physical and the chemical stability of the protein, and to achieve isotonicity.
2. Chemical and physical instability of proteins in aqueous media is usually the reason to dry the protein solution.

   Freeze-drying is then the preferred technology, as other drying techniques do not give rapidly reconstitutable dry forms for the formulation and/or because elevated temperatures necessary for drying jeopardize the integrity of the protein. Lyoprotectants protect the proteins from degradation during the freeze-drying process.

   The collapse temperature (Tc) should not be exceeded (a few degrees below Te or Tg/Tg′), as otherwise collapse of the cake occurs. Collapse slows down the freeze-drying process rate, and collapsed material does not rapidly dissolve upon adding water for reconstitution.
3. Because the protein will degrade through the Maillard reaction, as glucose is a reducing sugar. This is true for both liquid and lyophilized formulations.
4. Because of the hostile environment in the GI tract regarding protein stability and the poor absorption characteristics of proteins (high molecular weight/often hydrophilic).
5. Both the extent and rate of uptake into the blood circulation are affected. When changing from IV to SC administration, the AUC (area under the curve) and the absorption rate are reduced.
6. Information that should be available
   - The desired pharmacokinetic profile (e.g., information on the PK/PD relationship/circadian rhythm)
   - Chemical and physical stability of the protein on long-term storage at body/ambient temperature
   - Availability of a biosensor system (stability in vivo, precision/accuracy)
   - Availability of a reliable pump system (see Table 5.9)
7. A preservative is included to neutralize contaminations in containers. A multi-dose formulation needs a preservative. Examples of preservatives used in protein formulations are phenol, meta-cresol, benzyl alcohol, and chlorobutanol. A disadvantage of preservatives is that they may interact with the protein, affecting their own and/or the protein's performance.
8. Surfactants reduce adsorption to interfaces and by doing so prevent aggregation. Examples of commonly used surfactants are polysorbate 80 and 20. A disadvantage of surfactants is that too high concentrations may cause denaturation (unfolding) of the protein. A disadvantage of polysorbates is that they can hydrolyze, which reduces their stabilizing potential and may lead to insoluble degradation products (a.o. fatty acids).

REFERENCES

Arakawa T, Kita Y, Carpenter JF (1991) Protein-solvent interactions in pharmaceutical formulation. Pharm Res 8:285–291

Bahrenburg S, Karow AR, Garidel P (2015) Buffer-free therapeutic antibody preparations provide a viable alternative to conventionally buffered solutions: from protein buffer capacity prediction to bioprocess applications. Biotechnol J 10:610–622

Chang BS, Hershenson S (2002) Practical approaches to protein formulation development. In: Carpenter JF, Manning MC (eds) Rational design of stable protein formulations–theory and practice. Kluwer Academic/Plenum, New York, pp 1–20

Chi E, Krishnan S, Randolph TW, Carpenter JF (2003) Physical stability of proteins in aqueous solution: mechanism and driving forces in nonnative protein aggregation. Pharm Res 20:1325–1336

Constantino HR, Pikal MJ (2004) Lyophilization of biopharmaceuticals. AAPS Press, Arlington

Geidobler R, Winter G (2013) Controlled ice nucleation in the field of freeze-drying: fundamentals and technology review. Eur J Pharm Biopharm 85:214–222

Hawe A, Wiggenhorn M, van de Weert M, Garbe JHO, Mahler H-C, Jiskoot W (2012) Forced degradation of therapeutic proteins. J Pharm Sci 101:895–913

Heilmann K (1984) Therapeutic systems. Rate controlled delivery: concept and development. Georg Thieme Verlag, Stuttgart

Hizentra Infusion Guide. https://www.hizentra.com/common/pdf/Hizentra-Step-by-step-infusion-guide.pdf. Accessed Nov 2017

Hovorka R (2011) Closed-loop insulin delivery: from bench to clinical practice. Nat Rev Endocrinol 7:385–395

Jiskoot W, Crommelin DJA (2005) Methods for structural analysis of protein pharmaceuticals. AAPS Press, Arlington

Jiskoot W, Nejadnik MR, Sediq AS (2017) Potential issues with the handling of biologicals in a hospital. J Pharm Sci 106:1688–1689

Jorgensen J, Nielsen HM (eds) (2009) Delivery technologies for biopharmaceuticals: peptides, proteins, nucleic acids and vaccines. Wiley, Chichester

Kamerzell TJ, Esfandiary R, Joshi SB, Middaugh CR, Volkin DB (2011) Protein–excipient interactions: mechanisms and biophysical characterization applied to protein formulation development. Adv Drug Deliv Rev 63:1118–1159

Kinnunen HM, Mrsny RJ (2014) Improving the outcomes of biopharmaceutical delivery via the subcutaneous route by understanding the chemical, physical and physiological properties of the subcutaneous injection site. J Control Release 182:22–32

Maberly GF, Wait GA, Kilpatrick JA, Loten EG, Gain KR, Stewart RDH, Eastman CJ (1982) Evidence for insulin degradation by muscle and fat tissue in an insulin resistant diabetic patient. Diabetologia 23:333–336

Manning MC, Chou DK, Murphy BM, Payne RW, Katayama DS (2010) Stability of protein pharmaceuticals: an update. Pharm Res 27:544–575

Manning MC, Patel K, Borchardt RT (1989) Stability of proteins. Pharm Res 6:903–918

Martos A, Koch W, Jiskoot W, Wuchner K, Winter G, Friess W, Hawe A (2017) Trends on analytical characterization of polysorbates and their degradation products in biopharmaceutical formulations. J Pharm Sci 106:1722–1735

Mensink MA, Frijlink HW, van der Voort Maarschalk K, Hinrichs W (2017) How sugars protect proteins in the solid state and during drying (review): mechanisms of stabilization in relation to stress conditions. Eur J Pharm Biopharm 114:288–295

Moeller EH, Jorgensen L (2009) Alternative routes of administration for systemic delivery of protein pharmaceuticals. Drug Discov Today Technol 5:89–94

Nejadnik MR, Randolph TW, Volkin DB, Schöneich C, Carpenter JF, Crommelin DJA, Jiskoot W (2018) Post-production handling and administration of protein pharmaceuticals and potential instability issues. J Pharm Sci 107(8):2013–2019

Nguyen TH, Ward C (1993) Stability characterization and formulation development of alteplase, a recombinant tissue plasminogen activator. In: Wang YJ, Pearlman R (eds) Stability and characterization of protein and peptide drugs. Case histories. Plenum Press, New York, pp 91–134

Patton JS, Bukar JG, Eldon MA (2004) Clinical pharmacokinetics and pharmacodynamics of inhaled insulin. Clin Pharmacokinet 43:781–801

Pearlman R, Bewley TA (1993) Stability and characterization of human growth hormone. In: Wang YJ, Pearlman R (eds) Stability and characterization of protein and peptide drugs. Case histories. Plenum Press, New York, pp 1–58

Pikal MJ (1990) Freeze-drying of proteins. Part I: process design. BioPharm 3:18–27

Pristoupil TI (1985) Haemoglobin lyophilized with sucrose: effect of residual moisture on storage. Haematologia 18:45–52

Richter WF, Bhansali SG, Morris ME (2012) Mechanistic determinants of biotherapeutics absorption following sc administration. AAPS J 14:559–570

Runge A, Brown A (2016) https://diatribe.org/fda-approval-medtronic-minimed-670g-hybrid-closed-loop-system

Sacha GA, Saffell-Clemmer W, Abram K, Akers MJ (2010) Practical fundamentals of glass, rubber, and plastic sterile packaging systems. Pharm Dev Technol 15(1):6–34. https://doi.org/10.3109/10837450903511178

Sacha G, Rogers JA, Miller RL (2015) Pre-filled syringes: a review of the history, manufacturing and challenges. Pharm Dev Technol 20:1–11. https://doi.org/10.3109/10837450.2014.982825

Schaepelynck P, Darmon P, Molines L, Jannot-Lamotte MF, Treglia C, Raccah D (2011) Advances in pump technology: insulin patch pumps, combined pumps and glucose sensors, and implanted pumps. Diabetes Metab 37:S85–S93

Schersch K, Betz O, Garidel P, Muehlau S, Bassarab S, Winter G (2010) Systematic investigation of the effect of lyophilizate collapse on pharmaceutically relevant proteins I: stability after freeze-drying. J Pharm Sci 99:2256–2278

Sediq AS, van Duijvenvoorde RB, Jiskoot W, Nejadnik MR (2016) Subvisible particle formation during stirring. J Pharm Sci 105:519–529

Supersaxo A, Hein WR, Steffen H (1990) Effect of molecular weight on the lymphatic absorption of water-soluble compounds following subcutaneous administration. Pharm Res 7:167–169

Tomlinson E (1987) Theory and practice of site-specific drug delivery. Adv Drug Deliv Rev 1:87–198

Trevitt S, Simpson S, Wood A (2016) Artificial pancreas device systems for the closed-loop control of type 1 diabetes: what systems are in development? J Diabetes Sci Technol 10:714–723

Vemuri S, Yu CT, Roosdorp N (1993) Formulation and stability of recombinant alpha1-antitrypsin. In: Wang YJ, Pearlman R (eds) Stability and characterization of protein and peptide drugs. Plenum Press, New York, pp 263–286

Vlieland ND, Gardarsdottir H, Bouvy ML, Egberts TCG, van den Bemt BJF (2016) The majority of patients do not store their biologic disease-modifying antirheumatic drugs within the recommended temperature range. Rheumatology 55:704–709

Vlieland ND, Nejadnik MR, Gardarsdottir H, Romeijn AS, Sediq S, Bouvy ML, Egberts ACG, van den Bemt BJF,

Jiskoot W (2018) The impact of inadequate temperature storage conditions on aggregate and particle formation in drugs containing tumor necrosis factor-alpha inhibitors. Pharm Res 35:42

Weinbuch D, Hawe A, Jiskoot W, Friess W (2018) In: Mahler HC, Warne NW (eds) Challenges in protein product development. AAPS advances in the pharmaceutical sciences series. AAPS Press/Springer, New York, pp 3–22

Zbacnik TJ, Holcomb RE, Katayama DS, Murphy BM, Payne RW, Coccaro RC, Evans GJ, Matsuura JE, Henry CS, Manning MC (2017) Role of buffers in protein formulations. J Pharm Sci 106:713–733

Zölls S, Tantipolphan R, Wiggenhorn M, Winter G, Jiskoot W, Friess W, Hawe A (2012) Particles in therapeutic protein formulations–part I. Overview of analytical methods. J Pharm Sci 101:914–935

FURTHER READING

Carpenter JF, Manning MC (2002) Rational design of stable protein formulations–theory and practice. Kluwer Academic/Plenum, New York

Mahler H-C, Jiskoot W (2012) Analysis of aggregates and particles in protein pharmaceuticals. Wiley, Hoboken

Mahler HC, Warne NW (2018) Challenges in protein product development. AAPS advances in the pharmaceutical sciences series. AAPS Press/Springer, New York, p 2018

Manning MC, Liu J, Li T, Holcomb RE (2018) Rational design of liquid formulations of proteins. Adv Protein Chem Struct Biol 112:1–59

6 Pharmacokinetics and Pharmacodynamics of Therapeutic Peptides and Proteins

Bernd Meibohm

INTRODUCTION

The rational use of drugs and the design of effective dosage regimens are facilitated by the appreciation of the central paradigm of clinical pharmacology that there is a defined relationship between the administered dose of a drug, the resulting drug concentrations in various body fluids and tissues, and the intensity of pharmacologic effects caused by these concentrations (Meibohm and Derendorf 1997). This dose-exposure-response relationship and thus the dose of a drug required to achieve a certain effect are determined by the drug's pharmacokinetic and pharmacodynamic properties (Fig. 6.1).

Pharmacokinetics describes the time course of the concentration of a drug in a body fluid, preferably plasma or blood, that results from the administration of a certain dosage regimen. It comprises all processes affecting drug absorption, distribution, metabolism, and excretion. Simplified, pharmacokinetics characterizes "*what the body does to the drug*." In contrast, pharmacodynamics characterizes the intensity of a drug effect or toxicity resulting from certain drug concentrations in a body fluid, usually at the assumed site of drug action. It can be simplified to *what the drug does to the body* (Fig. 6.2) (Holford and Sheiner 1982; Derendorf and Meibohm 1999).

The understanding of the dose-concentration-effect relationship is crucial to any drug—including peptides and proteins—as it lays the foundation for dosing regimen design and rational clinical application. General pharmacokinetic and pharmacodynamic principles are to a large extent equally applicable to protein and peptide drugs as they are to traditional small molecule-based therapeutics. Deviations from some of these principles and additional challenges with regard to the characterization of the pharmacokinetics and pharmacodynamics of therapeutic peptides and proteins, however, arise from some of their specific properties:

(a) Their definition by the production process in a living organism rather than a chemically exactly defined structure and purity as it is the case for small-molecule drugs
(b) Their structural similarity to endogenous structural or functional proteins and nutrients
(c) Their intimate involvement in physiologic processes on the molecular level, often including regulatory feedback mechanisms
(d) The analytical challenges to identify and quantify them in the presence of a myriad of similar molecules
(e) Their large molecular weight and macromolecule character (for proteins)

This chapter will highlight some of the major pharmacokinetic properties and processes relevant for the majority of therapeutic peptides and proteins and will provide examples of well-characterized pharmacodynamic relationships for peptide and protein drugs. The clinical pharmacology of monoclonal antibodies, including special aspects in their pharmacokinetics and pharmacodynamics, will be discussed in further detail in Chap. 8. For a more general discussion on pharmacokinetic and pharmacodynamic principles, the reader is referred to several textbooks and articles that review the topic in extensive detail (see Further Reading).

B. Meibohm (✉)
Department of Pharmaceutical Sciences, University of Tennessee Health Science Center, College of Pharmacy, Memphis, TN, USA
e-mail: bmeibohm@uthsc.edu

D. J. A. Crommelin et al. (eds.), *Pharmaceutical Biotechnology*, https://doi.org/10.1007/978-3-030-00710-2_6

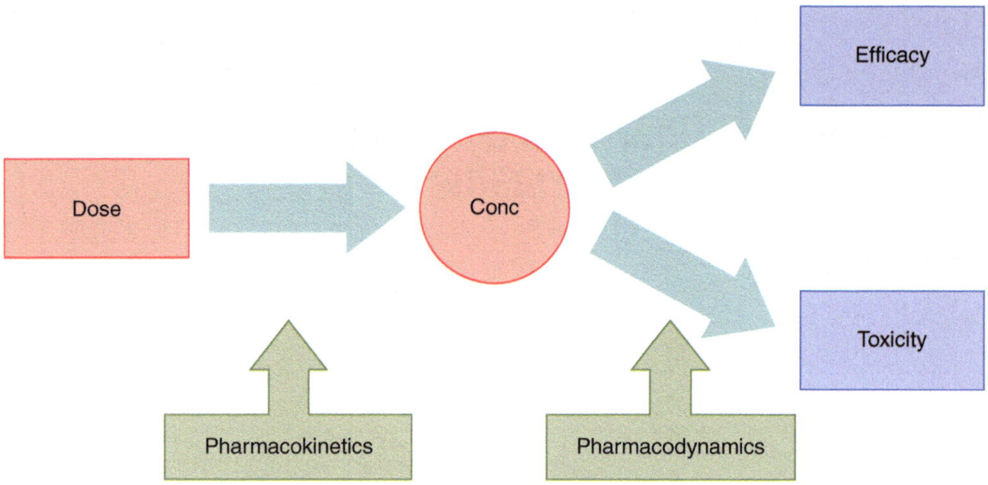

Figure 6.1 ■ The central paradigm of clinical pharmacology: the dose-concentration-effect relationship

PHARMACOKINETICS OF THERAPEUTIC PROTEINS

The in vivo disposition of peptide and protein drugs may often be predicted to a large degree from their physiological function (Tang and Meibohm 2006). Peptides, for example, which frequently have hormone activity, usually have short elimination half-lives, which is desirable for a close regulation of their endogenous levels and thus function. Insulin, for example, shows dose-dependent elimination with a relatively short half-life of 26 and 52 min at 0.1 and 0.2 U/kg, respectively. Contrary to that, proteins that have transport tasks such as albumin or long-term immunity functions such as immunoglobulins have elimination half-lives of several days, which enables and ensures the continuous maintenance of physiologically necessary concentrations in the bloodstream (Meibohm and Derendorf 2004). This is, for example, reflected by the elimination half-life of antibody drugs such as the anti-epidermal growth factor receptor antibody cetuximab, an IgG1 chimeric antibody for which a half-life of approximately 7 days has been reported (Herbst and Langer 2002).

■ Absorption of Therapeutic Proteins

Enteral Administration

Peptides and proteins, unlike conventional small-molecule drugs, are generally not therapeutically active upon oral administration (Fasano 1998; Mahato et al. 2003; Tang et al. 2004). The lack of systemic bioavailability is mainly caused by two factors: (1) high gastrointestinal enzyme activity and (2) low permeability through the gastrointestinal mucosa. In fact, the substantial peptidase and protease activity in the gastrointestinal tract makes it the most efficient body compartment for peptide and protein metabolism. Furthermore, the gastrointestinal mucosa presents a major absorption barrier for water-soluble macromolecules such as peptides and proteins (Tang et al. 2004). Thus, although various factors such as permeability, stability, and gastrointestinal transit time can affect the rate and extent of orally administered proteins, molecular size is generally considered the ultimate obstacle (Shen 2003).

Since oral administration is still a highly desirable route of delivery for protein drugs due to its convenience, cost-effectiveness, and painlessness, numerous strategies to overcome the obstacles associated with oral delivery of proteins have recently been an area of intensive research. Suggested approaches to increase the oral bioavailability of protein drugs include encapsulation into micro- or nanoparticles thereby protecting proteins from intestinal degradation (Lee 2002; Mahato et al. 2003; Shen 2003). Other strategies are chemical modifications such as amino acid backbone modifications and chemical conjugations to improve the resistance to degradation and permeability of the protein drug (Diao and Meibohm 2013). Coadministration of protease inhibitors has also been suggested for the inhibition of enzymatic degradation (Pauletti et al. 1997; Mahato et al. 2003). More details on approaches for oral delivery of therapeutic peptides and proteins are discussed in Chap. 5.

Parenteral Administration

Most peptide and protein drugs are currently formulated as parenteral formulations because of their poor oral bioavailability. Major routes of administration include intravenous (IV), subcutaneous (SC), and intramuscular (IM) administration. In addition, other non-oral administration pathways are utilized, including nasal, buccal, rectal, vaginal, transdermal, ocular, and pulmonary drug delivery (see Chap. 5).

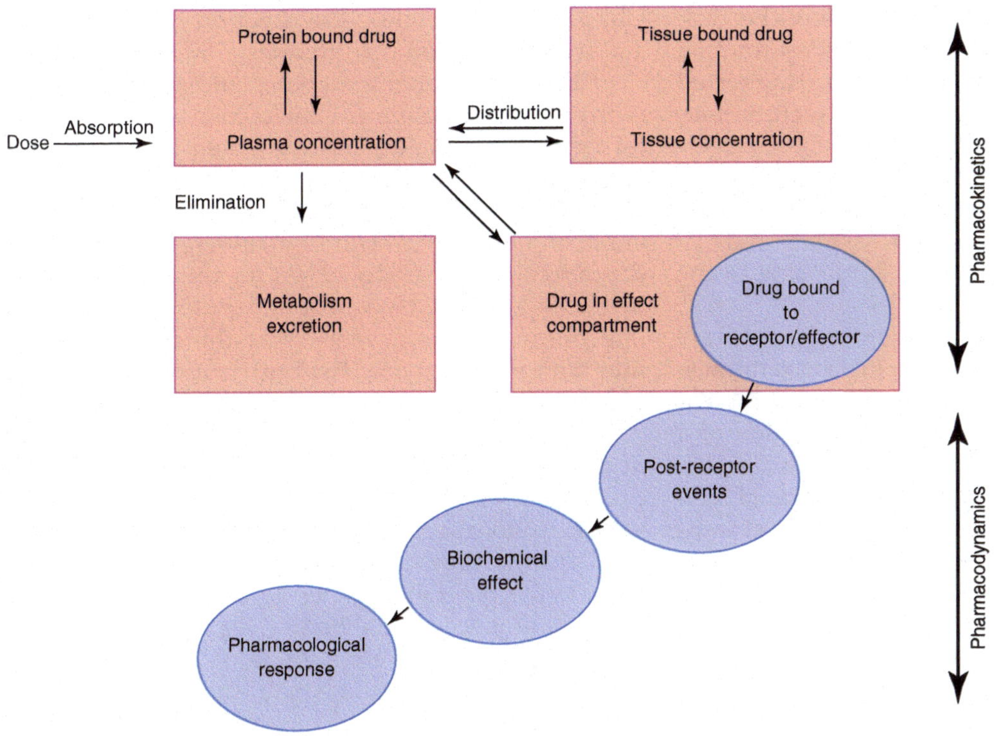

Figure 6.2 ■ Physiological scheme of pharmacokinetic and pharmacodynamic processes

IV administration of peptides and proteins offers the advantage of circumventing presystemic degradation, thereby achieving the highest concentration in the biological system. Therapeutic proteins given by the IV route include, among many others, the tissue plasminogen activator (t-PA) analogues alteplase and tenecteplase, the recombinant human erythropoietin epoetin-α, and the granulocyte colony-stimulating factor filgrastim (Tang and Meibohm 2006).

IV administration as either a bolus dose or constant rate infusion, however, may not always provide the desired concentration-time profile depending on the biological activity of the product. In these cases, IM or SC injections may be more appropriate alternatives. For example, luteinizing hormone-releasing hormone (LH-RH) in bursts stimulates the release of follicle-stimulating hormone (FSH) and luteinizing hormone (LH), whereas a continuous baseline level will suppress the release of these hormones (Handelsman and Swerdloff 1986). To avoid the high peaks from an IV administration of leuprorelin, an LH-RH agonist, a long-acting monthly depot injection of the drug is approved for the treatment of prostate cancer and endometriosis (Periti et al. 2002). A recent study comparing SC versus IV administration of epoetin-α in patients receiving hemodialysis reports that the SC route can maintain the hematocrit in a desired target range with a lower average weekly dose of epoetin-α compared to IV (Kaufman et al. 1998). In addition, SC injections have become increasingly popular as they allow self-administration by the patient, especially with the introduction of microneedles and pen devices, and thus not only circumvent the need to intravenous access, but also have increased patient acceptance and overall lower administration cost.

One of the potential limitations of SC and IM administration, however, are the presystemic degradation processes frequently associated with these administration routes, resulting in a reduced systemic bioavailability compared to IV administration. No correlation between the molecular weight of a therapeutic protein and its systemic bioavailability has so far been described in any species (Richter et al. 2012), and clinically observed bioavailability seems to be product-specific based on physicochemical properties and structure.

Bioavailability assessments for therapeutic proteins may be challenging if the protein exhibits the frequently encountered nonlinear pharmacokinetic behavior. Classic bioavailability assessments comparing systemic exposures quantified as area-under-the-concentration-time curve (AUC) resulting from extravascular versus IV administration assume linear pharmacokinetics, i.e., a drug clearance independent of concentration and the administration pathway. As this is not the case for many therapeutic proteins, especially those that undergo target-mediated drug disposition (see respective section in this chapter), bioavailability assessments using the classic approach can result in substantial bias (Limothai and Meibohm 2011). Potential approaches suggested to minimize or overcome these effects include bioavailability assessments at doses at which the target- or receptor-mediated processes are saturated or to compare concentration-time profiles with similar shape and magnitude for extravascular and IV administration by modulating the input rate in the IV experiment.

The pharmacokinetically derived apparent absorption rate constant k_{app} for protein drugs administered via these administration routes is the combination of absorption into the systemic circulation and presystemic degradation at the absorption site, i.e., the sum of a true first-order absorption rate constant k_a and a first-order degradation rate constant. The true absorption rate constant k_a can then be calculated as

$$k_a = F \cdot k_{app}$$

where F is the systemic bioavailability compared to IV administration. A rapid apparent absorption, i.e., large k_{app}, can thus be the result of a slow true absorption and a fast presystemic degradation, i.e., a low systemic bioavailability (Colburn 1991).

Other potential factors that may limit the rate and/or extent of uptake of proteins after SC or IM administration include variable local blood flow, injection trauma, and limitations of uptake into the systemic circulation related to effective capillary pore size, diffusion, and convective transport.

Several therapeutic proteins including anakinra, etanercept, insulin, and pegfilgrastim, but also monoclonal antibodies such as adalimumab, omalizumab or alirocumab are administered as SC injections. Following a SC injection, therapeutic peptides and proteins may enter the systemic circulation either via blood capillaries or through lymphatic vessels (Porter and Charman 2000). There appears to be a defined relationship between the molecular weight of the protein and the proportion of the dose absorbed by the lymphatics (see Fig. 5.13) (Supersaxo et al. 1990). In general, peptides and proteins larger than 16 kDa are predominantly absorbed into the lymphatics, whereas those under 1 kDa are mostly absorbed into the blood circulation. While diffusion is the driving force for the uptake into blood capillaries, transport of larger proteins through the interstitial space into lymphatic vessels is mediated by convective transport with the interstitial fluid following the hydrostatic and osmotic pressure differences (see paragraphs on distribution). The fraction of insulin (5.2 kDa), for example, that has been described to undergo absorption through the lymphatic system is approximately 20% (see Chap. 5 and 18), while this fraction is approaching 100% for monoclonal antibodies (150 kDa).

For monoclonal antibodies and fusion proteins with antibody Fc fragment, interaction with the neonatal Fc receptor (FcRn) has also been identified as a potential absorption process (Roopenian and Akilesh 2007). In this context, FcRn prevents the monoclonal antibody or fusion protein from undergoing lysosomal degradation (see Chap. 8 for details) and thereby increases systemic bioavailability, but may also facilitate transcellular transport from the absorption site into the vascular space. The contribution of this pathway to overall absorption, however, is limited.

Since lymph flow and interstitial convective transport are substantially slower than blood flow and diffusion processes, larger proteins taken up into lymphatic vessels usually show a delayed and prolonged absorption process after SC administration that can even become the rate-limiting step in their overall disposition. For monoclonal antibodies, for example, the time of the maximum concentration (t_{max}) was substantially delayed after SC administration, ranging from 1.7 to 13.5 days, with frequent values around 6–8 days (Zhao et al. 2013). A related model-based analysis suggests that lymphatic flow rate is the most influential factor for t_{max} of SC administered monoclonal antibodies.

Preferential uptake into lymphatic vessel after SC administration is of particular importance for those agents whose therapeutic targets are lymphoid cells (i.e., interferons and interleukins). Studies with recombinant human interferon α-2a (rhIFN α-2a) indicate that following SC administration, high concentrations of the recombinant protein are found in the lymphatic system, which drains into regional lymph nodes (Supersaxo et al. 1988). Due to this targeting effect, clinical studies show that palliative low-to-intermediate-dose SC recombinant interleukin-2 (rIL-2) in combination with rhIFN α-2a can be administered to patients in the ambulatory setting with efficacy and safety profiles comparable to the most aggressive IV rIL-2 protocol against metastatic renal cell cancer (Schomburg et al. 1993).

More recently, charge has also been described as an important factor in the SC absorption of proteins: While the positive and negative charges from collagen and hyaluronan in the extracellular matrix seem to be of similar magnitude, additional negative charges of proteoglycans may lead to a negative interstitial charge (Richter et al. 2012). This negative net charge and the associated ionic interactions with SC-administered proteins result in a slower transport for more positively rather than negatively charged proteins, as could be shown for several monoclonal antibodies (Mach et al. 2011).

■ Distribution of Therapeutic Proteins

Distribution Mechanisms and Volumes

The rate and extent of protein distribution is largely determined by the molecule size and molecular weight, physiochemical properties (e.g., charge, lipophilicity), binding to structural or transport proteins, and their dependency on active transport processes to cross biomembranes. Since most therapeutic proteins have high molecular weights and are thus large in size, their apparent volume of distribution is usually small and limited to the volume of the extracellular space due to their limited mobility secondary to impaired passage through biomembranes (Zito 1997). In addition, there is a mutual exclusion between therapeutic proteins and the structural molecules of the extracellular matrix. This fraction of the interstitial space that is not available for distribution is expressed as the excluded volume (Ve). It is dependent on the molecular weight and charge of the macromolecule and further limits extravascular distribution. For albumin (MW 66 kDa), the Ve has been reported as ~50% in muscle and skin (Ryman and Meibohm 2017). Active tissue uptake and binding to intra- and extravascular proteins, however, can substantially increase the apparent volume of distribution of protein drugs, as reflected by the relatively large volume of distribution of up to 2.8 L/kg for interferon β-1b (Chiang et al. 1993).

In contrast to small-molecule drugs, protein transport from the vascular space into the interstitial space of tissues is largely mediated by convection rather than diffusion, following the unidirectional fluid flux from the vascular space through paracellular pores into the interstitial tissue space (Fig. 6.3). The subsequent removal from the interstitial space is accomplished by lymph drainage back into the systemic circulation (Flessner et al. 1997). This underlines the unique role the lymphatic system plays in the disposition of therapeutic proteins as already discussed in the section on absorption. The fact that the transfer clearance from the vascular to the interstitial space is smaller than the transfer clearance from the interstitial space to the lymphatic system results in lower protein concentrations in the interstitial space compared to the vascular space, thereby further limiting the apparent volume of distribution for therapeutic proteins. For endogenous and exogenous immunoglobulin G antibodies, for example, the tissue: blood concentration ratio is in the range of 0.1–0.5, i.e. antibody concentrations are substantially lower in the tissue interstitial fluid than in plasma (Ryman and Meibohm 2017). For brain tissue, the ratio is even in the range of 0.01 or lower, but may be higher in cases of compromised blood-brain barrier (Kingwell 2016).

Another, but much less prominent pathway for the movement of protein molecules from the vascular to the interstitial space is transcellular migration via endocytosis (Baxter et al. 1994; Reddy et al. 2006).

Besides the size-dependent sieving of macromolecules through the capillary walls, charge may also play an important role in the biodistribution of proteins. It has been suggested that the electrostatic attraction between positively charged proteins and negatively charged cell membranes might increase the rate and extent of tissue distribution. Most cell surfaces are negatively charged because of their abundance of glycosaminoglycans in the extracellular matrix.

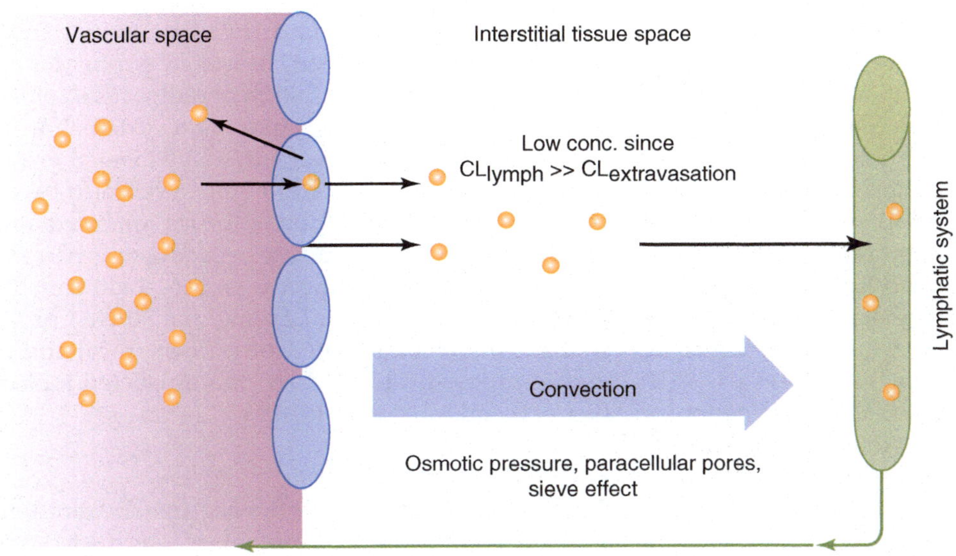

Figure 6.3 ■ Distribution mechanisms of therapeutic proteins: convective extravasation rather than diffusion as major distribution process. $CL_{extravasation}$ transfer clearance from the vascular to the interstitial, CL_{lymph} transfer clearance from the interstitial space to the lymphatic system

After IV administration, peptides and proteins usually follow a biexponential plasma concentration-time profile that can best be described by a two-compartment pharmacokinetic model (Meibohm 2004). A biexponential concentration-time profile has, for example, been described for clenoliximab, a macaque-human chimeric monoclonal antibody specific to the CD4 molecule on the surface of T lymphocytes (Mould et al. 1999). Similarly, secukinumab, a human monoclonal antibody that binds and neutralizes interleukin 17A for the treatment of psoriasis, exhibited biphasic pharmacokinetics after IV administration (Bruin et al. 2017). The central compartment in this two-compartment model represents primarily the vascular space and the interstitial space of well-perfused organs with permeable capillary walls, including the liver and the kidneys. The peripheral compartment is more reflective of concentration-time profiles in the interstitial space of slowly equilibrating tissues.

The central compartment in which proteins initially distribute after IV administration has thus typically a volume of distribution equal or slightly larger than the plasma volume, i.e., 3–8 L. The total volume of distribution frequently comprises with 14–20 L not more than two to three times the initial volume of distribution (Colburn 1991; Dirks and Meibohm 2010). An example for such a distribution pattern is the t-PA analogue tenecteplase. Radiolabeled ^{125}I-tenecteplase was described to have an initial volume of distribution of 4.2–6.3 L and a total volume of distribution of 6.1–9.9 L with liver as the only organ that had a significant uptake of radioactivity. The authors concluded that the small volume of distribution suggests primarily intravascular distribution for tenecteplase, consistent with the drug's large molecular weight of 65 kDa (Tanswell et al. 2002).

Epoetin-α, for example, has a volume of distribution estimated to be close to the plasma volume at 0.056 L/kg after an IV administration to healthy volunteers (Ramakrishnan et al. 2004). Similarly, volume of distribution for darbepoetin-α has been reported as 0.062 L/kg after IV administration in patients undergoing dialysis (Allon et al. 2002), and distribution of thrombopoietin has also been reported to be limited to the plasma volume (~3 L) (Jin and Krzyzanski 2004).

It should be stressed that pharmacokinetic calculations of volume of distribution may be problematic for many therapeutic proteins (Tang et al. 2004; Straughn 2006). Noncompartmental determination of volume of distribution at steady state (V_{ss}) using statistical moment theory assumes first-order disposition processes with elimination occurring from the rapidly equilibrating or central compartment (Perrier and Mayersohn 1982; Straughn 1982; Veng-Pedersen and Gillespie 1984). These basic assumptions, however, are not fulfilled for numerous therapeutic proteins, as proteolysis and receptor-mediated elimination in peripheral tissues may constitute a substantial fraction of the overall elimination process. If therapeutic proteins are eliminated from slowly equilibrating tissues at a rate greater than their distribution process, substantial error in the volume of distribution assessment may occur. A recent simulation study could show that if substantial tissue elimination exists, a V_{ss} determined by noncompartmental methods will underestimate the "true" V_{ss} and that the magnitude of error tends to be larger the more extensively the protein is eliminated by tissue routes (Meibohm 2004; Straughn 2006; Tang and Meibohm 2006).

These challenges in characterizing the distribution of therapeutic proteins can only be overcome by determining actual protein concentrations in the tissue by biopsy or necropsy or via biodistribution studies with radiolabeled compound and/or imaging techniques.

Biodistribution studies are imperative for small organic synthetic drugs, since long residence times of the radioactive label in certain tissues may be an indication of tissue accumulation of potentially toxic metabolites. Because of the possible reutilization of amino acids from protein drugs in endogenous proteins, such a safety concern does not exist for therapeutic proteins. Therefore, biodistribution studies for protein drugs are usually only performed to assess drug targeting to specific tissues or to detect the major organs of elimination.

If a biodistribution study with radiolabeled protein is performed, either an external label such as ^{125}I can be chemically coupled to the protein if it contains a suitable amino acid such as tyrosine or lysine, or internal labeling can be used by growing the production cell line in the presence of amino acids labeled with ^{3}H, ^{14}C, ^{35}S, etc. The latter method, however, is not routinely used because of the prohibition of radioactive contamination of fermentation equipment (Meibohm and Derendorf 2004). Moreover, internally labeled proteins may be less desirable than iodinated proteins because of the potential reutilization of the radiolabeled amino acid fragments in the synthesis of endogenous proteins and cell structures. Irrespective of the labeling method, but more so for external labeling, the labeled product should have demonstrated physicochemical and biological properties identical to the unlabeled molecule (Bennett and McMartin 1978).

Protein Binding of Therapeutic Proteins

Another factor that can influence the distribution of therapeutic peptides and proteins is binding to endogenous protein structures. Physiologically active endogenous peptides and proteins frequently interact with specific binding proteins involved in their transport and regulation. Furthermore, interaction with binding proteins may enable or facilitate cellular uptake processes and thus affect the drug's pharmacodynamics.

It is a general pharmacokinetic principle, which is also applicable to proteins, that only the free, unbound fraction of a drug substance is accessible to distribution and elimination processes as well as interactions with its target structures at the site of action, for example, a receptor or ion channel. Thus, protein binding may affect the pharmacodynamics, but also disposition properties of therapeutic proteins. Specific binding proteins have been identified for numerous protein drugs, including recombinant human DNase for use as mucolytic in cystic fibrosis (Mohler et al. 1993), growth hormone (Toon 1996), and recombinant human vascular endothelial growth factor (rhVEGF) (Eppler et al. 2002).

Protein binding not only affects the unbound fraction of a protein drug and thus the fraction of a drug available to exert pharmacological activity, but many times it also either prolongs protein circulation time by acting as a storage depot or it enhances protein clearance. Recombinant cytokines, for example, may after IV administration encounter various cytokine-binding proteins including soluble cytokine receptors and anti-cytokine antibodies (Piscitelli et al. 1997). In either case, the binding protein may either prolong the cytokine circulation time by acting as a storage depot or it may enhance the cytokine clearance.

Growth hormone, as another example, has at least two binding proteins in plasma (Wills and Ferraiolo 1992). This protein binding substantially reduces growth hormone elimination with a tenfold smaller clearance of total compared to free growth hormone, but also decreases its activity via reduction of receptor interactions.

Ectodomain shedding is another source of binding proteins circulating in plasma where the extracellular domain of membrane-standing receptors is cleaved and released into the circulation (Hayashida et al. 2010). For therapeutic proteins targeting these receptors, the shed ectodomain constitutes a binding reservoir that by being in the vascular space is often more easily accessible than the intact membrane-standing receptor on target cells in the extravascular space. Thus, shed antigen can limit the disposition of a therapeutic protein and can inactivate a fraction of the administered therapeutic protein by preventing it from accessing its intended target (Ryman and Meibohm 2017). Different patients may have vastly different shed antigen concentrations and thus different effects, as shown for CD52, the target for alemtuzumab (Albitar et al. 2004).

Apart from these specific bindings, peptides and proteins may also be nonspecifically bound to plasma proteins. For example, metkephamid, a met-enkephalin analogue, was described to be 44–49% bound to albumin (Taki et al. 1998), and octreotide, a somatostatin analogue, is up to 65% bound to lipoproteins (Chanson et al. 1993).

Distribution Via Receptor-Mediated Uptake

Aside from physicochemical properties and protein binding of therapeutic proteins, site-specific receptor-mediated uptake can also substantially influence and contribute to the distribution of therapeutic proteins, as well as to elimination and pharmacodynamics (see section on "Target-Mediated Drug Disposition").

The generally low volume of distribution should not necessarily be interpreted as low tissue penetration. Receptor-mediated specific uptake into the target organ, as one mechanism, can result in therapeutically effective tissue concentrations despite a relatively small volume of distribution. Nartograstim, a recombinant derivative of the granulocyte colony-stimulating factor (G-CSF), for example, is characterized by a specific, dose-dependent, and saturable tissue uptake into the target organ bone marrow, presumably via receptor-mediated endocytosis (Kuwabara et al. 1995).

■ Elimination of Therapeutic Proteins

Therapeutic proteins are generally subject to the same catabolic pathways as endogenous or dietetic proteins. The end products of protein metabolism are thus amino acids that are reutilized in the endogenous amino acid pool for the de novo biosynthesis of structural or functional proteins in the human body (Meibohm 2004). Detailed investigations on the metabolism of proteins are relatively difficult because of the myriad of potential molecule fragments that may be formed, and are therefore generally not conducted. Non-metabolic elimination pathways such as renal or biliary excretion are negligible for most proteins. If biliary excretion occurs, however, it is generally followed by subsequent metabolic degradation of the compound in the gastrointestinal tract.

Proteolysis

In contrast to small-molecule drugs, metabolic degradation of peptides and therapeutic proteins by proteolysis can occur unspecifically nearly everywhere in the body. Due to this unspecific proteolysis of some proteins already in blood as well as potential active cellular uptake, the clearance of protein drugs can exceed cardiac output, i.e., >5 L/min for blood clearance and >3 L/min for plasma clearance (Meibohm 2004). The clearance of peptides or proteins in this context describes the irreversible removal of active substance

Molecular weight (kDa)	Elimination site	Predominant elimination mechanisms
<0.5	Blood, liver	Extracellular hydrolysis Passive lipoid diffusion
0.5–1	Liver	Carrier-mediated uptake Passive lipoid diffusion
1–60	Kidney	Glomerular filtration and subsequent degradation processes (see Fig. 6.4)
50–200	RES, endothelial cells (skin, muscle, gut), liver	Receptor-mediated endocytosis Pinocytosis
200–400	Immune system	Opsonization
>400	Phagocytic cells	Phagocytosis

Based on Meijer and Ziegler (1993) and Eigenmann et al. (2017)
Other determining factors are size, charge, lipophilicity, functional groups, sugar recognition, vulnerability for proteases, aggregation to particles, formation of complexes with opsonization factors, etc. As indicated, mechanisms may overlap. Endocytosis may occur at any molecular weight range; *RES* reticuloendothelial system

Table 6.1 ■ Molecular weight as major determinant of the elimination mechanisms of peptides and proteins

from the vascular space, which includes besides metabolism also cellular uptake. The metabolic rate for protein degradation generally increases with decreasing molecular weight from large to small proteins to peptides (Table 6.1), but is also dependent on other factors such as size, charge, lipophilicity, functional groups, and glycosylation pattern as well as secondary and tertiary structure.

Proteolytic enzymes such as proteases and peptidases are ubiquitous throughout the body. Sites capable of extensive peptide and protein metabolism are not only limited to the liver, kidneys, and gastrointestinal tissue, but also include blood and vascular endothelium as well as other organs and tissues. As proteases and peptidases are also located within cells, intracellular uptake is per se more an elimination rather than a distribution process (Tang and Meibohm 2006). While peptidases and proteases in the gastrointestinal tract and in lysosomes are relatively unspecific, soluble peptidases in the interstitial space and exopeptidases on the cell surface have a higher selectivity and determine the specific metabolism pattern of an organ. The proteolytic activity of subcutaneous and particularly lymphatic tissue, for example, results in a partial loss of activity of SC compared to IV administrated interferon-γ.

Gastrointestinal Protein Metabolism

As pointed out earlier, the gastrointestinal tract is a major site of protein metabolism with high proteolytic enzyme activity due to its primary function to digest dietary proteins. Thus, gastrointestinal metabolism is one of the major factors limiting systemic bioavailability of orally administered protein drugs. The metabolic activity of the gastrointestinal tract, however, is not limited to orally administered proteins. Parenterally administered peptides and proteins may also be metabolized in the intestinal mucosa following intestinal secretion. At least 20% of the degradation of endogenous albumin, for example, has been reported to take place in the gastrointestinal tract (Colburn 1991).

Renal Protein Metabolism

The kidneys are a major site of protein metabolism for smaller-sized proteins that undergo glomerular filtration. The size-selective cutoff for glomerular filtration is approximately 60 kDa, although the effective molecule radius based on molecular weight and conformation is probably the limiting factor (Edwards et al. 1999). Glomerular filtration is most efficient, however, for proteins smaller than 30 kDa (Kompella and Lee 1991). Peptides and small proteins (<5 kDa) are filtered very efficiently, and their glomerular filtration clearance approaches the glomerular filtration rate (GFR, ~120 mL/min in humans). For molecular weights exceeding 30 kDa, the filtration rate falls off sharply. In addition to size selectivity, charge selectivity has also been observed for glomerular filtration where anionic macromolecules pass through the capillary wall less readily than neutral macromolecules, which in turn pass through less readily than cationic macromolecules (Deen et al. 2001).

The importance of the kidneys as elimination organ could, for example, be shown for interleukin-2, macrophage colony-stimulating factor (M-CSF), and interferon-α (McMartin 1992; Wills and Ferraiolo 1992).

Renal metabolism of peptides and small proteins is mediated through three highly effective processes (Fig. 6.4). As a result, only minuscule amounts of intact protein are detectable in urine.

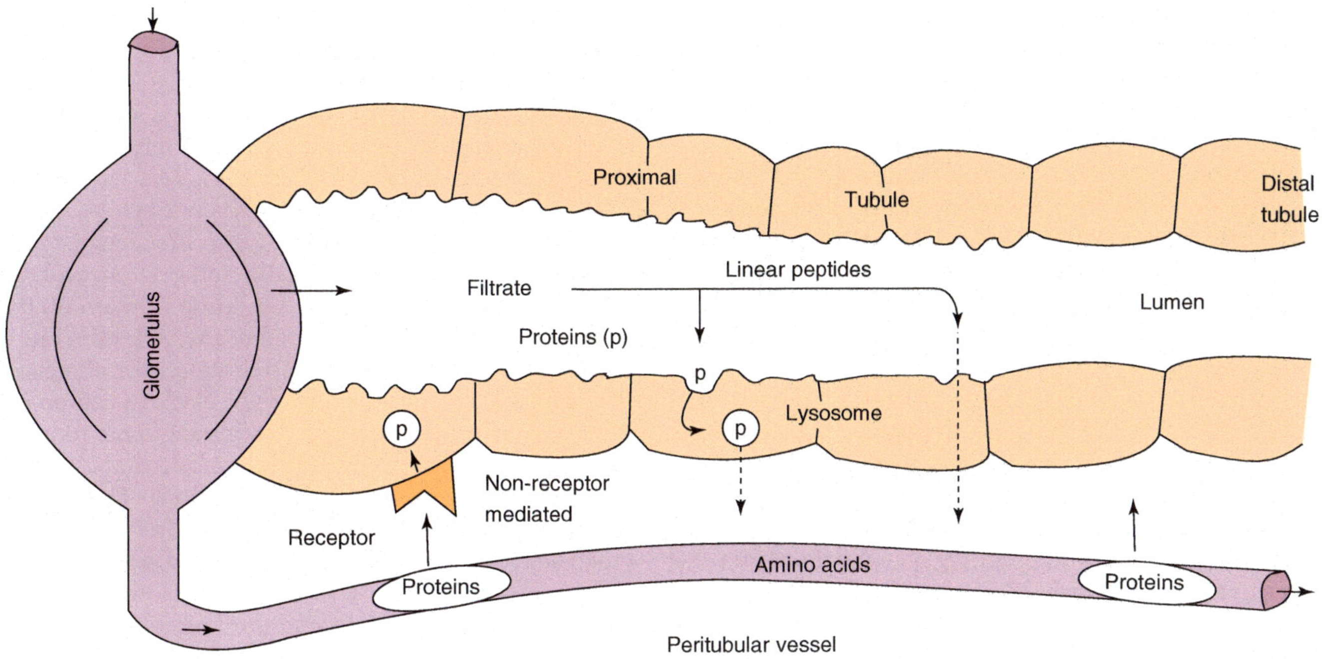

Figure 6.4 ■ Pathways of renal metabolism of peptides and proteins: glomerular filtration followed by either (1) intraluminal metabolism or (2) tubular reabsorption with intracellular lysosomal metabolism and (3) peritubular extraction with intracellular lysosomal metabolism (modified from Maack et al. 1985)

The first mechanism involves glomerular filtration of larger, complex peptides and proteins followed by reabsorption into endocytic vesicles in the proximal tubule and subsequent hydrolysis into small peptide fragments and amino acids (Maack et al. 1985). This mechanism of elimination has been described for IL-2 (Anderson and Sorenson 1994), IL-11 (Takagi et al. 1995), growth hormone (Johnson and Maack 1977), and insulin (Rabkin et al. 1984).

The second mechanism entails glomerular filtration followed by intraluminal metabolism, predominantly by exopeptidases in the luminal brush border membrane of the proximal tubule. The resulting peptide fragments and amino acids are reabsorbed into the systemic circulation. This route of disposition applies to small linear peptides such as glucagon and LH-RH (Carone and Peterson 1980; Carone et al. 1982). Recent studies implicate the proton-driven peptide transporters PEPT1 and especially PEPT2 as the main route of cellular uptake of small peptides and peptide-like drugs from the glomerular filtrate (Inui et al. 2000). These high-affinity transport proteins seem to exhibit selective uptake of di- and tripeptides, which implicates their role in renal amino acid homeostasis (Daniel and Herget 1997).

For both mechanisms, glomerular filtration is the dominant, rate-limiting step as subsequent degradation processes are not saturable under physiologic conditions (Maack et al. 1985; Colburn 1991). Under pathologic conditions or very high doses of the therapeutic protein, however, renal tubular reuptake processes may be overwhelmed, resulting in dose-dependent increases in urinary excretion of filtered proteins, as observed for the humanized monoclonal antibody Fab fragment (48 kDa) idarucizumab. The likely underlying mechanism is saturation of megalin and cubilin receptors on the apical membranes of renal tubular cells (Glund et al. 2018).

Due to this limitation of renal elimination, the renal contribution to the overall elimination of proteins is dependent on the proteolytic activity for these proteins in other body regions. If metabolic activity for these proteins is high in other body regions, there is only minor renal contribution to total clearance, and it becomes negligible in the presence of unspecific degradation throughout the body. If the metabolic activity is low in other tissues or if distribution to the extravascular space is limited, however, the renal contribution to total clearance may approach 100%.

The involvement of glomerular filtration in the renal metabolism of therapeutic proteins implies that the pharmacokinetics of therapeutic proteins below the molecular weight or hydrodynamic volume cutoff size for filtration will be affected by renal impairment. Indeed, it has been reported that the systemic exposure and elimination half-life increases with decreasing glomerular filtration rate for recombinant human interleukin-10 (18 kDa), recombinant human growth hormone (22 kDa), and the recombinant human IL-1 receptor antagonist anakinra (17.3 kDa). Consistent with these theoretical considerations is also the observation that for monoclonal antibodies (150 kDa) such as rituximab, cetuximab, bevacizumab, trastuzumab and elotuzumab, no effect of renal impairment on their disposition has been reported (Meibohm and Zhou 2012; Berdeja et al. 2016).

The third mechanism of renal metabolism is peritubular extraction of peptides and proteins from postglomerular capillaries with subsequent intracellular metabolism. Experiments using radioiodinated growth hormone (^{125}I-rGH) have demonstrated that while reabsorption into endocytic vesicles at the proximal tubule is still the dominant route of disposition, a small percentage of the hormone may be extracted from the peritubular capillaries (Krogsgaard Thomsen et al. 1994). Peritubular transport of proteins and peptides from the basolateral membrane has also been shown for insulin (Nielsen et al. 1987).

Hepatic Protein Metabolism

Aside from renal and gastrointestinal metabolism, the liver may also play a major role in the metabolism of therapeutic proteins, especially for larger proteins. Exogenous as well as endogenous proteins undergo proteolytic degradation to dipeptides and amino acids that are reused for endogenous protein synthesis. Proteolysis usually starts with endopeptidases that attack in the middle part of the protein, and the resulting oligopeptides are then further degraded by exopeptidases. The rate of hepatic metabolism is largely dependent on the specific amino acid sequence of the protein (Meibohm 2004).

The major prerequisite for hepatic protein metabolism is the uptake of proteins in the different liver cell types. Small peptides may cross the hepatocyte membrane via simple passive diffusion if they have sufficient hydrophobicity. Peptides of this nature include cyclosporin (cyclic peptide) (Ziegler et al. 1988). Other cyclic and linear peptides of small size (<1.4 kDa) and hydrophobic nature (containing aromatic amino acids), such as cholecystokinin-8 (CCK-8; 8 amino acids), are taken up by the hepatocytes by carrier-mediated transport (Ziegler et al. 1988), in the case of CCK-8 by the organic anion-transporting polypeptide OATP-8 (SLCO1B3) (Ismair et al. 2001). After internalization into the cytosol, these peptides are usually metabolized by microsomal enzymes or cytosolic peptidases.

Uptake of larger peptides and proteins can either be facilitated through pinocytosis or by receptor-mediated endocytosis. Pinocytosis is an unspecific fluid-phase endocytosis, in which molecules are taken up into cells by forming invaginations of cell membrane around extracellular fluid, that are subsequently taken up as membrane vesicles.

Receptor-mediated endocytosis is a clathrin-mediated endocytosis process via relatively unspecific, promiscuous membrane receptors (McMahon and Boucrot 2011). In receptor-mediated endocytosis, circulating proteins are recognized by specific receptor proteins. The receptors are usually integral membrane glycoproteins with an exposed binding domain on the extracellular side of the cell membrane. After the binding of the circulating protein to the receptor, the complex is already present or moves in clathrin-coated pit regions, and the membrane invaginates and pinches off to form an endocytotic coated vesicle that contains the receptor and ligand (internalization). The vesicle coat consists of proteins (clathrin, adaptin, and others), which are then removed by an uncoating adenosine triphosphatase (ATPase). The vesicle parts, the receptor, and the ligands dissociate and are targeted to various intracellular locations. Some receptors, such as the low-density lipoprotein (LDL), asialoglycoprotein, and transferrin receptors, are known to undergo recycling. Since sometimes several hundred cycles are part of a single receptor's lifetime, the associated receptor-mediated endocytosis is of high capacity. Other receptors, such as the interferon receptor, undergo degradation. This degradation leads to a decrease in the concentration of receptors on the cell surface (receptor downregulation). Others, such as insulin receptors, for example, undergo both recycling and degradation (Kompella and Lee 1991).

For glycoproteins, receptor-mediated endocytosis through sugar-recognizing C-type lectin receptors is an efficient hepatic uptake mechanism if a critical number of exposed sugar groups (mannose, galactose, fucose, N-acetylglucosamine, N-acetylgalactosamine, or glucose) is exceeded (Meijer and Ziegler 1993). Important C-type lectin receptors in the liver are the asialoglycoprotein receptor on hepatocytes and the mannose and fucose receptors on Kupffer and liver endothelial cells (Smedsrod and Einarsson 1990; Bu et al. 1992). The high-mannose glycans in the first kringle domain of t-PA, for example, have been implicated in its hepatic clearance via these receptors (Cumming 1991).

The low-density lipoprotein receptor-related protein (LRP) is a member of the LDL receptor family responsible for endocytosis of several important lipoproteins, proteases, and protease-inhibitor complexes in the liver and other tissues (Strickland et al. 1995).

Uptake of proteins by liver cells is followed by transport to an intracellular compartment for metabolism. Proteins internalized into vesicles via an endocytotic mechanism undergo intracellular transport towards the lysosomal compartment near the center of the cell. There, the endocytotic vehicles fuse with or mature into lysosomes, which are specialized acidic vesicles that contain a wide variety of hydrolases capable of degrading all biological macromolecules. Proteolysis is started by endopeptidases (mainly cathepsin D) that act on the middle part of the proteins. Oligopeptides—as the result of the first step—are further degraded by exopeptidases. The resulting amino acids and dipeptides reenter the metabolic pool of the cell. The hepatic metabolism of glycoproteins may occur more slowly than the naked protein because protecting oligosaccharide chains need to be removed first. Metabolized proteins and peptides in lysosomes from hepatocytes, hepatic sinusoidal cells, and Kupffer cells may be released into the blood. Degraded proteins in hepatocyte lysosomes can also be delivered to the bile canaliculus and excreted by exocytosis.

Besides intracellular degradation, a second intracellular pathway for proteins is the direct shuttle or transcytotic pathway (Kompella and Lee 1991). In this case, the endocytotic vesicle formed at the cell surface traverses the cell to the peribiliary space, where it fuses with the bile canalicular membrane, releasing its contents by exocytosis into bile. This pathway bypasses the lysosomal compartment completely. It has been described for polymeric immunoglobulin A but is not assumed to be a major elimination pathway for most protein drugs.

Target-Mediated Protein Metabolism

Therapeutic proteins frequently bind with high affinity to membrane-associated receptors on the cell surface if the receptors are the target structure to which the therapeutic protein is directed. This binding can lead to receptor-mediated uptake by endocytosis and subsequent intracellular lysosomal metabolism. The associated drug disposition behavior in which the binding to the pharmacodynamic target structure affects the pharmacokinetics of a drug compound is termed "target-mediated drug disposition" (Levy 1994).

For conventional small-molecule drugs, receptor binding is usually negligible compared to the total amount of drug in the body and rarely affects their pharmacokinetic profile. In contrast, a substantial fraction of a therapeutic protein can be bound to its pharmacologic target structure, for example, a receptor. Target-mediated drug disposition can affect distribution as well as elimination processes. Most notably, receptor-mediated protein metabolism is a frequently encountered elimination pathway for many therapeutic proteins (Meibohm 2004).

Receptor-mediated uptake and metabolism via interaction with these generally high-affinity, low-capacity binding sites is not limited to a specific organ or tissue type. Thus, any tissue including the therapeutically targeted cells that express receptors for the drug can contribute to the elimination of the therapeutic protein (Fig. 6.5) (Zhang and Meibohm 2012).

Since the number of protein drug receptors is limited, receptor-mediated protein metabolism can usually be saturated within therapeutic concentrations, or more specifically at relatively low molar ratios between the protein drug and the receptor (Mager 2006). As a consequence, the elimination clearance of these protein drugs is not constant but dose dependent and decreases with increasing dose. Thus, receptor-mediated elimination constitutes a major source for nonlinear pharmacokinetic behavior of numerous protein drugs, i.e., systemic exposure to the drug increases more than proportional with increasing dose (Tang et al. 2004).

Recombinant human macrophage colony-stimulating factor (M-CSF), for example, undergoes besides linear renal elimination a nonlinear elimination pathway that follows Michaelis-Menten kinetics and is linked to a receptor-mediated uptake into macrophages. At low concentrations, M-CSF follows linear pharmacokinetics, while at high concentrations nonrenal elimination pathways are saturated resulting in nonlinear pharmacokinetic behavior (Fig. 6.6) (Bauer et al. 1994).

Nonlinearity in pharmacokinetics resulting from target-mediated drug disposition has also been observed for several monoclonal antibody therapeutics, for instance for the anti-HER2 humanized monoclonal antibody trastuzumab. Trastuzumab is approved for the combination treatment of HER2 protein overexpressing metastatic breast cancer. With increasing dose level, the mean terminal half-life of trastuzumab increases and the clearance decreases, leading to overproportional increases in systemic exposure with increasing dose (Tokuda et al. 1999). Since trastuzumab is rapidly internalized via receptor-mediated endocytosis after binding to HER2, its target structure on the cell surface, saturation of this elimination pathway is the likely cause for the observed dose-dependent pharmacokinetics (Kobayashi et al. 2002).

Modulation of Protein Disposition by the FcRn Receptor

Immunoglobulin G (IgG)-based monoclonal antibodies and their derivatives as well as albumin conjugates constitute important classes of therapeutic proteins with many members currently being under development or in therapeutic use. Interaction with the neonatal Fc receptor (FcRn) constitutes a major component in the drug disposition of IgG molecules (Roopenian and Akilesh 2007). FcRn has been well-described in the transfer of passive humoral immunity from a mother to her fetus by transferring IgG

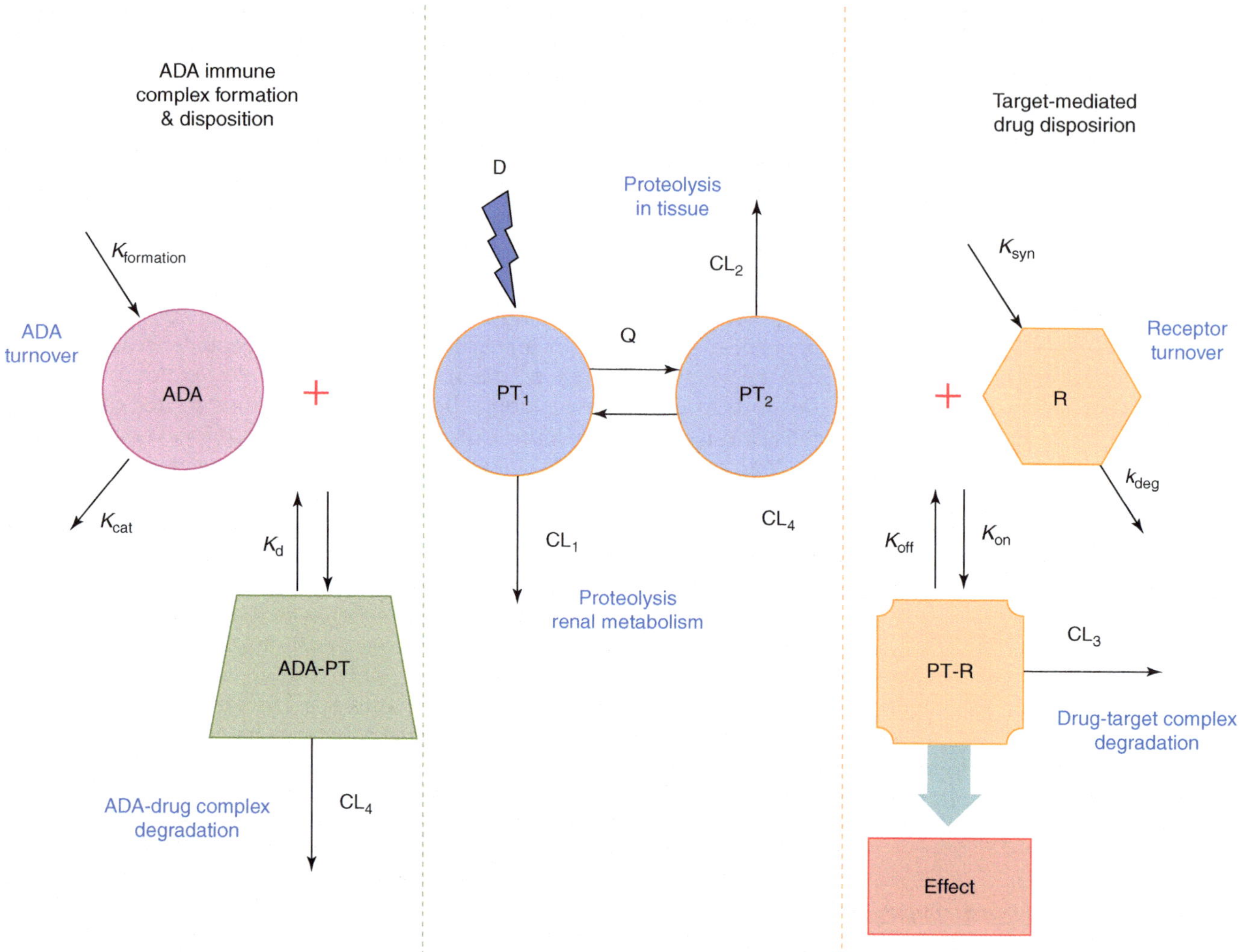

Figure 6.5 ■ Example of multiple clearance pathways affecting the pharmacokinetics of a typical therapeutic protein. Depicted is a two-compartment pharmacokinetic model with intravenous administration of a dose (*D*), concentrations of the therapeutic protein in the central (PT_1) and peripheral (PT_2) compartment, and interdepartmental clearance Q. The pharmacokinetic model includes two clearance pathways, one from the central compartment (CL_1) representative of, for example, renal metabolism or proteolytic degradation through the reticuloendothelial system and a second proteolytic degradation pathway from the peripheral compartment (CL_2) representative of, for example, proteolytic degradation through a receptor-mediated endocytosis pathway. Added to these two clearance pathways is on the right side a target-mediated disposition pathway that constitutes interaction of the therapeutic protein with its pharmacologic target receptor, which is in a homeostatic equilibrium of synthesis and degradation (synthesis rate k_{syn} and degradation rate constant k_{deg}). The dynamic equilibrium for the formation of the resulting therapeutic protein-receptor complex (*PT-R*) is determined through the association rate constant k_{on} and the dissociation rate constant k_{off}. The formation of PT-R does not only elicit the pharmacologic effect, but also triggers degradation of the complex. Thus, target binding and subsequent PT-R degradation constitute an additional clearance pathway for the therapeutic protein (CL_3). The left side of the graphic depicts the effect of an immune response to the therapeutic protein resulting in anti-drug antibody (*ADA*) formation. Again, the circulating concentration of the ADA is determined by a homeostatic equilibrium between its formation rate ($k_{formation}$) and a catabolic turnover process (rate constant k_{cat}). The ADA response results in the formation of immune complexes with the drug (*ADA-PT*). Dependent on the size and structure of the immune complexes, endogenous elimination pathways though the reticuloendothelial system may be triggered, most likely via Fcγ-mediated endocytosis. Thus, immune complex formation and subsequent degradation may constitute an additional clearance pathway (CL_4) for therapeutic proteins (from Chirmule et al. 2012)

across the placenta. More importantly, interaction with FcRn in a variety of cells, including endothelial cells and monocytes, macrophages, and other dendritic cells, protects IgG from lysosomal catabolism and thus constitutes a salvage pathway for IgG molecules that have been internalized in these cells types. This is facilitated by intercepting IgG in the endosomes and recycling it to the systemic circulation (Wang et al. 2008). The interaction with the FcRn receptor thereby prolongs the elimination half-life of

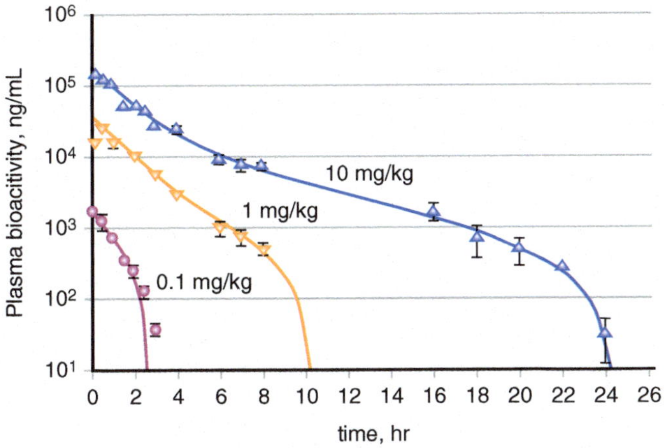

Figure 6.6 ■ Nonlinear pharmacokinetics of macrophage colony-stimulating factor (M-CSF), presented as measured (*triangles* and *circles*; mean ± SE) and modeled plasma bioactivity-time curves (*lines*) after intravenous injection of 0.1 mg/kg ($n = 5$), 1.0 mg/kg ($n = 3$), and 10 mg/kg ($n = 8$) in rats. Bioactivity is used as a substitute for concentration (from Bauer et al. 1994, with permission from American Society for Pharmacology and Experimental Therapeutics)

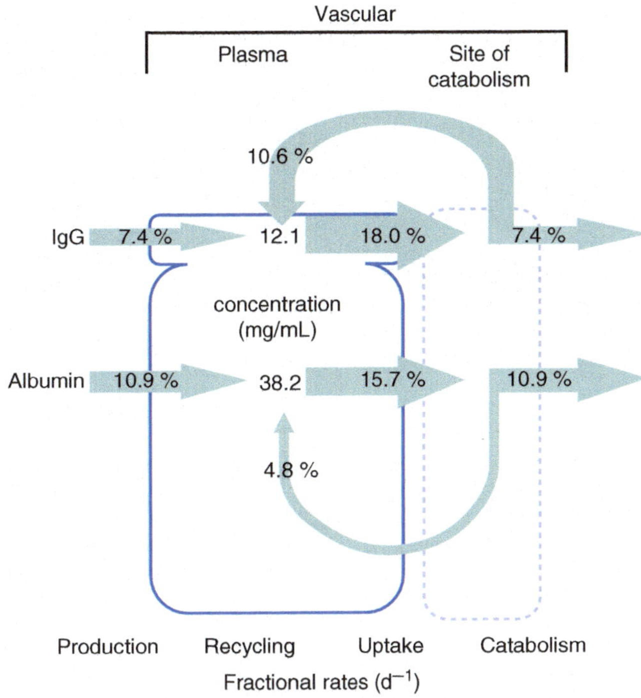

Figure 6.7 ■ Effect of FcRn-mediated recycling on IgG and albumin turnover in humans expressed as fractional rates. Shown are homeostatic plasma concentrations (12.1 and 38.2 mg/mL), fractional catabolic rates (7.4 and 10.9%/day), the FcRn-mediated fractional recycling rates (10.6 and 4.8%/day), and the fractional production rates (7.4 and 10.9%/day). The figure is to scale: areas for plasma amounts and arrow widths for rates (from Kim et al. 2007, with permission from Elsevier)

IgG, with a more pronounced effect the stronger the binding of the Fc fragment of the antibody is to the receptor: Based on the affinity of this binding interaction, human IgG1, IgG2, and IgG4 have a half-life in humans of 18–21 days, whereas the less strongly bound IgG3 has a half-life of only 7 days, and murine IgG in humans has a half-life of 1–2 days (Dirks and Meibohm 2010).

Similar to IgG, FcRn is also involved in the disposition of albumin molecules. The kinetics of IgG and albumin recycling are illustrated in Fig. 6.7. For IgG1, approximately 60% of the molecules taken up into lysosomes are recycled, for albumin 30%. As FcRn is responsible for the extended presence of IgG, albumin, and other Fc- or albumin-conjugated proteins in the systemic circulation, modulation of the interaction with FcRn allows to deliberately control the half-life of these molecules (Kim et al. 2007).

Immunogenicity and Protein Pharmacokinetics

The antigenic potential of therapeutic proteins may lead to antibody formation against the therapeutic protein during chronic therapy. This is especially of concern if animal-derived proteins are applied in human clinical studies, but also if human proteins are used in animal studies during preclinical drug development. Chapter 7 discusses in detail the phenomenon of immunogenicity and its consequences for the pharmacotherapy with therapeutic proteins.

The formation of anti-drug antibodies (ADA) against a therapeutic protein may not only modulate or even obliterate the biological activity of a protein drug, but may also modify its pharmacokinetic profile. In addition, ADA-drug complex formation may lead to immune complex-mediated toxicity, particularly if the complexes get deposited in a specific organ or tissue. Glomerulonephritis has, for example, been observed after deposition of ADA-protein drug complexes in the renal glomeruli of Cynomolgus monkeys after intramuscular administration of rhINF-γ. Similar to other circulating immune complexes, ADA-protein drug complexes may trigger the regular endogenous elimination pathways for these complexes, which consist of uptake and lysosomal degradation by the reticuloendothelial system. This process has been primarily described for the liver and the spleen and seems to be mediated by Fcγ receptors.

The ADA formation may either lead to the formation of neutralizing or non-neutralizing ADA. Neutralizing ADA bind at or near the target-binding domain of the therapeutic protein and interfere with its ability to bind to its target receptor, thereby reducing its biologic activity. Non-neutralizing ADA bind to regions of the therapeutic protein that are more distant to the target-binding domain and do not interfere with its target binding. Independent on whether

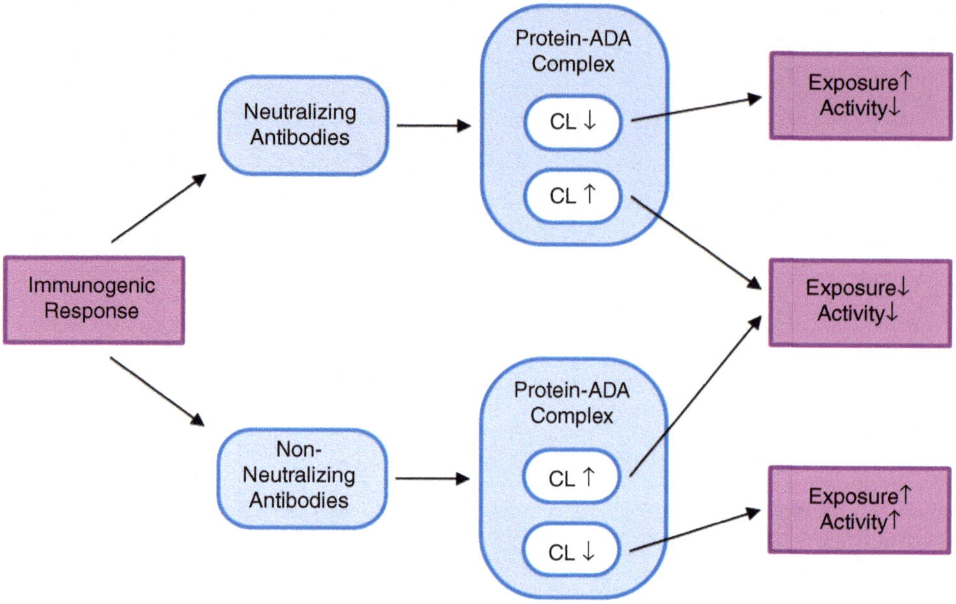

Figure 6.8 ■ Effect of anti-drug antibody (ADA) formation on the pharmacokinetics and pharmacodynamics of therapeutic proteins. *CL* clearance

ADA are neutralizing or non-neutralizing, they can both modulate the therapeutic protein's pharmacokinetics: Clearing ADA increase the clearance of the therapeutic protein, whereas sustaining ADA decrease the clearance of the therapeutic protein (Fig. 6.8). For clearing ADA, the immune complex formation triggers elimination via the reticuloendothelial system, which constitutes an additional elimination pathway for the protein (Fig. 6.5). This increase in clearance for the protein results in a decreased systemic exposure and reduced elimination half-life, which ultimately leads to reduced activity also for non-neutralizing ADA. A clearing effect of ADA is often observed for large therapeutic proteins such as monoclonal antibodies (Richter et al. 1999).

For sustaining ADA, the immune complex formation does not trigger the regular endogenous elimination processes, but serves as a storage depot for the protein, thereby reducing its clearance, increasing its systemic exposure, prolonging its half-life, and thereby increasing its activity in case of non-neutralizing ADA. This behavior has often been described for small therapeutic proteins where the immune complex formation, for example, prevents glomerular filtration and subsequent tubular metabolism. The elimination half-life of the therapeutic protein is then often increased to approach that of IgG (Chirmule et al. 2012).

Whether ADA-protein drug complex formation results in clearing or sustaining effects seems to be a function of its physicochemical and structural properties, including size, antibody class, ADA-antigen ratio, characteristics of the antigen, and location of the binding epitopes. For example, both an increased and decreased clearance is possible as ADA effect for the same protein, dependent on the dose level administered. At low doses, protein-antibody complexes delay clearance because their elimination is slower than the unbound protein. In contrast, at high doses, higher levels of protein-antibody complex result in the formation of larger aggregates, which are cleared more rapidly than the unbound protein.

The enhancement of the clearance of the cytokine interleukin-6 (IL-6) via administration of cocktails of three anti-IL-6 monoclonal antibodies was suggested as a therapeutic approach in cytokine-dependent diseases like multiple myeloma, B-cell lymphoma, and rheumatoid arthritis (Montero-Julian et al. 1995). The authors could show that, while the binding of one or two antibodies to the cytokine led to stabilization of the cytokine, simultaneous binding of three anti-IL-6 antibodies to three distinct epitopes induced rapid uptake of the complex by the liver and thus mediated a rapid elimination of IL-6 from the systemic circulation.

It should be emphasized that ADA formation is a polyclonal and usually relatively unspecific immune response to the therapeutic protein, with formation of different antibodies with variable binding affinities and epitope specificities, and that this ADA formation with its multiple-involved antibody species is different in different patients. Thus, reliable prediction of ADA formation and effects remains elusive at the current time (Chirmule et al. 2012).

The immunogenicity of therapeutic proteins is also dependent on the route of administration.

Extravascular injection is known to stimulate antibody formation more than IV application, which is most likely caused by the increased immunogenicity of protein aggregates and precipitates formed at the injection site. Further details on these aspects of immunogenicity are discussed in Chap. 7.

Species Specificity and Allometric Scaling

Peptides and proteins often exhibit distinct species specificity with regard to structure and activity. Peptides and proteins with identical physiological function may have different amino acid sequences in different species and may have no activity or be even immunogenic if used in a different species. The extent of glycosylation and/or sialylation of a protein molecule is another factor of species differences, e.g., for interferon-α or erythropoietin, which may not only alter its efficacy and immunogenicity (see Chap. 7) but also the drug's clearance.

Projecting human pharmacokinetic behavior for therapeutic proteins based on data in preclinical species is often performed using allometric approaches. Allometry is a methodology used to relate morphology and body function to the size of an organism. Allometric scaling is an empirical technique to predict body functions based on body size. Allometric scaling has found wide application in drug development, especially to predict pharmacokinetic parameters in humans based on the corresponding parameters in several animal species and the body size differences among these species and humans. Multiple allometric scaling approaches have been described with variable success rates, predominantly during the transition from preclinical to clinical drug development (Dedrick 1973; Boxenbaum 1982). In the most frequently used approach, pharmacokinetic parameters between different species are related via body weight using a power function:

$$P = a \cdot W^b$$

where P is the pharmacokinetic parameter scaled, W is the body weight in kg, a is the allometric coefficient, and b is the allometric exponent. a and b are specific constants for each parameter of a compound. General tendencies for the allometric exponent are 0.75 for clearances and flow rates, 1 for volumes of distribution, –0.25 for biologic rate constants, and 0.25 for half-lives. More recently, allometric approaches are being complemented by physiologically based pharmacokinetic modeling.

For most traditional small-molecule drugs, allometric scaling is often imprecise, especially if hepatic metabolism is a major elimination pathway and/or if there are interspecies differences in metabolism. For peptides and proteins, however, allometric scaling has frequently proven to be much more precise and reliable if their disposition is governed by relatively unspecific proteolytic degradation pathways. The reason is probably the similarity in handling peptides and proteins among different mammalian species (Wills and Ferraiolo 1992). Clearance and volume of distribution of numerous therapeutically used proteins like growth hormone or t-PA follow a well-defined, weight-dependent physiologic relationship between lab animals and humans. This allows relatively precise quantitative predictions for their pharmacokinetic behavior in humans based on preclinical findings (Mordenti et al. 1991).

Figure 6.9, for example, shows allometric plots for the clearance and volume of distribution of a

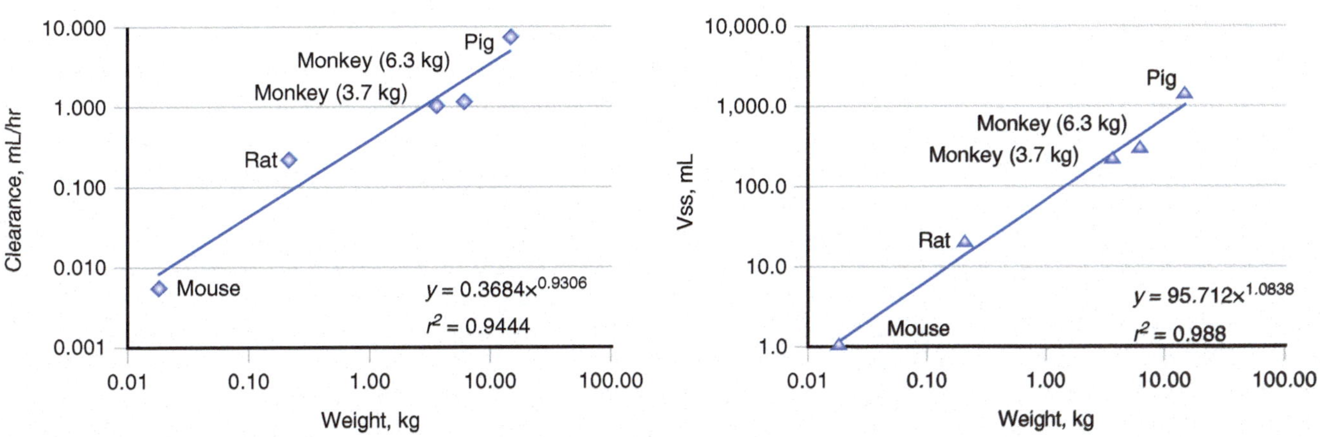

Figure 6.9 ■ Allometric plots of the pharmacokinetic parameter clearance and volume of distribution at steady state (V_{ss}) for the P-selectin antagonist rPSGL-Ig. Each data point within the plot represents an averaged value of the respective pharmacokinetic parameter in one of five species: mouse, rat, monkey (3.7 kg), monkey (6.3 kg), and pig, respectively. The *solid line* is the best fit with a power function to relate pharmacokinetic parameters to body weight (Khor et al. 2000; with permission from American Society for Pharmacology and Experimental Therapeutics)

P-selectin antagonist, P-selectin glycoprotein ligand-1, for the treatment of P-selectin-mediated diseases such as thrombosis, reperfusion injury, and deep vein thrombosis. The protein's human pharmacokinetic parameters could accurately be predicted using allometric power functions based on data from four species: mouse, rat, monkey, and pig (Khor et al. 2000).

Recent work on scaling the pharmacokinetics of monoclonal antibodies has suggested that allometric scaling from one nonhuman primate species, in this case the Cynomolgus monkey, using an allometric exponent of 0.85 might be superior to traditional allometric scaling approaches (Deng et al. 2011).

In any case, successful allometric scaling seems so far largely limited to unspecific protein elimination pathways. Once interactions with specific receptors are involved in drug disposition, for example, in receptor-mediated processes or target-mediated drug disposition, then allometric approaches oftentimes have large prediction error margins or even fail to scale drug disposition of therapeutic proteins across species due to differences in binding affinity and specificity, as well as expression and turnover kinetics of the involved receptors and targets in different species. In this situation, it becomes especially important to only consider for scaling preclinical pharmacokinetic data from "relevant" animal species for which the therapeutic protein shows cross-reactivity between animal and human receptors or targets. Dong et al. (2011) provided practical examples how unspecific and receptor-mediated elimination pathways for the same therapeutic protein can independently be scaled to improve human clearance predictions.

It needs to be emphasized that allometric scaling techniques are useful tools for predicting a dose that will assist in the planning of dose-ranging studies, including first-in-man studies, but are not a replacement for such studies. The advantage of including such dose prediction in the protocol design of dose-ranging studies is that a smaller number of doses need to be tested before finding the final dose level. Interspecies dose predictions simply narrow the range of doses in the initial pharmacological efficacy studies, the animal toxicology studies, and the human safety and efficacy studies. More recently, physiologically–based pharmacokinetic modeling has become more widely used to make more mechanistically based and accurate predictions of human pharmacokinetic behavior of therapeutic proteins (Diao and Meibohm 2015; Glassman and Balthasar 2016).

Chemical Modifications for Optimizing the Pharmacokinetics of Therapeutic Proteins

In recent years, approaches modifying the molecular structure of therapeutic proteins have repeatedly been applied to affect the immunogenicity, pharmacokinetics, and/or pharmacodynamics of protein drugs (Kontermann 2012). These approaches include the addition, deletion, or exchange of selected amino acids within the protein's sequence, synthesis of truncated proteins with a reduced amino acid sequence, glycosylation or deglycosylation, and covalent linkage to polymers (Veronese and Caliceti 2006). The latter approach has been used for several therapeutic proteins by linking them to monomethoxy polyethylene glycol (PEG) molecules of various chain lengths in a process called PEGylation (Caliceti and Veronese 2003).

The conjugation of high polymeric mass to protein drugs is generally aimed at preventing the protein being recognized by the immune system as well as reducing its elimination via glomerular filtration or proteolytic enzymes, thereby prolonging the oftentimes relatively short elimination half-life of endogenous proteins. Conjugation of protein drugs with PEG chains increases their molecular weight, but because of the attraction of water molecules by PEG even more their hydrodynamic volume, this in turn results in a reduced renal clearance and restricted volume of distribution. PEGylation can also shield antigenic determinants on the protein drug from detection by the immune system through steric hindrance (Walsh et al. 2003). Similarly, amino acid sequences sensitive towards proteolytic degradation may be shielded against protease attack. By adding a large, hydrophilic molecule to the protein, PEGylation can also increase drug solubility (Molineux 2003).

PEGylation has been used to improve the therapeutic properties of numerous therapeutic proteins including interferon-α, asparaginase, and filgrastim. More details on the general concept of PEGylation and its specific application for therapeutic proteins can be found in Chap. 27.

The therapeutic application of L-asparaginase in the treatment of acute lymphoblastic leukemia has been hampered by its strong immunogenicity with allergic reactions occurring in 33–75% of treated patients in various studies. The development of pegaspargase, a PEGylated form of L-asparaginase, is a successful example for overcoming this high rate of allergic reactions towards L-asparaginase using PEG conjugation techniques (Graham 2003). Pegaspargase is well-tolerated compared to L-asparaginase, with 3–10% of the treated patients experiencing clinical allergic reactions.

Pegfilgrastim is the PEGylated version of the granulocyte colony-stimulating factor filgrastim, which is administered for the management of chemotherapy-induced neutropenia. PEGylation minimizes filgrastim's renal clearance by glomerular filtration, thereby making neutrophil-mediated clearance

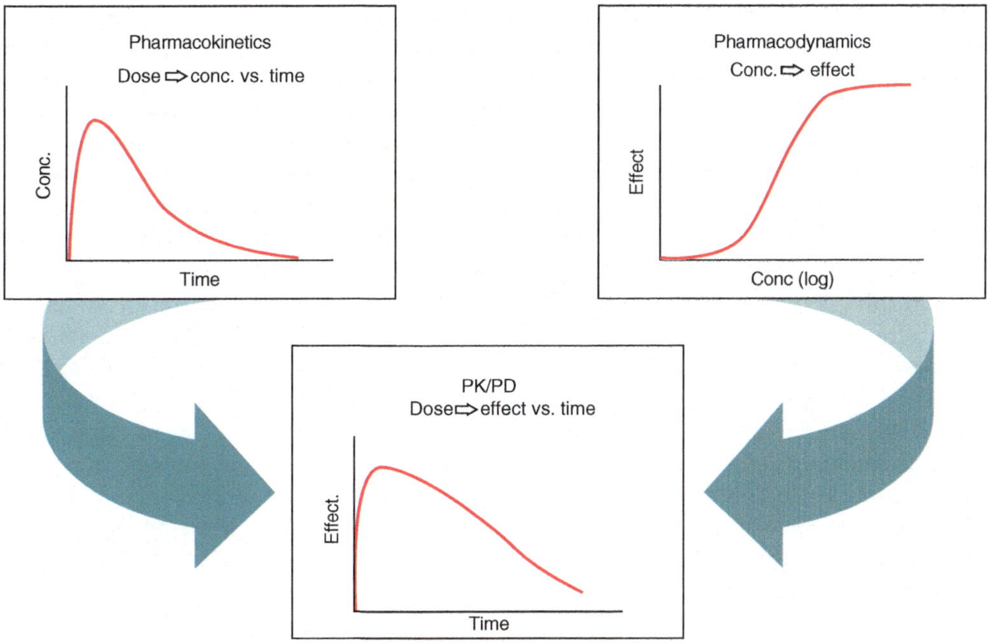

Figure 6.10 ■ General concept of PK/PD modeling. Pharmacokinetic-pharmacodynamic (PK/PD) modeling combines a pharmacokinetic model component that describes the time course of drug in plasma and a pharmacodynamic model component that relates the plasma concentration to the drug effect in order to describe the time course of the effect intensity resulting from the administration of a certain dosage regimen (from Derendorf and Meibohm 1999)

the predominant route of elimination. Thus, PEGylation of filgrastim results in so-called self-regulating pharmacokinetics since pegfilgrastim has a reduced clearance and thus prolonged half-life and more sustained duration of action in a neutropenic compared to a normal patient because only few mature neutrophils are available to mediate its elimination (Zamboni 2003).

The hematopoietic growth factor darbepoetin-α is an example of a chemically modified endogenous protein with altered glycosylation pattern. It is a glycosylation analogue of human erythropoietin, with two additional N-linked oligosaccharide chains (five in total) (Mould et al. 1999). The additional N-glycosylation sites were made available through substitution of five amino acid residues in the peptide backbone of erythropoietin, thereby increasing the molecular weight from 30 to 37 kDa. Darbepoetin-α has a substantially modified pharmacokinetic profile compared to erythropoietin, resulting in a threefold longer serum half-life that allows for reduced dosing frequency. More details on hematopoietic growth factors, including erythropoietin and darbepoetin-α, are provided in Chap. 24.

PHARMACODYNAMICS OF THERAPEUTIC PROTEINS

Therapeutic proteins are usually highly potent compounds with steep dose-effect curves as they are targeted therapies towards a specific, well-described pharmacologic structure or mechanism. Thus, a careful characterization of the concentration-effect relationship, i.e., the pharmacodynamics, is especially desirable for therapeutic proteins (Tabrizi and Roskos 2006). Combination of pharmacodynamics with pharmacokinetics by integrated pharmacokinetic-pharmacodynamic modeling (PK/PD modeling) adds an additional level of complexity that allows furthermore characterization of the dose-exposure-response relationship of a drug and a continuous description of the time course of effect intensity directly resulting from the administration of a certain dosage regimen (Fig. 6.10) (Meibohm and Derendorf 1997; Derendorf and Meibohm 1999).

PK/PD modeling is a technique that combines the two classical pharmacologic disciplines of pharmacokinetics and pharmacodynamics. It integrates a pharmacokinetic and a pharmacodynamic model component into one set of mathematical expressions that allows the description of the time course of effect intensity in response to administration of a drug dose. This so-called integrated PK/PD model allows deriving pharmacokinetic and pharmacodynamic model parameters that characterize the dose-concentration-effect relationship for a specific drug based on measured concentration and effect data. In addition, it allows simulation of the time course of effect intensity for dosage regimens of a drug beyond actually measured data, within the constraints of the validity of the model assumptions for the simulated condition. Addition of a statistical model component describing inter- and intraindividual variation in model parameters allows expanding PK/PD models to describe time courses of effect intensity not only for individual subjects, but also for whole populations of subjects.

Integrated pharmacokinetic-pharmacodynamic (PK/PD) modeling approaches have widely been applied for the characterization of therapeutic proteins (Tabrizi and Roskos 2006). Embedded in a model-informed drug development paradigm, modeling and simulation based on integrated PK/PD does not only provide a comprehensive summary of the available data, but also enables to test competing hypotheses regarding processes altered by the drug, allows making predictions of drug effects under new conditions, and facilitates to estimate inaccessible system variables (Meibohm and Derendorf 1997; Mager et al. 2003).

Mechanism-based PK/PD modeling appreciating the physiological events involved in the elaboration of the observed effect has been promoted as superior modeling approach as compared to empirical modeling, especially because it does not only describe observations but also offers some insight into the underlying biological processes involved and thus provides flexibility in extrapolating the model to other clinical situations (Levy 1994; Derendorf and Meibohm 1999; Suryawanshi et al. 2010). Since the molecular mechanism of action of a therapeutic protein is generally well-understood, it is often straightforward to transform this available knowledge into a mechanism-based PK/PD modeling approach that appropriately characterizes the real physiological process leading to the drug's therapeutic effect.

The relationship between exposure and response may be either simple or complex, and thus obvious or hidden. However, if no simple relationship is obvious, it would be misleading to conclude a priori that no relationship exists at all rather than that it is not readily apparent (Levy 1986).

The application of PK/PD modeling is beneficial in all phases of preclinical and clinical drug development and has been endorsed by the pharmaceutical industry, academia, and regulatory agencies (Peck et al. 1994; Lesko et al. 2000; Sheiner and Steimer 2000; Meibohm and Derendorf 2002; Lesko 2007). Thus, PK/PD concepts and model-based drug development play a pivotal role especially in the drug development process for biologics, and their widespread application supports a scientifically driven, evidence-based, and focused product development for therapeutic proteins (Zhang et al. 2008; Mould and Meibohm 2016).

While a variety of PK/PD modeling approaches has been employed for biologics, we will in the following focus on five classes of approaches to illustrate the challenges and complexities, but also opportunities to characterize the pharmacodynamics of therapeutic proteins:

- Direct link PK/PD models
- Indirect link PK/PD models
- Indirect response PK/PD models
- Cell life span models
- Complex response models

It should not be unmentioned, however, that PK/PD models for therapeutic proteins are not only limited to continuous responses as shown in the following, but are also used for binary or graded responses. Binary responses are responses with only two outcome levels where a condition is either present or absent, e.g., dead versus alive. Graded or categorical responses have a set of predefined outcome levels, which may or may not be ordered, for example, the categories "mild," "moderate," and "severe" for a disease state. Lee et al. (2003), for example, used a logistic PK/PD modeling approach to link cumulative AUC of the anti-TNF-α protein etanercept with a binary response, the American College of Rheumatology response criterion of 20% improvement (ARC20) in patients with rheumatoid arthritis.

Direct Link PK/PD Models

The concentration of a therapeutic protein is usually only quantified in plasma, serum, or blood, while the magnitude of the observed response is determined by the concentration of the protein drug at its effect site, the site of action in the target tissue (Meibohm and Derendorf 1997). Effect site concentrations, however, are usually not accessible for measurement, and plasma, serum, or blood concentrations are usually used as their substitute. The relationship between the drug concentration in plasma and at the effect site may either be constant or undergo time-dependent changes. If equilibrium between both concentrations is rapidly achieved or the site of action is within plasma, serum, or blood, there is practically a constant relationship between both concentrations with no temporal delay between plasma and effect site. In this case, measured plasma concentrations can directly serve as input for a pharmacodynamic model (Fig. 6.11). The most frequently used direct link pharmacodynamic model is a sigmoid E_{max} model:

$$E = \frac{E_{max} \cdot C^n}{EC_{50}^n + C^n}$$

with E_{max} as maximum achievable effect, C as drug concentration in plasma, and EC_{50} the concentration of the drug that produces half of the maximum effect. The Hill coefficient n is an empirical shape factor that allows for an improved fit of the relationship to the observed data. As represented by the equation for the sigmoid E_{max} model, a direct link model directly connects measured concentration to the observed effect without any temporal delay (Derendorf and Meibohm 1999).

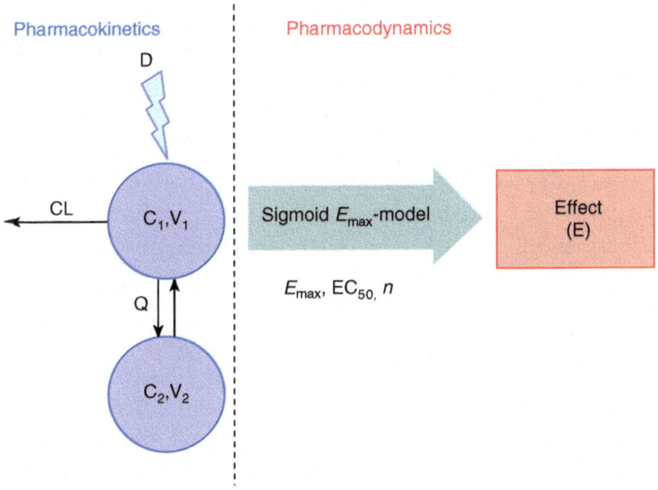

Figure 6.11 ■ Schematic of a typical direct link PK/PD model. The PK model is a typical two-compartment model with a linear elimination clearance from the central compartment (*CL*) and a distributional clearance (*Q*). C_1 and C_2 are the concentrations in the central and peripheral compartments, and V_1 and V_2 are their respective volumes of distribution. The effect (*E*) is directly linked to the concentration in the central compartment C_1 via a sigmoid E_{max} model. The sigmoid E_{max} relationship is characterized by the pharmacodynamic parameters E_{max}, the maximum achievable effect, EC_{50}, the concentration of the drug that produced half of the maximum effect, and the Hill coefficient *n* as via the sigmoid E_{max} equation

A direct link model was, for example, used to relate the serum concentration of the antihuman immunoglobulin E (IgE) antibody CGP 51901 for the treatment of seasonal allergic rhinitis to the reduction of free IgE via an inhibitory E_{max} model (Fig. 6.12) (Racine-Poon et al. 1997). It should be noted that the peak and trough concentrations and effects are directly related and thus occur at the same times, respectively, without time delay. Similarly, a direct link model was used to relate the effect of recombinant interleukin-10 (IL-10) on the ex vivo release of the pro-inflammatory cytokines TNF-α and interleukin-1β in LPS-stimulated leukocytes (Radwanski et al. 1998). In the first case, the site of action and the sampling site for concentration measurements of the therapeutic protein were identical, i.e., in plasma, and so the direct link model was mechanistically well justified. In the second case, the effect was dependent on the IL-10 concentration on the cell surface of leukocytes where IL-10 interacts with its target receptor. Again sampling fluid and effect site were in instant equilibrium.

■ Indirect Link PK/PD Models

The concentration-effect relationship of many protein drugs, however, cannot be described by direct link PK/PD models, but is characterized by a temporal dissociation between the time courses of plasma concentration and effect. In this case, plasma concentration maxima occur before effect maxima; effect intensity may increase despite decreasing plasma concentrations and may persist beyond the time when drug concentrations in plasma are no longer detectable. The relationship between measured concentration and observed effect follows a counterclockwise hysteresis loop. This phenomenon can either be caused by an indirect response

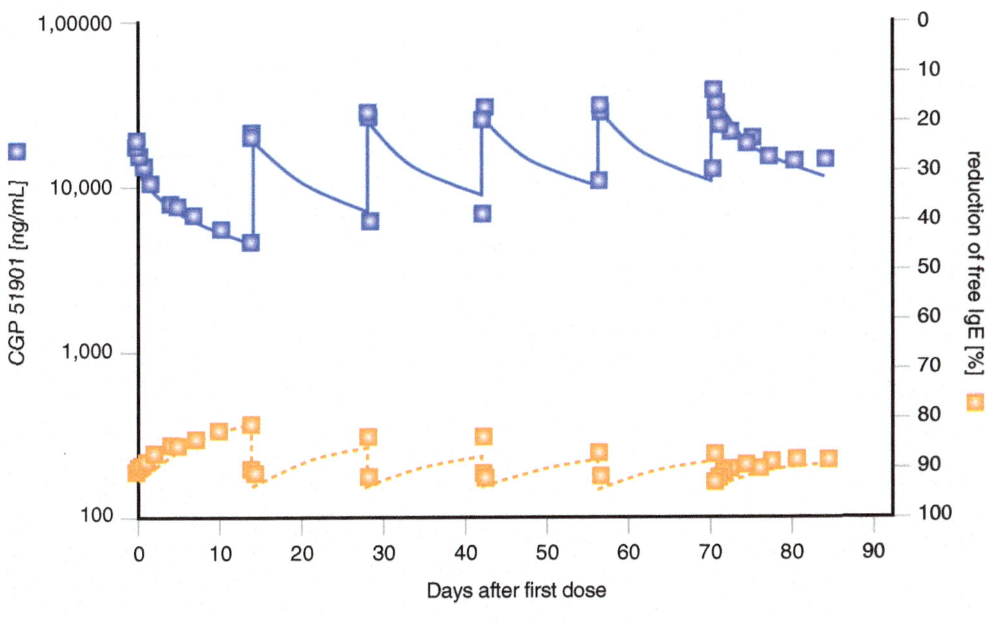

Figure 6.12 ■ Observed (Blue square) and model-predicted (Blue solid line) serum concentration of the antihuman IgE antibody CGP 51901 and observed (Orange square) and model-predicted (Orange dashed line) reduction of free IgE in one representative patient, given six IV doses of 60 mg biweekly. The predictions were modeled with a direct link PK/PD model (modified from Racine-Poon et al. 1997; with permission from Macmillan Publishers Ltd.)

mechanism (see section "Indirect Response PK/PD Models") or by a distributional delay between the drug concentrations in plasma and at the effect site.

The latter one can conceptually be described by an indirect link model, which attaches a hypothetical effect compartment to a pharmacokinetic compartment model (Fig. 6.13). The effect compartment addition to the pharmacokinetic model does not account for mass balance, i.e., no actual mass transfer is implemented in the pharmacokinetic part of the PK/PD model. Instead, drug transfer with respect to the effect compartment is defined by the time course of the effect itself (Sheiner et al. 1979; Holford and Sheiner 1982). The effect-compartment approach, however, is necessary, as the effect site can be viewed as a small part of a pharmacokinetic compartment that from a pharmacokinetic point of view cannot be distinguished from other tissues within that compartment. The concentration in the effect compartment represents the active drug concentration at the effect site that is slowly equilibrating with the plasma and is usually linked to the effect via an E_{max} model.

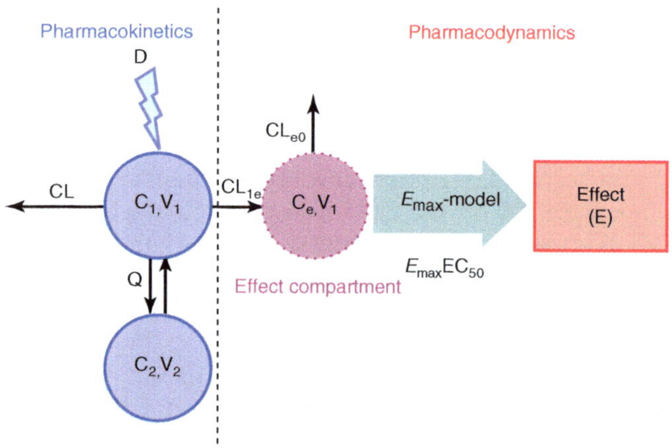

Figure 6.13 Schematic of a typical indirect link PK/PD model. A hypothetical effect compartment is linked to the central compartment of a two-compartment pharmacokinetic model. The concentration in the effect compartment (C_e) drives the intensity of the pharmacodynamic effect (E) via an E_{max} relationship. CL_{1e} is the transfer clearance from the central to the effect compartment, CL_{e0} the equilibrium clearance for the effect compartment. All other PK and PD parameters are identical to those used in Fig. 6.11

Although this PK/PD model is constructed with tissue distribution as the reason for the delay of the effect, the distribution clearance to the effect compartment can be interpreted differently, including other reasons of delay, such as transduction processes and secondary post-receptor events.

Human regular U-500 insulin has recently been developed for insulin-resistant and high-dose insulin-treated patients to provide the ability of administering large doses (500 U/mL) at one-fifth the volume of that of the previously highest concentrated dosage form, human regular U-100 insulin. In order to explore the effect-time course after administration of once-daily, twice-daily and thrice-daily administration of U-500 insulin, a PK/PD model was developed based on single dose euglycemic clamp studies in healthy individuals and patients with type I diabetes. Insulin concentrations were related to glucose infusion rate as measure of pharmacodynamic effect via an effect compartment model (de la Peña et al. 2014). Model-based simulations of the different administration frequencies at steady state (Fig. 6.14) suggest that BID and TID dosing may

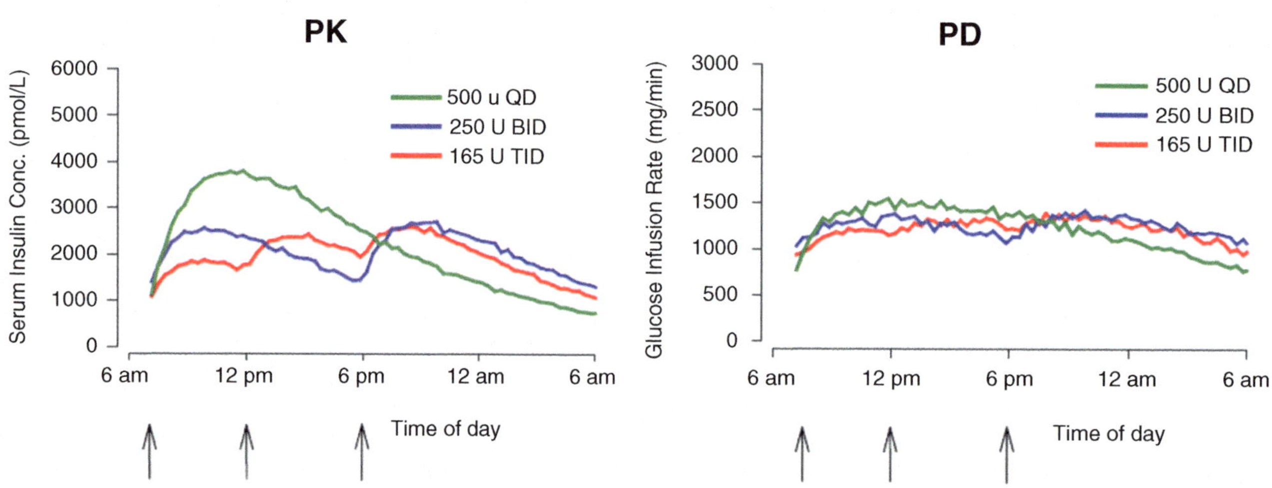

Figure 6.14 PK/PD model-based simulations of different dosing regimens of U-500 insulin during 24 h at steady-state: 500 U QD (*green*), 250 U BID (*blue*), 165 U TID (*red*). Arrows represent dose administration times: for QD at 7 am, BID at 7 am and 6 pm, and TID at 7 am, 12 noon, and 6 pm. The PK panel on the left shows the resulting serum insulin concentration-time profiles, the PD panel on the right side the time course of the glucose infusion rate needed to maintain euglycemia (from de la Peña et al. 2014)

provide adequate insulin action throughout the day, but QD dosing leads to fluctuations in effect that may increase the risk for hypoglycemia and may thus not be adequate for use as basal insulin therapy.

■ Indirect Response PK/PD Models

The effect of most therapeutic proteins, however, is not mediated via a direct interaction between drug concentration at the effect site and response systems but frequently involves several transduction processes that include at their rate-limiting step the stimulation or inhibition of a physiologic process, for example the synthesis or degradation of a molecular response mediator like a hormone or cytokine. In these cases, the time courses of plasma concentration and effect are also dissociated resulting in counterclockwise hysteresis for the concentration-effect relationship, but the underlying cause is not a distributional delay as for the indirect link models, but a time-consuming indirect response mechanism (Meibohm and Derendorf 1997).

Indirect response models generally describe the effect on a representative response parameter via the dynamic equilibrium between increase or synthesis and decrease or degradation of the response, with the former being a zero-order and the latter a first-order process (Fig. 6.15). The response itself can be modulated in one of four basic variants of the model. In each variant, the synthesis or degradation process of the response is either stimulated or inhibited as a function of the drug concentration. A stimulatory or inhibitory E_{max} model is used to describe the drug effect on the synthesis or degradation of the response (Dayneka et al. 1993; Sharma and Jusko 1998; Sun and Jusko 1999).

As indirect response models appreciate the underlying physiological events involved in the elaboration of the observed drug effect, their application is often preferred in PK/PD modeling as they have a mechanistic basis on the molecular and/or cellular level that often allows for extrapolating the model to other clinical situations.

An indirect response model was, for example, used in the evaluation of SB-240563, a humanized monoclonal antibody directed towards IL-5 in monkeys (Zia-Amirhosseini et al. 1999). IL-5 appears to play a significant role in the production, activation, and maturation of eosinophils. The delayed effect of SB-240563 on eosinophils is consistent with its mechanism of action via binding to and thus inactivation of IL-5. It was modeled using an indirect response model with inhibition of the production of response (eosinophil count) (Fig. 6.16). The obtained low EC_{50} value for reduction of circulating eosinophils combined with a long terminal half-life of the therapeutic protein of 13 days suggests the possibility of an infrequent dosing regimen for SB-240563 in the pharmacotherapy of disorders with increased eosinophil function, such as asthma.

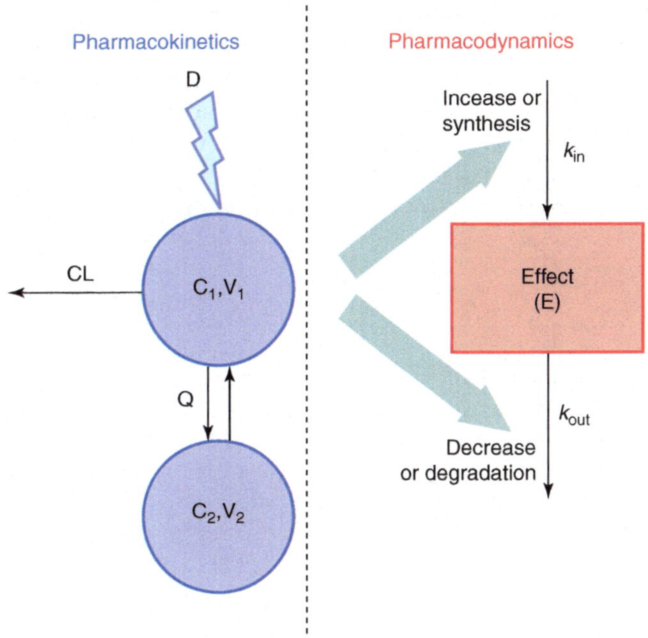

Indirect response model subtypes

Subtype I: inhibition of synthesis (k_{in})

$$\frac{dE}{dt} = k_{in} \cdot \left(1 - \frac{C_1}{EC_{50} + C_1}\right) - k_{out} \cdot E$$

Subtype II: inhibition of degradation (k_{out})

$$\frac{dE}{dt} = k_{in} - k_{out} \cdot \left(1 - \frac{C_1}{EC_{50} + C_1}\right) \cdot E$$

Subtype III: stimulation of synthesis (k_{in})

$$\frac{dE}{dt} = k_{in} \cdot \left(1 + \frac{E_{max} \cdot C_1}{EC_{50} + C_1}\right) - k_{out} \cdot E$$

Subtype IV: stimulation of degradation (k_{out})

$$\frac{dE}{dt} = k_{in} - k_{out} \cdot \left(1 + \frac{E_{max} \cdot C_1}{EC_{50} + C_1}\right) \cdot E$$

Figure 6.15 ■ Schematic of a typical indirect response PK/PD model. The effect measure (E) is maintained by a dynamic equilibrium between an increase or synthesis and a decrease or degradation process. The former is modeled by a zero-order process with rate constant k_{in}, the latter by a first-order process with rate constant k_{out}. Thus, the rate of change in effect (dE/dt) is expressed as the difference between synthesis rate (k_{in}) and degradation rate (k_{out} times E). Drug concentration (C_1) can stimulate or inhibit the synthesis or the degradation process for the effect (E) via an E_{max} relationship using one of four subtypes (model I, II, III or IV) of the indirect response model. The pharmacokinetic model and all other PK and PD parameters are identical to those used in Fig. 6.11

Indirect response models were also used for the effect of growth hormone on endogenous IGF-1 concentration (Sun et al. 1999), as well as the effect of epoetin-α on two response parameters, free ferritin concentration and soluble transferrin receptor concentration (Bressolle et al. 1997). Similarly, a modified indirect response model was used to relate the concentration of the humanized anti-factor IX antibody SB-249417 to factor IX activity in Cynomolgus monkeys as well as humans (Benincosa et al. 2000; Chow et al. 2002). The drug effect in this model was introduced by interrupting the natural degradation of factor IX by sequestration of factor IX by the antibody.

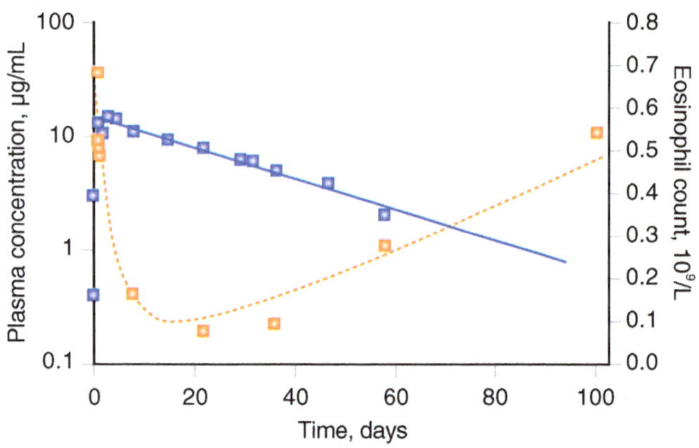

Figure 6.16 ■ Model-predicted and observed plasma concentration (observed, *blue circles*; predicted, *solid blue line*) and eosinophil count (observed, *orange squares*; predicted, *dashed orange line*) following SC administration of 1 mg/kg of the anti-IL-5 humanized monoclonal antibody SB-240563 in a Cynomolgus monkey. A mechanism-based indirect response PK/PD model was used to describe eosinophil count as a function of SB-240563 plasma concentration. The reduction in eosinophil count in peripheral blood (as effect *E*) was modeled as a reduction of the recruitment of eosinophils from the bone, i.e., an inhibition of the production rate k_{in} using the indirect response model of subtype I (see Fig. 6.15) (Zia-Amirhosseini et al. 1999; with permission from American Society for Pharmacology and Experimental Therapeutics)

■ Cell Life Span Models

A sizable number of therapeutic proteins exert their pharmacologic effect through direct or indirect modulation of blood and/or immune cell types. For these kinds of therapeutics, cell life span models have been proven useful to capture their exposure-response relationship and describe and predict drug effects (Perez-Ruixo et al. 2005). Cell life span models are mechanism-based, physiologic PK/PD models that are established based on the sequential maturation and life span-driven cell turnover of their affected cell types and progenitor cell populations. Cell life span models are especially widely used for characterizing the dose-concentration-effect relationships of hematopoietic growth factors aimed at modifying erythropoiesis, granulopoiesis, or thrombopoiesis (Perez-Ruixo et al. 2005; Agoram et al. 2006). The fixed physiologic time span for the maturation of precursor cells is the major reason for the prolonged delay between drug administration and the observed response, i.e., change in the cell count in peripheral blood. Cell life span models accommodate this sequential maturation of several precursor cell populations at fixed physiologic time intervals by a series of transit compartments linked via first- or zero-order processes with a common transfer rate constant.

A cell life span model was, for example, used to describe the effect of a multiple dose regimen of erythropoietin (EPO) 600 IU/kg given once weekly by SC injection (Ramakrishnan et al. 2004). The process of erythropoiesis and the applied PK/PD approach including a cell life span model are depicted in Figs. 6.17

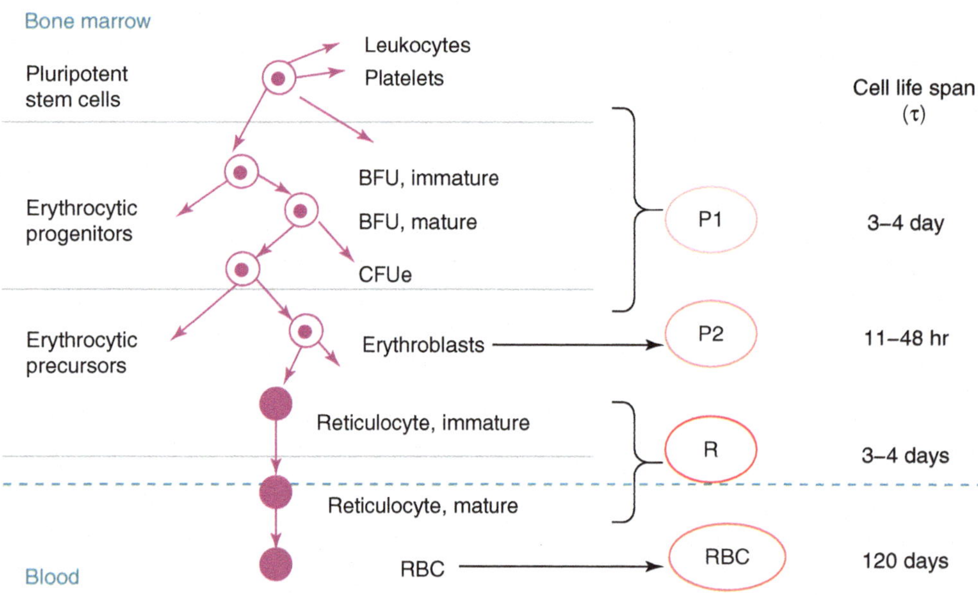

Figure 6.17 ■ Process of erythropoiesis. Erythropoietin stimulates the proliferation and differentiation of the erythrocyte progenitors (*BFU* burst-forming unit erythroid, *CFUe* colony-forming unit erythroid) as well as the erythroblasts in the bone marrow. The life spans (τ) of the various cell populations are indicated at the right (from Ramakrishnan et al. 2004, with permission from John Wiley & Sons, Inc. Copyright American College of Clinical Pharmacology 2004)

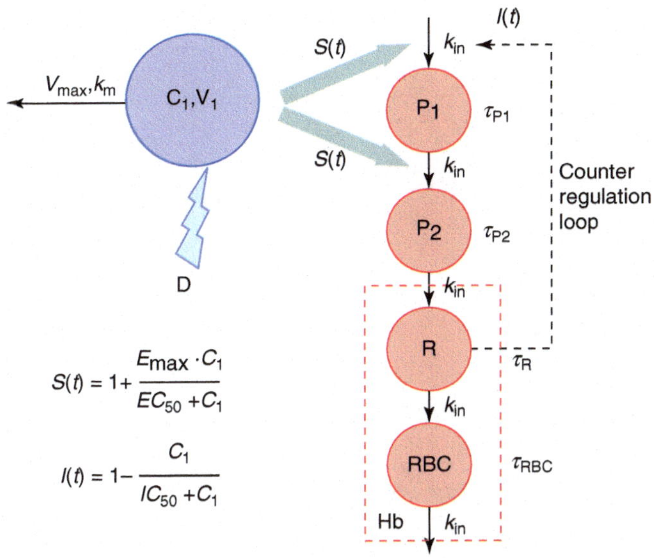

Figure 6.18 ■ A PK/PD model describing the disposition of recombinant human erythropoietin and effects on reticulocyte count, red blood cell count, and hemoglobin concentration. The PK model is a one-compartment model with Michaelis-Menten type elimination (K_m, V_{max}) from the central compartment. The PD model is a cell life span model with four sequential cell compartments, representing erythroid progenitor cells (P_1), erythroblasts (P_2), reticulocytes (*R*), and red blood cells (*RBC*). τ_{P1}, τ_{P2}, τ_R, and τ_{RBC} are the corresponding cell life spans, k_{in} the common zero-order transfer rate between cell compartments. The target parameter hemoglobin in the blood (*Hb*) is calculated from the reticulocyte and red blood cell count and the hemoglobin content per cell. The effect of erythropoietin is modeled as a stimulation of the production of both precursor cell populations (P_1 and P_2) in the bone marrow with the stimulation function *S*(*t*). E_{max} is the maximum possible stimulation of reticulocyte production by erythropoietin, EC_{50} the plasma concentration of erythropoietin that produced half-maximum stimulation. A counter-regulatory feedback loop represents the feedback inhibition of reticulocytes on their own production by reducing the production rate of cells in the P_1 compartment via the inhibitory function *I*(*t*). IC_{50} is the reticulocyte count that produced half of complete inhibition (modified from Ramakrishnan et al. 2004)

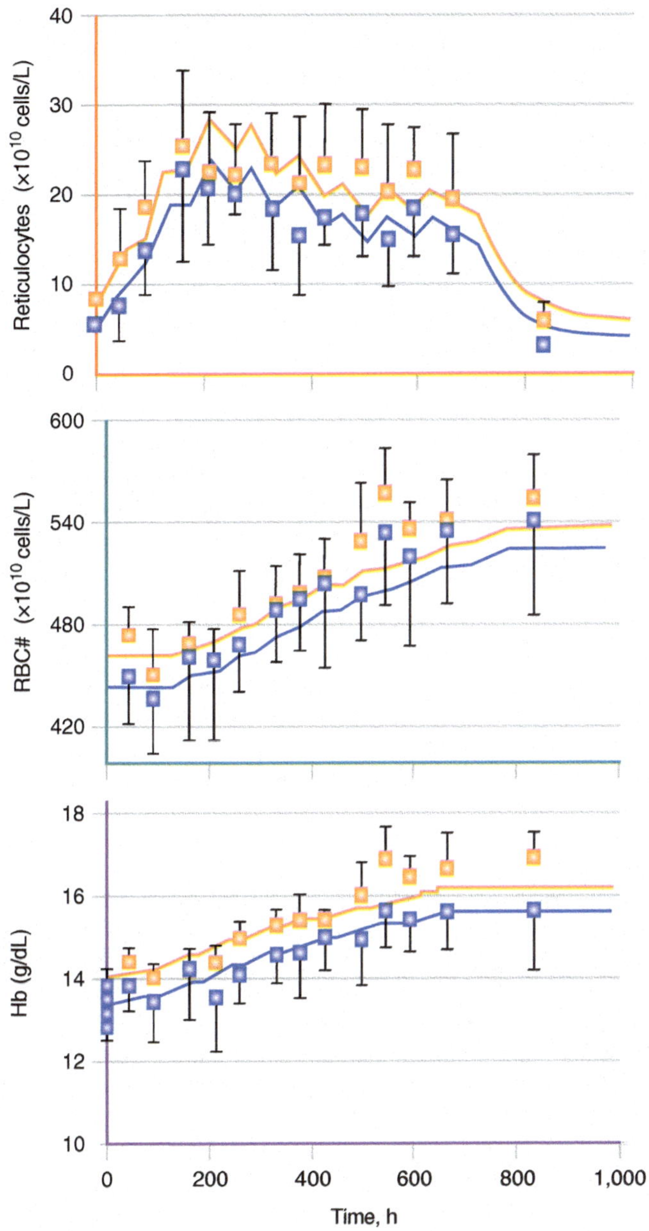

Figure 6.19 Reticulocyte, red blood cell (*RBC*), and hemoglobin (*Hb*) time courses after multiple SC dosing of 600 IU/kg/week recombinant human erythropoietin. *Orange* and *blue squares* represent data for males and females, whereas the *orange* and *blue lines* for the reticulocytes are model fittings. The *lines* in the RBC and Hb panels are the predictions using the model-fitted curves for the reticulocytes and the life span parameters (from Ramakrishnan et al. 2004, with permission from John Wiley & Sons, Inc. Copyright American College of Clinical Pharmacology 2004)

and 6.18, respectively. EPO is known to stimulate the production and release of reticulocytes from the bone marrow. The EPO effect was modeled as stimulation of the maturation of two progenitor cell populations (P1 and P2 in Fig. 6.17), including also a feedback inhibition between erythrocyte count and progenitor proliferation. Development and turnover of the subsequent populations of reticulocytes and erythrocytes was modeled, taking into account their life spans as listed in Fig. 6.17. The hemoglobin concentration as pharmacodynamic target parameter was calculated from erythrocyte and reticulocyte counts and hemoglobin content per cell. Figure 6.19 shows the resulting time courses in reticulocyte count, erythrocyte count, and hemoglobin concentration.

■ Complex Response Models

Since the effect of most therapeutic proteins is mediated via complex regulatory physiologic processes including feedback mechanisms and/or tolerance phenomena, some PK/PD models that have been described

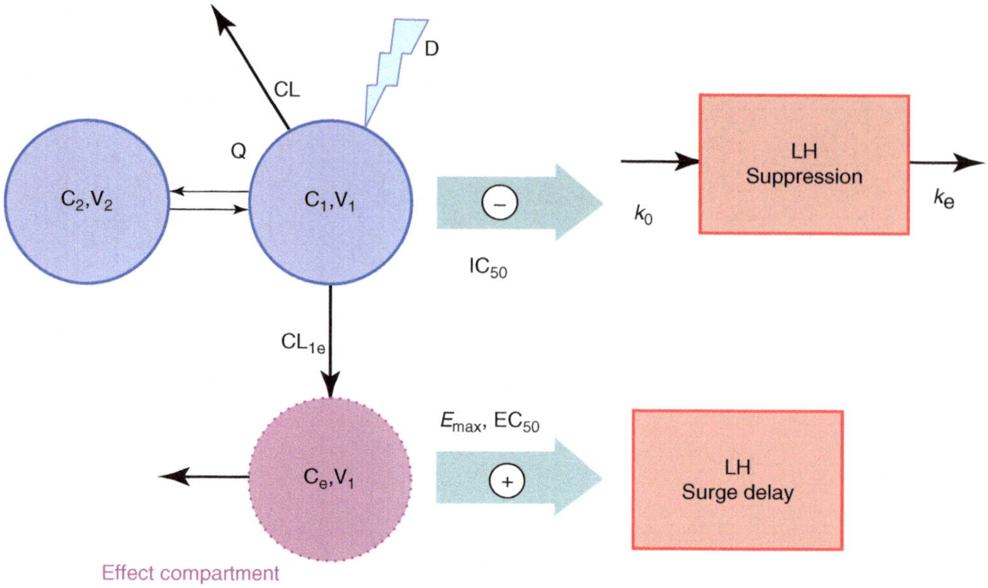

$$\frac{dLH}{dt} = k_0 \cdot \left(1 - \frac{C_1^{\,n}}{IC_{50}^{n} + C_1^{\,n}}\right) \cdot \left(1 + \frac{SA}{\left(\frac{t - \left(T_0 + \frac{E_{max} \cdot C_e}{EC_{50} + C_e}\right)}{SW}\right)^4 + 1}\right) - k_e \cdot LH$$

Figure 6.20 ■ A PK/PD model for the combined effect of the luteinizing hormone-releasing hormone (LH-RH) antagonist cetrorelix on luteinizing hormone (*LH*) suppression and delay of the LH surge. The PK model is a two-compartment model identical to the model described in Fig. 6.11. The PD model consists of two components: an indirect response model of subtype I to model the suppression of LH by cetrorelix and an indirect link model that models the delay in LH surge as a function of the cetrorelix concentration in a hypothetical effect compartment. Both PD model components are combined in the provided mathematical expression that describes the rate of change in LH concentration (dLH/d*t*) as a function of both processes. LH is the LH concentration, k_0 and k_e are the zero-order production rate and first-order elimination rate constants for LH at baseline, C_1 and C_e are the cetrorelix concentrations in plasma and a hypothetical effect compartment, respectively, SA is the LH surge amplitude, *t* is the study time in terms of cycle day, T_0 is the study time in terms of cycle day at which the peak occurs under baseline conditions, SW is the width of the peak in time units, IC_{50} is the cetrorelix concentration that suppresses LH levels by 50%, n is the Hill factor fixed at 2, E_{max} is the maximum delay in LH surge, and EC_{50} is the cetrorelix concentrations that produces half of E_{max}. Baseline data analysis indicated that the slope of the surge peak and SW were best fixed at values of 4 and 24 h, respectively. Other PK and PD parameters are identical to those used in Fig. 6.13 (modified from Nagaraja et al. 2000)

for protein drugs are much more sophisticated than the four classes of models previously discussed.

One example of such a complex modeling approach has been developed for the therapeutic effects of the luteinizing hormone-releasing hormone (LH-RH) antagonist cetrorelix (Nagaraja et al. 2000, 2003; Pechstein et al. 2000). Cetrorelix is used for the prevention of premature ovulation in women undergoing controlled ovarian stimulation in in vitro fertilization protocols. LH-RH antagonists suppress the LH levels and delay the occurrence of the preovulatory LH surge, and this delay is thought to be responsible for postponing ovulation. The suppression of LH was modeled in the PK/PD approach with an indirect-response model approach directly linked to cetrorelix plasma concentrations (Fig. 6.20) (Nagaraja et al. 2003). The shift in LH surge was linked to cetrorelix concentration with a simple E_{max} function via a hypothetical effect compartment to account for a delay in response via complex signal transduction steps of unknown mechanism of action. Figure 6.21 shows the application of this PK/PD model to characterize the LH suppression and LH surge delay after subcutaneous administration of cetrorelix to groups of 12 women at different dose levels. The analysis revealed a marked dose–response relationship for the LH surge and thus predictability of drug response to cetrorelix (Nagaraja et al. 2000).

Another example for a complex PK/PD model is the cytokinetic model used to describe the effect of

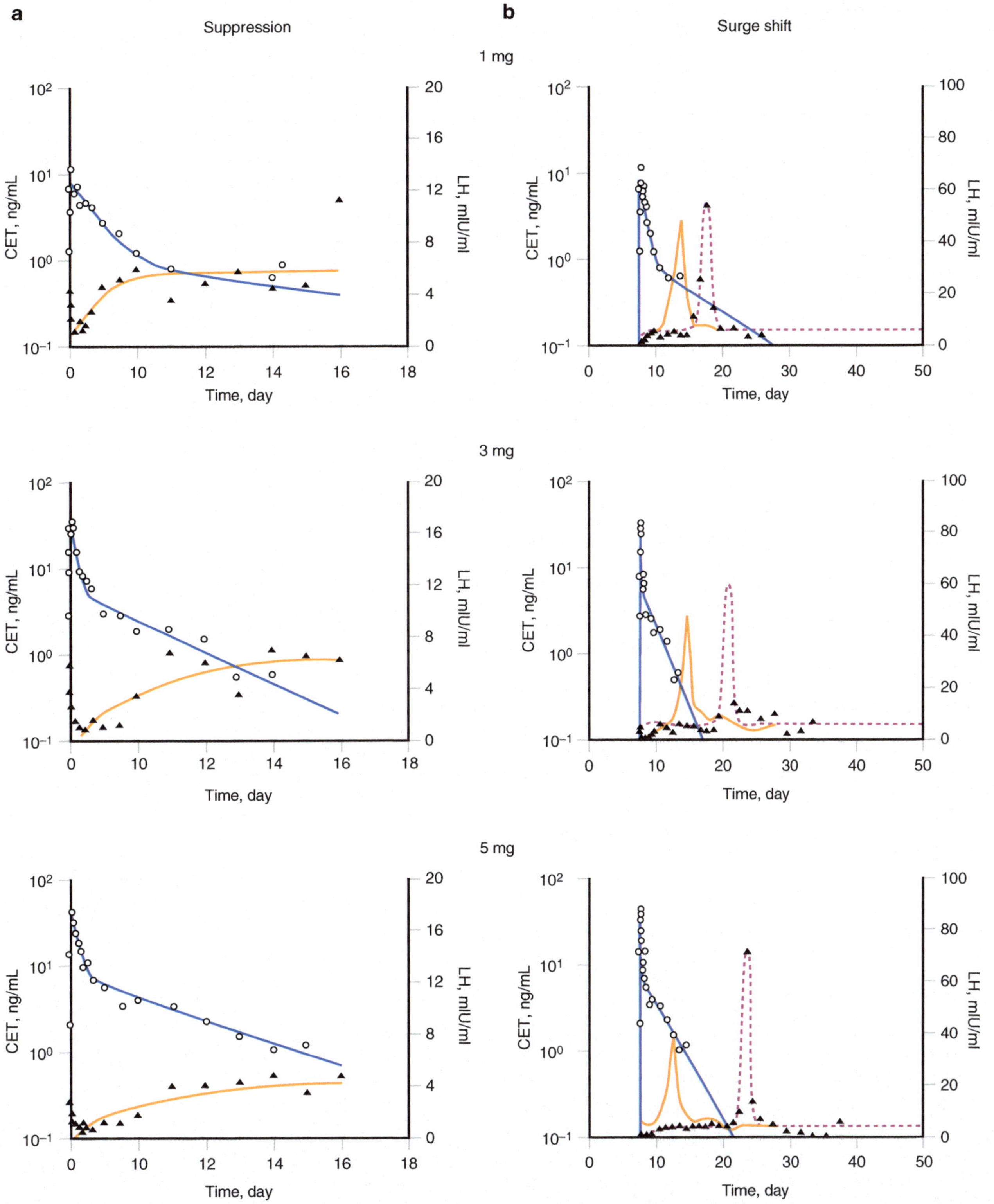

Figure 6.21 ■ Pharmacokinetic and pharmacodynamic relationship between cetrorelix (CET;○) and LH concentrations (▲) after single doses of 1, 3, and 5 mg cetrorelix in representative subjects. Cetrorelix and LH concentrations were modeled using the PK/PD model presented in Fig. 6.20. *Left panel*: LH suppression. *Right panel*: LH suppression and LH surge profiles. The *solid blue line* represents the model-fitted cetrorelix concentration, the *dashed purple line* the model-fitted LH concentration, and the *solid orange line* in the *right panels* the pretreatment LH profile (not fitted). The cetrorelix-dependent delay in LH surge is visible as the rightward shift of the LH surge profile under cetrorelix therapy compared to the respective pretreatment LH profile (from Nagaraja et al. 2000, with permission from Macmillan Publishers Ltd.)

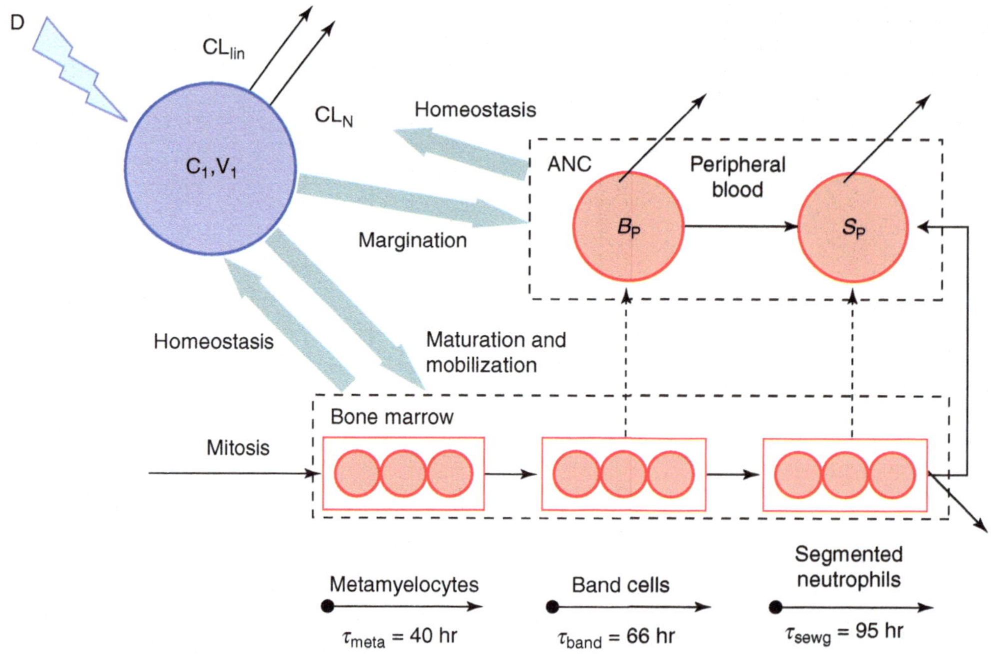

Figure 6.22 ■ A PK/PD model describing the granulopoietic effects of pegfilgrastim. The PK model is a one-compartment model with two parallel elimination pathways, a first-order elimination process (CL_{lin}) and a neutrophil-mediated elimination process (CL_N). C_1 and V_1 are the concentrations in the PK compartment and the corresponding volume of distribution. The PD model is a cytokinetic model similar to the cell life span model in Fig. 6.18. Three maturation stages of neutrophils and their respective life spans (t_{meta}, t_{band}, t_{seg}) are included in the model, metamyelocytes, band cells, and segmented neutrophils. Each maturation stage is modeled by three sequential transit compartments. Serum concentrations of pegfilgrastim stimulate mitosis and mobilization of band cells and segmented neutrophils in bone marrow, decrease maturation times for postmitotic cells in marrow, and affect margination of the peripheral blood band cell (B_P) and segmented neutrophil (S_P) populations, the sum of which is the total absolute neutrophil count (*ANC*). Changes in neutrophil counts in peripheral blood provide feedback regulation of pegfilgrastim clearance (modified from Roskos et al. 2006)

pegfilgrastim on the granulocyte count in peripheral blood (Roskos et al. 2006; Yang 2006). Pegfilgrastim is a PEGylated form of the human granulocyte colony-stimulating factor (G-CSF) analogue filgrastim. Pegfilgrastim, like filgrastim and G-CSF, stimulates the activation, proliferation, and differentiation of neutrophil progenitor cells and enhances the functions of mature neutrophils (Roskos et al. 2006). Pegfilgrastim is mainly used as supportive care to ameliorate and enhance recovery from neutropenia secondary to cancer chemotherapy regimens. As already discussed in the section on PEGylation, pegfilgrastim follows target-mediated drug disposition with saturable receptor-mediated endocytosis by neutrophils as major elimination pathway (CL_N) and a parallel first-order process as minor elimination pathway (CL_{lin}; Fig. 6.22). The clearance for the receptor-mediated pathway is determined by the absolute neutrophil count (ANC), the sum of the peripheral blood band cell (B_p) and segmented neutrophil (S_p) populations.

A maturation-structured cytokinetic model of granulopoiesis was established to describe the relationship between pegfilgrastim serum concentration and neutrophil count (Fig. 6.22). The starting point is the production of metamyelocytes from mitotic precursors. Subsequent maturation stages are captured as band cells and segmented neutrophils in the bone marrow. Each maturation stage is modeled by three sequential transit compartments. Pegfilgrastim concentrations are assumed to increase ANC by stimulating mitosis and mobilization of band cells and segmented neutrophils from the bone marrow into the systemic circulation. Pegfilgrastim also promotes rapid margination of peripheral blood neutrophils, i.e., adhesion to blood vessels; this effect is modeled as an expansion of neutrophil dilution volume.

Figure 6.23 shows observed and modeled pegfilgrastim concentration-time and ANC-time profiles after escalating single SC dose administration of pegfilgrastim. The presented PK/PD model for pegfilgrastim allowed determining its EC_{50} for the effect on ANC. Based on this EC_{50} value and the obtained pegfilgrastim plasma concentrations, it was concluded that a 100 μg/kg dose was sufficient to reach the maximum therapeutic effect of pegfilgrastim on ANC (Roskos et al. 2006; Yang 2006).

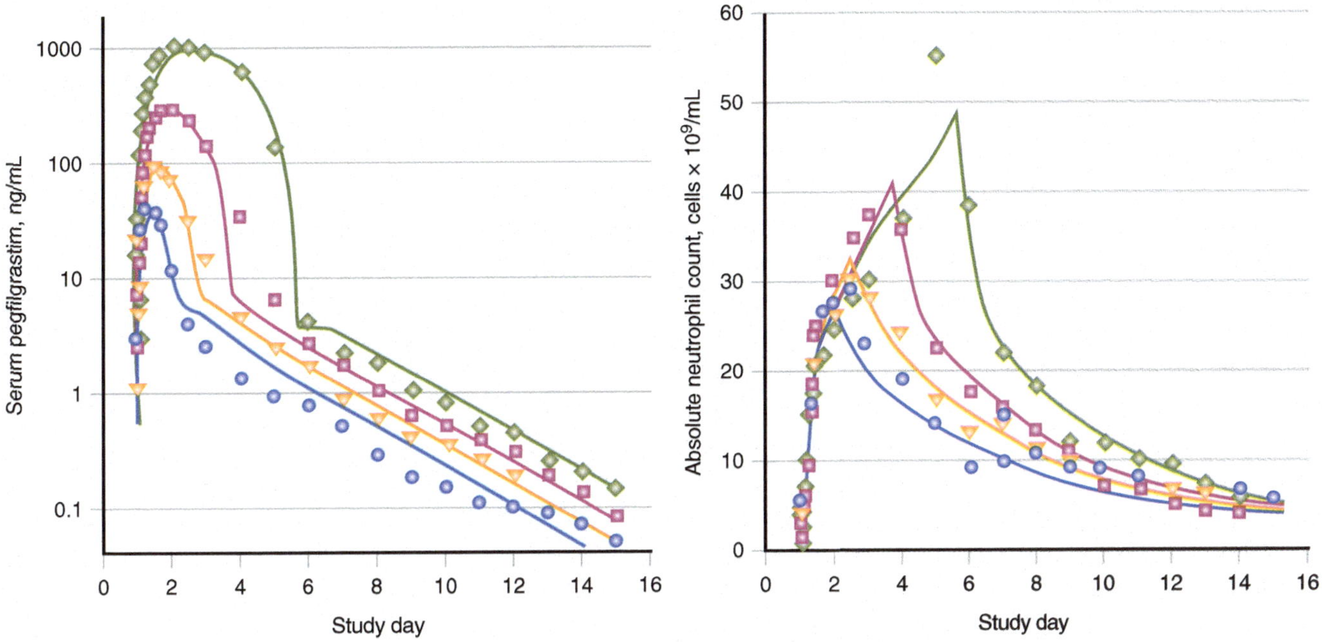

Figure 6.23 ■ Pegfilgrastim concentration time course and absolute neutrophil count (ANC) time profiles in healthy subjects after a single SC administration of 30, 60, 100, and 300 μg/kg pegfilgrastim (n = 8/dose group). Measured data are presented by symbols as mean ± SEM. Lines represent modeled time courses based on the cytokinetic PK/PD model presented in Fig. 6.22 (from Roskos et al. 2006, with permission from John Wiley & Sons, Inc. Copyright American College of Clinical Pharmacology 2006)

CONCLUSION

The pharmacokinetic and pharmacodynamic characteristics of peptides and proteins form the basis for their therapeutic application. Appreciation of the pharmacokinetic and pharmacodynamic differences between therapeutic biologics and traditional small-molecule drugs will empower the drug development scientist as well as the healthcare provider to handle, evaluate, and apply these compounds in an optimal fashion during the drug development process as well as during applied pharmacotherapy. Rationale, scientifically based drug development and pharmacotherapy based on the use of pharmacokinetic and pharmacodynamic concepts will undoubtedly propel the success and future of therapeutic proteins and might ultimately contribute to provide the novel medications that may serve as the key for the aspired "precision medicine" in the healthcare systems of the future (Dugger et al. 2018).

SELF-ASSESSMENT QUESTIONS

Questions

1. What are the major elimination pathways for protein drugs after administration?
2. Which pathway of absorption is rather unique for proteins after SC injection?
3. What is the role of plasma binding proteins for natural proteins?
4. How do the sugar groups on glycoproteins influence hepatic elimination of these glycoproteins?
5. In which direction might elimination clearance of a protein drug change when antibodies against the protein are produced after chronic dosing with the protein drug? Why?
6. What is the major driving force for the transport of proteins from the vascular to the extravascular space?
7. Why are therapeutic proteins generally not active upon oral administration?
8. Many therapeutic proteins exhibit Michaelis-Menten type, saturable elimination kinetics. What are the underlying mechanisms for this pharmacokinetic behavior?
9. Explain counterclockwise hysteresis in plasma concentration-effect plots.
10. Why is mechanism-based PK/PD modeling a preferred modeling approach for therapeutic proteins?

Answers

1. Proteolysis, glomerular filtration followed by intraluminal metabolism or tubular reabsorption with intracellular lysosomal degradation, receptor-

mediated endocytosis followed by metabolism in the skin, muscle, liver and possibly other organs and tissues.
2. Biodistribution from the injection site into the lymphatic system.
3. Plasma proteins may act as circulating reservoirs for the proteins that are their ligands. Consequently, the protein ligands may be protected from elimination and distribution.
4. In some cases, the sugar groups are recognized by hepatic receptors (e.g., galactose by the galactose receptor), facilitating receptor-mediated uptake and metabolism.
5. Clearance may increase or decrease by forming antibody-protein complexes. A decrease of clearance occurs when the antibody-protein complex is eliminated slower than free protein. An increase of clearance occurs when the protein-antibody complex is eliminated more rapidly than the unbound protein, such as when reticuloendothelial uptake is stimulated by the complex.
6. Protein extravasation, i.e., transport from the blood or vascular space to the interstitial tissue space, is predominantly mediated by convection. Protein molecules follow the fluid flux from the vascular space through pores between adjacent cells into the interstitial space. Drainage of the interstitial space through the lymphatic system allows therapeutic proteins to distribute back into the vascular space.
7. The gastrointestinal mucosa is a major absorption barrier for hydrophilic macromolecule such as proteins. In addition, therapeutic peptides and proteins are degraded by the extensive peptidase and protease activity in the gastrointestinal tract. Both processes minimize the oral bioavailability of therapeutic proteins.
8. Receptor-mediated endocytosis is the most frequent cause of nonlinear pharmacokinetics in therapeutic proteins. Its occurrence becomes even more prominent if the therapeutic protein undergoes target-mediated drug disposition, i.e., if the receptor-mediated endocytosis is mediated via the pharmacologic target of the therapeutic protein. As the binding to the target is usually of high affinity, and the therapeutic protein is often dosed to saturate the majority of the available target receptors for maximum pharmacologic efficacy, saturation of the associated receptor-mediated endocytosis as elimination pathway is frequently encountered.
9. Counterclockwise hysteresis is an indication of the indirect nature of the effects seen for many protein drugs. It can be explained by delays between the appearance of drug in plasma and the appearance of the pharmacodynamic response. The underlying cause may either be a distributional delay between the drug concentrations in plasma and at the effect site (modeled with an indirect link PK/PD model) or by time-consuming post-receptor events that cause a delay between the drug-receptor interaction and the observed drug effect, for example, the effect on a physiologic measure or endogenous substance.
10. Therapeutic proteins are often classified as "targeted therapies" where the drug compound acts on one specific, well-defined response pathway. This well-documented knowledge on the mechanism of action can relatively easily be translated into a mechanism-based PK/PD modeling approach that incorporates the major physiological processes relevant for the pharmacologic effect. The advantage of mechanism-based as compared to empirical PK/PD modeling is that mechanism-based models are usually more robust and allow more reliable simulations beyond the actually measured data.

REFERENCES

Agoram B, Heatherington AC, Gastonguay MR (2006) Development and evaluation of a population pharmacokinetic-pharmacodynamic model of darbepoetin alfa in patients with nonmyeloid malignancies undergoing multicycle chemotherapy. AAPS J 8(3):E552–E563

Albitar M, Do KA, Johnson MM et al (2004) Free circulating soluble CD52 as a tumor marker in chronic lymphocytic leukemia and its implication in therapy with anti-CD52 antibodies. Cancer 101(5):999–1008

Allon M, Kleinman K, Walczyk M et al (2002) Pharmacokinetics and pharmacodynamics of darbepoetin alfa and epoetin in patients undergoing dialysis. Clin Pharmacol Ther 72(5):546–555

Anderson PM, Sorenson MA (1994) Effects of route and formulation on clinical pharmacokinetics of interleukin-2. Clin Pharmacokinet 27(1):19–31

Bauer RJ, Gibbons JA, Bell DP, Luo ZP, Young JD (1994) Nonlinear pharmacokinetics of recombinant human macrophage colony-stimulating factor (M-CSF) in rats. J Pharmacol Exp Ther 268(1):152–158

Baxter LT, Zhu H, Mackensen DG, Jain RK (1994) Physiologically based pharmacokinetic model for specific and nonspecific monoclonal antibodies and fragments in normal tissues and human tumor xenografts in nude mice. Cancer Res 54(6):1517–1528

Benincosa LJ, Chow FS, Tobia LP et al (2000) Pharmacokinetics and pharmacodynamics of a humanized monoclonal antibody to factor IX in cynomolgus monkeys. J Pharmacol Exp Ther 292(2):810–816

Bennett HP, McMartin C (1978) Peptide hormones and their analogues: distribution, clearance from the circulation, and inactivation in vivo. Pharmacol Rev 30(3):247–292

Berdeja J, Jagannath S, Zonder J, Badros A, Kaufman JL, Manges R, Gupta M, Tendolkar A, Lynch M, Bleickardt E, Paliwal P, Vij R (2016) Pharmacokinetics and safety of elotuzumab combined with lenalidomide and dexamethasone in patients with multiple myeloma and various levels of renal impairment: results of a phase Ib study. Clin Lymphoma Myeloma Leuk 16(3):129–138

Boxenbaum H (1982) Interspecies scaling, allometry, physiological time, and the ground plan of pharmacokinetics. J Pharmacokinet Biopharm 10(2):201–227

Bressolle F, Audran M, Gareau R, Pham TN, Gomeni R (1997) Comparison of a direct and indirect population pharmacodynamic model: application to recombinant human erythropoietin in athletes. J Pharmacokinet Biopharm 25(3):263–275

Bruin G, Loesche C, Nyirady J, Sander O (2017) Population pharmacokinetic modeling of secukinumab in patients with moderate to severe psoriasis. J Clin Pharmacol 57(7):876–885

Bu G, Williams S, Strickland DK, Schwartz AL (1992) Low density lipoprotein receptor-related protein/alpha 2-macroglobulin receptor is an hepatic receptor for tissue-type plasminogen activator. Proc Natl Acad Sci U S A 89(16):7427–7431

Caliceti P, Veronese FM (2003) Pharmacokinetic and biodistribution properties of poly(ethylene glycol)-protein conjugates. Adv Drug Deliv Rev 55(10):1261–1277

Carone FA, Peterson DR (1980) Hydrolysis and transport of small peptides by the proximal tubule. Am J Phys 238(3):F151–F158

Carone FA, Peterson DR, Flouret G (1982) Renal tubular processing of small peptide hormones. J Lab Clin Med 100(1):1–14

Chanson P, Timsit J, Harris AG (1993) Clinical pharmacokinetics of octreotide. Therapeutic applications in patients with pituitary tumours. Clin Pharmacokinet 25(5):375–391

Chiang J, Gloff CA, Yoshizawa CN, Williams GJ (1993) Pharmacokinetics of recombinant human interferon-beta ser in healthy volunteers and its effect on serum neopterin. Pharm Res 10(4):567–572

Chirmule N, Jawa V, Meibohm B (2012) Immunogenicity to therapeutic proteins: impact on PK/PD and efficacy. AAPS J 14(2):296–302

Chow FS, Benincosa LJ, Sheth SB et al (2002) Pharmacokinetic and pharmacodynamic modeling of humanized anti-factor IX antibody (SB 249417) in humans. Clin Pharmacol Ther 71(4):235–245

Colburn W (1991) Peptide, peptoid, and protein pharmacokinetics/pharmacodynamics. In: Garzone P, Colburn W, Mokotoff M (eds) Petides, peptoids, and proteins, 3rd edn. Harvey Whitney Books, Cincinnati, pp 94–115

Cumming DA (1991) Glycosylation of recombinant protein therapeutics: control and functional implications. Glycobiology 1(2):115–130

Daniel H, Herget M (1997) Cellular and molecular mechanisms of renal peptide transport. Am J Phys 273(1 Pt 2):F1–F8

Dayneka NL, Garg V, Jusko WJ (1993) Comparison of four basic models of indirect pharmacodynamic responses. J Pharmocokinet Biopharm 21(4):457–478

De la Peña A, Ma X, Reddy S, Ovalle F, Bergenstal RM, Jackson JA (2014) Application of PK/PD modeling and simulation to dosing regimen optimization of high-dose human regular U-500 insulin. J Diabetes Sci Technol 8(4):821–829

Dedrick RL (1973) Animal scale-up. J Pharmacokinet Biopharm 1(5):435–461

Deen WM, Lazzara MJ, Myers BD (2001) Structural determinants of glomerular permeability. Am J Physiol Renal Physiol 281(4):F579–F596

Deng R, Iyer S, Theil FP et al (2011) Projecting human pharmacokinetics of therapeutic antibodies from nonclinical data: what have we learned? MAbs 3(1):61–66

Derendorf H, Meibohm B (1999) Modeling of pharmacokinetic/pharmacodynamic (PK/PD) relationships: concepts and perspectives. Pharm Res 16(2):176–185

Diao L, Meibohm B (2013) Pharmacokinetics and pharmacokinetic-pharmacodynamic correlations of therapeutic peptides. Clin Pharmacokinet 52(10):855–868

Diao L, Meibohm B (2015) Tools for predicting the PK/PD of therapeutic proteins. Expert Opin Drug Metab Toxicol 11(7):1115–1125

Dirks NL, Meibohm B (2010) Population pharmacokinetics of therapeutic monoclonal antibodies. Clin Pharmacokinet 49(10):633–659

Dong JQ, Salinger DH, Endres CJ, Gibbs JP, Hsu CP, Stouch BJ, Hurh E, Gibbs MA (2011) Quantitative prediction of human pharmacokinetics for monoclonal antibodies: retrospective analysis of monkey as a single species for first-in-human prediction. Clin Pharmacokinet 50(2):131–142

Dugger SA, Platt A, Goldstein DB (2018) Drug development in the era of precision medicine. Nat Rev Drug Discov 17(3):183–196

Edwards A, Daniels BS, Deen WM (1999) Ultrastructural model for size selectivity in glomerular filtration. Am J Phys 276(6 Pt 2):F892–F902

Eigenmann MJ, Fronton L, Grimm HP, Otteneder MB, Krippendorff BF (2017) Quantification of IgG monoclonal antibody clearance in tissues. MAbs 9(6):1007–1015

Eppler SM, Combs DL, Henry TD et al (2002) A target-mediated model to describe the pharmacokinetics and hemodynamic effects of recombinant human vascular endothelial growth factor in humans. Clin Pharmacol Ther 72(1):20–32

Fasano A (1998) Novel approaches for oral delivery of macromolecules. J Pharm Sci 87(11):1351–1356

Flessner MF, Lofthouse J, el Zakaria R (1997) In vivo diffusion of immunoglobulin G in muscle: effects of binding, solute exclusion, and lymphatic removal. Am J Phys 273(6 Pt 2):H2783–H2793

Glassman PM, Balthasar JP (2016) Physiologically-based pharmacokinetic modeling to predict the clini-

cal pharmacokinetics of monoclonal antibodies. J Pharmacokinet Pharmacodyn 43(4):427–446
Glund S, Gan G, Moschetti V, Reilly P, Honickel M, Grottke O, Van Ryn J (2018) The renal elimination pathways of the dabigatran reversal agent idarucizumab and its impact on dabigatran elimination. Clin Appl Thromb Hemost 24(5):724–733
Graham ML (2003) Pegaspargase: a review of clinical studies. Adv Drug Deliv Rev 55(10):1293–1302
Handelsman DJ, Swerdloff RS (1986) Pharmacokinetics of gonadotropin-releasing hormone and its analogs. Endocr Rev 7(1):95–105
Hayashida K, Bartlett AH, Chen Y, Park PW (2010) Molecular and cellular mechanisms of ectodomain shedding. Anat Rec 293(6):925–937
Herbst RS, Langer CJ (2002) Epidermal growth factor receptors as a target for cancer treatment: the emerging role of IMC-C225 in the treatment of lung and head and neck cancers. Semin Oncol 29(1 Suppl 4):27–36
Holford NH, Sheiner LB (1982) Kinetics of pharmacologic response. Pharmacol Ther 16(2):143–166
Inui K, Terada T, Masuda S, Saito H (2000) Physiological and pharmacological implications of peptide transporters, PEPT1 and PEPT2. Nephrol Dial Transplant 15(Suppl 6):11–13
Ismair MG, Stieger B, Cattori V et al (2001) Hepatic uptake of cholecystokinin octapeptide by organic anion-transporting polypeptides OATP4 and OATP8 of rat and human liver. Gastroenterology 121(5):1185–1190
Jin F, Krzyzanski W (2004) Pharmacokinetic model of target-mediated disposition of thrombopoietin. AAPS PharmSci 6(1):E9
Johnson V, Maack T (1977) Renal extraction, filtration, absorption, and catabolism of growth hormone. Am J Phys 233(3):F185–F196
Kaufman JS, Reda DJ, Fye CL et al (1998) Subcutaneous compared with intravenous epoetin in patients receiving hemodialysis. Department of Veterans Affairs Cooperative Study Group on Erythropoietin in Hemodialysis Patients. N Engl J Med 339(9):578–583
Khor SP, McCarthy K, DuPont M, Murray K, Timony G (2000) Pharmacokinetics, pharmacodynamics, allometry, and dose selection of rPSGL-Ig for phase I trial. J Pharmacol Exp Ther 293(2):618–624
Kim J, Hayton WL, Robinson JM, Anderson CL (2007) Kinetics of FcRn-mediated recycling of IgG and albumin in human: pathophysiology and therapeutic implications using a simplified mechanism-based model. Clin Immunol 122(2):146–155
Kingwell K (2016) Drug delivery: new targets for drug delivery across the BBB. Nat Rev Drug Discov 15(2):84–85
Kobayashi H, Shirakawa K, Kawamoto S et al (2002) Rapid accumulation and internalization of radiolabeled herceptin in an inflammatory breast cancer xenograft with vasculogenic mimicry predicted by the contrast-enhanced dynamic MRI with the macromolecular contrast agent G6-(1B4M-Gd)(256). Cancer Res 62(3):860–866
Kompella U, Lee V (1991) Pharmacokinetics of peptide and protein drugs. In: Lee V (ed) Peptide and protein drug delivery. Marcel Dekker, New York, pp 391–484
Kontermann R (2012) Therapeutic proteins: strategies to modulate their plasma half-lives. Wiley, Weinheim
Krogsgaard Thomsen M, Friis C, Sehested Hansen B et al (1994) Studies on the renal kinetics of growth hormone (GH) and on the GH receptor and related effects in animals. J Pediatr Endocrinol 7(2):93–105
Kuwabara T, Uchimura T, Kobayashi H, Kobayashi S, Sugiyama Y (1995) Receptor-mediated clearance of G-CSF derivative nartograstim in bone marrow of rats. Am J Phys 269(1 Pt 1):E1–E9
Lee HJ (2002) Protein drug oral delivery: the recent progress. Arch Pharm Res 25(5):572–584
Lee H, Kimko HC, Rogge M et al (2003) Population pharmacokinetic and pharmacodynamic modeling of etanercept using logistic regression analysis. Clin Pharmacol Ther 73(4):348–365
Lesko LJ (2007) Paving the critical path: how can clinical pharmacology help achieve the vision? Clin Pharmacol Ther 81(2):170–177
Lesko LJ, Rowland M, Peck CC, Blaschke TF (2000) Optimizing the science of drug development: opportunities for better candidate selection and accelerated evaluation in humans. J Clin Pharmacol 40(8):803–814
Levy G (1986) Kinetics of drug action: an overview. J Allergy Clin Immunol 78(4 Pt 2):754–761
Levy G (1994) Mechanism-based pharmacodynamic modeling. Clin Pharmacol Ther 56(4):356–358
Limothai W, Meibohm B (2011) Effect of dose on the apparent bioavailability of therapeutic proteins that undergo target-mediated drug disposition. AAPS J 13(S2)
Maack T, Park C, Camargo M (1985) Renal filtration, transport and metabolism of proteins. In: Seldin D, Giebisch G (eds) The kidney. Raven Press, New York, pp 1773–1803
Mach H, Gregory SM, Mackiewicz A et al (2011) Electrostatic interactions of monoclonal antibodies with subcutaneous tissue. Ther Deliv 2(6):727–736
Mager DE (2006) Target-mediated drug disposition and dynamics. Biochem Pharmacol 72(1):1–10
Mager DE, Wyska E, Jusko WJ (2003) Diversity of mechanism-based pharmacodynamic models. Drug Metab Dispos 31(5):510–518
Mahato RI, Narang AS, Thoma L, Miller DD (2003) Emerging trends in oral delivery of peptide and protein drugs. Crit Rev Ther Drug Carrier Syst 20(2-3):153–214
McMahon HT, Boucrot E (2011) Molecular mechanism and physiological functions of clathrin-mediated endocytosis. Nat Rev Mol Cell Biol 12(8):517–533
McMartin C (1992) Pharmacokinetics of peptides and proteins: opportunities and challenges. Adv Drug Res 22:39–106
Meibohm B (2004) Pharmacokinetics of protein- and nucleotide-based drugs. In: Mahato RI (ed) Biomaterials for delivery and targeting of proteins and nucleic acids. CRC Press, Boca Raton, pp 275–294
Meibohm B, Derendorf H (1997) Basic concepts of pharmacokinetic/pharmacodynamic (PK/PD) modelling. Int J Clin Pharmacol Ther 35(10):401–413
Meibohm B, Derendorf H (2002) Pharmacokinetic/pharmacodynamic studies in drug product development. J Pharm Sci 91(1):18–31

Meibohm B, Derendorf H (2004) Pharmacokinetics and pharmacodynamics of biotech drugs. In: Kayser O, Muller R (eds) Pharmaceutical biotechnology: drug discovery and clinical applications. Wiley, Weinheim, pp 147–172

Meibohm B, Zhou H (2012) Characterizing the impact of renal impairment on the clinical pharmacology of biologics. J Clin Pharmacol 52(1 Suppl):54S–62S

Meijer D, Ziegler K (1993) Biological barriers to protein delivery. Plenum Press, New York

Mohler M, Cook J, Lewis D et al (1993) Altered pharmacokinetics of recombinant human deoxyribonuclease in rats due to the presence of a binding protein. Drug Metab Dispos 21(1):71–75

Molineux G (2003) Pegylation: engineering improved biopharmaceuticals for oncology. Pharmacotherapy 23(8 Pt 2):3S–8S

Montero-Julian FA, Klein B, Gautherot E, Brailly H (1995) Pharmacokinetic study of anti-interleukin-6 (IL-6) therapy with monoclonal antibodies: enhancement of IL-6 clearance by cocktails of anti-IL-6 antibodies. Blood 85(4):917–924

Mordenti J, Chen SA, Moore JA, Ferraiolo BL, Green JD (1991) Interspecies scaling of clearance and volume of distribution data for five therapeutic proteins. Pharm Res 8(11):1351–1359

Mould DR, Davis CB, Minthorn EA et al (1999) A population pharmacokinetic-pharmacodynamic analysis of single doses of clenoliximab in patients with rheumatoid arthritis. Clin Pharmacol Ther 66(3):246–257

Mould DR, Meibohm B (2016) Drug development of therapeutic monoclonal antibodies. BioDrugs 30(4):275–293

Nagaraja NV, Pechstein B, Erb K et al (2000) Pharmacokinetic and pharmacodynamic modeling of cetrorelix, an LH-RH antagonist, after subcutaneous administration in healthy premenopausal women. Clin Pharmacol Ther 68(6):617–625

Nagaraja NV, Pechstein B, Erb K et al (2003) Pharmacokinetic/pharmacodynamic modeling of luteinizing hormone (LH) suppression and LH surge delay by cetrorelix after single and multiple doses in healthy premenopausal women. J Clin Pharmacol 43(3):243–251

Nielsen S, Nielsen JT, Christensen EI (1987) Luminal and basolateral uptake of insulin in isolated, perfused, proximal tubules. Am J Phys 253(5 Pt 2):F857–F867

Pauletti GM, Gangwar S, Siahaan TJ, Jeffrey A, Borchardt RT (1997) Improvement of oral peptide bioavailability: peptidomimetics and prodrug strategies. Adv Drug Deliv Rev 27(2-3):235–256

Pechstein B, Nagaraja NV, Hermann R et al (2000) Pharmacokinetic-pharmacodynamic modeling of testosterone and luteinizing hormone suppression by cetrorelix in healthy volunteers. J Clin Pharmacol 40(3):266–274

Peck CC, Barr WH, Benet LZ et al (1994) Opportunities for integration of pharmacokinetics, pharmacodynamics, and toxicokinetics in rational drug development. J Clin Pharmacol 34(2):111–119

Perez-Ruixo JJ, Kimko HC, Chow AT et al (2005) Population cell life span models for effects of drugs following indirect mechanisms of action. J Pharmacokinet Pharmacodyn 32(5-6):767–793

Periti P, Mazzei T, Mini E (2002) Clinical pharmacokinetics of depot leuprorelin. Clin Pharmacokinet 41(7):485–504

Perrier D, Mayersohn M (1982) Noncompartmental determination of the steady-state volume of distribution for any mode of administration. J Pharm Sci 71(3):372–373

Piscitelli SC, Reiss WG, Figg WD, Petros WP (1997) Pharmacokinetic studies with recombinant cytokines. Scientific issues and practical considerations. Clin Pharmacokinet 32(5):368–381

Porter CJ, Charman SA (2000) Lymphatic transport of proteins after subcutaneous administration. J Pharm Sci 89(3):297–310

Rabkin R, Ryan MP, Duckworth WC (1984) The renal metabolism of insulin. Diabetologia 27(3):351–357

Racine-Poon A, Botta L, Chang TW et al (1997) Efficacy, pharmacodynamics, and pharmacokinetics of CGP 51901, an anti-immunoglobulin E chimeric monoclonal antibody, in patients with seasonal allergic rhinitis. Clin Pharmacol Ther 62(6):675–690

Radwanski E, Chakraborty A, Van Wart S et al (1998) Pharmacokinetics and leukocyte responses of recombinant human interleukin-10. Pharm Res 15(12):1895–1901

Ramakrishnan R, Cheung WK, Wacholtz MC, Minton N, Jusko WJ (2004) Pharmacokinetic and pharmacodynamic modeling of recombinant human erythropoietin after single and multiple doses in healthy volunteers. J Clin Pharmacol 44(9):991–1002

Reddy ST, Berk DA, Jain RK, Swartz MA (2006) A sensitive in vivo model for quantifying interstitial convective transport of injected macromolecules and nanoparticles. J Appl Physiol 101(4):1162–1169

Richter WF, Bhansali SG, Morris ME (2012) Mechanistic determinants of biotherapeutics absorption following SC administration. AAPS J 14(3):559–570

Richter WF, Gallati H, Schiller CD (1999) Animal pharmacokinetics of the tumor necrosis factor receptor-immunoglobulin fusion protein lenercept and their extrapolation to humans. Drug Metab Dispos 27(1):21–25

Roopenian DC, Akilesh S (2007) FcRn: the neonatal Fc receptor comes of age. Nat Rev Immunol 7(9):715–725

Roskos LK, Lum P, Lockbaum P, Schwab G, Yang BB (2006) Pharmacokinetic/pharmacodynamic modeling of pegfilgrastim in healthy subjects. J Clin Pharmacol 46(7):747–757

Ryman JT, Meibohm B (2017) Pharmacokinetics of monoclonal antibodies. CPT: Pharmacometrics Syst Pharmacol 6(9):576–588

Schomburg A, Kirchner H, Atzpodien J (1993) Renal, metabolic, and hemodynamic side-effects of interleukin-2 and/or interferon alpha: evidence of a risk/benefit advantage of subcutaneous therapy. J Cancer Res Clin Oncol 119(12):745–755

Sharma A, Jusko W (1998) Characteristics of indirect pharmacodynamic models and applications to clinical drug responses. Br J Clin Pharmacol 45:229–239

Sheiner LB, Stanski DR, Vozeh S, Miller RD, Ham J (1979) Simultaneous modeling of pharmacokinetics and pharmacodynamics: application to d-tubocurarine. Clin Pharmacol Ther 25(3):358–371

Sheiner LB, Steimer JL (2000) Pharmacokinetic/pharmacodynamic modeling in drug development. Annu Rev Pharmacol Toxicol 40:67–95

Shen WC (2003) Oral peptide and protein delivery: unfulfilled promises? Drug Discov Today 8(14):607–608

Smedsrod B, Einarsson M (1990) Clearance of tissue plasminogen activator by mannose and galactose receptors in the liver. Thromb Haemost 63(1):60–66

Straughn AB (1982) Model-independent steady-state volume of distribution. J Pharm Sci 71(5):597–598

Straughn AB (2006) Limitations of noncompartmental pharmacokinetic analysis of biotech drugs. In: Meibohm B (ed) Pharmacokinetics and pharmacodynamics of biotech drugs. Wiley, Weinheim, pp 181–188

Strickland DK, Kounnas MZ, Argraves WS (1995) LDL receptor-related protein: a multiligand receptor for lipoprotein and proteinase catabolism. FASEB J 9(10):890–898

Sun YN, Jusko WJ (1999) Role of baseline parameters in determining indirect pharmacodynamic responses. J Pharm Sci 88(10):987–990

Sun YN, Lee HJ, Almon RR, Jusko WJ (1999) A pharmacokinetic/pharmacodynamic model for recombinant human growth hormone effects on induction of insulin-like growth factor I in monkeys. J Pharmacol Exp Ther 289(3):1523–1532

Supersaxo A, Hein W, Gallati H, Steffen H (1988) Recombinant human interferon alpha-2a: delivery to lymphoid tissue by selected modes of application. Pharm Res 5(8):472–476

Supersaxo A, Hein WR, Steffen H (1990) Effect of molecular weight on the lymphatic absorption of water-soluble compounds following subcutaneous administration. Pharm Res 7(2):167–169

Suryawanshi S, Zhang L, Pfister M, Meibohm B (2010) The current role of model-based drug development. Expert Opin Drug Discovery 5(4):311–321

Tabrizi M, Roskos LK (2006) Exposure-response relationships for therapeutic biologics. In: Meibohm B (ed) Pharmacokinetics and pharmacodynamics of biotech drugs. Wiley, Weinheim, pp 295–330

Takagi A, Masuda H, Takakura Y, Hashida M (1995) Disposition characteristics of recombinant human interleukin-11 after a bolus intravenous administration in mice. J Pharmacol Exp Ther 275(2):537–543

Taki Y, Sakane T, Nadai T et al (1998) First-pass metabolism of peptide drugs in rat perfused liver. J Pharm Pharmacol 50(9):1013–1018

Tang L, Meibohm B (2006) Pharmacokinetics of peptides and proteins. In: Meibohm B (ed) Pharmacokinetics and pharmacodynamics of biotech drugs. Wiley, Weinheim, pp 17–44

Tang L, Persky AM, Hochhaus G, Meibohm B (2004) Pharmacokinetic aspects of biotechnology products. J Pharm Sci 93(9):2184–2204

Tanswell P, Modi N, Combs D, Danays T (2002) Pharmacokinetics and pharmacodynamics of tenecteplase in fibrinolytic therapy of acute myocardial infarction. Clin Pharmacokinet 41(15):1229–1245

Tokuda Y, Watanabe T, Omuro Y et al (1999) Dose escalation and pharmacokinetic study of a humanized anti-HER2 monoclonal antibody in patients with HER2/neu-overexpressing metastatic breast cancer. Br J Cancer 81(8):1419–1425

Toon S (1996) The relevance of pharmacokinetics in the development of biotechnology products. Eur J Drug Metab Pharmacokinet 21(2):93–103

Veng-Pedersen P, Gillespie W (1984) Mean residence time in peripheral tissue: a linear disposition parameter useful for evaluating a drug's tissue distribution. J Pharmacokinet Biopharm 12(5):535–543

Veronese FM, Caliceti P (2006) Custom-tailored pharmacokinetics and pharmacodynamics via chemical modifications of biotech drugs. In: Meibohm B (ed) Pharmacokinetics and pharmacodynamics of boptech drugs. Wiley, Weinheim, pp 271–294

Walsh S, Shah A, Mond J (2003) Improved pharmacokinetics and reduced antibody reactivity of lysostaphin conjugated to polyethylene glycol. Antimicrob Agents Chemother 47(2):554–558

Wang W, Wang EQ, Balthasar JP (2008) Monoclonal antibody pharmacokinetics and pharmacodynamics. Clin Pharmacol Ther 84(5):548–558

Wills RJ, Ferraiolo BL (1992) The role of pharmacokinetics in the development of biotechnologically derived agents. Clin Pharmacokinet 23(6):406–414

Yang BB (2006) Integration of pharmacokinetics and pharmacodynamics into the drug development of pegfilgrastim, a pegylated protein. In: Meibohm B (ed) Pharmacokinetics and pharmacodynamics of biotech drugs. Wiley, Weinheim, pp 373–394

Zamboni WC (2003) Pharmacokinetics of pegfilgrastim. Pharmacotherapy 23(8 Pt 2):9S–14S

Zhang Y, Meibohm B (2012) Pharmacokinetics and pharmacodynamics and therapeutic peptides and proteins. In: Kayzer O, Warzecha H (eds) Pharmaceutical biotechnology: drug discovery and clinical applications. Wiley, Weinheim, pp 337–368

Zhang L, Pfister M, Meibohm B (2008) Concepts and challenges in quantitative pharmacology and model-based drug development. AAPS J 10(4):552–559

Zhao L, Ji P, Li Z, Roy P, Sahajwalla CG (2013) The antibody drug absorption following subcutaneous or intramuscular administration and its mathematical description by coupling physiologically based absorption process with the conventional compartment pharmacokinetic model. J Clin Pharmacol 53(3):314–325

Zia-Amirhosseini P, Minthorn E, Benincosa LJ et al (1999) Pharmacokinetics and pharmacodynamics of SB-240563, a humanized monoclonal antibody directed to human interleukin-5, in monkeys. J Pharmacol Exp Ther 291(3):1060–1067

Ziegler K, Polzin G, Frimmer M (1988) Hepatocellular uptake of cyclosporin A by simple diffusion. Biochim Biophys Acta 938(1):44–50

Zito SW (1997) Pharmaceutical biotechnology: a programmed text. Technomic, Lancaster

FURTHER READING

General Pharmacokinetics and Pharmacodynamics

Atkinson A, Abernethy D, Daniels C, Dedrick R, Markey S (2006) Principles of clinical pharmacology. Academic, San Diego

Bonate PL (2011) Pharmacokinetic-pharmacodynamic modeling and simulation. Springer, New York

Derendorf H, Meibohm B (1999) Modeling of pharmacokinetic/pharmacodynamic (PK/PD) relationships: concepts and perspectives. Pharm Res 16(2):176–185

Gabrielsson J, Hjorth S (2012) Quantitative pharmacology. Swedish Academy of Pharmaceutical Sciences, Stockholm

Gibaldi M, Perrier D (1982) Pharmacokinetics. Marcel Dekker, New York

Holford NH, Sheiner LB (1982) Kinetics of pharmacologic response. Pharmacol Ther 16(2):143–166

Rowland M, Tozer TN (2011) Clinical pharmacokinetics and pharmacodynamics: concepts and applications. Lippincott Williams & Wilkins, Baltimore

Pharmacokinetics and Pharmacodynamics of Peptides and Proteins

Diao L, Meibohm B (2013) Pharmacokinetics and pharmacokinetic-pharmacodynamic correlations of therapeutic peptides. Clin Pharmacokinet 52(10): 855–868

Diao L, Meibohm B (2015) Tools for predicting the PK/PD of therapeutic proteins. Expert Opin Drug Metab Toxicol 11(7):1115–1125

Kontermann R (2012) Therapeutic proteins: strategies to modulate their plasma half-lives. Wiley, Weinheim

Meibohm B (2006) Pharmacokinetics and pharmacodynamics of biotech drugs. Wiley, Weinheim

Mould DR, Meibohm B (2016) Drug development of therapeutic monoclonal antibodies. BioDrugs 30(4):275–293

Ryman JT, Meibohm B (2017) Pharmacokinetics of monoclonal antibodies. CPT: Pharmacometrics Syst Pharmacol 6(9):576–588

Tang L, Persky AM, Hochhaus G, Meibohm B (2004) Pharmacokinetic aspects of biotechnology products. J Pharm Sci 93(9):2184–2204

7 Immunogenicity of Therapeutic Proteins

Wim Jiskoot, Theo Rispens, and Grzegorz Kijanka

INTRODUCTION

Proteins were first used as medicines at the end of the nineteenth century when antisera from animals were introduced for the treatment of serious infections, such as diphtheria and tetanus. However, because such antisera were loaded with proteins foreign to the patients' immune system, they often led to serious and sometimes even fatal side effects. In general, persons who had been treated had a warning in their passports or identification cards to alert physicians for a possible anaphylactic reaction after re-challenge with an antiserum.

In the 1920s porcine and bovine insulin products were introduced to treat diabetes. Many patients receiving these insulins developed antibodies neutralizing the protein (anti-drug antibodies, ADA). At first, this had been explained by the animal origin of the products. However, reduction of immunogenicity of these products following improvements in the production methods and increasing purity strongly indicated that the protein's animal origin was not the only factor leading to their immunogenicity. In the second half of the twentieth century, a number of human proteins from natural sources such as plasma derived clotting factors and growth hormone produced from pituary glands of cadavers was introduced into the clinic. These products were given mainly to children with an innate deficiency who therefore lacked the natural immune tolerance. Consequently, their immune response was also interpreted as a response to foreign proteins. The correlation between the factor VIII gene defects and level of deficiency with the immune response in hemophilia patients confirmed this explanation (Fakharzadeh and Kazazian Jr 2000). However, similar to the animal derived insulins, improved purification protocols led to reduced immunogenicity levels for some of the human protein products.

The true breakthrough in availability of therapeutic proteins occurred in the 1980s when recombinant DNA technologies allowed large-scale production of highly purified proteins. In 1982 human insulin was marketed as the first recombinant DNA derived protein for human use. Since then dozens of recombinant proteins have entered the market and some of these products, such as the interferons and the epoetins, are among the most widely used medicines in the world. However, although these proteins were developed as close copies of human endogenous proteins, nearly all of them induce ADA, sometimes even in a majority of patients (Table 7.1). Importantly, most of these products are used in patients who do not have an innate deficiency and thus one can assume that they developed immune tolerance to the protein.

The initial assumption was that the production by recombinant technology in non-human host cells and the downstream processing modified the proteins and the immunological response was the classical response to a foreign protein. However, in some cases circumventing B-cell tolerance might be the basis for the antibody response to human homologues. This phenomenon is not yet completely understood but appears to be different from the immune response against foreign antigens used in vaccines. On the other hand, for therapeutic monoclonal antibodies, there are usually determinants present in the molecule that are foreign to the recipient (see section "Issues Specifically Related to Monoclonal Antibodies").

W. Jiskoot (✉) · G. Kijanka
Division of BioTherapeutics, Leiden Academic Centre for Drug Research (LACDR), Leiden University, Leiden, The Netherlands
e-mail: w.jiskoot@lacdr.leidenuniv.nl

T. Rispens
Department of Immunopathology, Sanquin, Amsterdam, The Netherlands
e-mail: t.rispens@sanquin.nl

D. J. A. Crommelin et al. (eds.), *Pharmaceutical Biotechnology*, https://doi.org/10.1007/978-3-030-00710-2_7

Therapeutic protein	Immunogenicity rate (%)	Reference
Growth hormone	7–22	Rougeot et al. (1991)
Factor VIII	3–35	Oldenburg et al. (2015)
Insulin	14–44	Fineberg et al. (2007)
Interferon beta	2–47	Bertolotto et al. (2004)
Monoclonal antibodies	0–89	Harding et al. (2010)
Interleukin-2	20–100	Prümmer (1997)

Table 7.1 ■ Non-exhaustive list of recombinant proteins showing immune reactions upon administration

The clinical manifestations of both types of reaction are very different. The typical vaccine-like response to foreign proteins occurs within days to weeks. Often a single injection is sufficient to induce a substantial ADA response. In general, high levels of neutralizing antibodies are induced and a re-challenge leads to a booster reaction, indicating a memory response.

However, the development of an immune response against certain recombinant human proteins may require months, sometimes years of chronic treatment. Moreover, secreted antibodies often do not neutralize the injected therapeutic protein and sometimes even do not manifest any apparent clinical effects. Additionally, in some cases these ADA, especially when produced in low or moderate amounts, tend to disappear shortly after the treatment has been stopped and sometimes even during treatment (Perini et al. 2001). Also, this response does not appear to generate immunological memory. In patients treated with recombinant human interferon β (rhIFNβ) or recombinant human growth hormone, the therapy often can be paused to allow the ADA levels to decline and then restarted without boosting of ADA titers (Schellekens and Casadevall 2004; Perini et al. 2001).

In contrast, the ADA response against therapeutic monoclonal antibodies such as adalimumab and infliximab follows a more classical pattern (Brandse et al. 2016; Bartelds et al. 2011), with ADA detected as early as 2 weeks after starting the treatment. Moreover, the vast majority of these ADA is neutralizing (van Schie et al. 2015a, 2017); and intermittent infliximab treatment is associated with more immunogenicity (Han and Cohen 2004).

THE IMMUNE RESPONSE

The therapeutic proteins currently available cover the whole spectrum, from completely foreign (e.g., bacteria-derived asparaginase) to completely human (e.g., recombinant human interferon α-2b (rhIFNα-2b)) as well as unnatural proteins, such as fusion proteins (e.g., etanercept), truncated antibodies (e.g., Fab fragments, nanobodies) and PEGylated proteins (e.g., PEGylated rhIFNα with PEG defined as polyoxyethylene glycol).

Foreign proteins elicit antibodies by the classical pathway, which includes ingestion and cleaving of the proteins into peptides by macrophages and dendritic cells, presentation of peptides by the MHC (major histocompatibility complex)-II system and activation of B-cells, and affinity maturation and isotype switching of the B-cells by helper CD4⁺ T-cells. Furthermore, they induce memory B-cells (see Chap. 14 for details).

It is much less clear how B-cell tolerance is circumvented. One of the theories to explain antibody formation against a self(-like) therapeutic protein was that aggregated protein induced exclusively T-cell independent B-cell activation via crosslinking of B-cell receptors by protein aggregates resembling bacterial or viral structures (Moore and Leppert 1980; Bachmann et al. 1993). Such structures present repetitive epitopes in a highly regular pattern, allowing rapid recognition as foreign substance and inducing a response without engaging $CD4^+$ T-cells. However, since this mechanism was first proposed, numerous preclinical and clinical observations have indicated involvement of $CD4^+$ T-cells in the antibody response against therapeutic self(-like) proteins. During $CD4^+$ T-cell independent responses, mostly low-affinity IgMs are produced, but in patients and in animal models mostly IgGs have been observed. Efficient isotype switching is one of the hallmarks of a $CD4^+$ T-cell response. However, production of non-neutralizing antibodies in part of the patients suggests impaired affinity maturation.

Another indication of a $CD4^+$ T-cell dependent mechanism is the observation that certain HLA alleles correlate with a higher probability of ADA formation against, e.g., rhIFNβ, epoetin and anti-TNF (tumor necrosis factor) mAb (Barbosa et al. 2006; Moss et al. 2013; Praditpornsilpa et al. 2009; Fijal et al. 2008). Moreover, in several animal models $CD4^+$ T-cell depletion resulted in almost complete abolishment of antibody production (reviewed by Jiskoot et al. 2016). Nevertheless, full explanations for immunogenicity occurrence in only part of the patients receiving the protein, the frequent formation of non-neutralizing antibodies, and the apparent lack of immunological memory are still missing.

FACTORS INFLUENCING ANTIBODY FORMATION TO THERAPEUTIC PROTEINS

Figure 7.1 depicts the different factors that influence immunogenicity (Schellekens 2002a; Hermeling et al. 2004). These factors will be discussed below.

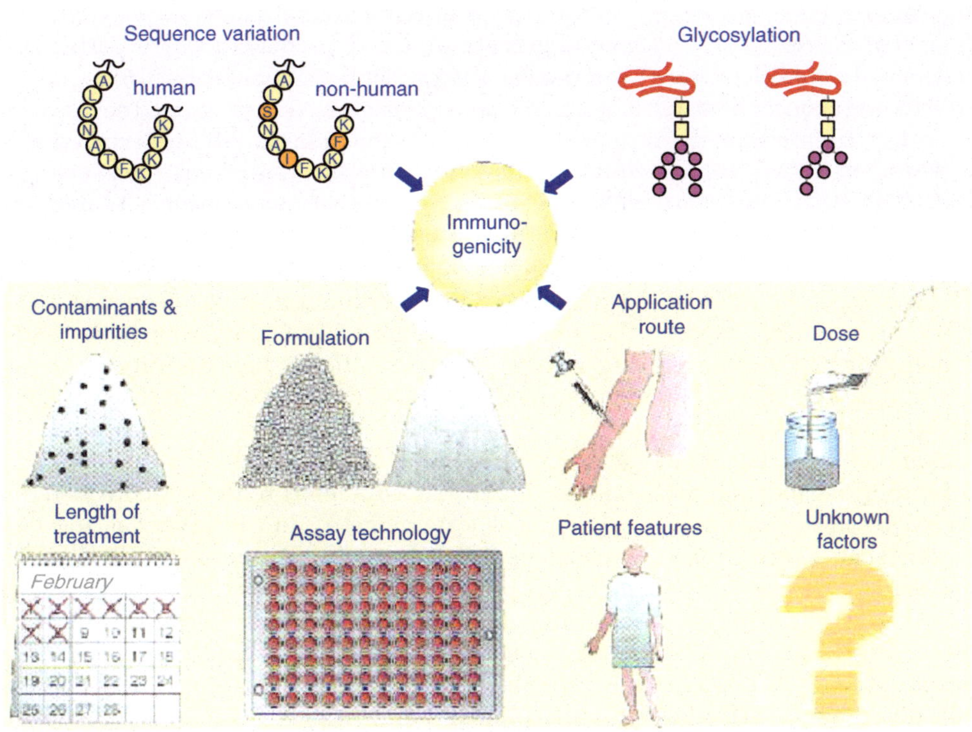

Schellekens, Nature Reviews Drug Discovery, 2002

Figure 7.1 ■ Factors influencing immunogenicity

■ Structural Factors

The similarity of a therapeutic protein's sequence to that of the human counterpart is one of the factors determining the probability of an ADA response against the therapeutic protein. However, the degree of non-self that is necessary to induce a vaccine-type response is highly dependent on the protein involved and the site of the divergence from the natural sequence of the endogenous protein. For instance, single mutations in inulin can lead to a new epitope and an ADA response, whereas other mutations have no influence at all; and consensus IFNα, in which more than 10% of the amino acids diverge from the nearest naturally occurring IFNα subtype, is not more immunogenic than the IFNα-2 homologue. Moreover, some unnatural proteins, such as etanercept, are relatively poorly immunogenic.

Glycosylation is another important structural factor for the immunogenicity of therapeutic proteins. There is little evidence that modified glycosylation, e.g., by expressing human glycoproteins in plant cells or other non-human eukaryotic hosts, may induce an immune response (Singh 2011). However, the level of glycosylation has a clear effect. For instance, rhIFNβ produced in *E. coli* (non-glycosylated) is much more immunogenic than rhIFNβ produced in mammalian cells. This may be explained by the higher hydrophobicity, causing higher aggregation levels in the non-glycosylated *E. coli*-derived product.

Futhermore, in certain populations, pre-existing IgE antibodies to non-human glycans present on cetuximab resulted in severe anaphylactic reactions (Chung et al. 2008).

■ Impurities

Impurities are considered to be important risk factors for the immunogenicity of therapeutic protein products. Among the clinically relevant impurities, protein aggregates have received most attention; the presence of aggregates is widely accepted as one of the most important risk factors for immunogenicity. Aggregation may be triggered by a variety of factors, such as thermal stress, pH shift, agitation, freeze-thawing and UV irradiation. Importantly, aggregates may be induced at every step of the production process as well as during storage, shipment, and product administration (cf. Chap. 5). Aggregation is believed to be one of the main causes of immunogenicity of e.g., human growth hormone and rhIFNβ-1b (Moore and Leppert 1980; Barnard et al. 2013). However, aggregation is not the only risk factor and products containing small amounts of aggregates might also be very immunogenic.

Chemical modification of human proteins e.g., oxidation, might lead to formation of neo-epitopes which might be recognized by a patient's immune system and trigger ADA. Moreover, as demonstrated in numerous animal studies, antibodies induced by chemically modified proteins can be cross-reactive with unmodified protein (Jiskoot et al. 2016).

Besides aggregates and chemically modified proteins, substances derived from the production process, such as host cell components, resins from chromatographic columns, enzymes used to activate the product and monoclonal antibodies used for affinity purification, may end up in the final product. Impurities may also be introduced by components of the formulation, may leak from the container and sealing of the product or may be introduced during the fill and finish steps. These impurities may be immunogenic by themselves and thereby elicit an immune response different from that to the therapeutic protein. Moreover, lipopolysaccharides from bacterial host cells and G-C rich bacterial host cell DNA are examples of impurities that can act as adjuvants. Antibodies induced by impurities may lead to general immune reactions such as skin reactions, allergies, anaphylaxis and serum sickness.

■ Formulation

Recombinant human therapeutic proteins are often highly biologically active and the doses may be at the μg level, making it a technological challenge to formulate the product and keep it stable with a reasonable shelf-life (cf. Chap. 5). The importance of designing a proper formulation in avoiding immunogenicity is highlighted in two historical cases. In the case of rhIFNα-2a, a large difference in immunogenicity was noted among different formulations (Fig. 7.2). A freeze-dried formulation, containing human serum albumin as a stabilizer that according to its instructions could be kept at room temperature, was more immunogenic in a clinical study than other formulations. It appeared that at room temperature rhIFNα-2a became partly oxidized. This led to the formation of aggregates, which most likely were responsible for the immune response (Ryff 1997). Interestingly, studies in animal models have confirmed that aggregates induced by oxidation are particularly immunogenic degradants (Jiskoot et al. 2016).

In the second case, an ADA-mediated severe form of anemia (pure red cell aplasia; PRCA) occurred after the formulation of an epoetin-α product was changed (Casadevall et al. 2002). Human serum albumin was replaced by glycine and polysorbate 80. How this formulation change led to a higher incidence of immunogenicity is still not certain, but it has been postulated that the new formulation is slightly less stable, resulting in aggregate formation when the product is not appropriately handled (Schellekens and Jiskoot 2006).

■ Route of Administration

Historically the subcutaneous route was considered to be the most immunogenic and intravenous the least immunogenic among administration routes used for therapeutic proteins (Schellekens 2002b). However, head-to-head comparison of administration routes is challenging, as the treatment regimen and/or the formulation have to be adjusted to compensate for altered pharmacokinetics and usually decreased bioavailability upon subcutaneous injection (Richter et al. 2012), all of which may influence the risk of an immune response. Subcutaneous formulations usually differ from intravenous ones because subcutaneous administration generally requires lower injection volumes. Overall, the influence of the administration route on immunogenicity seems to be strongly product dependent. Whereas for some products the subcutaneous route indeed seems to be associated with a higher immunogenicity risk as compared to the intravenous route, for others the influence of administration route seems to be negligible (Hamuro et al. 2017). Nevertheless, immunogenicity may occur after administration of a therapeutic protein via any route of application.

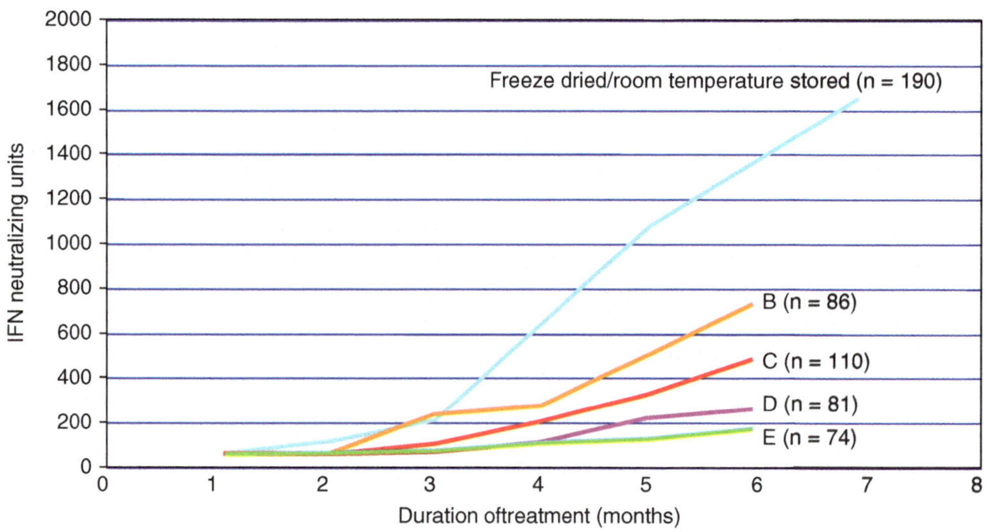

Figure 7.2 ■ Immunogenicity differences between rhIFNα-2a formulations in patients (figure adapted from Ryff 1997)

Dose

The effect of the dose is not quite clear. There are studies with the lowest incidence of ADA formation in the highest dose group (Maini et al. 1999; Food and Drug Administration 2002; Ross et al. 2000). However, such data should be interpreted with caution. In the highest dose group the higher therapeutic protein levels in the circulation may interfere with the assay, or the measured ADA level may be lower by increased immune complex formation.

Patient Features

Several patient related factors may influence the incidence of ADA formation. For example, many of the patients receiving monoclonal antibodies are immune compromised by diseases such as cancer or by immune suppressive treatment. These patients are less likely to produce ADA than patients with a normal immune status. An opposite effect can happen in patients suffering from chronic infections (like hepatitis): these patients may be more prone to development of ADA, as observed for rhIFNα-2 (Antonelli and Dianzani 1999).

There are several indications that circumventing B-cell tolerance is HLA-type dependent. This may explain, at least in part, why some individuals or populations do and others do not produce ADA when treated with the same product. For instance, associations between HLA-type and ADA formation were reported for infliximab (Billiet et al. 2015).

In many patients treated with therapeutic proteins, ADA are found before the start of the treatment (Gorovits et al. 2016). These so-called pre-existing ADA might be formed against structures, e.g., common glycans that closely resemble epitopes present in the therapeutic protein. In many of these patients the pre-existing ADA do not seem to have any impact on therapy safety or efficacy. However, since some patients who are tested positive for pre-existing ADA might be more susceptible to acute side effects or development of high titers of ADA, pre-existing ADA are considered as an immunogenicity risk factor.

Assays for Antibodies

Assays are probably an important factor influencing the reported incidence of ADA induction by therapeutic proteins. In the published studies with rhIFNα-2 in patients with viral infections the incidence of ADA induction varied from 0% to more than 60% positive patients. A similar variation has been seen with rhIFNβ (van Beers et al. 2010). This variation must be assay related. Evaluations of the performance of different test laboratories with blind panel testing showed a more than 50-fold difference in titers found in the same sera. Thus, any reliable comparison between different groups of patients when looking for a clinical effect of ADA or studying factors influencing immunogenicity can only be made if the antibody quantification is done with a well-validated assay in the same laboratory.

This situation persisted for evaluation of antibody formation against TNF inhibitors (infliximab, adalimumab), resulting in incidence rates varying from 0 to 87% in case of adalimumab (Vincent et al. 2013). Several factors account for these large discrepancies between studies, but one factor in particular was found to be of prime importance: drug interference. In particular, for therapeutic monoclonal antibodies high doses are used resulting in high concentrations of the therapeutic antibody in the blood. Then serum samples will contain considerable amounts of therapeutic protein that may interfere with the detection of ADA. Accordingly, many efforts have been made to design assays that overcome this interference, resulting in assays that are 'drug-tolerant' to variable degrees (Bloem et al. 2015).

The relationship between therapeutic antibody concentrations and ADA is important, not only for the detection of ADA, but also for the impact of ADA on efficacy. Often the main consequence of ADA formation is the reduction of 'active' protein concentrations. Thus, small amounts of ADA without a noticeable effect on the protein concentrations may be detected with a modern drug-tolerant assay but these ADA have no impact on efficacy (van Schouwenburg et al. 2013a).

Recommendations for Antibody Assays

There is a lack of standardization of assay methodology, and only a few reference and/or standard antibody preparations are available. Nevertheless, a number of papers appeared with recommendations for setting up and validating immunoassays for immunogenicity testing (Mire-Sluis et al. 2004; Shankar et al. 2008, 2014). A brief discussion of these recommendations follows below.

A single assay may not be sufficient to evaluate the immunogenicity of a new therapeutic protein. A number of assays may have to be used in conjunction. Most antibody assay strategies are based on a two-tier approach: a screening + confirmation assay to identify the ADA positive sera, followed by further characterization, e.g. determination of the ADA titer, affinity and isotype. Especially quantification may be useful, given that ADA levels can vary widely across individuals and the potential clinical impact of an ADA response usually relates to the extent of antibody formation.

In general, the screening assay is a binding assay, often a bridging type of assay (either ELISA –enzyme-linked immunosorbent assay (cf. Chap. 3) or electrochemoluminescence) with the radio-immune-precipitation methodology as an alternative. Screening assays are designed for optimal sensitivity to avoid false negatives, and often, the cut-point (i.e., threshold positive/negative) for the assay is set at a 5% false positive level by using a panel of normal human sera and/or untreated patient sera representative of the groups to be treated. The results would have to be evaluated in conjunction with a confirmatory assay that evaluates those samples found positive in the screening assay. The confirmatory assay may be the same screening assay, in which excess unlabeled therapeutic protein is added to evaluate if the signal is reduced. Moreover, a more strict confirmatory cut-point is defined to make sure that only 'true' positive samples are identified as such.

One issue that complicates cut-point determination is the possible existence of pre-existing antibodies. In rare cases (e.g., cetuximab, see above) these might have clinical consequences. More often, pre-existing antibodies towards a therapeutic protein may be detected in a (small) fraction of individuals without a clear clinical impact (Xue and Rup 2013). This needs to be dealt with on a case by case basis (Gorovits et al. 2016). One common type of pre-existing antibodies that is found in most rheumatoid arthritis patients but also in a few percent of the general population is the so-called 'rheumatoid factor', low-affinity antibodies binding to the Fc portion of human IgG. There is no evidence for these antibodies being relevant in immunogenicity assessment and measures should be taken to avoid their measurement (van Schie et al. 2015b). Antibodies to PEG groups attached to proteins are another commonly observed phenomenon, although their accurate measurement is still in its infancy, hampering the evaluation of their potential risk (Krishna et al. 2015; Schellekens et al. 2013).

The assay for neutralizing antibodies is in general a modification of the potency assay for the therapeutic protein product. The potency assay is in most cases an *in vitro* cell based assay. A predefined amount of product is added to the serum and a reduction of activity is then evaluated in the bioassay. An appropriate alternative is the competitive ligand binding assay, which evaluates reduction in target binding (Finco et al. 2011). The latter type of assays is much easier to set up and validate, and may be preferred unless there is a risk of antibodies formed to the therapeutic protein that neutralize its activity via a mechanism other than preventing target binding.

ISSUES SPECIFICALLY RELATED TO MONOCLONAL ANTIBODIES

The first generation of monoclonal antibodies was of murine origin. They induced an immune response in the majority of patients, as foreign proteins should trigger a classical vaccine-type immune response. This so-called HAMA response (human antibodies to murine antibodies) was a major restriction in the clinical success of these murine antibodies. Over the years, however, methods were introduced to (fully) humanize monoclonal antibodies (cf. Chap. 8). Recombinant DNA technology was used to exchange the murine constant parts of the immune globulin chains with their human counterparts resulting in chimeric monoclonal antibodies. The next step was to graft murine complementarity determining regions (CDRs), which determine the specificity, into a human immune globulin backbone creating humanized monoclonal antibodies. The final step was the development of transgenic animals, phage display technologies and other developments allowing the production of fully human monoclonal antibodies. The assumption that human monoclonal antibodies would have no immunogenicity proved wrong. Although humanization has reduced the immunogenicity, even completely human monoclonal antibodies may induce antibodies, as illustrated in Fig. 7.3.

As discussed, multiple factors may cause the immunogenicity of human therapeutic proteins including monoclonal antibodies. One of them is aggregation. In fact, in classical studies done more than 40 years ago aggregated immunoglobulin preparations were used to break B-cell tolerance (Weigle 1971). More recently, several preclinical studies have indicated that aggregates enhance the immunogenicity of monoclonal antibodies (reviewed by Jiskoot et al. 2016). However, also mAb products containing very low amounts of aggregates may be highly immunogenic. In contrast to other recombinant human proteins, monoclonal antibodies, even when fully human, may expose foreign epitopes in their complementarity-determining regions (CDR). Analysis of several monoclonal antibodies indeed confirmed that, in most cases, foreign $CD4^+$ T cells epitopes are found primarily within the CDR sequence (Harding et al. 2010).

Monoclonal antibodies have properties that may contribute to their immunogenicity. They can activate T-cells by themselves and may boost the immune response by their Fc functions such as macrophage activation and complement activation. Indeed, removal or modification of specific sugar units from N-linked glycosyl chains from the Fc part of the immunoglobulin may reduce Fc function and lead to a diminished immunogenicity (Liu 2015).

The molecule to which an antibody binds also influences its immunogenicity. Monoclonal antibodies targeting cell bound antigens generally induce a higher level of ADA than those targeting soluble targets (Harding et al. 2010). Monoclonal antibodies directed to antigens on immune cells with the purpose of inducing immune suppression also suppress an immunological response.

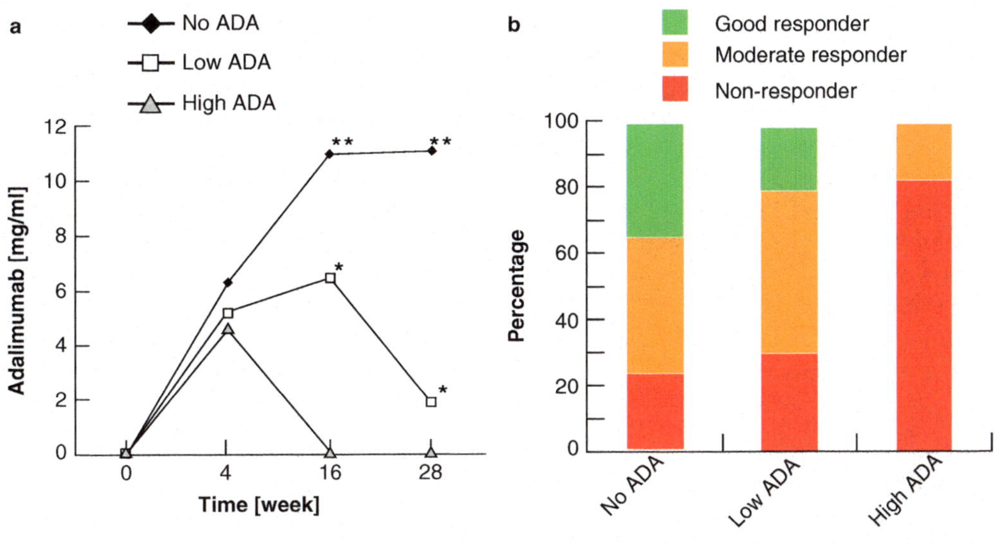

Figure 7.3 ■ Impact of immunogenicity on the serum level and treatment efficacy of fully human monoclonal antibody adalimumab. (**a**) The concentration of adalimumab in serum is altered by the presence of ADA. Low ADA titer corresponds to 12–100 AU/mL, high ADA titer corresponds to >100 AU/mL of ADA. $^*p < 0.05$, $^{**}p < 0.01$. (**b**) In patients with high ADA titers treatment is hampered to a higher extent than in patients with moderate or no ADA (figure adapted from Bartelds et al. 2011)

Although for a number of therapeutic proteins more injections and higher doses are associated with a higher immune response, for therapeutic antibodies this may not apply. In fact, lower doses and episodic treatment are usually associated with more antibody formation (Han and Cohen 2004). Although this may in part be the result of ADA assays not detecting antibodies in the presence of high therapeutic protein concentrations (see previous section), transient antibody formation has been reported for both infliximab and adalimumab, using drug-tolerant assays to measure the ADA response (van de Casteele et al. 2013; van Schouwenburg et al. 2013b). A phenomenon called 'high-dose tolerance' might be operational, where soluble antigen overwhelms the immune system.

Another important aspect when studying the immunogenicity of monoclonal antibodies is timing of the blood sampling of patients. These products may have a relatively long half-life (up to several weeks) and the circulating product may interfere with the detection of induced antibodies and may lead to false negative results. Sampling sera up to 20 weeks after the patient has received the last injection may be necessary to avoid the interference of circulating therapeutic monoclonal antibodies. Also natural antibodies, soluble receptors and immune complexes may interfere with assays and lead to either false positive or false negative results.

CLINICAL EFFECTS OF INDUCED ANTIBODIES

The list of protein products with clinically relevant immunogenicity-related side effects is growing (Schellekens 2002a; Malucchi and Bertolotto 2008). The most common consequence is loss of efficacy. Sometimes this loss can be overcome by increasing the dose or changing to another product.

Clinical consequence	Examples of therapeutic proteins
Loss of efficacy	• Animal and recombinant human (rh) insulin • Factor VIII (both natural and rh) • Rh Interferon alpha 2 • Rh Interferon beta • Rh Interleukin 2 • Human chorionic gonadotropin • Monoclonal antibodies
Neutralization of endogenous protein	• Rh megakaryocyte-derived growth factor • Epoetin
No apparent biological consequence	• Rh growth hormone • Rh insulin
General immune effects 1. Allergy 2. Serum sickness 3. Anaphylaxis 4. Injection site reactions	• Various therapeutic proteins

Table 7.2 ■ Examples of clinical consequences of immunogenicity of therapeutic proteins (adopted from Schellekens 2002a; Malucchi and Bertolotto 2008)

The most dramatic and undisputed complication occurs when the antibodies to the product cross-neutralize an endogenous factor with an important biological function. This has been described for a megakaryocyte growth and differentiation factor which induced antibodies cross-reacting with endogenous thrombopoietin (see Table 7.2). Volunteers and patients in a clinical trial developed severe thrombocytopenia and needed platelet transfusions. Because of this complication, the product was withdrawn from further development.

Another example is the upsurge of PRCA (see above) associated with a formulation change of epoetin-α marketed outside the USA. The antibodies induced by the product neutralized the residual endogenous erythropoietin in these patients, resulting in a severe anemia that could only be treated with blood transfusions.

ADA can also influence the side effects of therapeutic proteins. The consequences are dependent on the cause of the side effects. If the adverse effects are the results of the intrinsic activity of the protein, antibodies may reduce the side effects, as it is the case with rhIFNα-2. Sometimes the mitigation of the side effects is even the first clinical sign of the induction of ADA.

With some products the side effects are caused by the ADA formation. This is in general the case when the product is administered in relatively high doses, such as with some monoclonal antibodies. Symptoms caused by immune complexes, such as delayed type hypersensitivity and serum sickness, are related to the level of antibodies induced.

The general effects caused by an immune reaction to a therapeutic protein such as acute anaphylaxis, hypersensitivity, skin reaction, serum sickness etc. are relatively common when large amounts of non-human proteins are administered. These effects are relatively rare for recombinant human proteins administered in relatively low amounts, but they are still relatively common during treatment with high doses of monoclonal antibodies.

IMMUNOGENICITY RISK ASSESSMENT AND REDUCTION

The occurrence of immunogenicity is seldom a result of a single risk factor (cf. Fig. 7.1). Rather, several factors working synergistically may trigger immunogenicity. For example, the higher immunogenicity of interferon beta 1b (Betaferon) than interferon beta 1a (Avonex) is most likely the combined result of differences in treatment regimen and product quality (Bertolotto et al. 2004). Moreover, the immune mechanisms leading to antibody induction by therapeutic proteins are still not completely understood. Consequently, based on our current knowledge it is impossible to fully predict the immunogenicity of a new product in a patient population, let alone in individual patients. However, immunogenicity risk assessment and potential mitigation strategies are required by authorities for all new products. The most commonly used tools for assessing the relative immunogenicity risk are summarized in Table 7.3.

Tools to Assess Immunogenicity

According to current knowledge, $CD4^+$ T-cells are key players in immunogenicity. Therefore, one of the most commonly used approaches to assess immunogenicity risk is an *in silico* analysis of $CD4^+$ T-cell epitopes, i.e., short peptides within the protein sequence capable of binding to MHC II molecules. Multiple algorithms have been developed for this purpose (reviewed by Jawa et al. 2013). Generally speaking, the more high-affinity $CD4^+$ T-cell epitopes a protein contains, the higher is the expected risk of immunogenicity. Recent developments in understanding of the immune system allowed improving *in silico* prediction algorithms. Instead of assessing the overall/total number of $CD4^+$ T-cell epitopes, nowadays epitopes for effector and regulatory $CD4^+$ T-cells can be discriminated (Cousens et al. 2014). Combined anal-

Assessment tool		Pros	Cons
In silico	• $CD4^+$ T-cell epitope prediction • Regulatory T-cell epitope prediction	1. Fast and cheap 2. Useful as a first step of immunogenicity assessment 3. Allows design or selection of less immunogenic protein variant	1. Tendency to be over-predictive 2. Results based exclusively on primary sequence 3. The quality of results depends on degree of understanding of studied process 4. Translational power limited
In vitro	• Dendritic cell uptake and activation • $CD4^+$ T-cell activation • MHC II binding	1. Relatively fast and cheap 2. Enable studying formulated products (assessing factors other than primary sequence) 3. Some assays may allow studying biological effect	1. Quality of results strongly dependent on assay format 2. Cells from a large set of representative donors required 3. Focus on isolated immune cells 4. Translational power limited
In vivo	• Non-transgenic rodents • Transgenic rodents • Non-human primates	1. (Usually) presence of complete, functional immune system 2. Immune processes similar to those in patients 3. Various factors influencing immunogenicity can be studied 4. In some models, studying biological effect possible	1. Time-consuming and expensive 2. Translational power depends on protein and animal model 3. Immune system of used model differs from that of patient to various extents (non-transgenic mice vs transgenic mice)

Table 7.3 ■ Tools used for assessing protein immunogenicity (adopted from Brinks et al. 2013; Kijanka et al. 2012)

ysis of effector and regulatory $CD4^+$ T-cell analysis may be more reliable than analysis of total $CD4^+$ T-cell epitopes. However, as these approaches rely exclusively on the primary sequence of the protein and do not take into consideration other factors such as protein folding, posttranslational modifications, presence of impurities and complexity of the interaction between different immune cells, their prediction power is limited especially for self(-like) proteins.

Another approach is represented by a number of *in vitro* tools, such as $CD4^+$ T-cell stimulation and MHC II binding tests. Although, similarly to *in silico* tools, these assays do not fully represent the complexity of the immune system, they do allow assessing the impact of formulation related factors on immunogenicity risk. Thus, they can be used for validation of *in silico* results and to measure relative immunogenicity of different protein variants or different formulations of the same protein.

A third type of immunogenicity assessment tool is a set of *in vivo* models ranging from wild type and transgenic mice to non-human primates (Jiskoot et al. 2016; Brinks et al. 2013). The main benefit of *in vivo* models is that the complexity of an animal's immune system is similar to that of patients. Thus, they might be used not only to assess the immunogenicity, but also to study immune mechanisms and to provide insight into the possible clinical effects of immunogenicity.

Reducing Immunogenicity

Several strategies are being applied to reduce immunogenicity. At an early stage of development, one may alter the amino acid sequence of the lead candidate molecule in order to remove potentially immunogenic or aggregate prone sequences (Griswold and Bailey-Kellogg 2016). Once the drug substance has been chosen, the immunogenicity can be reduced by redesigning the formulation and/or treatment regimen. As discussed previously, improvement in quality of the first therapeutic protein products resulted in considerable reduction of immunogenicity. Many protein therapeutics, especially mAbs, are used in combination with immunosuppressant medicines. Medicines such as methotrexate, rapamicin or aziothioprine can strongly inhibit formation of antibodies, but patients might be more prone to infections or malignancy (de Mattos et al. 2015). Another strategy is an induction of specific tolerance towards the protein. It has been observed that administration of high dose(s) of factor VIII may induce tolerance in hemophilia patients with antibodies to factor VIII (Aledort 1994). Another, recently proposed strategy for specific tolerance induction is co-administration of peptides recognized by regulatory T-cells (Tregitopes) with the protein of interest. These Tregitopes activate the suppressing (or regulatory) T-cells, which may result in tolerance towards the administered therapeutic protein (Jawa et al. 2013).

CONCLUSIONS

The most important points of this chapter are summarized in the following bullet points:

- Immunogenicity of therapeutic proteins is a commonly occurring phenomenon
- The clinical consequences can widely vary
- Validated detection methods are essential to study the immunogenicity of therapeutic proteins
- The prediction of immunogenicity in patients based on physico-chemical characterization and animal studies is not easy
- There is still a lot to be learned about why and how patients produce antibodies to therapeutic proteins

The growing awareness of the importance of immunogenicity of therapeutic proteins is illustrated by the adoption of a standard requirement in regulatory dossiers for new proteins and biosimilars to evaluate their immunogenicity in clinical trials (cf. Chap. 12).

SELF-ASSESSMENT QUESTIONS

Questions

1. Which factors contribute to unwanted immunogenicity of therapeutic proteins?
2. What are possible clinical consequences of antibody formation against biopharmaceuticals in patients?
3. Why do aggregates of recombinant human proteins induce antibodies that cross-react with the (non-aggregated) protein?
4. Explain the fundamental difference between (a) antibody formation in children with growth hormone deficiency treated against with recombinant human growth hormone and (b) antibody formation against epoetin in patients with chronic renal failure.
5. Give an example of a case that demonstrates that the formulation of a biopharmaceutical can affect the immune response.
6. Give at least 3 approaches that can be followed to reduce the immunogenicity of a biopharmaceutical.
7. Why is standardization of assays for detection of ADA important?
8. Why are ADA titers against a monoclonal antibody more difficult to determine accurately than antibodies against interferon?

Answers

1. See Fig. 7.1.
2. Reduction of therapeutic efficacy, (seldom) enhancement of efficacy, anaphylactic reactions, cross-reactivity with endogenous protein.
3. Aggregates can circumvent B-cell tolerance against native (like) epitopes; the more 'native like' the aggregate, the more likely cross-reactivity of the elicited antibodies with the monomer will occur.
4. (a) is the classical immune response versus (b) circumventing B-cell tolerance.
5. The examples given in the text are epoetin and interferon α.
6. Design another formulation, remove aggregates, change the glycosylation pattern of the protein or use amino acid mutants, use human(ized) versions of the proteins or select another route of administration. NB. Some of these approaches will lead to a new drug substance, which has implications for the way authorities will judge the procedure to be followed for obtaining marketing approval.
7. Different assay formats and blood sampling schedules give different answers and thus hamper direct comparison between studies. Therefore, it is difficult to compare the results obtained with different products that are tested for immunogenicity in different labs.
8. Monoclonal antibodies are often administered in high doses and have a long circulation time (days/weeks). This will likely cause interference with the ADA assay by the circulating therapeutic antibodies (resulting in false negatives or underestimation of antibody titers). Another possibility for interference is the occurrence of cross-reactivity of the reagents in the test for the ADA and the administered monoclonal antibody. With interferon a different situation is encountered: interferons are rapidly cleared and administered in low doses (microgram range); therefore, interferons will less likely interfere with the measurement of anti-IFN antibodies.

REFERENCES

Aledort L (1994) Inhibitors in hemophilia patients: current status and management. Am J Hematol 47:208–217

Antonelli G, Dianzani F (1999) Development of antibodies to interferon beta in patients: technical and biological aspects. Eur Cytokine Netw 10:413–422

Bachmann MF, Rohrer UH, Kündig TM, Bürki K, Hengartner H, Zinkernagel RM (1993) The influence of antigen organization on B cell responsiveness. Science 262:1448–1451

Barbosa MD, Vielmetter J, Chu S, Smith DD, Jacinto J (2006) Clinical link between MHC class II haplotype and interferon-beta (IFN-β) immunogenicity. Clin Immunol 118:42–50

Barnard JG, Babcock K, Carpenter JF (2013) Characterization and quantitation of aggregates and particles in interferon-β products: potential links between product quality attributes and immunogenicity. J Pharm Sci 102:915–928

Bartelds GM, Krieckaert CL, Nurmohamed MT, van Schouwenburg PA, Lems WF, Twisk JW, Dijkmans BA, Aarden L, Wolbink GJ (2011) Development of antidrug antibodies against adalimumab and association with disease activity and treatment failure during long-term follow-up. JAMA 305:1460–1468

Bertolotto A, Deisenhammer F, Gallo P, Sölberg Sørensen P (2004) Immunogenicity of interferon beta: differences among products. J Neurol 251:II15–II24

Billiet T, Vande Casteele N, Van Stappen T, Princen F, Singh S, Gils A, Ferrante M, Van Assche G, Cleynen I, Vermeire S (2015) Immunogenicity to infliximab is associated with HLA-DRB1. Gut 64:1344–1345

Bloem K, van Leeuwen A, Verbeek G, Nurmohamed MT, Wolbink GJ, van der Kleij D, Rispens T (2015) Systematic comparison of drug-tolerant assays for anti-drug antibodies in a cohort of adalimumab-treated rheumatoid arthritis patients. J Immunol Methods 418:29–38

Brandse JF, Mathôt RA, van der Kleij D, Rispens T, Ashruf Y, Jansen JM, Rietdijk S, Löwenberg M, Ponsioen CY, Singh S, van den Brink GR, D'Haens GR (2016) Pharmacokinetic features and presence of antidrug antibodies associate with response to infliximab induction therapy in patients with moderate to severe ulcerative colitis. Clin Gastroenterol Hepatol 14:251–258

Brinks V, Weinbuch D, Baker M, Dean Y, Stas P, Kostense S, Rup B, Jiskoot W (2013) Preclinical models used for immunogenicity prediction of therapeutic proteins. Pharm Res 30:1719–1728

Casadevall N, Nataf J, Viron B, Kolta A, Kiladjian JJ, Martin-Dupont P, Michaud P, Papo T, Ugo V, Teyssandier I, Varet B, Mayeux P (2002) Pure red-cell aplasia and antierythropoietin antibodies in patients treated with recombinant erythropoietin. N Engl J Med 346:469–475

Chung CH, Mirakhur B, Chan E, Le QT, Berlin J, Morse M, Murphy BA, Satinover SM, Hosen J, Mauro D, Slebos RJ, Zhou Q, Gold D, Hatley T, Hicklin DJ, Platts-Mills TA (2008) Cetuximab-induced anaphylaxis and IgE specific for galactose-α-1,3-galactose. N Engl J Med 358:1109–1117

Cousens L, Najafian N, Martin WD, De Groot AS (2014) Tregitope: immunomodulation powerhouse. Hum Immunol 75:1139–1146

de Mattos BR, Garcia MP, Nogueira JB, Paiatto LN, Albuquerque CG, Souza CL, Fernandes LG, Tamashiro WM, Simioni PU (2015) Inflammatory bowel disease: an overview of immune mechanisms and biological treatments. Mediat Inflamm 2015:1–11

Fakharzadeh SS, Kazazian HH Jr (2000) Correlation between factor VIII genotype and inhibitor development in hemophilia A. Semin Thromb Hemost 26:167–172

Fijal B, Ricci D, Vercammen E, Palmer PA, Fotiou F, Fife D, Lindholm A, Broderick E, Francke S, Wu X,

Colaianne J, Cohen N (2008) Case–control study of the association between select HLA genes and anti-erythropoietin antibody-positive pure red-cell aplasia. Pharmacogenomics 9:157–167

Finco D, Baltrukonis D, Clements-Egan A, Delaria K, Gunn GR 3rd, Lowe J, Maia M, Wong T (2011) Comparison of competitive ligand-binding assay and bioassay formats for the measurement of neutralizing antibodies to protein therapeutics. J Pharm Biomed Anal 54:351–358

Fineberg SE, Kawabata TT, Finco-Kent D, Fountaine RJ, Finch GL, Krasner AS (2007) Immunological responses to exogenous insulin. Endocr Rev 28:625–652

Food and Drug Administration (2002) Adalimumab. 2002. Pharmacology reviews: adalimumab product approval information—licensing action. Available from http://www.accessdata.fda.gov/drugsatfda_docs/nda/2008/125057s110TOC.cfm. Accessed 4 Nov 2017

Gorovits B, Clements-Egan A, Birchler M, Liang M, Myler H, Peng K, Purushothama S, Rajadhyaksha M, Salazar-Fontana L, Sung C, Xue L (2016) Pre-existing antibody: biotherapeutic modality-based review. AAPS J 18:311–320

Griswold KE, Bailey-Kellogg C (2016) Design and engineering of deimmunized biotherapeutics. Curr Opin Struct Biol 39:79–88

Hamuro L, Kijanka G, Kinderman F, Kropshofer H, Bu DX, Zepeda M, Jawa V (2017) Perspectives on subcutaneous route of administration as an immunogenicity risk factor for therapeutic proteins. J Pharm Sci 106:2946–2954

Han PD, Cohen RD (2004) Managing immunogenic responses to infliximab: treatment implications for patients with Crohn's disease. Drugs 64:1767–1777

Harding FA, Stickler MM, Razo J, DuBridge RB (2010) The Immunogenicity of humanized and fully human antibodies: residual immunogenicity resides in the CDR regions. MAbs 2:256–265

Hermeling S, Crommelin DJ, Schellekens H, Jiskoot W (2004) Structure-immunogenicity relationships of therapeutic proteins. Pharm Res 21:897–903

Jawa V, Cousens LP, Awwad M, Wakshull E, Kropshofer H, De Groot AS (2013) T-cell dependent immunogenicity of protein therapeutics: preclinical assessment and mitigation. Clin Immunol 149:534–555

Jiskoot W, Kijanka G, Randolph TW, Carpenter JF, Koulov AV, Mahler HC, Joubert MK, Jawa V, Narhi LO (2016) Mouse models for assessing protein immunogenicity: lessons and challenges. J Pharm Sci 105:1567–1575

Kijanka G, Jiskoot W, Sauerborn M, Schellekens H, Brinks V (2012) Immunogenicity of therapeutic proteins in pharmaceutical formulation development of peptides and proteins. CRC Press, Boca Raton, pp 297–322

Krishna M, Palme H, Duo J, Lin Z, Corbett M, Dodge R, Piccoli S, Myler H, Pillutla R, Desilva B (2015) Development and characterization of antibody reagents to assess anti-PEG IgG antibodies in clinical samples. Bioanalysis 7:1869–1883

Liu L (2015) Antibody glycosylation and its impact on the pharmacokinetics and pharmacodynamics of monoclonal antibodies and Fc-fusion proteins. J Pharm Sci 104:1866–1884

Maini R, St Clair EW, Breedveld F, Furst D, Kalden J, Weisman M, Smolen J, Emery P, Harriman G, Feldmann M, Lipsky P (1999) Infliximab (chimeric anti-tumour necrosis factor α monoclonal antibody) versus placebo in rheumatoid arthritis patients receiving concomitant methotrexate: a randomised phase III trial. Lancet 354:1932–1939

Malucchi S, Bertolotto A (2008) Clinical aspects of immunogenicity to biopharmaceuticals. Immunog Biopharm 47:27–56

Mire-Sluis AR, Barrett YC, Devanarayan V, Koren E, Liu H, Maia M, Parish T, Scott G, Shankar G, Shores E, Swanson SJ, Taniguchi G, Wierda D, Zuckerman LA (2004) Recommendations for the design and optimization of immunoassays used in the detection of host antibodies against biotechnology products. J Immunol Methods 289:1–16

Moore WV, Leppert P (1980) Role of aggregated human growth hormone (hGH) in development of antibodies to hGH. J Clin Endocrinol Metab 51:691–697

Moss AC, Brinks V, Carpenter JF (2013) Review article: Immunogenicity of anti-TNF biologics in IBD - the role of patient, product and prescriber factors. Aliment Pharmacol Ther 38:1188–1197

Oldenburg J, Lacroix-Desmazes S, Lillicrap D (2015) Alloantibodies to therapeutic factor VIII in hemophilia A: the role of von Willebrand factor in regulating Factor VIII immunogenicity. Haematologica 100:149–156

Perini P, Facchinetti A, Bulian P, Massaro AR, Pascalis DD, Bertolotto A, Biasi G, Gallo P (2001) Interferon-beta (INF-Beta) antibodies in interferon-beta1a- and interferon-beta1b-treated multiple sclerosis patients. Prevalence, kinetics, cross-reactivity, and factors enhancing interferon-beta immunogenicity in vivo. Eur Cytokine Netw 12:56–61

Praditpornsilpa K, Kupatawintu P, Mongkonsritagoon W, Supasyndh O, Jootar S, Intarakumthornchai T, Pongskul C, Prasithsirikul W, Achavanuntakul B, Ruangkarnchanasetr P, Laohavinij S, Eiam-Ong S (2009) The association of anti-R-HuEpo-associated pure Red cell aplasia with HLA-DRB1*09-DQB1*0309. Nephrol Dial Transplant 24:1545–1549

Prümmer O (1997) Treatment-induced antibodies to interleukin-2. Biotherapy 10:15–24

Richter WF, Bhansali SG, Morris ME (2012) Mechanistic determinants of biotherapeutics absorption following sc administration. AAPS J 14:559–570

Ross C, Clemmesen KM, Svenson M, Sørensen PS, Koch-Henriksen N, Skovgaard GL, Bendtzen K (2000) Immunogenicity of interferon-beta in multiple sclerosis patients: influence of preparation, dosage, dose Frequency, and route of administration. Ann Neurol 48:706–712

Rougeot C, Marchand PM, Dray F, Girard F, Job JC, Pierson M, Ponte C, Rochiccioli P, Rappaport R (1991) Comparative study of biosynthetic human growth hormone immunogenicity in growth hormone deficient children. Horm Res 35:76–81

Ryff JC (1997) Clinical investigation of the immunogenicity of interferon-alpha 2a. J Interf Cytokine Res 17:S29–S33

Schellekens H (2002a) Bioequivalence and the immunogenicity of biopharmaceuticals. Nat Rev Drug Discov 1:457–462
Schellekens H (2002b) Immunogenicity of therapeutic proteins: clinical implications and future prospects. Clin Ther 24:1720–1740
Schellekens H, Casadevall N (2004) Immunogenicity of recombinant human proteins: causes and consequences. J Neurol 251:II4–II9
Schellekens H, Jiskoot W (2006) Erythropoietin-associated PRCA: still an unsolved mystery. J Immunotoxicol 3:123–130
Schellekens H, Hennink WE, Brinks V (2013) The immunogenicity of polyethylene glycol: facts and fiction. Pharm Res 30:1729–1734
Shankar G, Devanarayan V, Amaravadi L, Barrett YC, Bowsher R, Finco-Kent D, Fiscella M, Gorovits B, Kirschner S, Moxness M, Parish T, Quarmby V, Smith H, Smith W, Zuckerman LA, Koren E (2008) Recommendations for the validation of immunoassays used for detection of host antibodies against biotechnology products. J Pharm Biomed Anal 48:1267–1281
Shankar G, Arkin S, Cocea L, Devanarayan V, Kirshner S, Kromminga A, Quarmby V, Richards S, Schneider CK, Subramanyam M, Swanson S, Verthelyi D, Yim S (2014) Assessment and reporting of the clinical immunogenicity of therapeutic proteins and peptides—harmonized terminology and tactical recommendations. AAPS J 16:658–673
Singh SK (2011) Impact of product-related factors on immunogenicity of biotherapeutics. J Pharm Sci 100:354–387
van Beers MM, Jiskoot W, Schellekens H (2010) On the role of aggregates in the immunogenicity of recombinant human interferon beta in patients with multiple sclerosis. J Interf Cytokine Res 30:767–775
van de Casteele N, Gils A, Singh S, Ohrmund L, Hauenstein S, Rutgeerts P, Vermeire S (2013) Antibody response to infliximab and its impact on pharmacokinetics can be transient. Am J Gastroenterol 108:962–971
van Schie KA, Hart MH, de Groot ER, Kruithof S, Aarden LA, Wolbink GJ, Rispens T (2015a) The antibody response against human and chimeric anti-TNF therapeutic antibodies primarily targets the TNF binding region. Ann Rheum Dis 74:311–314
van Schie KA, Wolbink GJ, Rispens T (2015b) Cross-reactive and pre-existing antibodies to therapeutic antibodies. Effects on treatment and immunogenicity. MAbs 7:662–671
van Schie KA, Kruithof S, van Schouwenburg PA, Vennegoor A, Killestein J, Wolbink G, Rispens T (2017) Neutralizing capacity of monoclonal and polyclonal anti-natalizumab antibodies: the immune response to antibody therapeutics preferentially targets the Antigen-binding site. J Allergy Clin Immunol 139:1035–1037
van Schouwenburg PA, Rispens T, Wolbink GJ (2013a) Immunogenicity of anti-TNF biologic therapies for rheumatoid arthritis. Nat Rev Rheumatol 9:164–172
van Schouwenburg PA, Krieckaert CL, Rispens T, Aarden L, Wolbink GJ, Wouters D (2013b) Long-term measurement of anti-adalimumab using pH-shift-anti-idiotype antigen binding test shows predictive value and transient antibody formation. Ann Rheum Dis 72:1680–1686
Vincent FB, Morand EF, Murphy K, Mackay F, Mariette X, Marcelli C (2013) Antidrug antibodies (ADA) to tumour necrosis factor (TNF)-specific neutralising agents in chronic inflammatory diseases: a real issue, a clinical perspective. Ann Rheum Dis 72:165–178
Weigle WO (1971) Recent observations and concepts in immunological unresponsiveness and autoimmunity. Clin Exp Immunol 9:437–447
Xue L, Rup B (2013) Evaluation of pre-existing antibody presence as a risk factor for posttreatment anti-drug antibody induction: analysis of human clinical study data for multiple biotherapeutics. AAPS J 15:893–896

SUGGESTED READING

Brinks V, Jiskoot W, Schellekens H (2011) Immunogenicity of therapeutic proteins: the use of animal models. Pharm Res 28:2379–2385
Filipe V, Hawe A, Schellekens H, Jiskoot W (2010) Aggregation and immunogenicity of therapeutic proteins. In: Wang W, Robert C (eds) Aggregation of therapeutic proteins. Wiley, Hoboken
Hermeling S, Crommelin DJA, Schellekens H, Jiskoot W (2007) Immunogenicity of therapeutic proteins. In: Gad SC (ed) Handbook of pharmaceutical biotechnology. Wiley, Hoboken, pp 911–931
Moussa EM, Panchal JP, Moorthy BS, Blum JS, Joubert MK, Narhi LO, Topp EM (2016) Immunogenicity of therapeutic protein aggregates. J Pharm Sci 105:417–430
Schellekens H, Crommelin D, Jiskoot W (2007) Immunogenicity of antibody therapeutics. In: Dübel S (ed) Handbook of therapeutic antibodies. Wiley, Weinheim, pp 267–276
Schellekens H (2010) The immunogenicity of therapeutic proteins. Discov Med 9:560–564

8

Monoclonal Antibodies: From Structure to Therapeutic Application

Rong Deng, C. Andrew Boswell, Wendy S. Putnam, Meina T. Tang, Amit Garg, Chunze Li, Shan Chung, and Sandhya Girish

INTRODUCTION

The exciting field of therapeutic monoclonal antibodies (MABs) had its origins when Köhler and Milstein presented their murine hybridoma technology in 1975 (Kohler and Milstein 1975). This technology provides a reproducible method for producing MABs with unique target selectivity in almost unlimited quantities. In 1984, both scientists received the Nobel Prize for their scientific breakthrough, and their work is viewed as a key milestone in the history of MABs as therapeutic modalities and their other applications. Although it took some time until the first therapeutic MAB received FDA approval in 1986 (Orthoclone OKT3, Chap. 25), MABs are now the standard of care in several disease areas. In particular, in oncology (Chap. 23), transplantation (Chap. 25), and inflammatory diseases (Chap. 26), patients now have novel life-changing treatment alternatives for diseases that had very limited or nonexistent medical treatment options before the emergence of MABs. Today, more than 75 MABs and MAB derivatives, including fusion proteins and MAB fragments, are available for a variety of indications (Table 8.1). The majority of approved biologic therapies are MABs, antibody-drug conjugates (ADCs), antibody fragments, and Fc fusion proteins. Technological evolutions have subsequently allowed much wider application of MABs thanks to the ability to generate mouse/human chimeric, humanized, and fully human MABs from antibodies (Abs) of pure murine origin. In particular, the reduction of the xenogenic portion of the MAB structure decreased the immunogenic potential of murine MABs, allowing their wider application. MABs are generally well-tolerated drugs because of their target selectivity, thus avoiding unnecessary exposure to, and consequently activity in, nontarget organs. This is particularly apparent in the field of oncology where MABs such as rituximab, trastuzumab, bevacizumab, cetuximab and immune-oncology MABs such as atezolizumab, pembrolizumab and nivolumab can offer a more favorable risk-benefit profile compared to common chemotherapeutic treatment regimens for some hematologic cancers and solid tumors.

The advent of MABs not only resulted in new drugs, but also triggered the development of an entirely new business model for drug research and development and the founding of hundreds of biotech companies focused on MAB development. Furthermore, the ability to selectively target disease-related molecules with MABs helped to launch a new era of targeted medicine and set new standards for successful drug research and development. The term translational medicine was coined to describe the use of biochemical, biological, and (patho)physiological understanding to find novel interventions to treat disease. During this process, biomarkers (e.g., genetic expression levels of marker genes, protein expression of target proteins, or molecular imaging) can be used to gain deeper understanding of the biological activities of drugs in a qualitative and, most importantly, quantitative sense, essentially encompassing the entire field of pharmacokinetics and pharmacodynamics (PK/PD). The application of these scientific methods, together with the principle of molecular-targeted medicine and the favorable PK and safety of MABs, may at least partly explain the higher success rates of biotechnologically derived products in reaching the market compared to chemically derived small molecule drugs.

This chapter addresses the following topics: Antibody structure and classes, currently approved MAB based therapeutics, mechanisms of action, clinical development and drug properties. In this sense, this

R. Deng · W. S. Putnam · M. T. Tang · A. Garg
C. Li · S. Girish (✉)
Clinical Pharmacology, Genentech Inc.,
South San Francisco, CA, USA
e-mail: sandhyag@gene.com

C. A. Boswell
Preclinical and Translational Pharmacokinetics,
Genentech Inc., South San Francisco, CA, USA

S. Chung
Bioanalytical Sciences, Genentech Inc.,
South San Francisco, CA, USA

D. J. A. Crommelin et al. (eds.), *Pharmaceutical Biotechnology*, https://doi.org/10.1007/978-3-030-00710-2_8

Name	Therapeutic area	Antibody/antibody derivatives		Target		PK					
		Type	Structure	Receptor/antigen	Type	Behavior[b]	Elimination/terminal half-life[c]	Clearance (CL)/apparent CL	Volume of distribution (V and apparent V)[d]	Route/dosing highlights
Abciximab	Cardiovascular/metabolism	Fragment	Chimeric Fab: +D31mVar-hIgG1	CD41	Cell-bound	Linear	0.29 days[e]	0.068 L/h/kg[f]	0.12 L/kg	IV bolus, mg/kg dose
Alirocumab	Cardiovascular/metabolism	MAB	hIgG1	PCSK9	Soluble	Nonlinear	17–20 days	NR	Central Vd: 0.04–0.05 L/kg	SC injection, flat mg dose
Dulaglutide	Cardiovascular/metabolism	Fusion protein	Disulfide-linked homo-dimer GLP-1 + modified hIgG4H (Fc)	GLP-1 R	Cell-bound	NR	5 days	0.75 mg dose: 0.111 L/h 1.5 mg dose: 0.107 L/h	0.75 mg dose: 19.2 L 1.5 mg dose: 17.4 L	SC injection, flat mg dose
Evolocumab	Cardiovascular/metabolism	MAB	hIgG2	PCSK9	Soluble	Nonlinear	11–17 days (effective $t_{1/2}$)	12 mL/h after 420 mg IV	3.3 L after 420 mg IV	SC injection, flat mg dose
Idarucizumab	Cardiovascular/metabolism	Fragment	Humanized IgG1 (Fab)	Dabigatran and its acyl-glucuronide metabolites	N/A	NR	Initial: 47 min; terminal:10.3 h	47.0 mL/min	8.9 L	IV infusion, flat gram dose
Antihemophilic factor (recombinant), Fc fusion protein	Hemophilia	Fusion protein	B-domain deleted human coagulation Factor VIII + hIgG1 Fc	NR	NR	NR	1–5 years: 12.7 h 6–11 years: 14.9 h 12–17 years: 16.4 h Adults: 19.7 h	1–5 years: 3.60 mL/h/kg 6–11 years: 2.78 mL/h/kg 12–17 years: 2.66 mL/h/kg Adults: 2.06 mL/h/kg	–5 years: 58.6 mL/kg 6–11 years: 52.1 mL/kg 12–17 years: 60.3 mL/kg Adults: 49.5 mL/kg	IV injection, individualized per label
Alprolix	Hemophilia	Fusion protein	Human coagulation Factor IX + hIgG1 (Fc)	N/A	N/A	NR	50 IU/kg: 86 h 100 IU/kg: 91 h	50 IU/kg dose: 3.3 mL/h/kg 100 IU/kg: 2.6 mL/h/kg	50 IU/kg: 327 mL/kg 100 IU/kg: 236 mL/kg	IV infusion, IU/kg dose
Emicizumab-kxwh	Hemophilia	MAB	Humanized bi-specific IgG4	Factor IXa and factor X	Soluble	Linear within dose range of 0.3–3.0 mg/kg	27.8 ± 8.1 days	CL/F: 0.24 L/day (apparent)	V/F: 11.4 L (apparent)	SC injection, mg/kg dose
Palivizumab	Infectious disease	MAB	Humanized IgG1	RSV F protein	Cell-bound	NR	20 days	NR	NR	IM injection, mg/kg dose
Bezlotoxumab	Infectious disease	MAB	hIgG1	*C. difficile* toxin B	Cell-bound	Linear	19 days	0.317 L/day	7.33 L	IV infusion, mg/kg dose
Obiltoxaximab[g]	Infectious disease	MAB	Chimeric: mVar-hIgG1 kappa	PA component *B. anthracis* toxin	Cell bound	Linear over 4–16 mg/kg dose range	15–23 days	NR	NR	IV infusion, mg/kg dose
Abatacept	Inflammation/autoimmunity	Fusion protein	hCTLA-4 ECD + hFc (hinge)	CD80, CD86	Cell-bound	Linear	13.1 days[h]	0.22 mL/h/kg[h]	0.07 L/kg	IV infusion, mg/kg dose
Adalimumab	Inflammation/autoimmunity	MAB	hIgG1	TNFα	Soluble, cell-bound	Linear	14.7–19.3 days[i]	9–12 mL/h[i]	5.1–5.75 L: *F* = 64%	SC injection, flat mg dose
Alefacept[j]	Inflammation/autoimmunity	Fusion protein	LFA-3 + hIgG1 (Fc)	CD2	Cell-bound	Nonlinear	11.3 days	0.25 (mL/h/kg)	IV: 94 mL/kg IM: *F* = 63%	IV infusion, flat mg dose

Belimumab	Inflammation/ autoimmunity	MAB	hIgG1	BLyS	Soluble, cell-bound	Linear	19.4 days	215 mL/day	5.29 L	IV infusion mg/ kg dose
Benralizumab	Inflammation/ autoimmunity	MAB	Humanized IgG1	IL-5Rα	Cell-bound	Linear at 20–200 mg range	15 days	70 kg patient: 0.29 L/day	70 kg patient: 5.7 L; SC: F ≈ 58%	SC injection, flat mg dose
Brodalumab	Inflammation/ autoimmunity	MAB	hIgG2	hIL-17RA	Cell-bound	Nonlinear	NR	CL/F: 3.0 ± 3.5 L/ day (apparent CL)	Vz/F: 8.9 ± 9.4 L (apparent Vz)	SC injection, flat mg dose
Canakinumab	Inflammation/ Autoimmunity	MAB	hIgG1	IL-1β	Soluble	Linear	26 days	0.174 L/day	6.01 L, *F* = 70%	SC injection, flat mg dose
Certolizumab pegol	Inflammation/ autoimmunity	Fragment	Humanized IgG1 (Fab) conjugated with PEG2MAL40K	TNFα	Soluble, cell-bound	Linear	14 days	9.21–14.38 mL/h	6–8 L, *F* = 76–88%	SC injection, flat mg dose
Daclizumab HYP	Inflammation/ autoimmunity	MAB	Humanized IgG1	CD25	Cell-bound	Linear	22 days	CL: 0.24 L/day CL/F: 0.274 L/ day (apparent CL)	6.41 L	SC injection, flat mg dose
Dupilumab[k]	Inflammation/ autoimmunity	MAB	hIgG4	IL-4Rα (common subunit IL-4R and IL-13R complexes)	Cell-bound	Nonlinear	NR	0.126 L/day	4.8 ± 1.3 L	SC injection, flat mg dose with loading dose
Eculizumab	Inflammation/ autoimmunity	MAB	Humanized IgG2/4 kappa	complement protein C5	Soluble	Linear	8–14.8 days	22 mL/h	7.7 L	IV infusion, flat mg dose
Efalizumab[l]	Inflammation/ autoimmunity	MAB	Humanized IgG1	CD11a	Cell-bound, internalized	Nonlinear	N/A	6.6 mL/kg/day[m]	58 mL/kg SC, *F* = 50%	SC injection, mg/kg dose
Etanercept	Inflammation/ autoimmunity	Fusion protein	TNF receptor + hIgG1 (Fc)	TNFα	Soluble, cell-bound	Linear	4 days[n]	120 mL/h; CL/F: 160 mL/hr[n]	*F*: 58%; Vd: 6–11 L	SC injection, flat mg dose
Golimumab	Inflammation/ autoimmunity	MAB	hIgG1	TNFα	Soluble, cell-bound	Linear	2 weeks	4.9–6.7 mL/day/ kg	Vd = 58–126 mL/kg; F = 53%	SC injection, flat mg dose
Infliximab	Inflammation/ autoimmunity	MAB	Chimeric: mVar-hIgG1	TNFα	Soluble, cell-bound	Linear	7.7–9.5 days	9.8 mL/h[o]	NR	IV infusion, mg/ kg dose
Ixekizumab	Inflammation/ autoimmunity	MAB	Humanized IgG4	IL-17A	Soluble, membrane bound	Linear	13 days	0.39 L/day	7.11 L	SC injection, flat mg dose with loading dose
Mepolizumab	Inflammation/ autoimmunity	MAB	Humanized IgG1, kappa	IL-5	Soluble	Linear	20 days (range 16–22 days)	70 kg patient: 0.28 L/day	70 kg patient: Vc = 3.6 L	SC injection, flat mg dose
Natalizumab	Inflammation/ autoimmunity	MAB	Humanized IgG4 kappa	α4 integrins	Cell-bound	NR	11 days	16 mL/h	NR	IV infusion, flat mg dose
Ocrelizumab	Inflammation/ autoimmunity	MAB	Humanized IgG1, glycosylated	CD20	Cell-bound	Nonlinear, linear over 400–2000 mg dose range	26 days	CL linear: 0.17 L/ day	Vc 2.78 L, Vp 2.68 L	IV infusion, flat mg dose

Table 8.1 ■ Therapeutic biologics (monoclonal antibodies, antibody fragments, fusion proteins and antibody-drug conjugates)[a]

Name	Therapeutic area	Antibody/antibody derivatives		Target		PK				
		Type	Structure	Receptor/ antigen	Type	Behavior[b]	Elimination/ terminal half-life[c]	Clearance (CL)/ apparent CL	Volume of distribution (V and apparent V)[d]	Route/dosing highlights
Omalizumab	Inflammation/ autoimmunity	MAB	Humanized IgG1, kappa	IgE	Soluble	Linear over 0.5 mg/kg	26 days (asthma) 24 days (CIU)	2.4 mL/day/kg (asthma); 3.0 mL/day/kg (CIU)	Apparent Vd = 78 ± 32 mL/kg; *F* = 62%	SC injection; Asthma: mg dose based on weight (kg) and IgE level (IU/mL), CIU: flat mg dose
Reslizumab	Inflammation/ autoimmunity	MAB	Humanized IgG4 kappa	IL-5	Soluble	Linear	24 days	7 mL/h	5 L	IV infusion,mg/kg dose
Rilonacept	Inflammation/ autoimmunity	Fusion protein	hIgG1	IL-1β	Soluble	NR	7.6 days	CL/F: 0.866 L/day	Vz/F: 9.73 L	SC injection, flat mg dose
Secukinumab	Inflammation/ autoimmunity	MAB	hIgG1 kappa	IL-17A	Soluble, cell-bound	Linear over 25–300 mg dose range	22–31 days	0.14–0.22 L/day	Vz: 7.10–8.60 L	SC injection, flat mg dose with loading dose
Siltuximab	Inflammation/ autoimmunity	MAB	Chimeric: mouse-human IgG1	IL-6	Soluble and cell-bound	Linear over a 2.8–11 mg/kg dose range	20.6 days range 14.2–29.7 days	0.23 L/day	70 kg male subject: 4.5 L	IV infusion, mg/kg dose
Tocilizumab	Inflammation/ autoimmunity	MAB	Humanized IgG1	IL-6R	Soluble, cell-bound	Nonlinear	Up to 13 days	12.5 mL/h	6.4 L	IV infusion, mg/kg dose
Ustekinumab[p]	Inflammation/ autoimmunity	MAB	hIgG1	IL-12, IL-23	Soluble	Linear	14.9–45.6 days	0.19 L/day	4.62 L	SC injection, flat mg dose
Vedolizumab	Inflammation/ Autoimmunity	MAB	Humanized IgG1	α4β7	Cell-bound	Linear and nonlinear	25 days at 300 mg	Linear CL: 0.157 L/day	5 L	IV infusion, flat mg dose
Alemtuzumab	Inflammation/ autoimmunity/ oncology	MAB	Humanized IgG1	CD52	Soluble	Nonlinear	MS: 14 days; CLL and NHL:11 h after single dose, 12 days following multiple doses[q]	NR	0.18 L/kg	IV infusion, flat mg dose
Rituximab	Inflammation/ autoimmunity/ oncology	MAB	Chimeric: mVar-hIgG1	CD20	Cell-bound	Linear	RA: 18 days (5.17–77.5 days); NHL: 22 days (6.1–52 days); CLL: 32 days (14–62 days)	RA: 0.335 L/day	RA: 3.1 L	IV infusion, mg/m^2 dose
Asfotase alfa	Metabolic disorder	Fusion protein/ enzyme	Human TNSALP catalytic domain + hIgG1(Fc)	Hydrolyzes phosphor-monoesters	N/A	Linear	5 days	NR	NR	SC injection, mg/kg dose
Atezolizumab	Oncology	MAB	Non-glycosylated humanized IgG1	PD-L1	Soluble, cell-bound	Linear over 1 mg/kg to 20 mg/kg	27 days	0.2 L/kg	6.9 L	IV infusion, flat mg dose

Avelumab	Oncology	MAB	hIGg1 lambda	PD-L1	Soluble, cell-bound	Linear over 10–20 mg/kg	6.1 days at 10 mg/kg	0.59 L/day	4.72 L	IV infusion, mg/kg dose
Bevacizumab	Oncology	MAB	Humanized IgG1	VEGF	Soluble	Linear	20 days	0.207–0.262 L/day	2.66–3.25 L	IV infusion, mg/kg dose
Brentuximab vedotin	Oncology	ADC	Chimeric mVar-hIgG1	CD30	Cell-bound	Linear over 1.2–2.7 mg/kg	4.43 days	1.76 L/day[r]	8.21 L	IV infusion, mg/kg dose
Catumaxomab[i] (EU only)	Oncology	MAB	Chimeric: rat-mouse tri-functional MAB	EpCAM and CD3	Cell-bound	NR	2.5 days (range: 0.7–17 days)	NR	NR	IP infusion, flat µg dose
Cetuximab	Oncology	MAB	Chimeric: mVar-hIgG1	EGFR	Soluble	Nonlinear	4.8 days	0.02–0.08 L/h/m^2	2–3 L/m^2	IV infusion, mg/m^2 dose
Daratumumab	Oncology	MAB	hIgG1 kappa	CD38	Cell-bound	Nonlinear	18 ± 9 days (mono-therapy) 23 ± 12 days (combination therapy)	171.4 ± 95.3 mL/day	Vc: 4.7 ± 1.3 L (mono-therapy) 4.4 ± 1.5 L (combination therapy)	IV infusion, mg/kg dose
Denosumab	Oncology	MAB	hIgG2	RANKL	Cell-bound	Linear	28 days	CL_{linear} = 3.25 mL/h/66 kg	Vc = 2.62 L/66 kg; Vss = 3.96 L/66 kg[s]	SC injection, flat mg dose
Dinutuximab	Oncology	MAB	Chimeric: mVar-hIgG1 kappa	GD2 glycolipid	Cell-bound	NR	10 days	0.21 L/day	5.4 L	IV infusion, mg/m^2/day dose
Durvalumab	Oncology	MAB	hIgG1 kappa	PD-L1	Soluble, cell-bound	Linear over dose range of 3–20 mg/kg	17 days	CLss: 8.24 mL/h (clearance decreases over time)	5.6 L	IV infusion, mg/kg dose
Elotuzumab	Oncology	MAB	Humanized IgG1	CD319 (SLAMF7)	Cell-bound	Nonlinear	NR	0.5 mg/kg dose: 17.5 mL/day/kg; 20 mg/kg dose: 5.8 mL/day/kg	NR	IV infusion, mg/kg dose with loading dose
Gemtuzumab ozogamicin	Oncology	ADC	Humanized IgG4 kappa (hP67.6) + *N*-acetyl-gamma-calicheamicin (cytotoxin)	CD33	Cell-bound	Nonlinear	t1/2 hp67.6 MAB: after 1st dose = 62 h, after 2nd dose = 90 h	CLss hp67.6 MAB: after 1st dose = 0.35 L/h, after 2nd dose = 0.15 L/h	V1 = 6.31 L, V2 = 15.1 L for hp67.6 MAB	IV infusion, mg/m^2 dose
Ibritumomab tiuxetan	Oncology	MAB	Murine IgG1+ tiuxetan (chelator)	CD20	Cell-bound	NR	47 h[t]	NR	NR	IV injection over 10 min, mci/kg dose
Inotuzumab ozogamicin	Oncology	ADC	Humanized IgG4 kappa + *N*-acetyl-gamma-calicheamicin (cytotoxin)	CD22	Cell-bound	Nonlinear	12.3 days	CLss, 0.0333 L/h	12 L for ADC	IV infusion, mg/m^2 dose

Table 8.1 ■ (continued)

Name	Therapeutic area	Antibody/antibody derivatives		Target		PK				
		Type	Structure	Receptor/ antigen	Type	Behavior[b]	Elimination/ terminal half-life[c]	Clearance (CL)/ apparent CL	Volume of distribution (V and apparent V)[d]	Route/dosing highlights
Ipilimumab	Oncology	MAB	hIgG1	CTLA-4	Cell-bound	Linear	15.4 days	16.8 mL/h	7.21 L	IV infusion, mg/ kg dose
Necitumumab	Oncology	MAB	hIgG1 kappa	EGFR	Cell-bound	Nonlinear	14 days (after 800 mg on days 1 and 8 of each 21-day cycle)	14.1 mL/h after 800 mg on days 1 and 8 of each 21-day cycle	7.0 L after 800 mg on Days 1 and 8 of each 21-day cycle	IV infusion, flat mg dose
Nivolumab	Oncology	MAB	hIgG4 kappa	PD-1	Cell-bound	Linear	25 days	8.2 mL/h	6.8 L	IV infusion, flat mg dose
Obinutuzumab	Oncology	MAB	Humanized IgG1 with reduced fucose content	CD20	Cell-bound	Linear within recommended dose range	CLL patients: 25.5 days NHL patients: 35.3 days	CLL: 0.11 L/day; NHL: 0.08 L/ day (both values after TMDD saturation)	CLL: 4.1 L NHL: 4.3 L	IV infusion, flat mg dose
Ofatumumab	Oncology	MAB	hIgG1 kappa	CD-20	Cell-bound	Nonlinear	14 days	0.01 L/h	1.7–5.1 L	IV infusion, flat mg dose
Olaratumab	Oncology	MAB	hIgG1	PDGFR-α	Cell-bound	NR	11 days (range 6–24 days)	0.56 L/day	7.7 L	IV infusion, mg/ kg dose
Panitumumab[u]	Oncology	MAB	hIgG2	EGFR	Cell-bound	Nonlinear	7.5 days	4.9 mL/day/kg	82 mL/kg	IV infusion, mg/ kg dose
Pembrolizumab	Oncology	MAB	hIgG4 kappa	PD-1	Cell-bound	Linear over 2–10 mg/kg dose range	22 days	252 mL/day after first dose, 195 mL/day at steady state (geometric mean)	6.0 L	IV infusion, flat mg dose
Pertuzumab	Oncology	MAB	Humanized IgG1	HER2	Cell-bound, shed	Linear over 2-25 mg/kg dose range	18 days[v]	0.235 L/day[v]	5.57 L	IV infusion, flat mg dose
Ramucirumab	Oncology	MAB	hIgG1	VEGFR2	Cell-bound	Linear	14 days	0.015 L/h	NR	IV infusion, mg/ kg dose
Tositumomab	Oncology	MAB (radiolabeled)	mIgG2α	CD20	Cell-bound	Nonlinear	NR	68.2 mL/h	NR	IV infusion, flat mg dose
Trastuzumab	Oncology	MAB	Humanized IgG1	HER2	Cell-bound, shed	Nonlinear	NR	0.173–0.283 L/ day (breast cancer) 0.189–0.337 L/ day (gastric cancer)[w]	6 L (breast cancer) 6.6 L (gastric cancer)	IV infusion, mg/ kg dose
Trastuzumab emtansine	Oncology	ADC	Humanized IgG1 + emtansine (cytotoxin)	HER2	Cell-bound, shed	Linear at dose ≥2.4 mg/kg	4 days for ADC	0.68 L/day For ADC	3.13 L for ADC	IV infusion, mg/ kg dose

Ziv-aflibercept	Oncology	Fusion protein	Human VEGF receptors 1 and 2 ligand-binding ECD + hIgG1 (Fc)	hVEGF-A, hVEGF-B, hPIGF	Soluble	Linear	6 days (range 4–7 days)	NR	NR	IV infusion, mg/kg dose
Aflibercept	Ophthalmology	Fusion protein	hVEGF receptors 1 and 2 ECDs + human IgG1 (Fc)	VEGF-A, PIGF	Soluble	NR	5–6 days after IV	NR	6 L after IV	Intravitreal, flat mg dose
Ranibizumab	Ophthalmology	Fragment	humanized IgG1κ	VEGF	Soluble	NR	9 days	NR	NR	Intravitreal injection, flat mg dose
Basiliximab	Transplantation	MAB	Chimeric: mVar-hIgG1	CD25	Cell-bound	NR	4.1 days[x]	75 mL/h[x]	5.5–13.9 L	IV bolus or infusion, flat mg dose
Belatacept	Transplantation	Fusion protein	hCTLA-4 ECD + hFc (hinge)	CD80, CD86	Cell-bound	Linear	9.8 days	0.49 mL/h/kg	0.11 L/kg	IV infusion, mg/kg dose
Daclizumab	Transplantation	MAB	humanized IgG1	CD25	Cell-bound	Linear	20 days	15 mL/h	5.9 L	IV infusion, mg/kg dose
Muromonab-CD3	Transplantation	MAB	mIgG2α	CD3	Cell-bound	NR	0.75 days[y]	NR	NR	IV bolus, flat mg dose

ADC antibody-drug conjugate, *CD* cluster of differentiation, *CDR* complementarity determining region, *CLL* chronic lymphocytic leukemia, *CTLA* cytotoxic T lymphocyte-associated antigen, *ECD*, extracellular domain, *EGFR* epidermal growth factor receptor, *CLss* clearance at steady-state, *F* bioavailability, *Fab* antigen-binding fragment, *Fc* constant fragment, *HER2* human epidermal growth factor receptor 2, *Ig* immunoglobulin, *IL* interleukin, *IM* intramuscular, *IV* intravenous, *LFA* lymphocyte function-associated antigen, *MAB* monoclonal antibody, *MS* multiple sclerosis, *mVar* murine variable, *NA* information not available or not found, *NHL* Non-Hodgkin lymphoma, *NR* information not reported, *PD-1* programmed cell death 1 receptor, *PDGFR* prostaglandin, *PIGF* phosphatidylinositol-glycan biosynthesis class F protein, *RA* rheumatoid arthritis, *RANKL* receptor activator of nuclear factor kappa-B ligand, *RSV* respiratory syncytial virus, *SC* subcutaneous, *TNSALP* tissue non-specific alkaline phosphatase, *TNF* tumor necrosis factor, *V1* volume of distribution of central compartment, *V2* volume of distribution of peripheral compartment, *Vc* volume of central compartment, *VEGF* vascular endothelial growth factor, *Vss* volume of distribution at steady state, *Vz* volume of distribution during the terminal phase

[a]Source: prescribing information (not shown) and/or additional references as shown
[b]Where PK are nonlinear, parameters are reported at usual clinical dose
[c]Terminal t1/2 reported for linear PK only
[d]Volume or apparent volume of distribution at steady state, unless otherwise indicated
[e]Kleiman et al. (1995) and Mager et al. (2003)
[f]Kleiman et al. (1995) and Mager et al. (2003)
[g]CDER (2015)
[h]Hervey and Keam (2006)
[i]Weisman et al. (2003)
[j]In 2011, manufacturing, distribution and sales of Amevive were halted during a supply disruption. According to the manufacturer, Astellas Pharma US, Inc., the decision to cease Amevive sales was neither the result of any specific safety concern nor of any FDA-mandated or voluntary product recall
[k]Kovarik et al. (2001) and Kovalenko et al. (2016)
[l]Withdrawn from market
[m]Joshi et al. (2006)
[n]Lee et al. (2003)
[o]Cornillie et al. (2001)
[p]Zhu et al. (2009)
[q]Morris et al. (2003)
[r]Younes et al. (2010)
[s]Gibiansky et al. (2012)
[t]Wiseman et al. (2001)
[u]Ma et al. (2009)
[v]Garg et al. (2014)
[w]Kirschbrown et al. (2017)
[x]Kovarik et al. (2001)
[y]Hooks et al. (1991)

chapter provides a general introduction to Chaps. 23, 25, and 26, where the currently marketed MABs and MAB derivatives including antibody fragments, fusion proteins and ADCs are discussed in the context of their therapeutic applications. Efalizumab (anti-CD11a), a MAB marketed as an anti-psoriasis drug in the US and EU, was chosen to illustrate the application of PK/PD principles in the drug development process.

ANTIBODY STRUCTURE AND CLASSES

Antibodies, or immunoglobulins (Igs), are roughly Y-shaped molecules or combinations of such molecules. There are five major classes of Ig: IgG, IgA, IgD, IgE, and IgM. Table 8.2 summarizes the characteristics of these molecules, particularly their structure (monomer, dimer, hexamer, or pentamer), molecular weight (ranging from ~150 to ~1150 kDa), and functions (e.g., activate complement, FcγR binding). Among these classes, IgGs and their derivatives form the framework for the development of therapeutic antibodies. Figure 8.1 depicts the general structural components of IgG and a conformational structure of efalizumab. An IgG molecule has four peptide chains, including two identical heavy (H) chains (50–55 kDa) and two identical light (L) chains (25 kDa), which are linked via disulfide (S–S) bonds at the hinge region. The first ~110 amino acids of both chains form the variable regions (V_H and V_L) and are also the antigen-binding regions. Each V domain contains three short stretches of

Property		IgA		IgG				IgM	IgD	IgE
Serum concentration in adult (mg/mL)		IgA1	IgA2	IgG1	IgG2	IgG3	IgG4			
		1.4–4.2	0.2–0.5	5–12	2–6	0.5–1	0.2–1	0.25–3.1	0.03–0.4	0.0001–0.0002
Molecular form		Monomer, dimer		Monomer				Pentamer, hexamer	Monomer	Monomer
Functional valency		2 or 4		2				5 or 10	2	2
Molecular weight (kDa)		160 (m), 300 (d)	160 (m), 350 (d)	150	150	160	150	950 (p)	175	190
Serum half-life (days)		5–7	4–6	21–24	21–24	7–8	21–24	5–10	2–8	1–5
% total IgG in adult serum		11–14	1–4	45–53	11–15	3–6	1–4	10	0.2	50
Function	Activate classical complement pathway	–		+	±	++	–	+++	–	–
	Activate alternative complement pathway	+	–	–	–	–	–	–	–	–
	Cross placenta	–		+	±	+	+	–	–	–
	Present on membrane of mature B cell	–		–	–	–	–	+	–	+
	Bind to Fc receptors of phagocytes	–		++	±	++	+	+	–	–
	Mucosal transport	++		–	–	–	–	+	–	–
	Induces mast cell degranulation	–		–	–	–	–	–	+	–
Biological properties		Secretory Ig, binds to polymeric Ig receptor		Placental transfer, secondary antibody for most response to pathogen, binds macrophage and other phagocytic cells by Fcγ receptor				Primary antibody response, some binding to polymeric Ig receptor, some binding to phagocytes	Mature B cell marker	Allergy and parasite reactivity, binds FcεR on mast cells and basophiles

Table 8.2 ■ Important properties of endogenous immunoglobulin subclass (Goldsby et al. 1999; Kolar and Capra 2003)

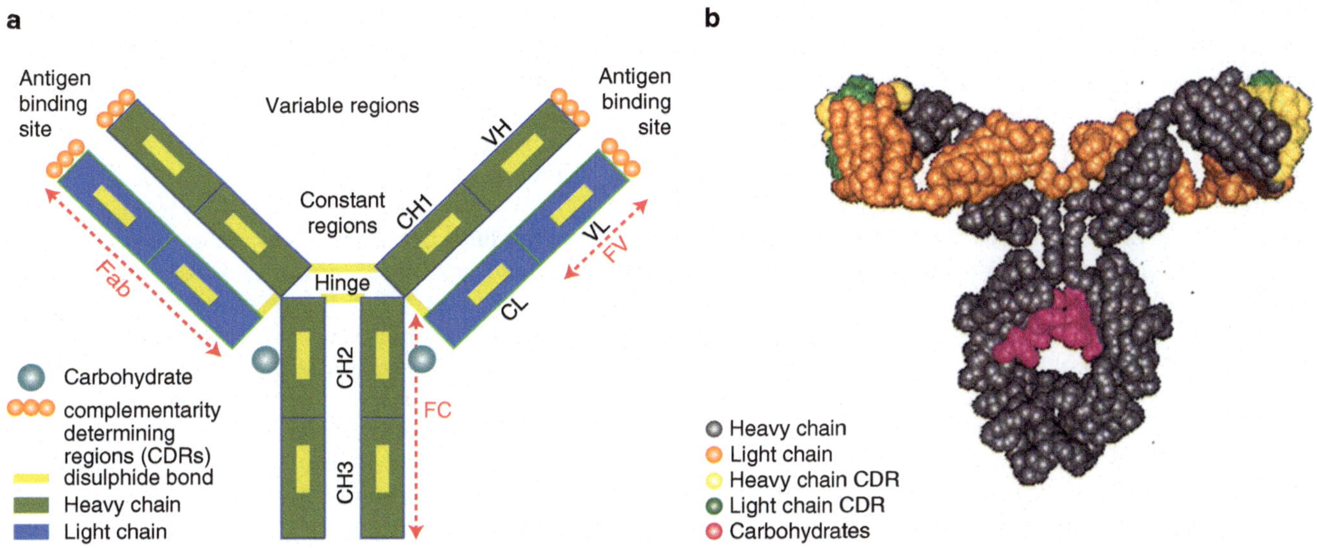

Figure 8.1 ■ (**a**) IgG1 antibody structure. Antigen is bound via the variable range of the antibody, whereas the Fc part of the IgG determines the mode of action (also called effector function). (**b**) Example of a conformational structure: efalizumab (anti-CD11a). *H chain* heavy chain consisting of VH, CH1, CH2, CH3; *L chain* light chain consisting of VL, CL; *VH, VL* variable light and heavy chain; *CHn, CL* constant light and heavy chain; *Fv* variable fraction; *Fc* crystallizable fraction; *Fab* antigen-binding fraction (http://people.cryst.bbk.ac.uk/~ubcg07s/gifs/IgG.gif)

peptide with hypervariable sequences (HV1, HV2, and HV3), known as complementarity determining regions (CDRs), i.e., the region that binds antigen. The remaining sequences of each light chain consist of a single constant domain (C_L). The remainder of each heavy chain contains three constant regions (C_{H1}, C_{H2}, and C_{H3}). Constant regions are responsible for effector recognition and binding. IgGs can be further divided into four subclasses (IgG1, IgG2, IgG3, and IgG4). The differences among these subclasses are also summarized in Table 8.2.

Murine, Chimeric, Humanized, and Fully Human MABs

The first therapeutic MABs were murine MABs produced via hybridomas; however, these murine MABs easily elicited formation of neutralizing human anti-mouse antibodies (HAMA) (Kuus-Reichel et al. 1994). With the advancement of technology, murine MABs have been engineered further to chimeric (mouse CDR, human Fc), humanized, and fully human MABs (Fig. 8.2). Murine MABs, chimeric MABs, humanized MABs, and fully human MABs have 0%, ~60–70%, ~90–95%, and ~100% sequence similarity to human MABs, respectively. Decreasing the xenogenic portion of the MAB potentially reduces the immunogenic risks of generating anti-drug antibodies (ADAs). Muromonab-CD3 (Orthoclone OKT3), a first-generation MAB of murine origin, has shown efficacy in the treatment of acute transplant rejection and was the first MAB licensed for use in humans. It is reported that 50% of the patients who received OKT3 produced

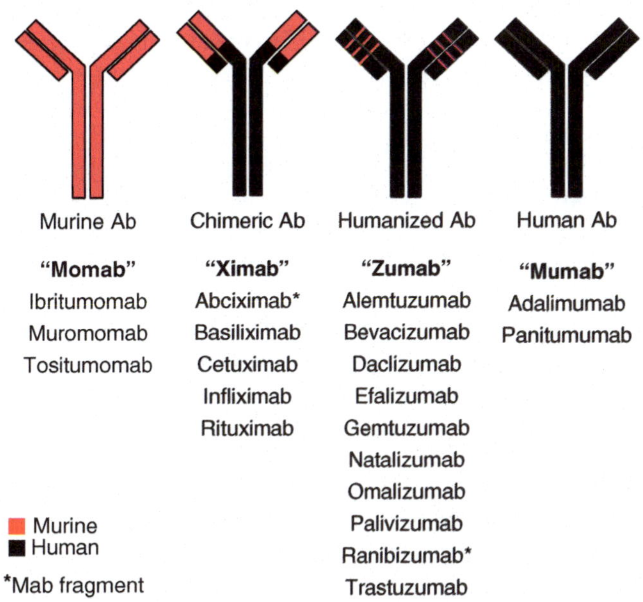

Figure 8.2 ■ Different generations of therapeutic antibodies

HAMA after the first dose. HAMA interfered with OKT3's binding to T cells, thus decreasing the therapeutic efficacy of the MAB (Norman et al. 1993). Later, molecular cloning and the expression of the variable region genes of IgGs facilitated the generation of engineered antibodies. A second generation of MABs, chimeric MABs, consists of human constant regions and mouse variable regions. The antigen specificity of a chimeric MAB is the same as the parental mouse antibody; however, the human Fc region renders a longer in vivo half-life than the parent murine MAB, and similar effector functions as a human antibody. Currently, there are 9 chimeric MABs, fragments and ADCs on the market (abciximab, basiliximab, cetuximab, dinutuximab, infliximab, obiltoxaximab, rituximab, siltuximab, and brentuximab vedotin). These MABs can still induce human anti-chimeric antibodies (HACA). For example, about 61% of patients who received infliximab had a HACA response associated with shorter duration of therapeutic efficacy and increased risk of infusion reactions (Baert et al. 2003). The development of ADAs appears to be different across indications. For example, 6 of 17 patients with systemic lupus erythematosus receiving rituximab developed high-titer HACA (Looney et al. 2004), whereas only 1 of 166 B cell depleted lymphoma patients developed HACA (McLaughlin et al. 1998). Humanized MABs contain significant portions of human sequence except the CDR which is still of murine origin. There are more than 25 humanized MABs (including ADCs) on the market (see Table 8.1). The incidence of ADAs (in this case, human anti-human antibodies or HAHAs), was greatly decreased for these humanized MABs. Trastuzumab has a reported a HAHA incidence of ~0.1% (1 of 903 cases) (Herceptin (Trastuzumab) Prescribing Information 2006), but daclizumab had HAHA rate as high as 34% (Zenapax (Daclizumab) Prescribing Information 2005). Another way to achieve full biocompatibility of MABs is to develop fully human antibodies, which can be produced by two approaches: through phage-display library or by using transgenic animals, such as the XenoMouse® or Trianni Mouse™ (Weiner 2006; Trianni.com 2018). Adalimumab is the first licensed fully human MAB generated using a phage-display library. Adalimumab was approved in 2002 and 2007 for the treatment of rheumatoid arthritis (RA) and Crohn's diseases, respectively (Humira (Adalimumab) Prescribing Information 2007). However, despite its fully human antibody structure, the incidence of HAHA was about 5% (58 of 1062 patients) in three randomized clinical trials with adalimumab (Cohenuram and Saif 2007; Humira (Adalimumab) Prescribing Information 2007). Panitumumab is the first approved fully human MAB generated using transgenic mouse technology. HAHA responses have been reported as less than 1% by an acid dissociation bridging enzyme-linked immunosorbent assay (ELISA) in clinical trial after chronic dosing with panitumumab to date (Vectibix (Panitumumab) Prescribing Information 2015; Cohenuram and Saif 2007). Of note, typically ADAs are measured using ELISA, and the reported incidence rates of ADAs for a given MAB can be influenced by the sensitivity and specificity of the assay. Additionally, the observed incidence of ADA positivity in an assay may also be influenced by several other factors, including sample handling, timing of sample collection, concomitant medications, and underlying disease. For these reasons, comparison of the incidence of ADAs to a specific MAB with the incidence of ADAs to another product may be misleading.

Key Structural Components of MABs

Proteolytic digestion of antibodies releases different fragments termed Fv (fragment variable), Fab (fragment antigen binding), and Fc (fragment crystallization) [reviewed by Wang et al. (2007)]. These fragments can also be generated by recombinant engineering. Treatment with papain generates two identical Fab's and one Fc. Pepsin treatment generates a F(ab')2 and several smaller fragments. Reduction of F(ab')2 will produce two Fab fragments. The Fv consists of the heavy chain variable domain (V_H) and the light chain variable domain (V_L) held together by strong noncovalent interaction. Stabilization of the Fv by a peptide linker generates a single chain Fv (scFv).

Modifying Fc Structures

The Fc regions of MABs play a critical role not only in their function but also in their disposition in the body. MABs elicit effector functions, including antibody-dependent cellular cytotoxicity (ADCC), antibody-dependent cellular phagocytosis (ADCP) and complement-dependent cytotoxicity (CDC), following interaction between their Fc regions and different Fcγ receptors and complement fixation (C1q, C3b). The CH2 domain and the hinge region joining CH1 and CH2 have been identified as the crucial regions for binding to FcγR (Presta 2002; Presta et al. 2002). Engineered MABs with enhanced or decreased ADCC, ADCP and CDC activity have been produced by manipulation of the critical Fc regions. Umana et al. (1999) engineered an anti-neuroblastoma IgG1 with enhanced ADCC activity compared with wild type (WT). Shields et al. (2001) demonstrated that selected IgG1 variants with improved binding to FcγRIIIA showed enhanced ADCC by peripheral blood monocyte cells and natural killer cells. These findings indicate that Fc-engineered antibodies may have important applications for improving therapeutic efficacy. It was found that the FcγRIIIA gene dimorphism generates two allotypes, FcγRIIIa-158V and FcγRIIIa-158F, and the polymorphism in FcγRIIIA is associated with favorable clinical response following rituximab administration in non-Hodgkin's lymphoma patients (Cartron et al. 2004; Dall'Ozzo et al. 2004). Recently, obinutuzumab, an anti-CD20 MAB with enhanced effector functions as compared to rituximab, was approved for the treatment of patients with previously untreated chronic lymphocytic leukemia (CLL) and patients with follicular lymphoma (FL) who relapsed after, or are refractory to, a rituximab-containing regimen. The efficacy of antibody-interleukin 2 fusion protein (Ab-IL2) was improved by reducing its interaction with Fc receptors (Gillies et al. 1999). In addition, the Fc portion of MABs also binds to FcRn (named based on its discovery in neonatal rats), an Fc receptor belonging to the major histocompatibility complex structure, which is involved in IgG transport and clearance (CL) (Junghans 1997). Engineered MABs with a decreased or increased FcRn binding affinity have been investigated for its potential to modify the pharmacokinetic behavior of MABs (see the section on Clearance for details).

■ Antibody Derivatives: F(ab')2, Fab, Antibody-Drug Conjugates and Fusion Proteins

The fragments of antibodies [Fab, F(ab')2, and scFv] have a shorter half-life compared with the corresponding full-sized antibodies. scFv can be further engineered into a dimer (diabody, ~60 kDa), or trimer (triabody, ~90 kDa). Two diabodies can be further linked together to generate a bispecific tandem diabody (tandab). A single Fab can be fused to a complete Fc engineered to form a single arm MAB, which is monovalent. Figure 8.3 illustrates the structure of different antibody fragments. Of note, abciximab, idarucizumab and ranibizumab are three Fabs approved by FDA. Abciximab is a chimeric Fab used for keeping blood from clotting that has a 20–30 min half-life in serum and 4-h half-life in platelets (Schror and Weber 2003). Ranibizumab, administrated via intravitreal injection, was approved for the treatment of macular degeneration in 2006 and exhibits a vitreous elimination half-life of 9 days (Albrecht and DeNardo 2006).

The half-life of Fc fragments is more similar to that of full-sized IgGs (Lobo et al. 2004). Therefore, Fc portions of IgGs have been used to form fusions with molecules such as cytokines, growth factor enzymes, or the ligand-binding region of receptor or adhesion molecules to improve their half-life and stability. There are ten Fc fusion proteins currently on the market [abatacept, aflibercept, alefacept, alprolix, antihemophilic factor (recombinant) Fc fusion protein, belatacept, dulaglutide, etanercept, rilonacept and ziv-aflibercept]. Etanercept, a dimeric fusion molecule consisting of the TNF-α receptor fused to the Fc region of human IgG1, has a half-life of approximately 70–100 h (Zhou 2005), which is much longer than that of the TNF-α receptor itself (30 min to ~2 h) (Watanabe et al. 1988).

Antibodies and antibody fragments can also be linked covalently with cytotoxic radionuclides or drugs to form radioimmunotherapeutic (RIT) agents or ADCs (Fig. 8.4), respectively. In each case, the antibody is used as a delivery mechanism to selectively target the cytotoxic moiety to tumors (Prabhu et al. 2011; Girish and Li 2015). For both ADCs and RIT agents, the therapeutic strategy involves selective delivery of a cytotoxin (drug or radionuclide) to tumors via the antibody. As targeted approaches, both technologies exploit the overexpression of target on the surface of the cancer cells and thereby minimize damage to normal tissues. Such approaches are anticipated to minimize the significant side effects encountered when cytotoxic small molecule drugs or radionuclides are administered as single agents, thus leading to enhanced therapeutic windows. However, important distinctions exist between these two therapeutic modalities. For example, ADCs usually require internalization into the endosomes and/or lysosomes for efficacy, while RIT agents are often able to emit beta or gamma radiation, even from the cell surface, to achieve cell killing following direct binding to membrane antigens. Furthermore, RIT can deliver high levels of radiation even with very low doses of radioimmunoconjugate. Importantly, most clinically successful ADC and RIT agents to date have been against hematologic tumors (Boswell and Brechbiel 2007). Trastuzumab emtansine is the only ADC approved in a solid tumor indication

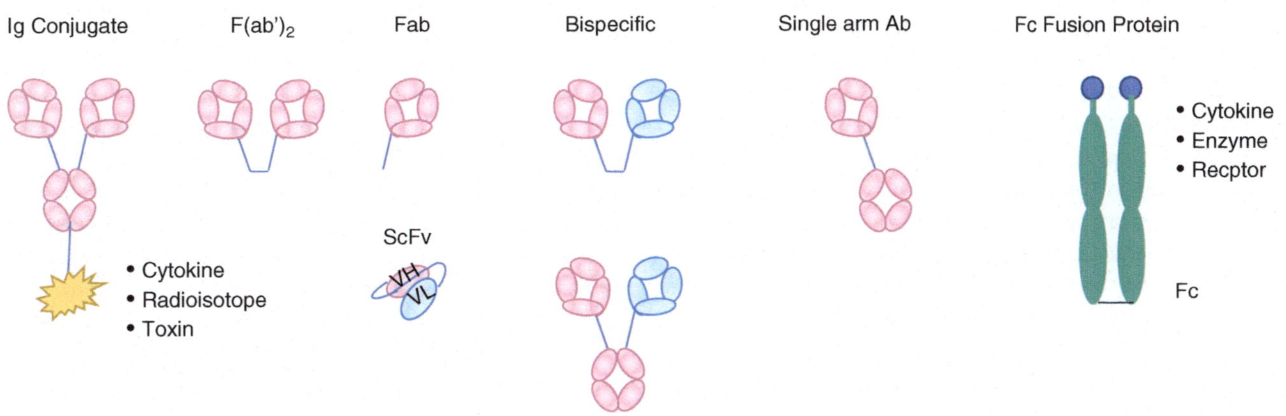

Figure 8.3 ■ Schematic representation of antibody derivatives: Ig conjugate, F(ab')2, Fab, scFv, bispecfic Ab, single arm Ab, and Fc fusion proteins

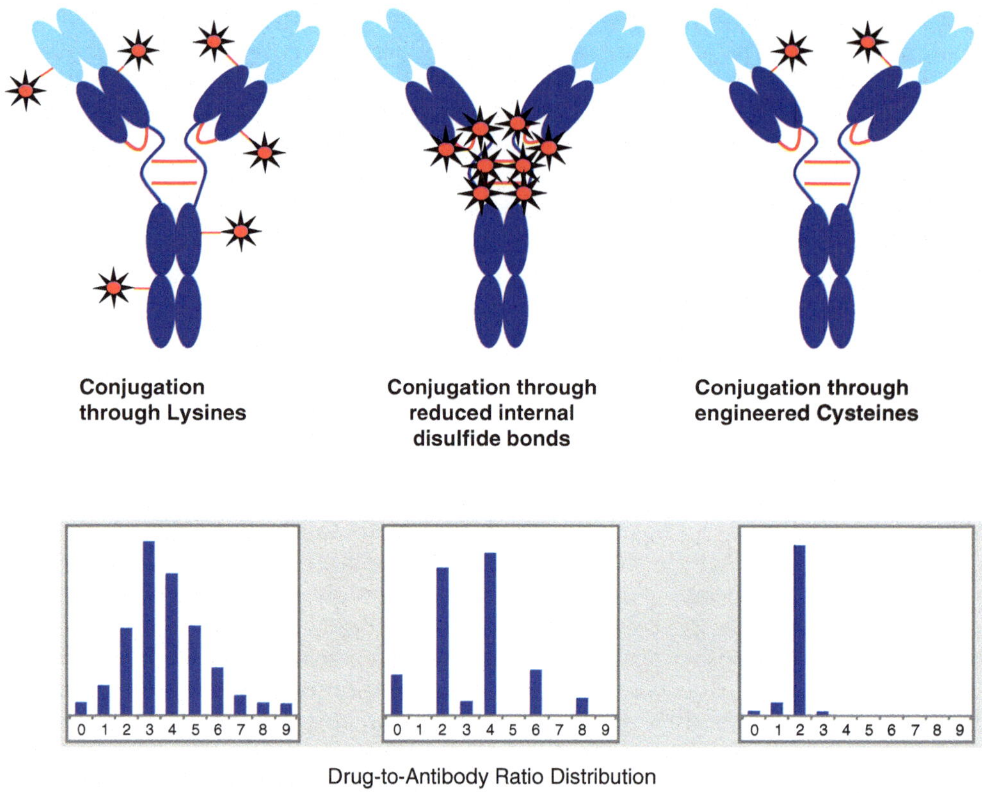

Figure 8.4 Schematic of ADC structures. ADCs are a heterogeneous mixture of different drug-to-antibody ratio (DAR) species, with individual molecules exhibiting a range of DARs (Adapted with permission from Kaur et al., Mass Spectrometry of Antibody-Drug Conjugates in Plasma and Tissue in Drug Development. In *Characterization of Protein Therapeutics Using Mass Spectrometry*, 2013. Guodong Chen, Ed., Springer Press, New York, NY, pp 279–304)

(LoRusso et al. 2011). Various impediments to the delivery of antibodies and other macromolecules to solid tumors have been widely discussed and studied, especially in the context of microspatial distribution (Thurber et al. 2008).

Currently, there are four ADCs on the market. Gemtuzumab ozogamicin (Dowell et al. 2001), an anti-CD33 MAB linked to the cytotoxic antitumor antibiotic drug calicheamicin, became the first approved ADC in 2000 when it was granted accelerated approval for the treatment of acute myelogenous leukemia. Calicheamicin binds to the minor groove of DNA, causing double-strand DNA breaks and resulting in inhibition of DNA synthesis. However, gemtuzumab ozogamicin was removed from the US market in June 2010 after subsequent confirmatory trials failed to verify clinical benefit and demonstrated safety concerns, including deaths. In September 2017, the FDA re-approved gemtuzumab ozogamicin with a lower recommended dose and a different schedule in combination with chemotherapy or on its own. Gemtuzumab ozogamicin's history underscores the importance of examining alternative dosing, scheduling, and administration of therapies for patients with cancer, especially in those who may be most vulnerable to the side effects of treatment. In August 2011, the FDA approved a second ADC, brentuximab vedotin, a CD30-directed MAB linked to the cytotoxic microtubule-disrupting agent MMAE, for treatment of Hodgkin's lymphoma and systemic anaplastic large-cell lymphoma. In February 2013, the FDA approved ado-trastuzumab emtansine, a human epidermal growth factor receptor (HER2)-targeted ADC for treatment of HER2-positive breast cancer (LoRusso et al. 2011). In August 2017, inotuzumab ozogamicin, a CD22-directed MAB linked to calicheamicin, was approved by FDA for the treatment of adults with relapsed or refractory B-cell precursor acute lymphoblastic leukemia.

The only current radioimmunotherapeutic agents licensed by the FDA are ibritumomab tiuxetan and tositumomab plus ^{131}I-tositumomab, both for non-Hodgkin's lymphoma. Both of the above intact murine MABs bind CD20 and carry a potent beta particle-emitting radioisotope (^{90}Y for ibritumomab/tiuxetan and ^{131}I for tositumomab). In the case of ibritumomab, the bifunctional chelating agent, tiuxetan, is used to covalently link the radionuclide to the MAB ibritumomab. However, another approved anti-CD20 MAB, rituximab, is included in the dosing regimen as a non-radioactive pre-dose to improve the biodistribution of the radiolabeled MAB. Despite impressive clinical results, radioimmunotherapeutic MABs have not generated considerable commercial success; various financial, regulatory, and commercial barriers have been cited as contributing factors to this trend (Boswell and Brechbiel 2007).

MAB THERAPEUTIC MECHANISMS OF ACTION (MOAS)

The pharmacological effects of antibodies are first initiated by the specific interaction between antibody and antigen. MABs generally exhibit exquisite specificity for the target antigen. The binding site on the antigen, called the epitope, can be linear or conformational and may comprise continuous or discontinuous amino acid sequences. The epitope is the primary determinant of the antibody's modulatory functions, and depending on the epitope, the antibody may exert antagonist or agonist effects, or it may be nonmodulatory. The epitope may also influence the antibody's ability to induce ADCC and CDC. MABs exert their pharmacological effects via multiple mechanisms that include direct modulation of the target antigen, CDC and ADCC, ADCP, apoptosis, delivery of a radionuclide or immunotoxin to target cells and T cell activation using bispecific constructs.

■ Direct Modulation of Target Antigen

Examples of direct modulation of the target antigen include anti-TNFα, anti-IgE, and anti-CD11a therapies that are involved in blocking and removal of the target antigen. Most MABs act through multiple mechanisms and may exhibit cooperativity with concurrent therapies.

■ Complement-Dependent Cytotoxicity (CDC)

The complement system is an important part of the innate (i.e., nonadaptive) immune system. It consists of many enzymes that form a cascade with each enzyme acting as a catalyst for the next. CDC results from interaction of cell-bound MABs with proteins of the complement system. CDC is initiated by binding of the complement protein, C1q, to the Fc domain. The IgG1 and IgG3 isotypes have the highest CDC activity, while the IgG4 isotype lacks C1q binding and complement activation (Presta 2002). Upon binding to immune complexes, C1q undergoes a conformational change, and the resulting activated complex initiates an enzymatic cascade involving complement proteins C2 to C9 and several other factors. This cascade spreads rapidly and ends in the formation of the membrane attack complex (MAC), which inserts into the membrane of the target cell and causes osmotic disruption and lysis of the target. Figure 8.5 illustrates the mechanism for CDC with rituximab (a chimeric MAB that targets the CD20 antigen) as an example.

■ Antibody-Dependent Cellular Cytotoxicity (ADCC)

ADCC is a mechanism of cell-mediated immunity whereby an effector cell of the immune system actively lyses a target cell that has been bound by specific antibodies. It is one of the mechanisms through which antibodies, as part of the humoral immune response, can act to limit and contain infection. Classical ADCC is mediated by natural killer (NK) cells, monocytes, or macrophages, but an alternate ADCC is used by eosinophils to kill certain parasitic worms known as helminths. ADCC is part of the adaptive immune response due to its dependence on a prior antibody response. The typical ADCC involves activation of NK cells, monocytes, or macrophages and is dependent on the recognition of antibody-coated infected cells by Fc receptors on the surface of these cells. The Fc receptors recognize the Fc portion of antibodies such as IgG, which bind to the surface of a pathogen-infected target cell. The Fc receptor that exists on the surface of NK cell is called CD16 or FcγRIII. Once bound to the Fc receptor of IgG, the NK cell releases cytokines such as IFN-γ and cytotoxic granules like perforin and granzyme that enter the target cell and promote cell death

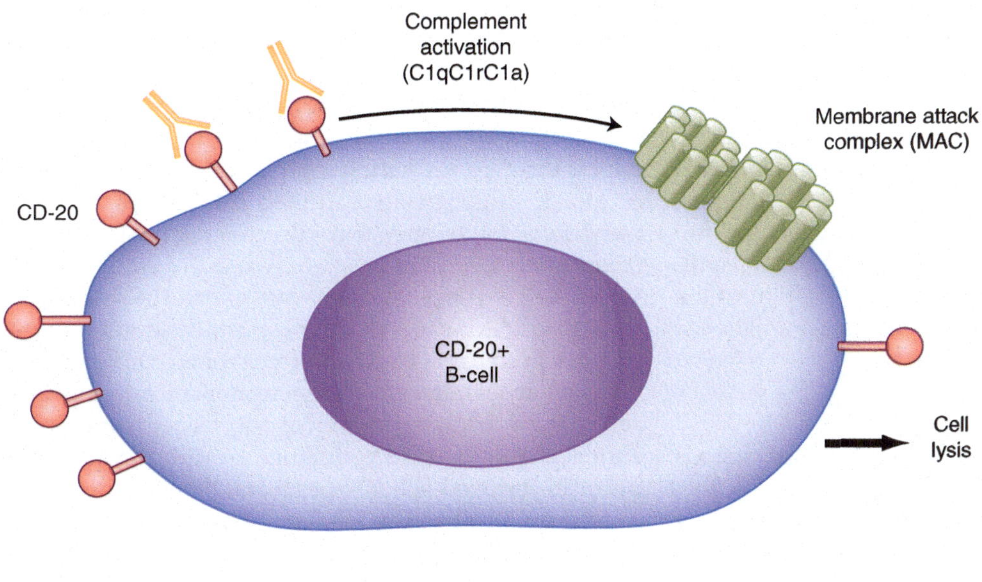

Figure 8.5 ■ An example of complement-dependent cytotoxicity (CDC), using a B cell lymphoma model, where the monoclonal antibody (MAB) rituximab binds to the receptor and initiates the complement system, also known as the "complement cascade." The end result is formation of a membrane attack complex (MAC), which leads to cell lysis and death

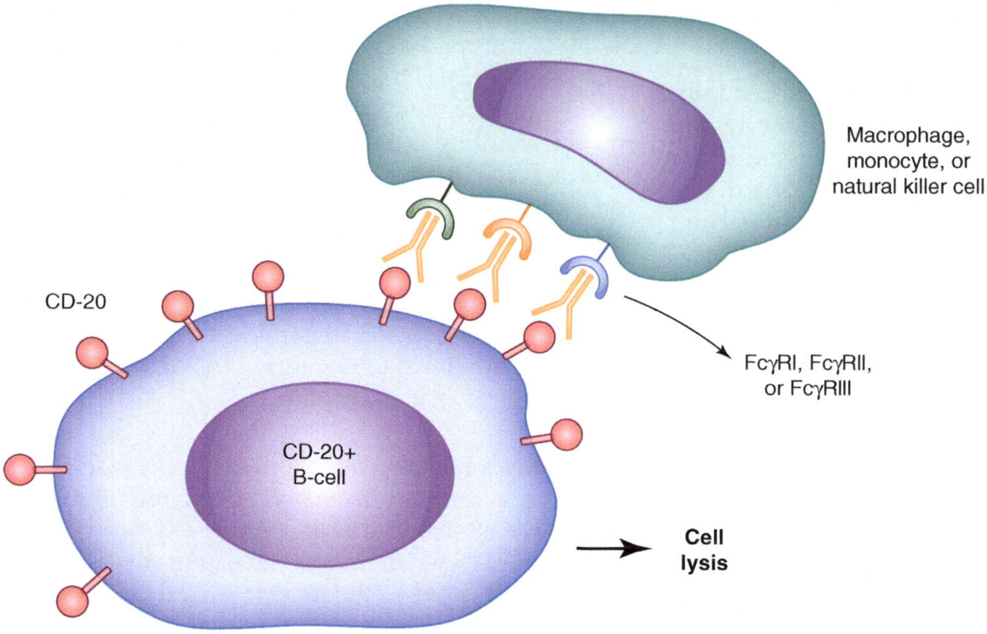

Figure 8.6 ■ An example of antibody-dependent cellular cytotoxicity (ADCC) and antibody-dependent cellular phagocytosis (ADCP). The monoclonal antibody (MAB) rituximab targets the CD20 antigen, which is expressed on a significant number of B cell malignancies. The Fc fragment of the MAB binds the Fc receptors found on effector cells such as monocytes, macrophages, and NK cells. These cells in turn either engulf the MAB-bound tumor cell (ADCP) or release cytotoxic agents such as perforin and granzymes, leading to destruction of the tumor cell (ADCC)

by triggering apoptosis. This is similar to, but independent of, responses by cytotoxic T cells. Figure 8.6 illustrates the mechanism for ADCC with rituximab as an example.

■ Antibody-Dependent Cellular Phagocytosis (ADCP)

ADCP is an immune effector function in which cells or particles opsonized with antibodies are engulfed by phagocytic effector cells, such as macrophages, following interactions between the Fc region of antibodies and Fcγ receptors on effector cells. In vivo, ADCP can be mediated by monocytes, macrophages, neutrophils and dendritic cells via all three types of activating Fcγ receptors: FcγRI, FcγRIIa, and FcγRIIIa. Studies have shown that MABs against tumor antigens induce phagocytosis of cancer cells in vitro, promote macrophage infiltration into tumors, and elicit macrophage-mediated destruction of tumors in mice (Weiskopf and Weissman 2015). ADCP is an important MOA of several antibody therapies for cancer, such as rituximab, obinutuzumab, and ocrelizumab. Engagement of Fcγ receptors expressed on phagocytic effector cells with antibodies bound to target cells triggers a signaling cascade leading to the engulfment of the antibody-opsonized tumor cells. Upon full engulfment, a phagosome is formed, which fuses with lysosomes, leading to acidification and digestion of the tumor cells. Figure 8.6 illustrates the mechanism for ADCP with rituximab as an example.

■ Apoptosis

MABs achieve their therapeutic effect through various mechanisms. In addition to the abovementioned effector functions, they can have direct effects in producing apoptosis or programmed cell death, which is characterized by nuclear DNA degradation, nuclear degeneration and condensation, and the phagocytosis of cell remains.

■ Targeted Delivery of Cytotoxic Drugs via ADCs

ADCs achieve their therapeutic effect through selectively delivering a potent cytotoxic agent to tumor cells (Girish and Li 2015). The MAB component enables the ADC to specifically bind to targeted cell surface antigens overexpressed on the tumor cells. After binding to the cell surface antigen, the ADC is internalized by the tumor cell, where it undergoes lysosomal degradation, leading to the release of the cytotoxic agent. Targeted delivery of cytotoxic drugs to tumors enables ADCs to potentially harness and improve their antitumor effect while minimizing their impact on normal tissues, thereby enhancing the benefit-risk profile.

■ $CD3^+$ T cell Activation Using Bispecific Constructs

CD3 bispecific constructs achieve their therapeutic effects through activating a patient's own $CD3^+$ T cells to attack target-positive tumor cells. CD3 bispecific constructs have one arm directed against the CD3 receptor on T cells and the other arm directed against a target cell surface antigen overexpressed by tumor cells (Mandikian et al. 2018). Simultaneous engagement of both arms results in formation of an immunologic synapse between a target tumor cell and a $CD3^+$ T cell, which leads to killing of the target tumor cells, either through direct killing by granzyme- and perforin-induced cell lysis or through cytokine release caused by T-cell activation.

TRANSLATIONAL MEDICINE/DEVELOPMENT PROCESS

The tight connection of basic to clinical sciences is an essential part of translational medicine, which aims to *translate* the knowledge of basic science into practical therapeutic applications for patients. This knowledge transfer is often referred to as the process of moving *from-bench-to-bedside*, emphasizing the transition of scientific advancements into clinical applications. This framework of translational medicine is applied during the discovery and drug development process of a specific MAB against a certain disease. It includes major steps such as identifying an important and viable pathophysiological target antigen to modify the disease in a beneficial way, producing MABs with structural elements providing optimal PK, preclinical safety and efficacy testing in relevant models, and finally clinical trials in patients. An overview of the development phases of the molecules comprising the preclinical activities is outlined in Fig. 8.7. Furthermore, the critical components of the entire MAB development process are explained in detail from a PK/PD perspective below.

■ Preclinical Safety Assessment of MABs

Preclinical safety assessment of MABs encounters unique challenges, as many of the classical evaluations employed for small molecules are not appropriate for protein therapeutics in general and MABs in particular. For example, in vitro genotoxicology tests such as the Ames and chromosome aberration assays are generally not conducted for MABs given their limited interaction with nuclear material and the lack of appropriate receptor/target expression in these systems. As MAB binding tends to be highly species specific, suitable animal models are often limited to nonhuman primates, and for this reason, many common in vivo models, such as rodent carcinogenesis bioassays and some safety pharmacology bioassays, are not viable for MAB therapeutic candidates. For general toxicology studies, cynomolgus and rhesus monkeys are most commonly employed and offer many advantages given their close phylogenetic relationship with humans; however, due to logistics, animal availability, and costs, group sizes tend to be much smaller than typically used for lower species, thus limiting statistical power. In some cases, alternative models are employed to enable studies in rodents. Rather than directly testing the therapeutic candidate, analogous MABs that can bind to target epitopes in lower species (e.g. mice) can be engineered and used as a surrogate MAB for safety evaluation (Clarke et al. 2004). Often the antibody framework amino acid sequence is modified to reduce antigenicity thus enabling longer-term studies (Albrecht and DeNardo 2006; Weiner 2006; Cohenuram and Saif 2007). Another approach is to use transgenic models that express the human receptor/target of interest (Bugelski et al. 2000), although results must be interpreted with caution as transgenic models often have altered physiology and typically lack historical background data for the model (Boswell et al. 2013). To address development issues that are specific to MABs and other

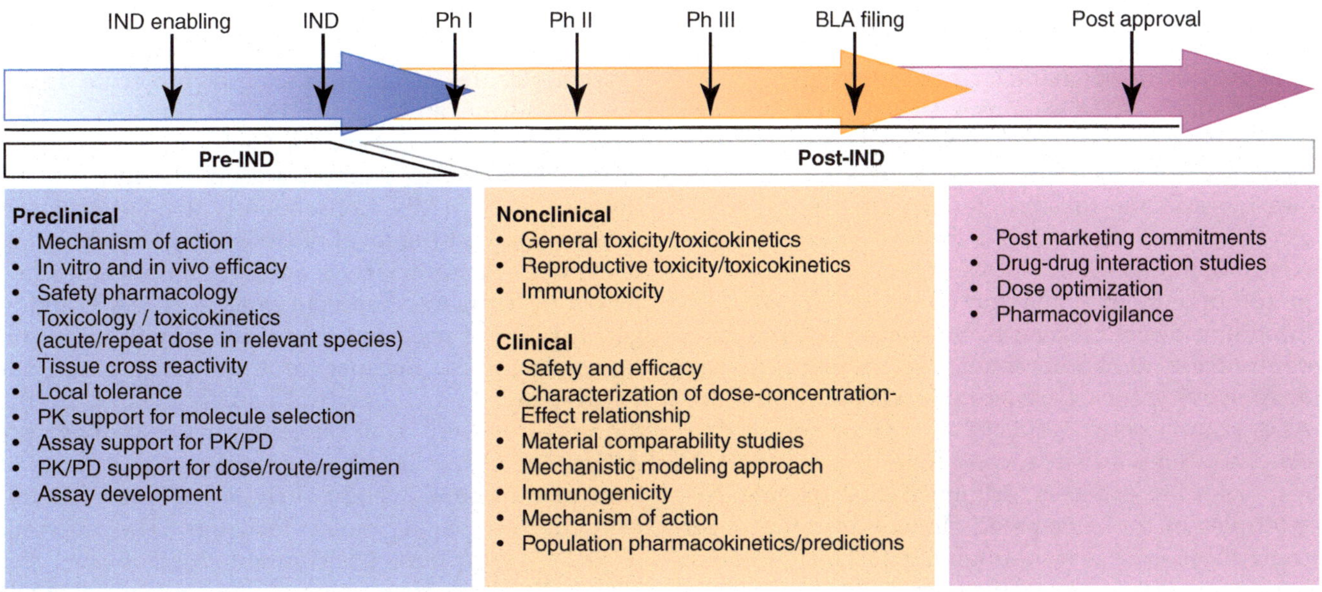

Figure 8.7 ■ Flowchart depicting high level PK/PD/toxicology study requirements during preclinical and clinical drug product development

protein therapeutics, the International Conference of Harmonization (ICH) has developed guidelines specific to the preclinical evaluation of biotechnology-derived pharmaceuticals (ICH 1997a, b).

For general safety studies, species selection is an important consideration given the exquisite species specificity often encountered with MABs. Model selection needs to be justified based on appropriate expression of the target epitope, appropriate binding affinity with the therapeutic candidate, and appropriate biologic activity in the test system. To aid in the interpretation of results, tissue cross-reactivity studies offer the ability to compare drug localization in both animal and human tissues. For MAB therapeutic candidates, a range of three or more dose levels are typically selected to attain pharmacologically relevant serum concentrations, to approximate levels anticipated in the clinic, and to provide information at doses higher than anticipated in the clinic. For most indications, it is important to include dose levels that allow identification of a no observable adverse effect level (NOAEL). If feasible, the highest dose should fall within the range where toxicity is anticipated; although, in practice, many MABs do not exhibit toxicity, and other factors limit the maximum dose. To best reflect human exposures, doses are often normalized and selected to match and exceed anticipated human therapeutic exposure in plasma, serum, or blood based upon the exposure parameters, area under the concentration-time curve (AUC), maximum concentration (C_{max}), or concentration immediately prior to next treatment (C_{trough}). The route of administration, dosing regimen, and dosing duration should be selected to best model the anticipated use in clinical trials (ICH 1997a, b).

To adequately interpret nonclinical study results, it is important to characterize ADA responses. For human MABs, ADA responses are particularly prominent in lower species but also evident in nonhuman primates albeit to a lesser degree, making these species more viable for chronic toxicity studies. ADAs can impact drug activity in a variety of ways. Neutralizing ADAs are those that bind to the therapeutic in a manner that prevents activity, often by inhibiting direct binding to the target epitope. Non-neutralizing antibodies may also indirectly impact drug activity, for example, rapid clearance of drug–ADA complexes can effectively reduce serum drug concentrations. In situations where prominent ADA responses are expected, administration of high-dose multiples of the anticipated clinical dose may overcome these issues by maintaining sufficient circulating concentrations of active drug when supported with sufficient safety margin. To properly interpret study results, it is important to characterize ADA incidence and magnitude, as the occurrence of ADA responses could mask toxicities. Alternatively, robust ADA responses may induce significant signs of toxicity, such as infusion-related anaphylaxis, that may not be predictive of human outcome where ADA formation is likely to be less of an issue. If ADA formation is clearly impacting circulating drug levels, ADA-positive individual animals are often removed from consideration when evaluating pharmacokinetic parameters to better reflect the anticipated PK in human populations.

Pharmacokinetics

A thorough and rigorous PK program in the early learning phase of preclinical drug development can provide a linkage between drug discovery and preclinical development. PK information can be linked to PD by mathematical modeling, which allows characterizing the time course of the effect intensity resulting from a certain dosing regimen. Antibodies often exhibit PK properties that are complex and different than those typically associated with small molecule drugs (Meibohm and Derendorf 2002). The PK of ADCs is more complex due to the presence of both an antibody component as well as a small molecule component. In the following sections, the basic characteristics of MAB and ADC PK are summarized in contrast to small molecule drugs.

The PK of antibodies and ADCs are very different from that of small molecules, as summarized in Table 8.3. Precise, sensitive, and accurate bioanalytical methods are essential for PK interpretation. However, for MABs, the immunoassays and bioassay methodologies are often less specific than assays used for small molecule drugs (e.g., LC/MS/MS). MABs are handled by the body very differently than are small molecules. In contrast to small molecule drugs, the typical metabolic enzymes and transporter proteins, such as cytochrome P450 and multidrug resistance (MDR) efflux pumps, are not involved in the disposition of MABs. Consequently, drug–drug interactions (DDI) at the level of these drug-metabolizing enzymes and transporters are not complicating factors in the drug development process of MABs and in general do not need to be addressed by in vitro and in vivo studies. Because of their large molecular weight, intact MABs are not usually cleared by the kidneys; however, renal clearance processes may play an important role in the elimination of molecules of smaller molecular weight such as Fab's and chemically derived small molecule drugs. The different *ADME* (*A*bsorption, *D*istribution, *M*etabolism, and *E*limination) processes comprising the PK of MABs are discussed separately to address their individual specifics.

Small Molecule Drugs	Monoclonal Antibodies	Antibody-Drug Conjugates
High potency and low specificity	Low potency and high specificity	High potency and high specificity
PK usually independent of PD	PK usually dependent of PD	Same as MAB
Binding generally nonspecific (can affect multiple enzymes)	Binding very specific for target protein or antigen	Same as MAB
Linear PK at low doses (usually therapeutic doses); nonlinear PK at high doses (after saturation of metabolic enzymes)	Nonlinear PK at low doses; linear PK at high doses after saturation of target	Same as MAB
Relatively short $t_{1/2}$ (hours)	Long $t_{1/2}$ (days or weeks)	Long $t_{1/2}$ of antibody; sustained delivery of small molecule (formation rate limited)
Oral delivery often possible	Need parenteral dosing. Subcutaeneous (SC) or intramusclular (IM) is possible	Need parenteral dosing. SC or IM has not been tested
Metabolism by cytochrome P450 or other phase I/ phase II enzymes	Catabolism by proteolytic degradation	Catabolism by proteolytic degradation; small molecule component can undergo excretion unchanged or metabolism by cytochrome P450 enzymes or other phase I/ phase II enzymes
Renal clearance often important	No renal clearance of intact antibody. May be eliminated by damaged kidneys. Antibody fragment might be eliminated by renal clearance.	Combination of mAb and small molecule; Released small molecule can be cleared renally and/or hepatically
High volume of distribution due to binding to tissues	Distribution usually limited to blood and extra-cellular space	Same as MAB
No immunogenicity	Immunogenicity may be seen	Same as MAB
Narrow therapeutic window	Large therapeutic window	Depends on potency of payload

Table 8.3 ■ Comparison of the pharmacokinetics between small molecule drugs, monoclonal antibodies and antibody-drug conjugates (Mould et al. 1999; Lobo et al. 2004; Roskos et al. 2004; Mould and Sweeney 2007; Kamath 2016)

Absorption

Most MABs are not administrated orally because of their limited gastrointestinal stability, lipophilicity, and size, all of which result in insufficient resistance against the hostile proteolytic gastrointestinal milieu and very limited permeation through the lipophilic intestinal wall. Therefore, intravenous (IV) administration is still the most frequently used route, which allows for immediate systemic delivery of a large volume of drug product and provides complete systemic availability. Subcutaneous (SC) administration, however, may offer a number of benefits over IV administration. Being less invasive and with a much shorter injection duration (2–7 min versus 30–90 min for IV infusion), and commonly with a fixed dose, SC dosing is expected to offer more convenience to patients compared to IV infusion. Additionally, IV infusion is typically administered in a hospital or physician's office; SC administration may allow self or healthcare professional-assisted home administration. Of note, 22 of the 75 FDA-approved MAB or MAB-derived therapies listed in Table 8.1 are administered by an extravascular route, either SC or IM. Aflibercept and ranibizumab are administered via intravitreal injection.

The absorption mechanisms of SC or IM administration are poorly understood. However, it is believed that the absorption of MABs after IM or SC injection is likely via lymphatic drainage due to its large molecular weight, leading to a slow absorption rate (see Chaps. 5 and 6). The bioavailability of MABs after SC or IM administration has been reported to be around 50–100% with maximal plasma concentrations observed 1–8 days following administration (Lobo et al. 2004). For example, following an IM injection, the bioavailability of alefacept was ~60% in healthy male volunteers; its C_{max} was threefold lower (0.96 versus 3.1 μg/mL), and its T_{max} was 30 times longer (86 versus 2.8 h) than a 30-min IV infusion (Vaishnaw and TenHoor 2002). Interestingly, differences in PK have also been observed between different sites of IM dosing. PAmAb, a fully humanized MAB against *Bacillus anthracis* protective antigen, has significantly different pharmacokinetics between IM-GM (gluteus maximus site) and IM-VL (vastus lateralis site) injection in healthy volunteers (Subramanian et al. 2005). The bioavailability of PAmAb is 50–54% for IM-GM injection and 71–85% for IM-VL injection (Subramanian et al. 2005). Of note, MABs appear to have greater bioavailability after SC administration in monkeys than in humans (Oitate et al. 2011). The mean bioavailability of adalimumab is 52–82% after a single 40 mg SC administration in healthy adult subjects, whereas it was observed to be 94–100% in monkeys. Similarly, the mean bioavailability of omalizumab is 66–71% after a single SC dose in patients with asthma versus 88–100% in monkeys (Oitate et al. 2011).

Although SC administration of MABs initially used low-volume injections (1–2 mL), in recent years, larger-volume injections (>2 mL) have been used, with and without permeation enhancers. SC injections of a viscous (5 cP) placebo buffer, characteristic of a high-concentration MAB formulation, at volumes of up to 3.5 mL had acceptable tolerability in healthy adult subjects at injection rates up to 3.5 mL/min (Dias et al. 2015a, b). Due to relatively large therapeutic doses (several hundred milligram), dosing volumes of high-concentration MABs may still be too large to facilitate a painless SC injection. Without co-injection of a permeation enhancer, large volume injections may produce swelling at the injection site, particularly in the thigh and arm. A permeation enhancer, such as recombinant human hyaluronidase (rHuPH20), reduces this swelling. Hyaluronidase is a 61-kD naturally-occurring enzyme that temporarily degrades hyaluronan in the skin and increases dispersion of the MAB over a greater area. Co-formulation of rHuPH20 with therapeutic proteins allows SC administration of larger injection volumes and potentially enhances absorption of the therapeutic protein into the systemic circulation (Frost 2007). Trastuzumab and rituximab have both been co-formulated with rHuPH20 to facilitate large-volume SC injections (Bittner et al. 2012). Trastuzumab is available as a 5-mL SC injection to be administered over 2–5 min, while rituximab is available at 11.7 or 13.4 mL injection volumes to be administered over 5 or 7 min, respectively.

Distribution

After reaching the bloodstream, MABs undergo biphasic elimination from serum, beginning with a rapid distribution phase. The volume of distribution of the rapid-distribution compartment is relatively small, approximating plasma volume. It is reported that the volume of the central compartment (Vc) is about 2–3 L, and the steady-state volume of distribution (Vss) is around 3.5–7 L for MABs in humans (Lobo et al. 2004; Roskos et al. 2004). The small Vc and Vss for MABs indicate that the distribution of MABs is restricted to the blood and extracellular spaces, which is in agreement with their hydrophilic nature and their large molecular weight, limiting access to the intracellular compartment surrounded by a lipid bilayer. Small volumes of distributions are consistent with relatively small tissue: blood ratios for most antibodies typically ranging from 0.1 to 0.5 (Baxter et al. 1995; Baxter et al. 1994; Berger et al. 2005). For example, the tissue-to-blood concentration ratios for a murine IgG1 MAB against the human ovarian cancer antigen CA125 in mice at 24 h after injection are 0.44, 0.39, 0.48, 0.34, 0.10, and 0.13 for the spleen, liver, lung, kidney, stomach, and muscle, respectively. Brain and cerebrospinal fluid are anatomically protected by blood–brain barriers. Although the blood-brain barrier was believed to be impaired in certain neurodegenerative disease states, recent work has brought this into question (Bien-Ly et al. 2015). Therefore, both compartments are very limited distribution compartments for MABs. For example, endogenous IgG levels in CSF were shown to be in the range of only 0.1–1% of their respective serum levels (Wurster and Haas 1994; Yadav et al. 2017; Yu et al. 2014).

It has been repeatedly noted that the reported Vss obtained by traditional non-compartmental or compartmental analysis may not be correct for MABs that primarily undergo catabolism within tissue (Lobo et al. 2004; Straughn et al. 2006; Tang et al. 2004). The rate and extent of MAB distribution will be dependent on the kinetics of MAB extravasation within tissue, distribution within tissue, and elimination from tissue. Convection, diffusion, transcytosis, binding, and catabolism are important determining factors for antibody distribution (Lobo et al. 2004). Therefore, Vss might be substantially greater than the plasma volume in particular for those MABs demonstrating high binding affinity in the tissue. Different research groups have reported effects of the presence of specific receptors (i.e., antigen sink) on the distribution of MABs (Danilov et al. 2001; Kairemo et al. 2001; Bumbaca et al. 2012). Danilov et al. (2001) found in rats that an anti-PECAM-1 (anti-CD31) MAB showed tissue-to-blood concentration ratios of 13.1, 10.9, and 5.96 for the lung, liver, and spleen, respectively, 2 h after injection. Therefore, the true Vss of the anti-PECAM-1 is likely to be 15-fold greater than plasma volume.

Another complexity to consider is that tissue distribution via interaction with target proteins (e.g., cell surface proteins) and subsequent internalization of the antigen-MAB complex may be dose dependent. For the murine analog MAB of efalizumab, M17, a pronounced dose-dependent distribution was demonstrated by comparing tissue-to-blood concentration ratios for liver, spleen, bone marrow, and lymph node after a tracer dose of radiolabeled M17 and a high-dose treatment (Coffey et al. 2005). The tracer dose of M17 resulted in substantially higher tissue-to-blood concentration ratios of 6.4, 2.8, 1.6, and 1.3 for the lung, spleen, bone marrow, and lymph node, respectively, in mice at 72 h after injection. In contrast, the saturation of the target antigen at the high-dose level reduced the tissue distribution to the target independent distribution and resulted consequently in substantially lower tissue-to-blood concentration ratios (less than 1).

FcRn may play an important role in the transport of IgGs from plasma to the interstitial fluid of tissue. Recently, the data from Yip et al. increased understanding of FcRn's role in antibody PK and catabolism at the tissue level (Yip et al. 2014). They reported that distribution of the wild-type IgG and the variant with enhanced binding for FcRn were largely similar to each other in mice, but vastly different for the low-FcRn-binding variant due to its very low systemic exposure and widespread catabolism, particularly in liver and spleen. Ferl et al. (2005) reported that a physiologically based pharmacokinetic (PBPK) model, including the kinetic interaction between the MAB and the FcRn receptor within intracellular compartments, could describe the biodistribution of an anti-CEA MAB in a variety of tissue compartments such as plasma, lung, spleen, tumor, skin, muscle, kidney, heart, bone, and liver. FcRn was also reported to mediate the crossing of placental barriers by IgG (Junghans 1997) and the vectorial transport of IgG into the lumen of intestine (Dickinson et al. 1999) and lung (Spiekermann et al. 2002).

Clearance

Antibodies are mainly cleared by catabolism and broken down into peptide fragments and amino acids, which can be recycled—to be used as energy supply or for new protein synthesis. Due to the small molecular weight of antibodies fragments (e.g., Fab and Fv), elimination of these fragments is faster than for intact IgGs, and they can be filtered through the glomerulus and reabsorbed and/or metabolized by proximal tubular cells of the nephron (Lobo et al. 2004). Murine monoclonal anti-digoxin Fab, F(ab')2, and IgG1 have half-lives of 0.41, 0.70, and 8.10 h in rats, respectively (Bazin-Redureau et al. 1997). Several studies reported that the kidney is the major route for the catabolism of Fab and elimination of unchanged Fab (Druet et al. 1978; McClurkan et al. 1993).

Typically, IgGs have serum half-lives of approximately 21 days, resulting from CL values of about 3–5 mL/day/kg, and Vss's of 50–100 mL/kg. The exception is IgG3, which has a half-life of only 7 days. The half-life of IgG is much longer than that of other Igs (IgA, 6 days; IgE, 2.5 days; IgM, 5 days; IgD, 3 days). The FcRn receptor has been demonstrated to be a primary determinant of the disposition of IgG antibodies (Ghetie et al. 1996; Junghans 1997; Junghans and Anderson 1996). FcRn, which protects IgG from catabolism and contributes to the long plasma half-life of IgG, was first postulated by Brambell in 1964 (Brambell et al. 1964) and cloned in the late 1980s (Simister and Mostov 1989a, b). FcRn is a heterodimer comprising of a β_2m light chain and a MHC class I-like heavy chain. The receptor is ubiquitously expressed in cells and tissues. Several studies have shown that IgG CL in β_2m knockout mice (Ghetie et al. 1996; Junghans and Anderson 1996) and FcRn heavy chain knockout mice (Roopenian et al. 2003) is increased 10 to 15-fold, with no changes in the elimination of other Igs. Figure 8.8 illustrates how the FcRn receptor protects IgG from catabolism and contributes to its long half-life. The FcRn receptor binds to IgG in a pH-dependent manner: binding to IgG at the acidic pH (6.0) of the endosome and releasing IgG at physiological pH (7.4). The unbound IgG proceeds to the lysosome and undergoes proteolysis.

It has been demonstrated that IgG half-life is dependent on its affinity to FcRn receptors. The shorter half-life of IgG3 was attributed to its low binding affinity to the FcRn receptor (Junghans 1997; Medesan et al. 1997). Murine MABs have serum half-lives of 1–2 days in human. The shorter half-life of murine antibodies in human is due to their low binding affinity to the human FcRn receptor. It is reported that human FcRn binds to human, rabbit, and guinea pig IgG, but not to rat, mouse, sheep, and bovine IgG; however, mouse FcRn binds to IgG from all of these species (Ober et al. 2001). Interestingly, human IgG1 has greater affinity to murine FcRn (Petkova et al. 2006), which indicates potential limitations of using mice as preclinical models for human IgG1 pharmacokinetic evaluations.

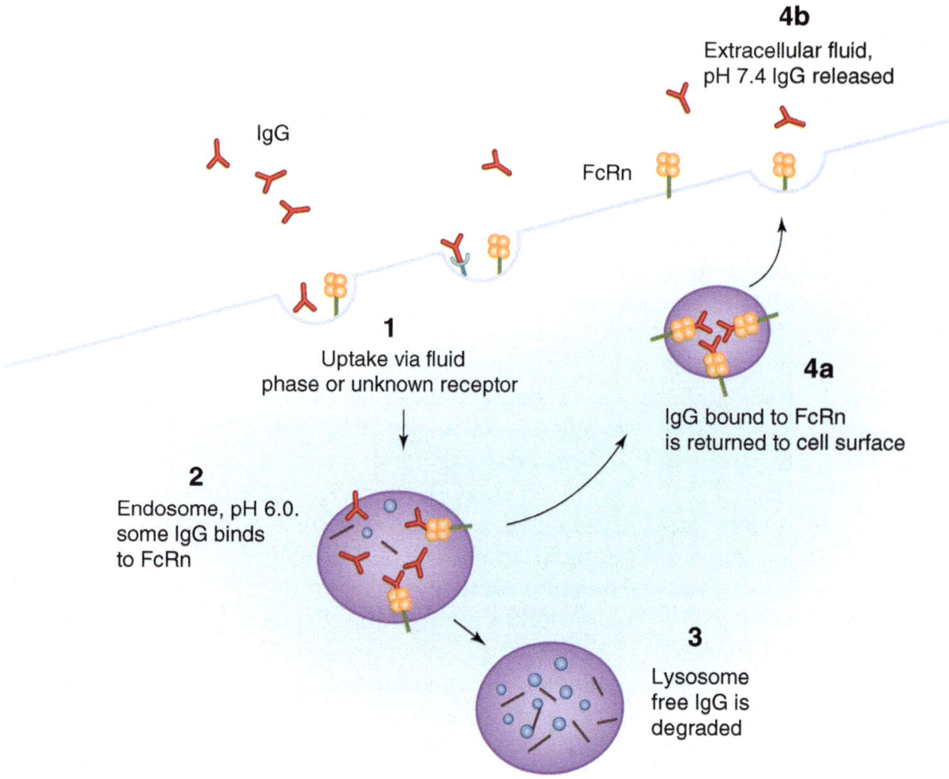

Figure 8.8 ■ Schematic disposition pathway of IgG antibodies via interaction with FcRn in endosomes. (1) IgGs enter cells by receptor-mediated endocytosis by binding of the Fc part to FcRn. (2) The intracellular vesicles (endosomes) fuse with lysosomes containing proteases. (3) Proteases degrade unbound IgG molecules, whereas IgGs bound to FcRn are protected. (4a) The intact IgG bound to FcRn is transported back to the cell surface and (4b) released back to the extracellular fluid

Ward's group confirmed that an engineered human IgG1 had disparate properties in murine and human systems (Vaccaro et al. 2006). Engineered IgGs with higher affinity to FcRn receptor have a two to three-fold longer half-life compared with WT in mice and monkeys (Hinton et al. 2006; Petkova et al. 2006). Two engineered human IgG1 mutants with enhanced binding affinity to human FcRn show a considerably extended half-life compared with WT in hFcRn transgenic mice (4.35 ± 0.53, 3.85 ± 0.55 days versus 1.72 ± 0.08 days) (Hinton et al. 2006; Petkova et al. 2006) found that the half-life of IgG1 FcRn mutants with increasing binding affinity to human FcRn at pH 6.0 is about 2.5-fold longer than the WT antibody in monkey (838 ± 187 h versus 336 ± 34 h).

Dose-proportional, linear CL has been observed for MAB against soluble antigens with low endogenous levels (such as TNF-α, IFN-α, VEGF, and IL-5). For example, linear PK has been observed for a humanized MAB directed to human interleukin-5 following IV administration over a 6000-fold dose range (0.05–300 mg/kg) in monkeys (Zia-Amirhosseini et al. 1999). The CL of rhuMAB against VEGF after IV dosing (2–50 mg/kg) ranged from 4.81 to 5.59 mL/day/kg and did not depend on dose (Lin et al. 1999). The mean total serum CL and the estimated mean terminal half-life of adalimumab were reported to range from 0.012 to 0.017 L/h and 10.0 to 13.6 days, respectively, for a 5-cohort clinical trial (0.5–10 mg/kg), with an overall mean half-life of 12 days (den Broeder et al. 2002). However, MABs against soluble antigens with high endogenous levels (such as IgE) exhibit nonlinear PK. The PK of omalizumab, an MAB against IgE, is linear only at doses greater than 0.5 mg/kg (Petkova et al. 2006; Xolair (Omalizumab) Prescribing Information 2006).

Elimination of MABs may also be impacted by interaction with the targeted cell-bound antigen, and this phenomenon was demonstrated by dose-dependent clearance and half-life. At low dose, MABs show a shorter half-life and a faster clearance due to receptor-mediated elimination. With increasing doses, receptors become saturated, the half-life gradually increases to a constant, and the CL gradually decreases to a constant. The binding affinity (K_d), antigen density, and antigen turnover rate may influence the receptor-mediated elimination. Koon et al. found a strong inverse correlation between CD25 cell expression and the apparent half-life of daclizumab (a MAB specifically binding to CD25) (Koon et al. 2006). It has been shown that the PK of murine antihuman CD3 antibodies may be determined by the disappearance of target antigen (Meijer et al. 2002). In monkeys and mice, clearance of SGN-40, a humanized anti-CD40 MAB, was much faster at low dose, suggesting nonlinear PK (Kelley et al. 2006). In addition, Ng et al. demonstrated that an anti-CD4 MAB (TRX-1) had ~fivefold faster CL at 1 mg/kg dose compared with 10 mg/kg dose (37.4 ± 2.4 versus 7.8 ± 0.6 mL/day/kg) in healthy volunteers (Ng et al. 2006). They also found that receptor-mediated CL via endocytosis became saturated at higher doses; nonspecific clearance of TRX-1 contributed 8.6, 27.1, and 41.7% of total CL when dose was 1, 5, and 10 mg/kg, respectively.

In addition to FcRn and antigen–antibody interaction, other factors may also contribute to MAB elimination (Roskos et al. 2004; Tabrizi et al. 2006; Lobo et al. 2004):

1. *Immunogenicity*: The elimination of MABs in humans may increase with increasing level of immunogenicity (Tabrizi et al. 2006; Ternant and Paintaud 2005).
2. *Degree and the nature of glycosylation*: The impact of glycosylation on the pharmacokinetics and effector functions of therapeutic IgG1 monoclonal antibodies has been previously reviewed (Putnam et al. 2010).
3. *Susceptibility to proteolysis*: Gillies and coworkers improved the circulating half-life of antibody-interleukin 2 immunocytokine by two-fold compared with wild type (1.0 h versus 0.54 h) by increasing the resistance to intracellular degradation (Gillies et al. 2002).
4. *Charge*: Deliberate modification of the isoelectric point (pI) of an antibody by approximately one pI unit or more can lead to noticeable differences in the PK of an intact antibody (Igawa et al. 2010; Li et al. 2014; Bumbaca Yadav et al. 2015). Using a humanized anti-IL-6 receptor IgG1 as an example, Igawa et al. showed that lowering the pI point from 9.2 to 7.2 by engineering the V region reduced the IgG elimination in cynomolgus monkeys (Igawa et al. 2010). In contrast, minor changes in the nature of ionic charge resulting in pI differences of less than approximately one pI unit are not expected to affect the biological function of MABs, including tissue retention and whole blood clearance (Boswell et al. 2010b; Khawli et al. 2010).
5. *Effector function*: Effector functions, such as interactions with FcγR, can also regulate elimination and PK of MABs (Mahmood and Green 2005). Mutation of the binding site of FcγR, for example, had dramatic effects on the clearance of an Ab-IL-2 fusion protein (Gillies et al. 1999).
6. *Concomitant medications*: Methotrexate reduced adalimumab apparent CL after single dose and multiple dosing by 29 and 44%, respectively, in patients with RA (Humira (Adalimumab) Prescribing Information 2007). In addition, azathioprine and mycophenolate mofetil were reported to reduce CL of basiliximab by approximately 22 and 51%, respectively (Simulect (Basiliximab) Prescribing Information 2005). The effects of small molecule drugs on the expression of Fcγ receptors could explain this finding. It has also been shown that methotrexate affects expression of FcγRI on monocytes significantly in RA patients (Bunescu et al. 2004).
7. *Off-target binding*: Although specificity to their targets is a major characteristic of MABs, they may have off-target binding that may result in atypical PK, such as faster CL and larger volume distribution. An anti-respiratory syncytial virus MAB, A4b4, developed by affinity maturation of palivizumab, had poor PK in rats and cynomolgus monkeys due to broad nonspecific tissue binding and sequestration (Wu et al. 2007). The rapid elimination of a humanized anti-human amyloid beta peptide MAB, anti-Aβ Ab2, in cynomolgus monkeys was linked to off-target binding to cynomolgus monkey fibrinogen (Vugmeyster et al. 2011). In addition, a humanized anti-fibroblast growth factor receptor 4 MAB had rapid CL in mice that was attributable to binding to mouse complement component 3 (Bumbaca et al. 2011). Other examples of MABs with off-target effects include MABs targeting Factor IXa/X (Sampei et al. 2013), interleukin-21 receptor (Vugmeyster et al. 2010). It is important to eliminate MABs with higher risk of failure at the discovery stage, to increase the success rate. As PK of these therapeutic proteins might be influenced by a large number of both specific and nonspecific factors, Dostalek et al. have proposed multiple pharmacokinetic de-risking tools for selection of MAB lead candidates (Dostalek et al. 2017).
8. *Body weight, age, disease state, and other demographic factors*: Individual characteristics can also change MAB PK (Mould and Sweeney 2007; Ryman and Meibohm 2017) (see Population Pharmacokinetics section).
9. *Albumin*: Albumin is often an indicator of disease status and a significant covariate affecting clearance for several MABs, including infliximab, pertuzumab, trastuzumab emtansine (Lu et al. 2014), and bevacizumab (Dirks and Meibohm 2010). It is believed that albumin, which binds to FcRn at different sites than IgG, is an indicator of increased number of FcRn (Dirks and Meibohm 2010; Fasanmade et al. 2010). Nevertheless, the correlation between the levels of albumin and the CL of pertuzumab and bevacizumab was moderate and dose modification was not recommended (Dirks and Meibohm 2010). Regardless, it has been suggested that serum albumin levels are a predictive factor for PK of infliximab and clinical response to the drug in patients with ulcerative colitis (Fasanmade et al. 2010).
10. *Disease state*: It has been reported that disease state can impact MAB PK. Lower exposure and faster CL for trastuzumab (Yang et al. 2013; Han et al.

2014), bevacizumab (Han et al. 2014), pertuzumab (Kang et al. 2013), and trastuzumab emtansine (Chen et al. 2017) in patients with gastric cancer (GC) versus breast cancer (BC) have been reported. Steady-state trastuzumab trough concentration (C_{trough}) in patients with metastatic GC is 24–63% lower than in BC (Yang et al. 2013). The underlying mechanism for faster CL of MABs in GC is unknown and warrants further research. Population PK analyses of ofatumumab were performed for various diseases with varying CD20 B-cell counts and indicated that target-mediated CL in CLL is greater than that in RA and FL, which is consistent with the higher B-cell count seen in CLL (Struemper et al. 2014). Diabetic comorbidity resulted in 28.7% higher CL/F for ustekinumab (Zhu et al. 2009). Infliximab CL is 40–50% higher in inflammatory bowel disease patients, which is likely due to protein losing enteropathy (Fasanmade et al. 2009). Recently, it has been observed that MABs in immune-oncology, such as pembrolizumab (Li et al. 2017) and nivolumab (Bajaj et al. 2017), have time-dependent CL. Sicker patients tend to have faster CL.

In summary, the association between baseline disease factors and PK complicates the interpretation of the exposure-efficacy analyses for MABs and ADCs in cancer patients, as only one-dose level is usually tested in the pivotal study. Although correction methods can be applied, the effect of disease severity on treatment exposure may result in an over-estimation of exposure–response relationships, i.e. visually a steep trend is seen when the true relationship is flat (Liu et al. 2015; Wang 2016).

THERAPEUTIC MAB–DRUG INTERACTIONS

MABs and other therapeutic proteins are increasingly combined with small molecule drugs to treat various diseases. Assessment of the potential for PK- and/or PD-based MAB–drug interactions is frequently incorporated into the drug development process (Girish et al. 2011). The exposure and response of concomitantly administered drugs can be altered by MABs (MAB as perpetrator), and other drugs can effect the PK and PD of therapeutic MABs (MAB as victim).

Several different mechanisms have been proposed for MAB–drug interactions. Various cytokines and cytokine modulators can influence the expression and activity of cytochrome P450 (CYP) enzymes and drug transporters (Lee et al. 2010). Therefore, if a therapeutic MAB is a cytokine or cytokine modulator, it can potentially alter the systemic exposure and/or clinical response of concomitantly administered drugs that are substrates of CYPs or transporters (Huang et al. 2010), particularly those with narrow therapeutic windows. For example, an increase in cyclosporin A (CsA) trough level was observed when given in combination with muromonab (Vasquez and Pollak 1997). Similarly, basiliximab has been shown to increase CsA and tacrolimus level when used in combination (Sifontis et al. 2002). In diseases states such as infection or inflammation, cytokines or cytokine modulators can also normalize previously changed activity of CYPs or transporters, thereby altering the exposure of co-administered drugs. Examples include tocilizumab coadministered with omeprazole and tocilizumab coadministered with simvastatin. At present, in vitro and preclinical systems have shown limited value in predicting a clinically relevant effect of cytokine-mediated therapeutic protein (TP)-DDI, and clinical evidence is preferred for informing the evolving risk assessment for TP-DDI (Huang et al. 2010; Slatter et al. 2013). To determine the necessity for a dedicated clinical DDI study, a four-step approach was proposed by the IQ Consortium/FDA TP-DDI workshop (San Diego 2012) in assessing TP-DDI risk for cytokines or cytokine modulators on CYP enzymes. This includes stepwise investigations of: (1) the disease effect on cytokine levels and CYP expression; (2) TP mechanism and its impact on cytokine-mediated DDI; (3) DDI liability of the concurrently used small molecule drugs; and (4) the above overall driving force in determining appropriate clinical TP-DDI strategies (Kenny et al. 2013). To date, a few dedicated clinical DDI studies have been performed for MABs that specifically target cytokines or cytokine receptors, e.g., tocilizumab (Schmitt et al. 2011), sirukumab (Zhuang et al. 2015), daclizumab HYP (Tran et al. 2016), and dupilumab (Davis et al. 2018). However, the overall impact of these cytokine-blocking MABs on PK of the CYP substrates (MAB as a perpetrator) were minimal (no effect, e.g., daclizumab HYP, ustekinumab, and dupilumab) or moderate (18–57% reduction in AUC for CYP 2C19 or 3A4 substrates, e.g., tocilizumab and sirukumab) and have not been implicated in dose justification for the relevant concurrent medicines.

MAB–drug interactions can also occur when a therapeutic MAB is administered with a concomitant drug that can alter the formation of ADAs. This may in turn alter MAB clearance from the systemic circulation. For example, methotrexate (MTX) reduced the apparent CL of adalimumab by 29 and 44% after single and repeated dosing (Humira (Adalimumab) Prescribing Information 2007). MTX also had similar effect on infliximab (Maini et al. 1998). PD-based interactions can result from alteration of target biology, such as the site of expression, relative abundance of expression, and the pharmacology of the target (Girish et al. 2011). Examples include efalizumab in combination with triple immune-suppressant therapy (Vincenti et al. 2007) and anakinra in combination with etanercept (Genovese et al. 2004).

To date, evidence of therapeutic MAB–drug interactions via nonspecific clearance appears to be limited, although down-regulation of Fcγ receptors by MTX is observed in patients with RA. It is possible that changes in Fcγ receptors can affect MAB clearance in the presence of MTX (Girish et al. 2011).

ADCs can also interact with drugs or MABs via the mechanisms described above. However, evidence of ADC–drug or ADC–MAB interaction appears to be absent. Lu et al. reported lack of interaction between trastuzumab emtansine (T-DM1) and pertuzumab in patients with HER2-positive metastatic breast cancer (Lu et al. 2012). Similarly, no interaction was observed between T-DM1 and paclitaxel or T-DM1 and docetaxel (Lu et al. 2012). With the theoretical potential for, and current experiences with, MAB–drug interactions, a question and risk-based integrated approach depending on the mechanism of the MABs and patient population have been progressively adopted during drug development to address important questions regarding the safety and efficacy of MAB and drug combinations (Girish et al. 2011). Various in vitro test systems have been used to provide some insight into the MAB–drug interactions, such as isolated hepatocytes and liver microsomes. However, the interpretation of these in vitro data is difficult. More importantly, prospective predictions of drug interactions based on in vitro findings have not been feasible for MABs. Therefore, clinical methods are primarily used to assess MAB–drug interactions. Three common methods used are population PK, clinical cocktail studies, and less frequently, dedicated drug interaction studies. Details of various strategies used in pharmaceutical industry were reviewed in a 2011 AAPS white paper (Girish et al. 2011). Recently, PBPK modeling has been used as a tool to predict drug interactions for antibody-drug conjugates (Chen et al. 2015).

PREDICTION OF HUMAN PK/PD BASED ON PRECLINICAL INFORMATION

Prior to a first-in-human (FIH) clinical study, a number of preclinical in vivo and in vitro experiments are conducted to evaluate the PK/PD, safety, and efficacy of a new drug candidate. However, the ultimate goal is at all times to predict how these preclinical results on PK, safety, and efficacy data translate into a given patient population. Therefore, the objective of translational research is to predict PK/PD/safety outcomes in a target patient population, acknowledging the similarities and differences between preclinical and clinical settings.

Over the years, many theories and approaches have been proposed and used for scaling preclinical PK data to humans (Fig. 8.9). Allometric scaling, based on a power–law relationship between size of the body and physiological and anatomical parameters, is the simplest and most widely used approach (Dedrick 1973; Mahmood 2005, 2009). More recently, experimental efforts have been dedicated to accurate measurement of physiological parameters that are required for calculating drug concentrations at site of action and for physiologically based models (Boswell et al. 2010a, 2012, 2014). Physiologically based PK modeling (Shah and Betts 2012), species-invariant time method (Dedrick approach) (Oitate et al. 2011), and nonlinear mixed effect modeling based on allometry (Jolling et al. 2005; Martin-Jimenez and Riviere 2002) have also been used for interspecies scaling of PK. While no single scaling method has been shown to definitively predict human PK in all cases, especially for small molecule drugs (Tang and Mayersohn 2005), the PK for MABs can be predicted reasonably well, especially for MAB at doses where the dominant clearance route is likely to be independent of concentration. Most therapeutic MABs bind to nonhuman primate antigens more often than to rodent antigens, due to the greater sequence homology observed between nonhuman primates and humans. The binding epitope, in vitro binding affinity to antigen, binding affinity to FcRn, tissue cross-reactivity profiles, and disposition and elimination pathways of MABs are often comparable in nonhuman primates and humans. It has recently been demonstrated that clearance and distribution volume of MABs with linear PK in humans can be reasonably projected based on data from nonhuman primates alone, with a fixed scaling exponent ranging from 0.75 to 0.9 for CL and a fixed scaling exponent 1 for volume of distribution (Oitate et al. 2011; Ling et al. 2009; Wang and Prueksaritanont 2010; Deng et al. 2011; Dong et al. 2011). For MABs that exhibited nonlinear PK, the best predictive performance was obtained above doses that saturated the target of the MAB (Dong et al. 2011). Pharmacokinetic prediction for low doses of a MAB with nonlinear elimination remains challenging and will likely require further exploration of species difference in target expression level, target antibody binding and target kinetics, as well as strategic in vivo animal PK studies, designed with relevant dose ranges. Immunogenicity is an additional challenge for the prediction of MAB PK. Alterations in the PK profile due to immune-mediated clearance mechanisms in preclinical species cannot be scaled up to humans, since animal models are not predictive of human immune response to human MABs. Thus, either excluding ADA-positive animals from PK scaling

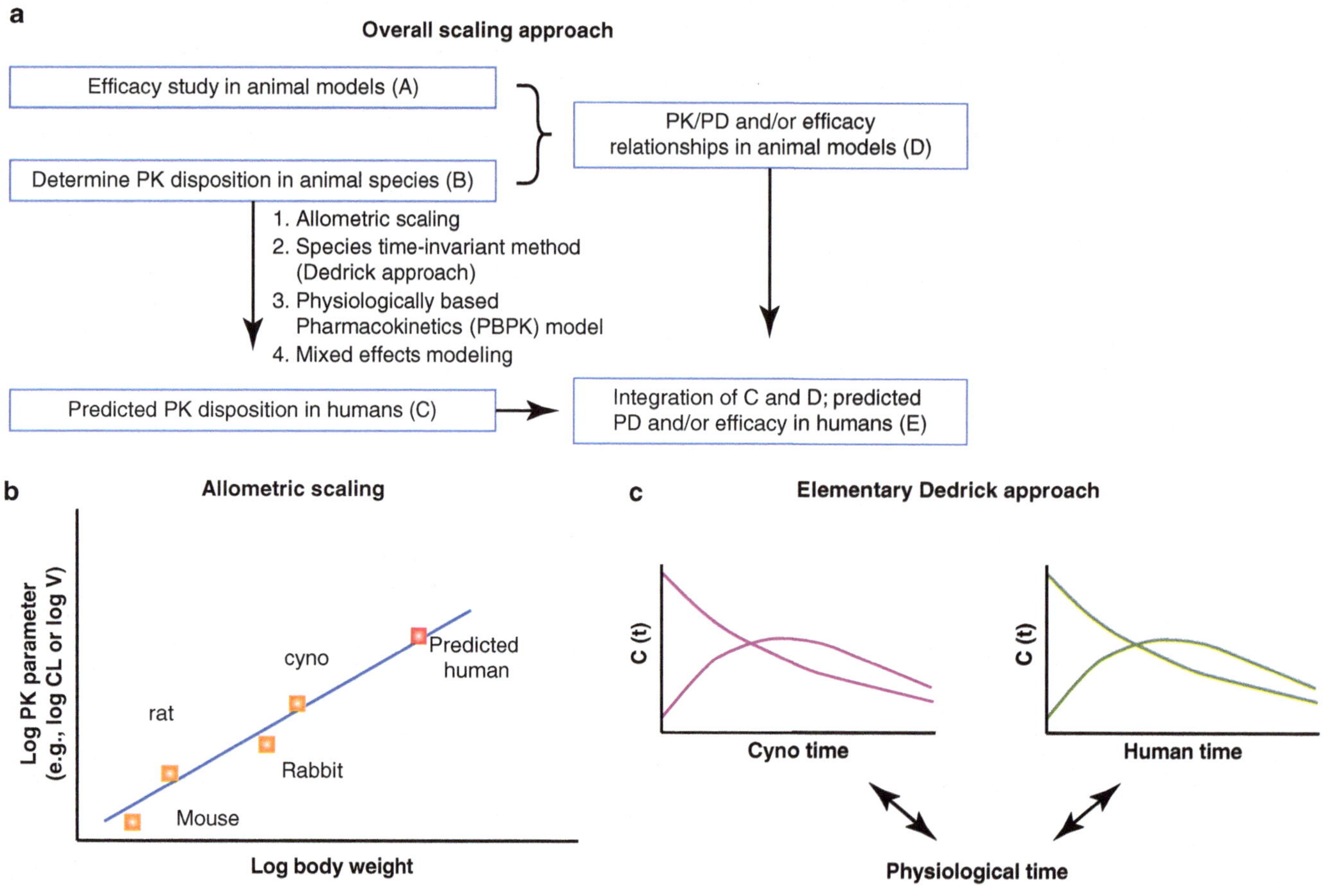

Figure 8.9 ■ PK/PD scaling approach from preclinical studies to humans. (**a**) Overall scaling approach. (**b**) Allometric scaling. (**c**) Elementary Dedrick approach

analysis or using only the early time points prior to ADAs observation in ADA-positive animals has been a standard practice in the industry.

Due to its complexity, any extrapolation of PD to humans requires more thorough consideration than for PK. Little is known about allometric relationships in PD parameters. It is expected that the physiological turnover rate constants of most general structures and functions among species should obey allometric principles, whereas capacity and sensitivity tend to be similar across species (Mager et al. 2009). Through integration of PK/PD modeling and interspecies scaling, PD effects in humans may be predicted if the PK/PD relationship is assumed to be similar between animal models and humans (Duconge et al. 2004; Kagan et al. 2010). For example, a PK/PD model was first developed to optimize the dosing regimen of a MAB against EGF/r3 using tumor-bearing nude mice as an animal model of human disease (Duconge et al. 2004). This PK/PD model was subsequently integrated with allometric scaling to calculate the dosing schedule required in a potential clinical trial to achieve a specific effect (Duconge et al. 2004).

In summary, species differences in antigen expression level, antigen–antibody binding and antigen kinetics, differences in FcRn binding between species, the immunogenicity, and other factors must be considered during PK/PD scaling of a MAB from animals to humans.

ROLE OF PK/PD IN CLINICAL DEVELOPMENT OF ANTIBODY THERAPEUTICS

Drug development has traditionally been performed in sequential phases, divided into preclinical as well as clinical phases I–IV. During the development phases of the molecules, the safety and PK/PD characteristics are established in order to select a compound for development and define a dosing regimen. This information-gathering process has been characterized as two successive learning–confirming cycles (Sheiner and Wakefield 1999; Sheiner 1997).

The first cycle (phases I and IIa) comprises learning about the dose regimen that is tolerated in healthy subjects and confirming that this dose regimen has shown drug-target engagement, acceptable tolerability and measurable clinical benefits in the targeted patients. An affirmative answer at this first cycle provides the justification for a larger and more costly second learn–confirm cycle (phases IIb and III), where the learning step is focused on defining the drug benefit/risk profile, whereas the confirm step is aimed at demonstrating acceptable benefit/risk in a large patient population (Meibohm and Derendorf 2002).

The drug development process at the clinical stage provides several opportunities for integration of PK/PD concepts. Clinical phase I dose escalation studies provide, from a PK/PD standpoint, the unique opportunity to evaluate the dose–concentration–effect relationship for therapeutic and toxic effects over a wide range of doses up to or even beyond the maximum tolerated dose under controlled conditions (Meredith et al. 1991). PK/PD evaluations at this stage of drug development can provide crucial information regarding the potency and tolerability of the drug in vivo and the verification and suitability of the PK/PD relationship established during preclinical studies.

Collecting robust data on the PK of the drug and PD or disease biomarkers that are indicative of drug pharmacology and disease progression/improvement is key to informing dose selection. Tocilizumab, omalizumab, and evolocumab are examples of MABs that utilized PK/PD or disease biomarker data to facilitate dose selection for pivotal trials, final doses and/or label revisions. In general, the strategy includes (1) understanding the PK profile and selecting clinical doses in the linear range, if possible; (2) identifying biomarkers having profiles correlated to clinically meaningful endpoints for PK/PD or exposure-response analyses, and (3) leveraging modeling and simulation approaches to predict the clinical outcome under different regimen scenarios, which is essential to determine the dose regimen for a pivotal trial or the final dose regimen on the label.

In the case of omalizumab, a dosing table for asthma patients was developed to select the dose based on an individual's pre-treatment serum IgE level and body weight. The dosing table was designed to achieve a serum-free IgE level associated with clinical improvement (Hochhaus et al. 2003). PK/PD modeling and simulation approaches were subsequently used to revise and expand the dosing table (Lowe et al. 2015; Honma et al. 2016). In the case of evolocumab, a high-level summary of the development program and dosing strategy follows.

Evolocumab is a recombinant, human IgG2 MAB that specifically binds to human proprotein convertase subtilisin/kexin type 9 (PCSK9). It prevents PCSK9 from interacting with the low density lipoprotein receptor (LDLR), thus upregulating LDLR, increasing uptake of circulating LDL-cholesterol (LDL-C) and reducing LDL-C concentration in plasma (Page and Watts 2015). Evolocumab is used as an adjunct to diet and maximally tolerated statin therapy for the treatment of adults with heterozygous familial hypercholesterolemia or clinical atherosclerotic cardiovascular disease. Its use is also indicated as an adjunct to diet and other LDL-lowering therapies for the treatment of patients with homozygous familial hypercholesterolemia.

The PK of evolocumab following multiple SC doses was evaluated in a Phase 1 study in subjects on a stable dose of statin over a dose range of 14–420 mg of evolocumab weekly, every 2 weeks, or every 4 weeks. Multiple doses of evolocumab resulted in nonlinear PK for the lower doses (up to 140 mg SC). Dose regimens of 140 mg and greater led to linear PK and concentrations associated with near complete suppression of PCSK9 (CDER 2014). Dose-dependent decreases in LDL-C levels were seen following treatment with evolocumab (CDER 2014) and this PD readout is also indicative of a meaningful clinical readout. There was a clear exposure-response relationship between evolocumab trough concentrations and LDL-C response (CDER 2014). These PK/PD data and the exposure-response relationship were used to support the final approved dose and dosing regimen.

■ Efalizumab Case Study (Raptiva®)

In the following sections, the recombinant humanized IgG1 MAB efalizumab is provided as a more detailed case study to understand the various steps during the development of therapeutic antibodies for various indications. Raptiva® received approval for the treatment of patients with psoriasis in more than 30 countries, including the United States and the European Union (Raptiva (Efalizumab) [Prescribing Information] 2004). However, it was withdrawn from the market when the use of efalizumab was found to be associated with an increased risk of progressive multifocal leukoencephalopathy (PML).

A summary of the preclinical program, the overall PK/PD data from multiple clinical studies, and the selection of the subcutaneous doses of efalizumab for the treatment of psoriasis will be discussed. Psoriasis is a chronic skin disease characterized by abnormal keratinocyte differentiation and hyperproliferation and by an aberrant inflammatory process in the dermis and epidermis. T cell infiltration and activation in the skin and subsequent T cell-mediated processes have been implicated in the pathogenesis of psoriasis (Krueger 2002). Efalizumab is a targeted inhibitor of T cell interactions (Werther et al. 1996). An extensive preclinical research program was conducted to study the safety and MOA of efalizumab. Multiple clinical studies were also conducted to investigate the efficacy, safety, PK, PD, and MOA of efalizumab in patients with psoriasis.

Preclinical Program of Efalizumab

A thorough and rigorous preclinical program provides a linkage between drug discovery and clinical development. At the preclinical stage, activities may include the evaluation of in vivo potency and intrinsic activity, the identification of bio-/surrogate markers, understanding of MOA, and characterization of nonclinical PK/PD, as well as dosage form/regimen selection and optimization. The role of surrogate molecules in assessing ADME of therapeutic antibodies is important as the antigen specificity of humanized MABs limits their utility in studies with rodents. Surrogate rodent MABs (mouse/rat) provide a means of gaining knowledge of PK and PD in a preclinical rodent model, facilitating dose optimization in the clinic.

In the case of efalizumab, to complete a more comprehensive safety assessment, a chimeric rat anti-mouse CD11a antibody, muM17, was developed and evaluated as a species-specific surrogate molecule for efalizumab. muM17 binds mouse CD11a with specificity and affinity similar to that of efalizumab to its human target antigen. In addition, pharmacological activities of muM17 in mice were demonstrated to be similar to those of efalizumab in humans (Clarke et al. 2004; Nakakura et al. 1993).

The preclinical ADME program for efalizumab consisted of PK, PD (CD11a down-modulation and saturation), and toxicokinetic data from PK, PD, and toxicology studies with efalizumab in chimpanzees and with muM17 in mice. The use of efalizumab in the chimpanzee and muM17 in mice for PK and PD and safety studies was supported by in vitro activity assessments. The preclinical data were used for PK and PD characterization, PD-based dose selection, and toxicokinetic support for confirming exposure in toxicology studies. Together, these data supported both the design of the preclinical program and its relevance to the clinical program.

The observed PD as well as the MOA of efalizumab and muM17 is attributed to binding CD11a present on cells and tissues. The binding affinities of efalizumab to human and chimpanzee CD11a on CD3 lymphocytes are comparable, supporting the use of chimpanzees as a preclinical model for human responses. CD11a expression has been observed to be greatly reduced on T lymphocytes in chimpanzees and mice treated with efalizumab and muM17, respectively. Expression of CD11a is restored as efalizumab and muM17 are eliminated from the plasma.

The disposition of efalizumab and of the mouse surrogate muM17 is mainly determined by the combination of both specific interactions with the ligand CD11a and by their IgG1 framework. The disposition is governed by the species specificity of the antibody for its ligand CD11a, the amount of CD11a in the system, and the administered dose. Binding to CD11a serves as a major pathway for clearance of these molecules, which leads to nonlinear PK depending on the relative amounts of CD11a and efalizumab or muM17 (Coffey et al. 2005).

Based on the safety studies, efalizumab was considered to be generally well tolerated in chimpanzees at doses up to 40 mg/kg/week IV for 6 months, providing an exposure ratio of 339-fold based on cumulative dose and 174-fold based on the cumulative AUC, compared with a clinical dose of 1 mg/kg/week. The surrogate antibody muM17 was also well tolerated in mice at doses up to 30 mg/kg/week SC. Overall, efalizumab was considered to have an excellent nonclinical safety profile, thereby supporting the use in adult patients. There was no signal for PML in the nonclinical studies, which subsequently led to withdrawal of efalizumab from the market.

Clinical Program of Efalizumab: PK/PD Studies, Assessment of Dose, Route, and Regimen

Efalizumab PK and PD data were available from ten studies in which more than 1700 patients with psoriasis received IV or SC efalizumab. In the phase I studies, PK and PD parameters were characterized by extensive sampling during treatment; in the phase III trials, steady-state trough levels were measured once or twice during the first 12-week treatment period for all the studies and during extended treatment periods for some studies. Several early phase I and II trials examined IV injection of efalizumab, and dose-ranging findings from these trials served as the basis for SC dosing levels used in several subsequent phase I and all phase III trials.

IV Administration of Efalizumab

The PK of MABs varies greatly, depending primarily on their affinity for and the distribution of their target antigen (Lobo et al. 2004). Efalizumab exhibited concentration-dependent nonlinear PK after administration of single IV doses of 0.03, 0.1, 0.3, 0.6, 1.0, 2.0, 3.0, and 10.0 mg/kg in a phase I study. This nonlinearity is directly related to specific and saturable binding of efalizumab to its cell surface receptor, CD11a, and has been described by a PK/PD model developed by Bauer et al. (1999), which was expanded to a PK/PD/efficacy model by Ng et al. (2005). The PK profiles of efalizumab following single IV doses with observed data and model predicted fit are presented in Fig. 8.10. Mean CL decreased from 380 to 6.6 mL/kg/day for doses of 0.03 mg/kg to 10 mg/kg, respectively. The volume of distribution of the central compartment

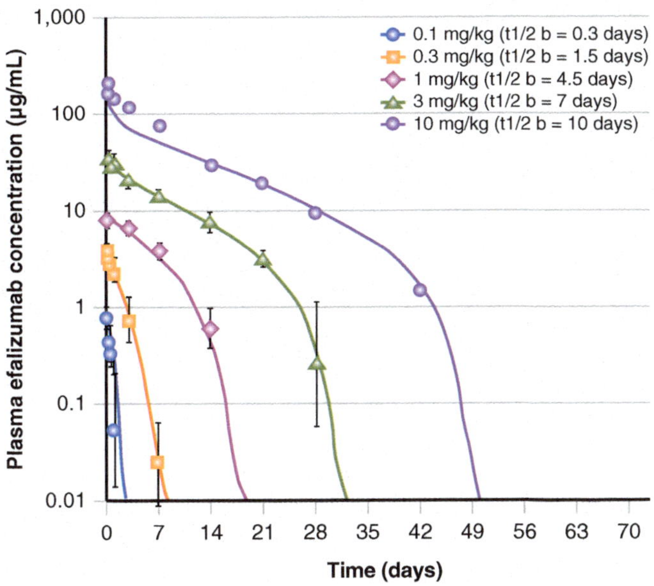

Figure 8.10 ■ Plasma concentration versus time profile for efalizumab following single IV doses in psoriasis patients (Ng et al. 2005)

(Vc) of efalizumab was 110 mL/kg at 0.03 mg/kg (approximately twice the plasma volume) and decreased to 58 mL/kg at 10 mg/kg (approximately equal to plasma volume), consistent with saturable binding of efalizumab to CD11a in the vascular compartment. Because of efalizumab's nonlinear PK, its half-life ($t_{1/2}$) is dose dependent.

In a phase II study of efalizumab, it was shown that at a weekly dosage of 0.1 mg/kg IV, patients did not maintain maximal down-modulation of CD11a expression and did not maintain maximal saturation. Also, at the end of 8 weeks of efalizumab treatment, 0.1 mg/kg/week IV, patients did not have statistically significant histological improvement and did not achieve a full clinical response. The minimum weekly IV dosage of efalizumab tested that produced histological improvements in skin biopsies was 0.3 mg/kg/week. This dosage resulted in submaximal saturation of CD11a binding sites but maximal down-modulation of CD11a expression. Improvements in patients' psoriasis were also observed, as determined by histology and by the Psoriasis Area and Severity Index (PASI) (Papp et al. 2001).

Determination of SC Doses

Although efficacy was observed in phase I and II studies with 0.3 mg/kg/week IV efalizumab, dosages of 0.6 mg/kg/week and greater (given for 7–12 weeks) provided more consistent T lymphocyte CD11a saturation and maximal PD effect. At dosages ≤0.3 mg/kg/week, large between-subject variability was observed, whereas at dosages of 0.6 or 1.0 mg/kg/week, patients experienced better improvement in PASI scores, with lower between-patient variability in CD11a saturation and down-modulation. Therefore, since the desired route of administration was SC, this IV dosage was used to estimate an appropriate minimum SC dose of 1 mg/kg/week (based on a 50% bioavailability) that would induce similar changes in PASI, PD measures, and histology. The safety, PK, and PD of a range of SC efalizumab doses (0.5–4.0 mg/kg/week administered for 8–12 weeks) were evaluated initially in two phase I studies (Gottlieb et al. 2003). To establish whether a higher SC dosage might produce better results, several phase III clinical trials assessed a 2.0 mg/kg/week SC dosage in addition to the 1.0 mg/kg/week dosage. A dose of 1.0 mg/kg/week SC efalizumab was selected as it produced sufficient trough levels in patients to maintain the maximal down-modulation of CD11a expression and binding-site saturation between weekly doses (Joshi et al. 2006). Figure 8.11 depicts the serum efalizumab levels, CD11a expression, and available CD11a binding sites on T lymphocytes (mean ± SD) after SC administration of 1 mg/kg efalizumab.

SC Administration of Efalizumab

The PK of SC efalizumab was well characterized following multiple SC doses of 1.0 and 2.0 mg/kg/week (Joshi et al. 2006; Mortensen et al. 2005). A phase I study that collected steady-state PK and PD data for 12 weekly SC doses of 1.0 and 2.0 mg/kg in psoriasis patients provided most of the pharmacologic data relevant to the product that was on the market prior to its withdrawal. Although peak serum concentration after the last dose (C_{max}) was observed to be higher for the 2.0 mg/kg/week (30.9 μg/mL) than for the 1.0 mg/kg/week dosage (12.4 μg/mL), no additional changes in PD effects were observed at the higher dosages (Mortensen et al. 2005). Following a dose of 1.0 mg/kg/week, serum efalizumab concentrations were adequate to induce maximal down-modulation of CD11a expression and a reduction in free CD11a binding sites on T lymphocytes (Fig. 8.12). Steady-state serum efalizumab levels were reached more quickly with the 1.0 mg/kg/week dosage at 4 weeks compared with the 2.0 mg/kg/week dosage at 8 weeks (Mortensen et al. 2005), which is in agreement with the average effective $t_{1/2}$ of 5.5 days for SC efalizumab 1.0 mg/kg/week (Boxenbaum and Battle 1995). The bioavailability was estimated at approximately 50%. Population PK analyses indicated that body weight was the most significant covariate affecting efalizumab SC clearance, thus supporting body weight-based dosing for efalizumab (Sun et al. 2005).

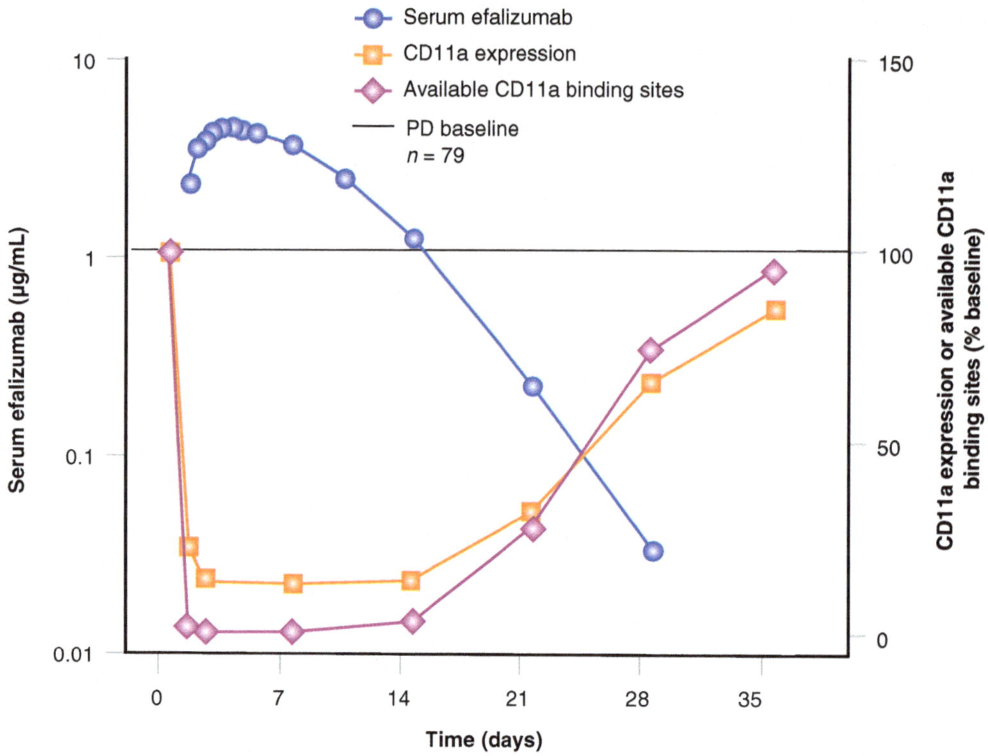

Figure 8.11 ■ PK/PD profile following efalizumab in humans (1 mg/kg SC) (Joshi et al. 2006)

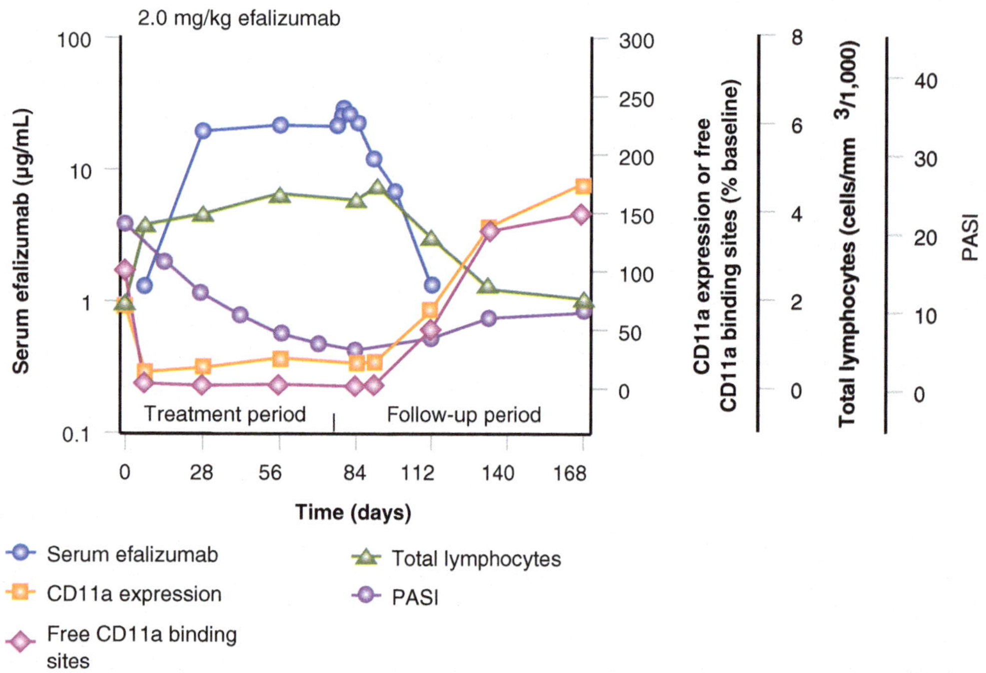

Figure 8.12 ■ Serum efalizumab, CD11a expression, and free CD11a binding sites on T lymphocytes, absolute lymphocyte counts, and Psoriasis Area and Severity Index (PASI) score (mean) following 1.0 mg/kg/week SC efalizumab for 12 weeks and 12 weeks post-treatment (Mortensen et al. 2005)

POPULATION PHARMACOKINETICS OF MONOCLONAL ANTIBODIES

Compared to many small molecule drugs, MABs typically exhibit less inter- and intra-subject variability of the standard PK parameters such as volume of distribution and clearance. However, it is possible that certain pathophysiological conditions may result into substantially increased intra- and inter-patient variability. In addition, patients are usually not very homogeneous; patients vary in sex, age, body weight; they may have concomitant disease and may be receiving multiple drug treatments. Even the diet, lifestyle, ethnicity, and geographic location can differ from a selected group of "normal" subjects. These covariates can have substantial influence on PK parameters. Therefore, good therapeutic practice should always be based on an understanding of both the influence of covariates on PK parameters as well as the PK variability in a given patient population. With this knowledge, dosage adjustments can be made to accommodate differences in PK due to genetic, environmental, physiological, or pathological factors, for instance, in case of compounds with a relatively small therapeutic index. The framework of application of population PK during drug development is summarized in the FDA guidance document entitled "Guidance for Industry—Population Pharmacokinetics" (FDA 1999).

For population PK data analysis, there are generally two reliable and practical approaches. One approach is the standard two-stage (STS) method, which estimates parameters from the plasma drug concentration data for an individual subject during the first stage. The estimates from all subjects are then combined to obtain a population mean and variability estimates for the parameters of interest. The method works well when sufficient drug concentration-time data are available for each individual patient; typically these data are gathered in phase 1 clinical trials. A second approach, nonlinear mixed effect modeling (NONMEM), attempts to fit the data and partition the differences between theoretical and observed values into random error terms. The influence of fixed effect (i.e., age, sex, body weight) can be identified through a regression model building process.

The original scope for the NONMEM approach was its applicability even when the amount of time-concentration data obtained from each individual is sparse and conventional compartmental PK analyses are not feasible. This is usually the case during the routine visits in phase III or IV clinical studies. Nowadays the NONMEM approach is applied far beyond its original scope due to its flexibility and robustness. It has been used to describe data-rich phase I and phase IIa studies or even preclinical data to guide and expedite drug development from early preclinical to clinical studies (Aarons et al. 2001; Chien et al. 2005).

There has been increasing interest in the use of population PK and PD analyses for different antibody products (i.e. antibodies, antibody fragments, or antibody fusion proteins) over the past 15 years (Dirks and Meibohm 2010; Agoram et al. 2007; Gibiansky and Frey 2012; Gibiansky and Gibiansky 2009; Nestorov et al. 2004; Zheng et al. 2011; Zhou et al. 2004; Yim et al. 2005; Hayashi et al. 2007; Lee et al. 2003). One example involving analysis of population plasma concentration data involved a dimeric fusion protein, etanercept. A one-compartment first-order absorption and elimination population PK model with interindividual and inter-occasion variability on CL, volume of distribution, and absorption rate constant, with covariates of sex and race on apparent CL and body weight on CL and volume of distribution, was developed for etanercept in rheumatoid arthritis adult patients (Lee et al. 2003). The population PK model for etanercept was further applied to pediatric patients with juvenile RA and established the basis of the 0.8 mg/kg once weekly regimen in pediatric patients with juvenile RA (Yim et al. 2005). Unaltered etanercept PK with concurrent methotrexate in patients with RA has been demonstrated in a phase IIIb study using a population PK modeling approach (Zhou et al. 2004). Thus, no etanercept dose adjustment is needed for patients taking concurrent MTX. A simulation exercise of using the final population PK model of subcutaneously administered etanercept in patients with psoriasis indicated that the two different dosing regimens (50 mg QWk versus 25 mg BIWk) provide a similar steady-state exposure (Nestorov et al. 2004). Therefore, their respective efficacy and safety profiles are likely to be similar as well.

An added feature is the development of a population model involving both PK and PD. Population PK/PD modeling has been used to characterize drug PK and PD with models ranging from simple empirical PK/PD models to advanced mechanistic models by using drug–receptor binding principles or other physiologically based principles. A mechanism-based population PK and PD binding model was developed for a recombinant DNA-derived humanized IgG1 MAB, omalizumab (Hayashi et al. 2007). Clearance and volume of distribution for omalizumab varied with body weight, whereas CL and rate of production of IgE were predicted accurately by baseline IgE, and overall, these covariates explained much of the interindividual variability. Furthermore, this mechanism-based population PK/PD model enabled the estimation of not only omalizumab disposition but also the binding with its target, IgE, and the rate of production, distribution, and elimination of IgE.

Recently, a platform population PK approach has been used to characterize MAB PK to improve the efficiency of study design, such as optimal dose regimens and PK sampling times. Davda et al. (2014) determined typical population PK values for four MABs with linear elimination using model-based meta-analysis, which can be utilized to prospectively optimize FIH study designs. A platform model describing PK properties of vc-MMAE antibody-drug conjugates based on 8 ADCs is reported by Kagedal et al. (2017). The model could be applied to predict PK-profiles of future vc-MMAE ADCs, estimate individual exposure for the subsequent exposure-response analysis, and optimize study design.

Population PK/PD analysis can capture uncertainty and the expected variability in PK/PD data generated in preclinical studies or early phases of clinical development. Understanding the associated PK or PD variability and performing clinical trial simulation by incorporating the uncertainty from the existing PK/PD data allows projecting a plausible range of doses for future clinical studies and final practical uses.

FUTURE PERSPECTIVE

The success of MABs as new therapeutic agents in several disease areas such as oncology, inflammatory diseases, autoimmune diseases, and transplantation has triggered growing scientific, therapeutic, and business interest in the MAB technology. The market for therapeutic MABs is one of the most dynamic sectors within the pharmaceutical industry. Further growth is expected by developing MABs towards other surface protein targets, which are not covered yet by marketed MABs. Particularly, the technological advancement in the area of ADCs and MAB fragments may overcome some of the limitations of MABs by providing highly potent drugs selectively to target compartments and to extend the distribution of the active moiety, which are typically not reached by MABs. ADCs hold great promise for selective drug delivery of potent drugs with unfavorable own selectivity to target cells (e.g., highly potent cytotoxic drugs). Several of such ADCs are under development to target different tumor types and are expected to reach the market in the next several years. Modification of the MAB structure allows adjusting the properties according to therapeutic needs (e.g., adjusting half-life, increasing volume of distribution, changing clearance pathways). By using modified MAB derivatives, optimized therapeutic agents might become available. For example, this technology has been successfully used for two antibody fragments marketed in inflammatory disease and anti-angiogenesis (abciximab, ranibizumab).

Bispecific antibodies represent another promising new methodological approach to antibody therapy. Technological refinements in antibody engineering have allowed the production of bispecific antibodies that are simultaneously directed towards two distinct target antigens (Holmes 2011). For instance, the CDR consisting of the variable domains (V_L and V_H) at the tip of one arm of an IgG may be asymmetrically designed to bind to a different target than that of the other arm (Fig. 8.1). Symmetrical formats in which each arm can bind two targets are also possible.

MABs have become a key part of the pharmaceutical armamentarium, especially in the oncology and immunology settings and will continue to be a focus area for drug discovery and development. More specifically, the recent approvals of MABs like pembrolizumab, nivolumab and atezolizumab in cancer immunotherapy have revolutionized cancer treatment paradigm. These MABs, either as monotherapy or in combinations with other cancer immunotherapies, including cancer vaccines, bispecifics and other modalities, offer tremendous promise for personalized medicine.

SELF-ASSESSMENT QUESTIONS

Questions

1. What are the structural differences among the five immunoglobulin classes?
2. What are key differences in PK/PD between MABs and small molecule drugs?
3. Why do IgGs typically show nonlinear PK in the lower plasma (serum) concentration range?
4. What is a surrogate MAB and how can it potentially be used in the drug development process of MABs?
5. Which other modes of actions apart from ADCC—antibody dependent cellular cytotoxicity are known for MABs? What are the key steps of ADCC?
6. Why do IgGs have a longer in vivo half-life compared with other Igs?
7. What are the development phases for antibody therapeutics? What major activities are involved in each phase?

Answers

1. The following structural properties distinguish MABs:
   The molecular form varies across the five immunoglobulin classes: IgG, IgD, and IgE are monomers; IgM forms a pentamer or hexamer, and IgA exists either as a monomer or dimer. Consequently, the molecular weights of various Igs differ (IgG 150–169 kD, IgA 160–300 kD, IgD 175 kD, IgE 190, IgM 950 kD).
2. Metabolism of MABs appears to be simpler than for small molecules. In contrast to small molecule drugs, the typical metabolic enzymes and transporter proteins, such as cytochrome P450, multidrug resistance (MDR) efflux pumps, are not involved in the disposition of MABs. Therefore, drug–drug interaction studies for those disposition processes are only part of the standard safety assessment for small molecules and not for MABs.
   MABs, which have a protein structure, are metabolized by proteases. These enzymes are ubiquitously available in mammalian organisms. In contrast, small molecule drugs are primarily metabolized in the liver.

Because of their large molecular weight, intact MABs are typically not cleared via the renal elimination route. However, renal clearance processes can play a major role in the elimination of small molecule drugs.

PK of MABs usually is dependent on the binding to the pharmacological target protein and shows nonlinear behavior as consequence of its saturation kinetics.

In general, MABs have a longer half-life (on the order of days and weeks) than small molecule drugs (typically on the order of hours).

The distribution of MABs is very restricted (volume of distribution in the range of 0.1 L/kg). As a consequence, MABs do have limited access to tissue compartments (e.g., brain) as potential target sites via passive, energy-independent distribution processes only.

3. At lower concentrations, MABs generally show nonlinear PK due to receptor-mediated clearance processes, which are characterized by small capacity of the clearance pathway and high affinity to the target protein. Consequently at these low concentrations, MABs exhibit typically shorter half-life. With increasing doses, these receptors become saturated, and the clearance as well as elimination half-life decreases until it becomes constant. The clearance in the higher concentration range, which is dominated by linear, non target-related clearance processes, is therefore also called nonspecific clearance in contrast to the target-related, specific clearance.
4. A surrogate MAB has similar antigen specificity and affinity in experimental animals (e.g., mice and rats) compared to those of the corresponding human antibody in humans. It is quite common that the antigen specificity limits ADME studies of humanized MABs in rodents. Studies using surrogate antibodies might lead to important information regarding safety, MOA, disposition of the drug, tissue distribution, and receptor pharmacology in the respective animal species, which might be too cumbersome and expensive to be conducted in nonhuman primates. Surrogate MABs (from mouse or rat) provide a means to gain knowledge of ADME and PD in preclinical rodent models and might facilitate the dose selection for clinical studies.
5. Apart from ADCC, MABs can exert pharmacological effects by multiple mechanisms that include direct modulation of the target antigen, complement-dependent cytotoxicity (CDC) and apoptosis. The key steps of ADCC are (1) opsonization of the targeted cells, (2) recognition of antibody-coated targeted cells by Fc receptors on the surface of monocytes, macrophages, natural killer cells, and other cells, and (3) destruction of the opsonized targets by phagocytosis of the opsonized targets and/or by toxic substances released after activation of monocytes, macrophages, natural killer cells, and other cells.
6. IgG can bind to neonatal Fc receptor (FcRn) in the endosome, which protects IgG from catabolism via proteolytic degradation. This protection results into a slower clearance and thus longer plasma half-life of IgGs. Consequently, changing the FcRn affinity allows adjustment of the clearance of MABs (higher affinity—lower clearance), which can be employed to tailor the PK of these molecules.
7. Pre-IND, phase I, II, III, and IV are the major development phases for antibody therapies. Safety pharmacology, toxicokinetics, toxicology, tissue cross-reactivity, local tolerance, PK support for candidate selection, assay support for PK/PD, and PK/PD support for dose/route/regimen are major activities in the pre-IND phase. General toxicity, reproductive toxicity, carcinogenicity, immunogenicity, characterization of dose–concentration–effect relationship, material comparability studies, mechanistic modeling approach, and population PK/predictions are major activities from phase I to phase III. Further studies might be performed as needed after the MAB got market authorization. These studies are called phase IV studies.

Acknowledgments Editorial and technical support was provided by AnshinBiosolutions, Corp.

REFERENCES

Aarons L, Karlsson MO, Mentre F, Rombout F, Steimer JL, van Peer A (2001) Role of modelling and simulation in Phase I drug development. Eur J Pharm Sci 13(2):115–122

Agoram BM, Martin SW, van der Graaf PH (2007) The role of mechanism-based pharmacokinetic-pharmacodynamic (PK-PD) modelling in translational research of biologics. Drug Discov Today 12(23-24):1018–1024. https://doi.org/10.1016/j.drudis.2007.10.002

Albrecht H, DeNardo SJ (2006) Recombinant antibodies: from the laboratory to the clinic. Cancer Biother Radiopharm 21(4):285–304. https://doi.org/10.1089/cbr.2006.21.285

Baert F, Noman M, Vermeire S, Van Assche G, DH G, Carbonez A, Rutgeerts P (2003) Influence of immunogenicity on the long-term efficacy of infliximab in Crohn's disease. N Engl J Med 348(7):601–608

Bajaj G, Wang X, Agrawal S, Gupta M, Roy A, Feng Y (2017) Model-based population pharmacokinetic analysis of nivolumab in patients with solid tumors. CPT Pharmacometrics Syst Pharmacol 6(1):58–66. https://doi.org/10.1002/psp4.12143

Bauer RJ, Dedrick RL, White ML, Murray MJ, Garovoy MR (1999) Population pharmacokinetics and pharmacodynamics of the anti-CD11a antibody hu1124 in human subjects with psoriasis. J Pharmacokinet Biopharm 27(4):397–420

Baxter LT, Zhu H, Mackensen DG, Jain RK (1994) Physiologically based pharmacokinetic model for specific and nonspecific monoclonal antibodies and fragments in normal tissues and human tumor xenografts in nude mice. Cancer Res 54(6):1517–1528

Baxter LT, Zhu H, Mackensen DG, Butler WF, Jain RK (1995) Biodistribution of monoclonal antibodies: scale-up from mouse to human using a physiologically based pharmacokinetic model. Cancer Res 55(20):4611–4622

Bazin-Redureau MI, Renard CB, Scherrmann JM (1997) Pharmacokinetics of heterologous and homologous immunoglobulin G, F(ab')2 and Fab after intravenous administration in the rat. J Pharm Pharmacol 49(3):277–281

Berger MA, Masters GR, Singleton J, Scully MS, Grimm LG, Soltis DA, Albone EF (2005) Pharmacokinetics, biodistribution, and radioimmunotherapy with monoclonal antibody 776.1 in a murine model of human ovarian cancer. Cancer Biother Radiopharm 20(6):589–602

Bien-Ly N, Boswell CA, Jeet S, Beach TG, Hoyte K, Luk W, Shihadeh V, Ulufatu S, Foreman O, Lu Y, DeVoss J, van der Brug M, Watts RJ (2015) Lack of widespread BBB disruption in Alzheimer's disease models: focus on therapeutic antibodies. Neuron 88(2):289–297. https://doi.org/10.1016/j.neuron.2015.09.036

Bittner B, Richter WF, Hourcade-Potelleret F, McIntyre C, Herting F, Zepeda ML, Schmidt J (2012) Development of a subcutaneous formulation for trastuzumab - nonclinical and clinical bridging approach to the approved intravenous dosing regimen. Arzneimittelforschung 62(9):401–409. https://doi.org/10.1055/s-0032-1321831

Boswell CA, Brechbiel MW (2007) Development of radioimmunotherapeutic and diagnostic antibodies: an inside-out view. Nucl Med Biol 34(7):757–778. https://doi.org/10.1016/j.nucmedbio.2007.04.001

Boswell CA, Ferl GZ, Mundo EE, Schweiger MG, Marik J, Reich MP, Theil FP, Fielder PJ, Khawli LA (2010a) Development and evaluation of a novel method for preclinical measurement of tissue vascular volume. Mol Pharm 7(5):1848–1857. https://doi.org/10.1021/mp100183k

Boswell CA, Tesar DB, Mukhyala K, Theil FP, Fielder PJ, Khawli LA (2010b) Effects of charge on antibody tissue distribution and pharmacokinetics. Bioconjug Chem 21(12):2153–2163. https://doi.org/10.1021/bc100261d

Boswell CA, Bumbaca D, Fielder PJ, Khawli LA (2012) Compartmental tissue distribution of antibody therapeutics: experimental approaches and interpretations. AAPS J 14(3):612–618. https://doi.org/10.1208/s12248-012-9374-1

Boswell CA, Mundo EE, Johnstone B, Ulufatu S, Schweiger MG, Bumbaca D, Fielder PJ, Prabhu S, Khawli LA (2013) Vascular physiology and protein disposition in a preclinical model of neurodegeneration. Mol Pharm 10(5):1514–1521. https://doi.org/10.1021/mp3004786

Boswell CA, Mundo EE, Ulufatu S, Bumbaca D, Cahaya HS, Majidy N, Van Hoy M, Schweiger MG, Fielder PJ, Prabhu S, Khawli LA (2014) Comparative physiology of mice and rats: radiometric measurement of vascular parameters in rodent tissues. Mol Pharm 11(5):1591–1598. https://doi.org/10.1021/mp400748t

Boxenbaum H, Battle M (1995) Effective half-life in clinical pharmacology. J Clin Pharmacol 35(8):763–766

Brambell FW, Hemmings WA, Morris IG (1964) A theoretical model of gamma-globulin catabolism. Nature 203:1352–1354

Bugelski PJ, Herzyk DJ, Rehm S, Harmsen AG, Gore EV, Williams DM, Maleeff BE, Badger AM, Truneh A, O'Brien SR, Macia RA, Wier PJ, Morgan DG, Hart TK (2000) Preclinical development of keliximab, a primatized anti-CD4 monoclonal antibody, in human CD4 transgenic mice: characterization of the model and safety studies. Hum Exp Toxicol 19(4):230–243. https://doi.org/10.1191/096032700678815783

Bumbaca Yadav D, Sharma VK, Boswell CA, Hotzel I, Tesar D, Shang Y, Ying Y, Fischer SK, Grogan JL, Chiang EY, Urban K, Ulufatu S, Khawli LA, Prabhu S, Joseph S, Kelley RF (2015) Evaluating the use of antibody variable region (Fv) charge as a risk assessment tool for predicting typical cynomolgus monkey pharmacokinetics. J Biol Chem 290(50):29732–29741. https://doi.org/10.1074/jbc.M115.692434

Bumbaca D, Wong A, Drake E, Reyes AE, Lin BC, Stephan JP, Desnoyers L, Shen BQ, Dennis MS (2011) Highly specific off-target binding identified and eliminated during the humanization of an antibody against FGF receptor 4. MAbs 3(4):376–386

Bumbaca D, Xiang H, Boswell CA, Port RE, Stainton SL, Mundo EE, Ulufatu S, Bagri A, Theil FP, Fielder PJ, Khawli LA, Shen BQ (2012) Maximizing tumour exposure to anti-neuropilin-1 antibody requires saturation of non-tumour tissue antigenic sinks in mice. Br J Pharmacol 166(1):368–377. https://doi.org/10.1111/j.1476-5381.2011.01777.x

Bunescu A, Seideman P, Lenkei R, Levin K, Egberg N (2004) Enhanced Fcgamma receptor I, alphaMbeta2 integrin receptor expression by monocytes and neutrophils in rheumatoid arthritis: interaction with platelets. J Rheumatol 31(12):2347–2355

Cartron G, Watier H, Golay J, Solal-Celigny P (2004) From the bench to the bedside: ways to improve rituximab efficacy. Blood 104(9):2635–2642

CDER (2014) Clinical pharmacology and biopharmaceutical reviews BLA 125522

CDER (2015) Addendum clinical pharmacology review BLA 125509. https://www.accessdata.fda.gov/drugsatfda_docs/nda/2016/125509Orig1s000ClinPharmR.pdf. Accessed May 8, 2018

Chen Y, Samineni D, Mukadam S, Wong H, Shen BQ, Lu D, Girish S, Hop C, Jin JY, Li C (2015) Physiologically based pharmacokinetic modeling as a tool to predict drug interactions for antibody-drug conjugates. Clin Pharmacokinet 54(1):81–93. https://doi.org/10.1007/s40262-014-0182-x

Chen SC, Kagedal M, Gao Y, Wang B, Harle-Yge ML, Girish S, Jin J, Li C (2017) Population pharmacokinetics of trastuzumab emtansine in previously treated patients with HER2-positive advanced gastric cancer (AGC). Cancer

Chemother Pharmacol 80(6):1147–1159. https://doi.org/10.1007/s00280-017-3443-1

Chien JY, Friedrich S, Heathman MA, de Alwis DP, Sinha V (2005) Pharmacokinetics/pharmacodynamics and the stages of drug development: role of modeling and simulation. AAPS J 7(3):E544–E559

Clarke J, Leach W, Pippig S, Joshi A, Wu B, House R, Beyer J (2004) Evaluation of a surrogate antibody for preclinical safety testing of an anti-CD11a monoclonal antibody. Regul Toxicol Pharmacol 40(3):219–226

Coffey GP, Fox JA, Pippig S, Palmieri S, Reitz B, Gonzales M, Bakshi A, Padilla-Eagar J, Fielder PJ (2005) Tissue distribution and receptor-mediated clearance of anti-CD11a antibody in mice. Drug Metab Dispos 33(5):623–629

Cohenuram M, Saif MW (2007) Panitumumab the first fully human monoclonal antibody: from the bench to the clinic. Anti-Cancer Drugs 18(1):7–15

Cornillie F, Shealy D, D'Haens G, Geboes K, Van Assche G, Ceuppens J, Wagner C, Schaible T, Plevy SE, Targan SR, Rutgeerts P (2001) Infliximab induces potent anti-inflammatory and local immunomodulatory activity but no systemic immune suppression in patients with Crohn's disease. Aliment Pharmacol Ther 15(4):463–473

Dall'Ozzo S, Tartas S, Paintaud G, Cartron G, Colombat P, Bardos P, Watier H, Thibault G (2004) Rituximab-dependent cytotoxicity by natural killer cells: influence of FCGR3A polymorphism on the concentration-effect relationship. Cancer Res 64(13):4664–4669

Danilov SM, Gavrilyuk VD, Franke FE, Pauls K, Harshaw DW, McDonald TD, Miletich DJ, Muzykantov VR (2001) Lung uptake of antibodies to endothelial antigens: key determinants of vascular immunotargeting. Am J Physiol Lung Cell Mol Physiol 280(6):L1335–L1347

Davda JP, Dodds MG, Gibbs MA, Wisdom W, Gibbs J (2014) A model-based meta-analysis of monoclonal antibody pharmacokinetics to guide optimal first-in-human study design. MAbs 6(4):1094–1102. https://doi.org/10.4161/mabs.29095

Davis JD, Bansal A, Hassman D, Akinlade B, Li M, Li Z, Swanson B, Hamilton JD, DiCioccio AT (2018) Evaluation of potential disease-mediated drug-drug interaction in patients with moderate-to-severe atopic dermatitis receiving dupilumab. Clin Pharmacol Ther. https://doi.org/10.1002/cpt.1058

Dedrick RL (1973) Animal scale-up. J Pharmacokinet Biopharm 1(5):435–461

Deng R, Iyer S, Theil FP, Mortensen DL, Fielder PJ, Prabhu S (2011) Projecting human pharmacokinetics of therapeutic antibodies from nonclinical data: what have we learned? MAbs 3(1):61–66

Dias C, Abosaleem B, Crispino C, Gao B, Shaywitz A (2015a) Erratum to: tolerability of high-volume subcutaneous injections of a viscous placebo buffer: a randomized, crossover study in healthy subjects. AAPS PharmSciTech 16(6):1500. https://doi.org/10.1208/s12249-015-0324-y

Dias C, Abosaleem B, Crispino C, Gao B, Shaywitz A (2015b) Tolerability of high-volume subcutaneous injections of a viscous placebo buffer: a randomized, crossover study in healthy subjects. AAPS PharmSciTech 16(5):1101–1107. https://doi.org/10.1208/s12249-015-0288-y

Dickinson BL, Badizadegan K, Wu Z, Ahouse JC, Zhu X, Simister NE, Blumberg RS, Lencer WI (1999) Bidirectional FcRn-dependent IgG transport in a polarized human intestinal epithelial cell line. J Clin Invest 104(7):903–911

Dirks NL, Meibohm B (2010) Population pharmacokinetics of therapeutic monoclonal antibodies. Clin Pharmacokinet 49(10):633–659. https://doi.org/10.2165/11535960-000000000-00000

Dong JQ, Salinger DH, Endres CJ, Gibbs JP, Hsu CP, Stouch BJ, Hurh E, Gibbs MA (2011) Quantitative prediction of human pharmacokinetics for monoclonal antibodies: retrospective analysis of monkey as a single species for first-in-human prediction. Clin Pharmacokinet 50(2):131–142. https://doi.org/10.2165/11537430-000000000-00000

Dostalek M, Prueksaritanont T, Kelley RF (2017) Pharmacokinetic de-risking tools for selection of monoclonal antibody lead candidates. MAbs 9(5):756–766. https://doi.org/10.1080/19420862.2017.1323160

Dowell JA, Korth-Bradley J, Liu H, King SP, Berger MS (2001) Pharmacokinetics of gemtuzumab ozogamicin, an antibody-targeted chemotherapy agent for the treatment of patients with acute myeloid leukemia in first relapse. J Clin Pharmacol 41(11):1206–1214

Druet P, Bariety J, Laliberte F, Bellon B, Belair MF, Paing M (1978) Distribution of heterologous antiperoxidase antibodies and their fragments in the superficial renal cortex of normal Wistar-Munich rat: an ultrastructural study. Lab Investig 39(6):623–631

Duconge J, Castillo R, Crombet T, Alvarez D, Matheu J, Vecino G, Alonso K, Beausoleil I, Valenzuela C, Becquer MA, Fernandez-Sanchez E (2004) Integrated pharmacokinetic-pharmacodynamic modeling and allometric scaling for optimizing the dosage regimen of the monoclonal ior EGF/r3 antibody. Eur J Pharm Sci 21(2-3):261–270

Fasanmade AA, Adedokun OJ, Ford J, Hernandez D, Johanns J, Hu C, Davis HM, Zhou H (2009) Population pharmacokinetic analysis of infliximab in patients with ulcerative colitis. Eur J Clin Pharmacol 65(12):1211–1228. https://doi.org/10.1007/s00228-009-0718-4

Fasanmade AA, Adedokun OJ, Olson A, Strauss R, Davis HM (2010) Serum albumin concentration: a predictive factor of infliximab pharmacokinetics and clinical response in patients with ulcerative colitis. Int J Clin Pharmacol Ther 48(5):297–308

FDA (1999) Guidance for industry: population pharmacokinetics

Ferl GZ, Wu AM, DiStefano JJ (2005) A predictive model of therapeutic monoclonal antibody dynamics and regulation by the neonatal Fc receptor (FcRn). Ann Biomed Eng 33(11):1640–1652

Frost GI (2007) Recombinant human hyaluronidase (rHuPH20): an enabling platform for subcutaneous drug and fluid administration. Expert Opin Drug Deliv 4(4):427–440. https://doi.org/10.1517/17425247.4.4.427

Garg A, Quartino A, Li J, Jin J, Wada DR, Li H, Cortes J, McNally V, Ross G, Visich J, Lum B (2014) Population pharmacokinetic and covariate analysis of pertuzumab, a HER2-targeted monoclonal antibody, and evaluation of a fixed, non-weight-based dose in patients with a variety of solid tumors. Cancer Chemother Pharmacol 74(4):819–829. https://doi.org/10.1007/s00280-014-2560-3

Genovese MC, Cohen S, Moreland L, Lium D, Robbins S, Newmark R, Bekker P, Study G (2004) Combination therapy with etanercept and anakinra in the treatment of patients with rheumatoid arthritis who have been treated unsuccessfully with methotrexate. Arthritis Rheum 50(5):1412–1419. https://doi.org/10.1002/art.20221

Ghetie V, Hubbard JG, Kim JK, Tsen MF, Lee Y, Ward ES (1996) Abnormally short serum half-lives of IgG in beta 2-microglobulin-deficient mice. Eur J Immunol 26(3):690–696

Gibiansky L, Frey N (2012) Linking interleukin-6 receptor blockade with tocilizumab and its hematological effects using a modeling approach. J Pharmacokinet Pharmacodyn 39(1):5–16. https://doi.org/10.1007/s10928-011-9227-z

Gibiansky L, Gibiansky E (2009) Target-mediated drug disposition model: relationships with indirect response models and application to population PK-PD analysis. J Pharmacokinet Pharmacodyn 36(4):341–351. https://doi.org/10.1007/s10928-009-9125-9

Gibiansky L, Sutjandra L, Doshi S, Zheng J, Sohn W, Peterson MC, Jang GR, Chow AT, Perez-Ruixo JJ (2012) Population pharmacokinetic analysis of denosumab in patients with bone metastases from solid tumours. Clin Pharmacokinet 51(4):247–260. https://doi.org/10.2165/11598090-000000000-00000

Gillies SD, Lan Y, Lo KM, Super M, Wesolowski J (1999) Improving the efficacy of antibody-interleukin 2 fusion proteins by reducing their interaction with Fc receptors. Cancer Res 59(9):2159–2166

Gillies SD, Lo KM, Burger C, Lan Y, Dahl T, Wong WK (2002) Improved circulating half-life and efficacy of an antibody-interleukin 2 immunocytokine based on reduced intracellular proteolysis. Clin Cancer Res 8(1):210–216

Girish G, Li C (2015) Clinical pharmacology and assay consideration for characterizing pharmacokinetics and understanding efficacy and safety of antibody-drug conjugates. In: Gorovits B, Shord S (eds) Novel methods in bioanalysis and characterization of antibody-drug conjugate. Future Science Ltd, London, pp 36–55

Girish S, Martin SW, Peterson MC et al (2011) AAPS workshop report: strategies to address therapeutic protein–drug interactions during clinical development. APPS J 3:405–416

Goldsby RA, Kindt TJ, Osborine BA, Kuby J (1999) Immunology, 4th edn. W.H. Freeman and Company, New York

Gottlieb AB, Miller B, Lowe N, Shapiro W, Hudson C, Bright R, Ling M, Magee A, McCall CO, Rist T, Dummer W, Walicke P, Bauer RJ, White M, Garovoy M (2003) Subcutaneously administered efalizumab (anti-CD11a) improves signs and symptoms of moderate to severe plaque psoriasis. J Cutan Med Surg 7(3):198–207

Han K, Jin J, Maia M, Lowe J, Sersch MA, Allison DE (2014) Lower exposure and faster clearance of bevacizumab in gastric cancer and the impact of patient variables: analysis of individual data from AVAGAST phase III trial. AAPS J 16(5):1056–1063. https://doi.org/10.1208/s12248-014-9631-6

Hayashi N, Tsukamoto Y, Sallas WM, Lowe PJ (2007) A mechanism-based binding model for the population pharmacokinetics and pharmacodynamics of omalizumab. Br J Clin Pharmacol 63(5):548–561. https://doi.org/10.1111/j.1365-2125.2006.02803.x

Herceptin (Trastuzumab) Prescribing Information (2006) South San Francisco, CA, USA

Hervey PS, Keam SJ (2006) Abatacept. BioDrugs 20(1):53–61

Hinton PR, Xiong JM, Johlfs MG, Tang MT, Keller S, Tsurushita N (2006) An engineered human IgG1 antibody with longer serum half-life. J Immunol 176(1):346–356

Hochhaus G, Brookman L, Fox H, Johnson C, Matthews J, Ren S, Deniz Y (2003) Pharmacodynamics of omalizumab: implications for optimised dosing strategies and clinical efficacy in the treatment of allergic asthma. Curr Med Res Opin 19(6):491–498. https://doi.org/10.1185/030079903125002171

Holmes D (2011) Buy buy bispecific antibodies. Nat Rev Drug Discov 10(11):798–800. https://doi.org/10.1038/nrd3581

Honma W, Gautier A, Paule I, Yamaguchi M, Lowe PJ (2016) Ethnic sensitivity assessment of pharmacokinetics and pharmacodynamics of omalizumab with dosing table expansion. Drug Metab Pharmacokinet 31(3):173–184. https://doi.org/10.1016/j.dmpk.2015.12.003

Hooks MA, Wade CS, Millikan WJ Jr (1991) Muromonab CD-3: a review of its pharmacology, pharmacokinetics, and clinical use in transplantation. Pharmacotherapy 11(1):26–37

Huang SM, Zhao H, Lee JI, Reynolds K, Zhang L, Temple R, Lesko LJ (2010) Therapeutic protein-drug interactions and implications for drug development. Clin Pharmacol Ther 87(4):497–503. https://doi.org/10.1038/clpt.2009.308

Humira (Adalimumab) Prescribing Information (2007) Chicago, IL, USA

ICH (1997a) ICH harmonized tripartite guideline M3: nonclinical safety studies for the conduct of human clinical trials for pharmaceuticals

ICH (1997b) ICH harmonized tripartite guideline S6: preclinical safety evaluation of biotechnology-derived pharmaceuticals

Igawa T, Tsunoda H, Tachibana T, Maeda A, Mimoto F, Moriyama C, Nanami M, Sekimori Y, Nabuchi Y, Aso Y, Hattori K (2010) Reduced elimination of IgG antibodies by engineering the variable region. Protein Eng Des Sel 23(5):385–392. https://doi.org/10.1093/protein/gzq009

Jolling K, Perez Ruixo JJ, Hemeryck A, Vermeulen A, Greway T (2005) Mixed-effects modelling of the interspecies pharmacokinetic scaling of pegylated human erythropoietin. Eur J Pharm Sci 24(5):465–475

Joshi A, Bauer R, Kuebler P, White M, Leddy C, Compton P, Garovoy M, Kwon P, Walicke P, Dedrick R (2006) An overview of the pharmacokinetics and pharmacodynamics of efalizumab: a monoclonal antibody approved for use in psoriasis. J Clin Pharmacol 46(1):10–20

Junghans RP (1997) Finally! The Brambell receptor (FcRB). Mediator of transmission of immunity and protection from catabolism for IgG. Immunol Res 16(1):29–57

Junghans RP, Anderson CL (1996) The protection receptor for IgG catabolism is the beta2-microglobulin-containing neonatal intestinal transport receptor. Proc Natl Acad Sci U S A 93(11):5512–5516

Kagan L, Abraham AK, Harrold JM, Mager DE (2010) Interspecies scaling of receptor-mediated pharmacokinetics and pharmacodynamics of type I interferons. Pharm Res 27(5):920–932. https://doi.org/10.1007/s11095-010-0098-6

Kagedal M, Gibiansky L, Xu J, Wang X, Samineni D, Chen SC, Lu D, Agarwal P, Wang B, Saad O, Koppada N, Fine BM, Jin JY, Girish S, Li C (2017) Platform model describing pharmacokinetic properties of vc-MMAE antibody-drug conjugates. J Pharmacokinet Pharmacodyn 44(6):537–548. https://doi.org/10.1007/s10928-017-9544-y

Kairemo KJ, Lappalainen AK, Kaapa E, Laitinen OM, Hyytinen T, Karonen SL, Gronblad M (2001) In vivo detection of intervertebral disk injury using a radiolabeled monoclonal antibody against keratan sulfate. J Nucl Med 42(3):476–482

Kamath AV (2016) Translational pharmacokinetics and pharmacodynamics of monoclonal antibodies. Drug Discov Today Technol 21-22:75–83. https://doi.org/10.1016/j.ddtec.2016.09.004

Kang YK, Ryu MH, Yoo C, Ryoo BY, Kim HJ, Lee JJ, Nam BH, Ramaiya N, Jagannathan J, Demetri GD (2013) Resumption of imatinib to control metastatic or unresectable gastrointestinal stromal tumours after failure of imatinib and sunitinib (RIGHT): a randomised, placebo-controlled, phase 3 trial. Lancet Oncol 14(12):1175–1182. https://doi.org/10.1016/S1470-2045(13)70453-4

Kelley SK, Gelzleichter T, Xie D, Lee WP, Darbonne WC, Qureshi F, Kissler K, Oflazoglu E, Grewal IS (2006) Preclinical pharmacokinetics, pharmacodynamics, and activity of a humanized anti-CD40 antibody (SGN-40) in rodents and non-human primates. Br J Pharmacol 148(8):1116–1123

Kenny JR, Liu MM, Chow AT, Earp JC, Evers R, Slatter JG, Wang DD, Zhang L, Zhou H (2013) Therapeutic protein drug-drug interactions: navigating the knowledge gaps-highlights from the 2012 AAPS NBC roundtable and IQ consortium/FDA workshop. AAPS J 15(4):933–940. https://doi.org/10.1208/s12248-013-9495-1

Khawli LA, Goswami S, Hutchinson R, Kwong ZW, Yang J, Wang X, Yao Z, Sreedhara A, Cano T, Tesar D, Nijem I, Allison DE, Wong PY, Kao YH, Quan C, Joshi A, Harris RJ, Motchnik P (2010) Charge variants in IgG1: isolation, characterization, in vitro binding properties and pharmacokinetics in rats. MAbs 2(6):613–624. https://doi.org/10.4161/mabs.2.6.13333

Kirschbrown WP, Quartino AL, Li H, Mangat R, Wada DR, Garg A, Jin JY, Lum BL (2017) Development of a population pharmacokinetic (PPK) model of intravenous (IV) trastuzumab in patients with a variety of solid tumors to support dosing and treatment recommendations. J Clin Oncol 35(Suppl):2525

Kleiman NS, Raizner AE, Jordan R, Wang AL, Norton D, Mace KF, Joshi A, Coller BS, Weisman HF (1995) Differential inhibition of platelet aggregation induced by adenosine diphosphate or a thrombin receptor-activating peptide in patients treated with bolus chimeric 7E3 Fab: implications for inhibition of the internal pool of GPIIb/IIIa receptors. J Am Coll Cardiol 26(7):1665–1671. https://doi.org/10.1016/0735-1097(95)00391-6

Kohler G, Milstein C (1975) Continuous cultures of fused cells secreting antibody of predefined specificity. Nature 256(5517):495–497

Kolar GR, Capra JD (2003) Immunoglobulins: structure and function. In: Paul WE (ed) Fundamental immunology, 5th edn. Lippincott Williams & Wilkins, Philadelphia

Koon HB, Severy P, Hagg DS, Butler K, Hill T, Jones AG, Waldmann TA, Junghans RP (2006) Antileukemic effect of daclizumab in CD25 high-expressing leukemias and impact of tumor burden on antibody dosing. Leuk Res 30(2):190–203

Kovalenko P, DiCioccio AT, Davis JD, Li M, Ardeleanu M, Graham N, Soltys R (2016) Exploratory population PK analysis of dupilumab, a fully human monoclonal antibody against IL-4ralpha, in atopic dermatitis patients and normal volunteers. CPT Pharmacometrics Syst Pharmacol 5(11):617–624. https://doi.org/10.1002/psp4.12136

Kovarik JM, Nashan B, Neuhaus P, Clavien PA, Gerbeau C, Hall ML, Korn A (2001) A population pharmacokinetic screen to identify demographic-clinical covariates of basiliximab in liver transplantation. Clin Pharmacol Ther 69(4):201–209

Krueger JG (2002) The immunologic basis for the treatment of psoriasis with new biologic agents. J Am Acad Dermatol 46(1):1–23

Kuus-Reichel K, Grauer LS, Karavodin LM, Knott C, Krusemeier M, Kay NE (1994) Will immunogenicity limit the use, efficacy, and future development of therapeutic monoclonal antibodies? Clin Diagn Lab Immunol 1(4):365–372

Lee H, Kimko HC, Rogge M, Wang D, Nestorov I, Peck CC (2003) Population pharmacokinetic and pharmacodynamic modeling of etanercept using logistic regression analysis. Clin Pharmacol Ther 73(4):348–365

Lee JI, Zhang L, Men AY, Kenna LA, Huang SM (2010) CYP-mediated therapeutic protein-drug interactions: clinical findings, proposed mechanisms and regulatory implications. Clin Pharmacokinet 49(5):295–310. https://doi.org/10.2165/11319980-000000000-00000

Li B, Tesar D, Boswell CA, Cahaya HS, Wong A, Zhang J, Meng YG, Eigenbrot C, Pantua H, Diao J, Kapadia SB, Deng R, Kelley RF (2014) Framework selection can influence pharmacokinetics of a humanized therapeutic

antibody through differences in molecule charge. MAbs 6(5):1255–1264. https://doi.org/10.4161/mabs.29809
Li H, Yu J, Liu C, Liu J, Subramaniam S, Zhao H, Blumenthal GM, Turner DC, Li C, Ahamadi M, de Greef R, Chatterjee M, Kondic AG, Stone JA, Booth BP, Keegan P, Rahman A, Wang Y (2017) Time dependent pharmacokinetics of pembrolizumab in patients with solid tumor and its correlation with best overall response. J Pharmacokinet Pharmacodyn 44(5):403–414. https://doi.org/10.1007/s10928-017-9528-y
Lin YS, Nguyen C, Mendoza JL, Escandon E, Fei D, Meng YG, Modi NB (1999) Preclinical pharmacokinetics, interspecies scaling, and tissue distribution of a humanized monoclonal antibody against vascular endothelial growth factor. J Pharmacol Exp Ther 288(1):371–378
Ling J, Zhou H, Jiao Q, Davis HM (2009) Interspecies scaling of therapeutic monoclonal antibodies: initial look. J Clin Pharmacol 49(12):1382–1402. https://doi.org/10.1177/0091270009337134
Liu J, Wang Y, Zhao L (2015) Assessment of exposure-response (E-R) and cse-control (C-C) analyses in oncology using simulation based approach. In: Am Conf. Pharmacometrics Ann Meeting
Lobo ED, Hansen RJ, Balthasar JP (2004) Antibody pharmacokinetics and pharmacodynamics. J Pharm Sci 93(11):2645–2668
Looney RJ, Anolik JH, Campbell D, Felgar RE, Young F, Arend LJ, Sloand JA, Rosenblatt J, Sanz I (2004) B cell depletion as a novel treatment for systemic lupus erythematosus: a phase I/II dose-escalation trial of rituximab. Arthritis Rheum 50(8):2580–2589
LoRusso PM, Weiss D, Guardino E, Girish S, Sliwkowski MX (2011) Trastuzumab emtansine: a unique antibody-drug conjugate in development for human epidermal growth factor receptor 2-positive cancer. Clin Cancer Res 17(20):6437–6447. https://doi.org/10.1158/1078-0432.CCR-11-0762
Lowe PJ, Georgiou P, Canvin J (2015) Revision of omalizumab dosing table for dosing every 4 instead of 2 weeks for specific ranges of bodyweight and baseline IgE. Regul Toxicol Pharmacol 71(1):68–77. https://doi.org/10.1016/j.yrtph.2014.12.002
Lu D, Burris HA, Wang B, Dees EC, Cortes J, Joshi A, Gupta M, Yi JH, Chu YW, Shih T, Fang L, Girish S (2012) Drug interaction potential of trastuzumab emtansine (T-DM1) combined with pertuzumab in patients with HER2-positive metastatic breast cancer. Curr Drug Metab 13(7):911–922
Lu D, Girish S, Gao Y, Wang B, Yi JH, Guardino E, Samant M, Cobleigh M, Rimawi M, Conte P, Jin JY (2014) Population pharmacokinetics of trastuzumab emtansine (T-DM1), a HER2-targeted antibody-drug conjugate, in patients with HER2-positive metastatic breast cancer: clinical implications of the effect of covariates. Cancer Chemother Pharmacol 74(2):399–410. https://doi.org/10.1007/s00280-014-2500-2
Ma P, Yang BB, Wang YM, Peterson M, Narayanan A, Sutjandra L, Rodriguez R, Chow A (2009) Population pharmacokinetic analysis of panitumumab in patients with advanced solid tumors. J Clin Pharmacol 49(10):1142–1156. https://doi.org/10.1177/0091270009344989
Mager DE, Mascelli MA, Kleiman NS, Fitzgerald DJ, Abernethy DR (2003) Simultaneous modeling of abciximab plasma concentrations and ex vivo pharmacodynamics in patients undergoing coronary angioplasty. J Pharmacol Exp Ther 307(3):969–976. https://doi.org/10.1124/jpet.103.057299
Mager DE, Woo S, Jusko WJ (2009) Scaling pharmacodynamics from in vitro and preclinical animal studies to humans. Drug Metab Pharmacokinet 24(1):16–24
Mahmood I (2005) Prediction of concentration-time profiles in humans. Pine House Publisher, Rockville
Mahmood I (2009) Pharmacokinetic allometric scaling of antibodies: application to the first-in-human dose estimation. J Pharm Sci 98(10):3850–3861. https://doi.org/10.1002/jps.21682
Mahmood I, Green MD (2005) Pharmacokinetic and pharmacodynamic considerations in the development of therapeutic proteins. Clin Pharmacokinet 44(4):331–347
Maini RN, Breedveld FC, Kalden JR, Smolen JS, Davis D, Macfarlane JD, Antoni C, Leeb B, Elliott MJ, Woody JN, Schaible TF, Feldmann M (1998) Therapeutic efficacy of multiple intravenous infusions of anti-tumor necrosis factor alpha monoclonal antibody combined with low-dose weekly methotrexate in rheumatoid arthritis. Arthritis Rheum 41(9):1552–1563. https://doi.org/10.1002/1529-0131(199809)41:9<1552::AID-ART5>3.0.CO;2-W
Mandikian D, Takahashi N, Lo AA, Li J, Eastham-Anderson J, Slaga D, Ho J, Hristopoulos M, Clark R, Totpal K, Lin K, Joseph SB, Dennis MS, Prabhu S, Junttila TT, Boswell CA (2018) Relative target affinities of T-cell-dependent bispecific antibodies determine biodistribution in a solid tumor mouse model. Mol Cancer Ther 17(4):776–785. https://doi.org/10.1158/1535-7163.MCT-17-0657
Martin-Jimenez T, Riviere JE (2002) Mixed-effects modeling of the interspecies pharmacokinetic scaling of oxytetracycline. J Pharm Sci 91(2):331–341
McClurkan MB, Valentine JL, Arnold L, Owens SM (1993) Disposition of a monoclonal anti-phencyclidine Fab fragment of immunoglobulin G in rats. J Pharmacol Exp Ther 266(3):1439–1445
McLaughlin P, Grillo-Lopez AJ, Link BK, Levy R, Czuczman MS, Williams ME, Heyman MR, Bence-Bruckler I, White CA, Cabanillas F, Jain V, Ho AD, Lister J, Wey K, Shen D, Dallaire BK (1998) Rituximab chimeric anti-CD20 monoclonal antibody therapy for relapsed indolent lymphoma: half of patients respond to a four-dose treatment program. J Clin Oncol 16(8):2825–2833
Medesan C, Matesoi D, Radu C, Ghetie V, Ward ES (1997) Delineation of the amino acid residues involved in transcytosis and catabolism of mouse IgG1. J Immunol 158(5):2211–2217
Meibohm B, Derendorf H (2002) Pharmacokinetic/pharmacodynamic studies in drug product development. J Pharm Sci 91(1):18–31
Meijer RT, Koopmans RP, ten Berge IJ, Schellekens PT (2002) Pharmacokinetics of murine anti-human CD3

antibodies in man are determined by the disappearance of target antigen. J Pharmacol Exp Ther 300(1): 346–353

Meredith PA, Elliott HL, Donnelly R, Reid JL (1991) Dose-response clarification in early drug development. J Hypertens Suppl 9(6):S356–S357

Morris EC, Rebello P, Thomson KJ, Peggs KS, Kyriakou C, Goldstone AH, Mackinnon S, Hale G (2003) Pharmacokinetics of alemtuzumab used for in vivo and in vitro T-cell depletion in allogeneic transplantations: relevance for early adoptive immunotherapy and infectious complications. Blood 102(1):404–406. https://doi.org/10.1182/blood-2002-09-2687

Mortensen DL, Walicke PA, Wang X, Kwon P, Kuebler P, Gottlieb AB, Krueger JG, Leonardi C, Miller B, Joshi A (2005) Pharmacokinetics and pharmacodynamics of multiple weekly subcutaneous efalizumab doses in patients with plaque psoriasis. J Clin Pharmacol 45(3):286–298

Mould DR, Sweeney KR (2007) The pharmacokinetics and pharmacodynamics of monoclonal antibodies--mechanistic modeling applied to drug development. Curr Opin Drug Discov Devel 10(1):84–96

Mould DR, Davis CB, Minthorn EA, Kwok DC, Elliott MJ, Luggen ME, Totoritis MC (1999) A population pharmacokinetic-pharmacodynamic analysis of single doses of clenoliximab in patients with rheumatoid arthritis. Clin Pharmacol Ther 66(3):246–257

den Broeder A, van de Putte L, Rau R, Schattenkirchner M, Van Riel P, Sander O, Binder C, Fenner H, Bankmann Y, Velagapudi R, Kempeni J, Kupper H (2002) A single dose, placebo controlled study of the fully human anti-tumor necrosis factor-alpha antibody adalimumab (D2E7) in patients with rheumatoid arthritis. J Rheumatol 29(11):2288–2298

Nakakura EK, McCabe SM, Zheng B, Shorthouse RA, Scheiner TM, Blank G, Jardieu PM, Morris RE (1993) Potent and effective prolongation by anti-LFA-1 monoclonal antibody monotherapy of non-primarily vascularized heart allograft survival in mice without T cell depletion. Transplantation 55(2):412–417

Nestorov I, Zitnik R, Ludden T (2004) Population pharmacokinetic modeling of subcutaneously administered etanercept in patients with psoriasis. J Pharmacokinet Pharmacodyn 31(6):463–490

Ng CM, Joshi A, Dedrick RL, Garovoy MR, Bauer RJ (2005) Pharmacokinetic-pharmacodynamic-efficacy analysis of efalizumab in patients with moderate to severe psoriasis. Pharm Res 22(7):1088–1100

Ng CM, Stefanich E, Anand BS, Fielder PJ, Vaickus L (2006) Pharmacokinetics/pharmacodynamics of nondepleting anti-CD4 monoclonal antibody (TRX1) in healthy human volunteers. Pharm Res 23(1):95–103

Norman DJ, Chatenoud L, Cohen D, Goldman M, Shield CF 3rd (1993) Consensus statement regarding OKT3-induced cytokine-release syndrome and human antimouse antibodies. Transplant Proc 25(2 Suppl 1):89–92

Ober RJ, Radu CG, Ghetie V, Ward ES (2001) Differences in promiscuity for antibody-FcRn interactions across species: implications for therapeutic antibodies. Int Immunol 13(12):1551–1559

Oitate M, Masubuchi N, Ito T, Yabe Y, Karibe T, Aoki T, Murayama N, Kurihara A, Okudaira N, Izumi T (2011) Prediction of human pharmacokinetics of therapeutic monoclonal antibodies from simple allometry of monkey data. Drug Metab Pharmacokinet 26(4): 423–430

Page MM, Watts GF (2015) Evolocumab in the treatment of dyslipidemia: pre-clinical and clinical pharmacology. Expert Opin Drug Metab Toxicol 11(9):1505–1515. https://doi.org/10.1517/17425255.2015.1073712

Papp K, Bissonnette R, Krueger JG, Carey W, Gratton D, Gulliver WP, Lui H, Lynde CW, Magee A, Minier D, Ouellet JP, Patel P, Shapiro J, Shear NH, Kramer S, Walicke P, Bauer R, Dedrick RL, Kim SS, White M, Garovoy MR (2001) The treatment of moderate to severe psoriasis with a new anti-CD11a monoclonal antibody. J Am Acad Dermatol 45(5):665–674

Petkova SB, Akilesh S, Sproule TJ, Christianson GJ, Al Khabbaz H, Brown AC, Presta LG, Meng YG, Roopenian DC (2006) Enhanced half-life of genetically engineered human IgG1 antibodies in a humanized FcRn mouse model: potential application in humorally mediated autoimmune disease. Int Immunol 18(12):1759–1769

Prabhu S, Boswell CA, Leipold D, Khawli LA, Li D, Lu D, Theil FP, Joshi A, Lum BL (2011) Antibody delivery of drugs and radionuclides: factors influencing clinical pharmacology. Ther Deliv 2(6):769–791

Presta LG (2002) Engineering antibodies for therapy. Curr Pharm Biotechnol 3(3):237–256

Presta LG, Shields RL, Namenuk AK, Hong K, Meng YG (2002) Engineering therapeutic antibodies for improved function. Biochem Soc Trans 30(4):487–490

Putnam WS, Prabhu S, Zheng Y, Subramanyam M, Wang YM (2010) Pharmacokinetic, pharmacodynamic and immunogenicity comparability assessment strategies for monoclonal antibodies. Trends Biotechnol 28(10):509–516. https://doi.org/10.1016/j.tibtech.2010.07.001

Raptiva (Efalizumab) [Prescribing Information] (2004) South San Francisco, Calif: Genentech, Inc

Roopenian DC, Christianson GJ, Sproule TJ, Brown AC, Akilesh S, Jung N, Petkova S, Avanessian L, Choi EY, Shaffer DJ, Eden PA, Anderson CL (2003) The MHC class I-like IgG receptor controls perinatal IgG transport, IgG homeostasis, and fate of IgG-Fc-coupled drugs. J Immunol 170(7):3528–3533

Roskos LK, Davis CG, Schwab GM (2004) The clinical pharmacology of therapeutic monoclonal antibodies. Drug Dev Res 61:108–120

Ryman JT, Meibohm B (2017) Pharmacokinetics of monoclonal antibodies. CPT Pharmacometrics Syst Pharmacol 6(9):576–588. https://doi.org/10.1002/psp4.12224

Sampei Z, Igawa T, Soeda T, Okuyama-Nishida Y, Moriyama C, Wakabayashi T, Tanaka E, Muto A, Kojima T, Kitazawa T, Yoshihashi K, Harada A, Funaki M, Haraya K, Tachibana T, Suzuki S, Esaki K, Nabuchi Y, Hattori K (2013) Identification and multidimensional optimization of an asymmetric bispecific IgG antibody

mimicking the function of factor VIII cofactor activity. PLoS One 8(2):e57479. https://doi.org/10.1371/journal.pone.0057479
Schmitt C, Kuhn B, Zhang X, Kivitz AJ, Grange S (2011) Disease-drug-drug interaction involving tocilizumab and simvastatin in patients with rheumatoid arthritis. Clin Pharmacol Ther 89(5):735–740. https://doi.org/10.1038/clpt.2011.35
Schror K, Weber AA (2003) Comparative pharmacology of GP IIb/IIIa antagonists. J Thromb Thrombolysis 15(2):71–80
Shah DK, Betts AM (2012) Towards a platform PBPK model to characterize the plasma and tissue disposition of monoclonal antibodies in preclinical species and human. J Pharmacokinet Pharmacodyn 39(1):67–86. https://doi.org/10.1007/s10928-011-9232-2
Sheiner LB (1997) Learning versus confirming in clinical drug development. Clin Pharmacol Ther 61(3):275–291
Sheiner L, Wakefield J (1999) Population modelling in drug development. Stat Methods Med Res 8(3):183–193
Shields RL, Namenuk AK, Hong K, Meng YG, Rae J, Briggs J, Xie D, Lai J, Stadlen A, Li B, Fox JA, Presta LG (2001) High resolution mapping of the binding site on human IgG1 for Fc gamma RI, Fc gamma RII, Fc gamma RIII, and FcRn and design of IgG1 variants with improved binding to the Fc gamma R. J Biol Chem 276(9):6591–6604
Sifontis NM, Benedetti E, Vasquez EM (2002) Clinically significant drug interaction between basiliximab and tacrolimus in renal transplant recipients. Transplant Proc 34(5):1730–1732
Simister NE, Mostov KE (1989a) Cloning and expression of the neonatal rat intestinal Fc receptor, a major histocompatibility complex class I antigen homolog. Cold Spring Harb Symp Quant Biol 54(Pt 1):571–580
Simister NE, Mostov KE (1989b) An Fc receptor structurally related to MHC class I antigens. Nature 337(6203):184–187
Simulect (Basiliximab) Prescribing Information (2005) East Hanover, NJ, USA
Slatter JG, Wienkers LC, Dickmann LC (2013) Drug interactions of cytokines and anticytokine therapeutic proteins. Drug-drug interactions for therapeutics biologics. Wiley, Hoboken
Spiekermann GM, Finn PW, Ward ES, Dumont J, Dickinson BL, Blumberg RS, Lencer WI (2002) Receptor-mediated immunoglobulin G transport across mucosal barriers in adult life: functional expression of FcRn in the mammalian lung. J Exp Med 196(3):303–310
Straughn JM, Oliver PG, Zhou T, Wang W, Alvarez RD, Grizzle WE, Buchsbaum DJ (2006) Anti-tumor activity of TRA-8 anti-death receptor 5 (DR5) monoclonal antibody in combination with chemotherapy and radiation therapy in a cervical cancer model. Gynecol Oncol 101(1):46–54. https://doi.org/10.1016/j.ygyno.2005.09.053
Struemper H, Sale M, Patel BR, Ostergaard M, Osterborg A, Wierda WG, Hagenbeek A, Coiffier B, Jewell RC (2014) Population pharmacokinetics of ofatumumab in patients with chronic lymphocytic leukemia, follicular lymphoma, and rheumatoid arthritis. J Clin Pharmacol 54(7):818–827. https://doi.org/10.1002/jcph.268
Subramanian GM, Cronin PW, Poley G, Weinstein A, Stoughton SM, Zhong J, Ou Y, Zmuda JF, Osborn BL, Freimuth WW (2005) A phase 1 study of PAmAb, a fully human monoclonal antibody against Bacillus anthracis protective antigen, in healthy volunteers. Clin Infect Dis 41(1):12–20
Sun YN, Lu JF, Joshi A, Compton P, Kwon P, Bruno RA (2005) Population pharmacokinetics of efalizumab (humanized monoclonal anti-CD11a antibody) following long-term subcutaneous weekly dosing in psoriasis subjects. J Clin Pharmacol 45(4):468–476
Tabrizi MA, Tseng CM, Roskos LK (2006) Elimination mechanisms of therapeutic monoclonal antibodies. Drug Discov Today 11(1-2):81–88
Tang H, Mayersohn M (2005) Accuracy of allometrically predicted pharmacokinetic parameters in humans: role of species selection. Drug Metab Dispos 33(9):1288–1293
Tang L, Persky AM, Hochhaus G, Meibohm B (2004) Pharmacokinetic aspects of biotechnology products. J Pharm Sci 93(9):2184–2204. https://doi.org/10.1002/jps.20125
Ternant D, Paintaud G (2005) Pharmacokinetics and concentration-effect relationships of therapeutic monoclonal antibodies and fusion proteins. Expert Opin Biol Ther 5(Suppl 1):S37–S47
Thurber GM, Schmidt MM, Wittrup KD (2008) Antibody tumor penetration: transport opposed by systemic and antigen-mediated clearance. Adv Drug Deliv Rev 60(12):1421–1434. https://doi.org/10.1016/j.addr.2008.04.012
Tran JQ, Othman AA, Wolstencroft P, Elkins J (2016) Therapeutic protein-drug interaction assessment for daclizumab high-yield process in patients with multiple sclerosis using a cocktail approach. Br J Clin Pharmacol 82(1):160–167. https://doi.org/10.1111/bcp.12936
Trianni.com (2018) http://trianni.com/technology/mouse/. Accessed May 8, 2018
Umana P, Jean-Mairet J, Moudry R, Amstutz H, Bailey JE (1999) Engineered glycoforms of an antineuroblastoma IgG1 with optimized antibody-dependent cellular cytotoxic activity. Nat Biotechnol 17(2):176–180
Vaccaro C, Bawdon R, Wanjie S, Ober RJ, Ward ES (2006) Divergent activities of an engineered antibody in murine and human systems have implications for therapeutic antibodies. Proc Natl Acad Sci U S A 103(49):18709–18714
Vaishnaw AK, TenHoor CN (2002) Pharmacokinetics, biologic activity, and tolerability of alefacept by intravenous and intramuscular administration. J Pharmacokinet Pharmacodyn 29(5-6):415–426
Vasquez EM, Pollak R (1997) OKT3 therapy increases cyclosporine blood levels. Clin Transpl 11(1):38–41
Vectibix (Panitumumab) Prescribing Information (2015) Thousand Oaks, CA, USA
Vincenti F, Mendez R, Pescovitz M, Rajagopalan PR, Wilkinson AH, Butt K, Laskow D, Slakey DP, Lorber MI, Garg JP, Garovoy M (2007) A phase I/II

randomized open-label multicenter trial of efalizumab, a humanized anti-CD11a, anti-LFA-1 in renal transplantation. Am J Transplant 7(7):1770–1777. https://doi.org/10.1111/j.1600-6143.2007.01845.x

Vugmeyster Y, Guay H, Szklut P, Qian MD, Jin M, Widom A, Spaulding V, Bennett F, Lowe L, Andreyeva T, Lowe D, Lane S, Thom G, Valge-Archer V, Gill D, Young D, Bloom L (2010) In vitro potency, pharmacokinetic profiles, and pharmacological activity of optimized anti-IL-21R antibodies in a mouse model of lupus. MAbs 2(3):335–346

Vugmeyster Y, Szklut P, Wensel D, Ross J, Xu X, Awwad M, Gill D, Tchistiakov L, Warner G (2011) Complex pharmacokinetics of a humanized antibody against human amyloid beta peptide, anti-abeta Ab2, in nonclinical species. Pharm Res 28(7):1696–1706. https://doi.org/10.1007/s11095-011-0405-x

Wang Y (2016) Special considerations for modeling exposure response for biologics. In: Am Soc Clin Pharmacol and Therapeutics Ann Meeting

Wang W, Prueksaritanont T (2010) Prediction of human clearance of therapeutic proteins: simple allometric scaling method revisited. Biopharm Drug Dispos 31(4):253–263. https://doi.org/10.1002/bdd.708

Wang W, Singh S, Zeng DL, King K, Nema S (2007) Antibody structure, instability, and formulation. J Pharm Sci 96(1):1–26

Watanabe N, Kuriyama H, Sone H, Neda H, Yamauchi N, Maeda M, Niitsu Y (1988) Continuous internalization of tumor necrosis factor receptors in a human myosarcoma cell line. J Biol Chem 263(21):10262–10266

Weiner LM (2006) Fully human therapeutic monoclonal antibodies. J Immunother 29(1):1–9

Weiskopf K, Weissman IL (2015) Macrophages are critical effectors of antibody therapies for cancer. MAbs 7(2):303–310. https://doi.org/10.1080/19420862.2015.1011450

Weisman MH, Moreland LW, Furst DE, Weinblatt ME, Keystone EC, Paulus HE, Teoh LS, Velagapudi RB, Noertersheuser PA, Granneman GR, Fischkoff SA, Chartash EK (2003) Efficacy, pharmacokinetic, and safety assessment of adalimumab, a fully human anti-tumor necrosis factor-alpha monoclonal antibody, in adults with rheumatoid arthritis receiving concomitant methotrexate: a pilot study. Clin Ther 25(6):1700–1721

Werther WA, Gonzalez TN, O'Connor SJ, McCabe S, Chan B, Hotaling T, Champe M, Fox JA, Jardieu PM, Berman PW, Presta LG (1996) Humanization of an anti-lymphocyte function-associated antigen (LFA)-1 monoclonal antibody and reengineering of the humanized antibody for binding to rhesus LFA-1. J Immunol 157(11):4986–4995

Wiseman GA, White CA, Sparks RB, Erwin WD, Podoloff DA, Lamonica D, Bartlett NL, Parker JA, Dunn WL, Spies SM, Belanger R, Witzig TE, Leigh BR (2001) Biodistribution and dosimetry results from a phase III prospectively randomized controlled trial of Zevalin radioimmunotherapy for low-grade, follicular, or transformed B-cell non-Hodgkin's lymphoma. Crit Rev Oncol Hematol 39(1-2):181–194

Wu H, Pfarr DS, Johnson S, Brewah YA, Woods RM, Patel NK, White WI, Young JF, Kiener PA (2007) Development of motavizumab, an ultra-potent antibody for the prevention of respiratory syncytial virus infection in the upper and lower respiratory tract. J Mol Biol 368(3):652–665. https://doi.org/10.1016/j.jmb.2007.02.024

Wurster U, Haas J (1994) Passage of intravenous immunoglobulin and interaction with the CNS. J Neurol Neurosurg Psychiatry 57(Suppl):21–25

Xolair (Omalizumab) Prescribing Information (2006) South San Francisco, CA, USA & East Hanover, NJ, USA

Yadav DB, Maloney JA, Wildsmith KR, Fuji RN, Meilandt WJ, Solanoy H, Lu Y, Peng K, Wilson B, Chan P, Gadkar K, Kosky A, Goo M, Daugherty A, Couch JA, Keene T, Hayes K, Nikolas LJ, Lane D, Switzer R, Adams E, Watts RJ, Scearce-Levie K, Prabhu S, Shafer L, Thakker DR, Hildebrand K, Atwal JK (2017) Widespread brain distribution and activity following i.c.v. infusion of anti-beta-secretase (BACE1) in nonhuman primates. Br J Pharmacol 174(22):4173–4185. https://doi.org/10.1111/bph.14021

Yang J, Zhao H, Garnett C, Rahman A, Gobburu JV, Pierce W, Schechter G, Summers J, Keegan P, Booth B, Wang Y (2013) The combination of exposure-response and case-control analyses in regulatory decision making. J Clin Pharmacol 53(2):160–166. https://doi.org/10.1177/0091270012445206

Yim DS, Zhou H, Buckwalter M, Nestorov I, Peck CC, Lee H (2005) Population pharmacokinetic analysis and simulation of the time-concentration profile of etanercept in pediatric patients with juvenile rheumatoid arthritis. J Clin Pharmacol 45(3):246–256. https://doi.org/10.1177/0091270004271945

Yip V, Palma E, Tesar DB, Mundo EE, Bumbaca D, Torres EK, Reyes NA, Shen BQ, Fielder PJ, Prabhu S, Khawli LA, Boswell CA (2014) Quantitative cumulative biodistribution of antibodies in mice: effect of modulating binding affinity to the neonatal Fc receptor. MAbs 6(3):689–696. https://doi.org/10.4161/mabs.28254

Younes A, Bartlett NL, Leonard JP, Kennedy DA, Lynch CM, Sievers EL, Forero-Torres A (2010) Brentuximab vedotin (SGN-35) for relapsed CD30-positive lymphomas. N Engl J Med 363(19):1812–1821. https://doi.org/10.1056/NEJMoa1002965

Yu YJ, Atwal JK, Zhang Y, Tong RK, Wildsmith KR, Tan C, Bien-Ly N, Hersom M, Maloney JA, Meilandt WJ, Bumbaca D, Gadkar K, Hoyte K, Luk W, Lu Y, Ernst JA, Scearce-Levie K, Couch JA, Dennis MS, Watts RJ (2014) Therapeutic bispecific antibodies cross the blood-brain barrier in nonhuman primates. Sci Transl Med 6(261):261ra154. https://doi.org/10.1126/scitranslmed.3009835

Zenapax (Daclizumab) Prescribing Information (2005) Nutley, NJ, USA

Zheng Y, Scheerens H, Davis JC Jr, Deng R, Fischer SK, Woods C, Fielder PJ, Stefanich EG (2011) Translational pharmacokinetics and pharmacodynamics of an FcRn-variant anti-CD4 monoclonal antibody from preclinical model to phase I study. Clin Pharmacol Ther 89(2):283–290. https://doi.org/10.1038/clpt.2010.311

Zhou H (2005) Clinical pharmacokinetics of etanercept: a fully humanized soluble recombinant tumor necrosis factor receptor fusion protein. J Clin Pharmacol 45(5):490–497

Zhou H, Mayer PR, Wajdula J, Fatenejad S (2004) Unaltered etanercept pharmacokinetics with concurrent methotrexate in patients with rheumatoid arthritis. J Clin Pharmacol 44(11):1235–1243. https://doi.org/10.1177/0091270004268049

Zhu Y, Hu C, Lu M, Liao S, Marini JC, Yohrling J, Yeilding N, Davis HM, Zhou H (2009) Population pharmacokinetic modeling of ustekinumab, a human monoclonal antibody targeting IL-12/23p40, in patients with moderate to severe plaque psoriasis. J Clin Pharmacol 49(2): 162–175. https://doi.org/10.1177/0091270008329556

Zhuang Y, de Vries DE, Xu Z, Marciniak SJ Jr, Chen D, Leon F, Davis HM, Zhou H (2015) Evaluation of disease-mediated therapeutic protein-drug interactions between an anti-interleukin-6 monoclonal antibody (sirukumab) and cytochrome P450 activities in a phase 1 study in patients with rheumatoid arthritis using a cocktail approach. J Clin Pharmacol 55(12):1386–1394. https://doi.org/10.1002/jcph.561

Zia-Amirhosseini P, Minthorn E, Benincosa LJ, Hart TK, Hottenstein CS, Tobia LA, Davis CB (1999) Pharmacokinetics and pharmacodynamics of SB-240563, a humanized monoclonal antibody directed to human interleukin-5, in monkeys. J Pharmacol Exp Ther 291(3):1060–1067

9

Genomics, Other "OMIC" Technologies, Precision Medicine, and Additional Biotechnology-Related Techniques

Robert D. Sindelar

INTRODUCTION

Today's regulatory approved medicines look very different than those of the last century. Biologics, especially monoclonal antibodies (mAbs) and recombinant replacement proteins are becoming the preferred therapeutic entities. The industry pipeline has begun a profound shift in that direction. The products resulting from the techniques and processes of biotechnology continue to grow at an exponential rate, and the expectations are that an even greater percentage of drug development and clinically-utilized pharmaceuticals worldwide will be classified as biologics. A recent Pharmaceutical Research and Manufacturers of America report (PhRMA 2017) notes that there are currently about 7000 medicines in clinical development globally and 80% in the pipeline have the potential to be first-in-class treatments. Most pertinent to this textbook, the majority of these medicines in development were impacted directly or indirectly by biotechnologies at one or more points during their lifetime via: target identification, and/or lead identification, and/or lead optimization, and/or clinical development and evaluation and/or product production.

Pharmaceutical biotechnology techniques are at the core of most methodologies used today for drug discovery and development of both biologics and small molecules. Genetic discovery leads to the underlying disease mechanism elucidation and target discovery. This leads to drug lead discovery and lead optimization, followed by clinical development and hopefully, regulatory approval and clinical use. While recombinant DNA technology and hybridoma techniques are the major methods utilized in pharmaceutical biotechnology through most of its historical timeline, our ever-widening understanding of human cellular function and disease processes, now down to the individual cell has resulted in a wealth of additional and innovative biotechnologies in order to harvest the information found in the human genome. These technological advances will provide a better understanding of the relationship between genetics and biological function, unravel the underlying causes of disease, explore the association of genomic variation and drug response, enable personalized and precision medicine, enhance pharmaceutical research, and fuel the discovery and development of new and novel biopharmaceuticals. These revolutionary technologies and additional biotechnology-related techniques are improving the very competitive and costly process of drug development of new medicinal agents, diagnostics, and medical devices. Some of the technologies and techniques described in this chapter are both well established and commonly used applications of biotechnology, producing clinically-utilized medicines as well as potential therapeutic products now in the developmental pipeline. New techniques are emerging at a rapid and unprecedented pace and their full impact on the future of molecular medicine will turn dreams into realities.

Central to any meaningful discussion of pharmaceutical biotechnology and modern personalized and precision health care are the "OMIC" technologies. The completion 17+ years ago of the Human Genome Project (HGP), one of the great feats of exploration in human history has provided a wealth of new knowledge that continues to grow exponentially as more genes are sequenced at greater resolution and gene editing techniques have been developed with much greater precision. Researchers are turning increasingly to the task of converting the DNA sequence data into information that will improve, and

R. D. Sindelar (✉)
Faculty of Pharmaceutical Sciences and The Centre for Health Evaluation & Outcomes Sciences (CHEOS), The University of British Columbia (UBC), Vancouver, BC, Canada

Global Drug Commercialization Centre (GDCC)-China and GDCC-worldwide, Chengdu, China
e-mail: robert.sindelar@ubc.ca

D. J. A. Crommelin et al. (eds.), *Pharmaceutical Biotechnology*, https://doi.org/10.1007/978-3-030-00710-2_9

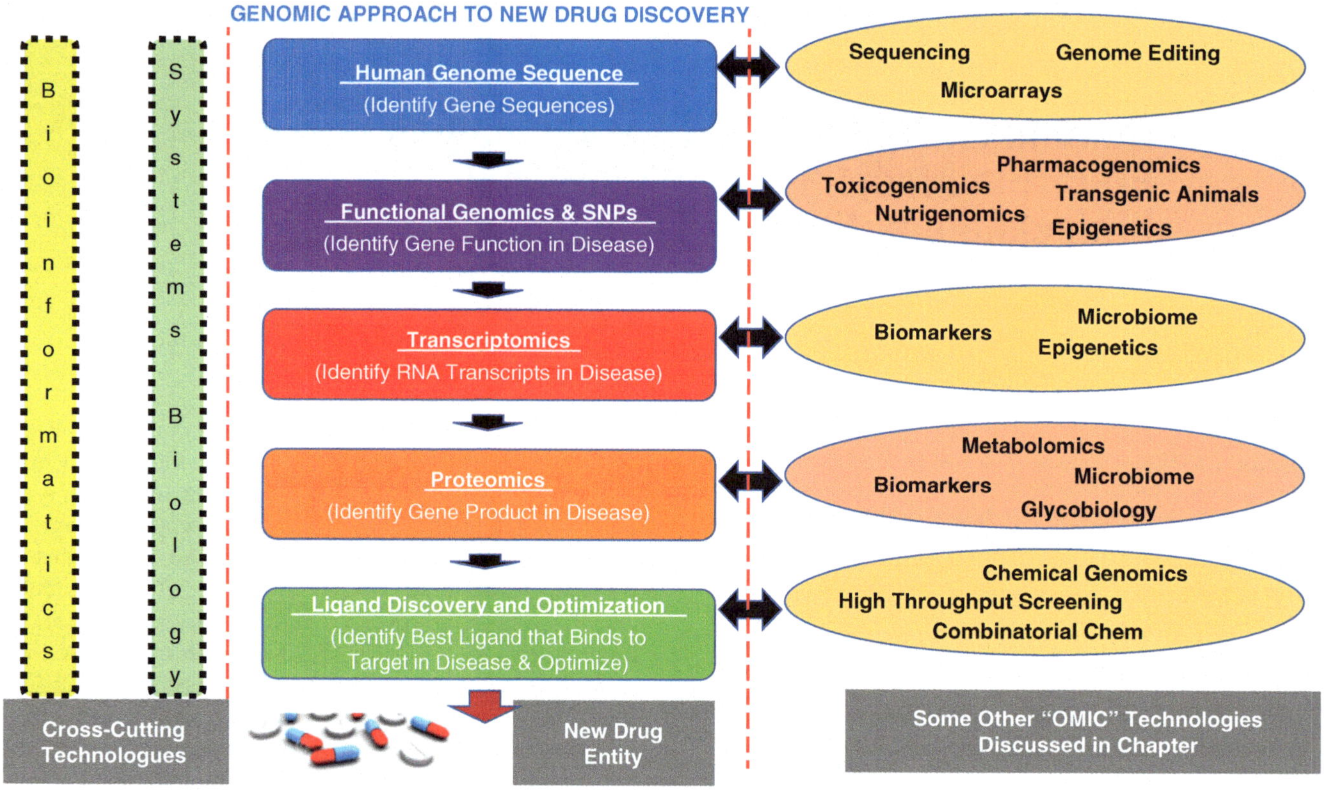

Figure 9.1 ■ The genomic strategy for new drug discovery

even revolutionize, drug discovery (see Fig. 9.1) and patient-centered pharmaceutical care. Pharmaceutical scientists are poised to take advantage of a broad range of omics technologies, most discussed in this chapter, to create a new drug discovery, development, and clinical translation paradigm. These additional techniques in biotechnology and molecular biology are being rapidly exploited to bring new drugs to market and each topic will be introduced in this chapter.

It is not the intention of this author to detail each and every biotechnology technique exhaustively, since numerous printed and web specialized resources already meet that need. Rather, this chapter will illustrate and enumerate various biotechnologies that should be of key interest to pharmacy students, practicing pharmacists, and pharmaceutical scientists because of their effect on many aspects of pharmacy, drug discovery, and drug development.

AN INTRODUCTION TO "OMIC" TECHNOLOGIES

Since the discovery of DNA's overall structure in 1953, the world's scientific community has rapidly gained a detailed knowledge of the genetic information encoded by the DNA of a cell or organism so that today we are "personalizing" this information with greater precision. In the 1980s and 1990s, biotechnology techniques produced novel therapeutics and a wealth of information about the mechanisms of various diseases such as cancer at the genetic and molecular level, yet the etiologies of other complex diseases such as obesity and heart disease remained poorly understood. However, today researchers utilizing exciting and groundbreaking "OMIC" technologies and working closely with clinicians in a "bedside-to-benchtop-back to the bedside" paradigm are making serious progress not only toward a molecular-level understanding of the etiology of complex diseases but to clearly identify that there are actually many genetically different diseases called by the single name of cancer, diabetes, depression, etc. Later in this chapter, we will explore the concepts of phenotype. Important here is that most human diseases are manifested through very complex phenotypes that result from genetic, environmental, and other factors. In a large part, the answers were hidden in what was unknown about the human genome. Despite the increasing knowledge of DNA structure and function in the 1990s, the genome, the entire collection of genes and all other functional and nonfunctional DNA sequences in the nucleus of an organism, had yet to be sequenced. DNA may well be the largest, naturally occurring molecule known. Successfully meeting the challenge of sequencing the entire human genome is one of history's great scientific achievements and has opened a path of discovery unprecedented in biology and medicine (Venter et al. 2001; The International Human Genome Sequencing Consortium 2001). While the genetic code for transcription and translation has been known for years, sequencing the human genome provided a blueprint for all human proteins and the sequences of all regulatory elements that govern the developmental interpretation of the genome. The potential significance includes identifying genetic determinants of common and rare diseases, providing a methodology for their diagnosis including clinically-useful biomarkers, suggesting interesting new molecular sites for intervention (see Fig. 9.1), and the development of new biotechnologies to bring about their more detailed study and eventual eradication. Unlocking the secrets of the human genome and the technologies to edit the genome is leading to a paradigm shift in medicines research and clinical practice toward better disease understanding and taxonomy, and true personalized precision medicine at the molecular level.

■ Genomics

An organism's complete set of DNA is called it genome. The term genomics is the comprehensive analysis and understanding of DNA structure and function and broadly refers to the analysis of all genes within the genome of an organism. Sequencing the human genome and the genomes of many other organisms has led to an in-depth understanding of not only DNA structure and function but also a fundamental understanding of human biology and disease at the molecular level. While it is a complex and complicated journey from acquiring a DNA sample to sequencing the exact order of bases in a DNA strand, a multitude of technologies and approaches along with exponential enhancements in instrumentation and computation have been employed to sequence genomic DNA faster and less expensively. Many industry analysts predicted a tripling of pharmaceutical R&D productivity due to the sequencing of the human genome, but it is the next-generation of whole genome sequencing technology and the continually reduced cost of sequencing that is driving genomic technology into the clinic (Jacob et al. 2013). While the causation of rare diseases was commonly pursued via genetic testing, clinical medicine has historically assessed risk of common diseases in their patients based upon family history. However, the price of whole-genome and whole-exome sequencing (a sequencing technique for sequencing all of the protein-coding genes in a genome) has fallen to the level where these methods are now more commonly used in clinical medicine for many diseases, both rare and common.

Likewise, the field of genomics is having a fundamental impact on modern drug discovery and development. While validation of viable drug targets identified by genomics has been challenging, great progress has occurred (Dugger et al. 2017). No matter whether it is a better understanding of disease or improved drug discovery, the genomic revolution has been the foundation for an explosion in "OMIC" technologies that find applications in research to address poorly treated and neglected diseases.

Structural Genomics and the Human Genome Project

Genetic analysis initially focused on the area of structural genomics, essentially, the characterization of the macromolecular structure of a genome utilizing computational tools and theoretical frameworks. Structural genomics intersects the techniques of DNA sequencing, cloning, PCR, protein expression, crystallography, and big data analysis. It focuses on the physical aspects of the genome through the construction and analysis of gene sequences and gene maps. To understand the significant new advances developing today in the field of biotechnology, it is valuable to better understand structural genomics and the impact of the Human Genome Project. Proposed in the late 1980s, the publicly funded Human Genome Project (HGP) or Human Genome Initiative (HGI) was officially sanctioned in October 1990 to map the structure and to sequence human DNA (US DOE 2018). For historical context, as described in Table 9.1, HGP structural genomics was envisioned to proceed through increasing levels of genetic resolution: detailed human genetic linkage maps [approximately 2 megabase pairs (Mb = million base pairs) resolution], complete physical maps (0.1 Mb resolution), and ultimately complete DNA sequencing of the approximately three billion base pairs (23 pairs of chromosomes) in a human cell nucleus [1 base pair (bp) resolution]. Projected for completion in 2003, the goal of the project was to learn not only what was contained in the genetic code but also how to "mine" the genomic information to cure or help prevent the estimated 4000 genetic diseases afflicting humankind. The project would identify all the genes in the human genome, determine the base pair sequence and store the information in databases, create new tools and improve existing tools for data analysis, and address the ethical, legal, and societal issues (ELSI) that may arise from the project. Earlier than projected, a milestone in genomic science was reached on June 26, 2000, when researchers at the privately funded Celera Genomics and the publicly funded International Human Genome Sequencing Consortium (the international collaboration associated with the HGP) jointly announced that they had completed sequencing 97–99% of the human genome. The journal *Science* rated the mapping of the human genome

Human genome project goals	Base pair resolution
Detailed genetic linkage map	2 Mb
Comments: poorest resolution; depicts relative chromosomal locations of DNA markers, genes, or other markers and the spacing between them on each chromosome	
Complete physical map	0.1 Mb
Comments: instead of relative distances between markers, maps actual physical distance in base pairs between markers; lower resolution = actual observance of chromosomal banding under microscope; higher resolution is "restriction map" generated in presence of restriction enzymes	
Complete DNA sequence	1 bp
Comments: the ultimate goal; determine the base sequence of the genes and markers found in mapping techniques along with the other segments of the entire genome; techniques commonly used include DNA amplification methods such as cloning, PCR and other techniques described in Chap. 1 along with novel sequencing and bioinformatics techniques	

Mb megabase = 1 million base pairs, *bp* base pair

Table 9.1 The increasing levels of genetic resolution obtained from structural genomic studies of the HGP

as its "breakthrough of the year" in its December 22, 2000, issue. The two groups published their results in 2001 (Venter et al. 2001; The International Human Genome Sequencing Consortium 2001).

While both research groups employed the original cloning-based Sanger technique for DNA sequencing (now >35 years old), the genomic DNA sequencing approaches of the HGP and Celera Genomics differed. HGP chopped the human DNA sequence into segments of ever decreasing size. Each DNA segment was further divided or blasted into smaller fragments. Each small fragment was individually sequenced and the sequenced fragments assembled according to their known relative order. The Celera researchers broke the whole genome into many small fragments at once. Each fragment was sequenced and assembled in order by identifying where they overlapped. Each of the two sequencing approaches required unprecedented computer resources (the field of bioinformatics is described later in this chapter).

Regardless of genome sequencing strategies, the collective results are impressive. More than 27 million high-quality sequence reads provided fivefold coverage of the entire human genome. Genomic studies identified over one million single-nucleotide polymorphisms (SNPs), binary elements of genetic variability (SNPs are described later in this chapter). While original estimates of the number of human genes in the genome varied consistently between 80,000–120,000, the genome researchers unveiled a number far short of biologist's predictions; 32,000 (Venter et al. 2001; The International Human Genome Sequencing Consortium 2001). Within months, others suggested that the human genome possesses between 65,000 and 75,000 genes (Wright et al. 2001). Approximately 20,000 genes is the number now most often cited (Madhusoodanan 2014). The HGP provided the foundation for rapid growth of sequencing methodologies, instrumentation, sequencing reagents and bioinformatics approaches that have advanced genome sciences to today's state-of-the-art.

Next-Generation Genome Sequencing (NGS) Including Whole-Genome Sequencing (WGS) and Whole-Exome Sequencing (WES)

The full spectrum of human genetic variation ranges from large chromosomal changes down to the single base pair alterations. The challenge for genomic scientists is to discover the full extent of genomic structural variation, referred to as genotyping, so that the variations and genetic coding may be associated with the encoded trait or traits displayed by the organism (the phenotype). And they wish to do this using as little DNA material as possible, in as short time and for the least cost, all important characteristics of a useful point-of-care clinical technology. The discovery and genotyping of structural variation has been at the core of understanding disease associations as well as identifying possible new drug targets (Hasin et al. 2017). Efficiency of DNA sequencing (sequencing technology is now 40 years old) has facilitated these studies. In the 1.5 decades since the completion of the HGP, sequencing efficiency has increased by approximately 100,000-fold and the cost of a single genome sequence has decreased from nearly $1 million in 2007 to $500–$1000 U.S. depending on the size of the sequence and the reagents utilized (Wetterstrand 2017). The move toward low-cost, high-throughput sequencing is essential for the implementation of genomics into precision medicine and is altering the clinical landscape.

Next-generation genome sequencing methodologies, which differ from the original cloning-based Sanger technique, are massively parallel high-throughput, imaging-based systems with vastly increased speeds and data output. There is no clear definition for *next-generation genome sequencing, also known generally as NGS*, but most are characterized by the direct and parallel sequencing of large numbers of amplified and fragmented DNA without vector-based cloning (Levy and Myers 2016). The fragmented DNA tends to have sequence reads of 30–400 base pairs.

There are now numerous examples of single cell as well as some single nucleic acid -molecule techniques utilizing commercially available DNA sequencers (Shendure et al. 2017; Smaglik 2017). These are techniques effectively creating a "genetic microscope" is poised to revolutionize the fields of oncology and immunology where each cell may be different (Smaglik 2017). Differing from high-throughput sequencing methods, single-cell genomics focuses on each cell independently. Research efforts to begin to genetically profile the millions of every single cell type of the human body may be a formidable task more daunting than the HGP.

There is great excitement surrounding whole-genome sequencing (WGS), a next-generation sequencing development that delivers a comprehensive view of the entire genome effectively achieving the last base pair resolution goal of the HGP (as listed in Table 9.1). Largely used as a research tool until recently, WGS (also known as full genome sequencing, complete genome sequencing, or entire genome sequencing) is a process of determining all of the 3 billion DNA nucleotides of an individual's DNA sequence, including noncoding sequences at a single time (Benjak et al. 2015). This entails sequencing all of an individual's chromosomal DNA as well as the DNA contained in the mitochondria. The most comprehensive method for analyzing the genome, the ability to manage the large volume of data generated during analysis and the rapidly dropping sequencing costs have helped translate this methodology into the clinic (Caspar et al. 2017). A powerful tool whose development has been driven by human research and now initial clinical use, WGS is equally useful for sequencing any species including microorganisms, livestock and plants.

The most widely utilized targeted genome sequencing approach is exon sequencing which investigates only the protein-coding regions of the genome (does not include the non-protein-coding sequences of the genome) (Hehir-Kwa et al. 2015). Humans have about 233,000 exons constituting <2% of the human genome, and current research suggests that most known Mendelian and common polygenic disease-related variants are in the exons. Thus, this sequencing approach is a cost-effective alternative to WGS that produces smaller and more manageable data sets for faster analysis. Together, all the exons in a genome are known as the exome and their entire sequencing at one time is called whole-exome sequencing (WES). Note that because DNA variations outside of the exons can affect gene activity and protein production leading to genetic disorders, WES is not always an effective sequencing approach. WGS and WES are valuable methods for researchers and are now being introduced in clinics.

Progress is being made on "dynamic 3D genomics." Many genome sequencing techniques are being used in combination with imaging methods such as fluorescence in situ hybridization (FISH) for probing a genome's 3D architecture. As researchers continue to manipulate genome structure, combining genomics and imaging will deepen our understanding of the effects of regional proximity of specific gene sequences on biological processes.

Functional Genomics, Comparative Genomics and Biobanks

Functional genomics is the subfield of genomics that attempts to answer questions about the function of specific DNA sequences at the levels of transcription and translation, i.e., genes, RNA transcripts, and protein products (Adams et al. 2016). Research to relate genomic sequence data determined by structural genomics with observed biological function is predicted to fuel new drug discoveries through a better understanding of what genes do, how they are regulated, and the direct relationship between genes and their activity. The DNA sequence information itself rarely provides definitive information about the function and regulation of that particular gene. After genome sequencing, a functional genomic approach is the next step in the knowledge chain to identify functional gene products that are potential biotech drug leads and new drug discovery targets (see Fig. 9.1).

To relate functional genomics to therapeutic clinical outcomes, the human genome sequence must reveal the thousands of genetic variations among individuals that will become associated with diseases or symptoms in the patient's lifetime. Sequencing alone is not the solution, simply the end of the beginning of the genomic medicine era. Determining gene functionality in any organism opens the door for linking a disease to specific genes or proteins, which become targets for new drugs, methods to detect organisms (i.e., new diagnostic agents), and/or biomarkers (the presence or change in gene expression profile that correlates with the risk, progression, or susceptibility of a disease). Success with functional genomics will facilitate the ability to observe a clinical problem, take it to the benchtop for structural and functional genomic analysis, and return personalized solutions to the bedside in the form of new therapeutic interventions and medicines.

The face of biology has changed forever with the sequencing of the genomes of numerous organisms. Biotechnologies applied to the sequencing of the human genome are also being utilized to sequence the genomes of comparatively simple organisms as well as other mammals. Often, the proteins encoded by the genomes of more simple organisms and the regulation of those genes closely resemble the proteins and gene regulation in humans. Now that the sequencing of the entire genome is a reality, the chore of sorting through human, pathogen, and other organism diversity factors and correlating them with genomic data to provide real pharmaceutical benefits is an active area of research. Comparative genomics is the field of genomics that studies the relationship of genome structure and function across different biological species or strains and thus, provides information about the evolutionary processes that act upon a genome (Lawrie and Petrov 2014). Comparative genomics exploits both similarities and differences in the regulatory regions of genes, as well as RNA and proteins of different organisms to infer how selection has acted upon these elements.

Since model organisms are much easier to maintain in a laboratory setting, researchers are actively pursuing "comparative" genomic studies between multiple organisms. Unlocking genomic data for each of these organisms provides valuable insight into the molecular basis of inherited human disease. As an example, *S. cerevisiae*, a yeast, is a good model for studying cancer and is a common organism used in rDNA methodology. It is well known that women who inherit a gene mutation of the *BRCA1* gene have a high risk, perhaps as high as 85%, of developing breast cancer before the age of 50 (Paul and Paul 2014). The first diagnostic product generated from genomic data was the *BRCA1* test for breast cancer predisposition. The gene product of *BRCA1* is a well-characterized protein implicated in both breast and ovarian cancer. Evidence had accumulated suggesting that the Rad9 protein of *S. cerevisiae* was distantly, but significantly, related to the *BRCA1* protein. Thus, *S. cerevisiae* in the lab was well studied during the development of *BRCA1* diagnostics. Similarly, studying *C. elegans*, an unsegmented vermiform, has provided much of our early knowledge of apoptosis, the normal biological process of programmed cell death. Greater than 90 % of the proteins identified thus far from a common laboratory animal, the mouse, have structural similarities to known human proteins.

Similarly, mapping the whole of a human cancer cell genome is pinpointing the genes involved in cancer and aids in the understanding of cell changes and treatment of human malignancies utilizing the techniques of both functional and comparative genomics (Friedman et al. 2015). In cancer cells, small changes in the DNA sequence can cause the cell to make a protein that doesn't allow the cell to function as it should. These proteins can make cells grow quickly and cause damage to neighboring cells, becoming cancerous. The genome of a cancer cell can also be used to stratify cancer cells identifying one type of cancer from another or identifying a subtype of cancer within that type, such as HER2+ breast cancer. Understanding the cancer genome is a step toward improved cancer drug therapy and personalized oncology (Moody et al. 2010).

A valuable resource for performing functional and comparative genomics is the "biobank," a collection of biological samples for reference purposes (Schneider et al. 2016). Repositories of this type also might be referred to as biorepositories or named after the type of tissue depending on the exact type of specimens (i.e., tissue banks). Genomic techniques are fostering the creation of DNA and RNA banks, the collection, storage, and analysis of hundreds of thousands of specimens containing analyzable DNA and/or RNA. All nucleated cells, including cells from blood, hair follicles, buccal swabs, cancer biopsies, and urine specimens, are suitable nucleic acid samples for analysis in the present or at a later date. Note that traditional biopsy is an invasive procedure to obtain a sample of tissue (i.e., cancer cells, heart tissue, liver tissue, etc.) and is not always feasible. New techniques have been developed that allow a less invasive test on a sample of blood called "liquid biopsy". For example, a liquid biopsy can be conducted on a cancer patient to look for cancer cells from a tumor that are circulating in the blood, but also for pieces of DNA or RNA from tumor cells that are in the blood sample (Kwapisz 2017). DNA banks are proving to be valuable tools for genetics research. While in its broadest sense such repositories could incorporate any collection of plant or animal samples, some of the most developed biobanks in the world are devoted to research on various types of cancer. While DNA and RNA banks devoted to cancer research have grown the fastest, there also has been an almost explosive growth in biobanks specializing in research on autism, schizophrenia, Alzheimers, heart disease, diabetes, and many other diseases.

■ "OMICS"-Enabling Technology: Bioinformatics in the Big Data Era

Recent technological advances in structural genomics, functional genomics, transcriptomics, proteomics, pharmacogenomics, metabolomics and other "OMIC" techniques have generated an enormous volume of genetic and biochemical data to store and analyze. The continually lowering cost of data generation is leading to the "big data" era. The term "big data" addresses the challenges of data capture, data storage, data analysis, data search, data mining, data visualization and data sharing of data sets that are so voluminous and complex that traditional data processing and software are incapable of doing the job. In this case, data mining refers to the bioinformatics approach of "sifting" through volumes of raw data, identifying and extracting relevant information, and developing useful relationships among them (Murdoch and Detsky 2013). Big data development has focused on the creation and enhancement of predictive analytic methods that extract value from large data sets. New observations are generated that spot trends and correlations that would otherwise be lost in the volume of data being analyzed.

Living in an era of faster computers, bigger and better data storage, and improved methods of data analysis fostered the information superhighway that facilitated the HGP and the "OMIC" revolution. Scientists applied advances in information technology, innovative software algorithms, and massive parallel computing to the ongoing research in biotechnology areas such as genomics to give birth to the fast-growing field of bioinformatics (Greene et al. 2014). Bioinformatics, the interdisciplinary field to analyze and interpret biological information, is essential to accelerating the rate of biotechnology-related discovery. Now, technological advances in high throughput profiling of biological systems including next-generation sequencing techniques coupled with the unprecedented ability to data mine and analyze in the big data environment provides scientists with the essential tools required to accelerate the rate of discovery that will improve health, well-being, and patient care. Bioinformatics is the application of computer technologies to the biological sciences with the object of discovering new knowledge and interconnections. With bioinformatics, a researcher can now better exploit the tremendous flood of genomic, transcriptomic and proteomic data, and more cost-effectively data mine for a drug discovery "needle" in that massive data "haystack." We can now examine the relationship of DNA sequence to structure and function cross-cut with measurements of mRNA expression, transcription factor binding, protein synthesis, metabolite concentrations and phenotype (to be explained later in this chapter).

Modern drug discovery and the commensurate need to better understand and define disease is utilizing bioinformatics techniques to gather information from multiple sources [such as functional genomic studies, proteomics, phenotyping, patient electronic health records (EHRs; sometimes referred to as electronic medical records, EMRs), and bioassay results including toxicology studies], integrate the data, apply life science developed algorithms, and generate useful target identification and drug lead identification data (Premsrirut 2017). The term "Reverse Informatics" has been used to describe the drug discovery informatics tool that regenerates data in a structured format from primary literature so that it can be easily synchronized with other data sets and mined to identify new drug targets. As seen in Fig. 9.2, the hierarchy of information

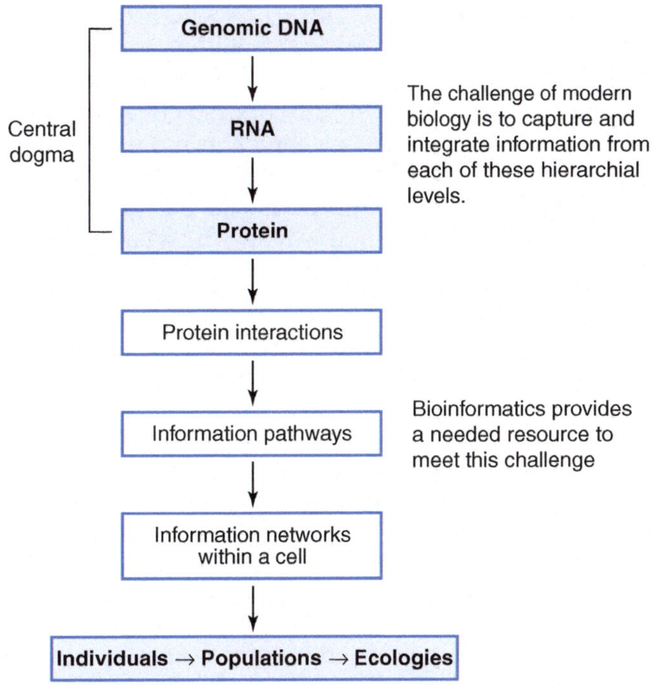

Figure 9.2 ■ The information challenges of systems biology in the genomic era

collection goes well beyond the biodata contained in the genetic code that is transcribed and translated. A recent National Research Council report for the US National Academies entitled "Toward Precision Medicine: Building a Knowledge Network for Biomedical Research and a New Taxonomy of Disease" calls for a new data network that integrates emerging research on the molecular basis of diseases with the clinical data from individual patients to drive the development of a more accurate taxonomy of disease that ultimately improves disease diagnosis and patient outcomes (U.S. National Academies 2011). The report notes that challenges include both scientific (technical advances needed to correlate genetic and environmental findings with incidence of disease) and legal and ethical challenges (privacy issues, EHRs, etc.).

The entire encoded human DNA sequence alone requires computer storage of approximately 10^9 bits of information: the equivalent of a thousand 500-page books! GenBank (managed by the National Center for Biotechnology Information, NCBI, of the National Institutes of Health, http://www.ncbi.nlm.nih.gov) and the European Molecular Biology Laboratory (EMBL, https://www.embl.org/) are two of the many centers worldwide that collaborate on collecting nucleic acid sequences. These databanks (both public and private) store tens of millions of sequences. Among the largest data sets are The Cancer Genome Atlas (TCGA, https://www.genome.gov/17516564/the-cancer-genome-atlas/) and the Encyclopedia of DNA

Elements (ENCODE, https://www.encodeproject.org). Once stored, analyzing the volumes of data (i.e., comparing and relating information from various sources) to identify useful and/or predictive characteristics or trends, such as selecting a group of drug targets from all proteins in the human body, presents a Herculean task. This approach has the potential of changing the fundamental way in which basic science is conducted and valid biological conclusions are reached (The Cancer Genome Atlas Research Network 2014; Davis et al. 2018).

With OMICS, health care has experienced an explosion in biomedical knowledge fostering dramatic innovations in therapy and expanded capacities to treat challenging medical conditions. The system has lagged in adjusting to new discoveries, disseminating data in real time and learning from each and every health care intervention. The concept of a "continuous learning health care system" has begun to be proposed as a paradigm to apply the resources and tools at hand in new science, bioinformatics and big data, and the transformation of the care culture to produce high-quality health care informed by constantly collected and analyzed information and data (IOM (Institute of Medicine) 2013). Likewise, rapidly expanding areas that will likely be very important by time the 6th edition of this textbook is written are Artificial Intelligence (AI) as applied to health care and delivery, and Digital Medicine, the intersection of wearable sensor technologies, mobile computing, the internet and the incentives for healthy living. Thus, the profession of pharmacy and the pharmaceutical sciences must readily recognize that optimal patient-centered care requires an effective integration of data and information (drug and patient information) into a system now known as "pharmacy informatics" (Goundrey-Smith 2013). Patient information includes data from genomics, proteomics, other OMIC technologies, individual patient characteristics, patient safety, evidence-based medicine, and EHRs. Drug information includes that found in the primary literature, drug information databases, internet resources, hospital information systems, pharmacy information systems, drug discovery literature, and pharmacogenomic studies. Pharmacy informatics integrates and uses knowledge, information, technology and automation in the precision medication optimization process. While it is well beyond the scope of this chapter to explore continuous learning health care systems, AI, Digital Medicine and Pharmacy Informatics further, these are becoming important areas for pharmacists and pharmaceutical scientists to be well informed and knowledgeable.

Transcriptomics

Remember that the central dogma of molecular biology is DNA to RNA via the process of transcription and RNA to protein via the process of translation (Fig. 9.2). The transcriptome is the collection of all RNA transcribed elements for a given genome, not only the collection of transcripts that are subsequently translated into proteins (mRNAs). Noncoding transcripts such as noncoding microRNAs (miRNAs) are part of the transcriptome and are described in detail in our chapter on nucleic acid therapies. The term transcript*omics* refers to the OMIC technology that examines the complexity of RNA transcripts of an organism under a variety of internal and external conditions reflecting the genes that are being actively expressed at any given time (with the exception of mRNA degradation phenomena such as transcriptional attenuation). Therefore, the transcriptome can vary within individual cells with external environmental conditions, while the genome is roughly fixed for a given cell line (excluding mutations) (Jiang et al. 2015; Kolodziejczyk et al. 2015). The variances between distinct cells can have profound functional effects. Whole transcriptome analysis can help identify the relationship of sequence to function by exploring genetic networks underlying cellular, physiological, biochemical and biological systems. This approach is important to modern biomarker discovery. The transcriptomes of stem cells and cancer cells are of particular interest to better understand the processes of cellular differentiation and carcinogenesis.

Many OMICS methods are currently being optimized with respect to analysis speed and ease, resolution and accuracy, and the number of genes that can profiled in a transcriptomics approach. High-throughput techniques based on microarray technology are used to examine the expression level of mRNAs in a given cell population. Recently, single-cell mRNA sequencing techniques have been developed to provide high-resolution transcriptomic analysis of specific individual cells. "Spatial transcriptomics" is the integration of gene transcription data into a spatial coordinate system mapped upon various tissue atlases. This type of approach is critical for the in-depth understanding of individual cell identity and function within the tissue context. The international Human Cell Atlas (HCA; https://www.humancellatlas.org/) and the U.S. NIH hosted Human BioMolecular Atlas Program (HuBMAP; https://commonfund.nih.gov/hubmap), both creating comprehensive reference maps of all human cells, include technological components that incorporate spatial transcriptomic mapping as explicit goals.

Proteomics, Structural Proteomics, and Functional Proteomics

Proteomics is the study of an organism's complete complement of proteins. Proteomics seeks to define the function and correlate that with expression profiles of all proteins encoded within an organism's genome or "proteome" (Altelaar et al. 2013). Defining protein composition in both the healthy state and in the disease state is a key step in understanding the function of biological systems. The application of functional proteomics in the process of drug discovery has created a field of research referred to as pharmacoproteomics that tries to compare whole protein profiles of healthy persons versus patients with disease. This analysis may point to new and novel targets for drug discovery and precision medicine. While functional genomic research is providing an unprecedented information resource for the study of biochemical pathways at the molecular level, a vast array of the human genes identified in sequencing the human genome are being analyzed to determine if they are functionally important in various disease states (i.e., the druggable genome). These key proteins when identified serve as potential new sites for therapeutic intervention (see Fig. 9.1) (Zhang et al. 2014). The transcription and translation of approximately 20,000 human genes can produce hundreds of thousands of proteins due to posttranscriptional regulation and posttranslational modification of the protein products (Cf. Chap. 2). The number, type, and concentration may vary depending on cell or tissue type, disease state, and other factors. The protein's function(s) is dependent on the primary, secondary, and tertiary structure of the protein and the molecules they interact with. Less than 40 years old, the concept of proteomics requires determination of the structural, biochemical, and physiological repertoire of all proteins.

Proteomics is a greater scientific challenge than genomics due to the intricacy of protein expression and the complexity of 3D protein structure (structural proteomics) as it relates to biological activity (functional proteomics). Protein expression, isolation, purification, identification, and characterization are among the key procedures utilized in proteomic research. To perform these procedures, technology platforms such as 2D gel electrophoresis, mass spectrometry, chip-based microarrays (discussed later in this chapter), X-ray crystallography, protein nuclear magnetic resonance (nmr), and phage displays are employed. The Human Proteome Project (HPP, https://hupo.org/human-proteome-project) is an international project organized by the Human Proteome Organization (HUPO; https://hupo.org/) that aims to revolutionize our understanding of the human proteome via a multinational harmonized research effort to map the entire human proteome utilizing currently available and emerging techniques. Successful completion of this multi-year project will enrich and focus our understanding of human biology at the cellular level and lay a foundation for development of new and novel diagnostic, therapeutic, and preventive medical applications (Omenn et al. 2016).

Pharmaceutical scientists are finding that many of the proteins identified by proteomic research are entirely novel, possessing unknown or little known functions. This scenario offers not only a unique opportunity to identify previously unknown molecular targets from drug design, but also to develop new biomarkers and ultrasensitive diagnostics to address unmet clinical needs.

Often, multiple genes and their protein products are involved in a single disease process. Since few proteins act alone, studying protein interactions will be paramount to a full understanding of functionality (see systems biology later in this chapter). Also, many abnormalities in cell function may result from overexpression of a gene and/or protein, underexpression of a gene and/or protein, a gene mutation causing a malformed protein, and posttranslational modification changes that alter a protein's function. Therefore, the real value of human genome sequence data will only be realized after every protein coded by the approximately 20,000 genes has a function assigned to it with the completion of the HPP (Wiktorowicz and Brasier 2016).

"OMICS"-Enabling Technology: Microarrays

The biochips known as microarrays are multiplex lab-on-a-chip assays used in high-throughput screening of biological materials (Schumacher et al. 2015). The initial microarrays were DNA or oligonucleotide microarrays that are a collection of hundreds to thousands of immobilized nucleic acid sequences or oligonucleotides in a grid created with specialized equipment that can be simultaneously examined to conduct expression analysis. These gene chips would contain representatives of a particular set of gene sequences (i.e., sequences coding for all human cytochrome P450 isozymes) or may contain sequences representing all genes of an organism. They are finding greater clinical use with the Roche Diagnostics AmpliChip™ CYP 450 an example of one of the first FDA-approved (approved in 2005) microarrays available (Chau and Thomas 2015). This specific gene chip is used to determine a patient's genotype with respect to two genes that govern drug metabolism, CYP2D6 (4 phenotypes based on

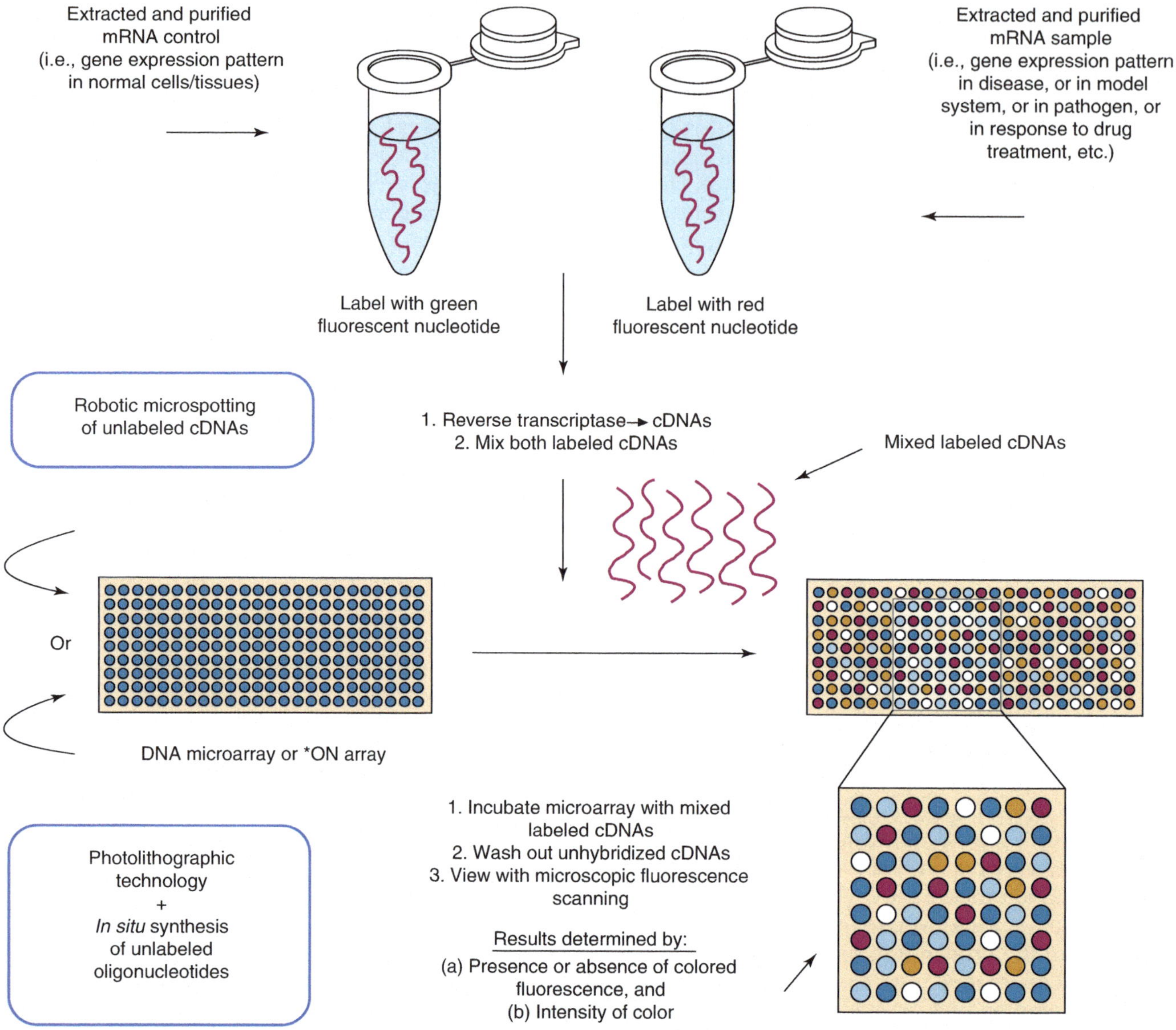

Figure 9.3 ■ Principle of operation of a representative DNA microarray or oligonucleotide (*ON) microarray

rate of metabolism, over 90 variants) and CYP2C19 (2 phenotypes based on rate of metabolism, mainly 3 variants). The results obtained may be useful to a physician to select the appropriate drug and/or dosage for a given patient in the areas of cardiovascular disease, high blood pressure, depression, and others (according to the company).

Commonly, arrays are prepared on nonporous supports such as glass microscope slides or silicon thin-film cells. DNA microarrays generally contain high-density microspotted cDNA sequences approximately 1 kb in length representing thousands of genes. The field was advanced significantly when technology was developed to synthesize closely spaced oligonucleotides on glass wafers using semiconductory industry photolithographic masking techniques (see Fig. 9.3). Oligonucleotide microarrays contain closely spaced synthetic gene-specific oligonucleotides representing thousands of gene sequences. Microarrays can provide expression analysis for mRNAs. Screening of DNA variation is also possible. Thus, biochips can provide polymorphism detection and genotyping as well as hybridization-based expression monitoring. Microarray analysis has gained increasing significance as a direct result of the genome sequencing studies. Array technology is a logical tool for studying functional genomics since the results obtained may link function to expression. Microarray technology's potential to study key areas of molecular medicine and drug discovery is unlimited at this stage of development. For example, gene expression levels of thousands of mRNA species may be studied simultaneously in normal versus cancer cells, each incubated with potential anticancer drug candidates.

Researchers have developed many types of microarrays beyond the initial DNA or oligonucleotide arrays such as: protein, peptide, tissue, cellular, chemical compound, antibody, carbohydrate, phenotype, and microarrays of lysates or serum (Schumacher et al. 2015). The principles are the same, while the immobilized collections differ accordingly.

"OMICS"-Enabled Technology: Brief Introduction to Biomarkers

Biomarkers or biological markers are clinically relevant biological measures used as indicators of normal biological processes, a disease state, predisposition to a disease, disease progression or pharmaceutical response to a therapeutic intervention (Zhao et al. 2015). The significance of biotechnology produced biomarkers has been recognized by the research community, pharma industry and now the clinic. Detection of or concentration change of a biomarker may indicate a particular disease state (e.g., the presence of a certain antibody may indicate an infection), physiology, or toxicity. A change in expression or state of a protein or other OMIC-related biomarkers may correlate with the risk of or progression of a disease, with the susceptibility of the disease to a given treatment or the drug's safety profile (Anderson and Kodukula 2014). Biomarkers may be used alone or in combination. Implemented in the form of a medical device, a measured biomarker becomes an in vitro diagnostic tool (Drabovich et al. 2015). While it is well beyond this chapter to provide a detailed discussion of biomarkers, it is important to note that OMIC technologies including OMIC-enabled technologies such as microarrays are being developed as clinical measuring devices for biomarkers. Biomarkers enable focused characterization of patient populations undergoing clinical trials or drug therapy and may accelerate drug development. Modern drug discovery often simultaneously involves biomarker discovery and diagnostic development (Zhao et al. 2015). Drug development scientists are hopeful that the development of appropriate biomarkers will facilitate "go" and "no go" decisions during a preclinical and clinical development processes. Biomarker discovery is closely tied to the other applications of genomics previously described in this chapter. As an indicator of normal biological processes, pathogenic processes, or pharmacological responses to therapeutic intervention, biomarkers may serve as a substitute for a clinical end point and thus be a surrogate end point (Zhao and Brasier 2015). Biomarkers are now available for a wide range of diseases and conditions. A recent PubMed search of the term "biomarker" as key word filtered on clinical trials and publications in the last 10 years yielded almost 500 entries (Zhao et al. 2015). Approximately 60% were disease-related such as Alzheimer's and Parkinson's disease, cardiac injury, lung injury, acute kidney injury, various cancers and a host of other diseases and pathological conditions. Another 20% were prognostic or predictive in nature.

A "theranostic" is a rapid diagnostic, possibly a microarray, measuring a clinically significant biomarker, which may identify patients most likely to benefit or be harmed by a new medication. Bundled with a new drug (and likely developed in parallel with that drug), the theranostic's diagnosis of the requisite biomarker (e.g., the overexpression of the HER2 gene product in certain breast cancer patients) influences the physician's therapeutic decisions [i.e., prescribing the drug trastuzumab (Herceptin) for HER2 receptor-positive breast cancer patients]. Thus, the diagnostic and the therapy are distinctly coupled = theranostic. The theranostic predicts clinical success of the drug. In the PubMed study quoted above, approximately 8% of all the publications found included HER2 testing highlighting the utility of biomarkers for appropriate patient selection. This example used to introduce the concept of a theranostic is possibly the best example of precision medicine (see later in this chapter), achieving the best medical outcomes by choosing treatments that work well with a person's genomic profile or with certain OMIC characteristics.

Metabolomics and Metabonomics

The human metabolome consists of the complete set of small molecules that are involved in the energy transmission in the cells by interacting with other biological molecules following metabolic pathways (Lindon and Nicholson 2014; Mastrangelo et al. 2014). These metabolites may be metabolic intermediates, hormones and other signaling molecules, and secondary metabolites (Patti et al. 2012). The techniques and processes for identifying clinically significant biomarkers of human disease and drug safety have fostered the systematic study of the unique chemical fingerprints that specific cellular processes leave behind, specifically their small molecule metabolite profiles. Thus, while genomics and proteomics do not tell the whole story of what might be happening within a cell, metabolic profiling can give an instantaneous snapshot of the physiology of that cell.

Metabolomics is a powerful tool kit for the analysis of phenotype, by: (1) providing diagnostic patterns via fingerprinting a complex mixture of metabolites in the metabolome, (2) measuring the absolute concentration of targeted metabolites, (3) determining the relative abundance of selected portions of the metabolome, and (4) tracing the biochemical fate of individual metabolites. High-performance liquid chromatography coupled with sophisticated nuclear magnetic resonance (NMR) and mass spectrometry (MS) techniques is used to separate and quantify complex metabolite mixtures found in biological fluids to get a picture of the metabolic continuum of an organism influenced by an internal and external environment (Bingol et al. 2016). The field of "metabonomics" is the holistic study of the metabolic continuum at the equivalent level to the study of genomics and proteomics. However, unlike genomics and proteomics, microarray technology is little used since the molecules assayed in metabonomics are small molecule end products of gene expression and resulting protein function. The term metabolomics has arisen as the metabolic composition of a cell at a specified time, whereas the term metabonomics includes both the static metabolite composition and concentrations and the full-time course fluctuations. Coupling the information being collected in biobanks, large collections of patient's biological samples and medical records, with metabonomic and metabolomic studies, will not only detect why a given metabolite level is increasing or decreasing but may reliably predict the onset of disease. Also, the techniques are finding use in drug safety screening, identification of clinical biomarkers, and systems biology studies (see below).

In oncology, metabolomic studies may be able to interrogate cancer cells for the optimal window for therapeutic intervention based upon metabolite concentrations. Scientists have created a number of metabolomics databases to may offer guidance on how metabolomics can be used to study cancer (Wishart et al. 2016). The largest such database, the Human Metabolome Database (HMDB; http://www.hmdb.ca/) contains over 114,000 metabolite entries including both water soluble and lipid soluble metabolites that are considered either abundant in the human metabolome (>1 uM) or relatively rare (<1 uM) plus greater than 5000 protein sequences linked to the metabolites (Wishart et al. 2018). Each entry contains 130 data fields devoted to chemical, clinical, enzymatic or biochemical data on the metabolites and many fields are linked to related databases (such as GenBank, DrugBank, PubChem, etc.).

Glycomics and Glycobiology

The novel scientific field of glycomics, or glycobiology, may be defined most simply as the study of the structure, synthesis, and biological function of all glycans (may be referred to as oligosaccharides or polysaccharides, depending on size) and glycoconjugates in simple and complex systems (Cummings and Pierce 2014; Rudd et al. 2017). The application of glycomics or glycobiology is sometimes called glycotechnology to distinguish it from biotechnology (referring to glycans rather than proteins and nucleic acids). However, many in the biotech arena consider glycobiology one of the research fields encompassed by the term biotechnology. In the postgenomic era, the intricacies of protein glycosylation, the mechanisms of genetic control, and the internal and external factors influencing the extent and patterns of glycosylation are important to understanding protein function and proteomics. Like proteins and nucleic acids, glycans are biopolymers. While once referred to as the last frontier of pharmaceutical discovery, recent advances in the biotechnology of discovering, cloning, and harnessing sugar cleaving and synthesizing enzymes have enabled glycobiologists to analyze and manipulate complex carbohydrates more easily (Tang et al. 2014).

Many of the proteins produced by animal cells contain attached sugar moieties, making them glycoproteins. The majority of protein-based medicinal agents contain some form of posttranslational modification that can profoundly affect the biological activity of that protein. Bacterial hosts for recombinant DNA could produce the animal proteins with identical or nearly identical amino acid sequences. However, early work in bacteria lacked the ability to attach sugar moieties to proteins (a process called glycosylation). New methodologies may help overcome this issue (cf. Chaps. 1, 2, and 4). Many of the non-glycosylated proteins differ in their biological activity as compared to the native glycoprotein. The production of animal proteins that lacked glycosylation provided an unexpected opportunity to study the functional role of sugar molecules on glycoproteins. Glycoengineering of yeast to humanize *N*-glycosylation pathways resulted in therapeutic glycoprotein expression in yeasts (Wildt and Gerngross 2005).

The complexity of the field can best be illustrated by reviewing the building blocks of glycans, the simple carbohydrates called saccharides or sugars and their derivatives (i.e., amino sugars). Simple carbohydrates can be attached to other types of biological molecules to form glycoconjugates including glycoproteins (predominantly protein), glycolipids and proteoglycans (about 95% polysaccharide and 5% protein). While carbohydrate chemistry and biology have been active areas of research for centuries, advances in biotechnology have provided techniques and added energy to the study of glycans. Oligosaccharides found conjugated to proteins (glycoproteins) and lipids (glycolipids) display a tremendous structural diversity. The linkages of the monomeric units in proteins and in nucleic acids are generally consistent in all such molecules. Glycans, however, exhibit far greater variability in the linkage

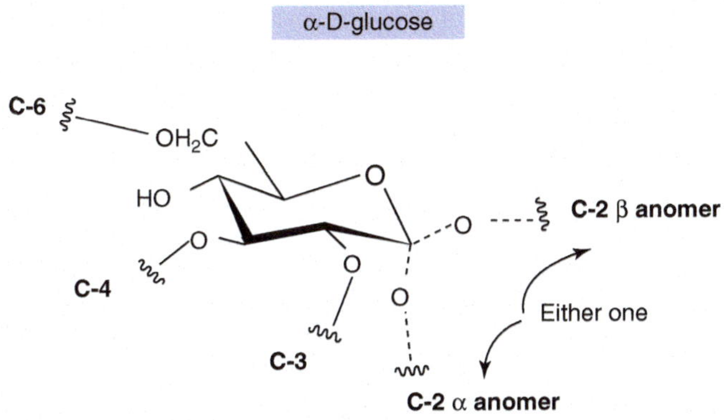

Figure 9.4 ■ Illustration of the common linkage sites to create biopolymers of glucose. Linkages at four positions: C-2, C-3, C-4, and C-6 and also can take one of two possible anomeric configurations at C-2 (α and β)

between monomeric units than that found in the other biopolymers. As an example, Fig. 9.4 illustrates the common linkage sites to create polymers of glucose. Glucose can be linked at four positions: C-2, C-3, C-4, and C-6 and also can take one of two possible anomeric configurations at C-2 (α and β). It is estimated that for a 10-mer (oligomer of length 10), the number of structurally distinct linear oligomers for each of the biopolymers is for DNA (with 4 possible bases), 1.04×10^6; for protein (with 20 possible amino acids), 1.28×10^{13}; and for oligosaccharide (with eight monosaccharide types), 1.34×10^{18}.

Glycosylation and Medicine

Patterns of glycosylation significantly affect the biological activity of proteins (Wildt and Gerngross 2005; Costa et al. 2014). Many of the therapeutically used recombinant DNA-produced proteins are glycosylated including erythropoietin, glucocerebrosidase, and tissue plasminogen activator. Without the appropriate carbohydrates attached, none of these proteins will function therapeutically as does the parent glycoprotein. Glycoforms (variations of the glycosylation pattern of a glycoprotein) of the same protein may differ in physicochemical and biochemical properties. For example, erythropoietin has one O-linked and three N-linked glycosylation sites. The removal of the terminal sugars at each site destroys in vivo activity and removing all sugars results in a more rapid clearance of the molecule and a shorter circulatory half-life (Jiang et al. 2014). Yet, the opposite effect is observed for the deglycosylation of the hematopoietic cytokine granulocyte-macrophage colony-stimulating factor (GM-CSF) (Höglund 1998). In that case, removing the carbohydrate residues increases the specific activity six-fold. The sugars of glycoproteins are known to play a role in the recognition and binding of biomolecules to other molecules in disease states such as asthma, rheumatoid arthritis, cancer, HIV infection, the flu, and other infectious diseases.

■ Lipidomics

Lipids, the fundamental components of membranes, play multifaceted roles in cell, tissue, and organ physiology. The research area of lipidomics is a lipid-targeted metabolomics approach focused on the comprehensive large-scale study of pathways and networks of cellular lipids in biological systems (Zhao et al. 2015b). The metabolome would include the major classes of biological molecules: proteins (and amino acids), nucleic acids, and carbohydrates. The "lipidome" would be a subset of the metabolome that describes the complete lipid profile within a cell, tissue, or whole organism. In lipidomic research, a vast amount of information (structures, functions, interactions, and dynamics) quantitatively describing alterations in the content and composition of different lipid molecular species is accrued after perturbation of a cell, tissue, or organism through changes in its physiological or pathological state.

Abnormal lipid metabolism is implicated in a number of human lifestyle-related diseases. The study of lipidomics is important to a better understanding of many metabolic diseases, as lipids are believed to play a role in obesity, atherosclerosis, stroke, hypertension, diabetes, respiratory disease and cancer (Zhao et al. 2015a). Lipidomics research may help identify potential biomarkers for establishing preventative or therapeutic interventions against human disease.

Progress of modern lipidomics and lipid profiling has been greatly accelerated by the development of sensitive analytical techniques such as electrospray ionization (ESI) and matrix-assisted laser desorption/ionization (MALDI). Currently, the isolation and subsequent analysis of lipid mixtures is hampered by extraction and analytical limitations due to characteristics of lipid chemistry.

■ Nutrigenetics and Nutrigenomics

The well-developed tools and techniques of genomics and bioinformatics have been applied to the investigation of the intricate interaction of mammalian diet and genetic makeup. It is critically important to study the effects of genetic variation on dietary responses and the role of nutrients and bioactive food components in gene expression. Nutrigenetics involves the influence of genetic variation on nutrition. Whereas nutrigenomics or nutritional genomics has been defined as the influence of nutrition on genome stability, epigenome modifications, transcriptomic alterations, and proteomic changes. This appears to result from gene expression and/or gene variation (e.g., SNP analysis) on a nutrient's absorption, distribution, metabolism, elimination, or biological effects (Ferguson et al. 2016). This includes how nutrients impact on the production and action of specific gene products and how the expressed proteins in turn affect the response to nutrients. Nutrigenomic studies aim to develop predictive means to optimize nutrition, with respect to an individual's genotype. Areas of study include dietary supplements, common foods and beverages, mother's milk, as well as diseases such as cardiovascular disease, obesity, and diabetes. Nutrigenomics is thought to be a critical science for personalized health and especially public health (Berná et al. 2014).

Microbiome

The human microbiome (or sometimes called the human microbiota) is the collection of bacteria, viruses and fungi and their genomes colonizing the human body. These microorganisms reside primarily in the gut and the rest of the GI tract, but importantly also live on the skin and in the mouth and saliva, in the nostrils, in the eyes, in the genital areas on the body, and in our hair. Led by the tremendous advances in OMICS technology, there has recently been tremendous growth and understanding in the collective knowledge of the human microbiome (Cénit et al. 2014). As humans, we share our body space with symbiotic, pathogenic and commensal microorganisms as an ecological community. Sometimes called the "Second Genome" and the Forgotten Organ," the human microbiome contributes more protein-coding genes than the human host. The human microbiome is estimated to contain 10 times the number of cells and >140 times the number of genes that our human bodies contain (please see Fig. 9.5).

There is little doubt that the microbiome plays a critical role in human health and disease and may influence nearly all aspects of human biology through (a) host-microbe interaction(s) (Ji and Nielsen 2015; Tuddenham and Sears 2015). Analysis of the functional interactions between the human host and its microbi-

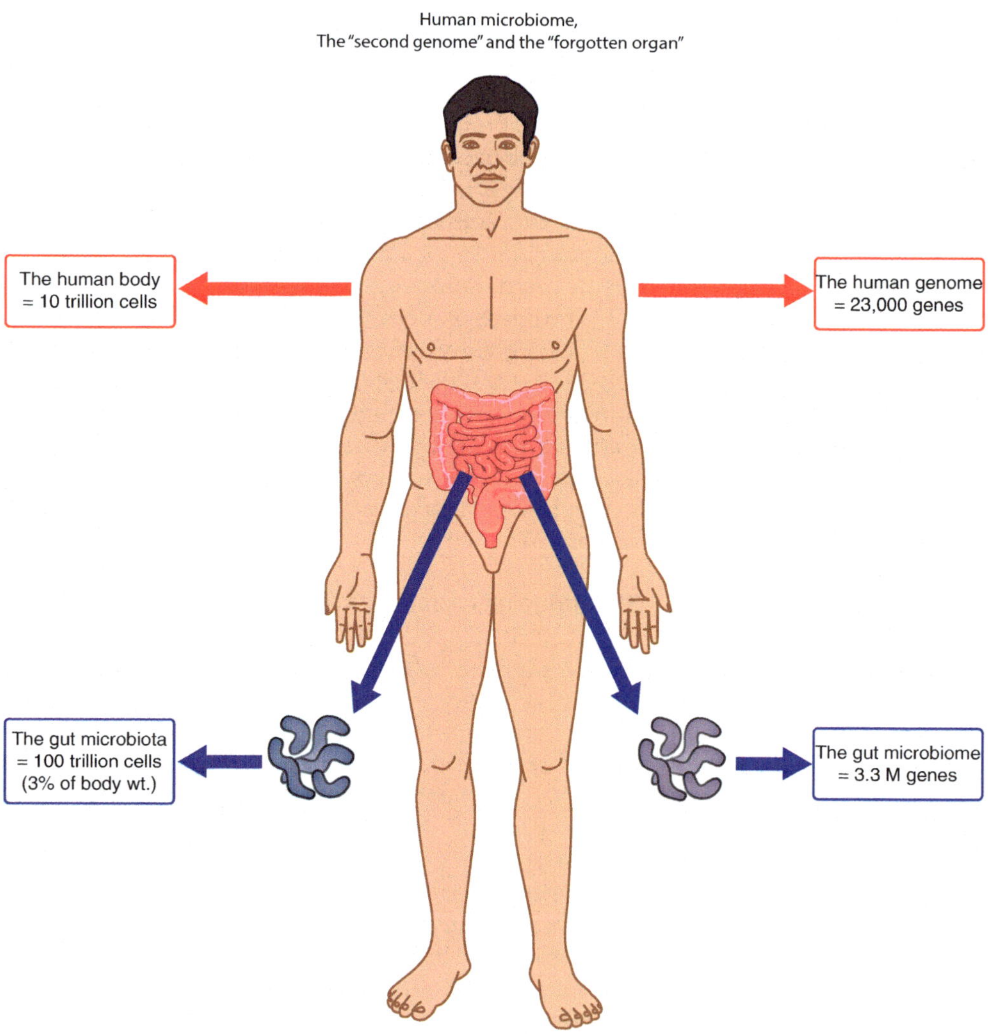

Figure 9.5 ■ The human microbiome emphasizing the gut microbiome. Millions of microbes/cm² on your body. There are more microbes in your intestines than there are human cells in your body

ome under a variety of conditions will provide a better mechanistic understanding of the role of the microbiome in health and disease states and is expected to lead to new diagnostic, prognostic and treatment interventions. There is strong evidence that diet can influence microbiome composition and function. Diet is known to influence the progression and severity of symptoms of pathogenic states such as inflammatory bowel disease, Crohn's disease, ulcerative colitis, some CNS disorders (such as Parkinson's disease and Alzheimer's) and many other immune-mediated and metabolic diseases. The gut microbiome of an obese twin differs from a lean twin. Research will pave the way for new and novel therapeutic strategies to combat these diseases. There is great promise in the dietary manipulation of the gut microbiome as an approach to treat associated disease as well as maintain good health.

The Human Microbiome Project (HMP; https://commonfund.nih.gov/hmp) is sponsored by the U.S. NIH and is dedicated to the study of the human "supraorganism" composed of both human and non-human cells composing the microbiome. The role of human genome polymorphisms in therapeutic outcomes is well established and is discussed in the next section of this chapter on pharmacogenetics and pharmacogenomics. To date, much less is known about the impact of our microbiome or "second genome" genetic polymorphisms in therapeutic outcomes. The microbiome influences the metabolism of drugs and their metabolites (Spanogiannopoulos et al. 2016; Yadav et al. 2017). Orally administered drugs encounter the gut microbiome prior to reaching many host tissues responsible for metabolism and first-pass metabolism. Thus, the goal of true precision medicine cannot be achieved until we better understand our microbial guests.

■ Pharmacogenetics and Pharmacogenomics

It has been noted for decades that patient response to the administration of a drug was highly variable within a diverse patient population. Efficacy as determined in clinical trials is based upon a standard dose range derived from large population studies. Better understanding of the molecular interactions occurring within the pharmacokinetics phase of a drug's action, coupled with new genetics knowledge and then genomic knowledge of the human have advanced us closer to a rational means to optimize drug therapy. Optimization with respect to the patients' genotype, to ensure maximum efficacy with minimal adverse effects, is the goal. Environment, diet, age, lifestyle, and state of health all can influence a person's response to medicines, but understanding an individual's genetic makeup is thought to be the key to creating personalized drugs with greater efficacy and safety. Approaches such as the related pharmacogenetics and pharmacogenomics promise the advent of "precision medicine," in which drugs and drug combinations are optimized for each individual's unique genetic makeup. This chapter will only serve as an introduction, as entire classes are now offered and many books and review articles have been written about pharmacogenetics and pharmacogenomics (Brazeau and Brazeau 2011a; Lee et al. 2014; Zdanowicz 2017).

Single-Nucleotide Polymorphisms (SNPs)

While comparing the base sequences in the DNA of two individuals reveals them to be approximately 99.5% identical, base differences, or polymorphisms, are scattered throughout the genome. The best-characterized human polymorphisms are single-nucleotide polymorphisms (SNPs) occurring approximately once every 1000 bases in the three billion base pair human genome. The DNA sequence variation is a single nucleotide—A, T, C, or G—in the genome difference between members of a species (or between paired chromosomes in an individual). For example, two sequenced DNA fragments from different individuals, AAGTTCCTA to AAGTTC*T*TA, contain a difference in a single nucleotide. Commonly referred to as "snips," these subtle sequence variations account for most of the genetic differences observed among humans. Thus, they can be utilized to determine inheritance of genes in successive generations.

Research suggests that, in general, humans tolerate SNPs as a probable survival mechanism. This tolerance may result because most SNPs occur in noncoding regions of the genome. Identifying SNPs occurring in gene coding regions (cSNPs) and/or regulatory sequences may hold the key for elucidating complex, polygenic diseases such as cancer, heart disease, and diabetes and understanding the differences in response to drug therapy observed in individual patients. Some cSNPs do not result in amino acid substitutions in their gene's protein product(s) due to the degeneracy of the genetic code. These cSNPs are referred to as synonymous cSNPs. Other cSNPs, known as non-synonymous, can produce conservative amino acid changes, such as similarity in side chain charge or size or more significant amino acid substitutions.

While SNPs themselves do not cause disease, their presence can help determine the likelihood that an individual may develop a particular disease or malady. SNPs, when associated with epidemiological and pathological data, can be used to track susceptibilities to common diseases such as cancer, heart disease, and diabetes (Biesecker and Spinner 2013; Li et al. 2017). Biomedical researchers have recognized that discovering SNPs linked to diseases will lead potentially to the identification of new drug targets and diagnostic tests. The identification and mapping of hundreds of thousands of SNPs for use in large-scale association studies may turn the SNPs into biomarkers of disease and/or drug response. Genetic factors such as SNPs are believed to likely influence the etiology of diseases such as hypertension, diabetes, and lipidemias directly and via effects on known risk factors. For example, in the chronic metabolic disease type 2 diabetes, a strong association with obesity and its pathogenesis includes defects of both secretion and peripheral actions of insulin. The association between type 2 diabetes and SNPs in three genes was detected in addition to a cluster of new variants on chromosome 10q. However, heritability values range only from 30 to 70% as type 2 diabetes is obviously a heterogeneous disease etiologically and clinically. Thus, SNPs, in the overwhelming majority of cases, will likely not be indicators of disease development by themselves.

Pharmacogenetics Versus Pharmacogenomics

In simplest terms, pharmacogenomics is the whole genome application of pharmacogenetics, which examines the single gene interactions with drugs. Tremendous advances in biotechnology are causing a dramatic shift in the way new pharmaceuticals are discovered, developed, and monitored during patient use. Pharmacists will utilize the knowledge gained from genomics and proteomics to tailor drug therapy to meet the needs of their individual patients employing the fields of pharmacogenetics and pharmacogenomics (Brazeau and Brazeau 2011a; Lee et al. 2014; Papastergiou et al. 2017; Zdanowicz 2017).

Pharmacogenetics is the study of how an individual's genetic differences influence drug action, usage, and dosing (Drew 2016). A detailed knowledge of a patient's pharmacogenetics in relation to a particular drug therapy may lead to enhanced efficacy and greater safety. Pharmacogenetic analysis may identify the responsive patient population prior to administration, i.e., precision medicine. The field of pharmacogenetics is over 60 years old, but is undergoing renewed, exponential growth at this time. Of particular interest in the field of pharmacogenetics is our understanding of the genetic influences on drug pharmacokinetic profiles such as genetic variations affecting liver enzymes (i.e., cytochrome P450 group) and drug transporter proteins and the genetic influences on drug pharmacodynamic profiles such as the variation in receptor protein expression.

In contrast, pharmacogenomics is linked to the whole genome, not an SNP in a single gene. It is the study of the entire genome of an organism (i.e., human patient), both the expressed and the non-expressed genes in any given physiologic state. Pharmacogenomics combines traditional pharmaceutical sciences with annotated knowledge of genes, proteins, and single-nucleotide polymorphisms. It might be viewed as a logical convergence of the stepwise advances in genomics with the growing field of pharmacogenetics. Incorrectly, the definitions of pharmacogenetics and pharmacogenomics are often used interchangeably. Whatever the definitions, they share the challenge of clinical translation, moving from bench top research to bedside application for patient care.

Genome-Wide Association Studies (GWAS)

The methods of genome-wide association studies (GWAS), also known as whole genome association studies, are powerful tools to identify genetic loci that affect, for instance, drug response or susceptibility to adverse drug reactions (De et al. 2014; Visscher et al. 2017). These studies are an examination of the many genetic variations found in different individuals to determine any association between a variant (genotype) and a biological trait (phenotype). The majority of GWAS typically study associations between SNPs and drug response or SNPs and major disease. While the first GWAS was published only in 2005, they have emerged as important tools and driver in the vision for precision medicine. Challenges have included difficulties identifying the key genetic loci due to two or more genes with small and additive effects on the trait (epistasis), the trait caused by gene mutations at several different chromosomal loci (locus heterogeneity), environmental causes modifying expression of the trait or responsible for the trait, and undetected population structure in the study such as those arising when some study members share a common ancestral heritage (Brazeau and Brazeau 2011b). The practical use of this approach and its introduction into the everyday clinical setting remain a challenge, but will undoubtedly be aided by new next-generation sequencing techniques, enhanced bioinformatics capabilities, and better genomic understanding.

■ On the Path to Precision Medicine: A Brief Introduction

Much of modern medical care decision-making is based upon observations of successful diagnosis and treatment at the larger population level. There is an expectation, however, that health care is starting to undergo a revolutionary change as new genomic and other "OMIC" technologies become available to the clinic that will better predict, diagnose, monitor, and treat disease at the level of the specific patient. A goal is to match individual patients with the most effective and safest drugs and doses.

Genome sequencing and other genomic test are becoming more accessible through clinics, public health systems and direct-to-consumer genomic tests

(Filipski et al. 2017). The market place for direct-to-consumer genomic testing is in flux with several companies recently exiting the market for physician ordered testing and only 23 and Me remaining. Academic medical centers demonstrate the feasibility of routine clinical genotyping as a means of informing pharmacotherapeutic treatment selection in many therapeutic areas especially including oncology and infectious diseases.(Relling and Evans 2015). For example, at St. Jude's Hospital for Children in Memphis Tennessee, they routinely screen a panel of 20 genes that affect about 80 medications that are actionable in the clinic. Likewise, demonstration projects in pharmacogenomics entered pharmacy practice in several settings (Frick et al. 2016). Pharmacy education curricula are evolving to prepare graduates practice in a precision medicine environment. This approach is entirely consistent with the concept of patient-centered care to improve patient outcomes.

Modern genomics, transcriptomics, proteomics, metabolomics, pharmacogenomics, epigenomics (to be discussed later in this chapter), and other technologies, implemented in the clinic in faster and less expensive instrumentation and methodologies, are now being introduced to identify genetic variants, better inform health care providers about their individual patient, tailor evidence-based medical treatment, and suggest rational approaches toward preventative care. The hopes and realities of precision medicine (sometimes referred to as part of "molecular medicine"), pharmacotherapy informed by a patient's individual genomic and proteomic information, are global priorities. As a pharmaceutical biotechnology text, our limited discussion here will focus on precision medicine in a primarily pharmacogenomic and pharmacogenetic context. However, other genomic-type technologies including GWAS, next-generation sequencing, proteomics, and metabolomics will be crucial for the successful implementation of precision medicine. The hope is that "OMIC" science will bring predictability to the optimization of drug selection and drug dosage to assure safe and effective pharmacotherapy (Fig. 9.6).

Personalized Medicine, P4 Medicine, and Precision Medicine

One of the early rewards expected from the completion of the HGP was to pinpoint specific genes of the ~23,000 discovered that caused common diseases. While most diseases are now recognized as polygenic with more complex systems interactions than single gene diseases, the data acquired from the HGP has the potential to forever transform health care. Genome-based medicine has been called personalized medicine or molecular medicine and is the next logical step in the evolution of medicine and direct patient care. The in-depth knowledge of an individual's genetics, when coupled with molecular-level understanding of disease mechanisms, and biological systems characteristics of wellness can focus a specific patient's health care in a "personalized" way.

Leroy Hood of the Institute for Systems Biology coined the term "P4 Medicine." He and his colleagues recognized that medicine was undergoing a revolution as a result of the rapid advances in OMICS technologies and the wealth of information being generated (Cesario et al. 2014; Sagner et al. 2017). One area of OMICS study, systems biology (described in greater detail later in this chapter) was starting to focus on the incredible complexity of biological systems, both normal and diseased. Taking a systems approach to the study of disease coupled with OMIC technologies allows an individual to single genes, single molecules, single cells, single organs be analyzed as single genes, single molecules, single cells, single organs, etc. Recognizing that the current medical framework used to guide health care and manage chronic disease is largely ineffective, they proposed a new way to personalize medicine. A medicine paradigm that is *Preventative, Predictive, Personalized and Participatory (i.e., P4)* would hold great promise to improve patient health outcomes by harnessing modern biotechnologies and a better understanding of the mechanisms of disease into evidence-based health interventions.

The term "Precision Medicine" has become commonly used at the time of release of the 5th edition of this textbook and effectively is interchangeable with personalized medicine, molecular medicine and to some extent, P4 medicine. The goal of precision medicine is to enable clinicians to employ the most appropriate course of action for each individual patient managing the extreme complexity of each patient given all of the tools now available in the health care system: OMICS technology data, disease mechanisms, the electronic health record, public health information, big data, etc. (Aronson and Rehm 2015; Beckmann and Lew 2016). Thus, OMICS data, histopathological profiling of a patient's disease state together with the potential response of a particular patient to a particular treatment regimen all influence medical decisions. To be successful, precision medicine must be conducted in an ecosystem that is a continuously learning health care system (described earlier in this chapter) and links clinicians, medical laboratories, research enterprises and health information systems. Precision medicine has the potential to profoundly impact the practice of medicine at all levels (ambulatory and primary care, secondary care, tertiary care and clinical education). Possibly the best way to consider precision medicine is to consider patients no longer "passengers' on an airplane, but now they are "co-pilots."

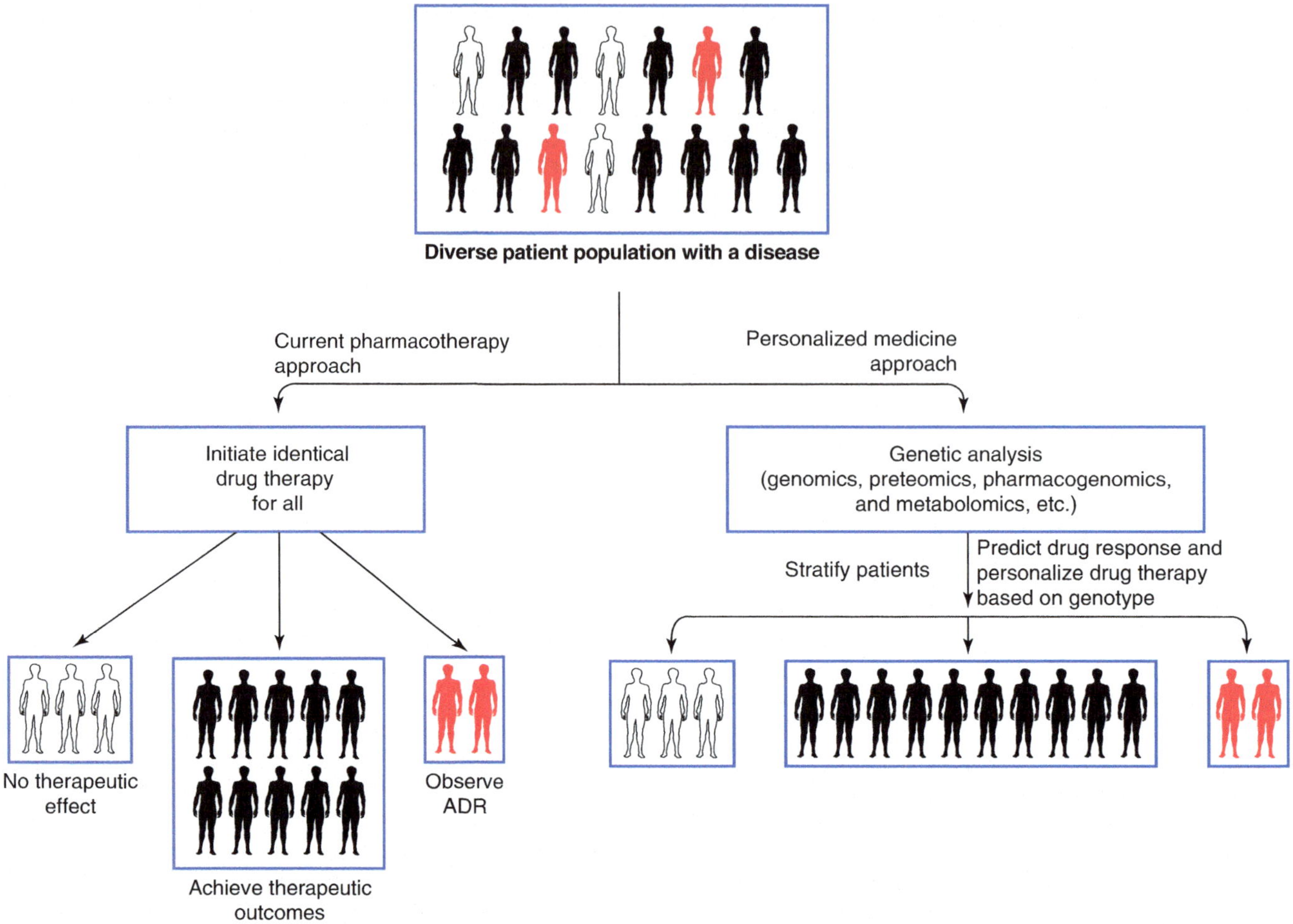

Figure 9.6 ■ The role of "OMIC" technologies in precision medicine

Implementing Precision Medicine

Optimized precision medicine utilizing pharmacogenomic knowledge would not only spot disease before it occurs in a patient or detect a critical variant that will influence treatment but should increase drug efficacy upon pharmacotherapy and reduce drug toxicity. Also, it would facilitate the drug development process (see Fig. 9.1) including improving clinical development outcomes, reducing overall cost of drug development, and leading to development of new diagnostic tests that impact on therapeutic decisions (Hollebecque et al. 2014; Hyman et al. 2015). Individualized optimized pharmacotherapy would first require a detailed genetic analysis of a patient, assembling a comprehensive list of SNPs. Pharmacogenomic tests most likely in the form of microarray technology and based upon clinically validated biomarkers would be administered to pre-identify responsive patients before dosing with a specific agent. Examples of such microarray-based diagnostics are the FDA-approved AmpliChip P450 from Roche to screen a patient for the presence of any of 27 SNPs in CYP2D6 and CYP2C19, the Infiniti 2C9 & VKORC1 Multiplex Assay for warfarin therapy from AutoGenomics, and the Pathwork Tissue of Origin test of 15 common malignant tumor types to better focus treatment options. The impact of the patient's SNPs on the use of new or existing drugs would thus be predicted and individualized drug therapy would be identified that assures maximal efficacy and minimal toxicity (Hayes et al. 2014).

Precision medicine would also require knowledge of an individual patient's genomic profile to help identify potential drug responders and nonresponders. This might be accomplished by testing for the presence or absence of critical biomarkers that may be associated with prediction of response rates. The US FDA provides an online list of all FDA-approved drugs with pharmacogenomic information in their labels (black boxes). Some, but not all, of the labels include specific actions to be taken based on genetic information. The drug labels contain information on genomic biomarkers that may be predictive of drug exposure and clinical response rate, risk of adverse reactions, genotype-specific dosing, susceptibility to a specific mechanism of drug action, or polymorphic drug target and disposition genes. Rather than reproducing this table in whole or part in this text, the reader may access it in its constantly updated form at https://www.fda.gov/Drugs/ScienceResearch/ucm572698.htm (Accessed Jan 25, 2018)

It is well understood that beyond genomics and proteomics, a patient's behavioral and environmental factors influence clinical outcomes and susceptibility to disease. Emerging fields of nutrigenomics and envirogenomics are studying these additional layers of complexity. Precision medicine will become especially important in cases where the cost of testing is less than either the cost of the drug or the cost of correcting adverse drug reactions caused by the drug. Pharmaceutical care would begin by identifying a patient's susceptibility to a disease, then administering the right drug to the right patient at the right time. For example, the monoclonal antibody trastuzumab (Herceptin) is a personalized breast cancer therapy specifically targeted to the HER2 gene product (25–30% of human breast cancers overexpress the human epidermal growth factor receptor, HER2 protein). Exhibiting reduced side effects as compared to standard chemotherapy due to this protein target specificity, trastuzumab is not prescribed to treat a breast cancer patient unless the patient has first tested positive for HER2 overexpression. While currently an immunohistochemical assay, not a sophisticated DNA microarray assay, the example shows the power of such future tests.

The success of targeted therapy for precision medicine has fostered the concept that the era of the blockbuster drug may be over and will be replaced by the "niche buster" drug, a highly effective medicine individualized for a small group of responding patients identified by genomic and proteomic techniques. The market for precision medicine is expected to increase from $39 billion U.S. in 2015 to $94 billion U.S. by 2024 (Global Market Insights 2017). Also, while numerous articles predicted that pharmacogenomics would revolutionize medicine, the initial predictions have not been lived up to the hype due to statistical, scientific, and commercial hurdles. With more than 11 million SNP positions believed to be present in the human population, large-scale detection of genetic variation holds the key to successful precision medicine (Ahmed et al. 2016; Chambliss and Chan 2016). Correlation of environmental factors, behavioral factors, genomic and proteomic factors (including pharmacogenomic and metabolomic factors), and phenotypical observables across large populations remains a daunting data-intensive challenge. Yet, pharmacogenetics and pharmacogenomics are having an impact on modern medicine.

Human Genomic Variation Affecting Drug Pharmacokinetics

Genetic variation associated with drug metabolism and drug transport, processes resulting from products of gene expression (metabolic enzymes and transport proteins, respectively) play a critical role in determining the concentration of a drug in its active form at the site of its action and also at the site of its possible toxic action(s). Thus, pharmacogenetic and pharmacogenomic analysis of drug metabolism and drug transport is important to a better clinical understanding of and prediction of the effect of genetic variation on drug effectiveness and safety (Patel 2015; Bitto et al. 2016; Hertz and Rae 2016).

It is well recognized that specific drug metabolic phenotypes may cause adverse drug reactions. For instance, some patients lack an enzymatically active form, have a diminished level, or possess a modified version of CYP2D6 (a cytochrome P450 allele) and will metabolize certain classes of pharmaceutical agents differently to other patients expressing the native active enzyme. All pharmacogenetic polymorphisms examined to date differ in frequency among racial and ethnic groups. For example, CYP2D6 enzyme deficiencies may occur in $\leq$2% Asian patients, $\leq$5% black patients, and $\leq$11% white patients (Chaudhry et al. 2014). A diagnostic test to detect CYP2D6 deficiency could be used to identify patients that should not be administered drugs metabolized predominantly by CYP2D6. Table 9.2 provides some selected examples of common drug metabolism polymorphisms and their pharmacokinetic consequences.

With the burgeoning understanding of the genetics of warfarin metabolism, warfarin anticoagulation therapy is becoming a leader in pharmacogenetic analysis for pharmacokinetic prediction (Beitelshees et al. 2015; Roden 2016). Adverse drug reactions (ADRs) for warfarin account for 15% of all ADRs in the USA, second only to digoxin. Warfarin dose is adjusted with the goal of achieving an INR (International Normalized Ratio = ratio of patient's prothrombin time as compared to that of a normal control) of 2.0–3.0. The clinical challenge is to limit hemorrhage, the primary ADR, while achieving the optimal degree of protection against thromboembolism. Deviation in the INR has been shown to be the strongest risk factor for bleeding complications. The major routes of metabolism of warfarin are by CYP2C9 and CYP3A4. Some of the compounds, which have been identified to influence positively or negatively warfarin's INR, include cimetidine, clofibrate, propranolol, celecoxib (a competitive inhibition of CYP2C9), fluvoxamine (an inhibitor of several CYP enzymes), various antifungals and antibiotics (e.g.,

Enzyme	Common variant	Potential consequence
CYP1A2	CYP1A2*1F	Increased inducibility
CYP1A2	CYP1A2*1K	Decreased metabolism
CYP2A6	CYP2A6*2	Decreased metabolism
CYP2B6	CYP2B6*5	No effect
CYP2B6	CYP2B6*6	Increased metabolism
CYP2B6	CYP2B6*7	Increased metabolism
CYP2C8	CYP2C8*2	Decreased metabolism
CYP2C9	CYP2C9*2	Altered affinity
CYP2C9	CYP2C9*3	Decreased metabolism
CYP2D6	CYP2D6*10	Decreased metabolism
CYP2D6	CYP2D6*17	Decreased metabolism
CYP2E1	CYP2E1*2	Decreased metabolism
CYP3A7	CYP3A7*1C	Increased metabolism
Flavin-containing monooxygenase 3	FMO3*2	Decreased metabolism
Flavin-containing monooxygenase 3	FMO3*4	Decreased metabolism
Data from references noted in the Pharmacogenomics section of Chap. 9		

Table 9.2 ■ Some selected examples of common drug metabolism polymorphisms and their pharmacokinetic consequences

miconazole, fluconazole, erythromycin), omeprazole, alcohol, ginseng, and garlic. Researchers have determined that the majority of individual patient variation observed clinically in response to warfarin therapy is genetic in nature, influenced by the genetic variability of metabolizing enzymes, vitamin K cycle enzymes, and possibly transporter proteins. The CYP2C9 genotype polymorphisms alone explain about 10 % of the variability observed in the warfarin maintenance dose. Figure 9.7 shows the proteins involved in warfarin action and indicates the pharmacogenomic variants that more significantly influence warfarin therapy optimal outcome.

Studies at both the basic research and clinical level involve the effect of drug transport proteins on the pharmacokinetic profile of a drug. Some areas of active study of the effect of genetic variation on clinical effectiveness include efflux transporter proteins (for bioavailability, CNS exposure, and tumor resistance) and neurotransmitter uptake transporters (as valid drug targets). Novel transporter proteins are still being identified as a result of the HGP and subsequent proteomic research. More study is needed on the characterization of expression, regulation, and functional properties of known and new transporter proteins to better assess the potential for prediction of altered drug response based on transporter genotypes.

Human Genomic Variation Affecting Drug Pharmacodynamics

Genomic variation such as factors influencing the expression of the protein target directly affects not only the pharmacokinetic profile of drugs, it also strongly influences the pharmacodynamic profile of drugs. Targets include the drug receptor involved in the response as well as the proteins associated with disease risk, pathogenesis, and/or toxicity including infectious disease. There are increasing numbers of prominent examples of inherited polymorphisms influencing drug pharmacodynamics. To follow on the warfarin example above (see Fig. 9.7), the major component of individual patient variation observed clinically in response to anticoagulant therapy is genetic in nature. However, the CYP2C9 genotype polymorphisms alone only explain about 10% of the variability observed in the warfarin maintenance dose. Warfarin effectiveness is also influenced by the genetic variability of vitamin K cycle enzymes. The drug receptor for warfarin is generally recognized as vitamin K epoxide reductase, the enzyme that recycles vitamin K in the coagulation cascade. Vitamin K epoxide reductase complex1 (VKORC1) has been determined to be highly variant with as much as 50% of the clinical variability observed for warfarin resulting from polymorphisms of this enzyme.

Associations have been implicated between drug response and genetic variations in targets for a variety of drugs including antidepressants (G-protein β3), antipsychotics (dopamine D2, D3, D4; serotonin 5HT2A, 5HT2C), sulfonylureas (sulfonylurea receptor protein), and anesthetics (ryanodine receptor) (Ahles and Engelhardt 2014; Thompson et al. 2014). In addition, similar associations have been studied for drug toxicity and disease polymorphisms including abacavir (major histocompatability proteins; risk of hypersensitivity), cisapride and terfenadine (HERG, KvLQT1, Mink, MiRP1; increased risk of drug-induced torsade de pointes), and oral contraceptives (prothrombin and factor V; increased deep vein thrombosis). Likewise, similar associations for efficacy are known such as statins (apolipoprotein E; enhanced survival prolongation with simvastatin) and tacrine (apolipoprotein E; clinical improvement of Alzheimer's symptoms).

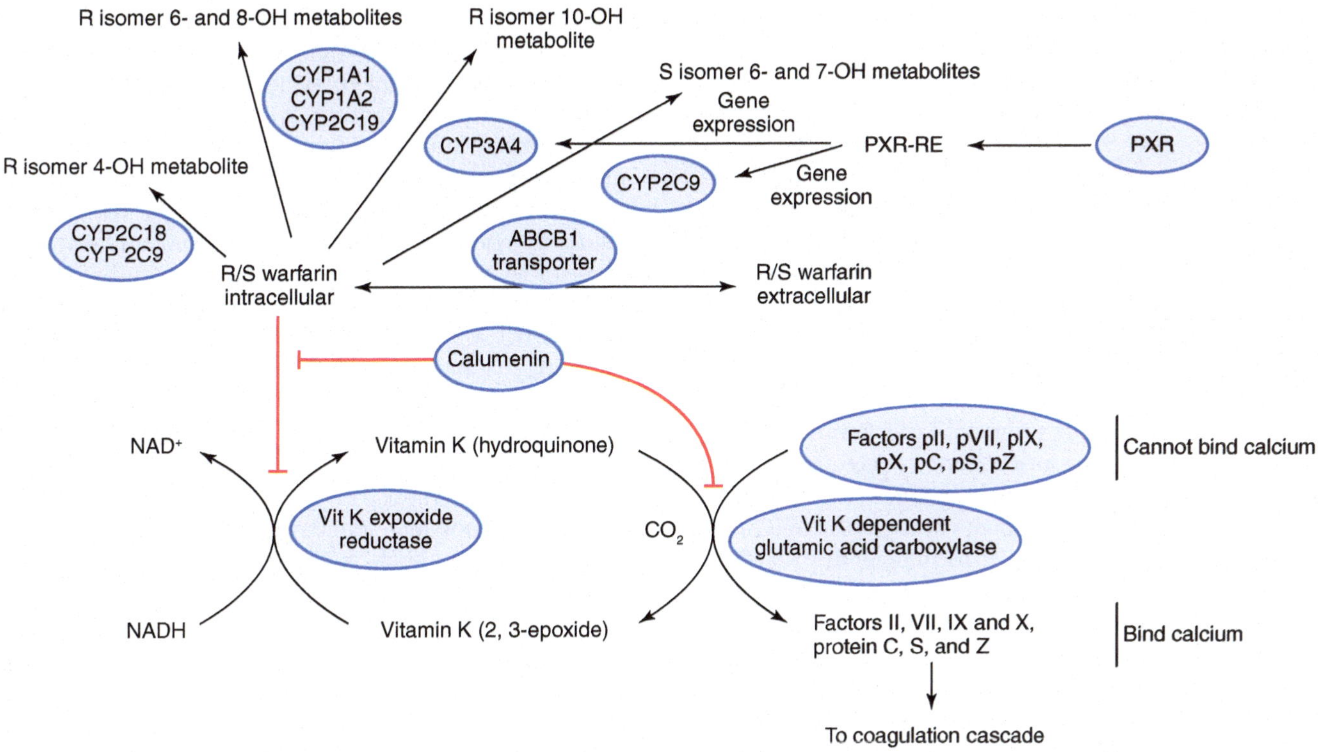

Figure 9.7 ■ Critical pharmacogenomic variants affecting warfarin drug action and ADR

Value of Precision Medicine in Disease

Due to the intimate role of genetics in carcinogenesis, precision medicine is rapidly becoming a success story in oncology based on genetic profiling using proteomic analyses of tumor biopsies (Sabatier et al. 2014; Blumenthal et al. 2016; Prasad et al. 2016). As described above, targeted cancer therapies such as trastuzumab (Herceptin) are successful and are viewed as the way of the future. Also, clinically important polymorphisms predict increased toxicity in patients with cancer being treated with chemotherapeutic drugs, for example, 6-mercaptopurine (thiopurine methyltransferase *2, *3A, and *3C variants), 5-fluorouracil (5-FU) (dihydropyrimidine dehydrogenase *2A variant), and irinotecan (UGT1A1*28 allele; FDA-approved Invader UGT1A1 Molecular Assay diagnostic available to screen for presence of this allele associated with irinotecan toxicity). Likewise, clinically important pharmacogenetics predicts efficacy in oncology patients treated with 5-FU (thymidylate synthase *2 and *3C variants).

A classic application of pharmacogenetics is our present understanding of the potentially fatal hematopoietic toxicity that occurs in some patients administered standard doses of the antileukemic agents azathioprine, mercaptopurine, and thioguanine (Chouchana et al. 2014). These drugs are metabolized by the enzyme thiopurine methyltransferase (TPMT) to the inactive S-methylated products. Gene mutations (polymorphisms) may occur in as many as 11 % of patients resulting in decreased TPMT-mediated metabolism of the thiopurine drugs. A diagnostic test for TPMT is now available and used clinically. Identified patients with poor TPMT metabolism may need their drug dose lowered 10 to 15-fold. Mechanisms of multidrug resistance to cancer drugs are influenced by genetic differences. A number of polymorphisms in the MDR-1 gene coding for P-glycoprotein, the transmembrane protein drug efflux pump responsible for multidrug resistance, have been identified. One, known as the T/T genotype and correlated with decreased intestinal expression of P-glycoprotein and increased drug bioavailability, has an allele frequency of 88% in African-American populations, yet only approximately 50% in Caucasian-American populations. Pharmacogenetic and pharmacogenomic analysis of patients is being actively studied in many disease states. However, a detailed discussion goes beyond what this introduction may provide. The reader is encouraged to read further in the pharmacogenetic/pharmacogenomic-related references available, some provided at the end of this chapter.

Challenges in Precision Medicine

There are many keys to success for precision medicine that hinge on continued scientific advancement. While it is great for the advancement of the OMIC sciences, some have questioned how good it is for individual patients, particularly if they are very health challenged, at this stage of its development due to potential exaggerated claims in the public press falling short of the predictive, preventative and participatory health care paradigm promised. Also, modern medicine may lack proven prevention interventions necessary to address certain genomic traits once discovered (van Rooij et al. 2012; Alyass et al. 2015; Beckmann and Lew 2016). There are also economic, societal, and ethical issues that must be addressed to successfully implement genetic testing-based individualized pharmacotherapy (Joly et al. 2014). It is fair to state that most drugs will not be effective in all patients all of the time. Thus, the pressure of payers to move from a "payment for product" to a "payment for clinically significant health outcomes" model is reasonable. The use of OMIC health technologies and health informatics approaches to stratify patient populations for drug effectiveness and drug safety is a laudable goal. However, the technologies are currently quite expensive and the resulting drug response predictability is now just being validated clinically. Cost-effectiveness and cost-benefit analyses are limited at this date (Hatz et al. 2014). Also, the resulting environment created by these technologies in the context of outcomes expectations and new drug access/reimbursement models will give rise to a new pharmaceutical business paradigm that is still evolving and not well understood.

Epigenetics and Epigenomics

DNA is the heritable biomolecule that contains the genetic information resulting in phenotype from parent to offspring. Modern genomics, GWAS and SNP analyses, confirm this and identify genetic variants that may be associated with a different phenotype. However, genome-level information alone does not generally predict phenotype at an individual level (Daxinger and Whitelaw 2012). For instance, researchers and clinicians have known for some time that an individual's response to a drug is affected by their genetic makeup (DNA sequence, genotype) and a set of disease and environmental characteristics working alone or in concert to determine that response. Research in animal models has suggested that in addition to DNA sequence, there are a number of other "levels" of information that influence transcription of genomic information. As you are aware, every person's body contains trillions of cells, all of which have essentially the same genome and, therefore, the same genes. Yet some cells are optimized for development into one or more of the 200+ specialized cells that make up our bodies: muscles, bones, brain, etc. For this to transpire from within the same genome, some genes must be turned on or off at different points of cell development in different cell types to affect gene expression, protein production, and cell differentiation, growth, and function. There is a rapidly evolving field of research known as epigenetics (or epigenomics) that can be viewed as a conduit between genotype and phenotype (Inbar-Feigenberg et al. 2013; Prokopuk et al. 2015). Epigenetics literally means "above genetics or over the genetic sequence." It is the factor or factors that influence cell behavior by means other than via a direct effect on the genetic machinery. Epigenetic regulation includes DNA methylation and covalent histone modifications (Fig. 9.8). They result without heritable changes in DNA sequence. Epigenomics is the merged science of genomics and epigenetics (Raghavachari 2012). Functionally, epigenetics acts to regulate gene expression, gene silencing during genomic imprinting, apoptosis, X-chromosome inactivation, and tissue-specific gene activation (such as maintenance of stem cell pluripotency).

The more we understand epigenetics and epigenomics, the more we are likely to understand those phenotypic traits that are not a result of genetic information alone. This should be facilitated by developments in single-cell epigenomics (Bheda and Schneider 2014; Kelsey et al. 2017). Single-cell epigenomics allows for the study of cellular heterogeneity at different time scales to effectively record a cell's past and predict its future functionality. Epigenetics is becoming relevant for public health (Rozek et al. 2014). Epigenetics/epigenomics may also explain low association predictors found in some pharmacogenetic/pharmacogenomic studies. Etiology of disease, such as cancer, likely involves both genetic variants and epigenetic modifications that could result from environmental effects (Dawson and Kouzarides 2012). Age also likely influences epigenetic modifications as studies of identical twins show greater differences in global DNA methylation in older rather than younger sets of twins (Feinberg et al. 2010). Abnormal epigenetic regulation is likely a feature of complex diseases such as diabetes, cancer, and heart disease (Chen and Zhang 2011; Raciti et al. 2014). Therefore, epigenetics targets are being explored for drug design, especially those observed in cancer (Schweiger et al. 2013). The first generation of FDA-approved epigenetics-based drugs is available with two DNA demethylating agents (5-azacytidine and decitabine) and two histone deacetylase (HDAC) inhibitors (vorinostat and romidepsin). These have been approved mainly for the treatment of blood cancers, in particularly myelodysplastic syndromes (MDS).

One of the most studied and best understood molecular mechanisms of epigenetic regulation is methylation of cytosine residues at specific positions in the DNA molecule (Fig. 9.8). Another mechanism of

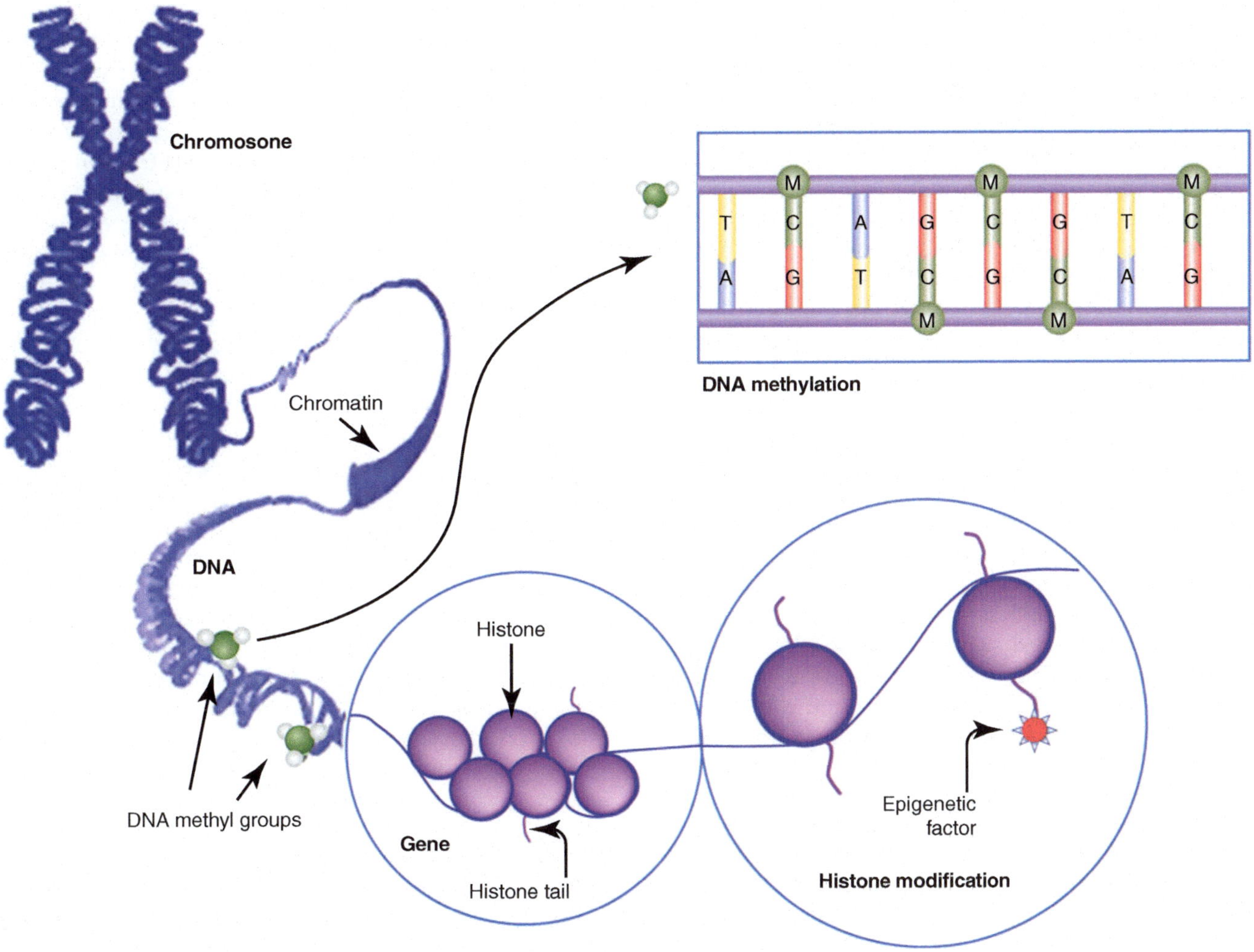

Figure 9.8 ■ Epigenetic regulation via DNA methylation, histone modifications, and chromatin structure

epigenomic control appears to occur at the level of chromatin. In the cell, DNA is wrapped around 8 different histone proteins to form chromatin. Packaging of DNA into chromatin can render large regions of the DNA inaccessible and prevent processes such as DNA transcription from occurring. Epigenetic regulation of histone proteins can be by chemical modification including acetylation, methylation, sumoylation and ubiquitylation. Each can cause structural changes in chromatin affecting DNA accessibility. Non-protein-coding RNAs, known as ncRNAs, have also been shown to contribute to epigenetic regulation as have mRNAs which can be processed and participate in various interference pathways (Collins and Schonfeld 2011).

■ Toxicogenomics

Toxicogenomics, related to pharmacogenomics, combines toxicology, genetics, molecular biology, and environmental health to elucidate the response of living organisms to stressful environments or xenobiotic agents based upon their genetic makeup (Chen et al. 2012). First described in 1999, the field is in its infancy, yet emerging rapidly. While toxicogenomics studies how the genome responds to toxic exposures, pharmacogenetics studies how an individual's genetic makeup affects his/her response to environmental stresses and toxins such as carcinogens, neurotoxins, and reproductive toxins. Toxicogenomics can be very useful in drug discovery and development as new drug candidates can be screened through a combination of gene expression profiling and toxicology to understand gene response, identify general mechanisms of toxicity, and possibly predict drug safety at a better cost (Khan et al. 2014). There have been suggestions that toxicogenomics may decrease the time needed for toxicological investigations of new drug candidates and reduce both cost and animal usage versus conventional toxicity studies.

Genomic techniques utilized in toxicogenomic studies include gene expression level profiling, SNP analysis of the genetic variation, proteomics, and/or metabolomic methods so that gene expression, protein production, and metabolite production may be studied (Raghavachari 2012). The rapid growth in next-generation DNA sequencing capability may drive a conversion from microarrays now most commonly used for SNP analysis) to NGS technology.

Toxicogenomic studies attempt to discover associations between the development of drug toxicities and genotype. Clinicians and researchers are attempting to correlate genetic variation in one population to the manifestations of toxicity in other populations to identify and then to predict adverse toxicological effects in clinical trials so that suitable biomarkers for these adverse effects can be developed (Chen et al. 2014). Using such methods, it would then theoretically possible to test an individual patient for his or her susceptibility to these adverse effects before prescribing a medication. Patients that would show the marker for an adverse effect would be switched to a different drug. Therefore, toxicogenomics will become increasingly more powerful in predicting toxicity as new biomarkers are identified and validated. Much of the new toxicogenomic technology is developing in the pharmaceutical industry and other corporate laboratories.

■ Other "OMIC" Technologies

Pharmaceutical scientists and pharmacists may hear about other "OMIC" technologies in which the "OMIC" terms derive from the application of modern genomic techniques to the study of various biological properties and processes. For example, interactomics is the data-intensive broad system study of the interactome, which is the interaction among proteins and other molecules within a cell. Proteogenomics has been used as a broadly encompassing term to describe the merging of genomics, proteomics, small molecules, and informatics. Cellomics has been defined as the study of gene function and the proteins they encode in living cells utilizing light microscopy and especially digital imaging fluorescence microscopy. The field of optogenetics is used by neuroscientists to turn on and off neurons selectively. This combination of genetics and optics utilizes visible light to control well-defined events in cells in living tissues that have been genetically modified to express light-sensitive ion channel, ion pump, or G-Protein coupled receptor.

■ "OMICS" Integrating Technology: Systems Biology

The Human Genome Project (HGP) and the development of bioinformatics technologies have catalyzed fundamental changes in the practice of modern biology and helped unveil a remarkable amount of information about many organisms and their complexity. Biology has become an information science defining all the elements in a complex biological system, simultaneously measuring thousands of data points and placing them in a database for comparative interpretation. As seen in Fig. 9.2, the hierarchy of information collection goes well beyond the biodata contained in the genetic code that is transcribed and translated. The heart of systems biology involves a generally complex interactive system with insightful views of cells, organisms and populations. This research area is often described as a noncompetitive or precompetitive technology by the pharmaceutical industry because it is believed to be a foundational technology that must be better developed to be successful at the competitive technology of drug discovery and development. It is the study of the interactions between the components of a biological system and how these interactions give rise to the function and behavior of that system (Schneider 2014; Karahalil 2016). Systems biology is essential for our understanding of how all the individual parts of intricate biological networks are organized and function in living cells. The biological system may involve enzymes and metabolites in a metabolic pathway or other interacting biological molecules affecting a biological process. Molecular biologists have spent the past 60+ years teasing apart cellular pathways down to the molecular level. Characterized by a cycle of theory, computational modeling, and experiments to quantitatively describe cells or cell processes, systems biology is a data-intensive endeavor that results in a conceptual framework for the analysis and understanding of complex biological systems in varying contexts (Eddy et al. 2013). Statistical mining, data alignment, probabilistic and mathematical modeling, and data visualization into networks are among the mathematical models employed to integrate the data and assemble the systems network (Fluck and Hofmann-Apitius 2014). New measurements are stored with existing data, including extensive functional annotations, in molecular databases, and model assembly provides libraries of network models.

As the biological interaction networks are extremely complex, so are graphical representations of these networks. After years of research, a set of guidelines known as the Systems Biology Graphical Notation (SBGN) has been drafted by a community of biochemists, modelers and computer scientists and is generally accepted to be the standard for graphical representation by all researchers. These standards, very similar to the block diagrams used by electrical engineers are designed to facilitate the interchange of systems biology information and storage. Due to the complexity of these diagrams depending on the interactions examined and the level of understanding, a figure related to systems biology has not been included in this chapter. However, the reader is referred to the following website authored by the SBGN organization for several excellent examples of complex systems biology-derived protein interaction networks: http://sbgn.github.io/sbgn/examples. The inability to visualize the complexity of biological systems has in the past impeded the identification and validation of new and novel drug targets. The accepted SBGN standards facilitate the efforts of pharmaceutical scientists to validate new and novel targets for drug design.

Since the objective is a model of all the interactions in a system, the experimental techniques that most suit systems biology are those that are system-wide and attempt to be as complete as possible. High-throughput "OMIC" technologies such as genomics, epigenomics, transcriptomics, proteomics, pharmacogenomics, metabolomics, microbiomics and toxicogenomics are used to collect quantitative data for the construction and validation of systems models. Pharmaceutical and clinical end points include systems level biomarkers, genetic risk factors, aspects of precision medicine, and drug target identification (Schneider and Klabunde 2013; Ebhardt et al. 2015; Medina 2013). In the future, application of systems biology approaches to drug discovery promises to have a profound impact on patient-centered medical practice, permitting a comprehensive evaluation of underlying predisposition to disease, disease diagnosis, and disease progression. Also, realization of precision medicine and systems medicine will require new analytical approaches such as systems biology to decipher extraordinarily large, and extraordinarily noisy, data sets.

"OMICS" Enabling Technology: Genome Editing (Also See Chap. 16)

Since the discovery of DNA's overall structure in 1953, the world's scientific community has rapidly gained a detailed knowledge of the genetic information encoded by the DNA of a cell or organism and have been correlating this structure with biological function. The exact base pair sequence of the genome, its genotype that includes the entire collection of genes and all other functional and nonfunctional DNA sequences in the nucleus of an organism, has a direct observable impact on the function of the organism or its phenotype.

In today's biology, genome editing (sometimes called genome engineering) makes specific changes to the DNA of a cell or organism and observes its impact. Genome editing effectively also occurs naturally in organisms including humans via endogenous DNA repair mechanisms (i.e., HDR, homologous directed repair; and NHEJ, non-homologous end-joining; natural mechanisms that repairs harmful breaks that occur in DNA) and the modifications of DNA that occur as a result of epigenetics. Researchers have wanted to modify DNA sequence since DNA's discovery to study the correlation of genomic structure to protein structure and to function. One early approach at editing a DNA sequence was site-directed mutagenesis, also called site-specific mutagenesis or oligonucleotide-directed mutagenesis. Site-directed mutagenesis at a single amino acid position in an engineered protein is called a point mutation. Therefore, site-directed mutagenesis techniques can aid in the examination at the molecular level of the relationship of protein 3D structure (resulting from a transcribed and translated mutated DNA sequence) and the function of the resulting new protein. Since the 1980s, researchers have used the process of HDR to exchange endogenous genomic DNA with exogenous donor DNA with varying success.

Key to genome editing is the ability to selectively and predictively modify the DNA sequence of the target organism an assure the integrity of the resulting edits. Major advances were achieved in the pioneering experiments using yeast meganucleases, a naturally occurring enzyme and engineered versions that can recognize and cut double-stranded DNA sequences of >14 base pairs. There has been explosive development in genome editing in the last decade for DNA targeted gene deletions, integrations, or modifications with the fundamental shift from yeast meganucleases to the latest prokaryotic nucleases used for precise genome manipulation. Genome editing nucleases are engineered enhanced nuclease enzymes or "sequence-specific molecular scissors" based upon native enzymes that specifically cut double stranded DNA in the target cell. They currently belong to one of three known nuclease categories: zinc-*f*inger *n*ucleases (ZFN; key to improved transgenic animal production and discussed later in this chapter), *t*ranscription *a*ctivator-*l*ike *e*ffector *n*ucleases (TALEN), and *c*lustered *r*egularly *i*nterspaced *s*hort *p*alindromic *r*epeats (CRISPR) and their associated proteins (such as Cas9). Genome editing nuclease-mediated mutagenesis can occur exogenously or endogenously if the nuclease targeting the user's gene of interest is delivered into a parental cell line, either by transfection, electroporation or viral vector delivery.

Applications of genome editing methodologies are extensive and include cell-line optimization (i.e., creation of cell lines that produce higher yields of targeted proteins including antibodies), functional genomics and target validation in drug discovery (i.e., creation of gene knockouts in multiple cell lines, the complete knockout of genes not amenable to RNAi), and cell-based screening (i.e., creation of knock-in cell lines with promoters, fusion tags or reporters integrated into endogenous genes. Unlocking the secrets of the human genome editing and improving upon specificity of the DNA cuts and repair have many implications including a paradigm shift in medical research and clinical practice toward better disease understanding and taxonomy, and true precision medicine at the molecular level. These genome editing techniques can introduce unintended genomic alterations cleaving DNA at an off-target site. Thus, genome editing is a very powerful technology that has also far-reaching economic, bioethical, and national security implications. It is expected that genome editing "drugs," enzyme systems that selectively bind, cleave and enable the direct editing of a specific DNA sequence, based upon these technologies and delivered into a cell in vivo, will be entering clinical trials soon.

The mechanism by which the nuclease genome editing tools including ZFN, TALEN and CRISPR tools can target and cleave specific double stranded DNA sequences are generally analogous with differences in binding recognition, associated proteins, specificity and ease of use. Figure 9.9 provides a very simple generalization of this analogous genome editing mechanism to facilitate understanding. However, there is an important difference that has vaulted CRISPR tools into the forefront of genome editing. Whereas ZFN and TALEN bind to DNA through a direct protein-DNA interaction, requiring the protein to be redesigned for each new target DNA site, the CRISPR-Cas system achieves target specificity through a small RNA that can easily be swapped for other RNAs targeting new sites.

Genome Editing Improvement with Zinc-Finger Nucleases and TALEN

Zinc finger nucleases (ZFNs) are zinc containing proteins that occur in several transcription factors (Carroll 2011; Gaj et al. 2013; Kim and Kim 2014). They are used in genome editing as engineered DNA-binding enzymes that enable targeted editing of the genome by creating double-strand breaks in DNA at user-specified locations. Double-strand breaks are important for site-specific mutagenesis as they stimulate the cell's endogenous DNA-repair mechanisms (homologous recombination and non-homologous end joining). Meganucleases had a distinct disadvantage because they cut the DNA strand at a specific location (specific sequence of base pairs) making them very selective. Unfortunately, there was little chance of finding or engineering the exact meganuclease requisite to cut a specific DNA sequence. The key discovery was finding a nuclease whose DNA recognition site and cleaving site were separate from each other. ZFN, TALEN and CRISPR meet this architecture. Thus, all three technologies are non-specific DNA cutting enzymes which can then be linked to specific DNA sequence recognizing peptides such as zinc fingers, transcription activator-like effectors (TALEs) and proteins such as Cas9. Scientists have identified a large number of zinc fingers that rec-

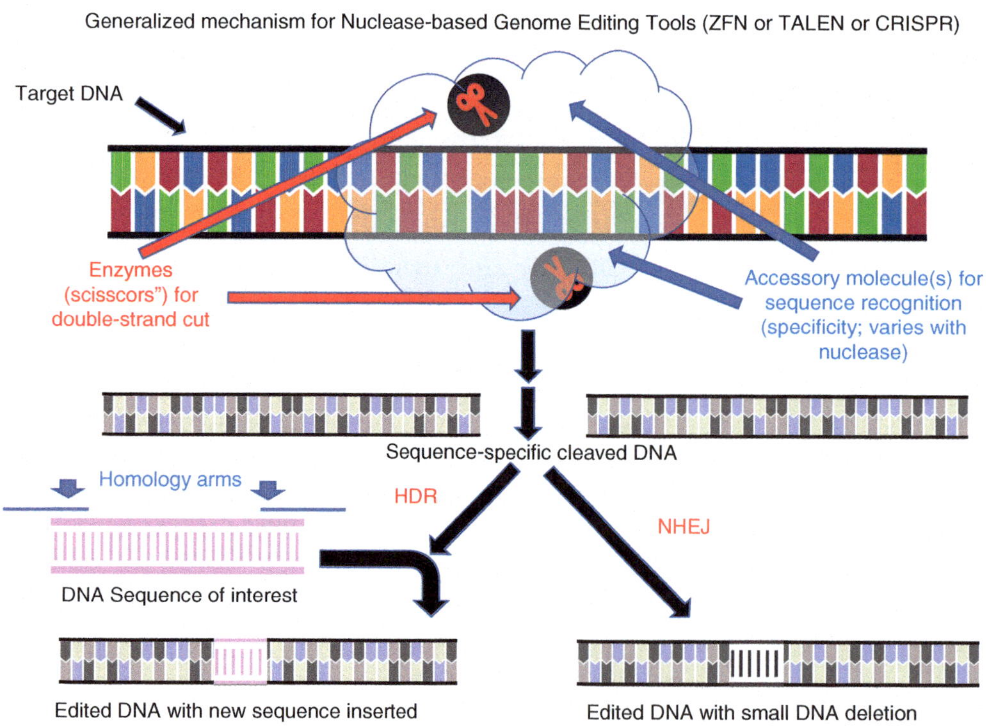

Figure 9.9 ■ A generalized depiction of the analogous genome editing mechanism for ZFN, TALEN and CRISPR tools. (*HDR* homologous directed repair, *NHEJ* non-homologous end-joining; natural mechanisms that repair harmful DNA strand breaks that occur in DNA)

ognize various nucleotide triplets and with some trial and error, ZFNs are able to recognize their targets with fairly high specificity. ZFN because of their mechanism has potential targetable sites in the average genome of every 500 bp. ZFN were quickly employed as genomic editing tools for the generation of mammalian transgenic animals with possibly the biggest impact in transgenic livestock species (i.e. pigs, cattle, etc.). Gene therapy applications were also explored.

TALEN (transcription activator-like effector nucleases) are engineered restriction enzymes generated by fusing a specific DNA-binding domain designed to bind any desired targeted DNA sequence, to a non-specific DNA cleaving domain that can create double strand breaks at the target site that can be repaired by error-prone non-homogenous end-joining (Gaj et al. 2013; Joung and Sander 2013; Kim and Kim 2014). The DNA sequence specific targeting can be engineered by using specific DNA-binding proteins excreted by the plant pathogen Xanthomanos app. These DNA binding domains are called TAL *e*ffectors (TAL*E*s) and consist of repeated domains, each of which contains a highly specific sequence of 34 amino acids, and recognize a single DNA nucleotide. Whereas ZFNs are entirely engineered in the laboratory, TALE proteins exist in nature and many are isolated for use as well as engineered once their precise DNA-binding code was deciphered. They can be effectively designed to bind any desired DNA sequence (with some limitations). TALEN are used in a similar way to the designed zinc finger nucleases. However, because of their different mechanism they have potential targetable sites approximately every 35 bp. TALEN was first used to efficiently produce knockout rats and extended to mice. They have been shown to be successful in generating genome edited mouse strains and transgenic large animal models of human disease. TALEN tools have also been studied for gene therapy applications with a number of pre-clinical applications including with modifying induced pluripotent stem cells in the laboratory (Garate et al. 2015).

Genome Editing with CRISPR Tools

While ZFN and TALEN are powerful genome editing tools, researchers have been looking for more precise genome alterations with high efficiency and ease of laboratory application. *C*lustered *r*egularly *i*nterspaced *s*hort *p*alindromic *r*epeats (CRISPR) and CRISPR-*as*sociated proteins (Cas) has proven to be the answer (Gaj et al. 2013; Harms et al. 2014; Kim and Kim 2014; Mojica and Montoliu 2016). Elements of an adaptive immune system against viruses found in most bacteria, they were recognized early after their discovery to be potential tools for genome editing. CRISPR sequences would be placed on each end of short stretches of DNA that bacteria and other prokaryotes have copied from invading viral phages, preserving a memory of the viruses that have attacked them in the past. These sequences are then transcribed into short RNAs and stored so that they can guide Cas proteins to matching viral sequences when exposed to the same phages in the future. The Cas proteins destroy the matching viral DNA by cutting it.

The initially identified CRISPRs were very simple systems, but were simplified further in the laboratories of Jennifer Doudna and Emmanuelle Charpentier and published in their 2012 milestone paper (Jinek et al. 2012). Literature to date often refers to "CRISPR-Cas9" as the genome-editing tool. There are numerous CRISPR systems now located in prokaryotes, each associated with a different set of CRISPR-associated proteins. This has become a very actively researched area as improvements, subtle variations are sought and limitations are explored. The most common current CRISPR tool, however, is derived from the CRISPR-Cas system isolated from *Streptococcus pyogenes* (the CRISPR-associated protein is Cas9). An excellent video depicting how CRISPR-Cas9 works can be found on the web at: https://www.statnews.com/2018/0404/how-crispr-works-visualized/.

In 2015, a second system, called CRISPR-Cpf1, which is even simpler and more specific (Zetsche et al. 2015) has been studied. The CRISPR-associated protein Cpf1 is simpler than systems with Cas as it requires only a single stranded RNA for base-specific recognition. Also smaller in size than Cas, Cpf1 is thus potentially easier to deliver into cells and tissues. The CRISPR-Cpf1 tool will likely have major implications for genome editing research and medical applications. New systems are continuing to be discovered and explored (Burstein et al. 2017).

Research facilities and drug discovery labs have benefited as genome editing techniques have been reduced to a relatively easy experiment with multiple suppliers of the enzymes, reagents and whole editing systems. Basic research into the mechanisms of DNA repair, functional genomics studies, and the creation of laboratory animals tailored with very specific gene alterations have proliferated as a result of the discovery of CRISPR tools and the refinement of ZFN and TALEN methodologies. CRISPR systems have provided molecular biology with powerful tools for genome editing both in the laboratory, but potentially also in live animals and humans (Kim and Kim 2014; Mojica and Montoliu 2016; Birling et al. 2017; Servick 2017; Sheridan 2017). Animal models of human genetic-related disorders and diseases are being created. Experiments have been designed for the production of interspecies chimeras. Transgenic animals are now being created with the ability to transcribe and translate human genes inserted into the host species into human proteins to facilitate xenotransplantation (discussed later in this chapter). Gene therapy applications, gene editing "drugs" for injection into the blood stream of patients, and studying gene function in human embryos (human embryo editing) have become possible. Although most of these are in a basic research stage, some have reached the pre-clinical stage or are even starting to be clinically studied. And this is likely only the "tip of the iceberg." A new journal has been created named "The CRISPR Journal" emphasizing the importance of this newer technology (see http://www.liebertpub.com/crispr). However, it must again be stated that genome editing is a very powerful technology that has also far-reaching economic, bioethical, and national security implications.

TRANSGENIC ANIMALS AND PLANTS AND GENE MODIFIED CELLS/TISSUES IN DRUG DISCOVERY, DEVELOPMENT, AND PRODUCTION

For thousands of years, man has selectively bred animals and plants either to enhance or to create desirable traits in numerous species. The explosive development of recombinant DNA technology, other OMIC technologies and genome editing tools have made it possible to engineer species possessing particular unique and distinguishing genetic characteristics. As described in Chap. 1, the genetic material of an animal or plant can be manipulated so that extra genes may be inserted (transgenes) or replaced (i.e., human gene homologs coding for related human proteins), or deleted (knockout). Theoretically, these approaches enable the introduction of virtually any gene into any organism. A greater understanding of specific gene regulation and expression, and the growing knowledge from functional genomics studies will contribute to important new discoveries made in relevant animal models. Such genetically altered species have found utility in a myriad of research and potential commercial applications including the generation of models of human disease, protein drug production, creation of organs and tissues for xenotransplantation, a host of agricultural uses, and drug discovery.

■ Transgenic Animals

The term transgenic animal describes an animal in which a foreign DNA segment (a transgene) is incorporated into their genome (Pinkert 2014). Later, the term was extended to also include animals in which their endogenous genomic DNA has had its molecular structure manipulated. While there are some similarities between transgenic technology and gene therapy, it is important to distinguish clearly between them. Technically speaking, the introduction of foreign DNA sequences into a living cell is called gene transfer. Thus, one method to create a transgenic animal involves gene transfer (transgene incorporated into the genome). Gene therapy is also a gene transfer procedure and, in a sense, produces a transgenic human (will be discussed in a later chapter). In transgenic animals, however, the foreign gene is transferred indiscriminately into all cells, including germline cells. The process of gene therapy differs generally from transgenesis since it involves a transfer of the desired gene in such a way that involves only specific somatic and hematopoietic cells, and not germ cells. Thus, unlike in gene therapy, the genetic changes in transgenic organisms are conserved in any offspring according to the general rules of Mendelian inheritance. Please note that the ability to use engineered nuclease tools to edit the genome of an embryo (a germline cell) will conserve the genetic changes in any subsequent somatic and new generations of germline cells. These tools are likely to become the predominant methods available to create new transgenic animals. The three production techniques described below may still be utilized to introduce the new DNA into what will become a transgenic animal if the engineered nuclease-based genome editing tools are used to build the mutated DNA to be inserted *ex vivo*. And they are important as they are used to produce numerous transgenic animals today. However, it is expected that new and improved in vivo genome editing tools will likely become the method of choice in the future.

The creation of transgenic animals is not new. They have been produced since the 1970s. However, modern biotechnology has greatly improved the methods of inducing the genetic transformation. While the mouse has been the most studied animal species, transgenic technology has been applied to a wide array of small and large mammals, fish (especially zebra fish), poultry, various lower animal forms such as insects, and numerous prokaryotes (Table 9.3). Transgenic animals have already made valuable research contributions to studies involving regulation of gene expression, the function of the immune system, genetic diseases, viral diseases, cardiovascular disease, and the genes responsible for the development of cancer. Transgenic animals have proven to be indispensable in drug lead identification, lead optimization, preclinical drug development, and disease modeling.

Production of Transgenic Animals by DNA Microinjection and Random Gene Addition

The production of transgenic animals has most commonly involved the microinjection (also called gene transfer) of 100–200 copies of exogenous transgene DNA into the larger, more visible male pronucleus

Year	Cloned animals
1996	Sheep (Dolly)
1998	Cattle (Noto and Kaga)
1998	Goat (Mira)
2000	Mouse (Cumulina)
2000	Pig (a family)
2000	Mouflon (Ombretta, endangered animal)
2001	Cat (Copy cat)
2001	Gaur (Noah, Asian wild ox)
2001	Rabbit
2002	Rat (Ralph)
2003	Mule (Idaho Gem)
2003	African wildcat (Ditteaux)
2003	Horse (Prometea)
2003	Deer (Dewey)
2004	Ferrets (Libby and Lilly)
2005	Wolves (Snuwolf and Snuwolffy)
2005	Dog (Snuppy)
2017	Monkey (Zhong Zhong and Hua Hua)

Table 9.3 ■ Some cloned animals

(as compared to the female pronucleus) of a recipient fertilized embryo (see Fig. 9.10) (Miao 2013; Polites et al. 2014; Bertolini et al. 2016). The transgene contains both the DNA encoding the desired target amino acid sequence along with regulatory sequences that will mediate the expression of the added gene. The microinjected eggs are then implanted into the reproductive tract of a female and allowed to develop into embryos. The foreign DNA generally becomes randomly inserted at a single site on just one of the host chromosomes (i.e., the founder transgenic animal is heterozygous). Thus, each transgenic founder animal (positive transgene incorporated animals) is a unique species. Interbreeding of founder transgenic animals where the transgene has been incorporated into germ cells may result in the birth of a homozygous progeny provided the transgene incorporation did not induce a mutation of an essential endogenous gene. All cells of the transgenic animal will contain the transgene if DNA insertion occurs prior to the first cell division. However, usually only 20–25% of the offspring contain detectable levels of the transgene. Selection of neonatal animals possessing an incorporated transgene can readily be accomplished either by the direct identification of specific DNA or mRNA sequences or by the observation of gross phenotypic characteristics.

Production of Transgenic Animals by Retroviral Infection

The production of the first genetically altered laboratory mouse embryos was by insertion of a transgene via a modified retroviral vector (More details are provided in a later chapter of this textbook). The nonreplicating viral vector binds to the embryonic host cells, allowing subsequent transfer and insertion of the transgene into the host genome (Miao 2013; Koo et al. 2014; Bertolini et al. 2016). Many of the experimental human gene therapy trials employ the same viral vectors. Advantages of this method of transgene production are the ease with which genes can be introduced into embryos at various stages of development, and the characteristic that only a single copy of the transgene is usually integrated into the genome. Disadvantages include possible genetic recombination of the viral vector with other viruses present, the size limitation of the introduced DNA (up to 7 kb of DNA, less than the size of some genes), and the difficulty in preparing certain viral vectors.

Production of Transgenic Animals by Homologous Recombination in Embryonic Stem Cells Following Microinjection of DNA

Transgenic animals can also be produced by the in vitro genetic alteration of pluripotent embryonic stem cells (ES cells) (see Fig. 9.11). ES cell technology is more efficient at creating transgenics than microinjection protocols (Miao 2013; Sanford and Doetschman 2014; Bertolini et al. 2016). ES cells, a cultured cell line derived from the inner cell mass (blastocyst) of a blastocyte (early preimplantation embryo), are capable of having their genomic DNA modified while retaining their ability to contribute to both somatic and germ cell lineages. The desired gene is incorporated into ES cells by one of several methods such as microinjection. This is followed by introduction of the genetically modified ES cells into the blastocyst of an early preimplantation embryo, selection, and culturing of targeted ES cells which are transferred subsequently to the reproductive tract of the surrogate host animal. The resulting progeny is screened for evidence that the desired genetic modification is present and selected appropriately. In mice, the process results in approximately 30 % of the progeny containing tissue genetically derived from the incorporated ES cells. Interbreeding of selected founder animals can produce species homozygous for the mutation.

While transforming embryonic stem cells is more efficient than the microinjection technique described first, the desired gene must still be inserted into the cultured stem cell's genome to ultimately produce the transgenic animal. The gene insertion could occur in a random or in a targeted process. Nonhomologous recombination, a random process, readily occurs if the desired DNA is introduced into the ES cell genome by a gene recombination process that does not require any sequence homology between genomic DNA and the foreign DNA. While most ES cells fail to insert the

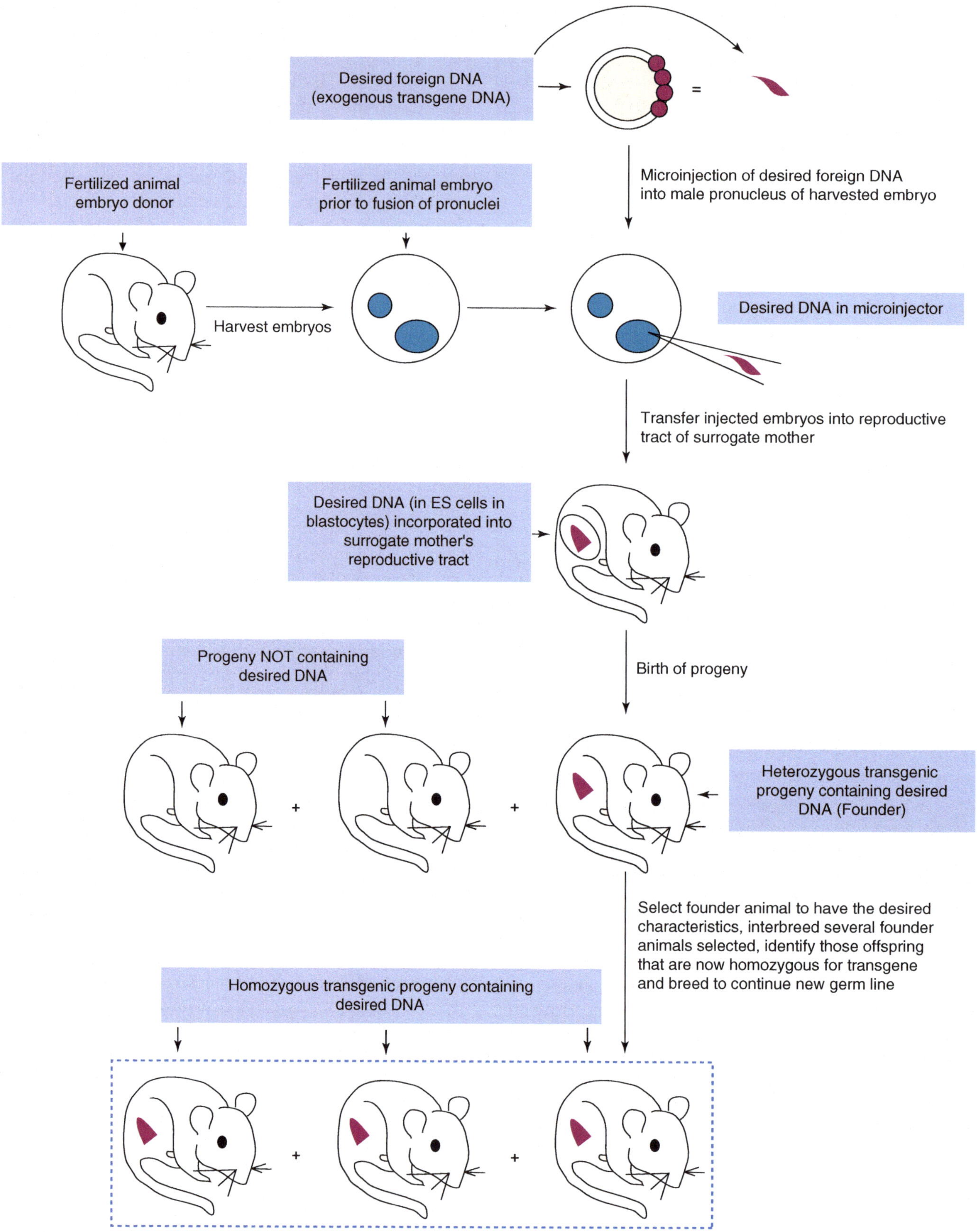

Figure 9.10 ■ Schematic representation of the production of transgenic animals by DNA microinjection that alters the DNA of all cells of the animal, both somatic and germline

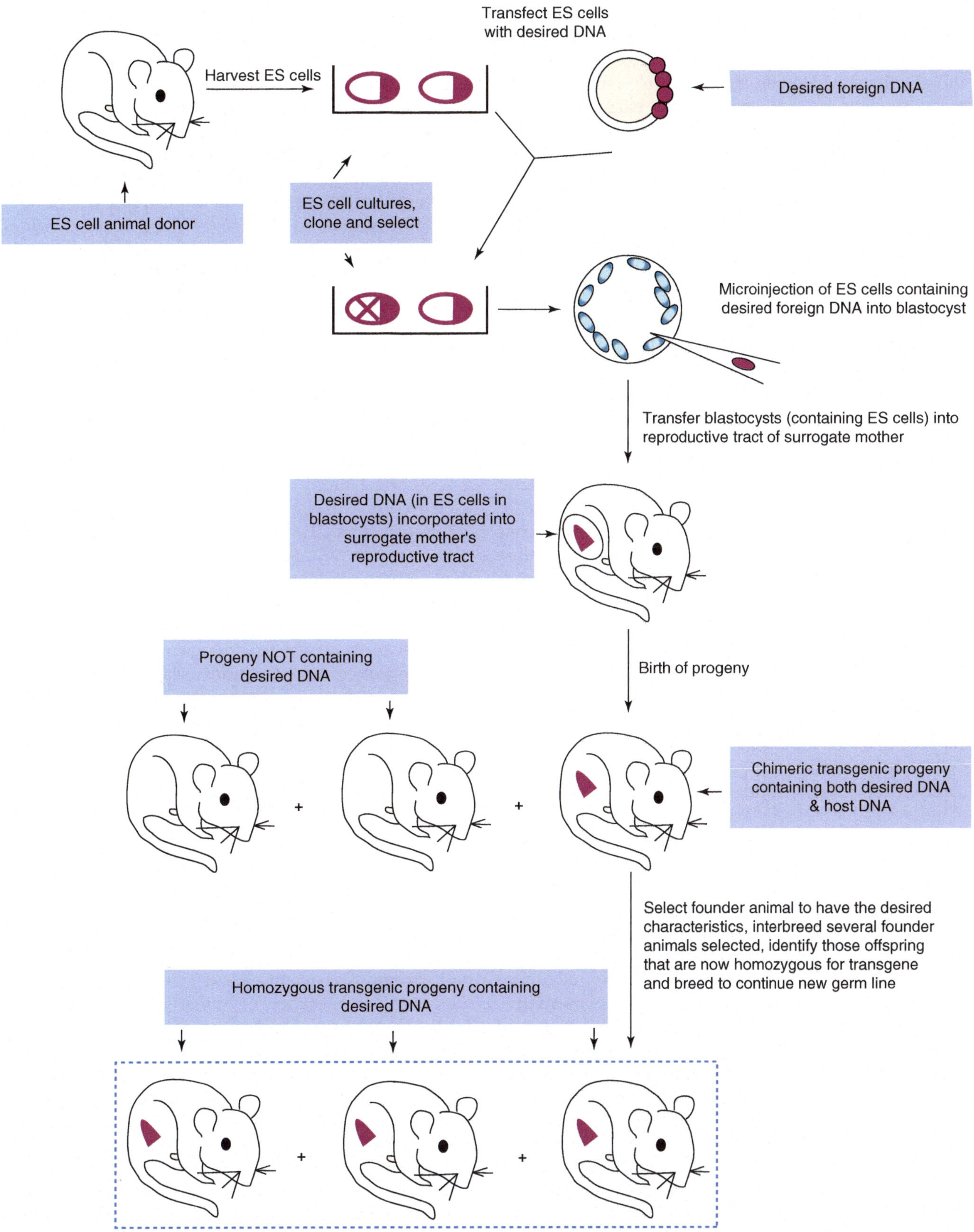

Figure 9.11 ■ Schematic representation of the production of transgenic animals by pluripotent embryonic stem cell methodology that alters the DNA of all cells of the animal, both somatic and germline

foreign DNA, some do. Those that do are selected and injected into the inner cell mass of the animal blastocyst and thus eventually lead to a transgenic species. In still far fewer ES cells, homologous recombination occurs by chance. Segments of DNA base sequence in the vector find homologous sequences in the host genome, and the region between these homologous sequences replaces the matching region in the host DNA. A significant advance in the production of transgenic animals in ES cells is the advent of targeted homologous recombination techniques.

Homologous-directed repair, while much rarer to this point in transgenic research than non-homologous end-joining, can be favored when the researcher carefully designs (engineers) the transferred DNA to have specific sequence homology to the endogenous DNA at the desired integration site and also carefully selects the transfer vector conditions. This targeted homologous recombination at a precise chromosomal position provides an approach to very subtle genetic modification of an animal or can be used to produce knockout mice (to be discussed later).

A modification of the procedure involves the use of hematopoietic bone marrow stem cells rather than pluripotent embryonic stem cells. The use of ES cells results in changes to the whole germ line, while hematopoietic stem cells modified appropriately are expected to repopulate a specific somatic cell line or lines (more similar to gene therapy).

The science of cloning and the resulting ethical debate surrounding it is well beyond the scope of this chapter. Yet it is important to place the concept of animal cloning within the pharmaceutically important context of transgenic animal production. The technique of microinjection (and its variations) has formed the basis for commercial transgenic animal production. While successful, the microinjection process is limited to the creation of only a small number of transgenic animals in a given birth. The slow process of conventional breeding of the resulting transgenic progeny must follow to produce a larger number of transgenic animals with the same transgene as the original organism. To generate a herd (or a flock, etc.), an alternative approach would be advantageous. The technique of nuclear transfer, the replacement of the nuclear genomic DNA of an oocyte (immature egg) or a single-cell fertilized embryo with that from a donor cell, is such an alternative breeding methodology. Animal "cloning" can result from this nuclear transfer technology. Judged a ground-breaking biotech achievement in 1997, creating the sheep Dolly, the first cloned mammal, from a single cell of a 6-year old ewe was a feat many had thought impossible. Dolly was born after nuclear transfer of the genome from an adult mammary gland cell. Since this announcement, commercial and exploratory development of nuclear transfer technology has progressed rapidly with various species cloned. It is important to note that the cloned sheep Dolly was NOT a transgenic animal. While Dolly was a clone of an adult ewe, she did not possess a transgene. However, cloning could be used to breed clones of transgenic animals or to directly produce transgenic animals (if prior to nuclear transfer, a transgene was inserted into the genome of the cloning donor). For example, human factor IX (a blood factor protein) transgenic sheep was generated by nuclear transfer from transfected fetal fibroblasts. Several of the resulting progeny were shown to be transgenic (i.e., possessing the human factor IX gene), and one was named Polly. Thus, animal cloning can be utilized not only for breeding but also for the production of potential human therapeutic proteins and other useful pharmaceutical products.

A major advance in the field was reported this year with the cloning of first primates, Zhong Zhong and sibling Hua Hua using the exact same technique used to clone the sheep Dolly some 20 years earlier (Nature Editors 2018). The cloning of genetically identical primates promises to be a major advancement in the ability to create models of human disease. Also, the use of mitochondrial replacement, a specialized form of in vitro fertilization used to edit the genes of mothers who carry genes for mitochondrial diseases has been approved for use under special cases in the UK. However, these impressive biomedical accomplishments have renewed concerns about reproductive cloning of humans.

■ Transgenic Plants

A variety of biotechnology genetic engineering techniques have been employed to create a wealth of transgenic plant species as mentioned in Chap. 4: cotton, maize, soybean, potato, petunia, tobacco, papaya, rose, and others (Ahmad et al. 2012; Rybicki 2014). Agricultural enhancements have resulted by engineering plants to be more herbicide tolerant, insect resistant, fungus resistant, virus resistant, and stress tolerant. Of importance for human health and pharmaceutical biotechnology, gene transfer technology is routinely used to manipulate bulk human protein production in a wide variety of transgenic plant species. It is significant to note that transgenic plants are attractive bulk bioreactors because their posttranslational modification processes often result in plant-derived recombinant human proteins with a similar glycosylation pattern to that found in the corresponding native human protein from a mammalian production system (cf. Chap. 2). Transplantation to the field followed by normal growth, harvest of the biomass, and downstream isolation and protein purification results in a valuable alternative crop for farming. Tobacco fields producing pharmaceutical grade human antibodies (sometimes referred to as "plantibodies") and edible vaccines contained in transgenic potatoes and tomatoes are not futuristic visions, but current research projects in academic and corporate laboratories and test fields. With antibody-based targeted therapeutics becoming increasingly important, the use of transgenic plants will likely continue to expand once research helps to solve problems related to the isolation of the active protein drug and issues concerning cross fertilization with non-genetically modified organisms (non-GMOs).

Biopharmaceutical Protein Production in Transgenic Animals and Plants: "Biopharming"

The use of transgenic animals and plants as bioreactors for the production of pharmaceutically important proteins may one day become an important use of engineered species once numerous practical challenges are addressed (Ahmad et al. 2012; Rybicki 2014; Bertolini et al. 2016; Lamas-Toranzo et al. 2017). Table 9.4 provides a list of some selected examples of biopharmaceuticals from transgenic animals and plants that have been studied in recent years. Utilizing conventional agronomic and farming techniques, transgenic animals and plants may offer the opportunity to produce practically unlimited quantities of biopharmaceuticals.

The techniques to produce transgenic animals have been used to develop animal strains that secrete high levels of important proteins in various end organs such as milk, blood, urine, and other tissues. During such large animal "gene farming," the transgenic animals serve as bioreactors to synthesize recoverable quantities of therapeutically useful proteins. Among the advantages of expressing protein in animal milk is that the protein is generally produced in sizable quantities and can be harvested manually or mechanically by simply milking the animal. Protein purification from the milk requires the usual separation techniques for proteins. In general, recombinant genes coding for the desired protein product are fused to the regulatory sequences of the animal's milk-producing genes. The animals are not endangered by the insertion of the recombinant gene. The logical fusion of the protein product gene to the milk-producing gene targets the transcription and translation of the protein product exclusively in mammary tissues normally involved in milk production and does not permit gene activation in other, non-milk-producing tissues in the animal. Transgenic strains are established and perpetuated by breeding the animals since the progeny of the original transgenic animal (founder animal) usually also produce the desired recombinant protein.

Yields of protein pharmaceuticals produced transgenically are expected to be 10–100 times greater than those achieved in recombinant cell culture. Protein yields from transgenic animals are generally good [conservative estimates of 1 g/l (g/L) with a 30% purification efficiency] with milk yield from various species per annum estimated at: cow = 10,000 L; sheep = 500 L; goat = 400 L; and pig = 250 L (Rudolph 1995). In addition, should the desired target protein require posttranslational modification, the large mammals used in milk production of pharmaceuticals would be a bioreactor capable of adding those groups (unlike a recombinant bacterial culture).

Using genetic engineering techniques to create transgenic plants, "pharming" for pharmaceuticals is producing an ever-expanding list of drugs and diagnostic agents derived from human genes. Some examples of human peptides and proteins under development in transgenic plants include TGF-beta, vitronectin, thyroid-stimulating hormone receptor, insulin, glucocerebrosidase, apolipoprotein A-1, and taliglucerase alfa. See Table 9.4 for additional examples.

For both animal species and plants, CRISPR tools and other nuclease-based genome editing techniques are transforming the biopharmaing area and will become the method of choice as we move forward (Lamas-Toranzo et al. 2017). Numerous livestock knockout animals have been created (knockout concept will be explained later in this chapter).

Xenotransplantation: Transplantable Transgenic Animal Organs

An innovative use of transgenics for the production of useful proteins is the generation of clinically transplantable transgenic animal organs, the controversial cross-species transplant. The success of human-to-human transplantation of heart, kidney, liver, and other vascularized organs (allotransplantation) created the significant expectation and need for donor organs. Primate-to-human transplantation (xenotransplantation) was successful, but ethical issues and limited number of donor animals were significant barriers. Transplant surgeons recognized early on that organs from the pig were a rational choice for xenotransplantation (due to physiological, anatomical, ethical, and supply reasons) if the serious hyperacute rejection could be overcome. Researchers in academia and industry have pioneered the transgenic engineering of pigs expressing both human complement inhibitory proteins and key human blood group proteins (antigens) including key immunogenic carbohydrates that are detected by the human immune system. Cloning and other genomic manipulation technologies have now produced transgenic pigs for xenotransplantation (Denner 2017; Waltz 2017). Pigs are a good donor spe-

Species	Protein product	Potential indication(s)
Cow	Collagen	Burns, bone fracture
Cow	Human fertility hormones	Infertility
Cow	Human serum albumin	Surgery, burns, shock, trauma
Cow	Lactoferrin	Bacterial GI infection
Goat	α-1-antiprotease inhibitor	Inherited deficiency
Goat	α-1-antitrypsin	Anti-inflammatory
Goat	Antithrombin III (ATryn)	Associated complications from genetic or acquired deficiency
Goat	Growth hormone	Pituitary dwarfism
Goat	Human fertility hormones	Infertility
Goat	Human serum albumin	Surgery, burns, shock, trauma
Goat	LAtPA2	Venous status ulcers
Goat	Monoclonal antibodies	Colon cancer
Goat	tPA2	Myocardial infarct, pulmonary embolism
Pig	Factor IX	Hemophilia
Pig	Factor VIII	Hemophilia
Pig	Fibrinogen	Burns, surgery
Pig	Human hemoglobin	Blood replacement for transfusion
Pig	Protein C	Deficiency, adjunct to tPA
Rabbit	Insulin-like growth factor	Wound healing
Rabbit	Interleukin-2	Renal cell carcinoma
Rabbit	Protein C	Deficiency, adjunct to tPA
Sheep	α–1-antitrypsin	Anti-inflammatory
Sheep	Factor VIII	Hemophilia
Sheep	Factor IX	Hemophilia
Sheep	Fibrinogen	Burns, surgery
Sheep	Protein C	Deficiency, adjunct to tPA
Tobacco	IgG	Systemic therapy (rabies virus, hepatitis B virus)
Tobacco	TGF-β2	Ovarian cancer
Tobacco	Vitronectin	Protease
Tobacco	RhinoR	Fusion of human adhesion protein and human IgA for common cold
Tomato Tomato Safflower	Beta-amyloid Vaccines Insulin	Study of Alzheimer's disease Infectious disease Diabetes
Carrot Corn	DTP subunit vaccine Meripase	Infectious disease Cystic fibrosis
Cherry Duckweed	Hep B surface antigen Lacteron	Hep B vaccine production Controlled release of α-interferon for hepatitis B and C
Potato	Poultry vaccine	Avian influenza (H5N1)

Data from references noted in this section of Chap. 9
Abbreviations: *tPA* tissue plasminogen activator, *LAtPA* long acting tissue plasminogen activator, *TGF-β3* tissue growth factor-beta, *DTP* diphtheria and tetanus and pertussis, *Hep B* hepatitis B

Table 9.4 ■ Some examples of human proteins that have been studied in transgenic animals and plants is provided to show the variety of what may become a viable techbnology in the future

cies for exploring human xenotransplantation because their organs are anatomically similar to human and pig breeding cycles are faster than primates. Cells, tissues, and organs from these sophisticated transgenic animals appear to be very resistant to the humoral immune system-mediated reactions of both primates and likely humans. These findings begin to pave the way for potential xenograft transplantation of animal components into humans with a lessened chance of acute rejection. A continuing concern is that many animals, such as pigs, have shorter life spans than humans, meaning that their tissues age at a quicker rate. Also, there have been concerns because pig organs harbor retroviruses that could be transmitted to humans. CRISPR tools have succeeded to inactivate all 62 copies of a retrovirus found in an experimental pig cell line (Niu et al. 2017). With hundreds of thousands of patients on waitlists for heart and kidney transplants, human xenotransplant trials may close.

■ Knockout Mice (and Knockout Rats)

While many species including mice, zebra fish, and nematodes have been transformed to lose genetic function for the study of drug discovery and disease modeling, mice have proven to be the most useful. Mice are the laboratory animal species most closely related to humans in which the knockout technique can be easily performed, so they are a favorite subject for knockout experiments and are the gold standard. While a mouse carrying an introduced transgene is called a transgenic mouse, transgenic technologies can also produce a knockout animal. A knockout mouse, also called a gene knockout mouse or a gene-targeted knockout mouse, is an animal in which an endogenous gene (genomic wild-type allele) has been specifically inactivated or "knocked out" by replacing it with a null allele (Morgan et al. 2012; Bradley et al. 2012; Ayadi et al. 2012). A null allele is a nonfunctional allele of a gene generated by either deletion of the entire gene or mutation of the gene resulting in the synthesis of an inactive protein. Recent advances in intranuclear gene targeting and embryonic stem cell technologies (as described above and in later chapters of this textbook) are expanding the capabilities to produce knockout mice routinely for studying certain human genetic diseases or elucidating the function of a specific gene product.

The procedure for producing knockout mice basically involves a four-step process. A null allele (i.e., knockout allele) is incorporated into one allele of murine embryonic stem (ES) cells. Incorporation is generally quite low; approximately one cell in a million has the required gene replacement. However, the process is designed to impart neomycin and ganciclovir resistance only to those ES cells in which homologous gene integration has resulted. This facilitates the selection and propagation of the correctly engineered ES cells. The resulting ES cells are then injected into early mouse embryos creating chimeric mice (heterozygous for the knockout allele) containing tissues derived from both host cells and ES cells. The chimeric mice are mated to confirm that the null allele is incorporated into the germ line. The confirmed heterozygous chimeric mice are bred to homogeneity producing progeny that are homozygous knockout mice. Worldwide, there are major mouse knockout programs and collectives that have attempted to pool results and to create a mutation in each of the approximately 20,000 protein-coding genes in the mouse genome using a combination of gene trapping and gene targeting in mouse embryonic stem (ES) cells. These consortia have changed over recent years with most agreeing to work together to achieve this goal in C57BL/6 mouse ES cells and called The International Mouse Phenotyping Consortium (IMPC; http://www.mousephenotype.org/). This is an exceptional source for background and technical information on knockout mice, links to the many consortia members and labs working in this area of research, and tools to access the approximately 17,000 knockout mice strains thus far created. This comprehensive and publicly available resource aids researchers examining the role of each gene in normal physiology and development and shed light on the pathogenesis of abnormal physiology and diseases. Continuing discoveries will further create better animal models of human monogenic and polygenic diseases such as cancer, diabetes, obesity, cardiovascular disease, and psychiatric and neurodegenerative diseases.

Rats have not routinely been bred as knockouts primarily due to not isolating rat ES cells necessary for the process until much later than mouse ES cells. Since the isolation of rat ES cells plus the development of the genome editing techniques for manipulating human genes now being applied to rats and other animal species, knockout rat stains have become available to the research community, but will not likely replace the important role of knockout ice. The whole field of animal models is rapidly evolving. There is little doubt that CRISPR tools and related techniques will create a boom in genetically modified mouse models. The many C57BL/6 mouse strains now available are revolutionizing drug discovery.

■ 3D-Cell Cultures and Organoids

With new biotechnology tools becoming increasingly available especially stem cell methodologies, researchers are continually trying to develop new and improved in vitro technologies to replace some animal models in their study of biology and the drug development process. One approach is to grow in the laboratory miniature versions of human organs that simulate the anatomical, physiological and mechanical properties of the real thing. Classic 2D-cell culture techniques were being enhanced for greater realistic microenvironment simulation by new "3D-cell culture" techniques (Ravi et al. 2015; van Duinen et al. 2015). Unlike in 2D-cell cultures where the cells are grown as thin layers in petri dishes, the cells in 3D-cell cultures are allowed to grow in all three dimensions usually in bioreactors creating cell colonies or spheroid-shaped accumulations of cells. These cultures are derived from one or a few cells from a specific tissue type or organ, or by manipulation of induced pluripotent stem cells (to be discussed in a later chapter in this textbook, Chap. 17). When the 3D-cell cultures are derived from specific organs, the in vitro 3D-organ cell culture that is created is known as an "organoid" (Fatehullah et al. 2016; Foley 2017; Sinha 2017). 3D-cell culturing has become a commonly used method in the study of cancer and cancer cell growth. Numerous organoids have been grown including brain, liver, lung, stomach, pancreas, ear, thyroid, GI, kidney, and testicular. 3D-cell cultures including organoids are transforming medical research and have many potential uses that are being explored. Besides cancer studies, uses include toxicity studies, modeling infectious disease in humans, personalized medicine, pre-clinical drug development, microbiome studies and regenerative medicine.

■ "On-a-Chip" Technology ("Organ-on-Chip")

Recent advances in systems biology, stem cell technology, materials science, 3D-cell culture (expansion of the classic 2-D cell culture techniques allowing greater cell-cell communication and interaction better mimicking true complex tissue architecture) and microfluidics (the physics and manipulation of extremely small amounts of fluids) have allowed researchers to develop miniature models of human "organs on a chip (OOC)." Basically, an artificial organ, the 3-D cell culture grown on a chip is linked to microfluid handing and sensor capabilities that together simulate the anatomical, physiological and mechanical properties and responses of entire organs and organ systems (Selimović et al., 2013; Zhang and Radisic 2017). The chip support framework is generally a silicon wafer or piece of plastic of only millimeters to a few square centimeters in size. A veryu good picture with structural diagrams for an organ-on-a-chip can be found on the web at: https://labiotech.eu/organs-on-chips-the-end-of-animal-testing-in-biotech/?nabe=6526793858416640:1&utm_referrer=https%3A%2F%2Fwww.google.com%2F.

Lab-on-a-chip devices were being developed to integrate one-or-more laboratory functions onto a single engineered chip that required minute amounts of sample fluid volume and reagents to complete the task. The field developed rapidly in the mid-1990s due to developments in microarray genomics applications, key improvements in micro-electromechanical systems engineering and the need for portable biological and chemical warfare agent detection systems. Academicv laboratories and pharmaceutical companies have embraced the use and further development of this in vitro technology to replace some animal models in the drug development process. Numerous organ systems have been created and tested including lung, liver, heart, artery and kidney chips that provide an alternative test system to traditional toxicity studies in laboratory animals (Chang et al. 2016; Skardal et al. 2016). The chips are characterized for use as both normal organ tissues as well as diseased organs. Researchers have been experimenting with the integration of multiple organ chips including up to 10 different organ chips into a single system that may in the future mimic the human body. With further development, "on-a-chip" technology may have a significant impact on high-throughput screening, toxicity testing, drug delivery and overall drug development. Another rapidly emerging area of tissue and organ research that impacts the production of organ-on-a-chip as well as a stand-alone tissue model technology is 3D-bioprinting (Mandrycky et al. 2016). 3D-bioprinting allows for the layer-by-layer deposition of biological materials in a printing-like approach to produce a range of cell types and resulting tissues. An in-depth exploration of the topic is beyond the context of this textbook. However, 3-D-bioprinting has been employed in the production of some organ-on-a-chip systems.

SYNTHETIC BIOLOGY

Modern biotechnology tools have allowed for a number of ways to study very complex biological systems. For example, as described above, systems biology examines complex biological systems as interacting and integrated complex networks. The new and developing field of study known as *synthetic biology* explores how to build artificial complex biological systems employing many of the same tools and experimental techniques favored by system biologists. Synthetic biology looks at both the strategic redesign and/or the fabrication of existing biological systems and the design and construction of biological components and systems that do not already exist in nature (Cameron et al. 2014; Church et al. 2014). The focus of synthetic biology is often on ways of taking parts of natural biological systems, characterizing and simplifying them, and using them as a component of a highly unnatural, engineered, biological system. Synthetic biology studies may provide a more detailed understanding of complex biological systems down to the molecular level. Being able to design and construct a complex system is also one very practical approach to understanding that system under various conditions. The levels a synthetic biologist may work at include the organism, tissue and organ, intercellular, intracellular, biological pathway, and down to the molecular level.

There are many exciting applications for synthetic biology that have been explored or hypothesized across various fields of scientific study including designed and optimized biological pathways, natural product manufacturing, new drug molecule synthesis, and biosensing. From an engineering perspective, synthetic biology could lead to the design and building of engineered biological systems that process information, modify existing chemicals, fabricate new molecules and materials, and maintain and enhance human health and our environment. Because of the obvious societal concerns that synthetic biology experiments raise, the broader science community has engaged in considerable efforts at developing guidelines and regulations and addressing the issues of intellectual property and governance and the ethical, societal, and legal implications. Several bioethics research institutes published reports on ethical concerns and the public perception of synthetic biology. A report from the United States Presidential Commission for the Study of Bioethical Issues called for enhanced federal oversight on this emerging technology.

In 2006, a research team, at the J. Craig Venter Institute constructed and filed a patent application for a synthetic genome of a novel synthetic minimal bacterium named *Mycoplasma laboratorium* (Glass et al. 2007). The team was able to construct an artificial chromosome of 381 genes, and the DNA sequence they have pieced together is based upon the bacterium Mycoplasma genitalium. The original bacterium had a fifth of its DNA removed and was able to live successfully with the synthetic chromosome in place. Venter's goal is to make cells that might take carbon dioxide out of the atmosphere and produce methane, used as a feedstock for other fuels.

Chang and coworkers published pioneering work utilizing a synthetic biology approach to assemble two heterologous pathways for the biosynthesis of plant-derived terpenoid natural products. Terpenoids are a highly diverse class of lipophilic natural products that have historically provided a rich source for discovery of pharmacologically active small molecules, such as the anticancer agent paclitaxel (Taxol) and the antimalarial artemisinin. Unfortunately, these secondary metabolites are typically produced in low abundance in their host organism, and their isolation consequently suffers from low yields and high consumption of natural resources. A key step is developing methods to carry out cytochrome P450 (P450)-based oxidation chemistry in vivo. Their work suggests that potentially, entire metabolic pathways can be designed in silico and constructed in bacterial hosts. Synthetic biology methods can modify a yeast to produce opioids from sugar (Höhne and Kabisch 2016).

BIOTECHNOLOGY AND DRUG DISCOVERY

Pharmaceutical scientists have taken advantage of every opportunity or technique available to aid in the long, costly, and unpredictable drug discovery process. In essence, Chap. 9 is an overview of some of the many applications of biotechnology and related techniques useful in target identification and validation, drug discovery or design, lead optimization, and development including pre-clinical and clinical studies. The techniques described throughout Chap. 9 have changed the way drug research is conducted, refining the process that optimizes the useful pharmacological properties of an identified novel chemical lead and minimizes the unwanted properties. The promise of genomics, transcriptomics, proteomics, microarrays, pharmacogenomics/genetics, epigenomics, precision medicine, metabonomics/metabolomics, microbiomics, toxicogenomics, glycomics, systems biology, genome editing, genetically engineered animals, and bioinformatics and big data has radically changed the new drug discovery paradigm. Figure 9.12 shows schematically the interaction of three key elements that are essential for modern drug discovery: new targets identified by genomics, proteomics, and related technologies; validation of the identified targets; rapid, sensitive bioassays utilizing high-throughput screening methods; and new molecule creation and optimization employing a host of approaches (Russell et al. 2013; Dopazo 2014; Eder and Herrling 2016; Vijaya Bhaskar Reddy et al. 2016). The key elements are underpinned at each point by bioinformatics and now big data. Several of the technologies, methods, and approaches listed in Fig. 9.12 have been described previously in this chapter. Others will be described below.

■ Modern Drug Screening and Synthesis

Traditionally, drug discovery programs relied heavily upon random screening followed by analog synthesis and lead optimization via structure-activity relationship studies. Discovery of novel, efficacious, and safer small molecule medicinal agents with appropriate "drug-like characteristics is an increasingly costly and complex process." Therefore, any method allowing for a reduction in time and money is extremely valuable. Advances in biotechnology have contributed to a greater understanding of the cause and progression of disease and have identified new therapeutic targets

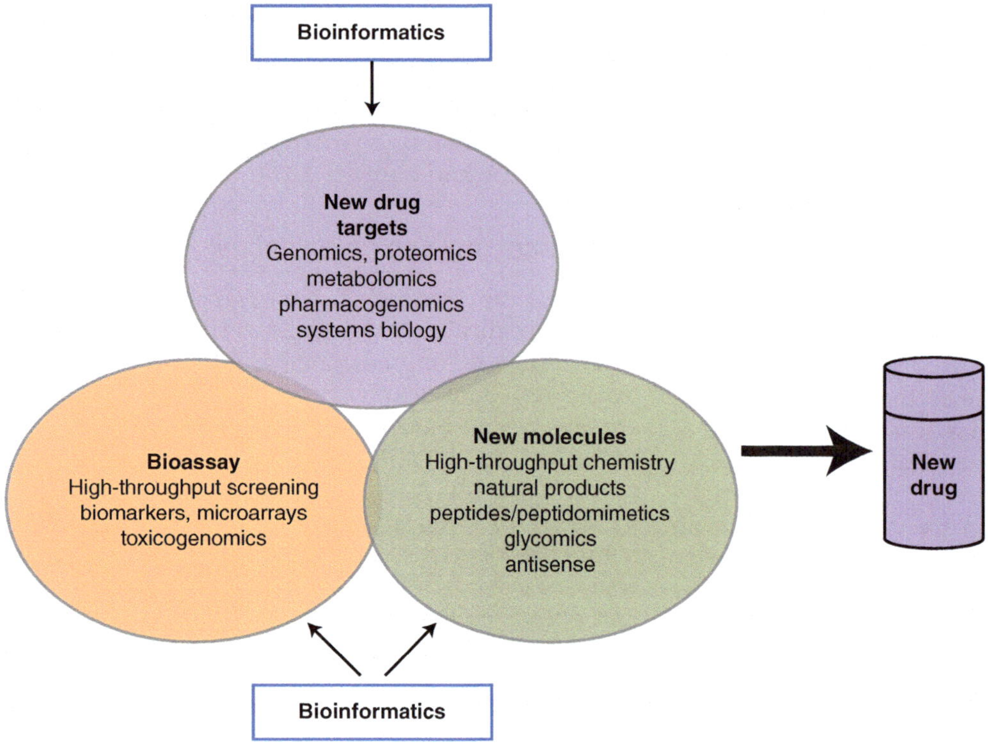

Figure 9.12 ■ Elements of modern drug discovery: impact of biotechnology

forming the basis of novel drug screens. New technical discoveries in the fields of proteomics for target discovery and validation and systems biology are expected to facilitate the discovery of new agents with novel mechanisms of action for diseases that were previously difficult or impossible to treat (Kell 2013). Proteins including monoclonal antibodies and RNA molecules have become popular and valuable drug leads and approved pharmaceutical products. Their discovery and development are facilitated by all of the technologies described in this chapter (Everett 2015). However, small molecule drugs are still highly desired. Therefore, in an effort to decrease the cost of identifying and optimizing useful, quality drug leads (both small molecule and biologic) against a pharmaceutically important target, researchers have developed newer approaches including high-throughput screening and high-throughput synthesis methods. Applications of biotechnology to in vitro screening include the improved preparation of (1) cloned membrane-bound receptors expressed in cell lines carrying few endogenous receptors; (2) immobilized preparations of receptors, antibodies, and other ligand-binding proteins; and (3) soluble enzymes and extracellular cell-surface expressed protein receptors. In most cases today, biotechnology contributes directly to the understanding, identification, and/or the generation of the drug target being screened (e.g., radioligand binding displacement from a cloned protein receptor).

Previously, libraries of synthetic compounds along with natural products from microbial fermentation, plant extracts, marine organisms, and invertebrates provide a diversity of molecular structures that were screened randomly. Screening can be made more directed if the compounds to be investigated are selected on the basis of structural information about the receptor or natural ligand. The development of sensitive radioligand binding assays and the access to fully automated, robotic screening techniques have accelerated the screening process.

High-throughput screening (HTS) provides for the bioassay of thousands of compounds in multiple assays at the same time. The process is automated with robots and utilizes multi-well microtiter plates. Today, companies can conduct 100,000 bioassays a day. In addition, modern drug discovery and lead optimization with DNA microarrays and other biotechnologies allow researchers to track hundreds to thousands of genes.

Traditionally, small drug molecules were synthesized by joining together structural pieces in a set sequence to prepare one product. One of the most powerful tools to optimize drug discovery is automated high-throughput synthesis. When conducted in a combinatorial approach, high-throughput synthesis provides for the simultaneous preparation of hundreds or thousands of related drug candidates. There are two overall approaches to high-throughput synthesis: combinatorial chemistry that randomly mixes various

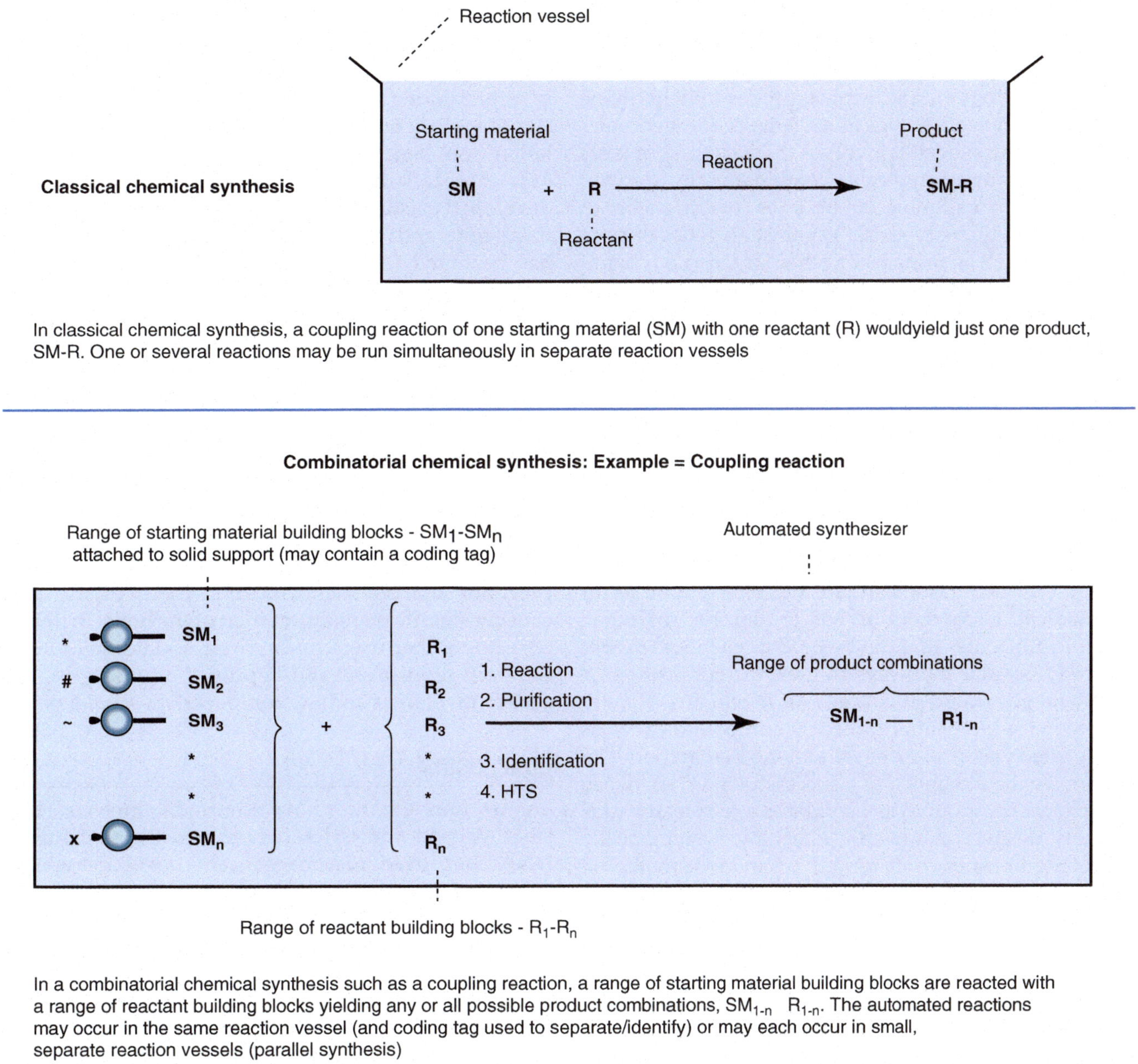

Figure 9.13 ■ A schematic representation of a coupling reaction: difference between classical chemical synthesis and combinatorial chemistry

reagents (such as many variations of reagent A with many variations of reagent B to give random mixtures of all products in a reaction vessel) and parallel synthesis that selectively conducts many reactions parallel to each other (such as many variations of reagent A in separate multiple reaction vessels with many variations of reagent B to give many single products in separate vessels) (Please see Fig. 9.13). Assigning the task to automated synthesizing equipment results in the rapid creation of large collections or libraries (as large as 10,000 compounds) of diverse molecules. Ingenious methods have been devised to direct the molecules to be synthesized, to identify the structure of the products, to purify the products via automation, and to isolate compounds. When coupled with high-throughput screening, thousands of compounds can be generated, screened, and evaluated for further drug discovery and development in a matter of weeks.

■ Chemical Genomics (Chemogenomics)

Having the ability to sequence the human genome coupled with the growth of proteomics now provides researchers with an abundance of potential new drug targets and the need to validate the roles of these newly identified human gene products. In modern drug discovery, chemical genomics (sometimes called chemogenomics or more generally included as a subset of chemical biology) uses chemical probes to help define the complexity of biological systems at the genomics and proteomics level. It involves the screening of large chemical libraries (typically combinatorially derived "druggable" small molecule libraries covering a broad expanse of "diversity space") against all genes or gene products, such as proteins or other targets (i.e., chemical universe screened against target universe) (Cong et al. 2012; Zanders 2012; Jung and Kwon 2015; Zhu et al. 2015). In Fig. 9.12, basically chemical genomics would occur when the "new molecules" to be tested in the "bioassay" developed from the "new drug targets" "OMIC approaches came from large chemical libraries typically of small molecules synthesized by high-throughput chemistry. As part of the U.S. National Institutes of Health (NIH) Roadmap for Biomedical Research, the National Center for Advanced Translational Medicine (NCATS) Chemical Genomics Center (NCGC) has led an effort to offer public sector biomedical researchers access to libraries of small organic molecules that can be used as chemical probes to study cellular pathways in greater depth (https://ncats.nih.gov/ncgc/about/goals). It remains difficult to predict which small molecule compounds will be most effective in a given situation. Researchers can maximize the likelihood of a successful match between a chemical compound, its usefulness as a research tool, and its desired therapeutic effect by systematically screening libraries containing thousands of small molecules. Drug candidates are expected from the correlations observed during functional analysis of the molecule—gene product interactions. Genomic profiling by the chemical library may also yield relevant new targets and mechanisms. The target universe will be well characterized when both the function of the receptor target has been recognized as well as a set of specific molecules that have the ability to bind to the target and modulate it. Chemical genomics has changed the drug discovery paradigm and the approach for the investigation of target pharmacology (see Figs. 9.1 and 9.12). It is expected to be a critical component of drug lead identification and proof of principle determination for selective modulators of complex enzyme systems including proteases, kinases, G-protein-coupled receptors, and nuclear receptors.

■ Drug Repurposing (Drug Repositioning or Drug Reprofiling)

In an effort to reduce the average 14-year time frame it takes to translate a new molecule into an approved drug, to improve the success rate and to lower the cost of drug discovery and development, drug repurposing has become a useful strategy. Drug repurposing, sometimes called drug repositioning or drug reprofiling, builds upon the existing knowledge of the pharmacology, formulation, toxicity, and human clinical testing of a known drug or drug candidates to quicken the translation from bench to bedside. This approach discovers new indications for approved or significantly developed existing agents thereby decreasing development time and cost (Bisson 2012). Drug repurposing has benefited from the rapid growth of proteomics, metabolomics, and other OMIC technologies to help define new pathways and drug targets the existing molecules will interact. Repurposing can occur at an early or late stage of drug development. The National Center for Advanced Translational Medicine (NCATS) supports research into drug repurposing (https://ncats.nih.gov/preclinical/repurpose/early; https://ncats.nih.gov/preclinical/repurpose/late). A classic example of a successful drug repurposing is the former sedative/hypnotic drug thalidomide used for nausea and to alleviate the symptoms of morning sickness in pregnant women. Removed from the market due to causing significant malformation of the limbs in infants born to mother users of the drug, today thalidomide has been repurposed and approved as a drug to treat certain myelomas and the complications from leprosy.

CONCLUSION

Tremendous advances have occurred in biotechnology since Watson and Crick determined the structure of DNA. Improved pharmaceuticals, novel therapeutic agents, unique diagnostic products, and new drug design tools have resulted from the escalating achievements of pharmaceutical biotechnology. While recombinant DNA technology and hybridoma techniques received most of the press in the late 1980s and early 1990s, a wealth of additional and innovative biotechnologies and approaches have been, and will continue to be, developed in order to enhance pharmaceutical research and transform our understanding of disease and its precision treatment. Genomics, transcriptomics, proteomics, microarrays, pharmacogenomics/genetics, epigenomics, precision medicine, metabonomics/metabolomics, microbiomics, toxicogenomics, glycomics, systems biology, genome editing, genetically engineered animals, and parallel high-throughput screening and drug lead synthesis are directly influencing the pharmaceutical sciences and are well positioned to significantly impact modern pharmaceutical care. Application of these, and yet to be discovered biotechnologies, will continue to reshape effective drug therapy as well as improve the competitive, challenging process of drug discovery and development of new medicinal agents and diagnostics. These extremely powerful technologies and there current and future applications present scientists, clinicians, policy makers and the public far-reaching economic, bioethical, and national security concerns that must be explored and addressed. Pharmacists, pharmaceutical scientists, and pharmacy students should be poised to take advantage of the products and techniques made available by the unprecedented scope and pace of discovery in biotechnology in the twenty-first century.

SELF-ASSESSMENT QUESTIONS

Questions

1. What were the increasing levels of genetic resolution of the human genome planned for study as part of the HGP?
2. What is functional genomics?
3. What is proteomics?
4. What are SNPs?
5. What is the difference between pharmacogenetics and pharmacogenomics?
6. Define metabonomics.
7. What is a DNA microarray?
8. What phase(s) of drug action is affected by genetic variation?
9. Define precision medicine.
10. What is a biomarker?
11. Define systems biology.
12. What is genome editing and what are the four genome editing nucleases?
13. What is the CRISPR-Cas9 tool
14. Why are engineered animal models valuable to pharmaceutical research?
15. What is a knockout mouse?

Answers

1. HGP structural genomics was envisioned to proceed through increasing levels of genetic resolution: detailed human genetic linkage maps [approx. 2 megabase pairs (Mb = million base pairs) resolution], complete physical maps (0.1 Mb resolution), and ultimately complete DNA sequencing of the approximately 3.5 billion base pairs (23 pairs of chromosomes) in a human cell nucleus [1 base pair (bp) resolution].
2. Functional genomics is an approach to genetic analysis that focuses on genome-wide patterns of gene expression, the mechanisms by which gene expression is coordinated, and the interrelationships of gene expression when a cellular environmental change occurs.
3. The research area called proteomics seeks to define the function and correlate that with expression profiles of all proteins encoded within a genome.
4. While comparing the base sequences in the DNA of two individuals reveals them to be approximately 99.9% identical, base differences, or polymorphisms, are scattered throughout the genome. The best-characterized human polymorphisms are single-nucleotide polymorphisms (SNPs) occurring approximately once every 1000 bases in the 3.5 billion base pair human genome.
5. Pharmacogenetics is the study of how an individual's genetic differences influence drug action, usage, and dosing. A detailed knowledge of a patient's pharmacogenetics in relation to a particular drug therapy may lead to enhanced efficacy and greater safety. While sometimes used interchangeably (especially in pharmacy practice literature), pharmacogenetics and pharmacogenomics are subtly different. Pharmacogenomics introduces the additional element of our present technical ability to pinpoint patient-specific DNA variation using genomic techniques. While overlapping fields of study, pharmacogenomics is a much newer term that correlates an individual patient's DNA variation (SNP level of variation knowledge rather than gene level of variation knowledge) with his or her response to pharmacotherapy.
6. The field of metabonomics is the holistic study of the metabolic continuum at the equivalent level to the study of genomics and proteomics.
7. The biochips known as DNA microarrays and oligonucleotide microarrays are a surface collection of hundreds to thousands of immobilized DNA sequences or oligonucleotides in a grid created with specialized equipment that can be simultaneously examined to conduct expression analysis.
8. Genomic variation affects not only the pharmacokinetic profile of drugs (via drug metabolizing enzymes and drug transporter proteins), it also strongly influences the pharmacodynamic profile of drugs via the drug target.
9. The goal of precision medicine is to enable clinicians to employ the most appropriate course of action for each individual patient managing the extreme complexity of each patient given all of the tools now available in the health care system: OMICS technology data, disease mechanisms, the electronic health record, public health information, big data, etc. Sometimes referred to as giving the right drug to the right patient in the right dose at the right time.
10. Biomarkers are clinically relevant substances used as indicators of a biologic state. Detection or concentration change of a biomarker may indicate a particular disease state physiology or toxicity. A change in expression or state of a protein biomarker may correlate with the risk or progression of a disease,

with the susceptibility of the disease to a given treatment or the drug's safety profile.

11. Systems biology is the study of the interactions between the components of a biological system, and how these interactions give rise to the function and behavior of that system.
12. Genome editing (sometimes called genome engineering) is the approach in modern biology to make specific changes to the DNA of a cell or organism and observing its impact. Key to genome editing is the ability to selectively and predictively modify the DNA sequence of the target organism an assure the integrity of the resulting edits. The four nucleases are meganucleases, ZFN, TALEN, and CRISPR.
13. Clustered *r*egularly *i*nterspaced *s*hort *p*alindromic *r*epeats (CRISPR) and CRISPR-*as*sociated proteins (Cas) are elements of an adaptive immune system against viruses found in most bacteria. They are used as sequence specific genome editing tools. There are numerous CRISPR systems found in prokaryotes, each associated with a different set of CRISPR-associated proteins. The most common current CRISPR tool is derived from the CRISPR-Cas system isolated from *Streptococcus pyogenes* (the CRISPR-associated protein is Cas9.
14. Engineered animal models are proving invaluable since small animal models of disease are often poor mimics of that disease in human patients. Genetic engineering can predispose an animal to a particular disease under scrutiny, and the insertion of human genes into the animal can initiate the development of a more clinically relevant disease condition.
15. A knockout mouse, also called a gene knockout mouse or a gene-targeted knockout mouse, is an animal in which an endogenous gene (genomic wild-type allele) has been specifically inactivated by replacing it with a null allele.

Acknowledgments I wish to acknowledge the tremendous contribution of Dr. Arlene Marie Sindelar, my wife, to some of the graphics found in figures in all five editions of this textbook.

REFERENCES

Adams R, Steckel M, Nicke B (2016) Functional genomics in pharmaceutical drug discovery. Handb Exp Pharmacol 232:25–41

Ahles A, Engelhardt S (2014) Polymorphic variants of adrenoceptors: pharmacology, physiology, and role in disease. Pharmacol Rev 66:598–637

Ahmad P, Ashraf M, Younis M, Hu X, Kumar A, Akram NA, Al-Qurainy F (2012) Role of transgenic plants in agriculture and biopharming. Biotechnol Adv 30:524–540

Ahmed S, Zhou Z, Zhou J, Chen S (2016) Pharmacogenomics of drug metabolizing enzymes and transporters: relevance to precision medicine. Genomics Proteomics Bioinformatics 14:298–313

Altelaar AF, Munoz J, Heck AJ (2013) Next-generation proteomics: towards an integrative view of proteome dynamics. Nat Rev Genet 14:35–48

Alyass A, Turcotte M, Meyre D (2015) From big data analysis to personalized medicine for all: challenges and opportunities. BMC Med Genet 8:33–44

Anderson DC, Kodukula K (2014) Biomarkers in pharmacology and drug discovery. Biochem Pharmacol 87:172–188

Aronson SJ, Rehm HL (2015) Building the foundation for genomics in precision medicine. Nature 526:336–342

Ayadi A, Birling MC, Bottomley J, Bussell J, Fuchs H, Fray M, Gailus-Durner V, Greenaway S, Houghton R, Karp N, Leblanc S, Lengger C, Maier H, Mallon AM, Marschall S, Melvin D, Morgan H, Pavlovic G, Ryder E, Skarnes WC, Selloum M, Ramirez-Solis R, Sorg T, Teboul L, Vasseur L, Walling A, Weaver T, Wells S, White JK, Bradley A, Adams DJ, Steel KP, Hrabě de Angelis M, Brown SD, Herault Y (2012) Mouse large-scale phenotyping initiatives: overview of the European Mouse Disease Clinic (EUMODIC) and of the Wellcome Trust Sanger Institute Mouse Genetics Project. Mamm Genome 23:600–610

Beckmann JS, Lew D (2016) Reconciling evidence-based medicine and precision medicine in the era of big data: challenges and opportunities. Genome Med 8:134

Beitelshees AL, Voora D, Lewis JP (2015) Personalized antiplatelet and anticoagulation therapy: applications and significance of pharmacogenomics. Pharmgenomics Pers Med 8:43–61

Benjak A, Sala C, Hartkoorn RC (2015) Whole-genome sequencing for comparative genomics and de novo genome assembly. Methods Mol Biol 1285:1–16

Berná G, Oliveras-López MJ, Jurado-Ruíz E, Tejedo J, Bedoya F, Soria B, Martín F (2014) Nutrigenetics and nutrigenomics insights into diabetes etiopathogenesis. Nutrients 6:5338–5369

Bertolini LR, Meade H, Lazzarotto CR, Martins LT, Tavares KC, Bertolini M, Murray JD (2016) The transgenic animal platform for biopharmaceutical production. Transgenic Res 25:329–343

Bheda P, Schneider R (2014) Epigenetics reloaded: the single-cell revolution. Trends Cell Biol 24:712–723

Biesecker LG, Spinner NB (2013) A genomic view of mosaicism and human disease. Nat Rev Genet 14:307–320

Bingol K, Bruschweller-Li L, Li D, Zhang B, Xie M, Bruschweiler R (2016) Emerging new strategies for successful metabolite identification in metabolomics. Bioanalysis 8:557–573

Birling MC, Schaefer L, André P, Lindner L, Maréchal D, Ayadi A, Sorg T, Pavlovic G, Hérault Y (2017) Efficient and rapid generation of large genomic variants in rats and mice using CRISMERE. Sci Rep 7:43331

Bisson WH (2012) Drug repurposing in chemical genomics: can we learn from the past to improve the future? Curr Top Med Chem 12:1883–1888

Bitto A, Pallio G, Messina S, Arcoraci V, Pizzino G, Russo GT, Pallio S, Squadrito F, Altavilla D (2016) Genomic variations affecting biological effects of statins. Curr Drug Metab 17:566–572

Blumenthal GM, Mansfield E, Pazdur R (2016) Next-generation sequencing in oncology in the era of precision medicine. JAMA Oncol 2:13–14

Bradley A, Anastassiadis K, Ayadi A, Battey JF, Bell C, Birling MC, Bottomley J, Brown SD, Bürger A, Bult CJ, Bushell W, Collins FS, Desaintes C, Doe B, Economides A, Eppig JT, Finnell RH, Fletcher C, Fray M, Frendewey D, Friedel RH, Grosveld FG, Hansen J, Hérault Y, Hicks G, Hörlein A, Houghton R, Hrabé de Angelis M, Huylebroeck D, Iyer V, de Jong PJ, Kadin JA, Kaloff C, Kennedy K, Koutsourakis M, Lloyd KC, Marschall S, Mason J, McKerlie C, McLeod MP, von Melchner H, Moore M, Mujica AO, Nagy A, Nefedov M, Nutter LM, Pavlovic G, Peterson JL, Pollock J, Ramirez-Solis R, Rancourt DE, Raspa M, Remacle JE, Ringwald M, Rosen B, Rosenthal N, Rossant J, Ruiz Noppinger P, Ryder E, Schick JZ, Schnütgen F, Schofield P, Seisenberger C, Selloum M, Simpson EM, Skarnes WC, Smedley D, Stanford WL, Stewart AF, Stone K, Swan K, Tadepally H, Teboul L, Tocchini-Valentini GP, Valenzuela D, West AP, Yamamura K, Yoshinaga Y, Wurst W (2012) The mammalian gene function resource: the International Knockout Mouse Consortium. Mamm Genome 23:580–586

Brazeau DA, Brazeau GA (2011a) Principles of the human genome and pharmacogenomics. American Pharmacists Association, Washington, DC, pp 1–10

Brazeau DA, Brazeau GA (2011b) Principles of the human genome and pharmacogenomics. American Pharmacists Association, Washington, DC, pp 11–34

Burstein D, Harrington LB, Strutt SC, Probst AJ, Anantharaman K, Thomas BC, Doudna JA, Ban Eld JF (2017) New CRISPR-Cas systems from uncultivated microbes. Nature 542:237–241

Cameron DE, Bashor CJ, Collins JJ (2014) A brief history of synthetic biology. Nat Rev Microbiol 12:381–390

Carroll D (2011) Genome engineering with zinc-finger nucleases. Genetics 188:773–782

Caspar SM, Dubacher N, Kopps AM, Maienberg J, Henggeler C, Matyas C (2017) Clinical sequencing: from raw data to diagnosis with lifetime value. Clin Genet 93(3):508–519

Cénit MC, Matzaraki V, Tigchelaar EF, Zhernakova A (2014) Rapidly expanding knowledge on the role of the gut microbiome in health and disease. Biochim Biophys Acta 1842:1981–1992

Cesario A, Auffray C, Russo P, Hood L (2014) P4 medicine needs P4 education. Curr Pharm Des 20:6071–6072

Chambliss AB, Chan DW (2016) Precision medicine: from pharmacogenomics to pharmacoproteomics. Clin Proteomics 13:25–33

Chang SY, Weber EJ, Ness KV, Eaton DL, Kelly EJ (2016) Liver and kidney on chips: microphysiological models to understand transporter function. Clin Pharmacol Ther 100:464–478

Chau SB, Thomas RE (2015) The amplichip: a review of itas analytic and clinical validity and clinical utility. Curr Drug Saf 10:113–124

Chaudhry SR, Muhammad S, Eidens M, Klemm M, Khan D, Efferth T, Weisshaar MP (2014) Pharmacogenetic prediction of individual variability in drug response based on CYP2D6, CYP2C9 and CYP2C19 genetic polymorphisms. Curr Drug Metab 15:711–718

Chen M, Zhang L (2011) Epigenetic mechanisms in developmental programming of adult disease. Drug Discov Today 16:1007–1018

Chen M, Zhang M, Borlak J, Tong W (2012) A decade of toxicogenomic research and its contribution to toxicological science. Toxicol Sci 130:217–228

Chen M, Bisgin H, Tong L, Hong H, Fang H, Borlak J, Tong W (2014) Toward predictive models for drug-induced liver injury in humans: are we there yet? Biomark Med 8:201–213

Chouchana L, Narjoz C, Roche D, Golmard JL, Pineau B, Chatellier G, Beaune P, Loriot MA (2014) Interindividual variability in TPMT enzyme activity: 10 years of experience with thiopurine pharmacogenetics and therapeutic drug monitoring. Pharmacogenomics 15:745–757

Church GM, Elowitz MB, Smolke CD, Voigt CA, Weiss R (2014) Realizing the potential of synthetic biology. Nat Rev Mol Cell Biol 15(4):289–294

Collins LJ, Schonfeld B (2011) The epigenetics of non-coding RNA. In: Tollefsbol T (ed) Handbook of epigenetics: the new molecular and medical genetics. Elsevier, London, pp 49–61

Cong F, Cheung AK, Huang SM (2012) Chemical genetics-based target identification in drug discovery. Annu Rev Pharmacol Toxicol 52:57–78

Costa AR, Rodrigues ME, Henriques M, Oliveira R, Azeredo J (2014) Glycosylation: impact, control and improvement during therapeutic protein production. Crit Rev Biotechnol 34:281–299

Cummings RD, Pierce JM (2014) The challenge and promise of glycomics. Chem Biol 21:1–15

Davis CA, Hitz BC, Sloan CA, Chan ET, Davidson JM, Gabdank I, Hilton JA, Ulugbek KJ, Baymuradov K, Narayanan AK (2018) The encyclopedia of DNA elements (ENCODE): data portal update. Nucleic Acids Res 41:D36–D42

Dawson MA, Kouzarides T (2012) Cancer epigenetics: from mechanism to therapy. Cell 150:12–27

Daxinger L, Whitelaw E (2012) Understanding transgenerational epigenetic inheritance via the gametes in mammals. Nat Rev Genet 13:153–162

De R, Bush WS, Moore JH (2014) Bioinformatics challenges in genome-wide association studies (GWAS). Methods Mol Biol 1168:63–81

Denner J (2017) Advances in organ transplant from pigs. Science 357:1238–1239

Dopazo J (2014) Genomics and transcriptomics in drug discovery. Drug Discov Today 19:126–132

Drabovich AP, Martinez-Morillo E, Diamandis EP (2015) Toward an integrated pipeline for protein biomarker development. Biochim Biophys Acta 1854:677–686

Drew L (2016) Pharmacogenetics: the right drug for you. Nature 537:S60–S62

Dugger SA, Platt A, Goldstein DB (2017) Drug development in the era of precision medicine. Nat Rev Drug Discov 17(3):183–196

Ebhardt HA, Root A, Sander C, Aebersold R (2015) Applications of targeted proteomics in systems biology and translational medicine. Proteomics 15:3193–3208

Eddy JA, Funk CC, Price ND (2013) Fostering synergy between cell biology and systems biology. Methods Mol Biol 1021:1–11

Eder J, Herrling PL (2016) Trends in modern drug discovery. Handb Exp Pharmacol 232:3–20

Everett JR (2015) Academic drug discovery: current status and prospects. Expert Opin Drug Discov 10:937–944

Fatehullah A, Tan SH, Barker N (2016) Organoids as an in vitro model of human development and disease. Nat Cell Biol 18:246–254

Feinberg AP, Irizarry RA, Fradin D, Aryee MJ, Murakami P, Aspelund T, Eirksdottir G, Harris TB, Launer L, Gudnason V, Fallin MD (2010) Personalized epigenomic signatures that are stable over time and covary with body mass index. Sci Transl Med 2:45–51

Ferguson LR, De Caterina R, Görman U, Allayee H, Kohlmeier M, Prasad C, Choi MS, Curi R, de Luis DA, Gil Á, Kang JX, Martin RL, Milagro FI, Nicoletti CF, Nonino CB, Ordovas JM, Parslow VR, Portillo MP, Santos JL, Serhan CN, Simopoulos AP, Velázquez-Arellano A, Zulet MA, Martinez JA (2016) Guide and position of the International Society of Nutrigenetics/Nutrigenomics on personalised nutrition: part 1 - fields of precision nutrition. J Nutrigenet Nutrigenomics 9:12–27

Filipski KK, Murphy JD, Helzlsouer KJ (2017) Updating the landscape of direct-to-consumer pharmacogenomic testing. Pharmgenomics Pers Med 10:229–232

Fluck J, Hofmann-Apitius M (2014) Text mining for systems biology. Mol Gen Genomics 289:727–734

Foley KE (2017) Organoids: a better *in vitro* model. Nat Methods 14:559–562

Frick A, Benton CS, Scolaro KL, McLaughlin JE, Bradley CL, Suzuki OT, Wang N, Wiltshire T (2016) Transitioning pharmacogenomics into the clinical setting: training future pharmacists. Pharmacogenomics 17:535–539

Friedman AA, Letai A, Fisher DE, Flaherty KT (2015) Precision medicine for cancer with next-generation functional diagnostics. Nat Rev Cancer 15:747–756

Gaj T, Gersbach CA, Barbas CF 3rd (2013) ZFN, TALEN, and CRISPR/Cas-based methods for genome engineering. Trends Biotechnol 31:397–405

Garate Z, Quintana-Bustamante O, Crane AM, Olivier E, Poirot L, Galetto R, Kosinski P, Hill C, Kung C, Agirre X, Orman I, Cer- rato L, Alberquilla O, Rodriguez-Fornes F, Fusaki N, Garcia- Sanchez F, Maia TM, Ribeiro ML, Sevilla J, Prosper F, Jin S, Mountford J, Guenechea G, Gouble A, Bueren JA, Davis BR, Segovia JC (2015) Generation of a high number of healthy erythroid cells from gene-edited pyruvate kinase deficiency patient-specifc induced pluripotent stem cells. Stem Cell Rep 5:1053–1066

Glass JI, Smith HO, Hutchison III CA, Alperovich NY, Assad-Garcia N (2007) Minimal bacterial genome. United States Patent Application 20070122826, May 31, 2007

Global Market Insights (2017) Precision medicine market worth over $96 Bn by 2024. https://www.gminsights.com/pressrelease/precision-medicine-market. Accessed 24 Jan 2018

Goundrey-Smith S (2013) Information technology in pharmacy. Springer, London

Greene CS, Tan J, Ung M, Moore JH, Cheng C (2014) Big data bioinformatics. J Cell Physiol 229:1896–1900

Harms DW, Quadros RM, Seruggia D, Ohtsuka M, Takahashi G, Montoliu L, Gurumurthy CB (2014) Mouse genome editing using the CRISPR/Cas system. Curr Protoc Hum Genet 83:1–27

Hasin Y, Seldin M, Lusis A (2017) Multi-omics approaches to disease. Genome Biol 18:1–15

Hatz MH, Schremser K, Rogowski WH (2014) Is individualized medicine more cost-effective? A systematic review. PharmacoEconomics 32:443–455

Hayes DF, Markus HS, Leslie RD, Topol EJ (2014) Personalized medicine: risk prediction, targeted therapies and mobile health technology. BMC Med 12:37–44

Hehir-Kwa JY, Pfundt R, Veltman JA (2015) Exome sequencing and whole genome sequencing for the detection of copy number variation. Expert Rev Mol Diagn 15:1023–1032

Hertz DL, Rae JM (2016) Pharmacogenetic predictors of response. Adv Exp Med Biol 882:191–215

Höglund M (1998) Glycosylated and non-glycosylated recombinant human granulocyte colony-stimulating factor (rhG-CSF)--what is the difference? Med Oncol 15:229–233

Höhne M, Kabisch J (2016) Brewing painkillers: a yeast cell factory for the production of opioids from sugar. Angew Chem Int Ed Engl 55:1248–1125

Hollebecque A, Massard C, Soria JC (2014) Implementing precision medicine initiatives in the clinic: a new paradigm in drug development. Curr Opin Oncol 26:340–346

Hyman DM, Solit DB, Arcila ME, Cheng DT, Sabbatini P, Baselga J, Berger MF, Ladanyi M (2015) Precision medicine at Memorial Sloan Kettering Cancer Center: clinical next-generation sequencing enabling next-generation targeted therapy trials. Drug Discov Today 20:1422–1428

Inbar-Feigenberg M, Choufani S, Butcher DT, Roifman M, Weksberg R (2013) Basic concepts of epigenetics. Fertil Steril 99:607–615

IOM (Institute of Medicine) (2013) Best care at lower cost: the path to continuously learning health care in America. The National Academies Press, Washington DC

Jacob HJ et al (2013) Genomics in clinical practice: lessons from the front lines. Sci Transl Med 5:1–5

Ji B, Nielsen J (2015) From next-generation sequencing to systematic modeling of the gut microbiome. Front Genet 6:219

Jiang J, Tian F, Cai Y, Qian X, Coatello CE, Ying W (2014) Site-specific qualitative and quantitative analysis of the N- and O-glycoforms in recombinant human erythropoietin. Anal Bioanal Chem 406:6265–6274

Jiang Z, Zhou X, Li R, Michal JJ, Zhang S, Dodson MV, Zhang Z, Harland RM (2015) Whole transcriptome analysis with sequencing: methods, challenges and potential solutions. Cell Mol Life Sci 72:3425–3439

Jinek M, Chylinski K, Fonfara I, Hauer M, Doudna JA, Charpentier E (2012) A programmable dual-RNA-guided DNA endonuclease in adaptive bacterial immunity. Science 337:816–821

Joly Y, Saulnier KM, Osien G, Knoppers BM (2014) The ethical framing of personalized medicine. Curr Opin Allergy Clin Immunol 14:404–408

Joung JK, Sander JD (2013) TALENs: a widely applicable technology for targeted genome editing. Nat Rev Mol Cell Biol 14:49–55

Jung HJ, Kwon HJ (2015) Target deconvolution of bioactive small molecules: the heart of chemical biology and drug discovery. Arch Pharm Res 38:1627–1641

Karahalil B (2016) Overview of systems biology and omics technologies. Curr Med Chem 23:4221–4230

Kell DB (2013) Finding novel pharmaceuticals in the systems biology era using multiple effective drug targets, phenotypic screening and knowledge of transporters: where drug discovery went wrong and how to fix it. FEBS J 280:5957–5980

Kelsey G, Stegle O, Reik W (2017) Single-cell epigenomics: recording the past and predicting the future. Science 358:69–75

Khan SR, Baghdasarian A, Fahlman RP, Michail K, Siraki AG (2014) Current status and future prospects of toxicogenomics in drug discovery. Drug Discov Today 19:562–578

Kim H, Kim JS (2014) A guide to genome engineering with programmable nucleases. Nat Rev Genet 15:321–334

Kolodziejczyk AA, Kim JK, Svensson V, Marioni JC, Teichmann SA (2015) The technology and biology of single-cell RNA sequencing. Mol Cell 58:610–620

Koo BC, Kwon MS, Kim T (2014) Retrovirus-mediated gene transfer. In: Pinkert CA (ed) Transgenic animal technology, 3rd edn. Elsevier, London, pp 167–194

Kwapisz D (2017) The first liquid biopsy test approved. Is it a new era of mutation testing for non-small cell lung cancer? Ann Transl Med 5:46

Lamas-Toranzo I, Guerrero-Sánchez J, Miralles-Bover H, Alegre-Cid G, Pericuesta E, Bermejo-Álvarez P (2017) CRISPR is knocking on barn door. Reprod Domest Anim 52(Suppl 4):39–47

Lawrie DS, Petrov DA (2014) Comparative population genomics: power and principles for the inference of functionality. Trends Genet Apr 30:133–139

Lee JW, Aminkeng F, Bhavsar AP, Shaw K, Carleton BC, Hayden MR, Ross CJ (2014) The emerging era of pharmacogenomics: current successes, future potential, and challenges. Clin Genet 86:21–28

Levy SE, Myers RM (2016) Advancements in next-generation Sequencing. Annu Rev Genomics Hum Genet 17:95–115

Li W, Li M, Pu X, Guo Y (2017) Distinguishing the disease-associated SNPs based on composition frequency analysis. Interdiscip Sci 9:459–467

Lindon JC, Nicholson JK (2014) The emergent role of metabolic phenotyping in dynamic patient stratification. Expert Opin Drug Metab Toxicol 10:915–919

Madhusoodanan J (2014) Human gene set shrinks again. The Scientist 28:17

Mandrycky C, Wang Z, Kim K, Kim DH (2016) 3D bioprinting for engineering complex tissues. Biotechnol Adv 34:422–434

Mastrangelo A, Armitage EG, Garcia A, Barbas C (2014) Metabolomics as a tool for drug discovery and personalized medicine. A review. Curr Top Med Chem 14:2627–2636

Medina MÁ (2013) Systems biology for molecular life sciences and its impact in biomedicine. Cell Mol Life Sci 70:1035–1053

Miao X (2013) Recent advances in the development of new transgenic animal technology. Cell Mol Life Sci 70:815–828

Mojica FJ, Montoliu L (2016) On the origin of CRISPR-Cas technology: from prokaryotes to mammals. Trends Microbiol 24:811–820

Moody SE, Boehm JS, Barbie DA, Hahn WC (2010) Functional genomics and cancer drug target discovery. Curr Opin Mol Ther 12:284–293

Morgan H, Simon M, Mallon AM (2012) Accessing and mining data from large-scale mouse phenotyping projects. Int Rev Neurobiol 104:47–70

Murdoch TB, Detsky AS (2013) The inevitable application of big data to health care. JAMA 3019:1351

Nature Editors (2018) Monkeys cloned in China. Nature 553:387–388

Niu D, Wei HJ, Lin L, George H, Wang T, Lee IH, Zhao HY, Wang Y, Kan Y, Shrock E, Lesha E, Wang G, Luo Y, Qing Y, Jiao D, Zhao H, Zhou X, Wang S, Wei H, Güell M, Church GM, Yang L (2017) Inactivation of porcine endogenous retrovirus in pigs using CRISPR-Cas9. Science 357:1303–1307

Omenn GS, Lane L, Lundberg EK, Beavis RC, Obverall CM, Deutsch EW (2016) Metrics for the human proteome project 2016: progress on identifying and characterizing the human proteome, including post-translational modifications. J Proteome Res 15:3951–3960

Papastergiou J, Tolios P, Li W, Li J (2017) The innovative canadian pharmacogenomic screening initiative in community pharmacy (ICANPIC) study. J Am Pharm Assoc 57:624–629

Patel JN (2015) Cancer pharmacogenomics: implications on ethnic diversity and drug response. Pharmacogenet Genomics 25:223–230

Patti GJ, Yanes O, Siuzdak G (2012) Metabolomics: the apogee of the omics trilogy. Nat Rev Mol Cell Biol 13:263–269

Paul A, Paul S (2014) The breast cancer susceptibility genes (BRCA) in breast and ovarian cancers. Front Biosci 19:605–618

PhRMA (2017) 2017 Industry profile: Medicines are Transforming the Trajectory of Disease. Available at http://phrma-docs.phrma.org/industryprofile/pdfs/2017IndustryProfile_MedicinesareTransforming.pdf. Accessed 11 Jan 2018

Pinkert CA (2014) Introduction to transgenic animal technology. In: Pinkert CA (ed) Transgenic animal technology, 3rd edn. Elsevier, London, pp 1–14

Polites HG, Johnson LW, Pinkert CA (2014) DNA microinjection, embryo handling, and germplasm preservation.

In: Pinkert CA (ed) Transgenic animal technology, 3rd edn. Elsevier, London, pp 17–70
Prasad V, Fojo T, Brada M (2016) Precision oncology: origins, optimism, and potential. Lancet Oncol 17:e81–e86
Premsrirut P (2017) Drug discovery in the age of big data. Drug Discov World 17:8–15
Prokopuk L, Western PS, Stringer JM (2015) Transgenerational epigenetic inheritance: adaptation through the germline epigenome? Epigenomics 7(5):829–846
Raciti GA, Nigro C, Longo M, Parrillo L, Miele C, Formisano P, Béguinot F (2014) Personalized medicine and type 2 diabetes: lesson from epigenetics. Epigenomics 6:229–238
Raghavachari N (2012) Overview of omics. In: Barh D, Blum K, Madigan MA (eds) OMICS-biomedical perspectives and applications. CRC Press, Boca Raton, pp 1–19
Ravi M, Paramesh V, Kaviya SR, Anuradha E, Solomon FD (2015) 3D cell culture systems: advantages and applications. J Cell Physiol 230:16–26
Relling MV, Evans WE (2015) Pharmacogenomics in the clinic. Nature 526:343–350
Roden DM (2016) Cardiovascular pharmacogenomics: current status and future directions. J Hum Genet 61:79–85
Rozek LS, Dolinoy DC, Sartor MA, Omenn GS (2014) Epigenetics: relevance and implications for public health. Annu Rev Public Health 35:105–122
Rudd P, Karlsson NG, Khoo K-H, Packer NH (2017) Glycomics and glycoproteomics. In: Varki A, Cummings RD, Esko JD, Stanley P, Hart GW, Aebi M, Darvill AG, Kinoshita T, Packer NH, Prestegard JH, Schnaar RL, Seeberger PH (eds) Essentials of glycobiology, 3rd edn. Cold Spring Harbor Laboratory Press, Cold Spring Harbor
Rudolph NS (1995) Advances continue in production of proteins in transgenic animal milk. Genet Eng News 15:8–9
Russell C, Rahman A, Mohammed AR (2013) Application of genomics, proteomics and metabolomics in drug discovery, development and clinic. Ther Deliv 4:395–413
Rybicki EP (2014) Plant-based vaccines against viruses. Virol J 11:205. https://doi.org/10.1186/s12985-014-0205-0
Sabatier R, Gonçalves A, Bertucci F (2014) Personalized medicine: present and future of breast cancer management. Crit Rev Oncol Hematol 91:223–233
Sagner M, McNeil A, Puska P, Auffray C, Price ND, Hood L, Lavie CJ, Han Z, Chen Z, Brahmachari SK, McEwen BS, Soares MB, Balling R, Epel E, Arena R (2017) The P4 health spectrum – a predictive, preventive, personalized and participatory continuum for promoting healthspan. Prog Cardiovasc Dis 59:506–521
Sanford LP, Doetschman T (2014) Gene targeting in embryonic stem cells, I: history and methodology. In: Pinkert CA (ed) Transgenic animal technology, 3rd edn. Elsevier, London, pp 109–140
Schneider MV (2014) Defining systems biology: a brief overview of the term and field. Drug Discov Today 19:140–144
Schneider HC, Klabunde T (2013) Understanding drugs and diseases by systems biology. Bioorg Med Chem Lett 23:1168–1176
Schneider D, Riegman PH, Cronin M, Negrouk A, Moch H, Balling R, Penault-Llorca F, Zatloukal K, Horgan D (2016) Accelerating the development and validation of new value-based diagnostics by leveraging biobanks. Public Health Genomics 19:160–169
Schumacher S, Muekusch S, Seitz H (2015) Up-to-date applications of microarrays and their way to commercialization. Microarrays 4:196–213
Schweiger MR, Barmeyer C, Timmermann B (2013) Genomics and epigenomics: new promises of personalized medicine for cancer patients. Brief Funct Genomics 12:411–421
Selimović S, Dokmeci MR, Khademhosseini A (2013) Organs-on-a-chip for drug discovery. Curr Opin Pharmacol 13:829–833
Servick K (2017) Embryo editing takes another step to clinic. Science 357:436–437
Shendure J, Balasubramanian S, Church GM, Gilbert W, Rogers J, Schloss JA, Waterston RH (2017) DNA sequencing at 40: past, present and future. Nature 550:345–353
Sheridan C (2017) CRISPR therapeutics push into human testing. Nat Biotechnol 35:3–5
Sinha G (2017) The organoid architect. Science 357:746–749
Skardal A, Shupe T, Atala A (2016) Organoid-on-a-chip and body-on-a-chip systems for drug screening and disease modeling. Drug Discov Today 21:1399–1411
Smaglik P (2017) The genetic microscope. Nature 545: S25–S27
Spanogiannopoulos P, Bess EN, Carmody RN, Turnbaugh PJ (2016) The microbial pharmacists within us: a metagenomic view of xenobiotic metabolism. Nat Microbiol 14:273–287
Tang H, Mayampurath A, Yu CY, Mechref Y (2014) Bioinformatics protocols in glycomics and glycoproteomics. Curr Protoc Protein Sci 76:1–7
The Cancer Genome Atlas Research Network (2014) Comprehensive molecular characterization of urothelial bladder carcinoma. Nature 507:315–322
The International Human Genome Sequencing Consortium (2001) Initial sequencing and analysis of the human genome. Nature 409:860–921
Thompson MD, Cole DE, Capra V, Siminovitch KA, Rovati GE, Burnham WM, Rana BK (2014) Pharmacogenetics of the G protein-coupled receptors. Methods Mol Biol 1175:189–242
Tuddenham S, Sears CL (2015) The intestinal microbiome and health. Curr Opin Infect Dis 28:464–470
U.S. DOE (2018) Human genome project information. Available at: http://web.ornl.gov/sci/techresources/Human_Genome/hg5yp/index.shtml. Accessed 11 Jan 2018
U.S. National Academies (2011) Toward precision medicine: building a knowledge network for biomedical research and a new taxonomy of disease. The National Academies Press, Washington, DC, pp 1–4
van Duinen V, Trietsch SJ, Joore J, Vulto P, Hankemeier T (2015) Microfluidic 3D cell culture: from tools to tissue models. Curr Opin Biotechnol 35:118–126

van Rooij T, Wilson DM, Marsh S (2012) Personalized medicine policy challenges: measuring clinical utility at point of care. Expert Rev Pharmacoecon Outcomes Res 12:289–295

Venter JC et al (2001) The sequence of the human genome. Science 291:1304–1351

Vijaya Bhaskar Reddy A, Yusop Z, Jaafar J, Madhavi V, Madhavi G (2016) Advances in drug discovery: impact of genomics and role of analytical instrumentation. Curr Drug Discov Technol 13:211–224

Visscher PM, Wray NR, Zhang Q, Sklar P, McCarthy MI, Brown MA, Yang J (2017) 10 years of GWAS discovery: biology, function, and translation. Am J Hum Genet 101:5–22

Waltz E (2017) When pig organs will fly. Nat Biotechnol 35:1133–1138

Wetterstrand KA (2017) DNA sequencing costs: data from the NHGRI genome sequencing program (GSP) Available at: www.genome.gov/sequencingcostsdata. Accessed 23 Dec 2017

Wiktorowicz JE, Brasier AR (2016) Introduction to clinical proteomics. Adv Exp Med Biol 919:435–441

Wildt S, Gerngross TU (2005) The humanization of N-glycosylation pathways in yeast. Nat Rev Microbiol 3:119–126

Wishart DS, Mandal R, Stanislaus AS, Ramirez-Gaona M (2016) Cancer metabolomics and the human metabolome database. Metabolites 6:1–17

Wishart DS, Feunang YD, Marcu A, Guo AC, Liang K, Vazquez-Fresno R, Sajed T, Johnson D, Li C, Karu N, Sayeeda Z, Lo E, Assempour N, Berjanski M, Singhai S, Arndt D, Liang Y, Badran H, Grant J, Serra-Cayuela A, Liu Y, Mandal R, Neveu V, Pon A, Knox C, Wilson M, Manach C, Scalbert A (2018) HMDB: the human metabolome database for 2018. Nucleic Acids Res 46:D608–D617

Wright FA et al (2001) A draft annotation and overview of the human genome. Genome Biol 2:1–18

Yadav M, Verma MK, Chauhan NS (2017) A review of metabolic potential of human gut microbiome in human nutrition. Arch Microbiol 200(2):203–217

Zanders ED (2012) Overview of chemical genomics and proteomics. Methods Mol Biol 800:3–10

Zdanowicz MM (2017) Pharmacogenomics: past, present, and future. In: Zdanowicz MM (ed) Concepts in pharmacogenomics. American Society of Health-systems Pharmacists, Bethesda, pp 3–18

Zetsche B, Gootenberg JS, Abudayyeh OO, Slaymaker IM, Makarova KS, Essletzbichler P, Volz SE, Joung J, van der Oost J, Regev A, Koonin EV, Zhang F (2015) Cpf1 is a single RNA-guided endo- nuclease of a class 2 CRISPR-Cas system. Cell 163:759–771

Zhang B, Radisic M (2017) Organ-on-a-chip devices advance to market. Lab Chip 17:2395–2420

Zhang HM, Nan ZR, Hui GQ, Liu XH, Sun Y (2014) Application of genomics and proteomics in drug target discovery. Genet Mol Res 13:198–204

Zhao Y, Brasier AR (2015) Qualification and verification of protein biomarker candidates. Adv Exp Med Biol 919:493–514

Zhao X, Modur V, Carayannopoulos LN, Laterza OF (2015) Biomarkers in pharmaceutical research. Clin Chem 61:1342–1353

Zhao YY, Cheng XL, Lin RC, Wei F (2015a) Lipidomics applications for disease biomarker discovery in mammal models. Biomark Med 9:153–168

Zhao YY, Miao H, Cheng XL, Wei F (2015b) Lipidomics: novel insight into the biochemical mechanism of lipid metabolism and dysregulation-associated disease. Chem Biol Interact 240:220–238

Zhu Y, Xiao T, Lei S, Zhou F, Wang MW (2015) Application of chemical biology in target identification and drug discovery. Arch Pharm Res 38:1642–1650

10

Dispensing Biotechnology Products: Handling, Professional Education, and Product Information

Robert D. Sindelar

INTRODUCTION

Preparation, dispensing, and patient education regarding appropriate use of pharmaceuticals are primarily the responsibility of the pharmacist. Traditionally, parenteral products have been available in ready-to-use containers or required appropriate dilution with sterile water or saline prior to use with no other special handling requirements. Hospital pharmacists, in particular, have prepared and dispensed parenteral products for individual patients for many years. While many pharmacists are skilled in handling parenteral products, biotechnology products present additional challenges since they are proteins subject to physical and chemical denaturation and thus require special handling techniques. These challenges will be explained in greater detail in this chapter. Practice issues with biotechnology products may be handled in slightly different ways depending on laws and pharmacy practice standards in each country. This chapter is written primarily from the view of practice in the United States since that is the primary experience of the original chapter authors.

PHARMACIST READINESS

To be prepared to provide pharmaceutical care services to patients who require therapy with biotechnology drugs, pharmacists must be well versed ands skilled in (1) knowledge about the tools of biotechnology; (2) an understanding of the therapeutic aspects of recombinant protein products; (3) a thorough familiarity with the side effects and patient education considerations; (4) a familiarity with the storage, handling, and reconstitution of proteins; and (5) the difficulty of handling expensive biotech drug reimbursement issues.

Pharmacists may view biotechnology drugs as quite different from traditional parenteral products and familiar oral dosage forms. However, in most respects, the services offered by pharmacists when preparing and dispensing biotechnology products are the same as those provided for traditional tablets or injectable products. To determine the knowledge and skills a pharmacist requires to work with biotechnology drugs, one must first consider who will be storing, preparing, dispensing, and administering the agent. Many agents will be prepared by a pharmacist or other health-care provider and the drug administered by a nurse, while the patient will prepare others and self-administered. Pharmacists who work in clinics or with home health-care providers need to understand how to store, prepare, and dispense the product to a nurse with instructions to maintain potency and sterility until the biotech drug is administered to the patient. The knowledge and skill set is similar but has some significant differences from the skills required by a community pharmacist who must be able to teach the patient how to store, reconstitute, and self-administer the biotechnology agent.

The decision as to who will store, prepare, and administer the drug is typically determined from a business perspective. For example, in the U.S., in order for a clinic to administer and be paid for a drug, the drug must not be "usually self-administered by the patients who take them" (Department of Health and Human Services 2018). The Medicare Benefit Policy manual, Chap. 13 outlines a process to make this determination. Drugs and biologicals are usually covered by U.S. Centers for Medicare & Medicaid Services (CMS) if they are of the type that cannot be self-administered, they are not excluded (i.e., immunizations), they are reasonable and necessary for the

Updated from the 4th Edition chapter authored by Peggy Piascik, Ph. D and Val Adams, PharmD

R. D. Sindelar (✉)
Faculty of Pharmaceutical Sciences and The Centre for Health Evaluation & Outcomes Sciences (CHEOS), The University of British Columbia (UBC), Vancouver, BC, Canada

Global Drug Commercialization Centre (GDCC)-China and GDCC-worldwide, Chengdu, China
e-mail: robert.sindelar@ubc.ca

D. J. A. Crommelin et al. (eds.), *Pharmaceutical Biotechnology*, https://doi.org/10.1007/978-3-030-00710-2_10

diagnosis or treatment of the illness or injury for which they are administered and they have not been determined by the FDA to be less than effective. In addition they must meet all the general requirements for coverage of items as incident to a physician's services. Generally, prescription and non-prescription drugs and biologicals purchased by or dispensed to a patient are not covered.

From a practical standpoint, drugs administered in the clinic are billed using a "J" code. What is a J-Code? J-Codes relate to permanent codes used in the U.S. CMS to report injectable drugs that ordinarily cannot be self-administered by patients such as chemotherapy drugs, immunosuppressive drugs and inhalation solutions as well as some orally administered drugs. Based on logistics, it is relatively safe to say that a drug that does not have a "J code" will be prepared and administered by the patient (see Table 10.3 for examples of biotechnology drugs with and without a J code). It is important, regardless of the product being dispensed, to ensure that the pharmacist and patient understand the use, dosage regimen, and potential adverse effects of the product. Patients who will be preparing and self-administering the drug must know the proper storage and handling instructions as well as receive specific training on the administration of the drug and proper disposal of unused medication. When patients do not understand the administration and monitoring requirements of biotechnology products, training sessions for patients and caregivers should be considered to ensure appropriate patient care.

As more novel protein products, in particular the monoclonal antibody drugs, have come to market and the indications for existing agents have expanded, pharmacists are increasingly required to deal with these protein pharmaceuticals. While the first protein/peptide recombinant products were used primarily in hospital settings, many of these agents are now commonplace in ambulatory settings. The traditional community pharmacy may now dispense products like colony-stimulating factors, growth hormone, and interferons to name a just a few.

Traditional routes of delivery for pharmaceuticals have been challenged by the unique characteristics of biotech product delivery. Community pharmacies may struggle to maintain sufficient inventory of high-cost products, with in-depth knowledge of the products and its characteristics and with product administration. Assisting patients with reimbursement issues is very important, but is also a time-consuming, complicated process. Physicians also have difficulty with inventory and with slow reimbursement. Managed care organizations may have difficulty tracking claims for these products. As a result, the majority of patients receiving biotech drugs are now managed by home health, home infusion, or specialty pharmacy services (Managed Care 2014). Specialty pharmacies have evolved to manage outpatient biotechnology therapies for patients (National Association of Specialty Pharmacy 2018; https://naspnet.org/). Specialty pharmacy, which once occupied only a small niche in the marketplace, has become a burgeoning industry. Pharmacists, regardless of their area of practice, should understand the place of specialty pharmacy within the industry, even though the field may be difficult to define. Collaborations between specialty pharmacies, retail settings, hospitals, and manufacturers are becoming increasingly commonplace. These collaborations can enhance patient access to specialty pharmaceuticals and the high-touch services a specialty pharmacy can provide, thereby improving patient care.

Specialty pharmacies are growing in size and scope, in part because an aging population requires more specialty drugs such as the biotech-produced protein pharmaceuticals and also infusion therapies for cancer treatment. These drugs are expensive and often require special training to be administered and to be used by the patient home. Often the medications also need to be stored under specific conditions. Because misuse can be costly, many insurers pay for the high-touch service via a specialty pharmacy to assure so that costly medication errors are minimized. Specialty pharmacists practicing within academic health systems are uniquely positioned to overcome restrictions to medication access, financial constraints, and provider burdens that often lead to obstacles for patients to start and maintain necessary treatments (Bagwell et al. 2017).

The services offered by these pharmacies go far beyond dispensing biotech products. These pharmacies have expertise in the following areas:

- Insurance coverage and drug costs
- Pipeline monitoring and management
- Utilization management
- Promoting adherence to drug regimen
- Disease state management
- One-on-one counseling
- Risk Evaluation and Mitigation Strategies (REMS) requirements

Payers, particularly managed care organizations, now contract with specialty pharmacies to provide biotech and other expensive agents to solve many of the problems these products pose for the payer. The specialty pharmacy market is expected to continue to grow within the overall pharmaceutical market, according to a report from the Healthcare Distribution Alliance Research Foundation (HDA Research Foundation 2018). In 2016, specialty pharmacy was 40% of the $450 billion pharmaceutical market, compared to 30% of the $318 billion market in 2012.

Specialty sales in 2016 rose 11% over 2015 sales, to $181 billion. Of the $181 billion in 2016 sales of specialty drugs, $45 billion in sales was in the oncology market, the largest single therapeutic category. Medications for autoimmune issues came in second at $37 billion. Both of these categories of medicines have a large number of biotech drugs. In 2016, the top three specialty drugs by plan cost cross medical and pharmacy claims were Humira®, Enbrel®, and Remicade® (Artemetrix 2017). The introduction of new gene therapy and CAR-T therapies will likely accelerate the growth in specialty pharmacies.

Types of Information Needed by Pharmacists

What types of information do pharmacists require to be confident providers of biotech drugs and services? For pharmacists who have been out of school for many years, a contemporary understanding of the immune system, autoimmune diseases, and mechanisms by which drugs modify the immune system is essential. Several appropriate books that can provide a basic background in immunology are listed in Table 10.1. Additionally, practitioners may enroll in organized courses or continuing education programs that can provide up-to-date information in the discipline of immunology. Current pharmacy students and recent graduates should be sufficiently trained in basic immunology as part of their professional curriculum.

Pharmacists dispensing and counseling on biotech drugs must recognize that biotechnology primarily refers to a set of tools that has allowed great strides to be made in basic research, the understanding of disease and development of new therapeutic agents. It is essential for pharmacists to have a basic understanding of recombinant DNA technology and monoclonal antibody technology. However, it is not necessary that pharmacy practitioners know how to use these tools in the laboratory but rather how the use of these tools provides new therapeutic agents and a greater understanding of disease processes.

Pharmacists may need to review or learn anew about protein chemistry and those characteristics that affect therapeutic activity, product storage, and routes of administration of these drugs. Apart from this textbook, several publications, videotapes, and continuing professional education programs from industry and academic institutions are available to pharmacists for learning about the technical aspects of product storage and handling. Pharmacists also need to become familiar with the drug delivery systems currently in use for biotech drugs as well as those that are in development (see Chap. 5).

Sources of Information for Pharmacists

Many pharmacists do not know where to obtain the information that will allow them to be good providers of products of biotechnology. This textbook provides much of the essential background information in one source.

An excellent source of information on biotechnology in general, and specific products in particular, is the biotech drug industry. Many manufacturer-sponsored programs describe approved biotech products and those likely to come to market in the near future. Manufacturer programs provide extensive information about the disease states for which their products are indicated as well as product-specific information. Manufacturers are prepared to help pharmacists in the most effective provision of products and services to hospital-based and ambulatory patients.

Cellular and Molecular Immunology. 9th ed.
Abbas AK, Lichtman AH, Pillai S. Philadelphia: Elsevier, 2017: 565 pp.
Softbound book providing basic immunology concepts and clinical issues. Includes access to online edition
Immunology: A Short Course. 7th ed.
Coico R, Sunshine G. New Jersey: John Wiley and Sons, Inc., 2015: 406 pp
Softbound elementary text with review questions for each chapter *Clinical Immunology, Principles and Practice.* 5th ed. Rich RR, Fleisher TA, Shearer WT, Schroeder, Jr. HW, Frew AJ, Weyand CM. Philadelphia: Elsevier, 2018: 1392 pp. Hardbound book based on evidence-based practices that result in improved patient care
Cancer Immunotherapy Principles and Practice
Butterfield LH, Kaufman HL, Marincola FM. New York: Demos Medical, Springer Publishing, 2017: 920 pp.
Hardbound, detailed overview of immunology and immunobiotechnology from the perspective of Immunotherapy advances.
Roitt's Essential immunology. 13th ed.
Delves, PJ, Martin, SJ, Burton, DR, Roitt, IM. Oxford; Boston: Wiley-Blackwell Publishing, 2017: 576 pp.
Softbound basic immunology textbook
Janeway's Immunobiology. 9th ed.
Murphy K, Weaver C. New York: Garland Science, 2016: 924 pp.
Softback text that presents immunology at the introductory level. Also available in e-book format

Table 10.1 ■ Selected texts to enhance immunology knowledge

Manufacturer	Professional services	Reimbursement hotline/ indigent patient programs	Manufacturer website
Amgen	1-800-772-6436	1-800-272-9376	www.amgen.com
Astellas Pharma	1-800-727-7003	1-800-477-6472	www.astellas.us
Baxter Healthcare	1-800-422-9837	1-800-548-4448	www.baxter.com
Bayer Healthcare	1-888-765-3846	1-800-288-8374	www.bayerhealthcare.com
Biogen Idec	1-800-456-2255	1-800-456-2255	www.biogenidec.com
BioMarin	1-800-983-4587	1-866-906-6100	www.bmrn.com
Bristol-Myers Squibb	1-800-332-2056	1-800-736-0003	www.bms.com
CSL Behring	1-800-504-5434		www.cslbehring.com
Eli Lilly	1-877-237-8197	1-800-545-5979	www.lilly.com
Genentech	1-800-821-8590	1-800-530-3083	www.gene.com
Genentech	1-800-821-8590	1-866-422-2377	www.genentechaccesssolutions.com
Genzyme	1-800-745-4447	1-800-745-4447	www.genzyme.com
GlaxoSmithKline	1-888-825-5249	1-888-825-5249	www.gsk.com
Janssen Biotech	1-800-526-7736	1-800-652-6227	www.janssenbiotech.com
Kite Pharma	1-844-454-KITE	1-844-454-KITE	www.kitepharma.com
Merck	1-800-444-2080	1-800-727-5400	www.merck.com
Novartis	1-888-669-6682	1-800-257-3273	www.novartis.com
Novo Nordisk	1-800-727-6500	1-877-668-6777	www.novomedlink.com
Pfizer	1-800-505-4426	1-866-706-2400	www.pfizer.com
Pfizer	1-800-505-4426	1-866-706-2400	www.pfizerhelpfulanswers.com
Roche	1-800-821-8590	1-800-285-2484	www.roche.com
Sanofi	1-800-981-2491	1-800-221-4025	www.sanofi.us
Sun Pharmaceuticals	1-877-208-3015		www.sunpharma.com

Table 10.2 Toll-free assistance numbers and websites for selected biopharmaceutical manufacturers in the USA and Canada

However, many pharmacists are unaware of these services and how to obtain them. A web search of specific products will lead to the product and manufacturer's websites where this information can be accessed.

The information provided by manufacturers can help pharmacists to confidently provide biotechnology products to their patients. The services provided generally fall into three categories: customer/medical services and support, educational materials, and reimbursement information. Manufacturers may have a separate number for reimbursement questions. Table 10.2 lists the manufacturer's toll-free assistance numbers and web addresses for obtaining product and reimbursement information in North America. Vaccines and insulin products are not included in this table since these products were previously available in a nonrecombinant form and pharmacists are generally well familiar with these products. Moreover, the recombinant forms of these products are generally not as costly as other types of biologic agents.

The Pharmacist and Handling of Biotech Drugs

The pharmacist is responsible for the storage, preparation, and dispensing of biotechnology drugs as well as patient education regarding the use of these products. In many cases, pharmacists must have additional training in order to be prepared for this role. This is especially true for pharmacists who practice in the ambulatory setting since these products are increasingly available for self-administration in the home. Pharmacies of the future may stock pumps, patches, timed-release tablets, liposomes, implants, and vials of tailored monoclonal antibodies. With advances in gene therapy and pharmacogenomics, it is possible that the pharmacist may eventually prepare and dispense precision medicine products tailored for specific patients.

This chapter discusses the general principles that pharmacists need to understand about storage, handling, preparation, administration of biotech products, and issues related to outpatient/home care. Specific examples will be discussed for illustrative purposes. Table 10.3 lists selected products along with

Generic name	Brand name	Storage temperature	Reconstitution solution	Stability after reconstitution RT	Stability after reconstitution Ref	Dilution/stability	J code[a]
Abatacept	Orencia®	2–8 °C	SWFI	24 h	24 h	24 h (further diluted in NS)	Yes
Adalimumab	Humira®	2–8 °C	RTU	NA	NA	NA	Yes
Alteplase	Activase®	2–25 °C	Dil	8 h	8 h	NA	Yes
Alteplase	Cathflo® Activase®	2–8 °C	SWFI	8 h	8 h	NA	Yes
Bevacizumab	Avastin®	2–8 °C	NS	NA	8 h	NA	Yes
Canakinumab	Ilaris®	2–8 °C	SWFI	24 h	24 h	NA	Yes
Cetuximab	Erbitux®	2–8 °C	RTU	NA	NA	NA	Yes
Darbepoetin alfa	Aranesp®	2–8 °C	RTU	NA	NA	NA	Yes
Denosumab	Prolia® Xgeva®	2–8 °C	RTU	NA	NA	NA	Yes
Dornase alfa	Pulmozyme®	2–8 °C	RTU	NA	NA	NA	Yes
Epoetin alfa SDV	Epogen® Procrit®	2–8 °C	SBWFI containing benzyl alcohol 0.9% in a 1:1 ratio	14 d (except for 40,000 units/mL vials which are stable for 7 d)	NA	Dilutions of 1:10 and 1:20 (1 part epoetin:19 parts sodium chloride): 18 h	Yes
Epoetin alfa MDV	Epogen® Procrit®	2–8 °C aie and between doses	RTU	NA	NA	Dilutions of 1:10 in $D_{10}W$ with human albumin 0.05 or 0.1%: 24 h	Yes
Erenumab-aooc	Aimovigv	2–8 °C	RTU	NA	NA	NA	No
Etanercept	Enbrel®	2–8 °C	SBWFI	NA	14 d	NA	Yes
Evolocumab	Rapatha®	2–8 °C	RTU	NA	NA	NA	Yes
Factor VIIa recombinant	NovoSeven® RT	2–25 °C	Histidine diluent	3 h	3 h	NA	No
Filgrastim	Neupogen®	2–8 °C	D_5W	24 h	14 d	24 h	Yes
Golimumab	Kinevet®	2–8 °C	RTU	NA	NA	NA	No
Infliximab	Remicade®	2–8 °C	SWFI	NA	NA	3 h	Yes
Interferon alfa- 2b	Intron®A	2–8 °C	SWFI		24 h	24 h (further diluted in NS)	Yes
Interferon-β1a prefilled syringe	Avonex®, Rebif®	2–8 °C	RTU	NA	NA	NA	Yes
Interferon-β1a reconstitutable vial	Avonex®, Rebif	2–8 °C	SWFI	NA	6 h	NA	Yes
Interferon-β1b	Betaseron®	25 °C	NaCl 0.54%	NA	3 h	NA	Yes
Ipilimumab	Yervoy®	2–8 °C	NS or D_5W	24 h	24 h	NA	Yes
Ixekizumab	Taltz®	2–8 °C	RTU	NA	5 d	NA	Yes
Ocrelizumab	Ocrevus®	2–8 °C	NaCl 0.9%	NA	NA	NA	No
Paclitaxel (protein bound)	Abraxane®	25 °C	NS	8 h	8 h	NA	Yes
Palivizumab	Synagis®	2–8 °C	RTU	NA	NA	NA	No
Peginterferon alfa-2a	Pegasys® Convenience Pack	2–8 °C	RTU	NA	NA	NA	No

Table 10.3 ■ Storage, stability, and reconstitution of selected biotechnology products

Generic name	Brand name	Storage temperature	Reconstitution solution	Stability after reconstitution RT	Ref	Dilution/stability	J code[a]
Peginterferon alfa-2b	PegIntron®	25 °C	SWFI	NA	24 h	NA	No
Peginterferon alfa-2b	Sylatron®	25 °C	SWFI	NA	24 h	NA	No
Peginterferon alfa-2b	Redipen®	2–8 °C	RTU	NA	24 h	NA	No
Pegfilgrastim	Neulasta®	2–8 °C	RTU	NA	NA	NA	Yes
Ramucirumab	Cyramza®	2–8 °C	NaCl 0.9%	4 h	24 h	24 h	Yes
Ranibizumab	Lucentis®	2–8 °C	RTU	NA	NA	NA	Yes
Redolizumab	Entyvio®	2–8 °C	NaCl 0.9%	12 h	24 h	12 h	Yes
Rituximab	Rituxan®	2–8 °C	NS or D_5W	24 h	24 h	NA	No
Secukinumab	Cosentyx®	2–8 °C	RTU	NA	NA	NA	No
Teriparatide	Forteo®	2–8 °C	RTU	NA	NA	NA	No
Tisagenlecleucel	Kymriah®	NA	In clinic	NA	NA	NA	No
Trastuzumab	Herceptin®	2–8 °C	SBWFI	NA	28 d	24 h (further diluted in NS)	Yes

Biologic products listed in the top 200 drugs in the US market by sales, 2017

Table key: *aie* after initial entry into vial, *d* days; *dil* supplied diluent, *h* hours, *mdv* applies only to multidose vials, *NA* not applicable/not available, *NS* normal saline, *Ref* under refrigeration, *RT* room temperature, *RTU* ready to use, *SBWFI* sterile bacterial water for injection, *SDV* applies only to single-dose vials, *SWFI* sterile water for injection

[a]Products have a J code for the first quarter of 2018 according to the document, 2018 ASP Drug Pricing Files Medicare Part B Drug Average Sales Price, listed on cms.gov (https://www.cms.gov/Medicare/Medicare-Fee-for-Service-Part-B-Drugs/McrPartBDrugAvgSalesPrice/2018ASPFiles.html)

Table 10.3 ■ (continued)

specific handling requirements for each. For specific products or recent updates to these requirements, contact the manufacturer. For additional information regarding drug handling and preparation, the pharmacist may consult publications such as the American Hospital Formulary Service (AHFS) Drug Information ONLINE (http://www.ahfsdruginformation.com/ahfs-clinical-drug-information/; and in print each year annually by the Association of Health-Systems Pharmacists) (AHFS 2018) or the *King Guide to Parenteral Admixture* (https://kingguide.net/collections/internet-edition) (King Guide 2018), an updated online guide to IV drug compatibility and stability (there are also print versions available for purchase). Pharmacy benefits management companies (PBMs) usually own specialty pharmacy companies and provide valuable information via their websites. The three largest specialty pharmacy companies in 2016 were CVS Specialty (CVS Health), Accredo/Freedom Fertility owned by Express Scripts, and Alliance Rx Walgreens Prime/Walgreens stores (Walgreens Boots Alliance) (Drug Channels 2018).

STORAGE

Biotech products have unique storage requirements when compared to the majority of products that pharmacists dispense. The shelf-life of these products is often considerably shorter than for traditional compounds (Cf. Chap. 5). For example, interferon-α2a (Roferon-A®, Roche Laboratories 2018) is only stable in a refrigerator in the ready-to-use solution for 2 years. After the first dose, cartridges may be stored at less than 25 °C for *up to* 28 days although refrigeration is recommended. Since most biologic products need to be kept at refrigerated temperatures (as discussed below), some pharmacies may need to increase cold storage space in order to accommodate the storage needs.

■ Temperature Requirements

Since biotech products are primarily proteins, they are subject to denaturation when exposed to extreme temperatures. In general, most biotech products are shipped by the manufacturer in gel ice containers and need to be stored at 2–8 °C (Banga and Reddy 1994; Rayfield et al. 2017). Once reconstituted, they should be stored under refrigeration until just prior to use. There are a few exceptions to this rule. For example, alteplase (tissue plasminogen activator, Activase®) lyophilized powder is stable at room temperature for several years at temperatures not to exceed 30 °C (86 °F). However, after reconstitution, the product should be used within 8 h (Genentech 2018b). For individual product temperature requirements, the product insert, product website, or the manufacturer should be contacted. Table 10.3 lists temperature requirements for selected frequently prescribed products.

The variability between products with respect to temperature is exemplified by granulocyte colony-stimulating factor (G-CSF, filgrastim, Neupogen®) (Amgen Inc 2018b) and erythropoietin (Epogen®) (Amgen Inc 2018a), which are stable in ready-to-use form at room temperature for 24 h and 14 days, respectively. Granulocyte macrophage colony-stimulating factor (GM-CSF, sargramostim, Leukine®) (Sanofi-Aventis 2018) is packaged as a lyophilized powder but still requires refrigeration and once reconstituted is stable at room temperature for 30 days or in the refrigerator for 2 years. Aldesleukin (interleukin-2, Proleukin®) is stable for 48 h at room temperature or under refrigeration (Prometheus Therapeutics and Diagnostics 2018). Interferon-β1b (Betaseron®) must be stored in a refrigerator and should be used within 3 h after reconstitution (Bayer HealthCare 2018). While most products require refrigeration to maintain stability due to denaturation by elevated temperatures, extreme cold such as freezing may be just as harmful to most products. The key is to avoid extremes in temperature whether it is heat or cold (Banga and Reddy 1994).

■ Storage in Dosing and Administration Devices

Many biotech products can adhere to either plastic or glass containers such as syringes, polyvinyl chloride (PVC) intravenous bags, infusion equipment, and glass intravenous bottles. The effectiveness of the product may be reduced by three- or fourfold due to adherence. In order to decrease the amount of adherence human serum albumin, (HSA) is usually added to the solutions. The relative loss through adherence is concentration dependent, i.e., the more concentrated the final solution, the less significant the adherence becomes. The amount of HSA added varies with the product (Banga and Reddy 1994; Finn et al. 2012). Some products that require the addition of HSA include filgrastim, sargramostim, aldesleukin, erythropoietin, and interferon-α. In the case of filgrastim, the addition of 2 mg/mL of HSA to the final solution is required for concentrations of 5–15 μg/mL (Amgen Inc 2018c). One milligram of HSA per 1 mL 0.9% sodium chloride injection is added to achieve a final concentration of 0.1% HSA for sargramostim concentrations of <10 μg/mL (Sanofi-Aventis 2018). For aldesleukin 0.1%, HSA is required for all concentrations (Prometheus Therapeutics and Diagnostics 2018). For erythropoietin, 2.5 mg HSA is present per mL in each single-dose and multidose vial (Amgen Inc 2018d). One milligram per milliliter of HSA is added to interferon-α-2b (Intron-A®) in single-dose and multidose vials and pens (RxList 2018).

For additional information or to find information for other products, check the current product information or contact the manufacturer.

■ Storage in IV Solutions

Biotech product stability may vary when stored in different types of containers and syringes. Some products are only stable in plastic syringes, e.g., somatropin and erythropoietin, while others are stable in glass, polyvinyl chloride, and polypropylene, e.g., aldesleukin. Batch prefilling of syringes is possible. However, it is important to make sure that the product you wish to provide in prefilled syringes is stable in the type of syringe you wish to use. This may present a challenge to specialty pharmacy programs. Determining how far in advance doses may be prepared is also an important consideration. G-CSF is stable in Becton Dickinson (B-D) disposable plastic syringes for up to 7 days (Amgen Inc 2018c), while erythropoietin is stable for up to 14 days (Amgen Inc 2018d). Aldesleukin is recommended to be administered in PVC although glass has been used in clinical trials with comparable results (Prometheus Therapeutics and Diagnostics 2018). Solutions are stable for 48 h when refrigerated. GM-CSF and G-CSF can be administered in either PVC or polypropylene (Sanofi-Aventis 2018).

■ Light Protection

Many biotech products are sensitive to light. Manufacturer's information usually suggests that products be protected from strong light until the product is used. Dornase-α (Pulmozyme®) is packaged in protective foil pouches by the manufacturer to protect it from light degradation and should be stored in these original light protective containers until use. For patients who travel, the manufacturer will provide special travel pouches on request (Genentech 2018a). Alteplase in the lyophilized form also needs to be protected from light but is not light sensitive when in solution (Genentech 2018b). Pharmacists must be aware of the specific storage requirements with respect to light for each of the products stocked in the pharmacy.

HANDLING

■ Mixing and Shaking

Improper handling of protein products can lead to denaturation. Shaking and severe agitation of most of these products will result in degradation (cf. Chap. 5). Therefore, special techniques must be observed in preparing biotech products for use. Biotech products should not be shaken when adding any diluent as this may cause the product to breakdown. Once the diluent is added to the container, the vial should be swirled rather than vigorously shaken. Some shaking during transport may be unavoidable and proper inspection of products should occur to make sure the products have not been damaged during transit. When a product is affected by excessive shaking, physical separation or frothing within the vial of liquid products can usually be observed. For lyophilized products, agitation is not harmful until the product has been or is reconstituted. In distributing individual products to patient or ward areas, pneumatic tubes should be avoided.

■ Travel Requirements

When patients travel with these products, certain precautions should be observed. The drugs should be stored in insulated, cool containers. This can be accomplished by using ice packs to keep the biotech drug at the proper temperature in warmer climates, whereas the insulated container in colder climates may be all that is required. When traveling in subfreezing weather, the products should be protected from freezing (temperatures below 2 °C). Keeping biotech drugs at proper temperature during automobile travel may present a problem with temperatures inside a parked car often exceeding 37 °C (100 °F) on a warm day. Patients and delivery personnel must take care not to leave products that are not in insulated containers inside the car, trunk, or glove compartment while shopping or making deliveries. When ice is used, care should be taken not to place the product directly on the ice. Dry ice should be avoided since it has the potential for freezing the product. When traveling by air, biotech products should be taken onto the plane in insulated packages and not placed in a cargo container. Airplane cargo containers may be cold enough to cause freezing (Banga and Reddy 1994).

PREPARATION

When preparing biotech products, aseptic technique must be employed as it is with traditional parenteral products. Sterile compounding procedures require clean facilities, specific training for operators, air quality evaluations, and a sound knowledge of sterilization and stability principles. USP 797 provides guidelines, procedures and compliance requirements for compounding sterile preparations. The product should be prepared in a clean room designed for this purpose with laminar airflow hoods, and other practices consistent with USP 797. Most of the products require reconstitution with sterile water or bacteriostatic water for injection depending on stability data. The compatibility of individual products varies and limited data is available. As mentioned previously, when adding diluent to these products, care should be taken not to shake them, but to swirl the container or roll it between the palms of the hands. In the case of lyophilized products, introduction of the diluent should be directed down the side of the vial and not directly on the powder to avoid denaturing the protein. It is important to mention that stability does not mean sterility. Biotech products require the same precautions as any other parenteral product. Sterility is particularly important when prefilling and premixing various doses for administration at home. Once the manufacturer's sterile packaging is entered, sterility can no longer be assured nor will the manufacturer be responsible for any subsequent related problems. Many biotech drugs are not compatible with preservative agents, and single-use vials do not contain a preservative. Individual manufacturers have not addressed the issue of sterility and each institution or organization must determine its own policy on this issue. Many of the currently available biotechnology-produced products are provided as single-dose vials and should not be reused. This does not, however, prevent preparing batches ("batching") of unit-of-use doses in order to be efficient. Many of the patients receiving these agents are likely to have suppressed immune systems and are vulnerable to infection. Therefore, a policy involving the maintenance of sterility of biotech products should be developed by each health-care organization, especially hospitals and specialty pharmacies. When products are made in a sterile environment under aseptic procedures, they should remain sterile until used and thus could be stored for as long as physical compatibility data dictates. However, most institutions have shorter expiration dates, which are generally 72 h or less, on reconstituted products. These expiration dates have been conservatively set due to lack of good sterility data to the contrary. Sterility studies should be performed in order to determine if reconstituted products could be stored for a longer period of time and still maintain sterility. For products reconstituted for home use, in the pharmacy sterile products area, a 7-day expiration date is used provided the product is stable and can be stored in the refrigerator. The American Society of Health-System Pharmacists has published a technical assistance bulletin on sterile products, which should be consulted for developing policies on storage of reconstituted parenteral products (American Society of Health-System Pharmacists 2017). Patients need to be informed about specific storage requirements and expiration dates to assure sterility and stability.

ADMINISTRATION

Prior to administering these products, pharmacists will need to use caution in reviewing dosing regimens. A potential source of medication error is the variation in units of measure for the various products. Some products are dosed in micrograms/kilogram (μg/kg) rather than milligrams/kilogram (mg/kg). Dosage calculations need to be carefully checked to avoid potential errors. Biotech products frequently receive approval for new indications after they have been on the market for a few years. The dosing regimen for these indications may be different than the original indication. Therefore, it is important to confirm the diagnosis and indication for products with multiple indications and dosing regimens. For example, adalimumab (Humira®) is dosed at 40 mg subcutaneously every other week to treat rheumatoid arthritis. The initial dose for plaque psoriasis is 80 mg subcutaneously, followed by a weekly dose of 40 mg. The initial dose for Crohn's disease is 160 mg subcutaneously, given as 4 injections on day 1 or 2 injections/day over 2 consecutive days, followed by an 80 mg dose 2 weeks later and a weekly maintenance dose of 40 mg every other week beginning on day 29 (AbbVie Inc 2018).

Another example of variations in dosing regimen is for the monoclonal antibody denosumab from Amgen Inc. For treatment of osteoporosis in postmenopausal females, the dose of denosumab (Prolia®; Amgen Inc 2018c) is 60 mg every month. For prevention of skeletal-related events in bone metastases from solid tumors, denosumab is administered 120 mg every 4 weeks (Xgeva®; Amgen Inc 2018d). The manufacturer recognizes the risk of errors in dosing and has given the product different names to help prevent mistakes in dosing regimens.

■ Routes of Administration

Biotech products are primarily administered parenterally although routes of administration may be used. For example, dornase alfa is administered by inhalation (Genentech 2018b). Some products may be given by either the intravenous or subcutaneous route, while others are restricted to the subcutaneous or intramuscular routes. In some cases, manufacturers have information on unapproved routes of administration or other unpublished information that may be available by contacting the individual manufacturer. In any case, the manufacturer should always be consulted in order to obtain supporting evidence for a particular route that is not approved, but may be more convenient for the patient. For example, G-CSF should be administered by the subcutaneous or intravenous route only, while GM-CSF is given by intravenous infusion, over a 2 h period (AHFS 2018). Aldesleukin is approved for intravenous administration only. However, subcutaneous administration has been used by some as an unlabeled route of administration (McDermott et al. 2005). Erythropoietin should only be administered by the intravenous or subcutaneous routes (Amgen Inc 2018d), while alteplase is only approved for the intravenous route (AHFS 2018; Genentech 2018a) Alteplase has also been administered by the intracoronary, intra-arterial, and intraorbital routes as well (AHFS 2018).

■ Filtration

Filtering biotech products is not generally recommended since most of these proteins will adhere to the filter. Some hospitals and home infusion companies routinely use in-line filters for all intravenous solutions to minimize the introduction of particulate matter into the patient. In the case of biotech products, they should be infused below the filter to avoid a potential decrease in the amount of drug delivered to the patient (Banga and Reddy 1994). Some manufacturers recommend infusing products using an in-line low protein-binding filter (≤1.2 μm).

■ Flushing Solutions

Biotechnology products are usually flushed with either saline or dextrose 5% in water. The product literature should be consulted and care should be taken to assure that the proper solution is used with each agent. In general, biotech drugs should not be administered with other drugs since, in most cases, data does not exist that demonstrates whether biotech products are compatible with other drugs or fluids.

■ Prophylaxis to Prevent Infusion Reactions

Some products have protocols to treat and/or prevent infusion reactions for repeat infusions. For example, the infliximab protocol to treat an infusion reaction includes reducing the infusion rate, initiating a normal saline infusion, use of symptomatic treatment (normally consisting of acetaminophen and diphenhydramine), and vital sign monitoring every 10 min until resolution of the reaction. For subsequent infusions, pretreatment with acetaminophen and diphenhydramine 90 min prior to the infusion is standard procedure. Patients who had severe reactions may receive corticosteroids (AbbVie Inc 2018).

BIOSIMILARS

The present state of the regulatory aspects of biosimilars (through FDA and EMA) is dealt with in Chap. 12. Making choices for health-care professionals is not new in the biotech market as it already contains several types of insulins, growth hormones, and second-generation products such as darbepoetin alfa (Aranesp®) and pegfilgrastim (Neulasta®). Pharmacists and formulary committees need to choose between a variety of biotech drugs produced in different cell lines with differences in physical properties but intended to produce the same therapeutic effect. The ability to achieve a similar therapeutic effect for patients with a particular chronic disease using a biosimilar product is only one important consideration of comparing biosimilar products to the innovator drug. Biosimilars will also differ from the innovator drug in the manufacturing process.

For example, a different cell line may be used to produce the recombinant protein. It is possible that the innovator and biosimilar drug may therefore differ in the immunogenicity of the product. Patients may be more or less likely to develop an immune response to the biosimilar agent. Health professionals will need to be involved in the clinical trials, patient monitoring, and postmarketing surveillance of biosimilars to determine the interchangeability of products and the patient care considerations that may be involved in using biosimilar agents.

OUTPATIENT/HOME CARE ISSUES

As mentioned previously, the management of patients in the outpatient and home settings is now an accepted aspect of health-care delivery. Home infusion and specialty pharmacy services dispense all forms of parenteral and enteral products including biotech drugs. These pharmacies have grown exponentially in the last 25 years due to cost savings for third-party payers, technological advances that allow these services to occur in the home, and patient preference to be treated at home rather than an in-patient setting.

■ Patient Assessment and Education

Before a patient can be a candidate for home therapy, an assessment of the patient's capabilities must occur. The patient, family member, or caregiver will need to be able to administer the medication and comply with all of the storage, handling, and preparation requirements. If the patient is incapable, then a caregiver (usually a relative, spouse, or friend) needs to be recruited to assist the patient. The pharmacy staff or other health professional may also make home visits to assist the patient in these tasks. The use of aseptic technique is usually new to the patients and in some cases may be overwhelming. The health-care provider must be sure that the patient or caregiver is competent and willing to follow these procedures. Self-instructional guides on specific products may be available from the manufacturer and, if so, should be provided to the patient providing they have the proper equipment for viewing.

Proper storage facilities will need to be available in the patient's home as well as a clean area for preparation and administration. Ideally, the patient will be able to prepare each dose immediately prior to the time of administration. If this is not possible, the pharmacy will have to prepare prefilled syringes and provide appropriate storage and handling requirements to the patient. The patient will also need to be educated regarding the proper handling of the syringes as well as other required supplies and materials such as needles, syringes, and alcohol wipes. Proper disposal of these hazardous wastes must also be reviewed. Specific issues related to patient teaching include rotating injection sites, product handling, drug storage including transporting and traveling with biotech drugs, expiration dates, refrigeration, cleansing the injection site with alcohol, disposal of needles and syringes, potential adverse effects, and expected therapeutic outcomes.

■ Monitoring

For patients who receive biotech drug therapy in the home, it is particularly important that close patient monitoring occurs. This will require frequent phone calls to the patient and periodic home visits. Monitoring parameters should include adverse events, progress to expected outcomes, assessment of administration technique, review of storage and handling procedures, and adherence to aseptic technique.

REIMBURSEMENT

Reimbursement issues include third-party billing information and availability of forms, cost-sharing programs that limit the annual cost of therapy, financial assistance programs for patients who would otherwise have difficulty paying for therapy, and reimbursement assurance programs that are designed to remove reimbursement barriers when reimbursement has been denied. Any detailed discussion of reimbursement issues is beyond the scope of this book and is subject to practice location. This discussion will deal only with the availability of information to pharmacists to appropriately handle reimbursement for products and services in the United States.

Pharmacists need to know current third-party payment policies including those conditions under which insurance companies will disallow claims. Some examples include off-label prescribing or administration of the product in the home rather than administration in a hospital or physician's office. Prior authorization is usually required particularly with managed care or prepaid plans. Manufacturers will often assist the patient by contacting the carrier to verify coverage, providing sample prior-approval letters, and following up on claims to determine the claim's status, and continuing to follow the case until it is resolved.

Manufacturers can also provide information that may convince the third-party payer to reconsider a denied claim. Some companies will intervene with the third-party payer to evaluate the case for denial and provide additional clinical documentation or coding information and will follow the appeal to conclusion. Pharmacists can act as facilitators to get qualified patients enrolled in programs to provide free medication to those who have insufficient insurance coverage or are otherwise unable to purchase the therapy.

Manufacturers' websites and toll-free numbers for reimbursement issues are provided in Table 10.2. Websites, toll-free numbers and email addresses can be found for a wide range of assistance programs on the WebMD site including programs run by pharmaceutical companies, by states and by non-profit groups (https://www.webmd.com/healthy-aging/patient-assistance-programs-for-prescription-drugs#1). A major program is the Partnership for Prescription Assistance website (https://www.pparx.org/) which provides information on a variety of patient assistance programs as well as the requirements to qualify for various programs. They are a program sponsored by drug companies, doctors, patient advocacy organizations, and civic groups.

EDUCATIONAL MATERIALS

Therapy with biotech drugs is a rapidly growing, ever-changing area of therapeutics, particularly as cell and gene therapy approaches enter the market. Pharmacists need to keep abreast of current information about existing agents such as new indications, management of adverse effects, results of studies describing drug interactions, or changes in information regarding product stability and reconstitution. Pharmacists will also be interested in the status of new agents as they move through the FDA approval process. Some good periodical sources of practical information about products of biotechnology are listed in Table 10.4. The Internet is a valuable site rich in up-to-date information concerning all aspects of pharmaceutical biotechnology. Sites include virtual libraries/catalogs, online journals (usually requiring a subscription), biomedical newsletters, and biotechnology-specific home pages. Since the number of biotech-related sites is constantly increasing, readers are encouraged to explore the web for useful options.

■ Educational Materials for Health Professionals

Manufacturer and specific product websites provide a variety of educational materials including continuing education programs for physicians, pharmacists, and nurses. These programs often focus on specific disease states as well as drug therapy. The programs sometimes include slides, videos, and brochures. Since most biotechnology products are parenteral products, several manufacturers have produced videotapes that show the proper procedure for product administration, storage, and handling. These instructional tapes are beneficial not just for patients but also for health professionals who may not be skilled in injection techniques.

■ Educational Materials for Patients

Detailed patient information booklets exist for many of the products both in print and by downloading from the Internet. Patient education materials can assist the patient and family members in learning more about his or her disease and how it will be treated. Education allows the patient to participate more actively in the therapy and to feel a greater level of control over the process. By contacting the manufacturer and acquiring patient educational materials, pharmacists can offer support to the patient in learning to use a new product. Dealing with a diagnosis of serious or chronic disease already overwhelms many patients. Learning about a new therapy, especially if it involves the necessity of self-injection, can cause additional stress for the patient and family.

Most commercially available biotech drugs now have individual websites to provide updated information to patients. These sites usually contain the following types of information: disease background, reimbursement information, dosing information, references, frequently asked questions, administration and storage information, and information specifically for health professionals. These websites also offer tools such as journals for patients to record administration of doses and monitoring information to assist health professionals in following the patient's progress. The websites also refer patients to disease-related associations and organizations whose services include a link to local chapters, meetings, and support groups. These groups may provide support to the patient while he or she adjusts to the diagnosis and treatment of a potentially serious disease.

2017 State of the Industry; PhRMA; http://phrma.org/industryprofile/
An *Introduction to Biotechnology*—Amgen; http://www.biotechnology.amgen.com/index.html
BioCentury News, BioCentury, Inc., San Carlos, CA; https://www.biocentury.com/
Bio/Technology, New York, nature Publishing Company; www.nature.com/nbt
BiotechNow Blog, Biotechnology Innovation Organization (BIO), Washington, D.C., https://www.bio.org/
BioWorld *Today*, Atlanta, Bioworld Publishing Group, newspaper; http://www.bioworld.com/
Genetic Engineering News, New York, GEN Publishing, bimonthly publication; https://www.genengnews.com/
"*The Pink Sheet*" Bridgewater, NJ, published weekly; https://pink.pharmaintelligence.informa.com/

Table 10.4 ■ Information sources for current trends in biotechnology

CONCLUDING REMARKS

The handling of biotechnology products requires similar skills and techniques as required for the preparation of other parenteral drugs, but there are often different nuances to the handling, preparation, and administration of biotechnology-produced pharmaceuticals. The pharmacist can become an educator regarding the pharmaceutical aspects of biotechnology products and can serve as a valuable resource to other health-care professionals. In addition, biotech products give the pharmacist the opportunity to provide enhanced patient care services since patient education and monitoring is required. To carry out this role successfully, the pharmacist will need to keep abreast of new developments as new literature and products become available.

SELF-ASSESSMENT QUESTIONS

Questions

1. What are some of the causes of pharmacist reluctance to handling biotech products?
2. In what areas of study do pharmacists and pharmacy students need to engage to be best prepared to provide pharmaceutical care services to patients receiving biotechnology therapeutic agents?
3. What resources are available to pharmacy practitioners to learn more about biotechnology and the drug products of biotechnology?
4. How do the storage requirements of biotech products differ from the majority of products pharmacists normally dispense?
5. What is the most common temperature for the storage of biotech pharmaceuticals?
6. Why is human serum albumin added to the solution of many biotech drugs?
7. Why should biotech products not be shaken when adding any diluent?
8. During travel, what precautions should also be observed with biotech products?
9. Should biotech products be filtered prior to administration?
10. What assessments must be done by the pharmacist before a patient can be considered a candidate for home therapy with a biotech product?
11. What types of professional services information are provided by manufacturers of biotech drugs?
12. What issues will the pharmacist need to consider when comparing innovator drugs to biosimilars?

Answers

1. Lack of understanding of the basics of biotechnology; lack of understanding of the therapeutics of recombinant protein products; unfamiliarity with the side effects and patient counseling information; lack of familiarity with the storage, handling, and reconstitution of proteins; and the difficulty of handling reimbursement issues.
2. Basic biotechnology/immunological methods; protein chemistry; therapeutics of biotechnology agents; and storage, handling, reconstitution, and administration of biotechnology products.
3. Biotechnology/immunology texts, continuing education programs, manufacturers' information and toll-free assistance, biotechnology-oriented journals, and the Internet.
4. The shelf-life of these products is often considerably shorter than has been the case with more traditional compounds. These products need to be kept at refrigerated temperatures. There are, of course, exceptions to this rule.
5. In general, most biotech products are shipped by the manufacturer in gel ice containers and need to be stored at 2–8 °C. Once reconstituted, they should be kept under refrigeration until just prior to use.
6. Most biotech products may adhere to either plastic or glass containers such as syringes and polyvinyl chloride (PVC) intravenous bags reducing effectiveness of the product. Human serum albumin is usually added to the solutions to prevent adherence.
7. Shaking may cause the product to breakdown (aggregation). Usually when this happens one can observe physical separation or frothing within the vial of liquid products.
8. They should be stored in insulated, cool containers. This can be accomplished by using ice packs to keep the biotech drug at the proper temperature in warmer climates, whereas the insulated container in colder climates may be all that is required. In fact, when traveling in subfreezing weather, the products should be protected from freezing.
9. Filtering biotech products is not generally recommended since most of the proteins will adhere to the filter.
10. Before a patient can be a candidate for home therapy, an assessment of the patient's capabilities must occur. The patient, family member, or caregiver will need to be able to inject the medication and comply with all of the storage, handling, and preparation requirements.
11. Medical information services provided by manufacturers of biotech drugs are similar to the product, medical and patient management services provided by drug companies for traditional drug products. Information provided via this service generally includes appropriate indications, side effects, contraindications to use, results of clinical trials, and investigational uses. Upon request, manufacturers can supply a product monograph

and selected research articles that provide valuable information about each product.

12. In addition to ensuring that the biosimilar drug produces the same therapeutic effect, differences in manufacturing that may affect the patient will need to be considered. The most significant of these is potential immunogenicity of the product.

REFERENCES

AbbVie Inc. (2018) Humira® information. Accessed at: https://www.humirapro.com. Accessed 25 May 2018

AHFS (2018) American hospital formulary service drug information. American Society of Health-System Pharmacists. Accessed at: http://www.ahfsdruginformation.com/ahfs-clinical-drug-information/. Accessed 25 May 2018

American Society of Health-System Pharmacists (2017) ASHP guidelines on compounding sterile preparations. Accessed at: https://www.ashp.org/-/media/assets/policy-guidelines/docs/guidelines/compounding-sterile-preparations.ashx. Accessed 25 May 2018

Amgen Inc. (2018a) Epogen® information. Accessed at: http://www.epogen.com/. Accessed 21 May 2018

Amgen Inc. (2018b) Neupogen® information. Accessed at: http://www.neupogenhcp.com. Accessed 21 May 2018

Amgen Inc. (2018c) Prolia® information. Accessed at: https://www.prolia.com/. Accessed 25 May 2018

Amgen Inc. (2018d) Xgeva® information. Accessed at: http://www.xgeva.com/. Accessed 25 May 2018

Artemetrix (2017) 2017 State of specialty management - specialty drug trend report. Accessed at: http://www.psgconsults.com/specialtyreport?gclid=EAIaIQobChMIlaeFxsWh2wIVDv5kCh0VGQENEAAYASAAEgIvDvD_BwE. Accessed 25 May 2018

Bagwell A, Kelley T, Carver A, Lee JB, Newman B (2017) Advancing patient care through specialty pharmacy services in an academic health system. J. Manag Care Spec Pharm 23:815–820

Banga AK, Reddy IK (1994) Biotechnology drugs: pharmaceutical issues. Pharm Times 60:68–76

Bayer HealthCare (2018) Betaseron® full prescribing information. https://www.betaseron.com/. Accessed 21 May 2018

Department of Health and Human Services (2018) CMS manual system, Pub 100–02 Medicare Benefit Policy, Chapter 15. Accessed at: https://www.cms.gov/Regulations-and-Guidance/Guidance/Manuals/Downloads/bp102c15.pdf. Accessed 08 May 2018

Drug Channels (2018) The top 15 specialty pharmacies of 2017: PBMs and payers still dominate. Accessed at: http://www.drugchannels.net/2018/03/the-top-15-specialty-pharmacies-of-2017.html. Accessed 25 May 2018

Finn TE, Nunez AC, Sunde M, Easterbrook-Smith SB (2012) Serum albumin prevents protein aggregation and amyloid formation and retains chaperone-like activity in the presence of physiological ligands. J Biol Chem 28:21530–21540

Genentech (2018a) Pulmozyme® information. Accessed at: https://www.pulmozyme.com/. Accessed 25 May 2018

Genentech (2018b) Activase® information. Accessed at: https://www.activase.com/. Accessed 21 May 2018

HDA Research Foundation (2018) Specialty Pharmaceutical Distribution Facts, Figures and Trends. Accessed at: https://www.hda.org/resources/2017-specialty-pharmaceutical-distribution. Accessed 22 May 2018

King Guide (2018) King guide to parenteral admixture. King Guide Publications, Inc. Accessed at: https://king-guide.net/collections/internet-edition. Accessed 25 May 2018

Managed Care (2014) Provider-administered drugs move to specialty pharmacy benefit. Manag Care 23:49

McDermott DF, Regan MM, Clark JI et al (2005) Randomized phase III trial of high-dose interleukin-2 versus subcutaneous interleukin-2 and interferon in patients with metastatic renal cell carcinoma. J Clin Oncol 23(1):133–141

National Association of Specialty Pharmacy (2018). Accessed at: https://naspnet.org/. Accessed 25 May 2018

Prometheus Therapeutics & Diagnostics (2018) Proleukin® information. Accessed at: https://www.proleukin.com/. Accessed 21 May 2018

Rayfield WJ, Kandula S, Khan H, Tugcu N (2017) Impact of freeze/thaw process on drug substance storage of therapeutics. J Pharm Sci 106:1944–1951

Roche Laboratories (2018) Summary of product characteristics. Accessed at: https://www.roche.com/products/product-details.htm?productId=1c3a82f3-ba8c-48d3-8ab0-dc7bda8e08d0. Accessed 24 May 2018

RxList (2018) Intron® information. Accessed at: https://www.rxlist.com/intron-a-drug.htm#description. Accessed 21 May 2018

Sanofi-Aventis (2018) Leukine® information. Accessed at: http://www.leukine.com/patient. Accessed 21 May 2018

SUGGESTED READING

See Tables 10.1, 10.2, and 10.4 for suggested readings

11 Economic Considerations in Medical Biotechnology

Amit S. Patel and Kartick P. Shirur

INTRODUCTION

The biotechnology revolution has coincided with another revolution in health care: the emergence of finance and economics as major issues in the use and success of new medical technologies. Health care finance has become a major social issue in nearly every nation, and the evaluation and scrutiny of the pricing and value of new treatments has become an industry unto itself. The most tangible effect of this change is the establishment of the so-called third hurdle for approval of new agents in many nations, after proving safety and efficacy. Beyond the traditional requirements for demonstrating the efficacy and safety of new agents, some nations and many private health care systems now demand data on the economic costs and benefits of new medicines. Although currently required only in a few countries, methods to extend similar prerequisites are being examined by the governments of most developed nations. Many managed care organizations in the USA now prefer that an economic dossier be submitted along with the clinical dossier to make formulary coverage decisions.

The licensing of new agents in most non-US nations has traditionally been accompanied by a parallel process of price and reimbursement approval, and the development of an economic dossier has emerged as a means of securing the highest possible rates of reimbursement. In recent years, sets of economic guidelines have been developed and adopted by the regulatory authorities of several nations to assist them in their decisions to reimburse new products. As many of the products of biotechnology are used to treat costly disorders and the products themselves are often costly to discover and produce, these new agents have presented new problems to those charged with the financing of medical care delivery. The movement to require an economic rationale for the pricing of new agents brings new challenges to those developing such agents. These requirements also provide firms with new tools to help determine which new technologies will provide the most value to society as well as contribute the greatest financial returns to those developing and marketing the products.

A. S. Patel (✉)
Department of Pharmacy, University of Mississippi, Oxford, MS, USA

Department of Pharmacy, Medical Marketing Economics, LLC, Oxford, MS, USA
e-mail: apatel@m2econ.com

K. P. Shirur
Medical Marketing Economics, LLC, Oxford, MS, USA

THE VALUE OF A NEW MEDICAL TECHNOLOGY

The task of determining the value of a new agent should fall somewhere within the purview of the marketing function of a firm. Although some companies have established health care economic capabilities within the clinical research structure of their organizations, it is essential that the group that addresses the value of a new product does so from the perspective of the market and not of the company or the research team. This is important for two reasons. First, evaluating the product candidate from the perspective of the user, and not from the team that is developing it, can minimize the bias that is inherent in evaluating one's own creations. Second, and most importantly, a market focus will move the evaluation away from the technical and scientifically interesting aspects of the product under evaluation and toward the real utility the product might bring to the medical care marketplace. Although the scientific, or purely clinical, aspects of a new product should never be ignored, when the time comes to measure the economic contribution of a new agent, those developing the new agent must move past these considerations. It is the tangible effects that a new treatment will have on the patient and the health care system that determine its value, not the technology supporting it. The phrase to keep in mind is "value in use."

D. J. A. Crommelin et al. (eds.), *Pharmaceutical Biotechnology*, https://doi.org/10.1007/978-3-030-00710-2_11

The importance of a marketing focus when evaluating the economic effects of a new agent, or product candidate, cannot be overstated. Failing to consider the product's value in use can result in overly optimistic expectations of sales performance and market acceptance. Marketing is often defined as the process of identifying and filling the needs of the market. If this is the case, then the developers of new pharmaceutical technologies must ask two questions: "What does the market need?" and "What does the market want?" Analysis of the pharmaceutical market in the first decade of the twenty-first century will show that the market needs and wants:

- Lower costs
- Controllable costs
- Predictable cost
- Improved outcomes

Note that this list does not include new therapeutic agents. From the perspective of many payers, authorities, clinicians, and buyers, a new agent, in and of itself, is a challenge. The effort required to evaluate a new agent and prepare recommendations to adopt or reject it takes time away from other efforts. For many in the health care delivery system, a new drug means more work—not that they are opposed to innovation, but newness in and of itself, regardless of the technology behind it, has no intrinsic value. The value of new technologies is in their efficiency and their ability to render results that are not available through other methods or at costs significantly lower than other interventions. Documenting and understanding the economic effects of new technologies on the various health care systems help the firm to allocate its resources more appropriately, accelerate the adoption of new technologies into the health care system, and reap the financial rewards of its innovation.

There are many different aspects of the term "value," depending upon the perspective of the individual or group evaluating a new product and the needs that are met by the product itself. When developing new medical technologies, it is useful to look to the market to determine the aspects of a product that could create and capture the greatest amount of value. Two products that have entered the market provide good examples of the different ways in which value is assessed.

Activase® (tPA, tissue plasminogen activator) from Genentech, one of the first biotechnology entrants in health care, entered the market priced at nearly ten times the price level of streptokinase, its nearest competitor. This product, which is used solely in the hospital setting, significantly increased the cost of medical treatment of patients suffering myocardial infarctions. But the problems associated with streptokinase and the great urgency of need for treatments for acute infarctions were such that many cardiologists believed that any product that proved useful in this area would be worth the added cost. The hospitals, which in the USA are reimbursed on a capitated basis for the bulk of such procedures, were essentially forced to subsidize the use of the agent, as they were unable to pass the added cost of tPA to many of their patients' insurers. The pricing of the product created a significant controversy, but the sales of Activase and its successors have been growing consistently since its launch. The key driver of value for tPA has been, and continues to be, the urgency of the underlying condition. The ability of the product to reduce the rate of immediate mortality is what drives its value. Once the product became a standard of care, incidentally, reimbursement rates were increased to accommodate it, making its economic value positive to hospitals.

An early biotechnology product that delivered a different type of value is the granulocyte-colony stimulating factor Neupogen® from Amgen, which was priced well below its economic value. The product's primary benefit is in the reduction of serious infections in cancer patients, who often suffer significant decreases in white blood cells due to chemotherapy. By bolstering the white blood cell count, Neupogen allows oncologists to use more efficacious doses of cytotoxic oncology agents while decreasing the rate of infection and subsequent hospitalization for cancer patients. It has been estimated that the use of Neupogen reduces the expected cost of treating infections by roughly $6000 U.S. per cancer patient per course of therapy. At a price of roughly $1400 per course of therapy, Neupogen not only provides better clinical care but also offers savings of approximately $4600 U.S. per patient. The economic benefits of the product have helped it to gain use rapidly with significantly fewer restrictions than products such as tPA, whose economic value is not as readily apparent.

These two very successful products both provide clear clinical benefits, but their sources of value are quite different. The value of a new product may come from several sources, depending on the needs of clinicians and their perceptions of the situations in which they treat patients. Value can come from the enhancement of the positive aspects of treatment as well. A product that has a higher rate of efficacy than current therapies is the most obvious example of such a case. But any product that provides benefits in an area of critical need, where few or no current treatments are available, will be seen as providing immediate value. This was, and remains, the case for tPA.

Some current treatments bring risk, either because of the uncertainty of their effects on the patient (positive or negative) or because of the effort or cost required to use or understand the treatments. A new product that

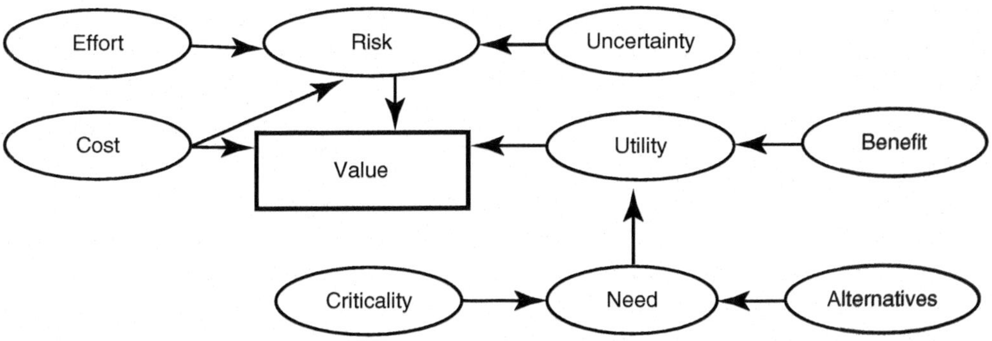

Figure 11.1 ■ Generalized model of value (Copyright © 2003, Medical Marketing Economics, LLC, Oxford, MS)

reduces this risk will be perceived as bringing new value to the market. In such cases, the new product removes or reduces some negative aspects of treatment. Neupogen, by reducing the chance of infection and reducing the average cost of treatment, brought new value to the marketplace in this manner. Any new product under development should be evaluated with these aspects of value in mind. A generalized model of value, presented in Fig. 11.1 below, can be used to determine the areas of greatest need in the marketplace for a new agent and to provide guidance in product development. By talking with clinicians, patients, and others involved in current treatments and keeping this model in mind, the shortcomings of those current approaches can be evaluated and the sources of new incremental value can be determined.

Understanding the source of the value brought to the market by a new product is crucial to the development of the eventual marketing strategy. Using Fig. 11.1 as a guide, the potential sources of value can be determined for a product candidate and appropriate studies, both clinical and economic, can be designed to measure and demonstrate that value.

AN OVERVIEW OF ECONOMIC ANALYSIS FOR NEW TECHNOLOGIES

A thorough economic analysis should be used to guide the clinical research protocol to ensure that the end points measured are commercially relevant and useful. The analysis should describe important elements of the market to the firm, helping decision makers to understand the way decisions are made and providing guidance in affecting those decisions. Later, the results of economic analyses should inform and guide marketing and pricing decisions as the product is prepared for launch, as well as help customers to use the product efficiently and effectively.

To prepare a thorough economic analysis, researchers must first have a comprehensive understanding of the flow of patients, services, goods, and money through the various health care systems. This process should begin as soon as the likely indications for a new product have been identified and continue throughout the product's development. The first step is to create basic economic models of the current treatment for the disorder(s) for which the product is likely to be indicated. This step will be used to fine-tune financial assumptions and clinical development process, to assure that the clinical protocols are designed to extract the greatest clinical and commercial potential from a product. Separate models should be prepared for each indication and level if the product is likely to be used to treat more than one indication and/or several different levels of the same indication (e.g., mild, moderate, and severe).

The purpose of the basic model is to provide a greater understanding of the costs associated with the disorder, and to identify areas and types of cost that provide the greatest potential for the product to generate cost savings. For example, the cost of a disorder that currently requires a significant amount of laboratory testing offers the potential for savings, and thus better pricing, if the new product can reduce or eliminate the need for tests. Similarly, some indications are well treated, but the incidence of side effects is sufficiently high to warrant special attention. When developing a new agent, it is as important to understand the source of the value to be provided as it is to understand the clinical effects of the agent.

PHARMACOECONOMICS

The field of economic evaluation of medical technologies goes by several names, depending on the discipline of the researchers undertaking the study and the type of technology being measured. For pharmaceutical and biotechnology products, the field has settled on the name of pharmacoeconomics, and an entire discipline has emerged to fill the needs of the area. Contributions to the development of the field have come from several disciplines, including economics, pharmacy administration, and many of the behavioral sciences.

Pharmacoeconomics has been defined as "the description and analysis of the costs of drug therapy to the health care systems and society" (Townsend 1987). Clinical studies assess the efficacy of a biotechnology product; likewise, pharmacoeconomic studies help to evaluate the efficiency of biotechnologically derived drug. In a complete pharmacoeconomic assessment, both the costs and consequences are identified, measured, and compared with other available medical interventions. The increase in the health care expenditure in the United States has resulted in excessive demand for cost-containment measures. Managed care organizations are striving hard to control drug spending and other health care-related costs. Payers are moving from an open formulary system to a more closed formulary system, leading to additional emphasis on pharmacoeconomic assessment. Additionally, several states in the United States have passed laws in an attempt to increase transparency of developmental costs for new drugs and cap price increases post launch.

Importance of Pharmacoeconomics

To understand the importance of pharmacoeconomics in the biotechnology industry, it is necessary to understand the differences between the biotechnology products and traditional pharmaceutical products. Szcus and Schneeweiss (2003) have highlighted these differences. They observed that biotechnologically derived products are more expensive than traditional pharmaceutical products and that many biotechnology products are termed "orphan drugs" as they are used in small- or moderate-size patient populations. At times these products could be the only option to treat underlying disease condition. Given the high production costs and selling prices of biotechnology products, it is critical for these products to demonstrate adequate cost-effectiveness to justify their high cost. Therefore, pharmacoeconomics analysis is one of the major tools for payers to differentiate between a high-priced traditional pharmaceutical products and costly biotechnology products in certain instances.

Pharmacoeconomic analysis plays a crucial role in disease management. Chang and Nash (1998) outlined the role of pharmacoeconomics in disease management, which includes evaluation and identification of cost-effective medications for the treatment of particular disease conditions. This information can be and is used by payers and hospital personnel to make potential formulary decisions. In such instances, drugs with unfavorable pharmacoeconomics evaluations are unlikely to remain on formularies or will be moved to a restricted status. In addition to formulary decisions, disease management programs often include clinical guidelines that are designed primarily on cost-effectiveness of medications Joshnson and Nash (1996). When communicated properly, economic analysis can lead physicians to change their prescribing behavior thus decreasing unexplained variation in the treatment of the same disease. Walkom et al. (2006) studied the role of pharmacoeconomics in formulary decision making and found growing importance of pharmacoeconomic evaluations in formulary decision making.

When used appropriately, pharmacoeconomics analysis should help us to answer questions such as:

- What drugs should be included in the outpatient formulary?
- Should these same drugs be included on a hospital formulary?
- What is the best drug for a particular disease in terms of efficacy and cost?
- What is the best drug for a pharmaceutical manufacturer to invest time and money?
- What are the relative cost and benefits of comparable treatment options?

To address the above questions, it becomes necessary for us to understand different costs considered in pharmacoeconomics analysis and the underlying techniques used to perform these pharmacoeconomic evaluations.

Understanding Costs

A comprehensive evaluation of relevant cost and consequences differentiates pharmacoeconomics from traditional cost-containment strategies and drug use evaluations. Costs are defined as the value of the resource consumed by a program or treatment alternative. Health economists use different costs in pharmacoeconomic evaluations, which can be grouped under direct costs, indirect costs, intangible costs, and opportunity costs.

In pharmacoeconomic evaluations, a comparison of two or more treatments extends beyond a simplistic comparison of drug acquisition cost. Including different costs, when appropriate, provides a more accurate estimate of the total economic impact of treatment alternatives and disease management programs in distinguished patients or populations.

Direct Costs

Direct costs are the resources consumed in the prevention or treatment of a disease. The direct costs are further divided into direct medical costs and direct nonmedical costs.

The direct medical costs include expenditures on drugs, medical equipment, laboratory testing, hospital supplies, physician visits, and hospitalization costs. Direct medical costs could be further divided into fixed costs and variable costs. Fixed costs generally represent the overhead costs and are relatively constant. Fixed costs include expenditures on rent, utilities, insurance, accounting, and other administrative activities. These costs are often not included in the pharmacoeconomic evaluations because their use or total cost is unlikely to change as a direct result of a specific intervention. On the other hand, variable costs are an integral part of pharmacoeconomic analysis. Variable costs include drugs, fees for professional services, and supplies. These variable costs increase or decrease depending on the volume.

Direct nonmedical costs are out-of-pocket costs paid by patients (or their caregivers) for nonmedical services which are generally outside health care sector. Direct nonmedical costs included expenditure on transportation to and from the hospital, clinic or physician office, additional trips to emergency rooms, expenses on special diet, family care expenses, and other various forms of out-of-pocket expenses.

Indirect Costs

Indirect costs are those costs that result from morbidity or mortality. Indirect costs assess the overall economic impact of an illness on a patient's life. Typical indirect costs include the loss of earnings due to temporary or permanent disability, loss of income to family member who gave up their job temporarily or permanently to take care of patient, and loss in productivity due to illness. Indirect medical costs are more related to patients and often unknown to or unappreciated by providers and payers.

Intangible Costs

Intangible costs are the most difficult to quantify in monetary terms. These costs represent the nonfinancial outcome of disease and medical care. The examples of intangible costs include pain, suffering, and emotional disturbance due to underlying conditions. Though these costs are identified in an economic analysis, they are not formally calculated. At times intangible costs are converted into a common unit of outcome measurement such as a quality-adjusted life-year (QALY).

Opportunity Costs

Opportunity costs are often discussed in the economic literature. Opportunity cost is defined as the value of the alternative that was forgone. In simple terms, suppose a person spends $100 to buy a drug to treat a particular disease condition, then the opportunity to use the same $100 to obtain a different medical intervention or treatment for the same disease condition, or for some nonmedical purpose, is lost. This is referred to as an opportunity cost. Although not often included in traditional pharmacoeconomic analysis, opportunity costs are often considered implicitly by patients when cost sharing (e.g., co-pays and coinsurance) is increased in a health benefit plan.

Method	Cost unit	Outcome unit
Cost of illness	Currency	Not assessed
Cost-minimization	Currency	Assumed to be equivalent in comparative groups
Cost-benefit	Currency	Currency
Cost-effectiveness	Currency	Natural units (life-years gained, mg/dL, blood glucose, mm Hg blood pressure)
Cost-utility	Currency	Quality-adjusted life-years or other utility

Table 11.1 ■ Economic evaluation methodologies

UNDERSTANDING PHARMACOECONOMIC METHODS

The purpose of this section is to provide an overview of pharmacoeconomic techniques currently used to evaluate drugs or treatment options. Table 11.1 represents the list of pharmacoeconomic methods. Selection of a particular technique depends on the objective of the study and outcome units which are compared. Grauer et al. (2003) stated that "the fundamental task of economic evaluation is to identify, measure, value and compare the costs and consequences of the alternatives being considered."

■ Cost of Illness (COI)

Cost of illness analysis is an important pharmacoeconomic tool to examine the economic burden of a particular disease. This technique takes into consideration the direct and indirect costs of a particular disease. A COI analysis thus identifies the overall cost of a particular disease in a defined population. Bootman et al. (1991) argue that COI analysis helps to evaluate the humanistic impact of disease and quantify the resources used in the treatment of disease prior to the discovery of new intervention. This information could be effectively used by pharmacoeconomic researchers to establish a baseline for comparison of new treatment or intervention. COI analysis is not used to compare two alternative treatment options, but to estimate the financial burden of the disease under consideration. Thus, the monetary benefits of prevention and treatment strategies could be measured against the baseline value estimated by cost of illness. In essence, a COI analysis provides the foundation for the measurement of the economic consequences of any treatment for the disorder in question. For example, Segel (2006) points out that a study on the cost-effectiveness of donepezil, published in 1999, relied on a COI study of Alzheimer's disease published a few years earlier. Without the initial COI study the cost-effectiveness work would have been exponentially more difficult and costly.

■ Cost-Minimization Analysis (CMA)

Cost-minimization analysis is the simplest pharmacoeconomic evaluation technique. The primary objective of the cost-minimization analysis is to determine the least costly alternative. CMA is used to compare two or more treatment alternatives that are equal in efficacy. An example of CMA would be a comparison of branded product to a generic equivalent. It is assumed that the outcomes associated with the two drugs are equivalent; therefore, costs alone could be compared directly. The cost included in this economic evaluation must extend beyond drugs acquisition cost and should include all relevant costs incurred for preparing and administering drugs.

Argenta et al. (2011) performed a CMA to evaluate the direct costs of venous thromboembolism treatment with unfractionated heparin (UFH) and enoxaparin from the institutional perspective. The drug acquisition costs, laboratory tests, hospitalization costs, and drug administration costs were included to estimate the medical cost. Statistically nonsignificant differences were observed between unfractionated heparin and enoxaparin groups in the number of bleeding events, blood transfusion, and death. The daily cost per patient for UFH was $12.63 U.S. and for enoxaparin was $9.87 U.S. Depending on the mean time of use, the total cost for UFH was $88.39 U.S. as compared to $69.11 U.S. for enoxaparin. Therefore, it was concluded that enoxaparin provided higher cost saving as compared to unfractionated heparin for the treatment of hospitalized patients with venous thromboembolism.

■ Cost-Benefit Analysis (CBA)

In cost-benefit analysis, costs and benefits are both measured in currency. In a CBA all the benefits obtained from the program or intervention are converted into some currency value (e.g., US dollars or euros). Likewise all program costs are identified and assigned a specific currency value. At times the costs are discounted to their present value. To determine the cost-benefit of a program, the costs are subtracted from the benefit. If the net benefit value is positive, then it can be concluded that the program is worth undertaking from an economic perspective.

The results of the CBA could be expressed either as cost-benefit ratio or a net benefit. For example, a cost associated with a medical program is $1000, and the outcome/benefit resulting from the program is $9000. Therefore, subtracting the cost $1000 from the benefits $9000 will yield net benefit of $8000. When comparing many treatment alternatives, an alternative with the greatest net benefit could be considered as most efficient in terms of use of resources. In CBA, all costs and benefits resulting from the program should be included.

A typical use of CBA is in the decision of whether a national health benefit should include the administration of a specific vaccine. In this case the cost of vaccinating the population and treating a smaller number of cases of the disease would be compared with the costs that would be incurred if the disease were not to be prevented. At times, however, it is much more difficult to assign a monetary value to benefits. For example, the benefit of a patient's satisfaction with the treatment or improvement in patient's quality of life is very difficult to convert to a monetary sum. This presents a considerable problem. At times these variables are considered as "intangible benefits," and the decision is left to the researcher to include in final analysis. Because of this CBA is seldom used as a pharmacoeconomic method to evaluate a specific treatment, although many who perform different types of analyses often mistakenly refer to their work as "cost-benefit."

■ Cost-Effectiveness Analysis (CEA)

Cost-effectiveness analysis is a method used to compare treatment alternatives or programs where cost is measured in currency and outcomes/consequences are measured in units of effectiveness or natural units. Therefore, cost-effectiveness analysis helps to establish and promote the most efficient drug therapy for the treatment of particular disease condition. The results of cost-effectiveness analysis are expressed as average cost-effectiveness ratios or as the incremental cost of one alternative over another. CEA is useful in comparing different therapies that have the same outcome units, such as an increase in life expectancy or decrease in blood pressure for hypertension drugs. CEA is a frequently used tool for evaluating different drug therapies to treat a particular disease condition. This type of analysis helps in determining the optimal alternative, which is not always the least costly alternative. CEA has an advantage that it does not require the conversion of health outcomes to monetary units.

CEA is often used to guide formulary management decisions. For example, consider a biotechnology product "X" that provides a 90% efficacy or cure rate for a specific disorder. The total treatment cost for 100 patients with product X is $750,000. Likewise assume that another biotechnology product "Y" prescribed for the same disorder shows 95% efficacy; however, the treatment cost of 100 patients with product Y is $1,000,000. The average cost-effectiveness ratio (ACER) of product X is calculated by dividing the cost $750,000 by the outcome, 90 cures, to yield an ACER of $8333 per cure. Similarly the ACER for product Y is $10,526 per cure. From this analysis, it is evident that using product Y would cost an additional $2192 per cure, which is the difference between ACERs of product Y and product X.

At times the incremental cost-effectiveness ratio (ICER) is important in drug selection decisions. From the above example, to calculate the ICER, total cost of product X ($750,000) is subtracted from total cost of product Y ($1,000,000). This is then divided by the cures from product X (90), subtracted from the cures resulting for product Y (95). Therefore, the incremental cost for each additional cure with product Y is $250,000 divided by 5 cures or $50,000 per cure. The incremental cost-effectiveness ratio poses the question of whether one additional cure is worth spending $50,000. The additional cost of cure might be justified by the severity of the disease or condition; this is a decision that is best made with the full knowledge of the economic implications. This provides an example of a situation in which the economic analysis is used to help guide the decision, but not to make the decision. Table 11.2 represents the ICER for product X and Y.

Good examples of CEAs are the recent comparisons of the use of proprotein convertase subtilisin/kexin type 9 (PCSK9) inhibitors Praluent® (alirocumab) and Repatha® (evolocumab) or ezetimibe with statin therapy. PCSK9 inhibitors were approved in 2015 to lower low-density lipoprotein levels in individuals with heterozygous familial hypercholesterolemia (FH) or artheroscclerotic cardiovascular disease (ASCVD). Annual acquisition costs of alirocumab and evolocumab were $14,600 U.S. and $14,100 U.S. respectively at launch, which were significantly higher than statins and ezetimibe, for which generic equivalents are available. Kazi et al. (2016) calculated the lifetime major adverse cardiovascular events (MACE), incremental cost per quality-adjusted life-year (QALY), and total cost to the US health care spending over 5 years. They estimated that adding PCSK9 inhibitors to statin therapy compared to ezetimibe prevented 316,300 MACE at a cost of $503,000 U.S. per QALY in heterozygous FH, and prevented 4.3 million MACE at a cost of $414,000 U.S. per QALY in ASCVD. Use of PCSK9 inhibitors would reduce costs for cardiovascular care by $29 billion U.S. over 5 years, but add drug costs worth $592 billion U.S. Since PCSK9 inhibitors cost four to five times higher than the generally accepted $100,000 U.S. per QALY threshold, the researchers concluded that annual acquisition costs of PCSK9 inhibitors would have to be reduced to $4536 U.S. in order for them to be cost-effective. Re-analysis of the model with recent data on ASCVD also shows that PCSK9 inhibitors are not cost-effective at 2017 prices (Kazi et al. 2017). Arrieta et al. (2017a, b) have made similar conclusions regarding the cost effectiveness of PCSK9 inhibitors compared to standard statin therapy.

Product	Efficacy (%)	No. of patients treated	Total costs ($)	ACER ($)	ICER ($)
Product X	90	100	750,000	8333	50,000
Product Y	95	100	1,000,000	10,526	

Table 11.2 ■ Incremental cost effectiveness ratio (ICER) for two products

■ Cost-Utility Analysis (CUA)

Cost-utility analysis was developed to factor quality of life into economic analysis by comparing the cost of the therapy/intervention with the outcomes measured in quality-adjusted life-years (QALY). The QALYs are calculated by multiplying the length of time in a specific health state by the utility of that health state—the utility of a specific health state is, in essence, the desirability of life in a specific health state compared with life in perfect health. A utility rating of 0.9 would mean that the health state in question is 90% as desirable as perfect health, while a utility rating of 0.5 would mean that health state is only half a desirable. Death is given a utility score of 0.0. The results of a CUA are expressed in terms of cost per QALY gained as a result of given treatment/intervention. CUA is beneficial when comparing therapies that produce improvements in different or multiple health outcomes. Cost per QALY can be measured and evaluated across several different treatment scenarios, allowing for comparisons of disparate therapies.

Goulart and Ramsey (2011) evaluated cost utility of Avastin® (bevacizumab) and chemotherapy versus chemotherapy alone for the treatment of advanced non-small-cell lung cancer (NSCLC). Avastin is currently approved for the treatment of NSCLC in combination with chemotherapy based on 2 months median survival proved in clinical trials. Researchers developed a model to determine quality-adjusted life-years and direct medical cost incurred due to treatment with bevacizumab in combination with chemotherapy. The utilities used in calculating QALY were obtained from the literature and costs were obtained from Medicare. The results of the study showed that bevacizumab is not cost-effective when added to chemotherapy. It was found that bevacizumab with chemotherapy increased the mean QALYs by only 0.13 (roughly the equivalent of 1.5 months of perfect health), at an incremental lifetime cost of $72,000 U.S. per patient. The incremental cost-utility ratio (ICUR) was found to be $560,000 U.S./QALY. The results of these analyses could be potentially used by payers while allocating resources for the treatment of NSCLC care. Table 11.3 represents the base case results of cost-utility analysis.

Outcomes	CPB	CP	Differences
Effectiveness			
Life expectancy (years)	1.24	1.01	0.23
Progression-free survival (years)	0.72	0.47	0.25
QALYs	0.66	0.53	0.13
Lifetime costs per patients (US$)[a]			
Drug utilization	70,284.75	646.96	69,637.79
Drug administration	4239.87	1495.24	2744.63
Fever and neutropenia	25.32	4.37	20.95
Severe bleeding	19.65	1.33	18.32
Other adverse events	39.06	32.09	6.97
Outpatient visits	1017.90	609.41	408.49
Progressive disease	40,283.71	41,500.96	−1217.25
Total	115,910.26	44,290.36	71,619.90
ICER (US$/life-years gained)			308,981.58
ICUR (US$/QALY gained)			559,609.48

CP carboplatin and paclitaxel, *CPB* carboplatin, paclitaxel, and bevacizumab, *ICER* incremental cost-effectiveness ratio, *ICUR* incremental cost-utility ratio, *QALYs* quality-adjusted life-years
[a]Cost in 2010 US dollars

Table 11.3 ■ Base case results of cost-utility analysis

SOURCES OF ECONOMIC VALUE

The economic value of the product may have elements besides the basic economic efficiency implied by the break-even level just discussed. Quality differences, in terms of reduced side effects, greater efficacy, or other substantive factors, can result in increases in value beyond the break-even point calculated in a simple cost comparison. Should these factors be present, it is crucial to capture their value in the price of the product, but how much value should be captured?

It is important to recognize that a product can provide a significant economic benefit in one indication but none in another. Therefore, it is prudent to perform these studies on all indications considered for a new product. A case in point is that of epoetin alfa (EPO). EPO was initially developed and approved for use in dialysis patients, where its principle benefit is to reduce, or even eliminate, the need for transfusion. Studies have shown that EPO doses that drive hematocrit levels to between 33 and 36% result in significantly lower total patient care costs than lower doses of EPO or none at all (Collins et al. 2000). The same product, when used to reduce the need for transfusion in elective surgery, however, has been shown not to be cost-effective (Coyle et al. 1999). Although EPO was shown to reduce the need for transfusion in this study, the cost of the drug far outweighed the savings from reduced transfusions as well as reductions in the transmission and treatment of blood-borne pathogens. Economic efficiency is not automatically transferred from one indication to another.

The lack of economic savings in the surgical indication does not necessarily mean that the product should not be used, only that users must recognize that in this indication use results in substantially higher costs while in dialysis it actually reduces the total cost of care.

FUTURE US HEALTH CARE CHANGES

Payers within the US health care system have begun to use similar methods of evaluation. Although it cannot be stated with certainty that the US system will adopt this approach to coverage wholeheartedly, the consistent news reports of new drugs costing tens, and hundreds, of thousands of dollars would indicate that the importance of delivering demonstrable value will increase in that market as well. Several states in the US have taken steps to control or increase transparency in drug pricing. New York state passed a law in 2017 which enables authorities to determine value-based prices for high-cost drugs, and then negotiate for additional rebates to achieve this price for its Medicaid program (Hwang et al. 2017). Other states have passed bills that require manufacturers to justify price increases above a certain threshold or publish research and development costs for new drugs (Sarpatwari et al. 2016).

In the pharmaceutical marketing environment of the foreseeable future, it is wise to first consider determining the true medical need for the intervention. Then, if the need is real, to consider surrendering some value to the market—pricing of the product at some point below its full economic value. This is appealing for several reasons:

- The measurement of economics is imprecise and the margin for error can be large.
- If the market is looking for lower costs, filling that need enhances the market potential of the product.
- From a public relations and public policy perspective, launching a new product with the message that it provides savings to the system can also provide positive press and greater awareness.

■ Biosimilars

Many drugs used to diagnose and treat diseases are biological products that until recently were available from a singular manufacturer. The first biosimilar (a product that is highly similar to the original biological product, described in more detail in Chap. 12 in this textbook) was Zarxio® (filgrastim-sndz), launched by Sandoz in 2015 as a biosimilar to Neupogen® (filgrastim). Subsequently, the biosimilars Inflectra® (infliximab-dyyb) and Renflexis™ (infliximab-abda) for Remicade® (infliximab) were launched in 2016 and 2017 respectively. Like generic alternatives launched at a discounted price to their branded counter-parts, Zarxio and Inflectra were launched at a 15% discount to Neupogen and Remicade respectively. Renflexis was priced at a 35% discount to Remicade and 20% discount to Inflectra.

Biomilars tend to take much longer than and may be more or equally expensive to develop as their original comparators. However, the current health care system and payers anticipate new biosimilars to be priced less than their original products; an expectation that developers and manufactures of biosimilars need to keep in mind as they pursue R&D of these products. Biosimilars have the potential to reduce overall health care costs spent on biological products compared to their original products; however, their pricing and value and ultimately commercial success remains to be examined. It remains to be seen if the recently approved, but yet to be launched biosimilars, Erelzi™ (etanercept-szzs), Amjevita™ (adalimumab-atta), Cyltezo™ (adalimumab-adbm), Mvasi™ (Bevacizumab-awwb), Ogivri™ (trastuzumab-dkst), and Ixifi™ (infliximab-qbtx) will also be priced at a discount to their reference products.

CONCLUSIONS

As societies continue to focus on the cost of health care interventions, we must all be concerned about the economic and clinical implications of the products we bring into the system. Delivering value, in the form of improved outcomes, economic savings, or both, is an important part of pharmaceutical science and marketing. Understanding the value that is delivered and the different ways in which it can be measured should be the responsibility of everyone involved with new product development. Further, all of this needs to be done with keeping the changing health care policy and regulatory landscape in mind.

■ Questions and Answers

1. When conducting pharmacoeconomic evaluations, typically the following costs are calculated or included in the analyses: direct, indirect, intangible and opportunity costs. Define these cost types and give examples to describe them.
   - Direct costs—They are the resources consumed in the prevention or treatment of a disease. Direct costs are further divided into:
     - Direct medical costs—These include expenditures on drugs, medical equipment, laboratory testing, hospital supplies, physician visits, and hospitalization costs. Direct medical costs are further divided into:
       - Variable costs—They are an integral part of pharmacoeconomic analysis. Variable costs increase or decrease depending on the volume, and include drugs, fees for professional services, and supplies.
       - Fixed costs—These include expenditures on rent, utilities, insurance, accounting, and other administrative activities. Fixed costs are <u>not included</u> in pharmacoeconomic evaluations because their use or total cost is unlikely to change as a direct result of a specific intervention.
     - Direct nonmedical costs—They are costs are out-of-pocket costs paid by patients (or their caregivers) for nonmedical services, and include expenditure on transportation to and from the hospital, clinic or physician office, additional trips to emergency rooms, expenses on special diet, family care expenses, and other various forms of out-of-pocket expenses.
   - Indirect costs—They are costs that result from morbidity or mortality. Indirect costs typically include the loss of earnings due to temporary or permanent disability, loss of income to family member who gave up their job temporarily or permanently to take care of patient, and loss in productivity due to illness.
   - Intangible costs—They represent the nonfinancial outcome of disease and medical care, and are the most difficult to quantify in monetary terms. Examples include pain, suffering, and emotional disturbance due to underlying conditions. Intangible costs are identified but not formally calculated in an economic analysis. At times they are converted into a common unit of outcome measurement such as a quality-adjusted life-year (QALY).
   - Opportunity costs—They are defined as the value of the alternative that was forgone due to the purchase of a medical treatment. Opportunity costs are *typically not included* in traditional pharmacoeconomic analysis.

2. List the five pharmacoeconomic techniques used to examine a new medical technology or treatment option?
   - Cost of Illness (COI)
   - Cost-Minimization Analysis (CMA)
   - Cost-Benefit Analysis (CBA)
   - Cost-Effectiveness Analysis (CEA)
   - Cost-Utility Analysis (CUA)
3. Cost-utility Analysis (CUA) includes outputs shown as QALY's. Define and describe QALY.
   - QALYs stand for Quality Adjusted Life Years. The QALYs are calculated by multiplying the length of time in a specific health state by the utility of that health state—the utility of a specific health state is, in essence, the desirability of life in a specific health state compared with life in perfect health. The results of a CUA are expressed in terms of cost per QALY gained as a result of given treatment/intervention.
4. Which method is used most often by insurance company payers to make product P&T formulary decisions? Why?
   - The cost-effectiveness analysis (CEA) is often used to guide formulary management decisions because:
     - The CEA does not require the conversion of health outcomes to monetary units.
     - The CEA helps in determining the optimal alternative, which may not always the least costly alternative.

REFERENCES

Argenta C, Ferreira MA, Sander GB, Moreira LB (2011) Short-term therapy with enoxaparin or unfractionated heparin for venous thromboembolism in hospitalized patients: utilization study and cost-minimization analysis. Value Health 14:S89–S92

Arrieta A, Page TF, Veledar E, Nasir K (2017a) Economic evaluation of PCSK9 inhibitors in reducing cardiovascular risk from health system and private payer perspectives. PLoS One 12(1):e0169761

Arrieta A, Hong JC, Khera R, Virani SS, Krumholz HM, Nasir K (2017b) Updated cost-effectiveness assessments of PCSK9 inhibitors from the perspectives of the health system and private payers: insights derived from the FOURIER trial. JAMA Cardiol 2(12):1369–1374

Bootman JL, Townsend JT, McGhan WF (1991) Principles of pharmacoeconomics. Harvey Whitney Books, Cincinnati

Chang K, Nash D (1998) The role of pharmacoeconomic evaluations in disease management. PharmacoEconomics 14(1):11–17

Collins AJ, Li S, Ebben J, Ma JZ, Manning W (2000) Hematocrit levels and associated Medicare expenditures. Am J Kidney Dis 36(2):282–293

Coyle D, Lee K, Laupacis A, Fergusson D (1999) Economic analysis of erythropoietin in surgery. Canadian Coordinating Office for Health Technology Assessment, Ottawa

Goulart B, Ramsey S (2011) A trial-based assessment of the utility of Bevacizumab and chemotherapy versus chemotherapy alone for advanced non-small cell lung cancer. Value Health 14:836–845

Grauer DW, Lee J, Odom TD, Osterhaus JT, Sanchez LA (2003) Pharmacoeconomics and outcomes: applications for patient care, 2nd edn. American College of Clinical Pharmacy, Kansas City

Hwang TJ, Kesselheim AS, Sarpatwari A (2017) Value-based pricing and state reform of prescription drug costs. JAMA 318(7):609–610

Joshnson N, Nash D (eds) (1996) The role of pharmacoeconomics in outcomes management. American Hospital Publishing, Chicago

Kazi DS, Moran AE, Coxson PG, Penko J, Ollendorf DA, Pearson SD, Tice JA, Guzman D, Bibbins-Domingo K (2016) Cost-effectiveness of PCSK9 inhibitor therapy in patients with heterozygous familial hypercholesterolemia or atherosclerotic cardiovascular disease. JAMA 316(7):743–753

Kazi DS, Penko J, Coxson PG, Moran AE, Ollendorf DA, Tice JA, Bibbins-Domingo K (2017) Updated cost-effectiveness analysis of PCSK9 inhibitors based on the results of the FOURIER trial. JAMA 318(8):748–750

Sarpatwari A, Avorn J, Kesselheim AS (2016) State initiatives to control medication costs — can transparency legislation help? N Engl J Med 374:2301–2304

Segel JE (2006) Cost-of-illness studies—a primer, RTI-UNC center of excellence in health promotion economics, Jan 2006. http://www.rti.org/pubs/coi_primer.pdf

Szcus TD, Schneeweiss S (2003) Pharmacoeconomics and its role in the growth of the biotechnology industry. J Commer Biotechnol 10(2):111–122

Townsend R (1987) Postmarketing drug research and development. Drug Intell Clin Pharm 21(1pt 2):134–136

Walkom E, Robertson J, Newby D, Pillay T (2006) The role of pharmacoeconomics in formulary decision-making: considerations for hospital and managed care pharmacy and therapeutics committees. Formulary 41:374–386

SUGGESTED READING

PHARMACOECONOMIC METHODS AND PRICING ISSUES

Bonk RJ (1999) Pharmacoeconomics in perspective. Pharmaceutical Products Press, New York

Drummond MF, O'Brien BJ, Stoddart GL, Torrance GW (1997) Methods for the economic evaluation of health care programmes, 2nd edn. Oxford University Press, Oxford

Kolassa EM (1997) Elements of pharmaceutical pricing. Pharmaceutical Products Press, New York

PHARMACOECONOMICS OF BIOTECHNOLOGY DRUGS

Dana WJ, Farthing K (1998) The pharmacoeconomics of high-cost biotechnology products. Pharm Pract Manag Q 18(2):23–31

Hui JW, Yee GC (1998a) Pharmacoeconomics of biotechnology drugs (part 1 of 2). J Am Pharm Assoc 38(1):93–97

Hui JW, Yee GC (1998) Pharmacoeconomics of biotechnology drugs (part 2 of 2). J Am Pharm Assoc 38(2):231–233

Reeder CE (1995) Pharmacoeconomics and health care outcomes management: focus on biotechnology (special supplement). Am J Health Syst Pharm 52:19,S4):S1–19,S4)S28

12 Regulatory Framework for Biosimilars

Vinod P. Shah and Daan J. A. Crommelin

INTRODUCTION

The term "biopharmaceuticals" is used to describe biotechnologically derived drug products. Biopharmaceuticals are protein-based macromolecules and include insulin, human growth hormone, the families of the cytokines and of the monoclonal antibodies, antibody fragments, and nucleotide-based systems such as antisense oligonucleotides, siRNA, and DNA preparations for gene delivery. A "generic" version of a biopharmaceutical may be introduced after patent expiration of the innovator's product. However, the generic paradigm as it has developed for low molecular weight actives over the years cannot be used for biopharmaceuticals. In the European Union and the US regulatory systems, the term "biosimilar" was coined for copies of brand name, new biopharmaceuticals. Different than for small molecule generic versions, in most cases, comparative clinical testing of the biosimilar product must include a robust evaluation of safety and confirmation of efficacy in appropriate patient populations.

The aim of this chapter is to provide a comprehensive view on current regulatory policies related to the approval of a biosimilar product in the EU and USA. Table 12.1 provides definitions of terms relevant to this chapter.

BACKGROUND

The mission of a regulatory authority is to "Assure that safe, effective, and high-quality drugs are marketed in the country and are available to the people." Safety of an innovator's drug product, be it a small molecule or biopharmaceutical, is established through preclinical studies in vitro and in animals and through controlled clinical studies in humans. Efficacy is established through clinical studies in patients. A description of drug quality is also part of the submitted dossier. In order to have a better understanding of the regulatory process involved, it is essential to appreciate the basic difference between small molecule drugs and macromolecular biopharmaceuticals (cf. Tables 12.2 and 12.3). Small molecules are chemically synthesized and can be fully characterized. On the other hand, most biopharmaceuticals are produced in a living system such as a microorganism, plant or animal cells and are difficult to fully characterize. The proteins are typically complex molecules and are unlikely to be shown to be structurally identical to a reference product. Differences in a manufacturing process may lead to alteration in the protein structure (Crommelin et al. 2003). Protein structures can differ in at least three ways: in their primary amino acid sequence, in (posttranslational) modification to those amino acids sequences (e.g., glycosylation), and in higher-order structure (folding patterns and (unwanted) aggregate formation. Advances in analytical sciences enable protein products to be extensively characterized with respect to their physicochemical and biological properties. However, current methodology may not detect all relevant structural and functional differences between two proteins and the interpretation of the impact of these differences is often unclear (Chaps. 2 and 3).

For the approval of a (small molecule) generic product, it must be pharmaceutically equivalent (same dosage form, strength of active, route of administration, and labeling as brand-name drug) and bioequivalent. Depending on the active, it should have the same in vitro dissolution, pharmacokinetic, pharmacodynamic, and clinical outcome profile as the brand name, innovation drug. For the more complex biological products, such a simple assessment of pharmaceutical equivalence and bioequivalence alone is not an option.

V. P. Shah (✉)
VPS Consulting, LLC, North Potomac, MD, USA
e-mail: dr.vpshah@comcast.net

D. J. A. Crommelin
Department of Pharmaceutics, Utrecht Institute for Pharmaceutical Sciences, Utrecht University, Utrecht, The Netherlands
e-mail: d.j.a.crommelin@uu.nl

D. J. A. Crommelin et al. (eds.), *Pharmaceutical Biotechnology*, https://doi.org/10.1007/978-3-030-00710-2_12

FDA	US Food and Drug Administration
EMA	European Medicines Agency
Low molecular weight drug	Classical medicinal product prepared by chemical synthesis
Generic product	Non-patented medicinal product of low molecular weight and therapeutically equivalent
Biopharmaceutical drug	The term "biopharmaceuticals" is used to describe biotechnologically derived drug products. Biopharmaceuticals are protein-based macromolecules and include insulin, human growth hormone, the families of the cytokines and of the monoclonal antibodies, antibody fragments, and nucleotide-based systems such as antisense oligonucleotides, siRNA, and DNA preparations for gene delivery[a]
Biosimilar product	A biosimilar is a biopharmaceutical product that is highly similar to an already approved biopharmaceutical product, notwithstanding minor differences in clinically inactive components, and for which there are no clinically meaningful differences between the biosimilar and the approved biopharmaceutical product in terms of safety, purity, and potency
Second-generation biopharmaceuticals	A second-generation biopharmaceutical product is derived from an approved biopharmaceutical product which has been deliberately modified to change one or more of the product's characteristics

[a]For the FDA, "biopharmaceuticals" are part of the "biological product" group, which also include viruses, sera, vaccines, and blood products

Table 12.1 ■ Definitions

Small, low molecular weight drugs	Biopharmaceuticals
Low molecular weight	High molecular weight
Simple chemical structure	Complex three-dimensional structure
Chemically synthesized	Produced by living organism
Easy characterization	Difficult to impossible to fully characterize
Synthetically pure	Often heterogeneous
Rarely produce immune response	Prone to eliciting an immune response

Table 12.2 ■ Difference between small, low molecular weight drugs and biopharmaceuticals

Generic (small molecule) product	Biosimilar product
Drug Price Competition and Patent Restoration Act of 1984	The Biologics Price Competition and Innovation Act of 2009 (BPCI Act)
Food Drug, and Cosmetic Act 505(j)	Public Health Service Act 351(k)
Pharmaceutical equivalent	Pharmaceutical equivalent
Bioequivalent	Non-clinical comparison (animal studies)
Pharmacokinetics	Physicochemical analysis
Pharmacodynamics	Clinical comparison (in humans)
Clinical comparison (not standard)	
In vitro analysis	

Table 12.3 ■ Drug approval for generic product and biosimilar product (FDA)

Both for a generic and for a biosimilar product, a complete set of information on Chemistry, Manufacturing, and Controls (CMC)section) is needed in the dossier submitted for approval to ensure that the drug substance and the drug product are pure, potent, and of high quality. The CMC section should include full analytical characterization, a description of the manufacturing process and test methods, and stability data. In addition to the establishment of safety and efficacy of the drug product, the approval process requires manufacturing of the drug product under controlled current good manufacturing practice (cGMP) conditions. The cGMP requirement ensures identity, potency, purity, and quality of the final product.

■ Characterization of Biosimilar Product (Details)

For biosimilars, a full comparison with the innovator's product characteristics (e.g., the primary, secondary, tertiary and quaternary structure, posttranslational modifications) and functional activity(ies) should be considered. A comprehensive understanding of all steps in the manufacturing process, process controls, and the use of a Quality-by-Design (cf. Chap. 4) approach will facilitate consistent manufacturing of a high-quality product.

As stated before, for complex proteins, the full characterization and assessment of equality of the biosimilar and innovator's product may not be possible with our present arsenal of analytical techniques (see Chap. 3). This means that for establishing biosimilarity, as a rule, clinical studies are required in the regulatory protocols described later on in this chapter.

Characterization of the active moiety and impurity/contaminant profiling plays an important role in the development process of a biosimilar drug product. The technological advances in instrumentation significantly improved identification and characterization of biotech products (Table 12.4 and Chap. 3). It is acknowledged that no one analytical method can fully characterize the biotech product. A collection of orthogonal analytical methods (Chap. 5) is needed to piece together a complete picture of a biotech product. Determining how a small, homogeneous protein is folded in absolute terms can be accomplished using crystal X-ray diffraction. This can be difficult, expensive, and nonrealistic to perform in the formulated drug product and on a routine basis. Moreover, X-ray diffraction analysis does not pick up low levels of conformational contaminants. The most basic aspect of assessing its identity is to determine its covalent, primary structure using liquid chromatography tandem mass spectrometry (LC/MS/MS), peptide mapping/amino acid sequencing (e.g., via the Edman-degradation protocol), and disulfide bond-locating methods. Through circular dichroism, Fourier transform infrared and fluorescence spectroscopy, immunological methods, chromatographic techniques, etc., differences in secondary and higher-order structures can be monitored. Selective analytical methods are used to determine the purity as well as impurities of the biotech product. Methods here include again chromatographic techniques and gel electrophoresis, capillary electrophoresis, isoelectric focusing, static and dynamic light scattering, and ultracentrifugation. Inadequate characterization can result in failure to detect product changes that can impact the safety and efficacy of a product. The characterization factors that impact safety and efficacy of the product should be identified in the product development process (cf. Chap. 3)

UV absorption spectroscopy
Circular dichroism spectroscopy
Fourier transform infrared spectroscopy (FTIR)
Fluorescence spectroscopy
Nuclead magnetic resonance spectroscopy (NMR)
Calorimetric approaches
Bio-assays
Immunochemical assays
Enzyme linked immunosorbent assay (ELISA)
Immunoprecipitation
Biosensor (Surface plasma resonance, SPR; quartz crystal microbalance, QCM)
Potency testing
In cell lines
In animals
Chromatographic techniques
Reverse phase high performance liquid chromatography, RP-HPLC
Size exclusion chromatography (SEC)
Hydrophobic interaction chromatography (HIC)
Ion-exchange chromatography (IEC)
Peptide mapping
Electrophoretic techniques
Sodium dodecyl sulfate polyacrylamide gel electrophoresis (SDS-PAGE)
Isoelectric focusing electrophoresis (IEF)
Capillary zone electrophoresis (CZE)
Field flow fractionaction (FFF) or asymmetrical flow field-flow fractionation (AF4)
Ultracentrifugation
Static and dynamic light scattering (SLS and DLS)
Electron microscopy
X-ray techniques
Mass spectrometry (MS)
Adapted from Crommelin et al. (2003)

Table 12.4 ■ Analytical techniques for monitoring protein structure

REGULATORY FRAMEWORK IN THE USA

FDA defines a generic drug as a copy that is the same as a brand-name drug in dosage form, strength, route of administration, quality, purity, safety, performance, and intended use. A generic product is a copy of the brand name, innovator's product, except for the inactive ingredients and/or formulations. The required dossier for market authorization focuses on only two aspects. The generic (small molecule) drug product should be pharmaceutically equivalent and bioequivalent to the brand-name product and is therefore therapeutically equivalent and interchangeable with the brand-name drug product. A generic product has the same active ingredient, and therefore, the safety and efficacy of the active ingredient is already established. The only question is the efficacy of the generic formulation, and this is assured by the bioequivalence study in healthy volunteers or patients.

In the case of small molecules, the identity of the active substance is established through a validated chemical synthesis route, full analysis of the active agent, impurity profiling, etc. In the case of biopharmaceuticals, this is, generally speaking, not possible. This biopharmaceutical product contains the active ingredient which is similar (but not necessarily equal) in characteristics to the reference product. For this reason, the generic biopharmaceutical products are referred to as biosimilar products (cf. Table 12.1).

Regulatory Pathway for Biosimilar Legal Framework

The Biologics Price Competition and Innovation Act of 2009 (BPCI Act) was enacted as part of the Affordable Care Act on March 23, 2010. The BPCI Act creates an abbreviated licensure pathway for biological products shown to be biosimilar to, or interchangeable with, an FDA-licensed biological referenced product. The objectives of the BPCI Act are conceptually similar to those of the Drug Price Competition and Patent Term Restoration Act of 1984, commonly referred to as the Hatch-Waxman Act that established abbreviated pathways for the approval of drug products under the Federal Food, Drug, and Cosmetic (FDC) Act. Section 351(k) of the Public Health Service (PHS) Act, added by the BPCI Act, sets forth the requirements for an application for a proposed biosimilar product and an application or a supplement for a proposed interchangeable product. A 351(k) application must contain information demonstrating that the biological product is biosimilar to a reference product based upon the data derived from analytical studies, animal studies, and clinical studies. To meet the *higher* standard of interchangeability, sufficient information must be provided to demonstrate biosimilarity. Interchangeable products may be substituted for the reference product without intervention of the prescribing health-care provider (note: this is the US interpretation of the term "interchangeable." It is interpreted differently in other parts of the world, e.g., in European countries). The BPCI Act also includes several exclusivity terms.

Biosimilar Drug Approval Process: the Principles

Approval of the biosimilar product is based on scientific considerations in demonstrating biosimilarity to a reference product. The scientific considerations will be on the basis of a risk-based "totality-of-the evidence" approach in comparing the proposed biosimilar (test) and the reference product. The term "totality-of-evidence" includes all data and information submitted in the application, including structural and functional characterization, nonclinical evaluation, human PK and PD data, clinical immunogenicity data, and comparative clinical study(ies) data.

Analytical studies serve as a foundation of a biosimilar development program. The reference product should be adequately characterized with respect to the critical quality attributes, clinically active components, mechanism of action and structure-function relationships. In addition, biochemical characterization, and functional characterization should be carried out. Once the reference product is characterized in detail, comparative tests between the reference product and the biosimilar product should be done.

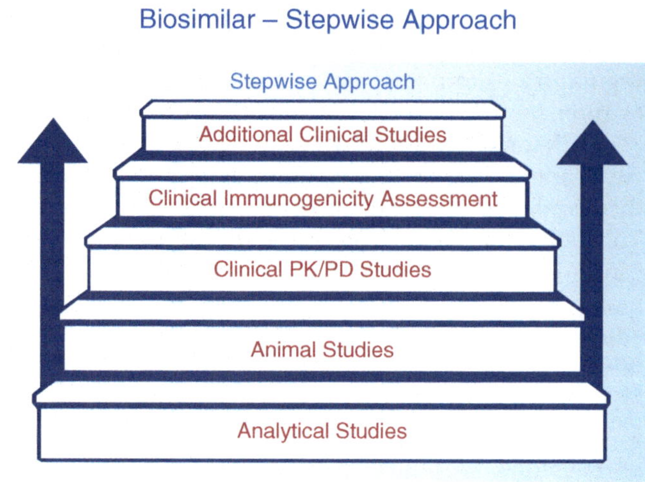

Figure 12.1 ■ (FDA/CDER Learn Program. FDA Continuing Education Course on Biosimilars. February 18, 2016) New figure-redraw

FDA recommends the use of a stepwise approach for the development of a biosimilar product: (1) Analytical Studies (2) Animal Studies (3) Clinical PK/PD Studies (4) Clinical Immunogenicity Assessment and (5) Additional Clinical Studies as necessary. This is shown schematically in Fig. 12.1. At each step, the sponsor should evaluate the level of residual uncertainty about the biosimilarity of the proposed biosimilar product to the reference product and identify the next step to address uncertainty. If there is a residual uncertainty about biosimilarity after conducting structural analyses, functional assays, animal testing, human PK and PD studies, and a clinical immunogenicity assessment, then additional clinical data may be needed to adequately address that uncertainty. A clinical study should be designed to investigate whether there are clinically meaningful differences between the biosimilar product and its reference product.

The requirements for approval of biosimilar products are based on the structural complexity and clinical knowledge of and experience with the reference biopharmaceutical product. For example, protein products such as growth hormone have known and relatively simple chemical structures. In addition, extensive manufacturing and clinical experience is available for these products. On the other hand, recFactor VIII is a large, highly complex molecule with several isoforms. Because of the varying complexity of biotech-derived products, the requirements for the approval process should be structured on a case-by-case basis. The following information is required for product approval:

- Structural information—primary, secondary, tertiary, and, if relevant, quaternary structure

information, including information regarding the glycosylation pattern, if relevant.
- Manufacturing process
- Quality attributes and clinical activities
- Pharmacokinetic-pharmacodynamic information, mechanism of drug action
- Clinical experience, efficacy and toxicity information

FDA prefers US-reference listed drug (RLD) for comparability studies—analytical, clinical and PK/PD, to demonstrate biosimilarity. For a PK/PD clinical study the most sensitive dose to detect and evaluate differences in the PK and PD profiles is suggested. FDA is encouraging a two-step process: approval of the biosimilar first and then interchangeability designation. To achieve designation of interchangeability, a special study should be designed in patients. The term interchangeable or interchangeability, in reference to a biological product means that in the USA—dependent on state laws- the biological product may be substituted for the reference product without the intervention of the health care provider who prescribed the reference product. The proposed interchangeable product "can be expected to produce the same clinical result as the reference product in a given patient." To support a demonstration of interchangeability, the sponsor must first show that the proposed product is biosimilar to the reference product. A dedicated switching study design and analysis is proposed for interchangeability designation (FDA 2017a). Up until March 2018 no biosimilar product has been designated as interchangeable.

Biosimilar products are different from second-generation biopharmaceuticals, e.g., pegylated G-CSF and interferon-alpha, and darbepoetin. The second-generation biopharmaceuticals have improved pharmacological properties/biological activity compared to an already approved biopharmaceutical product which has been deliberately modified. The second-generation products are marketed with the claim of clinical superiority. The second-generation biopharmaceuticals require a full New Drug Application (NDA) and are not interchangeable with the brand-name product.

FDA Guidance Documents on Biosimilars

The regulatory process for biosimilars is an evolutionary process. In April 2015 the FDA released two final guidance documents on biosimilar product development: (1) Scientific considerations in demonstrating biosimilarity to a reference product, (2) Quality considerations in demonstrating biosimilarity of a therapeutic protein product to a reference product (FDA 2015). In addition, FDA has published the guidance on Clinical pharmacology data to support a demonstration of biosimilarity to a reference product (FDA 2016a), draft guidance on Considerations in demonstrating interchangeability with a reference product (FDA 2017a), draft guidance on Labeling for biosimilar products (FDA 2016b) and guidance on Nonproprietary naming of biological products (FDA 2017b). These guidances are intended to assist sponsors in demonstrating that the proposed therapeutic protein product is biosimilar to a reference product under section 351(k) of the PHS Act.

Clinical Studies

As a rule, clinical studies are required to assure safety and efficacy of the biosimilar candidate product. The comparative clinical trial exercise is a stepwise procedure that should begin with pharmacokinetic and pharmacodynamic studies when necessary followed by clinical efficacy and safety trials. The choice of the design of the pharmacokinetic study, i.e., single dose and/or multiple doses, should be justified. Normally, comparative clinical trials are required for demonstration of clinical efficacy and safety. However, in certain cases, comparative pharmacokinetic/pharmacodynamic studies between the biosimilar product and the reference product using biomarkers may prove to be adequate.

Nonproprietary Naming (FDA 2017b)

The proper name for the approved biological product will include a core name (nonproprietary name) and an FDA-designated suffix. A distinguishing suffix that is devoid of meaning and composed of four lower case letters will be attached with a hyphen to the core name of each originator biological product, related biological product or biosimilar product. Use of shared core name will indicate a relationship among products, for example:
- replicamab-cznm,
- replicamab-jhxf.

This naming convention will facilitate pharmacovigilance for biological and biosimilar drug products.

At present the following biosimilars (not-interchangeable) are approved by FDA (see list in the Purple Book, FDA 2018): adalimumab-adbm Cyltezo; adalimumab-atto Amjevita; bevacizumab-awwb Mvasi; etanercept-szzs Erelzi; filgrastim-sndz Zarxio; infliximab-abda Renflexis; infliximab-dyyb Inflectra; infliximab-qbtx Ixifi; trastuzumab-dkst Ogivri

Labeling

- Information and data from a clinical study of a proposed biosimilar product should be described in its labeling only when necessary to inform safe and effective use by a health care practitioner.

EMA REGULATORY FRAMEWORK

The regulatory process for the approval of biopharmaceuticals and biosimilars in the EU follows a centralized (i.e., not a national competence of the member states) route through the European Medicines Agency (EMA). The EMA started issuing guidance documents on the regulatory process for biosimilars in 2004. The overarching guideline for biosimilar drug products is CHMP/437/04, revised in 2014. From 2006 on, EMA published a series of guidance documents on biosimilar medical products containing specific biotechnology-derived proteins as active substance, e.g., on recombinant erythropoietin, somatropin, granulocyte colony-stimulating factor (G-CSF), and human insulin. These guidelines define key concepts/principles of biotechnology-derived proteins and discuss quality issues and non-clinical and clinical issues and are regularly updated (EMA 2018a).

■ Status of Biosimilars in the EU

The EMA (EMA 2017) published an informative brochure on biosimilars explaining in detail its position on different aspects of the approval process and use of biosimilars. It also provides definitions on the terms interchangeability and substitution. It is not EMA but the individual EU countries that decide on interchangeability and substitution rules in their territory. Table 12.5 lists the biosimilars approved by the EMA (2018b)). This list is growing. The market share of biosimilars varies strongly per country and per biosimilar product (QuintilesIMS 2017). The advent of the biosimilars to the market led to questions on what grounds to choose, either for the originator's product or for the biosimilar product. The *European Journal of Hospital Pharmacists* published a document: "*Points to consider in the evaluation of biopharmaceuticals*", followed by '*How to select a biosimilar*' (2013) Health-care providers can use these publications to make a documented choice (Kraemer et al. 2008; Boone et al. 2013).

Nonproprietary Naming

'As required by EU law, every medicine will have an invented name (trade name or brand name) together with the active substance name (i.e., the INTERNATIONAL NONPROPRIETARY NAME, OR INN, which is assigned by WHO). For identifying and tracing biological medicines in the EU, medicines have to be distinguished by the trade name and batch number' (EMA 2017).

THE CHALLENGE AND THE FUTURE

A major problem today is the inadequate definition of the relationship between the complex structure and function of protein pharmaceuticals. Analytical tools are becoming increasingly sensitive and provide more detailed information regarding the molecular structure. This may allow for certain biopharmaceuticals to be shown to be pharmaceutically equivalent, therapeutically equivalent, and interchangeable on the basis of a validated analytical definition alone. For instance, for relatively small protein molecules like insulin, a well-characterized biopharmaceutical product, equivalence may be established using presently available analytical techniques (Table 12.4). But for larger and complex proteins, it is not possible to characterize the molecule in full detail and establish equivalence. In such a scenario, clinical safety and efficacy studies will be needed to establish equivalence.

Science-based regulatory policies are being developed. They are dynamic. They have evolved over the years and will continue to do so based on the development of superior analytical techniques to characterize the products, on introducing improved manufacturing practices and controls and on growing clinical and regulatory experience. Rigorous standards of ensuring product safety and efficacy must be maintained and, at the same time, unnecessary and/or unethical duplication trials must be avoided.

The approval of a biosimilar product should depend on the complexity of the molecule. A gradation scheme should be designed for the drug approval process rather than using a "one size fits all" model. From simple chemically synthesized molecules to highly complex molecules, e.g., from a chemically synthesized simple molecule such as acetaminophen to cyclosporine, to insulin, to human growth hormone, to interleukins, to erythropoietin type of growth factors, to albumin, to monoclonal antibodies, and to factor VIII, different regulatory regimens are required.

The regulatory processes for biosimilars are following an evolutionary route. We learn from new information coming in every day; we evaluate the data, adjust the rules, and develop new protocols to make sure that the patient keeps on receiving high-quality, safe and effective biopharmaceuticals.

SELF-ASSESSMENT QUESTIONS

Question 1: Human growth hormone has a molecular weight of around 22 kDa (see Chap. 20) and erythropoietin of 34 kDa (see Chap. 24). Why does the EMA request different clinical protocols for approval of a biosimilar product for these protein drugs?

Question 2: Can the US approved biosimilar product be interchanged with the brand name product?

Answer 1: Human growth hormone is a non-glycosylated protein with a well-established primary sequence; erythropoietin is heavily glycosylated with a

Biosimilar	CHMP positive opinion	Indication	Marketing Authorisation Holder	Authorised
Somatropin (Omnitrope®)	jun-03	Prader-Willi Syndrome, Dwarfism, Pituitary, Turner Syndrome	Sandoz	apr-06
Epoetin alfa (Abseamed®)	okt-08	Anemia, Kidney Failure, Chronic Cancer	Medice	aug-07
Epoetin alfa (Binocrit®)	jun-07	Anemia, Kidney Failure, Chronic Cancer	Sandoz	aug-07
Epoetin alfa (Epoetin Alfa Hexal®)	jun-07	Anemia, Kidney Failure, Chronic Cancer	Hexal	aug-07
Epoetin zeta (Retacrit®)	oct-07	Anemia, Kidney Failure, Chronic Blood Transfusion, Autologous Cancer	Hospira	dec-07
Epoetin zeta (Silapo®)	oct-07	Anemia, Kidney Failure, Chronic Blood Transfusion, Autologous Cancer	Stada	dec-07
Filgrastim (Ratiograstim®)	jul-08	Neutropenia, Hemato poietic Stem Cell Transplantation, Cancer	Ratiopharm	sep-08
Filgrastim (Tevagrastim®)	jul-08	Neutropenia, Hematopoietic Stem Cell Transplantation, Cancer	Teva	sep-08
Filgrastim (Filgrastim Hexal®)	nov-08	Neutropenia, Hematopoietic Stem Cell Transplantati on, Cancer	Hexal	feb-09
Filgrastim (Zarzio®)	nov-08	Neutropenia, Hematopoietic Stem Cell Transplantation, Cancer	Sandoz	feb-09
Filgrastim (Nivestim®)	mrt-10	Neutropenia, Hematopoietic Stem Cell Transplantation, Cancer	Hospira/Pfizer	jun-10
Infliximab (Remsima®)	jun-13	Spondylitis, AnkylosingArthritis, RheumatoidColitis, UlcerativeArthritis, PsoriaticCrohn Disease, Psoriasis	Celltrion	sep-13
Infliximab (Inflectra®)	jun-13	Spondylitis, AnkylosingArthritis, RheumatoidColitis, UlcerativeArthritis, PsoriaticCrohn Disease, Psoriasis	Hospira	sep-13
Follitropin alfa (Ovaleap®)	aug-13	Anovulation	Teva	sep-13
Filgrastim (Grastofil®)	jul-13	Neutropenia	Apotex	oct-13
Follitropin alfa (Bemfola®)	jan-14	Anovulation	Finox	mrt-14
Filgrastim (Accofil®)	jul-14	Neutropenia	Accord Healthcare	sep-14
Insulin glargine (Abasaglar®)	jun-14	Diabetes Mellitus	Eli Lilly	sep-14

Table 12.5 ■ EMA list of approved biosimilars, Jan 2018

Etanercept (Benepali®)	nov-15	Rheumatoid arthritis, psoriatic arthritis, axial spondyloarthritis and plaque psoriasis	Samsung Bioepis	jan-16
Infliximab (Flixabi®)	mrt-16	Rheumatoid arthritis, adult and paediatric Crohn's disease, ulcerative colitis, paediatric ulcerative colitis, ankylosing spondylitis, psoriatic arthritis and psoriasis	Samsung Bioepis	mei-16
Enoxaparin (Inhixa®)	jul-16	Prevention and treatment of various disorders related to blood clots	Techdow	sep-16
Enoxaparin (Thorinane®)	jul-16	Prevention and treatment of various disorders related to blood clots)	Pharmathen	sep-16
Insulin glargine (Lusduna®)	nov-16	Diabetes Mellitus	MSD	jan-17
Teriparatide (Movymia®)	nov-16	Osteoporosis	STADA Arzneimittel	jan-17
Teriparatide (Terrosa®)	nov-16	Osteoporosis	Gedeon Richter	jan-17
Rituximab (Truxima®)	dec-16	Non-Hodgkin's lymphoma, chronic lymphocytic leukaemia, rheumatoid arthritis, granulomatosis with polyangiitis and microscopic polyangiitis	Celltrion	feb-17
Adalimumab (Amgevita®)	jan-17	Rheumatoid arthritis, juvenile idiopathic arthritis, axial spondyloarthritis, psoriatic arthritis, psoriasis, paediatric plaque psoriasis, hidradenitis suppurativa, Crohn's disease, paediatric Crohn's disease, ulcerative colitis and uveitis.	Amgen	mrt-17
Adalimumab (Solymbic®)	jan-17	Rheumatoid arthritis, enthesitis-related arthritis, axial spondyloarthritis, psoriatic arthritis, psoriasis, hidradenitis suppurativa, Crohn's disease, ulcerative colitis and uveitis	Amgen	mrt-17
Etanercept (Erelzi®)	apr-17	Rheumatoid arthritis, juvenile idiopathic arthritis, psoriatic arthritis, axial spondyloarthritis, ankylosing spondylitis, non-radiographic axial spondyloarthritis, plaque psoriasis, paediatric plaque psoriasis.	Sandoz	jun-17
Rituximab (Riximyo®)	apr-17	Non-Hodgkin's lymphoma, rheumatoid arthritis, granulomatosis with polyangiitis and microscopic polyangiitis.	Sandoz	jun-17
Rituximab (Rixathon®)	apr-17	Non-Hodgkin's lymphoma, chronic lymphocytic leukaemia, rheumatoid arthritis, granulomatosis with polyangiitis and microscopic polyangiitis.	Sandoz	jun-17
Rituximab (Blitzima®)	may-17	Non-Hodgkin's lymphoma, chronic lymphocytic leukaemia, granulomatosis with polyangiitis and microscopic polyangiitis.	Celltrion	jun-17

Table 12.5 ■ (continued)

Rituximab (Rituzena®)	may-17	Non-Hodgkin's lymphoma, chronic lymphocytic leukaemia, granulomatosis with polyangiitis and microscopic polyangiitis.	Celltrion	jun-17
Rituximab (Ritemvia®)	may-17	Non-Hodgkin's lymphoma, granulomatosis with polyangiitis and microscopic polyangiitis.	Celltrion	jun-17
Insulin Lispro (Insulin lispro Sanofi®)	may-17	Diabetes mellitus.	Sanofi	jun-17
Adalimumab (Imraldi®)	jun-17	Rheumatoid Arthritis, Juvenile idiopathic arthritis, Axial spondyloarthritis, Psoriatic arthritis, Psoriasis, Paediatric plaque psoriasis, Hidradenitis suppurativa, Crohn's disease, Paediatric Crohn's disease, Ulcerative colitis, Uveitis.	Samsung Bioepis UK Limited	aug-17
Adalimumab (Cyltezo®)	sep-17	Rheumatoid Arthritis, Juvenile idiopathic arthritis, Axial spondyloarthritis, Psoriatic arthritis, Psoriasis, Paediatric plaque psoriasis, Hidradenitis suppurativa, Crohn's disease, Paediatric Crohn's disease, Ulcerative colitis, Uveitis.	Boehringer Ingelheim	nov-17
Trastuzumab (Ontruzant®)	sep-17	Metastatic breast cancer, Early breast cancer, Metastatic gastric cancer.	Samsung Bioepis UK Limited	Awaiting authorisation
Bevacizumab (Mvasi®)	nov-17	Fallopian Tube Neoplasms, Non-Small-Cell Lung Carcinoma, Ovarian Neoplasms, Renal Cell Carcinoma, Peritoneal Neoplasms, Breast Neoplasms	Amgen	Awaiting authorisation

Table 12.5 ■ (continued)

number of isoforms with more analytical challenges. The EMA guidance documents giving more details can be found on the EMA website.

Answer 2: No, it cannot be interchanged unless they do interchangeability studies and get FDA approval.

REFERENCES

Boone HN, van der Kuy H, Scott M, Mairs J, Krämer I, Vulto A, Janknegt R (2013) How to select a biosimilar. Eur J Hosp Pharm 20:275–228

Crommelin DJA, Storm G, Verrijk R, de Leede L, Jiskoot W, Hennink WE (2003) Shifting paradigms: biopharmaceuticals versus low molecular weight drugs. Int J Pharm 266:3–16

EMA (2017) http://www.ema.europa.eu/docs/en_GB/document_library/Leaflet/2017/05/WC500226648.pdf. Last accessed 18 Jan 2018

EMA (2018a) http://www.ema.europa.eu/ema/index.jsp?curl=pages/regulation/general/general_content_000408.jsp&mid=WC0b01ac058002958c. Last accessed Mar 2018

EMA (2018b) http://www.ema.europa.eu/ema/index.jsp?curl=pages%2Fmedicines%2Flanding%2Fepar_search.jsp&mid=WC0b01ac058001d124&searchTab=searchByAuthType&alreadyLoaded=true&isNewQuery=true&status=Authorised&keyword=Enter+keywords&searchType=name&taxonomyPath=&treeNumber=&searchGenericType=biosimilars&genericsKeywordSearch=Submit. Last accessed Mar 2018

FDA Guidances (2015) https://www.fda.gov/downloads/drugsguidancecomplianceregulatoryinformation/guidances/ucm291128.pdf. Last accessed 18 Jan 2018

FDA (2016a) https://www.fda.gov/downloads/Drugs/GuidanceComplianceRegulatoryInformation/Guidances/UCM397017.pdf. Last accessed 18 Jan 2018

FDA (2016b) https://www.fda.gov/downloads/Drugs/GuidanceComplianceRegulatoryInformation/Guidances/UCM493439.pdf. Last accessed 18 Jan 2018

FDA (2017a) https://www.fda.gov/downloads/Drugs/GuidanceComplianceRegulatoryInformation/Guidances/UCM537135.pdf

FDA (2017b) https://www.fda.gov/downloads/drugs/guidances/ucm459987.pdf. Last accessed 18 Jan 2018

FDA (2018) https://www.fda.gov/downloads/Drugs/DevelopmentApprovalProcess/HowDrugsareDevelopedandApproved/ApprovalApplications/TherapeuticBiologicApplications/Biosimilars/UCM560162.pdf. Last accessed 18 Jan 2018

Kraemer I, Tredree R, Vulto A (2008) Points to consider in the evaluation of biopharmaceuticals. EJHP Practice 14:73–76

QuintilesIMS (2017) The Impact of Biosimilar Competition in Europe. http://www.medicines-foreurope.com/wp-content/uploads/2017/05/IMS-Biosimilar-2017_V9.pdf

13

An Evidence-Based Practice Approach to Evaluating Biotechnologically Derived Medications

James P. McCormack

INTRODUCTION

Recent advances in pharmaceutical biotechnology have led to the development of many different therapeutic proteins. These technologies have given credence to the legitimate promise that we, at some point, may be able to more closely match some specific patients with the most effective and safe drugs at an individualized dose—personalized/precision medicine.

BACKGROUND

Despite the clear potential for these technologies, when it comes to treating patients within an evidence-based practice framework, a number of requirements come into the clinical decision making process with the use of these agents. Clinicians will need to consider all these requirements on a patient-by-patient basis if we are to fully realise the clinical potential of these therapeutic proteins.

These requirements can be separated into evidence and individual treatment decision issues. These are outlined in Table 13.1.

(A) *Evidence requirements*
Placebo controlled RCTs of these agents
RCTs comparing these agents directly to presently established therapy
RCTs of direct head-to head comparisons of monoclonal antibodies that are in the same class/used for the same indication
Cohort data with long term follow-up to estimate any on-going long-term safety issues
(B) *Patient-centered requirements*
The promotion of the concept of shared-decision making
Defining clear, specific and measureable individual patient outcomes
When possible starting with very low doses and/or continually adjusting doses based on individual response
A discussion of how to address the potential cost issues typically seen with these agents

Table 13.1 ■ Evidence and patient-centered requirements for making therapeutic decisions

At any clinical encounter where a treatment is to be recommended the obvious goal would be to "match individual patients with the most effective, and safest drugs and doses" (Sindelar 2013). Tailoring the correct medication and dose to an individual patient has been the goal and the approach of health care providers for millennia.

Over the last decade or so, much of this tailoring concept has been termed personalized medicine or precision medicine. Interestingly, these two terms have recently been co-opted by people interested in the fascinating and potentially very useful area of genomics. Despite this, it is important clinicians remember that pharmacogenomics is just one of a number of tools or approaches that can be useful as we appropriately attempt to tailor the use of medications in a more personalized way. Obviously, behavioural and environmental factors play an important role in the clinical outcomes associated with treatments and it is of value to remember these, and other similar factors, will likely never be importantly influenced by genomically-targeted medications.

Finally, the present-day personalized medicine discussion typically omits two of the most important aspects of true personalized medicine—first, patient's individual values and preferences and second, doses of medications need to be individualized based on a clear and objective review of an individual patient's response.

When it comes to these new "omic" technologies it is helpful to think through the issues outlined in Table 13.1 when trying to figure out where therapeutic proteins fit into the concept of evidence-based practice and true personalized medicine. Using six different recent examples, many of these issues will be examined. It is useful to breakdown these examples into two

J. P. McCormack (✉)
Faculty of Pharmaceutical Sciences, University of British Columbia, Vancouver, BC, Canada
e-mail: james.mccormack@ubc.ca

D. J. A. Crommelin et al. (eds.), *Pharmaceutical Biotechnology*, https://doi.org/10.1007/978-3-030-00710-2_13

specific therapeutic scenarios based on the overall treatment goals of the medication as this impacts the specific issues that require focus. These scenarios are prevention/risk reduction and symptom reduction.

TREATMENTS THAT REDUCE RISK

In prevention, one is taking a treatment to try to reduce the future chance of developing symptoms or of having an event such as a heart attack, stroke, hospitalization, or disease exacerbation.

Example 1: Palivizumab for Reducing the Risk of Severe RSV Infection in Children

Bronchiolitis and pneumonia in children are most commonly caused by the Respiratory Syncytial Virus (RSV). Most infants recover from this virus but serious complications can occur, especially in those with underlying medical conditions such as congenital heart disease. For those infants at higher risk of complications palivizumab (Synagis®), a monoclonal antibody produced by recombinant DNA technology, is used to reduce the risk of developing serious complications. The authors of a recent Cochrane review (Andabaka et al. 2013) state "there is evidence that palivizumab prophylaxis is effective in reducing the frequency of hospitalisations due to RSV infection" and to that end, "palivizumab prophylaxis was associated with a statistically significant reduction in RSV hospitalisations (RR 0.49, 95% CI 0.37–0.64) and a statistically non-significant reduction in all-cause mortality (RR 0.69, 95% CI 0.42–1.15) when compared to placebo". In other words palivizumab reduced the risk of RSV hospitalisations by approximately 50%.

So to properly use these numbers using an evidence-based practice framework, we need to know the baseline risk of RSV hospitalizations in these infants.

The patients studied were infants with serious medical conditions such as chronic lung disease, congenital heart disease, or those born preterm. In the placebo group, roughly 10% of the infants ended up being hospitalized for RSV over a 5-month period. Giving palivizumab reduces that risk by roughly 50%. Putting this into absolute numbers, the risk went from roughly 10% (in the placebo group) down to 5% (in the palivizumab group). This absolute 5% benefit means for every 20 children who got this agent (typically for 5 months) one benefited, or in other words 95% got no benefit from this treatment. To be fair, even if this treatment prevented all RSV hospitalizations, reducing a 10% risk down to 0% would still only mean 1 in 10 would benefit from treatment. In this example, unfortunately there is no way to predict which of these higher risk infants will benefit and there is also no way to titrate the dose to an effect. So when it comes to evidence-based practice we have evidence that this new medication has an effect in the population studied but this benefit needs to be balanced with the fact that 5-monthly injections will cost a total of roughly $10,000US for a 1 in 20 chance of benefiting. In addition, cohort studies would be required to determine the long-term effects of immunoprophylaxis on asthma, mortality and other important clinical outcomes. And finally, at present there are no studies comparing this agent to other potential treatments.

Example 2: Evolucumab for Hyperlipidemia and Reducing the Risk of Heart Disease

Another example of a risk reduction treatment is evolocumab (Repatha®) a monoclonal antibody (PCSK9 inhibitor) designed for the treatment of hyperlipidemia and recently approved to reduce the risks of heart attacks strokes and coronary revascularization. The study that evaluated the benefit of evolocumab was called the FOURIER study (Sabatine et al. 2017). The authors of this study investigated people with established heart disease, average age 63, and gave this agent for 2.2 years. Their primary outcome was the risk of a combined CVD endpoint - cardiovascular death, myocardial infarction, stroke, hospitalization for unstable angina, or coronary revascularization. The result was a reduction in the risk of combined CVD - hazard ratio of 0.85 (0.79–0.92) - or in other words a 15% relative benefit. Comparatively, these relative benefits (15%) are numerically less than that seen with statins and/or medications used for blood pressure (25–30%) but there are no head-to-head comparisons between these different treatments so comparisons are at best speculative.

Looking at the absolute numbers, 11.3% in the placebo group ended up with this CVD endpoint and this occurred in 9.8% of the group on evolocumab. This is a 1.6% absolute benefit or 63 people need to be treated to benefit one. As with palivizumab there can be no dosage titration because only a single dose has been studied and there is no endpoint to which to titrate. The cost of this agent is roughly $15,000 US a year for a 1 in 63 benefit and at present there is no information on the long-term benefits and harms of this agent. This is clearly an example where patient values and preferences will need to be taken into account via a shared-decision making process.

Example 3: Romosozumab or Alendronate for Fracture Prevention

Fractures increase morbidity and possibly mortality and there are some new biologic treatments that appear to reduce the risk of these fractures. An example of a very useful head to head study in this area is the ARCH study (Saag et al. 2017) where roughly 4100 subjects were randomized to receive either romosozumab (Evenity®) or alendronate in a blinded fashion for

12 months followed by both groups receiving alendronate alone for 12 more months. Over the 24 months, clinical fractures occurred in 9.7% of the romosozumab and 13% in the alendronate group—RR 0.73 (0.61, 0.88). This 27% relative benefit or 3.3% absolute benefit means that 30 people would need to take romosozumab over alendronate for 1 year for one additional person to benefit. Unfortunately, in this trial there was an increase in cardiovascular events in the subjects receiving romosozumab. In the romosozumab group, 2.5% had a serious cardiovascular event compared to 1.9% in the alendronate group. So for every 167 people taking romosozumab over alendronate, one would have a serious cardiovascular event. Because of this the FDA has at present decided not to approve this medication and is requiring the company to look at cardiovascular event data from all the clinical trials of this agent. There was also a 1.8% absolute increase in injection site reactions in the romosozumab group.

So in this scenario we have a new agent that is more effective at reducing fractures than the gold standard but it may also increase the risk of serious cardiovascular disease. If this agent is eventually approved, this is where shared decision-making becomes an essential part of the discussion. Does a 3.3% absolute reduction in fractures justify a 0.6% increase in serious cardiovascular events? Only an informed patient can participate in that sort of decision. On top of the benefits and harms discussion other considerations such as the requirement for injections, the lack of long-term follow-up data and the very likely fact that romosozumab will be considerably more expensive than generic alendronate need to be incorporated into the shared-decision.

In these three risk reduction examples, the only way clinicians and patients can make decisions about the use of these medications is to have a rough idea of the magnitude of the effect on clinically important endpoints and how these agents compare to either placebo or established therapies. This information, mixed with the cost and the potential long-term benefits and harms must be discussed with patients in the realm of a shared-decision.

TREATMENTS THAT REDUCE SYMPTOMS

In contrast to treatments that reduce risk, treatments for symptoms are used with the goal of reducing or eliminating disease-specific symptoms.

Example 4: Guselkumab Used in the Treatment of Plaque Psoriasis

Patients with moderate to severe psoriasis can experience not only physical discomfort but chronic psoriasis can lead to psychological distress secondary to the appearance of lesions over large portions of a person's body. In addition psoriasis is associated with the development of arthritis, worsened cardiovascular risk factors and other conditions like inflammatory bowel disease.

The VOYAGE 1 study is an example of a well-designed and informative trial of guselkumab (Tremfya®) for patients with moderate to severe psoriasis (Blauvelt et al. 2017). The VOYAGE 1 study had three arms—guselkumab (weeks 0–48), adalimumab (weeks 0–48), and a placebo arm (weeks 0–16) after which patients taking placebo crossed over to receive guselkumab from weeks 17–48. This very useful design answers two important questions: Is guselkumab better than placebo and is guselkumab better than an established therapy (adalimumab) from a similar class?

The main endpoint in this trial was a 90% or greater improvement in the Psoriasis Area Severity Index (PASI 90). This score is used to express the overall severity of psoriasis by combining erythema, induration and desquamation with the percentage of the affected area.

At week 16, roughly 3% of the placebo subjects had a PASI 90 score, whereas this occurred in 50% in the adalimumab arm and 73% in the guselkumab arm. The roughly absolute 25% advantage of guselkumab over adalimumab was maintained at week 24 and week 48. In other words, the 50% benefit in the adalimumab group means that for every two people given adalimumab one person will achieve a PASI 90 score. The 25% additional benefit for guselkumab over adalimumab means for every four people who get guselkumab instead of adalimumab one extra person will get a PASI 90 score. When one lowers the benefit threshold to a PASI 75, approximately 90% ended up with improvement in the guselkumab group.

In addition, overall quality of life was improved. A Dermatology Life Quality Index is a score from 0 to 30 with a higher score indicating more severe disease. These subjects started at ~13–14 on this scale. On placebo, this score remained essentially unchanged over the duration of the study. However, the score on this scale for subjects on these agents went down by between 9 and 11. For this scale a minimally important change is considered ~2–3. So not only do these agents clear up psoriatic lesions, this change is also associated with an impressive improvement in a subject's quality of life.

Over this 48-week trial, adverse effect data were collected and there were no greater numbers of people with regard to outcomes such as upper respiratory infections. Adverse events such as malignancies and major adverse coronary events occurred in less than 1% in all groups. While promising, this was only a 48-week study and any impact positively or negatively these agents might have on malignancies or cardiovascular disease may not be seen for years.

So in contrast to the first three examples, in this case we have a treatment that clearly provides clinically important benefits for the vast majority of people for an endpoint that is clear, specific and measureable (PASI score and quality of life). This allows clinicians and patients the opportunity to figure out if an individual patient gets a clinically important response from a therapeutic trial.

In addition, having an endpoint that is measurable in an individual patient allows clinicians and patients to evaluate different treatments and also to determine the lowest effective dose for an individual patient.

So how could clinicians and patients use this information? From this trial adalimumab is effective in roughly 50% of subjects so a reasonable approach could be to try adalimumab first as it is less expensive and there is likely more long term data as adalimiumab has been around longer than guselkumab. If an acceptable response is not seen, then one could switch to guselkumab. Regardless of which agent is chosen, once a response has been seen, the next step would be to find the lowest effective dose by either lowering the dose or increasing the interval of the injections and seeing what happens to patient response. This approach would hopefully reduce the cost and potentially reduce the risk of adverse events given the majority of adverse effects for medications are dose-related.

Example 5: Dupilumab for Uncontrolled Persistent Asthma

Roughly one-quarter of asthmatics have moderate to severe disease with an increased risk for exacerbations, hospitalizations and an impairment of quality of life. Dupilumab (Dupixent®) is an agent used for eczema but it has also recently been studied in subjects with moderate to severe asthma. Dupilumab was evaluated in 769 subjects with uncontrolled persistent asthma despite being on inhaled corticosteroids and a long acting beta-agonist (Wenzel et al. 2016). Subjects received either placebo or one of four different doses of dupilumab, for a total of 24 weeks.

The risk of a severe exacerbation over the 24-week study period was reduced from ~25% in the placebo group down to ~15% in those receiving a dupilumab every 4 weeks and to ~10% of subjects on the twice weekly doses of dupilumab. In other words 1 in 10 benefitted from monthly injections and 1 in 6 benefitted from every 2-week injections.

As with the plaque psoriasis study, these investigators also looked at the impact of this agent on quality of life using an Asthma Quality of Life Questionnaire. The score on this questionnaire ranges from 1 to 7 with higher scores indicating a better quality of life. Subjects started at a score of roughly 4 and the scores increased by 0.9 in the placebo group and by approximately 1.1–1.2 in the dupilumab group. A minimally important change on this scale is considered to be a change of 0.5. Interestingly, in contrast to the previously mentioned psoriasis study, the placebo group in this asthma study experienced a quality of life change (0.9) that would be considered clinically important. However, the difference between the treatment and placebo groups of ~0.2–0.3 (1.1 to 1.2 minus 0.9) on this 1–7 scale would not, on average, be considered clinically important. This makes evaluation of this agent on an individual basis much trickier because of the "benefit" seen in the placebo group and the minimal difference between placebo and dupilumab.

Overall, when given this medication, patients will on average experience what they perceive to be a benefit in their quality of life (as an improvement was seen in both the placebo and the active drug group). However, almost all of this improvement is secondary not to the impact of the medication, but likely a combination of regression to the mean, the natural history of the condition and possibly the placebo effect. For this reason, dose titration to symptom control in this example is not a reasonable approach. Dupilumab did however reduce the risk for severe exacerbations in roughly 1 in 5–10 people. Finally cost and the lack of long-term data would need to be given due consideration in the decision-making process.

Example 6: Enzyme Replacement for Fabry Disease

People with the genetic disorder Fabry disease lack the enzyme alpha-galactosidase A. This enzyme is responsible for the breakdown of certain lipid compounds (globotriaosylceramide) and without this enzyme these compounds build-up in blood vessels and affect the function of the eyes, skin, kidney, heart, gastrointestinal system, brain and nervous system. This build-up can lead to symptoms of pain in the hands and feet, cloudiness in the eye, a decreased ability to sweat, hearing loss, and dark red spots on the skin. In addition, life expectancy is also reduced. Two recombinant enzyme replacement therapies are available, agalsidase alfa (Replagal®) and agalsidase beta (Fabrazyme®).

One of the first studies of enzyme replacement randomized 58 patients to either agalsidase beta 1 mg/kg IV or placebo every 2 weeks for 20 weeks followed by open-label agalsidase beta for 6 months (Eng et al. 2001). The primary end point was the percentage of patients in each group who were free of microvascular endothelial deposits of globotriaosylceramide in renal-biopsy specimens. After 20 weeks, in the enzyme replacement arm, 31% patients had deposits but 100% had deposits in the placebo arm. Patients in the enzyme replacement arm also had lower scores on deposits in the heart and skin. Interestingly however, in this study, overall pain scores and quality of life scores were not different between the two groups. Infusion related adverse effects were higher in the enzyme group ~50% rigors, ~20% fevers, ~10% headache, ~15% chills than in the placebo group. A roughly 3-year follow-up study suggested that enzyme replacement therapy resulted in continuously decreased plasma globotriaosylceramide levels however this follow-up study was not designed to evaluate the impact of enzyme replacement on clinical relevant outcomes (Wilcox et al. 2004).

A recent Cochrane review (nine trials of either agalsidase alfa or beta in 351 subjects) concluded "Trials comparing enzyme replacement therapy to placebo show significant improvement with enzyme replacement therapy in regard to microvascular endothelial deposits of globotriaosylceramide and in pain-related quality of life" (ElDIb et al. 2016). Pain scores were reduced by ~2 points (a clinically relevant change) on a 10 point scale in studies of agalsidase alfa over a period of 6 months. However, the authors also stated "The long-term influence of enzyme replacement therapy on risk of morbidity and mortality related to Anderson-Fabry disease remains to be established."

So in this example we have patients with a specific enzyme deficiency that will clearly negatively impact their health over the long-term. We have evidence that enzyme replacement therapy reduces the surrogate marker of endothelial deposits and possibly leads to a reduction in pain but long-term impacts on clinical important outcomes may never truly be known because of the ethics of doing long-term placebo trials in these subjects. These unknowns make funding and medical decisions tricky because these enzyme replacements can cost in excess of $200,000US a year.

CONCLUSION

Using these examples, it is clear there is no single way to approach clinical decisions around the use of these "omic" technologies. However, even though these novel agents may have unique mechanisms, and in some cases clinically important benefits, they are yet just another treatment option. Given that, they should be incorporated into clinical practice just like any other treatment option, which is by using the best available evidence and balancing benefits and harms.

All of the requirements in Table 13.1 come into play as they would with any new medication entering the marketplace and clinical use. The individual decisions revolve very much around what the best available evidence shows and what condition is being treated. A personalized approach in each of these cases is crucial because each patient and response will be very unique. The benefits may be as small as one in 50–100 people benefitting, or in some cases 50–75% of people will derive a clinical benefit. These numbers are very much determined by the baseline risk of a patient and the overall effectiveness of the medication.

Regardless of condition, every decision needs to be informed by the best available evidence, which hopefully includes how these agents compare to not only placebo, but also how they compare to the gold standard treatments and other agents within in the same class.

To effectively use these agents, as with all medications, one needs to know what happens clinically in the placebo group, the magnitude of the change in the treatment group. Each of these examples bring to light the many different and unique aspects that need to be considered.

For medications like palivizumab, evolucumab and romosozumab clinicians need to be able to communicate the magnitude of the risk reduction to patients and to also discuss the adverse effects, the cost, the inconvenience and the fact that knowledge of the long-term effects is often fairly limited.

For agents like dupilumab and in particular guselkumab where one may be able to evaluate the individual response to a particular medication and dose, individualization and titration to the lowest effective dose becomes a key step in the overall use of these medications.

Finally, for medications like the enzyme replacement therapies for Fabry disease we may never know if life-long use of these treatments will actually lead to a clinically important improvement in quality of life or a reduction in negative clinical outcomes.

With these new "omic" technologies, there is certainly a possibility these new agents may be more effective or may in fact be the only effective treatment for a number of difficult to treat or uncommon conditions. However, every one of these new medications must be evaluated using the exact same principles of evidence-based practice presently used for all new and old treatments alike.

SELF-ASSESSMENT QUESTIONS

Questions

1. Is there anything unique about therapeutic proteins and how clinicians need to assess them?
2. If a medication produces a 25% relative reduction in the chance of developing heart disease does that mean 25% of people who take the medication benefit?
3. For any new medication that has an effect on symptoms, how does one go about figuring out the best dose for an individual patient?
4. When a new medication comes on the market there is often limited long-term safety data so how should a clinician deal with this problem?
5. Is cost an important issue when it comes to the new "omic" technologies?

Answers

1. Not really. As with all new therapeutic options they need to be evaluated with appropriately designed RCTs, and then the decision about their value should be based on a combination of evidence and patient-centered requirements.
2. No, any relative benefit needs to be applied to the baseline event rate in the placebo group. For instance if the baseline risk of a heart attack in the placebo group is 20% then applying a relative 25% benefit to the 20% baseline risk means that 15% of the treatment group end up getting a heart attack. The absolute risk difference is 20% minus 15% or an absolute benefit of 5% which translates to having to treat 20 people to benefit one.
3. One can (a) start with the dose used in the studies and then if a benefit is seen a dose titration down can be done to identify the lowest effective dose or, (b) start with a dose 1/4 to an 1/8th of that used in the initial clinical studies and then titrate the dose up to the dose that best controls the patients symptoms with a minimum of side effects.
4. In general, unless the new medication provides an important clinical benefit over other existing therapies it may be best to wait until longer-term adverse effect data is available before incorporating it into practice.
5. Cost is always an important issue when it comes to the selection of any therapeutic treatment. If a new agent doesn't provide a clinically important improvement over older treatments, then cost should be a determining factor in the selection process. If a new agent does provide a clinically relevant improvement in prevention or symptomatic treatment then the increased cost should be proportional to that increased benefit.

REFERENCES

Andabaka T, Nickerson JW, Rojas-Reyes MX, Rueda JD, Bacic Vrca V, Barsic B (2013) Monoclonal antibody for reducing the risk of respiratory syncytial virus infection in children. Cochrane Database Syst Rev 4:CD006602

Blauvelt A, Papp KA, Griffiths CEM et al (2017) Efficacy and safety of guselkumab, an anti-interleukin-23 monoclonal antibody, compared with adalimumab for the continuous treatment of patients with moderate to severe psoriasis: results from the phase III, double-blinded, placebo- and active comparator-controlled VOYAGE 1 trial. J Am Acad Dermatol 76:405–417

ElDib R, Gomaa H, Carvalho RP, Camargo SE, Bazan R, Barretti P, Barreto FC (2016) Enzyme replacement therapy for Anderson-Fabry disease. Cochrane Database Syst Rev 7:CD006663

Eng CM, Guffon N, Wilcox WR, Germain DP, Lee P, Waldek S et al (2001) Safety and efficacy of recombinant human alpha-galactosidase A replacement therapy in Fabry's disease. N Engl J Med 345:9–16

Saag KG, Petersen J, Brandi ML, Karaplis AC, Lorentzon M, Thomas T, Maddox J, Fan M, Meisner PD, Grauer A (2017) Romosozumab or alendronate for fracture prevention in women with osteoporosis. N Engl J Med 377:1417–1427

Sabatine MS, Giugliano RP, Keech AC, Honarpour N, Wiviott SD, Murphy SA, Kuder JF, Wang H, Liu T, Wasserman SM, Sever PS, Pedersen TR, FOURIER Steering Committee and Investigators (2017) Evolocumab and clinical outcomes in patients with cardiovascular disease. N Engl J Med 376:1713–1722

Sindelar RD (2013) Genomics, other "Omic" technologies, personalized medicine. In: Crommelin DJA, Sindelar RD, Meibohm B (eds) Pharmaceutical biotechnology, 4th edn. Springer, New York, pp 190–221

Wenzel S, Castro M, Corren J, Maspero J, Wang L, Zhang B, Pirozzi G, Sutherland ER, Evans RR, Joish VN, Eckert L, Graham NM, Stahl N, Yancopoulos GD, Louis-Tisserand M, Teper A (2016) Dupilumab efficacy and safety in adults with uncontrolled persistent asthma despite use of medium-to-high-dose inhaled corticosteroids plus a long-acting beta2 agonist: a randomised double-blind placebo-controlled pivotal phase 2b dose-ranging trial. Lancet 388:31–44

Wilcox WR, Banikazemi M, Guffon N, Waldek S, Lee P, Linthorst GE, Desnick RJ, Germain DP, International Fabry Disease Study Group (2004) Long-term safety and efficacy of enzyme replacement therapy for Fabry disease. Am J Hum Genet 75:65–74

14 Vaccines

Wim Jiskoot, Gideon F. A. Kersten, Enrico Mastrobattista, and Bram Slütter

INTRODUCTION

Since vaccination was documented by Edward Jenner in 1798, it has become the most successful means of preventing infectious diseases, saving millions of lives every year. Application of vaccines is currently not limited to the prevention of infectious diseases. Vaccines in the pipeline include, amongst others, therapeutic vaccines against allergies, cancer, and Alzheimer's disease.

Modern biotechnology has an enormous impact on current vaccine development. The elucidation of the molecular structures of pathogens and the tremendous progress made in immunology as well as developments in proteomics and bioinformatics have led to the identification of protective antigens and ways to deliver them. Together with technological advances, this has caused a move from empirical vaccine development to more rational approaches to develop effective and safe vaccines. In addition, modern methodologies may provide simpler and cheaper production processes for selected vaccine components.

Although vaccines resemble other biopharmaceuticals such as therapeutic proteins in some aspects, there are several important differences (Table 14.1). Unique features of vaccines include the low dose and frequency of administration, and the widely different vaccine categories (Table 14.2). Also, the target group is not only patients but basically every human being on the planet, with the emphasis on very young, healthy children. These differences have a huge impact on the requirements for vaccine admission on the market and release of vaccine batches, putting safety requirements on par with efficacy.

In the following section, immunological principles that are important for vaccine design are summarized. Subsequently, vaccine categories will be discussed, including current developments, especially in the field of therapeutic cancer vaccines. It is not our intent to provide a comprehensive review. Rather, we will explain current approaches to vaccine development and illustrate these approaches with representative examples. Routes of administration will be discussed in a separate section. In the last section, pharmaceutical aspects of vaccines, including issues related with production, formulation, characterization and storage, are dealt with.

IMMUNOLOGICAL PRINCIPLES

Introduction

As a reaction to infection, the human immune system launches a series of immunological responses with the goal of eliminating the pathogen. Innate immune cells will be the first to respond and will attempt to clear the pathogen through phagocytosis and/or lysis. As pathogens have developed strategies to evade the innate immune response, all vertebrates are capable of eliciting a highly specific response by virtue of their adaptive immune system. The adaptive immune system can generate humoral immunity and cell-mediated immunity (see Fig. 14.1 and Table 14.3). Antibodies, produced by B-cells, are the typical representatives of humoral immunity. An antibody belongs to one of four different immunoglobulin classes (IgM, IgG, IgA, or IgE) (cf. Chap. 8). Antibodies are able to prevent infection or disease through several mechanisms:

1. Binding of antibodies covers the pathogen with Fc (constant fragment), the "rear end" of immunoglobulins. Phagocytic cells, such as macrophages,

W. Jiskoot (✉) · B. Slütter
Division of BioTherapeutics, Leiden Academic Centre for Drug Research (LACDR), Leiden University, Leiden, The Netherlands
e-mail: w.jiskoot@lacdr.leidenuniv.nl; b.a.slutter@lacdr.leidenuniv.nl

G. F. A. Kersten
Institute for Translational Vaccinology, Bilthoven, The Netherlands
e-mail: gideon.kersten@intravacc.nl

E. Mastrobattista
Department of Pharmaceutics, Utrecht University, Utrecht, The Netherlands
e-mail: E.Mastrobattista@uu.nl

D. J. A. Crommelin et al. (eds.), *Pharmaceutical Biotechnology*, https://doi.org/10.1007/978-3-030-00710-2_14

Characteristic	Vaccines	Other biopharmaceuticals
Dose	Low (microgram range)	High (usually milligram range)
Frequency	Low (months –decades)	High (days – weeks)
Product group	Heterogeneous	Less heterogeneous
Characteristics	Sometimes ill-defined,	Mostly well-defined
Type of formulation	Usually a suspension or emulsion (liquid or lyophilized)	Usually a solution (liquid or lyophilized)
Indication	Mostly prophylactic	Therapeutic
Target group	Every human being	Patients
Number of active ingredients	>1 (antigen (s) and adjuvant(s))	1

Table 14.1 ■ Exemplary differences between vaccines and most other biopharmaceuticals

Vaccine (sub)type	Example(s)	Antigen	Disease	Prophylactic/ Therapeutic	Status of Develop ment*
Live					
Attenuated viruses	Poliovirus (Sabin)	Whole attenuated virus	Polio	P	2
	Rotavirus		Diarrhea	P	2
	Measles virus		Measles	P	2
	Mumps virus		Mumps	P	2
	Varicella zoster		Chickenpox	P	2
	Yellow fever virus		Yellow fever	P	2
Attenuated bacteria	BCG	Whole attenuated bacteria	Tuberculosis	p	2
	Salmonella typhi		Typhoid fever	P	2
Vectored	HIV antigens using vaccinia or adenoviral vectors	Multiple HIV antigens	AIDS	P	1
	Ebola antigens using adenoviral or vesicular stomatitis virus vectors	cAd3-EBO Z, VSV ZEBOV	Ebola virus disease	P	1
Human cells	Autologous dendritic cells (Provenge)	Prostate acid phosphatase (PAP)	Prostate cancer	T	2

Table 14.2 ■ Vaccine categories based on antigen source

Vaccine (sub)type	Example(s)	Antigen	Disease	Prophylactic/ Therapeutic	Status of Development*
Inactivated					
Whole virus	Poliovirus (2^{nd}generation)	Formaldehyde-inactivated poliovirus	Polio	P	2
	Rabies virus	Propriolactone-inactivated Pitman-Moore L503 rabies virus strain	Rabies	P	2
	Hepatitis A virus	Formaldehyde-inactivated Hepatitis A virus strain CR 326F antigen	Hepatitis	P	2
Whole bacteria	*Bordetella pertussis*	Heat or formaldehyde inactivated bacteria	Whooping cough	P	2
	Vibrio cholerae		Cholera	P	2
Human cells	Melacine	Melanoma cell extract	Melanoma	T	2
Subunits					
Proteins	Mosquirix	CSP-HBsAg fusion protein	Malaria	P	2
	Hepatitis B virus	HBsAg VLP	Hepatitis B	P	2
	Gardasil	HPV-6/11/16/18 VP1 VLPs	Cervical cancer	P	2
	Clostridium tetani	Tetanus toxoid	Tetanus	P	2
	Corynebacterium diphtheriae	Diphtheria toxoid	Diphtheria	P	2
Peptides	ISA101 synthetic long peptides (SLP)	HPV16 E6 and E7 T cell epitopes	Cervical cancer	T	1
Polysaccharides	*Haemophilis influenzae* type B (Hib)	Capsular polysaccharide	Invasive Hib disease	P	2
	Neisseria meningitidis	Capsular polysaccharides	Meningitis	P	2
	Streptococcus pneumoniae	Capsular polysaccharides, either free or conjugated to CRM197 diphtheria toxoid	Pneumonia, meningitis	P	2
Nucleic acids					
DNA	Influenza vaccine	H5N1, H1N1	Flu	P	1
	Human papilloma virus vaccine	HPV 16/18 fusion consensus antigens	Cervical cancer	T	1
	HIV vaccine	HIV-1 gag, env and pol	AIDS	T	1
RNA	Self-adjuvanted mRNA	PSA, PSCA, PSMA, STEAP1	Prostate cancer	T	1

* *1. Clinical evaluation, 2. Marketed product*

Abbreviations:

HIV: human immunodeficiency virus; HPV: human papillomavirus; cAd3 EBO-Z: Chimp adenovirus serotype 3-vectored Zaire ebolavirus antigens; VSV ZEBOV: Vesicular stomatitis virus-vectored Zaire ebolavirus antigens; CSP-HBsAg: circumsporozoite protein fused toHepatitis virus B surface antigen. VLP: virus-like particle; CRM197: genetically detoxified form of diphtheria toxin. H5N1, H1N1: influenza virus A subtypes, with differences in the surface antigens hemagglutinin (H) and Neuraminidase (N); HIV-1 gag, env and pol: the 3 major proteins of HIV-1, with gag being a polyprotein that is processed to matrix and core proteins, env a protein residing in the lipid envolope and pol the reverse transcriptase; PSA: prostate-specific antigen; PSCA: prostate stem cell antigen; PSMA: prostate-specific membrane antigen; STEAP1: prostate-specific metalloreductase

Table 14.2 ■ (continued)

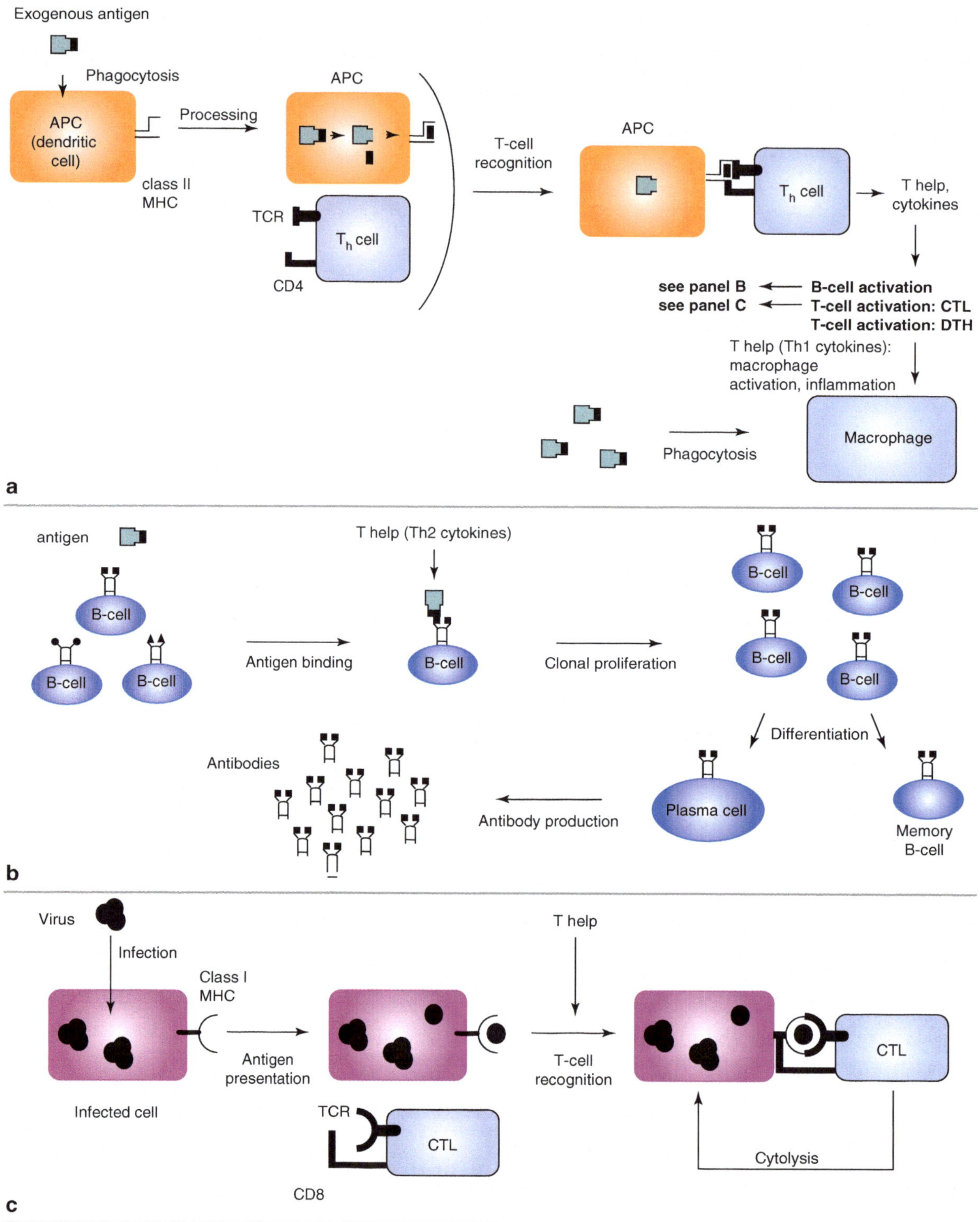

Figure 14.1 ■ Schematic representation of antigen-dependent immune responses. (**a**) Activation of T-helper cells (Th-cells). An antigen-presenting cell (APC), e.g., a dendritic cell, phagocytoses exogenous antigens (bacteria or soluble antigens) and degrades them partially. Antigen fragments are presented by MHC class II molecules to a CD4-positive Th-cell; the MHC-antigen complex on the APC is recognized by the T-cell receptor (TCR) and CD4 molecules on the Th-cell. The APC-Th-cell interaction leads to activation of the Th-cell. The activated Th-cell produces cytokines, resulting in the activation of macrophages (Th1 help), B cells (Th2 help; panel **b**), or cytotoxic T cells (panel **c**). (**b**) Antibody production. The presence of antigen and Th2-type cytokines causes proliferation and differentiation of B cells. Only B cells specific for the antigen become activated. The B cells, now called plasma cells, produce and secrete large amounts of antibody. Some B cells differentiate into memory cells. (**c**) Activation of cytotoxic T lymphocytes (CTLs). CTLs recognize nonself antigens expressed by MHC class I molecules on the surface of virally infected cells or tumor cells. Cytolytic proteins are produced by the CTL upon interaction with the target cell

express surface receptors for Fc. This allows targeting of the opsonized (antibody-coated) antigen to these cells, followed by enhanced phagocytosis.
2. Immune complexes (i.e., complexes of antibodies bound to target antigens) can activate complement, a system of proteins which then becomes cytolytic to bacteria, enveloped viruses, or infected cells.
3. Phagocytic cells may express receptors for complement factors associated with immune complexes. Binding of these activated complement factors enhances phagocytosis.

Immune response	Immune product	Accessory factors	Infectious agents
Humoral	IgG	Complement, neutrophils	Bacteria and viruses
	IgA	Alternative complement pathway	Microorganisms causing respiratory and enteric infections
	IgM	Complement, macrophages	(Encapsulated) bacteria
	IgE	Mast cells	Extracellular parasites
Cell mediated	CTL	Cytolytic proteins	Viruses, mycobacteria, intracellular parasites
	Th1	Macrophages	Mycobacteria, treponema (syphilis), fungi

Table 14.3 ■ Important immune products protecting against infectious diseases

4. Viruses can be neutralized by antibodies through binding at or near receptor binding sites on the virus surface. This may prevent binding to and entry into the host cell.

Antibodies are effective against many, but not all infectious microorganisms. They may have limited value when pathogens occupy intracellular niches (such as intracellular bacteria and parasites), which are not easily reached by antibodies. In this case cell-mediated immunity is required to clear the infected cells. T-cells are the major representative of cell-mediated immunity and can clear infections by the following mechanisms:

1. Cytotoxic T-lymphocytes (CTLs, also called cytotoxic T-cells) react with target cells and kill them by release of cytolytic proteins like perforin.
2. T-helper cells (Th1-type, see below) activate macrophages, allowing them to kill intracellular pathogens.

In contrast to the innate response, the adaptive immune response is very specific to the invading pathogen (Fig. 14.2). The adaptive immune system comprises B-cells and T-cells with a wide range of specificities, owing to the unique compositions of their B-cell receptor (BCR) and T-cell receptor (TCR). During an infection the innate immune system instructs those B- and T-cells that have BCRs and TCRs specific for the invading pathogen to proliferate and gain effector functions. When the infection is cleared, most of these B- and T-cells are obsolete and many will die by apoptosis. Antibodies produced by B-cells, however, can persist in the circulation for an extended period of time. Moreover, some of the B- and T-cells resist apop-

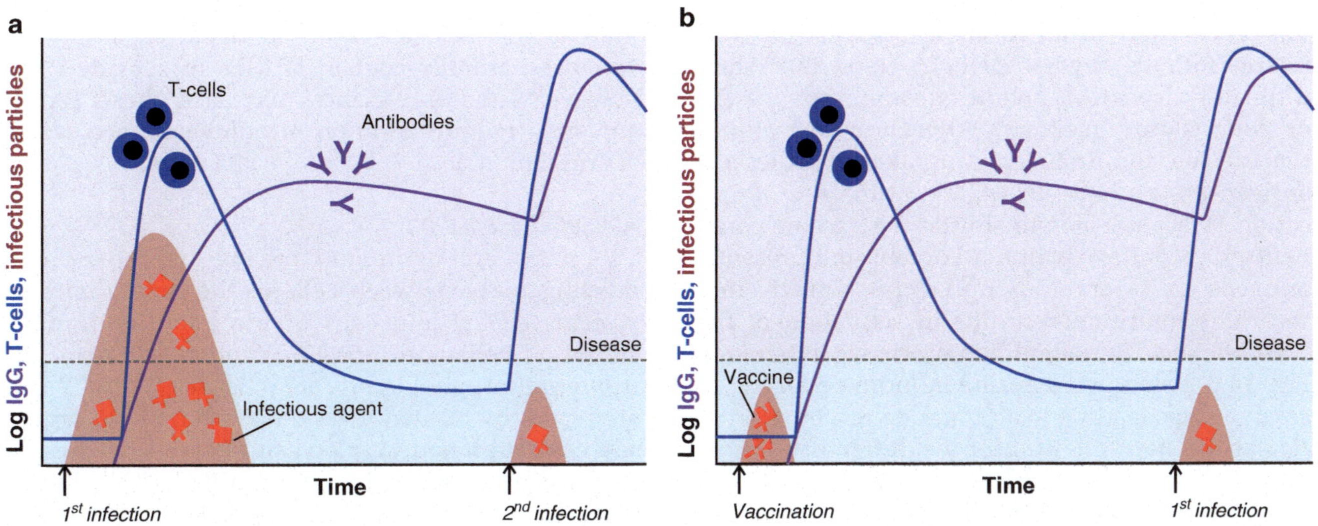

Figure 14.2 ■ Principle of adaptive immune responses following infection and vaccination. (**a**) Schematic representation of adaptive immune responses upon primary and secondary infection. Upon primary infection T- and B-cell responses take time to develop, allowing pathogens to proliferate and cause disease. Upon secondary infection, circulating antibodies and memory T-cells quickly respond, preventing proliferation and dissemination of the pathogen. (**b**) Application of a vaccine that induces an adaptive immune response like a natural infection, but without associated disease

tosis and can maintain themselves for many years as memory B- and T-cells. In contrast to their naive counterparts, these memory cells are rapidly activated and clonally expanded when they re-encounter the same pathogen on a later occasion. Therefore, unlike the primary response, the response after repeated infection is very fast and usually sufficiently strong to prevent reoccurrence of the disease (Fig. 14.2a).

Vaccination exploits the formation of this immunological memory by the adaptive immune system. The principle of vaccination is mimicking an infection in such a way that the natural specific defense mechanism of the host against the pathogen will be activated and immunological memory is established, but the host will remain free of the disease that normally results from a natural infection (Fig. 14.2b). This is effectuated by administration of antigenic components that consist of, are derived from, or are related to the pathogen. The immune response is highly specific: it discriminates not only between pathogen species but often also between different strains within one species (e.g., strains of meningococci, poliovirus, influenza virus). Albeit sometimes a hurdle for vaccine developers, this high specificity of the immune system allows an almost perfect balance between responsiveness to foreign antigens and tolerance to self-antigens.

Whereas prophylactic vaccines aim for immunological memory, the primary goal of therapeutic vaccines usually is induction of potent effector responses rather than memory. In the next paragraphs we will discuss the immunological principles leading to effector and memory responses.

■ Generation of an Immune Response and Immunological Memory

The generation of an immune response by vaccination follows several distinct steps that should ultimately lead to a potent effector response and/or long-lasting memory. After administration of the vaccine, the first step is uptake by professional antigen-presenting cells (APCs) at the site of application. APCs are able to shuttle the vaccine components to secondary lymphoid organs and present the antigens to T- and B-lymphocytes, which—under the right conditions—results in activation of these lymphocytes. This simplified process is illustrated in Fig. 14.3. Below we describe in more detail the successive steps leading to an immune response, in particular the steps relevant for the design of vaccines.

Activation of the Innate Immune System

Every immune reaction against a pathogen or a vaccine starts with activation of the innate immune system. Although the innate response itself does not lead to immunological memory, it is instrumental in activating and educating the adaptive immune system. Important constituents of the innate immune system are APCs like macrophages and dendritic cells (DCs), which reside in tissues. By continuously endocytosing extracellular material, they sample their environment for potential harmful materials. To distinguish harmful from innocuous substances, APCs are equipped with pattern recognition receptors (PRRs) that allow detection of conserved microbial and viral structures, called pathogen-associated molecular patterns (PAMPs) (Kawai and Akira 2009). Examples of PAMPs are viral RNA and bacterial cell wall constituents, such as lipopolysaccharide (LPS) and flagellin (Table 14.4). As pathogens occupy different cellular niches, PRRs can be found either on the cell surface and endosomes (for bacterial PAMPs) or in the cytoplasm (for viral PAMPs). Examples of PRRs are toll-like receptors (TLRs), C-type lectins and RIG-I-like receptors (Table 14.4).

PRR activation induces a maturation program, which switches APCs from an antigen sampling to an antigen presentation mode, which is critical for their role as intermediates for lymphocyte activation. PRR activation induces expression of MHC class I (MHCI) and MHC class II (MHCII) molecules, increasing the APCs' capacity to present antigen to T-cells. Moreover, APCs will gain expression of chemokine receptors (e.g., CCR7) that allow them to migrate to secondary lymphoid tissue. Finally, PRR stimulation induces upregulation of co-stimulatory molecules and pro-inflammatory cytokines, which provide import activation signals to T-cells during antigen presentation.

PRR activation is an essential step in the vaccination process and therefore important to consider when designing a vaccine. Live attenuated or inactivated vaccines naturally contain PAMPs to activate PRRs, however subunit vaccines may lack these PAMPs and may require addition of adjuvants (see section "Formulation").

Antigen Presentation

The peripheral lymphoid organs are the primary meeting place between cells of the innate immune system (APCs) and cells of the adaptive immune system (T-cells and B-cells). Whereas APCs are distributed throughout peripheral tissues, T- and B-cells are primarily located in secondary lymphoid organs, such as lymph nodes, spleen and Peyer's patches. An important reason for this is that, although the human body harbors a large number of lymphocytes (ca. 10^{12}), only few T- and B-cells will have a TCR or BCR that is specific for the antigen of interest. By concentrating lymphocytes in secondary lymphoid organs and having APCs presenting antigen there, the

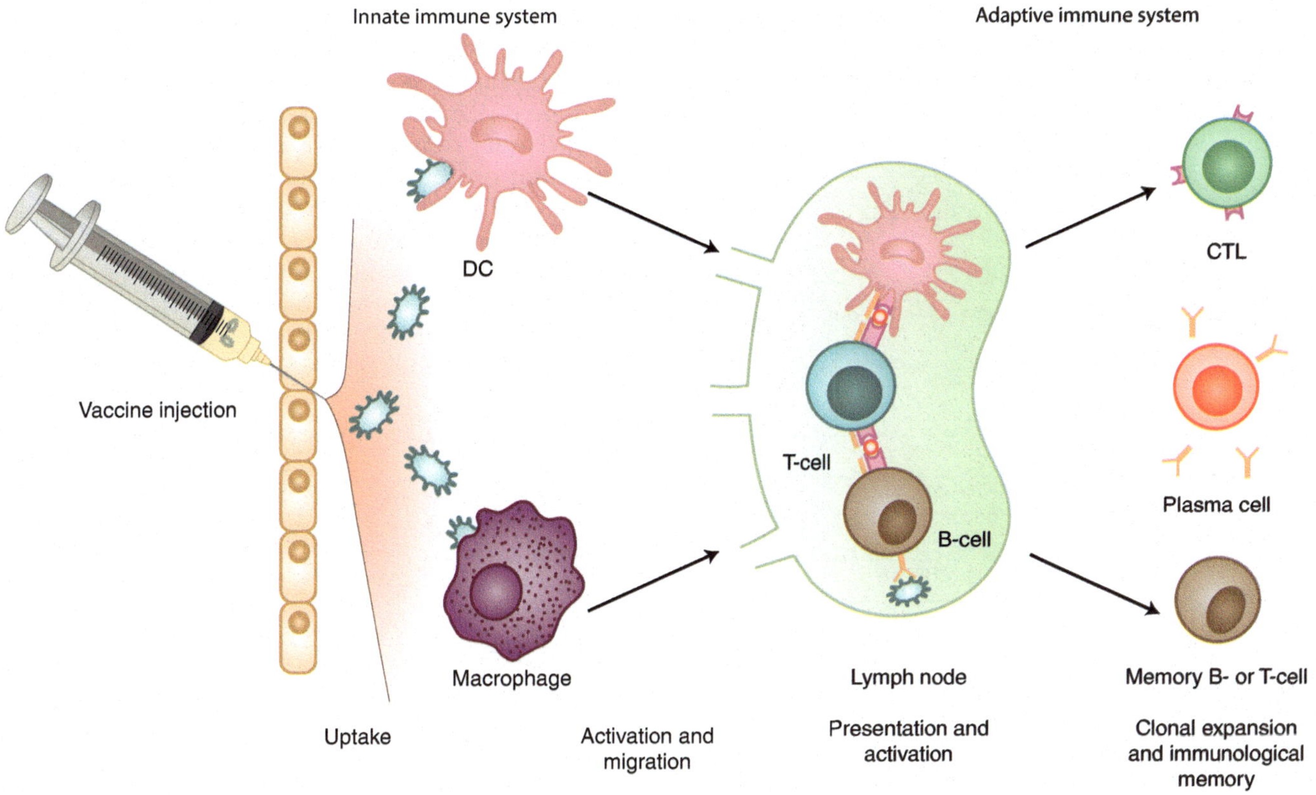

Figure 14.3 ■ Overview of the steps leading to immunity after administration of a vaccine. Upon subcutaneous or intramuscular administration, the vaccine components are taken up by phagocytic cells such as macrophages and dendritic cells (DCs) that reside in the peripheral tissue and express pattern recognition receptors (PRRs) that recognize pathogen-associated molecular patterns (PAMPs). Professional antigen-presenting cells (APCs) that have taken up antigens become activated and start migrating towards nearby lymph nodes. Inside the lymph nodes, the antigen processed by the APCs is presented to lymphocytes, which, when recognizing the antigen and receiving the appropriate co-stimulatory signals, become activated. These antigen-specific B- and T-cells clonally expand to produce multiple progenitors recognizing the same antigen. In addition, memory B- and T-cells are formed that provide long-term (sometimes lifelong) protection against infection with the pathogen

chance of antigen specific T- and B-cells encountering their cognate antigen is increased. Upon interaction with APCs, antigen specific T-cells and B-cells will be activated, provided that they acquire the appropriate signals.

The first of these signals is antigen presentation, which allows selection of antigen specific B- and T-cells. B-cells and T-cells recognize antigens in different ways. B-cells can recognize antigens in their native form as their BCR allows direct interaction with the antigen. Therefore, B-cell antigens do not require major processing. In fact, B-cells can take up antigens that are small enough to drain to lymph nodes without the help of APCs. To shuttle larger antigens to lymphoid tissue in their native form, APCs express receptors that allow presentation of intact antigens to B-cells (Batista and Harwood 2009).

Some antigens are able to directly stimulate antibody production by B-cells without T-cell involvement. These thymus-independent antigens include certain linear antigens that are not readily degraded in the body and have a repeating determinant, such as bacterial polysaccharides. Thymus-independent antigens do not induce immunological memory and are therefore less interesting from a vaccination standpoint. It is possible, however, to render these antigens thymus dependent by chemically coupling them to a protein carrier (see sections "B-cell and T-cell Activation" and "Polysaccharide Vaccines").

T-cells are unable to directly interact with antigen, but depend on the APCs to process antigens into peptide fragments (T-cell epitopes) and present them to the T-cells in the context of MHCI (to $CD8^+$ T-cells) or MHCII molecules ($CD4^+$ T-cells) on the APC surface. Whether antigens are presented on MHCI or MHCII molecules is dependent on the intracellular location of the antigen processing. Exogenous antigens, acquired by endocytosis, can undergo limited proteolysis in the endosome and associate with MHCII molecules (Fig. 14.1a). Loaded MHCII molecules return to the surface and can

PRR	PRR location	PAMP[b]	Source
TLR1–TLR2	Cell surface	Triacyl lipopeptides	Bacteria
TLR2–TLR6	Cell surface	Diacyl lipopeptides	Bacteria
		Zymosan	Fungus
TLR3	Endosome	dsRNA	Virus
TLR4	Cell surface	LPS	Bacteria
TLR5	Cell surface	Flagellin	Bacteria
TLR7	Endosome	Single stranded (ss) RNA	RNA viruses
TLR8	Endosome	ssRNA	RNA viruses
TLR9	Endosome	CpG DNA	Bacteria
RIG-I	Cytosol	ssRNA and short double stranded RNA	Viruses
MDA5	Cytosol	Long dsRNA	Viruses
LGP2 (helicase)	Cytosol	RNA	Viruses
NOD1/ NLRC1	Cytosol	iE-DAP	Bacteria
NOD2/ NLRC2	Cytosol	MDP	Bacteria
		ATP	Bacteria/ host
		Uric acid, CPPD, amyloid-β	Host
NALP1/ NLRP1	Cytosol	Anthrax lethal toxin	Bacteria
IPAF/NLRC4	Cytosol	Flagellin	Bacteria
NAIP5	Cytosol	Flagellin	Bacteria
Dectin-1	Cell surface	β-Glucan	Fungi

[a]Adapted from Kawai and Akira, Int. Immunol. 2009
[b]Several of the PAMPs listed here are used as vaccine adjuvants (see section "Formulation" and Table 14.6)

Table 14.4 ■ Examples of pattern recognition receptors (PRRs), their ligands (PAMPs) and source[a]

interact with $CD4^+$ T-helper cells. Endogenous antigens, such as viral or mutated proteins produced by the host cell, are generated by proteasomal processing in the cytosol. The resulting peptides can associate with MHCI in the endoplasmatic reticulum and can interact with ($CD8^+$) cytotoxic T-cells (Fig. 14.1c).

These different antigen presentation pathways have consequences for vaccine design. As T-cells only recognize processed antigen fragments, T-cell responses rely on continuous epitopes, which are linear peptide sequences (usually consisting of up to ten amino acid residues) of the protein (see Fig. 14.1a). In contrast, B-cell epitopes can be discontinuous epitopes comprising amino acid residues sometimes far apart in the primary sequence, which are brought together through the unique folding of the protein (see Fig. 14.1b). Antibody recognition of B-cell epitopes, whether continuous or discontinuous, is usually dependent on the conformation (=three-dimensional structure) of the antigen. For vaccines aimed to induce high levels of neutralizing antibodies (for instance, diphtheria and tetanus vaccines), one should take great care that the antigen remains in its native form. Vaccines that should induce CTL responses (e.g., some virus vaccines, cancer vaccines) will not necessarily require the antigen to be in its native form, as the antigen will have to be degraded before presentation anyway. A major challenge for these types of vaccines, however, is that MHCI presentation requires antigen to enter the cytosol rather than the endosomal compartment of an APC (see Fig. 14.1c). Professional APCs, especially DCs, have the capacity to transfer exogenously acquired antigens from the endosomal compartment into the MHCI processing pathway. The process is referred to as cross-presentation.

B-cell and T-cell Activation

Next to TCR stimulation through peptide loaded MHCI or MHCII molecules, the second signal T-cells require is co-stimulation via interaction of accessory and co-stimulatory molecules on the APCs (Fig. 14.4). This cell-cell interaction is essential for proper stimulation of lymphocytes, and without those accessory signals, antigen-specific T-cells will not proliferate and may become anergic (i.e., acquire a state of unresponsiveness). As co-stimulatory molecules, such as CD80/86, CD40 and ICAM-1, are upregulated on APCs after PRR stimulation, this signal functions as an additional safety check to prevent unwanted immune responses against self-antigens.

T-cells receiving TCR stimulation and co-stimulation will become activated, clonally expand and generate multiple progenitors all recognizing the same antigen. In contrast, T-cells can also receive co-inhibitory signals from the APC (e.g., PD1, CTLA4 activation). These signals reduce T-cell activation and provide a negative control mechanism against uncontrolled or unwanted T-cell responses.

Before and during clonal expansion, T-cells receive cytokine signals that influence their fate (signal 3). Cytokines can promote T-cell proliferation and also affect their effector function (See Fig. 14.4). For instance, interleukin 12 (IL-12) and type I interferon (IFN) are cytokines that are essential for the development of CTLs. Lack of these cytokines results in reduced proliferation of CTLs and a reduced capacity to kill target cells.

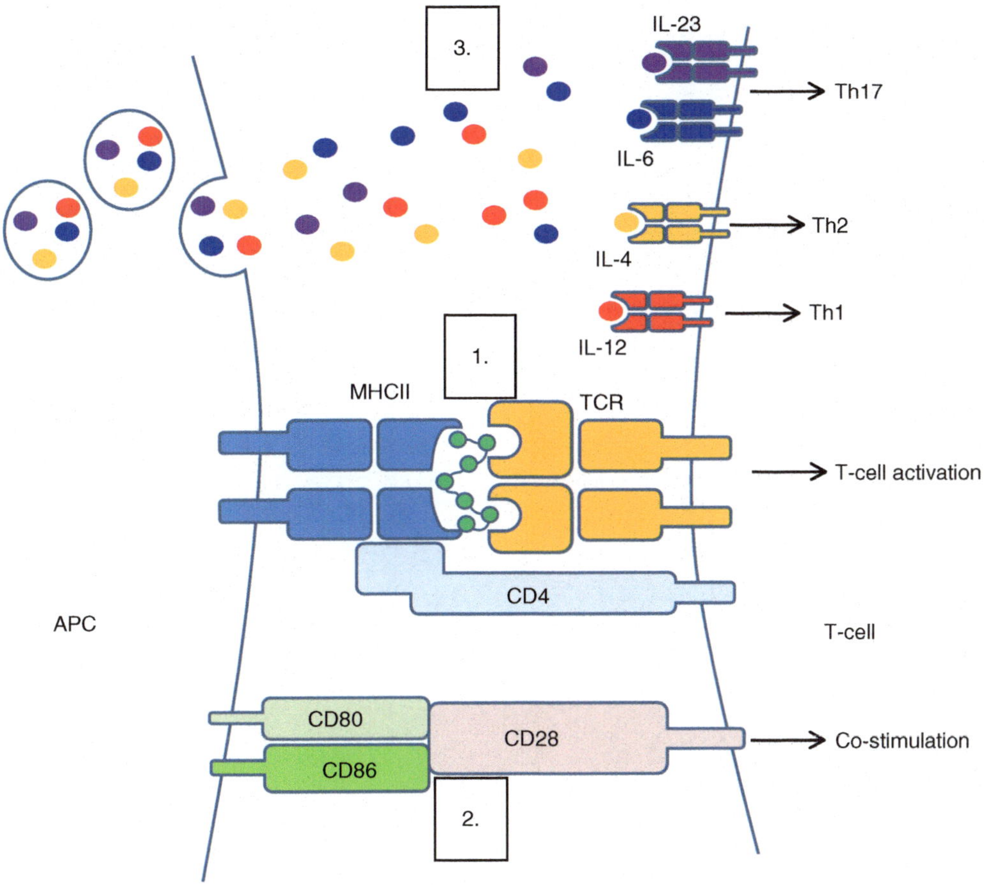

Figure 14.4 ■ The 3 signals of T-helper cell activation. 1. Antigen presentation. Peptides derived from a vaccine are loaded on MHCII molecules by the APC and presented to the T-cell receptor (TCR) on T-cells. 2. Co-stimulation. Activated APCs express co-stimulatory molecules, such as CD80/86 which support T-cell activation through interaction with CD28 on T-cells. 3. Cytokines. APCs can produce different cytokines depending on the type of PAMP that has activated the APC. These cytokines provide a third signal to the T-cell by engaging their cognate receptors on the T-cell surface. Whereas IL-12 (red) signaling leads to Th1 polarization of the CD4+ T-cell, IL-4 (yellow) signaling induces Th2 polarization and IL-6/IL23 (blue/purple) signaling provides a pathway towards Th17 CD4+ T-cells

Especially for the CD4+ T-helper cells the cytokine signal during priming is crucial, as T-helper cells can have various effector functions. For instance, in the presence of cytokines, such as IL-12 and type I IFN, CD4+ T-cells develop into T-helper 1 (Th1) cells. These cells produce cytokines, such as IFN-γ and tumor necrosis factor alfa (TNF-α), which potentiate the effector function of phagocytes and increase inflammation. Therefore, induction of memory Th1 cells is a major goal for vaccines that aim to protect against intracellular pathogens. T-helper 2 (Th2) cells develop under influence of IL-4 signaling. These Th2 cells produce another set of cytokines that prevent Th1 differentiation and support B-cell proliferation and differentiation. Th2 cells have therefore been associated with increased humoral responses. However, as the cytokines produced by Th2 cells have been linked to IgE production by B-cells, reducing the number of memory Th2 cells has become an important focus in the design of vaccines aiming to reduce allergic responses.

Next to Th1 and Th2 cells, various other T-helper subsets have been identified, each having unique functional properties. Th17 cells develop when CD4+ T-cells receive transforming growth factor beta (TGF-β), IL-6 and IL-23 signals, and produce IL-17 and IL-22. These cytokines support the defense of mucosal surfaces, but have also been linked to inflammatory disease, such as inflammatory bowel disease and psoriasis. Regulatory T-cells (Tregs) are subsets of CD4+ T-cells that play an important role in limiting inflammation through secretion of anti-inflammatory cytokines, such as IL-10 and TGF-β. Induction of Tregs may be of interest for vaccines that aim to reduce inflammation in autoimmune diseases.

One particular subset of Th-cells is devoted to providing help to B-cells, the so-called T-follicular helper cells (Tfhs). Under influence of IL-6 and IL-21, Tfhs upregulate molecules, such as C-X-C chemokine receptor type 5 (CXCR5), allowing them to migrate into B-cell zones. There, Tfhs can interact with B-cells that present cognate antigen on MHCII molecules. Only B-cells that receive co-stimulatory signals from Tfhs will be able to generate high-affinity IgG antibodies or mature into memory B-cells. This can have consequences for vaccine design, as vaccines that are aimed to generate B-cell memory need to contain both B-cell and T-cell epitopes in one entity. For instance, polysaccharides derived from *Haemophilus influenzae* type b, *Neisseria meningitidis*, or *Streptococcus pneumoniae* are targets for neutralizing antibodies, but require conju-

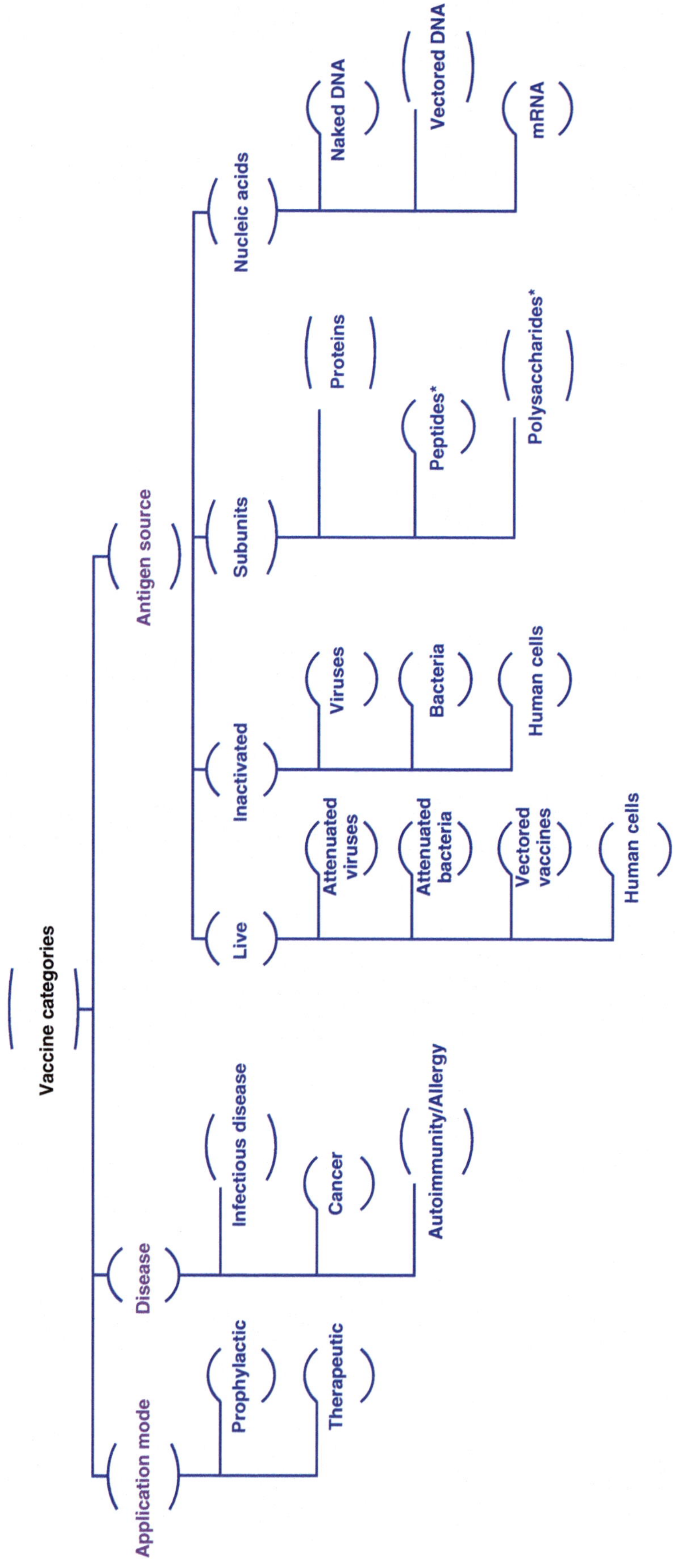

*either free or conjugated to a protein carrier

Figure 14.5 ■ Vaccine categories based on type of treatment, type of disease and antigen source

gation to a protein to allow T-cell help and development of B-cell memory.

VACCINE CATEGORIES

Vaccines can be classified based on whether they are aimed to prevent (prophylactic) or cure (therapeutic) a disease, the type of disease to treat (infectious diseases, allergy, autoimmune disease, cancer, etc.), or the antigen source used for vaccination (e.g., whole pathogens, subunits, peptides, or nucleic acids), as illustrated in Fig. 14.5. Below we first discuss vaccine categories based on antigen source. Next, current developments on therapeutic vaccines against cancer and other diseases are highlighted.

Classification Based on Antigen Source

Traditional vaccines originate from viruses or bacteria and can be divided in vaccines consisting of live attenuated pathogens and nonliving (inactivated) pathogens. In case the antigens that can convey immunity are known, specific subunits derived from the pathogen, such as proteins or polysaccharides, can be formulated into a vaccine. Nowadays such subunit vaccines can also be made recombinantly (in case of proteins), or by chemical conjugation to a carrier protein (in case of polysaccharides) to enhance the immune response to the antigenic components. Moreover, with our current knowledge on immune recognition, both B- and T-cell epitopes can be identified and synthetically made. Finally, nucleic acids form a separate class of antigen source, in which the DNA or RNA encoding the antigen(s) of interest is transfected into host cells to enable endogenous production and presentation of protein antigens. An overview of the various categories of vaccines and examples thereof is given in Table 14.2 and will be detailed in the sections below.

Live Attenuated Vaccines

Before the introduction of recombinant DNA (rDNA) technology, live vaccines were made by the attenuation of virulent microorganisms by serial passage and selection of mutant strains with reduced virulence or toxicity. Examples are vaccine strains for current vaccines such as oral polio vaccine, measles-mumps-rubella (MMR) combination vaccine, yellow fever vaccine and tuberculosis vaccine consisting of bacille Calmette-Guérin (BCG). An alternative approach is chemical mutagenesis. For instance, by treating *Salmonella typhi* with nitrosoguanidine, a mutant strain lacking some enzymes that are responsible for the virulence was isolated (Germanier and Fuer 1975).

Live attenuated vaccines have the advantage that after administration they may replicate in the host, similar to their pathogenic counterparts. This confronts the host with a larger and more sustained dose of antigen and PAMPs, which means that few and low doses are required. In general, the vaccines give long-lasting humoral and cell-mediated immunity.

Live attenuated vaccines also have drawbacks. Live viral vaccines bear the risk to revert to a virulent form, although this is unlikely when the attenuated seed strain contains several mutations. Nevertheless, for diseases such as viral hepatitis, AIDS and cancers, this drawback makes the use of traditional live vaccines virtually unthinkable. Furthermore, it is important to recognize that immunization of immune-deficient children or immunocompromised adults with live organisms can lead to serious complications. For instance, a child with T-cell deficiency may become overwhelmed with BCG and die. Similarly, patients using certain immunosuppressive drugs (e.g., cyclosporin, methotrexate) should not be vaccinated with live attenuated vaccines.

Genetically Attenuated Live Vaccines

Emerging insights in molecular pathogenesis of many infectious diseases make it possible to attenuate microorganisms more efficiently nowadays. By making multiple deletions, the risk of reversion to a virulent state during production or after administration can be virtually eliminated. A prerequisite for attenuation by genetic engineering is that the factors responsible for virulence and the life cycle of the pathogen are known in detail. It is also obvious that the protective antigens or epitopes must be known: attenuation must not result in reduced immunogenicity.

An example of an improved live vaccine obtained by homologous genetic engineering is the oral cholera vaccine Vaxchora. An effective cholera vaccine should induce a local, humoral response in order to prevent colonization of the small intestine. Initial trials with *Vibrio cholerae* cholera toxin (CT) mutants caused mild diarrhea, which was thought to be caused by the expression of accessory toxins. A natural mutant was isolated that was negative for these toxins. Next, CT was detoxified by rDNA technology. The resulting vaccine strain, called CVD 103, is well tolerated and challenge experiments with adult volunteers showed protection (Levine et al. 2017; Garcia et al. 2005).

Genetically attenuated live vaccines have the general drawbacks mentioned in the paragraph about classically attenuated live vaccines. For these reasons, it is not surprising that homologous engineering is mainly restricted to pathogens that are used as starting materials for the production of subunit vaccines (see the section "Subunit Vaccines," below).

Live Vectored Vaccines

A way to improve the safety or efficacy of vaccines is to use live, avirulent, or attenuated bacteria or viruses as a carrier to express protective antigens from a patho-

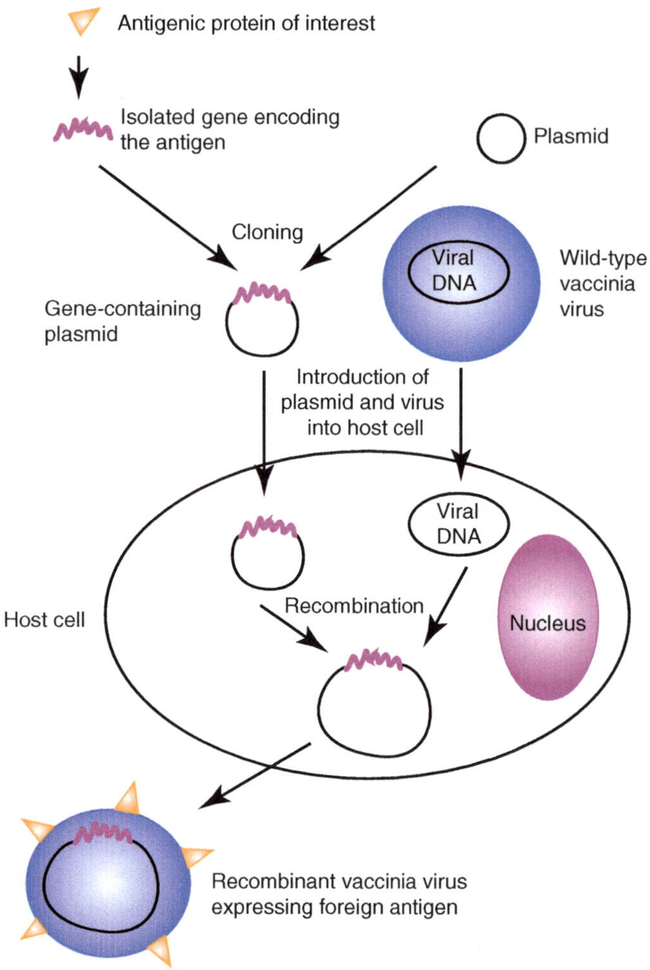

Figure 14.6 ■ Construction of recombinant vaccinia virus as a vector of foreign protein antigens. The gene of interest encoding an immunogenic protein is inserted into a plasmid. The plasmid containing the protein gene and wild-type vaccinia virus are then simultaneously introduced into a host cell line to undergo recombination of viral and plasmid DNA, after which the foreign protein is expressed by the recombinant virus

gen (see Table 14.2 for examples). Live vectored vaccines are created by recombinant technology, wherein one or more genes of the vector organism are replaced by one or more protective genes from the pathogen. Administration of such live vectored vaccines results in efficient and prolonged expression of the antigen-encoding genes either by the vaccinated individual's own cells or by the vector organism itself (e.g., in case of a bacterial vector).

Most experience has been acquired with vaccinia virus by using the principle that is schematically shown in Fig. 14.6. Advantages of vaccinia virus as vector include (1) its proven safety in humans as a smallpox vaccine, (2) the possibility for multiple immunogen expression, (3) the ease of production, (4) its relative heat resistance, and (5) its various possible administration routes. A multitude of live recombinant vaccinia vaccines with viral and tumor antigens have been constructed, several of which have been tested in the clinic (Njuguna et al. 2014; Buchbinder et al. 2017; Payne et al. 2017). It has been demonstrated that the products of genes coding for viral envelope proteins can be correctly processed and inserted into the plasma membrane of infected cells.

Adenoviruses can also be used as vaccine vectors (see also Chap. 16). Adenoviruses have several characteristics that make them suitable as vaccine vectors: (1) they can infect a broad range of both dividing and non-dividing mammalian cells, which expands possibilities to select production cell lines; (2) transgene expression is generally high and can be further increased by using heterologous promoter sequences; (3) adenovirus vectors are mostly replication deficient and do not integrate their genomes into the chromosomes of host cells, making these vectors very safe to use; and (4) upon parenteral administration, adenovirus vectors induce strong immunity and evoke both humoral and cellular responses against the expressed antigen. A number of clinical trials with human or chimpanzee adenovirus vectors (HAd5, ChAd3) expressing antigens of Ebola virus, human immunodeficiency virus (HIV), and severe acute respiratory syndrome (SARS) have been performed (Cohen and Frahm 2017).

A major limitation of the use of live vectored vaccines is the prevalence of preexisting immunity against the vector itself, which could neutralize the vaccine before the immune system can be primed. Such preexisting immunity has been described for adenoviral vectors, for which the prevalence of neutralizing antibodies can be as high as 90% of the total population. The use of human or nonhuman (e.g., chimpanzee) strains with no or low prevalence of preexisting immunity as live vectors is therefore recommended (Ahi et al. 2011; Wong et al. 2018).

Inactivated Vaccines

An early approach for preparing vaccines is the inactivation of whole bacteria or viruses. A number of chemical reagents (e.g., formaldehyde, glutaraldehyde, β-propriolactone) and heat are commonly used for inactivation. Examples of inactivated vaccines are whole cell pertussis, cholera, typhoid fever, and polio vaccines. Inactivation may result in the loss of relevant epitopes due to covalent changes or partial unfolding of antigens. Also, since these vaccines do not replicate in vivo, often a higher dose is needed to induce protection, as compared to live attenuated vaccines. This may increase the price.

Subunit Vaccines

Given the complexity and batch-to-batch variability of vaccines consisting of inactivated whole pathogens, the use of well-defined antigenic subunits of pathogens is desired. Such subunits can be antigens (proteins or polysaccharides) directly purified from the pathogen, recombinantly produced protein antigens, or synthetic peptides.

Diphtheria Toxoid and Tetanus Toxoid Vaccines

Some bacteria such as *Corynebacterium diphtheriae* and *Clostridium tetani* form toxins. Antibody-mediated immunity to the toxins is the main protection mechanism against the adverse effects of infections with these bacteria. Both toxins are proteins and are inactivated with formaldehyde for inclusion in vaccines. The immunogenicity of such toxoids is relatively low and is improved by adsorption of the toxoids to colloidal aluminum salts. This combination of an antigen and an adjuvant is still used in combination vaccines.

Polysaccharide Vaccines

Bacterial capsular polysaccharides consist of pathogen-specific multiple repeating carbohydrate epitopes, which are isolated from cultures of the pathogenic species. Plain capsular polysaccharides are thymus-independent antigens that are poorly immunogenic in infants and show poor immunological memory when applied in older children and adults. The immunogenicity of polysaccharides is highly increased when they are chemically coupled to carrier proteins containing T-cell epitopes. This coupling makes them T-cell dependent, which is due to the participation of Th-cells that are activated during the response to the carrier. Examples of such polysaccharide conjugate vaccines include meningococcal type C, pneumococcal, and *Haemophilus influenzae* type b (Hib) polysaccharide vaccines that are included in many national immunization programs.

Acellular Pertussis Vaccines

The relatively frequent occurrence of side effects of whole cell pertussis vaccine was the main reason to develop subunit pertussis vaccines. The development of such acellular pertussis vaccines in the 1980s exemplifies how a better insight into factors that are important for pathogenesis and immunogenicity can lead to improved vaccines: it was conceived that a subunit vaccine consisting of a limited number of purified immunogenic components and devoid of (toxic) bacterial LPS would significantly reduce undesired effects. Current licensed acellular pertussis vaccines contain one to four protein antigens. Although these vaccines are effective, they cannot prevent regular epidemics of whooping cough in many western countries. Short-lived immunity and vaccine induced selection of circulating strains resisting the primed immune system may contribute to this. Therefore, attempts are made to improve vaccination schemes and to develop new pertussis vaccines.

Recombinant Subunit Vaccines

To improve the yield, facilitate the production, and/or improve the safety of protein-based vaccines, protein antigens are nowadays often produced recombinantly, i.e., expressed by host cells that are safe to handle and/or allow high expression levels.

Heterologous hosts used for the expression of protein antigens include yeasts, bacteria, insect cells, plant cells, and mammalian cell lines. Hepatitis B surface antigen (HBsAg), which previously was obtained from plasma of infected individuals, has been expressed in baker's yeast, *Saccharomyces cerevisiae* (Vanlandschoot et al. 2002), and in mammalian cells, such as Chinese hamster ovary cells (Raz et al. 2001), by transforming the host cell with a plasmid containing the HBsAg-encoding gene. Both expression systems yield 22-nm HBsAg particles (also called virus-like particles or VLPs) that are structurally identical to the native virus. Advantages are safety, consistent quality, and high yields. The yeast-derived vaccine has become available worldwide and appears to be as safe and efficacious as the classical plasma-derived vaccine.

The two human papillomavirus (HPV) vaccines currently on the market are produced as recombinant proteins which, like HBsAg, assemble spontaneously into virus-like particles. Antigens for Gardasil, a quadrivalent HPV vaccine, are produced in yeast, whereas antigens for the bivalent vaccine Cervarix are produced in insect cells.

Recombinant Peptide Vaccines

After identification of a protective epitope, it is possible to incorporate the corresponding peptide sequence through genetic fusion into a carrier protein, such as HBsAg, hepatitis B core antigen, and β-galactosidase (Francis and Larche 2005). The peptide-encoding DNA sequence is synthesized and inserted into the carrier protein gene. An example of the recombinant peptide approach is a malaria vaccine based on a 16-fold repeat of the Asn-Ala-Asn-Pro sequence of a *Plasmodium falciparum* surface antigen. The gene encoding this peptide was fused with the HBsAg gene, and the fusion product was expressed by yeast cells (Vreden et al. 1991). Clinical trials with this candidate malaria vaccine demonstrated moderate efficacy in children and infants in Africa (RTS,S Clinical Trials Partnership 2015).

Genetic fusion of peptides with proteins offers the possibility to produce protective epitopes of toxic antigens derived from pathogenic species as part of nontoxic proteins expressed by harmless species. Furthermore, a uniform product is obtained in comparison with the variability of chemical conjugates (see the section "Synthetic Peptide Vaccines", below).

Synthetic Peptide Vaccines

In principle, a vaccine could consist of only the relevant epitopes instead of intact pathogens or proteins. Peptide epitopes are small enough to be produced synthetically and a peptide-based vaccine would be much better defined than traditional vaccines, making the concept of peptide vaccines attractive. However, it turned out to be difficult to develop these vaccines, and today there are no licensed peptide-based vaccines available yet. Nevertheless, important progress has been made, and some synthetic peptide vaccines have now entered the clinic, e.g., for immunotherapy of cancer (Melief and van der Burg 2008; van Poelgeest et al. 2013). To understand the complexity of peptide vaccines, one has to distinguish the different types of epitopes.

B-cell Epitope-Based Peptide Vaccines Epitopes recognized by antibodies or B-cells are very often conformation dependent (see above, section "Immunological Principles", and Van Regenmortel 2009). For this reason, it is difficult to identify them accurately and to synthesize them in the correct conformation. Manipulation of the antigen, such as digestion or the cloning of parts of the gene, will often affect B-cell epitope integrity. An accurate way of identifying epitopes is to elucidate the crystal structure of antigen-antibody complexes. This is difficult and time consuming, and although crystallography can reveal molecular interactions with unsurpassed detail, the molecular complex likely is much more dynamic in solution. Once the epitope is identified, synthesizing it as a functional peptide has proven to be difficult as well. The peptides need to be conformationally restrained. This can be achieved by cyclization of the peptide (Oomen et al. 2005) or by the use of scaffolds to synthesize complex peptide structures (Timmerman et al. 2007).

T-cell Epitope-Based Peptide Vaccines Regarding conformation, T-cell epitopes are less demanding because they are presented naturally as processed peptides by APCs to T-cells. As a result, T-cell epitopes are linear. Here, we discern $CD8^+$ epitopes (8–10 amino acid residues; MHC class I restricted) and $CD4^+$ epitopes (>12 amino acid residues; MHC class II restricted). The main requirement is that they fit into binding grooves of MHC molecules with high enough affinity. Studies with peptide-based cancer vaccines have shown that these should contain both $CD8^+$ and $CD4^+$ epitopes in order to elicit a protective immune response. Furthermore, minimal peptides that can be externally loaded on MHC molecules of cells have been shown to induce less robust responses than longer peptides that require intracellular processing after uptake by DCs. Another point to consider is the variable repertoire of MHC molecules in a patient population, implying that a T-cell epitope-based peptide vaccine should contain several T-cell epitopes in order to be effective in the majority of the vaccinated population. Following these concepts, clinical trials with overlapping long peptide vaccines have shown promising results in the immunotherapy of patients with HPV-induced malignancies (Melief and van der Burg 2008).

Nucleic Acid Vaccines

Immunization with nucleic acid vaccines involves the administration of genetic material, plasmid DNA or messenger RNA (mRNA), encoding the desired antigen. The encoded antigen is then expressed by the host cells and after which an immune response against the expressed antigen is raised. Nucleic acid vaccines offer the safety of subunit vaccines and the advantages of live recombinant vaccines. They can induce strong CTL responses against the encoded antigen. In addition, bacterial plasmids are ideal for activating innate immunity as TLR-9 expressed on many phagocytic cells can recognize unmethylated bacterial DNA (see section "Adjuvants"). The main disadvantage of nucleic acid immunization is the poor immunogenicity in man. Therefore, they often require, like subunit vaccines, adjuvants or delivery systems to boost the immune response against the DNA-encoded antigen(s). Nevertheless, DNA has proven to be very effective when used in combination with protein antigens in heterologous DNA-prime/protein-boost strategies. The long-term safety of nucleic acid vaccines remains to be established. The main pros and cons of nucleic acid vaccines are listed in Table 14.5. Examples of DNA vaccines that have been tested in clinical trials comprise plasmids encoding HIV-1 antigens and malaria antigens.

mRNA Vaccines

In recent years, mRNA vaccines have gained increasing attention mainly because of their excellent safety profile, transient, non-integrative protein expression and enhanced immunogenicity as compared to plasmid DNA vaccines. mRNA vaccination is typically applied in oncology for the expression of mixtures of tumor antigens, but can also be applied for personalized vaccines. Initially, mRNA-based vaccines coped with stability problems and poor expression levels. To enhance immunogenicity and prolong protein expression, mRNAs were either chemically modified (both backbone and nucleoside modifications), sequence optimized, or formulated in

Advantages	Disadvantages
Low intrinsic immunogenicity	Effects of long-term expression unknown
Induction of long-term immune responses	Formation of antinucleic acid antibodies possible
Induction of both humoral and cellular immune responses	Possible integration of the vaccine DNA into the host genome
Possibility of constructing multiple epitope plasmids	Concept restricted to peptide and protein antigens
Heat stability	Poor delivery
Ease of large-scale production	Poorly immunogenic in man

Table 14.5 ■ Advantages and disadvantages of nucleic acid vaccines

nanocarriers (e.g., protamine nanoparticles). These modifications resulted in slower degradation and enhanced immune activation primarily through TLR7 signaling. Optimized mRNA vaccines have been shown to elicit strong and balanced Th1/Th2 immune responses in animal models. This technology is currently being tested in clinical trials, e.g., for the treatment of prostate cancer (Kubler et al. 2015) and non-small cell lung carcinoma (Sebastian et al. 2014), and has demonstrated antigen-specific immune responses in most patients.

One drawback of mRNA-based vaccines is their transient nature, often leading to short antigen expression times, unfavorable for proper immune activation. This can be circumvented by making use of self-amplifying RNAs based on the alphavirus replication machinery. Four alphavirus genes responsible for RNA replication are co-expressed with the gene of interest encoding the desired antigen (Fig. 14.7). Transfection of this single RNA construct into cells leads to prolonged and 10–50-fold enhanced antigen expression.

Delivery of Nucleic Acid Vaccines

Since nucleic acids do not easily enter cells but require intracellular delivery in their intact form for their activity, therapeutic application of these biomacromolecules requires sophisticated delivery methods or systems. A detailed description of nucleic acid delivery systems can be found in Chap. 16 on gene therapy.

For vaccination purposes, naked nucleic acids (i.e., without a delivery system) can be administered to animals and humans via intramuscular injection. The favorable properties of muscle cells for DNA expression are probably due to their relatively low turnover rate, which prevents that plasmid DNA is rapidly dispersed in dividing cells. After intracellular uptake of the DNA, the encoded protein is expressed on the surface of host cells. After a single injection, the expression can last for more than a year. However, the use of naked DNA for vaccination requires high doses, most likely because of its poor delivery, and has so far shown poor immunogenicity in human trials.

Physical methods of DNA delivery can be used as well. These include ballistic approaches using a gene gun to inject DNA-coated gold nanoparticles into the epidermis, jet-injectors, electroporation and DNA tattooing (Samuels et al. 2017).

Delivery of nucleic acids with lipidic or polymeric nanocarriers can increase both the cellular uptake and immune activation. Nanocarriers protect the nucleic acids from premature degradation and enhance their cellular uptake by professional APCs. Besides synthetic nanocarriers, viruses can be used as vectors as well. A distinction can be made between replicating viruses and those that are replication incompetent. Examples of the latter are fowlpox and canarypox viruses that can infect mammalian cells, but are unable to replicate. Canarypox virus expressing HIV-1 rgp120 and rgp160 has been clinically tested as part of a heterologous prime/boost prophylactic HIV vaccine (O'Connell et al. 2016). Besides viruses, bacteria that replicate inside cells can also be used to deliver plasmid DNA into host cells for the expression of pathogen-derived antigens. Attenuated strains of *Shigella flexneri* and *Listeria monocytogenes* have been used for this purpose.

■ Therapeutic Vaccines

Most classical vaccine applications are prophylactic: they prevent an infectious disease from developing. Besides prophylactic applications, vaccines may be used to treat already established diseases, such as infectious diseases, cancer, and inflammatory disorders. Although the development of therapeutic vaccines is still in its infancy, especially in the field of cancer vaccines the insights and developments are rapidly progressing and some examples will be highlighted here.

Cancer Vaccines

Cancer is a collection of diseases characterized by uncontrolled cell division with the potential to invade and spread to other parts of the body. These characteristics are caused by gene mutations that are inherited or were accumulated during life by environmental factors. Such mutations may also lead to subtle changes in the antigenic repertoire of tumor cells as compared to healthy cells. This provides a basis for the development of therapeutic cancer vaccines aimed at inducing specific cellular immune responses and to a lesser extent humoral immune responses to pre-established cancer (Melief et al. 2015; van der Burg et al. 2016). A distinction can be made between so-called tumor-

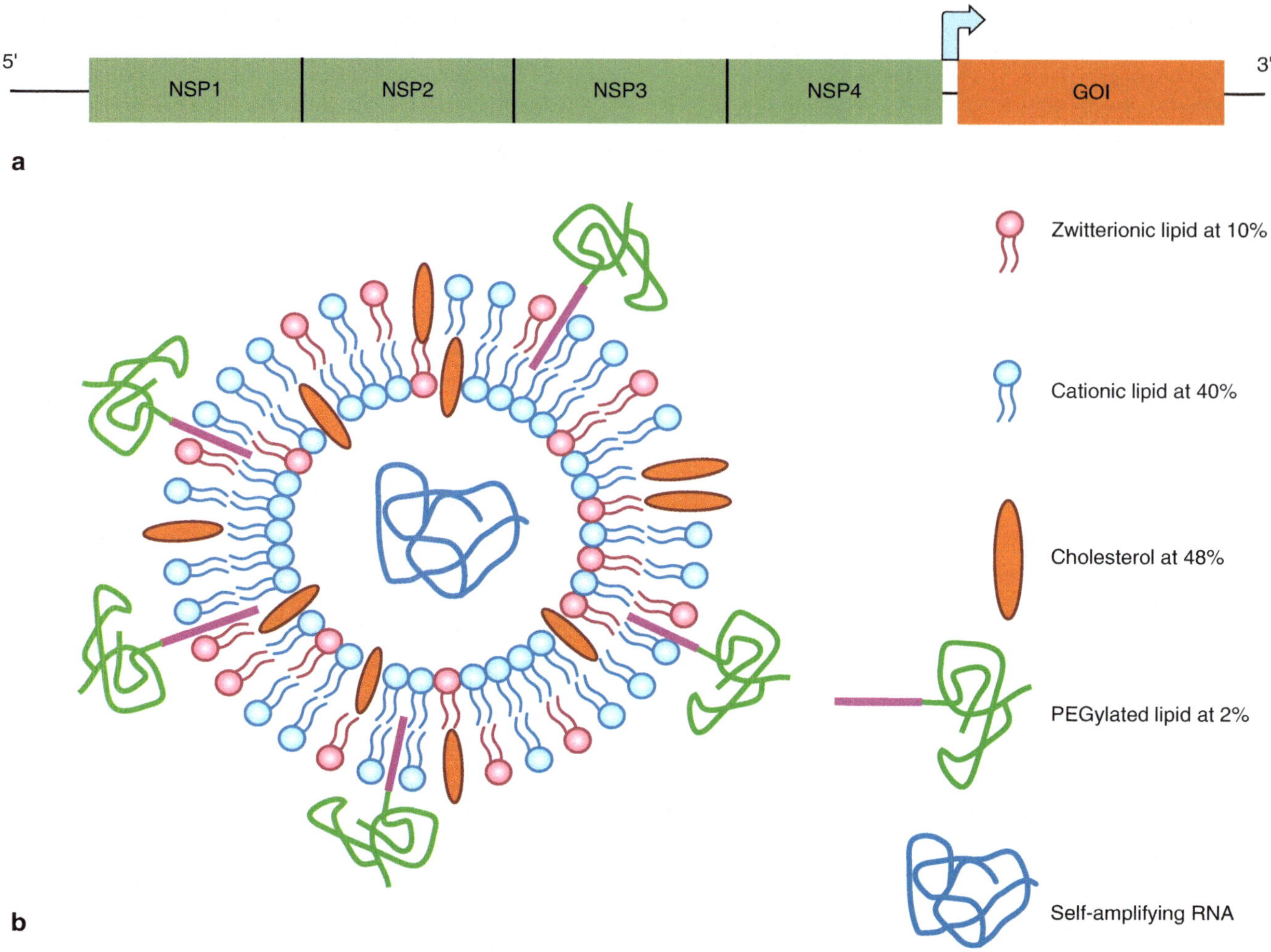

Figure 14.7 ■ Schematic illustration of an exemplary RNA vaccine. (**a**) Schematic illustration of an RNA construct encoding alphavirus-derived self-amplifying RNA. The RNA contains a 5′ cap, nonstructural genes for RNA replication (NSP1–4), a 26S subgenomic promoter (blue arrow), the gene of interest (GOI), and a 3′ polyadenylated tail. (**b**) Schematic illustration of a lipid nanoparticle encapsulating self-amplifying RNA, with the molar percentages of lipid components as indicated. Adapted from Geall et al. (2012)

associated antigens that are present in normal tissues, but over expressed in tumors, and neoantigens, which are newly formed tumor-specific antigens caused by somatic DNA mutations.

Tumor-Associated Antigen Vaccines

Initially, clinical trials with cancer vaccines focused on the use of a single tumor-associated antigen (e.g., melanoma-associated antigen-1, prostate-specific antigen, mucin-1, carcinoembryonic antigen), mixtures of ill-defined antigens from whole tumor cell lysates, or whole tumor cells. The latter can be autologous tumor cells directly isolated from the patients or allogeneic tumor cells that have been genetically modified to express cytokines (e.g., GM-CSF) or other immune-stimulating molecules. An advantage of using whole tumor cells is the presence of a wide array of tumor-specific antigens that could potentially lead to tumor-specific immune responses. A disadvantage is that ill-defined tumor cell lysates will mostly express self-antigens. Breaking immunological tolerance against these self-antigens can result in transient or persistent autoimmune reactions.

Neoantigen Vaccines

Neoantigens are preferred for use in cancer vaccines, as they are foreign protein sequences that are absent in healthy tissue. However, since most neoantigens are unique to an individual's tumor, neoantigen vaccination requires a personalized approach, in which the vaccine composition is adjusted to the patient's needs. This is a labor intensive and costly procedure which must be performed fast because the patient is waiting for treatment.

Various neoantigen vaccination platforms have entered the clinic for the treatment of various cancers. Synthetic long peptide (SLP) vaccines consist of sets of peptides containing both Th and CTL neoepitopes that need to be processed by professional APCs and cross presented on MHC class I in order to elicit antigen-specific cellular responses. An advantage of SLPs over synthetic peptide epitopes that can directly bind MHC class I molecules is that the need for antigen processing prevents T-cell anergy. Since the length of peptides that can be synthesized has its technical limitations, multiple SLPs need to be manufactured separately and combined to cover the breadth of neoantigens identified per individual. SLP vaccines have been successfully applied as therapeutic vaccines to treat cervical cancer as well as melanoma (Ott et al. 2017). Neoantigens can also be delivered as nucleic acids (both DNA and mRNA). An advantage of this approach is the intrinsic adjuvant properties of bacterially-derived plasmid DNA and mRNA and the ease at which multiple epitopes can be combined in a single construct. In addition, endogenous expression of antigen leads to efficient MHC class I presentation and subsequent $CD8^+$ T-cell induction.

Both SLP- and nucleic acid-based approaches can also be used for application in an ex vivo setting, in which patient-derived DCs are loaded with the antigen source and stimulated with cytokines before being administered to the patient (see also Chap. 17). Overall, the results with neoantigen vaccination look promising with reported partial and complete cancer regressions in several trials.

Other Therapeutic Vaccine Applications

Besides prevention of infectious diseases or treatment of cancer, vaccines are also being developed for other therapeutic applications. These include treatment of Alzheimer's disease, induction of tolerance against food components and prevention of drug abuse. Most of these vaccines are still in an experimental phase. A few of these developments will be highlighted below.

Tolerogenic Vaccines to Treat Allergy or Autoimmune Diseases

Vaccines can be designed to induce immunological tolerance via the generation of regulatory T-cells (Tregs) with the aim to durably suppress undesired immune responses. For example, patients with autoimmune diseases in which the immune system attacks self-antigens and causes irreversible damage of tissues and cells would benefit from a vaccine that could specifically induce tolerance to the self-antigens. For multiple sclerosis, the self-antigen is known and several vaccination approaches have been followed to induce tolerance. These range from injection of T-cell epitopes derived from self-antigens to vaccination with tolerogenic nanoparticles containing self-antigens and immunosuppressive drugs (Hunter et al. 2014; Northrup et al. 2016). Similarly, the administration of low doses of antigens, also called allergy-specific immunotherapy, to desensitize against food (e.g., shrimp, peanut, cow's milk) or other (e.g., birch pollen, house dust mite) allergies are applied (Shamji and Durham 2017; Berings et al. 2017). Although the mechanism of desensitization remains largely unknown, Tregs probably play an important role.

Vaccines Against Alzheimer's Disease

Alzheimer's disease is a neurodegenerative disease characterized by amyloid plaque formation in the brain caused by aggregated amyloid-β, cleavage products of amyloid precursor protein as well as other proteins. Vaccines that induce antibodies against the aggregated form of amyloid-β or against the microtubule-associated protein tau have been tested in clinical trials. Initial trials suffered from serious side effects due to T-cell activation, but later trials circumvented this problem and showed good safety profiles (Novak et al. 2017). From these studies we have learned that antibody responses play a role in slowing down disease progression. However, the immunology of Alzheimer's disease is complex and far from understood (Dansokho et al. 2016). Also, it may be very difficult to reverse the damage caused by plaque formation by vaccination and therefore early diagnosis and treatment of patients with Alzheimer's disease is important.

ROUTE OF ADMINISTRATION

■ Introduction

The immunological response to a vaccine is dependent on the route of administration. Most current vaccines are administered intramuscularly or subcutaneously. Parenteral immunization (here defined as administration via those routes where a conventional hypodermic needle is used) usually induces systemic immunity but has disadvantages compared to other routes, e.g., needle phobia, infections caused by needlestick injuries and needle re-use, required vaccine sterility and injection skills. Moreover, parenterally administered vaccines generally do not result in effective immune responses at mucosal surfaces. As mucosal surfaces are a common port of entry for many pathogens, induction of a mucosal secretory IgA response may prevent the attachment and entry of pathogens into the host. For example, antibodies against cholera need to be in the gut lumen to inhibit adherence to and colonization of the intestinal wall. Therefore, mucosal (e.g., oral, intranasal, or intravaginal) immunization may be preferred, because it may induce both mucosal and systemic immunity. For instance, orally administered live attenuated *Salmonella typhi* vaccine not only invades the mucosal lining of the gut but also infects cells of the phagocytic system throughout the body, thereby stimulating the production of both secretory and systemic antibodies. Additional advantages of mucosal immunization are the ease of administration and the avoidance of systemic side effects (Czerkinsky and Holmgren 2012; Holmgren and Czerkinsky 2005).

■ The Oral Route of Administration

From a receiver perspective, oral delivery of vaccines would be preferable in many cases, because it is vaccinee friendly. Up to now, however, only a limited number of oral vaccines (e.g., oral polio, cholera, typhoid fever, and rotavirus vaccines) have made it to the market. Most of these vaccines are based on attenuated versions of pathogens for which the route of administration is the same as the natural route of infection. The gut is relatively immune tolerant to prevent immune responses against food antigens. Therefore, a relatively high dose of antigen is required to induce significant responses. A replicating vaccine provides this more easily than an inactivated vaccine. In addition, oral bioavailability is usually very low because of (1) degradation of protein antigens in the gastrointestinal (GI) tract and (2) poor permeability of the wall of the GI tract in case of a passive transport process.

Still, for the category of oral vaccines, the abovementioned hurdles of degradation and permeation are not necessarily prohibitive. For oral immunization, only a (small) fraction of the antigen has to reach its target site to elicit an immune response. The target cells are lymphocytes and antigen-presenting accessory cells located in Peyer's patches (Fig. 14.8). The B-lymphocyte population includes cells that produce secretory IgA antibodies.

These Peyer's patches are macroscopically identifiable follicular structures located in the wall of the gastrointestinal tract. Peyer's patches are overlaid with microfold (M) cells that separate the luminal contents from the lymphocytes. These M cells have little lysosomal degradation capacity, are specialized in the uptake of particulate matter, and allow for antigen sampling and delivery to underlying APCs. Moreover, the density of mucus-producing goblet cells is lower in Peyer's patches than in surrounding parts of the GI tract. This reduces mucus production and facilitates access to the M cell surface for luminal contents (Delves and Roitt 2011), which is of particular importance for the uptake of nano- and microparticle based vaccines. Consequently, attempts to improve antigen delivery via the Peyer's patches and to enhance the immune response are made by using microspheres, liposomes, or modified live vectors, such as attenuated bacteria and viruses (Vela Ramirez et al. 2017). The latter have the additional advantage of replication induced dose increase.

■ Other Routes of Administration

Apart from the oral route, the nose, lungs, rectum, oral cavity, and skin have been selected as potential sites of non-invasive vaccine administration. Most vaccines administered via these routes are still under develop-

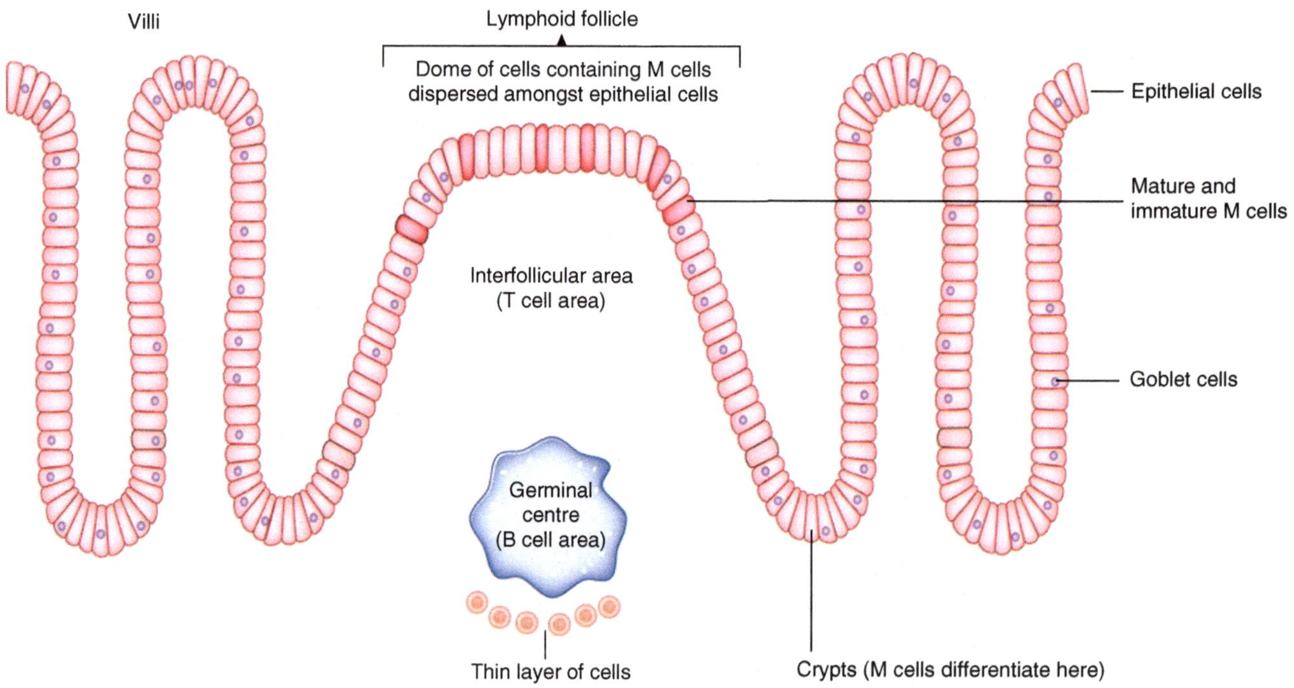

Figure 14.8 ■ Schematic diagram of the structure of intestinal Peyer's patches. M cells within the follicle-associated epithelium are enlarged for emphasis (from O'Hagan 1990)

ment. Today, only a nasal influenza vaccine is licensed (FluMist, branded as Fluenz in Europe).

Besides mucosal vaccines, a number of intradermal vaccine delivery systems have been developed. These include needle-free jet injection of vaccines in liquid form and intradermal delivery with microneedles (Kersten and Hirschberg 2004; van der Maaden et al. 2012; Hogan et al. 2015). Up to now, these products have not yet been registered although an influenza vaccine given intramuscularly with a fluid jet injector is licensed in the US. Intradermal jet injectors are in clinical development, e.g., for inactivated polio vaccine. The classical liquid jet injectors deliver small volumes (microliter range) of liquid vaccine formulation with a high velocity. Depending on fluid velocity and nozzle design, the vaccine is deposited intradermally or dispersed deeper, i.e., subcutaneously of intramuscularly. Current versions use prefilled disposable delivery units for single use to avoid contamination.

Another attractive, potentially pain free approach for intradermal vaccine delivery is the use of microneedles or microneedle arrays with small individual needles in the 100–1000 μm range. There are multiple microneedle types and formats, such as solid microneedle arrays on which the vaccine components are coated, hollow microneedles through which a liquid vaccine formulation can be delivered via a micropump or syringe, and dissolvable microneedles containing the antigen/adjuvant embedded in, e.g., a sugar or polymer matrix, which dissolves rapidly after application (Mitragotri 2005; Kis et al. 2012; van der Maaden et al. 2012). Examples are shown in Fig. 14.9.

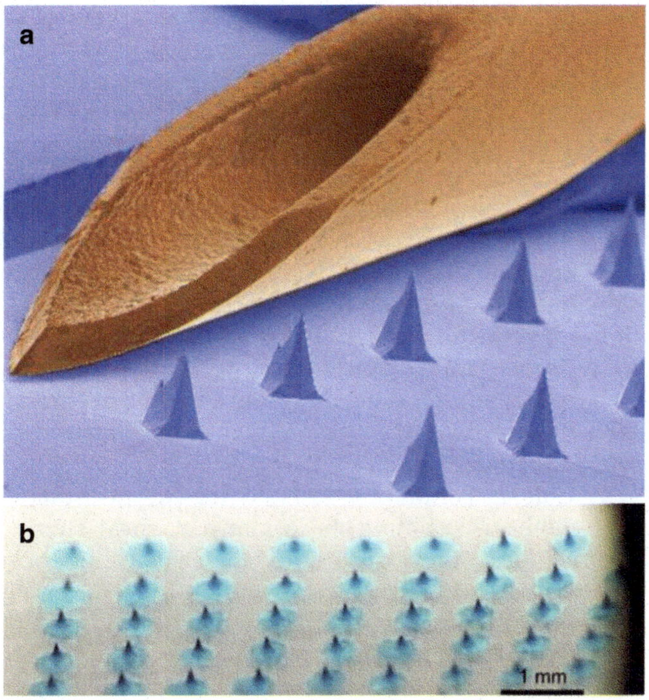

Figure 14.9 ■ (**a**) Hollow silicon microneedles, 300 μm in length, fabricated using a combination of wet and dry etch micromachining technologies (blue) and a 26-gauge syringe needle (brown) for comparison (Courtesy: Joe O'Brien & Conor O'Mahony, Tyndall National Institute). (**b**) Array of dissolvable microneedles, 280 μm in length at a density of 144 needles per cm^2, composed of sugars and polymers, fabricated in PDMS molds of master silicon microneedle arrays using a proprietary method (UK Patent Application Number 1107642.9) (Courtesy: Anne Moore, Anto Vrdoljak, School of Pharmacy, University College Cork)

PHARMACEUTICAL ASPECTS

■ Production

Except for synthetic peptides, the antigenic components of vaccines are derived from microorganisms or animal cells. For optimal expression of the required vaccine component(s), these microorganisms or animal cells can be genetically modified. Animal cells are used for the cultivation of viruses and for the production of some subunit vaccine components and have the advantage that the vaccine components are released into the culture medium. However, some viruses cause cell lysis and consequently the culture medium will contain high concentrations of host cell proteins and host cell DNA, requiring extensive purification steps.

Three stages can be discerned in the manufacture of cell-derived vaccines: (1) cultivation or upstream processing, (2) purification or downstream processing, and (3) formulation. For the first two stages, the reader is referred to Chap. 4 and formulation of biopharmaceuticals is addressed in Chap. 5. The following section deals with formulation aspects specifically related to vaccines.

■ Formulation

Adjuvants: Immune Potentiators and Delivery Systems

The formulation of the vaccine is one of the major determinants that influence the type of immune response that is elicited, as it determines the type of co-stimulatory molecules and cytokines that are expressed by APCs. Through their various PRRs, APCs are more or less capable of "sensing" the type of vaccine that is encountered. This determines the set of co-stimulatory signals and proinflammatory cytokines that APCs will generate when presenting the antigen to T-cells in the peripheral lymphoid organs (Pulendran and Ahmed 2011). For instance, pathogens or vaccines containing lipoproteins or peptidoglycans will trigger DCs via TLR-2, which predominantly generates a Th2 response, whereas stimulation of DCs through TLR-3, or TLR-9 is known to yield robust Th1 and CTL responses. Therefore, vaccines should be formulated in such a way that the appropriate T-cell response will be triggered. This can be done by presenting the antigen in its native format, as is the case for the live-attenuated vaccines, or by formulating the native antigen with adjuvants that stimulate the desired response.

Besides immune stimulatory molecules, a vehicle to deliver antigen to antigen presenting cells and B-cells may be crucial, especially for highly purified subunit antigens. Immune stimulatory molecules and delivery systems are called adjuvants. Adjuvants are defined as any material that can increase or modulate the immune response against an antigen. Adjuvants can stimulate the immune system by several, not mutually exclusive mechanisms (Guy 2007): (1) a depot effect leading to slow antigen release and prolonged antigen presentation, (2) attraction and stimulation of APCs by some local tissue damage and binding to PRRs present on or in APCs, and (3) delivery of the antigen to regional lymph nodes by improved antigen uptake, transport, and presentation by APCs.

Colloidal aluminum salts (hydroxide, phosphate) are widely used adjuvants in many classical vaccine formulations. A few other adjuvants, e.g., monophosphoryl lipid A in HPV vaccine and oil-in-water emulsions in influenza vaccines, have been introduced in marketed vaccines. Moreover, numerous adjuvants are in several stages of (pre)clinical testing or are used in veterinary vaccines. Table 14.6 shows some examples of well-known adjuvants.

Immune potentiators	Examples	Characteristics
Bacterial origin		
Triacyl lipopeptides	Pam3Cys; Pam3CSK4	TLR1–TLR2 agonists
Diacyl lipopeptides	Pam2Cys; MALP2	TLR2–TLR6 agonists
LPS analogs	MPL; RC-529	Endotoxins; TLR4 agonists
Cell wall components	Peptidoglycan; muramyl peptides	TLR2–TLR4 agonists
Flagellin		TLR5 agonist
CpG DNA		TLR9 agonist
Toxins	Cholera toxin B subunit; heat labile enterotoxin subunit B	
Viral origin		
Double stranded RNA	Poly(I:C); poly(rA:rU)	TLR3 agonists
Guanoside analogs	Imiquimod; resiquimod	TLR7–TLR8 agonists
Other origin		
Plant-derived	QuilA; QS21	Triterpene glycosides; crucial components of ISCOMs
Mineral	Aluminum hydroxide; aluminum phosphate	Colloidal suspensions; antigen adsorption is crucial
Synthetic lipids	Avridine; DDA	Used as liposome components
Delivery systems	*Examples*	*Characteristics*
Oil-in-water emulsions	AF03; MF59	
Water-in-oil emulsions	Montanide ISA 51; Montanide ISA 720	
Particulate carriers	Liposomes; virosomes; ISCOMs; polymeric nano- and microparticles; bacterial ghosts	Antigen association with carrier is crucial
Combination adjuvants	*Examples*	*Characteristics*
Miscellaneous	AS01; AS02; CAF01; Montanide ISA 51 plus GM-CSF	

[a]Adapted from Amorij et al. (2012)

Table 14.6 ■ Examples of adjuvants used in vaccine formulations[a]

Combination Vaccines

Since oral immunization is not possible for most available vaccines (see the section "Route of Administration" above), the strategy to mix individual vaccines in order to limit the number of injections has been common practice since many decades. Currently, vaccines are available containing up to six nonrelated antigens: diphtheria-tetanus-pertussis-hepatitis B-polio-Haemophilus *influenzae* type b vaccine. Another example is MMR vaccine, alone or in combination with varicella vaccine. Sometimes a vaccine contains antigens from several subtypes of a particular pathogen. Pneumococcal conjugate vaccine 13 (PCV13) is an example. This vaccine contains polysaccharides from 13 pneumococcal strains, conjugated to a carrier protein to provide T-helper cell recognition and, as a result, induce immunological memory.

Combining vaccine components sometimes results in pharmaceutical as well as immunological problems. For instance, formaldehyde-containing components may chemically react with other components; an unstable antigen may need freeze drying, whereas other antigens should not be frozen. Components that are not compatible can be mixed prior to injection, if there is no short-term incompatibility. To this end, dual-chamber cartridges (cf. Chap. 5) have been developed.

From an immunological point of view, the immunization schedules of the individual components of combination vaccines should match. Pertussis vaccine, for instance, should be given as early in life as possible, since whooping cough is most dangerous in very young children, whereas hepatitis B vaccine can be given later in life because it is mainly a sexually transmitted disease. Even when this condition of matching immunization schedules is met and the components are pharmaceutically compatible, the success of a combination vaccine is not warranted. Vaccine components in combination vaccines may exhibit a different behavior in vivo compared to separate administration of the components. For instance, enhancement (Paradiso et al. 1993) as well as suppression (Mallet et al. 2004) of humoral immune responses has been reported.

■ Characterization

Modern vaccines have to meet similar standards as other biotechnological pharmaceuticals and can be characterized with a combination of appropriate biochemical, physicochemical, and immunochemical techniques (cf. Chaps. 3 and 5). The use of state-of-the art analytical techniques for the design and release of new vaccines is gaining importance. Currently, animal experiments are needed for quality control of many vaccines but in vitro analytical techniques may eventually (partly) substitute tests in vivo. During the development of the production process of a vaccine component, a combination of suitable assays can be defined. These assays can subsequently be applied during its routine production.

Column chromatographic (HPLC) and electrophoretic techniques, such as gel electrophoresis and capillary electrophoresis, provide information about the purity, molecular weight, and other physicochemical properties of antigens. Physicochemical assays comprise mass spectrometry and spectroscopy, including circular dichroism and fluorescence spectroscopy. Information is obtained mainly about the molecular weight and the conformation of the antigen(s). Immunochemical assays, such as enzyme-linked immunoassays, are powerful methods for the quantification of the antigen(s). By using monoclonal antibodies (preferably with the same specificity as those of protective human antibodies) information can be obtained about the conformation and accessibility of the epitope to which the antibodies are directed. Moreover, the use of biosensors makes it possible to measure antigen-antibody interactions momentarily, allowing accurate determination of binding kinetics and affinity constants. Furthermore, since practically all vaccines are particulate in nature, it is sensible to use state-of-the-art particle sizing and counting methods to characterize them (Slütter and Jiskoot 2016).

■ Storage

Depending on their specific characteristics, vaccines are stored as solution or as a freeze-dried formulation, usually at 2–8 °C. Their shelf life depends on the composition and physicochemical characteristics of the vaccine formulation and on the storage conditions and typically is in the order of several years. The quality of the primary container can influence the long-term stability of vaccines, e.g., through adsorption or pH changes resulting from contact with the vial wall or vial stopper. The use of pH indicators or temperature- or time-sensitive labels ("vial vaccine monitors," which change color when too long exposed to too high temperatures) can avoid unintentional administration of an inappropriately stored vaccine.

CONCLUDING REMARKS

Despite the tremendous success of the classical vaccines, there are still many infectious diseases and other diseases (e.g., cancer) against which no effective vaccine exists. Although modern vaccines—like other biopharmaceuticals—are expensive, calculations may indicate cost-effectiveness for vaccination against many of these diseases. In addition, the growing resistance to the existing arsenal of antibiotics increases the need to develop vaccines against common bacterial infections. It is expected that novel vaccines against several of these diseases will become available, and in these cases, the preferred type of vaccine will be chosen from one of the different options described in this chapter.

SELF-ASSESSMENT QUESTIONS

■ Questions

1. Imagine three vaccine types against the same viral disease: (1) formaldehyde inactivated virus, (2) genetically attenuated live virus and (3) highly purified viral protein.
   (a) One vaccine is supplemented with an adjuvant. What is an adjuvant?
   (b) Which of the three vaccines should contain added adjuvant and why?
   (c) Vaccines 1 and 2 have almost the same antigen composition. Despite this, one vaccine can be given in a considerably lower dose than the other one to induce the same level of protection. Which one and why?
   (d) Which vaccine is able to induce cellular cytotoxic T-cell responses and why?
2. How do antibodies prevent infection or disease?
3. How does the immune system prevent unwanted T-cell responses against self-antigens and how does this affect vaccine design?
4. What is the definition of a subunit vaccine? Give three different types of subunit vaccines.
5. Mention at least three advantages and three disadvantages of nucleic acid vaccines. Give one advan-

tage and one disadvantage of RNA vaccines over DNA vaccines.
6. Mention at least three advantages of mucosal vaccination. What are M cells and why are they important in mucosal vaccination?
7. Mention two or more examples of currently available combination vaccines. Which pharmaceutical and immunological conditions have to be fulfilled when formulating combination vaccines?

Answers

1.
(a) An adjuvant is a vaccine component improving qualitatively and/or quantitatively the immune response against an antigen. Adjuvants act on the innate immune system.
(b) Vaccine 3, because it only contains pure antigen and lacks an innate immune stimulus. Vaccines 1 and 2 consist of complete viruses which in general contain innate immune potentiators, such as double stranded RNA.
(c) Vaccine 2 is a live vaccine. Therefore, it can replicate to some extent after administration, increasing the effective dose and extending the contact time with the immune system.
(d) Vaccine 2, because it infects cells. Infected cells produce progeny virus. This endogenous antigen source is partially processed and presented in MHC class 1 molecules to Th-cells. This results in induction of CD8 T-cells.

2. Antibodies are able to neutralize pathogens by at least four mechanisms:
   (a) Fc-mediated phagocytosis
   (b) Complement activation resulting in cytolytic activity
   (c) Complement-mediated phagocytosis
   (d) Competitive binding on sites that are crucial for the biological activity of the antigen
3. Besides antigen presentation through MHCI or MHCII molecules, T-cells require a second signal from an APC before they will proliferate. This second signal supplied by the APC is referred to as co-stimulation and only occurs when the APC has sensed danger, by detecting PAMPs. Therefore, an effective vaccine needs to contain both an antigen and a PAMP (often in the form of an adjuvant).
4. Subunit vaccines are vaccines that contain one or more individual components of a pathogen, e.g., proteins, oligosaccharides or peptide epitopes. These can be either isolated from the pathogen (in case of oligosaccharides, toxins or other protein antigens), recombinantly produced (in case of protein antigens) or synthesized (in case of peptide epitopes).
5. The advantages and disadvantages of nucleic acid vaccines are listed in Table 14.6. An advantage of RNA is that there is no risk of incorporation into host DNA. A disadvantage of RNA is that it is less stable than DNA.
6. Advantages of mucosal vaccination over vaccination by injection are that it:
   (a) avoids infections caused by needlestick injuries and needle re-use
   (b) is easier to perform and more vaccinee friendly
   (c) can induce mucosal immunity

   M cells are cells present in mucosal surfaces (such as the nasal cavity and the Peyer's patches in the gastrointestinal tract). M cells have little lysosomal degradation capacity, are specialized in the uptake of particulate matter, such as nano- and microparticulate vaccines. They can sample particulate antigens and deliver them to underlying APCs. The density of mucus-producing goblet cells is low in Peyer's patches and M cells do not produce mucus, which facilitates the access of (particulate) antigens to the M cell surface.
7. Examples of combination vaccines include diphtheria-tetanus-pertussis(−polio) vaccines and measles-mumps-rubella(−varicella) vaccines. Prerequisites for combining vaccine components are:
   (a) Pharmaceutical compatibility of vaccine components and additives
   (b) Compatibility of immunization schedules
   (c) No interference between immune responses to individual components

REFERENCES

Ahi YS, Bangari DS, Mittal SK (2011) Adenoviral vector immunity: its implications and circumvention strategies. Curr Gene Ther 11(4):307–320

Amorij JP, Kersten GF, Saluja V, Tonnis WF, Hinrichs WL, Slütter B, Bal SM, Bouwstra JA, Huckriede A, Jiskoot W (2012) Towards tailored vaccine delivery: needs, challenges and perspectives. J Control Release 161(2):363–376

Batista FD, Harwood NE (2009) The who, how and where of antigen presentation to B cells. Nat Rev Immunol 9(1):15–27

Berings M, Karaaslan C, Altunbulakli C, Gevaert P, Akdis M, Bachert C, Akdis CA (2017) Advances and highlights in allergen immunotherapy: on the way to sustained clinical and immunologic tolerance. J Allergy Clin Immunol 140(5):1250–1267

Buchbinder SP, Grunenberg NA, Sanchez BJ, Seaton KE, Ferrari G, Moody MA, Frahm N, Montefiori DC, Hay CM, Goepfert PA, Baden LR, Robinson HL, Yu X, Gilbert PB, McElrath MJ, Huang Y, Tomaras GD, Group HIVVTNS (2017) Immunogenicity of a novel

Clade B HIV-1 vaccine combination: results of phase 1 randomized placebo controlled trial of an HIV-1 GM-CSF-expressing DNA prime with a modified vaccinia Ankara vaccine boost in healthy HIV-1 uninfected adults. PLoS One 12(7):e0179597

Cohen KW, Frahm N (2017) Current views on the potential for development of a HIV vaccine. Expert Opin Biol Ther 17(3):295–303

Czerkinsky C, Holmgren J (2012) Mucosal delivery routes for optimal immunization: targeting immunity to the right tissues. Curr Top Microbiol Immunol 354:1–18

Dansokho C, Ait Ahmed D, Aid S, Toly-Ndour C, Chaigneau T, Calle V, Cagnard N, Holzenberger M, Piaggio E, Aucouturier P, Dorothee G (2016) Regulatory T cells delay disease progression in Alzheimer-like pathology. Brain 139(Pt 4):1237–1251

Delves PJ, Roitt IM (2011) Roitt's essential immunology, 12th edn. Wiley, Chichester

Donnelly JJ, Wahren B, Liu MA (2005) DNA vaccines: progress and challenges. J Immunol 175(2):633–639

Francis JN, Larche M (2005) Peptide-based vaccination: where do we stand? Curr Opin Allergy Clin Immunol 5(6):537–543

Garcia L, Jidy MD, Garcia H, Rodriguez BL, Fernandez R, Ano G, Cedre B, Valmaseda T, Suzarte E, Ramirez M, Pino Y, Campos J, Menendez J, Valera R, Gonzalez D, Gonzalez I, Perez O, Serrano T, Lastre M, Miralles F, Del Campo J, Maestre JL, Perez JL, Talavera A, Perez A, Marrero K, Ledon T, Fando R (2005) The vaccine candidate Vibrio cholerae 638 is protective against cholera in healthy volunteers. Infect Immun 73(5):3018–3024

Geall AJ, Verma A, Otten GR, Shaw CA, Hekele A, Banerjee K, Cu Y, Beard CW, Brito LA, Krucker T, O'Hagan DT, Singh M, Mason PW, Valiante NM, Dormitzer PR, Barnett SW, Rappuoli R, Ulmer JB, Mandl CW (2012) Nonviral delivery of self-amplifying RNA vaccines. Proc Natl Acad Sci U S A 109(36):14604–14609

Germanier R, Fuer E (1975) Isolation and characterization of Gal E mutant Ty 21a of Salmonella typhi: a candidate strain for a live, oral typhoid vaccine. J Infect Dis 131(5):553–558

Guy B (2007) The perfect mix: recent progress in adjuvant research. Nat Rev Microbiol 5(7):505–517

Hogan NC, Taberner AJ, Jones LA, Hunter IW (2015) Needle-free delivery of macromolecules through the skin using controllable jet injectors. Expert Opin Drug Deliv 12(10):1637–1648

Holmgren J, Czerkinsky C (2005) Mucosal immunity and vaccines. Nat Med 11(4 Suppl):S45–S53

Hunter Z, McCarthy DP, Yap WT, Harp CT, Getts DR, Shea LD, Miller SD (2014) A biodegradable nanoparticle platform for the induction of antigen-specific immune tolerance for treatment of autoimmune disease. ACS Nano 8(3):2148–2160

Kawai T, Akira S (2009) The roles of TLRs, RLRs and NLRs in pathogen recognition. Int Immunol 21(4):317–337

Kersten G, Hirschberg H (2004) Antigen delivery systems. Expert Rev Vaccines 3(4):453–462

Kis EE, Winter G, Myschik J (2012) Devices for intradermal vaccination. Vaccine 30(3):523–538

Kubler H, Scheel B, Gnad-Vogt U, Miller K, Schultze-Seemann W, Vom Dorp F, Parmiani G, Hampel C, Wedel S, Trojan L, Jocham D, Maurer T, Rippin G, Fotin-Mleczek M, von der Mulbe F, Probst J, Hoerr I, Kallen KJ, Lander T, Stenzl A (2015) Self-adjuvanted mRNA vaccination in advanced prostate cancer patients: a first-in-man phase I/IIa study. J Immunother Cancer 3:26

Levine MM, Chen WH, Kaper JB, Lock M, Danzig L, Gurwith M (2017) PaxVax CVD 103-HgR single-dose live oral cholera vaccine. Expert Rev Vaccines 16(3):197–213

Mallet E, Belohradsky BH, Lagos R, Gothefors L, Camier P, Carriere JP, Kanra G, Hoffenbach A, Langue J, Undreiner F, Roussel F, Reinert P, Flodmark CE, Stojanov S, Liese J, Levine MM, Munoz A, Schodel F, Hessel L, Hexavalent Vaccine Trial Study G (2004) A liquid hexavalent combined vaccine against diphtheria, tetanus, pertussis, poliomyelitis, Haemophilus influenzae type B and hepatitis B: review of immunogenicity and safety. Vaccine 22(11–12):1343–1357

Melief CJ, van der Burg SH (2008) Immunotherapy of established (pre)malignant disease by synthetic long peptide vaccines. Nat Rev Cancer 8(5):351–360

Melief CJ, van Hall T, Arens R, Ossendorp F, van der Burg SH (2015) Therapeutic cancer vaccines. J Clin Invest 125(9):3401–3412

Mitragotri S (2005) Immunization without needles. Nat Rev Immunol 5(12):905–916

Njuguna IN, Ambler G, Reilly M, Ondondo B, Kanyugo M, Lohman-Payne B, Gichuhi C, Borthwick N, Black A, Mehedi SR, Sun J, Maleche-Obimbo E, Chohan B, John-Stewart GC, Jaoko W, Hanke T (2014) PedVacc 002: a phase I/II randomized clinical trial of MVA.HIVA vaccine administered to infants born to human immunodeficiency virus type 1-positive mothers in Nairobi. Vaccine 32(44):5801–5808

Northrup L, Christopher MA, Sullivan BP, Berkland C (2016) Combining antigen and immunomodulators: emerging trends in antigen-specific immunotherapy for autoimmunity. Adv Drug Deliv Rev 98:86–98

Novak P, Schmidt R, Kontsekova E, Zilka N, Kovacech B, Skrabana R, Vince-Kazmerova Z, Katina S, Fialova L, Prcina M, Parrak V, Dal-Bianco P, Brunner M, Staffen W, Rainer M, Ondrus M, Ropele S, Smisek M, Sivak R, Winblad B, Novak M (2017) Safety and immunogenicity of the tau vaccine AADvac1 in patients with Alzheimer's disease: a randomised, double-blind, placebo-controlled, phase 1 trial. Lancet Neurol 16(2):123–134

O'Connell RJ, Excler JL, Polonis VR, Ratto-Kim S, Cox J, Jagodzinski LL, Liu M, Wieczorek L, McNeil JG, El-Habib R, Michael NL, Gilliam BL, Paris R, VanCott TC, Tomaras GD, Birx DL, Robb ML, Kim JH (2016) Safety and immunogenicity of a randomized phase 1 prime-boost trial with ALVAC-HIV (vCP205) and oligomeric glycoprotein 160 from HIV-1 strains MN and LAI-2 adjuvanted in alum or polyphosphazene. J Infect Dis 213(12):1946–1954

O'Hagan DT (1990) Intestinal translocation of particulates — implications for drug and antigen delivery. Adv Drug Deliv Rev 5(3):265–285

Oomen CJ, Hoogerhout P, Kuipers B, Vidarsson G, van Alphen L, Gros P (2005) Crystal structure of an Anti-meningococcal subtype P1.4 PorA antibody provides basis for peptide-vaccine design. J Mol Biol 351(5):1070–1080

Ott PA, Hu Z, Keskin DB, Shukla SA, Sun J, Bozym DJ, Zhang W, Luoma A, Giobbie-Hurder A, Peter L, Chen C, Olive O, Carter TA, Li S, Lieb DJ, Eisenhaure T, Gjini E, Stevens J, Lane WJ, Javeri I, Nellaiappan K, Salazar AM, Daley H, Seaman M, Buchbinder EI, Yoon CH, Harden M, Lennon N, Gabriel S, Rodig SJ, Barouch DH, Aster JC, Getz G, Wucherpfennig K, Neuberg D, Ritz J, Lander ES, Fritsch EF, Hacohen N, Wu CJ (2017) An immunogenic personal neoantigen vaccine for patients with melanoma. Nature 547(7662):217–221

Paradiso PR, Hogerman DA, Madore DV, Keyserling H, King J, Reisinger KS, Blatter MM, Rothstein E, Bernstein HH, Hackell J (1993) Safety and immunogenicity of a combined diphtheria, tetanus, pertussis and Haemophilus influenzae type b vaccine in young infants. Pediatrics 92(6):827–832

Payne RO, Silk SE, Elias SC, Miura K, Diouf A, Galaway F, de Graaf H, Brendish NJ, Poulton ID, Griffiths OJ, Edwards NJ, Jin J, Labbe GM, Alanine DG, Siani L, Di Marco S, Roberts R, Green N, Berrie E, Ishizuka AS, Nielsen CM, Bardelli M, Partey FD, Ofori MF, Barfod L, Wambua J, Murungi LM, Osier FH, Biswas S, McCarthy JS, Minassian AM, Ashfield R, Viebig NK, Nugent FL, Douglas AD, Vekemans J, Wright GJ, Faust SN, Hill AV, Long CA, Lawrie AM, Draper SJ (2017) Human vaccination against RH5 induces neutralizing antimalarial antibodies that inhibit RH5 invasion complex interactions. JCI Insight 2(21):96381

Pulendran B, Ahmed R (2011) Immunological mechanisms of vaccination. Nat Immunol 12(6):509–517

Raz R, Koren R, Bass D (2001) Safety and immunogenicity of a new mammalian cell-derived recombinant hepatitis B vaccine containing Pre-S1 and Pre-S2 antigens in adults. Isr Med Assoc J 3(5):328–332

RTS,S Clinical Trials Partnership (2015) Efficacy and safety of RTS,S/AS01 malaria vaccine with or without a booster dose in infants and children in Africa: final results of a phase 3, individually randomised, controlled trial. Lancet 386(9988):31–45

Samuels S, Marijne Heeren A, Zijlmans H, Welters MJP, van den Berg JH, Philips D, Kvistborg P, Ehsan I, Scholl SME, Nuijen B, Schumacher TNM, van Beurden M, Jordanova ES, Haanen J, van der Burg SH, Kenter GG (2017) HPV16 E7 DNA tattooing: safety, immunogenicity, and clinical response in patients with HPV-positive vulvar intraepithelial neoplasia. Cancer Immunol Immunother 66(9):1163–1173

Sebastian M, Papachristofilou A, Weiss C, Fruh M, Cathomas R, Hilbe W, Wehler T, Rippin G, Koch SD, Scheel B, Fotin-Mleczek M, Heidenreich R, Kallen KJ, Gnad-Vogt U, Zippelius A (2014) Phase Ib study evaluating a self-adjuvanted mRNA cancer vaccine (RNActive(R)) combined with local radiation as consolidation and maintenance treatment for patients with stage IV non-small cell lung cancer. BMC Cancer 14:748

Shamji MH, Durham SR (2017) Mechanisms of allergen immunotherapy for inhaled allergens and predictive biomarkers. J Allergy Clin Immunol 140(6): 1485–1498

Slütter B, Jiskoot W (2016) Sizing the optimal dimensions of a vaccine delivery system: a particulate matter. Expert Opin Drug Deliv 13(2):167–170

Timmerman P, Puijk WC, Meloen RH (2007) Functional reconstruction and synthetic mimicry of a conformational epitope using CLIPS technology. J Mol Recognit 20(5):283–299

van der Burg SH, Arens R, Ossendorp F, van Hall T, Melief CJ (2016) Vaccines for established cancer: overcoming the challenges posed by immune evasion. Nat Rev Cancer 16(4):219–233

van der Maaden K, Jiskoot W, Bouwstra J (2012) Microneedle technologies for (trans)dermal drug and vaccine delivery. J Control Release 161(2):645–655

van Poelgeest MI, Welters MJ, van Esch EM, Stynenbosch LF, Kerpershoek G, van Persijn van Meerten EL, van den Hende M, Lowik MJ, Berends-van der Meer DM, Fathers LM, Valentijn AR, Oostendorp J, Fleuren GJ, Melief CJ, Kenter GG, van der Burg SH (2013) HPV16 synthetic long peptide (HPV16-SLP) vaccination therapy of patients with advanced or recurrent HPV16-induced gynecological carcinoma, a phase II trial. J Transl Med 11:88

Van Regenmortel MH (2009) What is a B-cell epitope? Methods. Mol Biol 524:3–20

Vanlandschoot P, Roobrouck A, Van Houtte F, Leroux-Roels G (2002) Recombinant HBsAg, an apoptotic-like lipoprotein, interferes with the LPS-induced activation of ERK-1/2 and JNK-1/2 in monocytes. Biochem Biophys Res Commun 297(3):486–491

Vela Ramirez JE, Sharpe LA, Peppas NA (2017) Current state and challenges in developing oral vaccines. Adv Drug Deliv Rev 114:116–131

Vreden SG, Verhave JP, Oettinger T, Sauerwein RW, Meuwissen JH (1991) Phase I clinical trial of a recombinant malaria vaccine consisting of the circumsporozoite repeat region of Plasmodium falciparum coupled to hepatitis B surface antigen. Am J Trop Med Hyg 45(5):533–538

Wong G, Mendoza EJ, Plummer FA, Gao GF, Kobinger GP, Qiu X (2018) From bench to almost bedside: the long road to a licensed Ebola virus vaccine. Expert Opin Biol Ther 18(2):159–173

SUGGESTED READING

Abbas AK, Lichtman AH, Pillai S (2014) Basic immunology: functions and disorders of the immune system, 4th edn. Elsevier/Saunders, Philadelphia

Delves PJ, Martin SJ, Burton DR, Roitt IM (2017) Roitt's essential immunology, 13th edn. Wiley, Hoboken

Plotkin SA, Orenstein WA, Offit PA, Edwards KM (2017) Vaccines, 7th edn. Elsevier, Cambridge

Pulendran B, Ahmed R (2011) Immunological mechanisms of vaccination. Nat Immunol 12(6):509–517

15 Oligonucleotides

Raymond M. Schiffelers, Erik Oude Blenke, and Enrico Mastrobattista

INTRODUCTION

Oligonucleotides are short chains of single stranded or double stranded (chemically modified) ribo- or deoxyribonucleotides. Their ability to bind to chromosomal DNA, mRNA, or non-coding RNA (ncRNA) through Watson-Crick and Hoogsteen base pairing offers possibilities for highly specific intervention in genome editing, gene transcription, mRNA translation, and RNA regulatory pathways for therapeutic applications.

In theory, a specific sequence of 15–17 bases occurs only once in the human genome, which would allow specific manipulation of single genes for oligonucleotides with a complementary sequence in this size range. In addition, therapeutic effects of oligonucleotides can be obtained through sequence-specific binding of transcription factors and intramolecular folding into structures that can bind to and interfere with the function of various biomolecules. Finally, cells display specific receptors for oligonucleotides. These receptors can activate a variety of immunological responses that can be of therapeutic value.

Oligonucleotides can be very potent molecules. Yet, interpretation of the mechanism of therapeutic action of a specific oligonucleotide sequence is not straightforward (Moulton 2017). Apart from the desired activity, oligonucleotides are inclined to display, sequence-specific, unintended effects. Partial sequence complementarity may affect binding to nucleic acids other than the targeted species (known as off-target effects). This is increasingly complex as new classes of intracellular nucleic acids continue to be discovered such as, for example, circular RNAs whose functional role is at present understood to a limited extent (Wilusz 2018). Stimulation of immune responses may also occur and binding to proteins and peptides can alter their activity.

Other characteristics of oligonucleotides also impede clear-cut application as therapeutics. They are sensitive to degradation by nucleases and their physicochemical characteristics lead to rapid excretion by the kidneys and induce uptake by macrophages hindering target tissue accumulation (Geary et al. 2015). In addition, spontaneous passage over cell membranes for these large and charged molecules for intracellular applications is difficult.

Over the years a number of different modifications have been developed that overcome (part of) these problems (Fig. 15.1) (Dirin and Winkler 2013). All of the clinically studied oligonucleotides contain one or more of these modified nucleotides. In this chapter, we describe the classes of therapeutic oligonucleotides, categorized according to their mechanism of action. We start with oligonucleotides that are designed to bind to proteins either through a specific sequence and intramolecular folding, known as aptamers/riboswitches, or by binding to nucleic acid receptors, in particular Toll-like receptors.

In the subsequent sections, we discuss oligonucleotides that act by binding to complementary nucleic acids inside the cell. First, we discuss oligonucleotides that regulate the translation from mRNA. After that oligonucleotides that correct mutated DNA by changing the DNA sequence or structure, or change mRNA by skipping unwanted mRNA fragments are introduced.

The challenges to apply these oligonucleotides as therapeutics are faced by essentially all classes: rapid clearance, poor stability, and limited cellular uptake. These issues are discussed in the final section of this chapter, together with approaches to overcome these challenges and perspectives for future developments.

R. M. Schiffelers (✉)
Laboratory Clinical Chemistry & Haematology, University Medical Center Utrecht, Utrecht, The Netherlands
e-mail: r.schiffelers@umcutrecht.nl

E. O. Blenke
Department of Pharmaceutics, Utrecht Institute for Pharmaceutical Sciences, Utrecht University, Utrecht, The Netherlands

E. Mastrobattista
Department of Pharmaceutics, Utrecht University, Utrecht, The Netherlands

D. J. A. Crommelin et al. (eds.), *Pharmaceutical Biotechnology*, https://doi.org/10.1007/978-3-030-00710-2_15

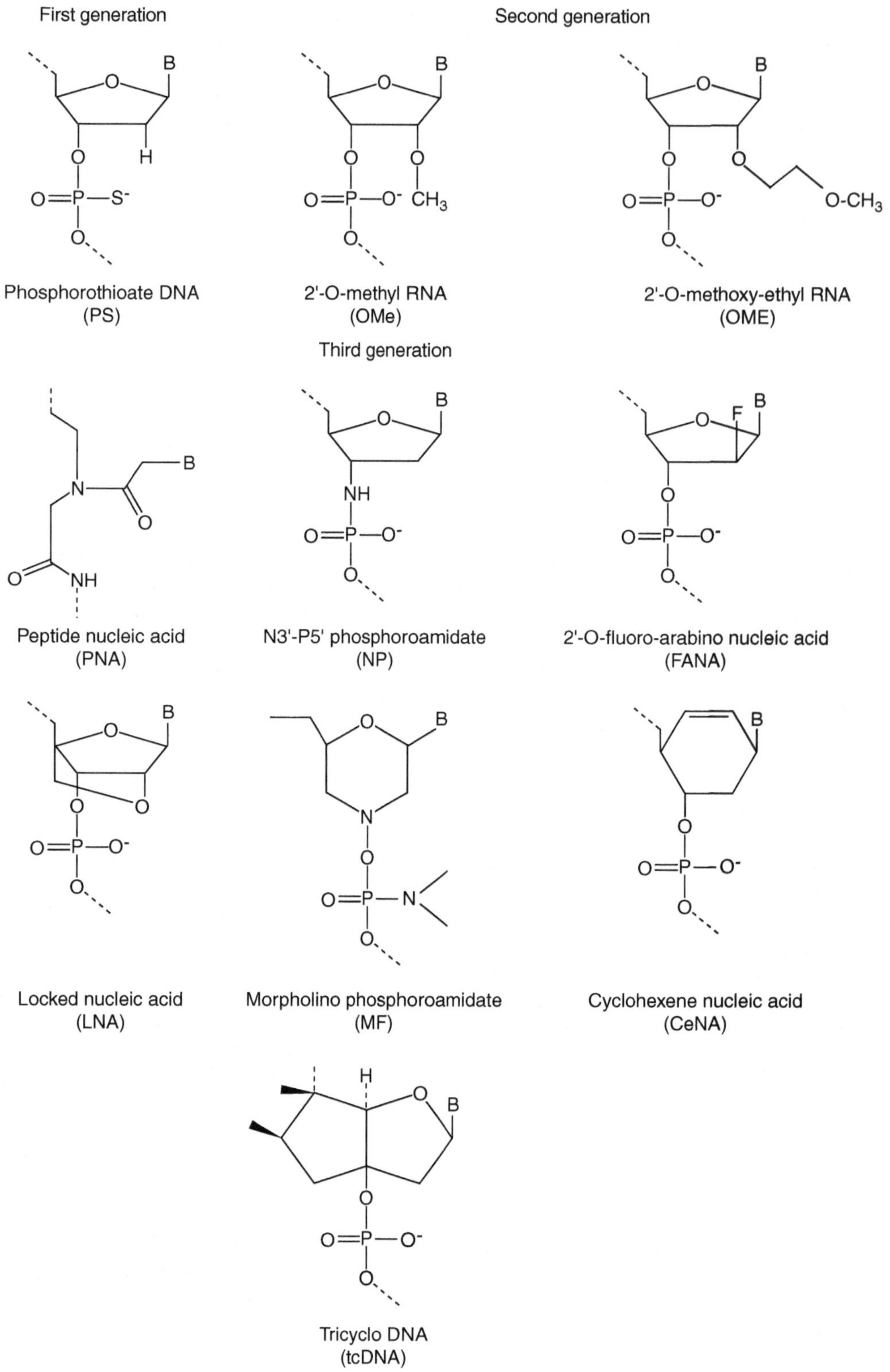

Figure 15.1 ■ Popular chemical modifications to improve nuclease resistance and distribution profile of oligonucleotides

DIRECT BINDING TO NON-NUCLEIC ACIDS

Some therapeutic oligonucleotides have applications that are not based on base pairing with endogenous nucleic acids. This can be the result from binding to specific immune receptors that recognize nucleic acids at unexpected locations (e.g., extracellular DNA) or specific structural qualities (e.g., CpG motifs). In addition, the ability of nucleic acids to fold into complex three-dimensional structures through internal regions of (partial) complementarity allows them to bind to virtually any molecule with nano- to picomolar affinity (Zhou et al. 2018). This high affinity is supported by data on their extreme specificity. A nucleic acid sequence specifically binding theophylline has a million times higher affinity for theophylline than caffeine, molecules which differ by only one methyl group (Zimmermann et al. 2000).

Aptamers/Riboswitches

Aptamers and riboswitches are single-stranded oligonucleotides of either DNA or RNA, generally about 60 nucleotides long, which fold into well-defined three-dimensional structures (Fig. 15.2). They bind to their target molecule by complementary shape interactions accompanied by charge and hydrophobic interactions and hydrogen bridges. The target can be small molecules or macromolecules. Aptamers are isolated artificially, whereas riboswitches occur naturally. Several viruses have been shown to encode small, structured RNAs that bind to viral or cellular proteins with high affinity and specificity. It was demonstrated that these RNAs could modulate the activity of proteins essential for viral replication or inhibit the activity of proteins involved in cellular antiviral responses. Also, the genomes of prokaryotes have been shown to contain nutrient responsive riboswitches to regulate gene expression. Synthetically, such compounds can be identified by subjecting a large diverse library of nucleic acid molecules to a panning procedure (Fig. 15.2). This selection process has been named SELEX (systematic evolution of ligands by exponential enrichment) (Stoltenburg et al. 2007). The resulting ligands are called aptamers. The SELEX process starts

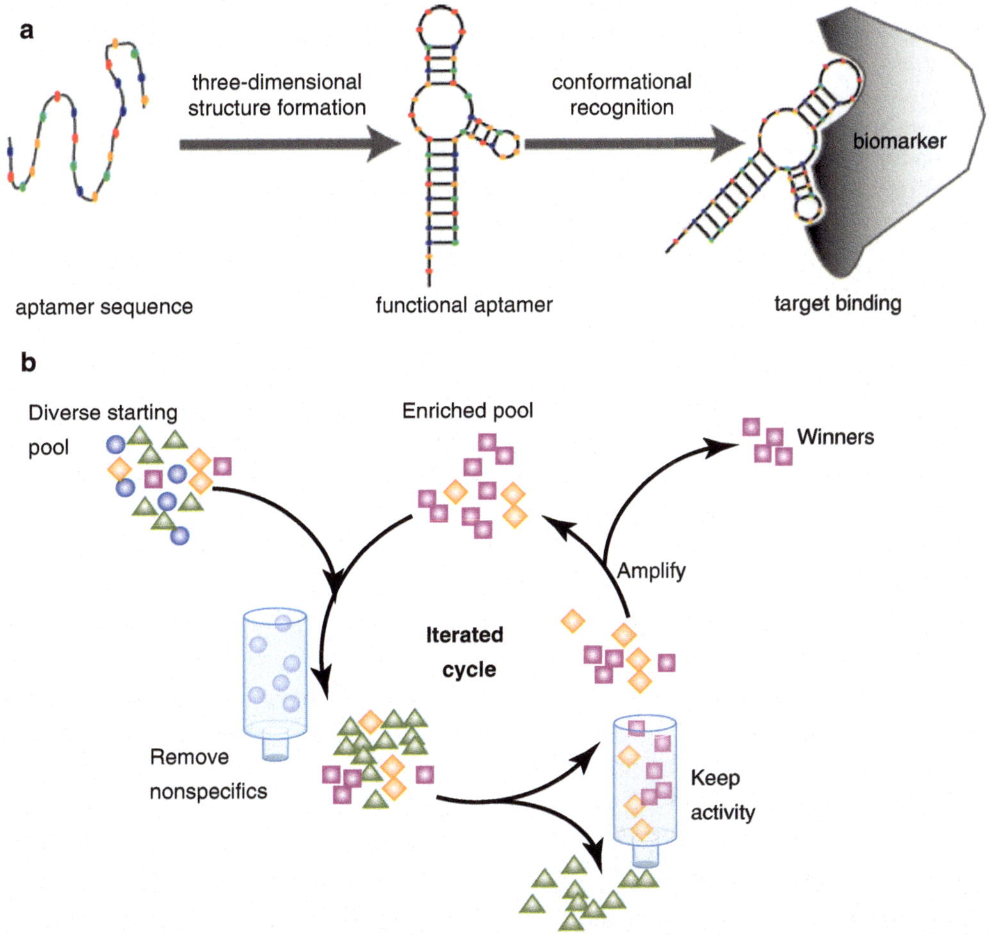

Figure 15.2 ■ Panel (**a**) Mechanism of action of specific protein binding by aptamers. Panel (**b**) General scheme for SELEX (systematic evolution of ligands by exponential enrichment)-based selection of aptamers. The SELEX process starts by generating a large library of randomized RNA sequences. This library contains up to 10^{15} different nucleic acid molecules that fold into different structures depending on their sequence. The library is incubated with the structure of interest and those RNAs present in the library that bind the protein are separated from those that do not. The obtained RNAs are then amplified by reverse transcriptase-PCR and in vitro transcribed to generate a pool of RNAs that have been enriched for those that bind the target of interest. This selection and amplification process is repeated (usually 8–12 rounds) under increasingly stringent binding conditions to promote Darwinian selection until the RNA ligands with the highest affinity for the target protein are isolated (in the Figure: winners). This molecular evolution process can also be performed with DNA, circumventing the need for reverse transcription before PCR and in vitro transcription

by generating a large library of randomized oligonucleotide sequences. For example, a library containing up to 10^{15} different RNA molecules that fold into different structures depending on their sequence. The library is incubated with the structure of interest, and those RNAs present in the library that bind the protein are separated from those that do not. The bound RNAs are liberated and subsequently amplified by reverse transcriptase-PCR. With error-prone amplification and transcription of a new pool of RNAs is created that is enriched for species that bind the target of interest. This selection and amplification process is repeated under increasingly stringent binding conditions to promote Darwinian selection until the ligands with the highest affinity for the target are isolated. This molecular evolution process can also be performed with DNA, circumventing the need for reverse transcription before PCR and in vitro transcription. Automation has reduced aptamer in vitro selection times from months to days, making aptamers suitable for application in high throughput target validation. Aptamers can bind to proteins for therapeutic use, like antibodies do. However, antibody selection requires a biological system for their production. The selection of aptamers is a chemical process, the oligonucleotides are selected and amplified in PCR-reactions, and therefore it can target in principle any protein. In contrast to antibodies, aptamers are prone to bind to functional domains of the target protein (for reasons unknown), such as substrate binding pockets or allosteric sites, thereby modulating the biological function of the molecule (Fig. 15.2). A common problem upon the therapeutic development of aptamers is that they can be so specific for the human version of a target protein that they have poor cross- reactivity with orthologs of the target from other animal species, making their preclinical evaluation difficult. Performing the SELEX procedure by switching between preclinical and clinical target favors selection of cross-reactive aptamers. This may overcome this problem.

Since SELEX is dependent on iterative rounds of enzymatic amplification, and in case of RNA aptamers reverse transcription, of the selected pool of aptamers. This requires the use of polymerases and therefore, for long it could only be used for selecting aptamers out of unmodified DNA and RNA molecules, with the concomitant disadvantage of rapid degradation in vivo. By applying directed evolution of natural polymerases to broaden their spectrum of substrates, synthesis and reverse transcription of completely synthetic nucleic acids, also called xeno nucleic acids (XNAs), has become possible (Pinheiro et al. 2012).

One aptamer targeting VEGF, pegaptanib (Macugen®), is marketed for wet age-related macular degeneration (Nimjee et al. 2017). The PEGylated aptamer (for PEGylation see also Chap. 27) is injected in the vitreous at a dose of 1.65 mg (0.3 mg of which is aptamer)/eye in 90 µl every 6 weeks. Adverse effects included endophthalmitis and bleeding events in the eye, related to the injection procedure. The compound also appeared to exhibit effects in diabetic retinopathy. To increase stability several nucleotides are 2′-O-methyl and 2′-O-fluoro modified and the aptamer is conjugated to polyethylene glycol, which stabilizes the aptamer in solution and facilitates clinical delivery.

The pegaptanib product was already approved in 2004. Given the experience with this clinical frontrunner and the fact that identification of aptamers binding a disease-associated protein of interest is relatively straightforward, an avalanche of aptamer-based therapeutics may be expected. In reality, pegaptanib is still the only approved aptamer therapeutic. A number of aptamers are in clinical development (Table 15.1). Yet clinical development has been halted for some, including pegnivacogin, which was in advanced Phase II studies (Povsic et al. 2016). Pegnivacogin is a modified 31-nucleotide RNA aptamer that binds to and inhibits factor IXa. It is conjugated to 40 kDa branched methoxy-polyethylene glycol. Severe allergic reactions occurred in a subset of patients (24 out of 1605 treated) with pre-existing PEG-antibodies. This indicates that the immunopriviliged environment of the eye may have been key to the clinical success of pegaptanib and requires careful consideration of PEGylation strategies for aptamers that are used systemically.

Stimulating Immune Responses

Differences in chemical structure between the genetic information of pathogenic microorganisms and mam-

Aptamer	Target	Indication
Pegaptanib (Macugen®)	VEGF	Age related macular degeneration
Avacincaptad pegol (Zimura®, ARC 1905)	Complement factor C5	Age related macular degeneration, idiopathic polypoidal choroidal vasculopathy
Pegpleranib (Fovista®, E10030)	Platelet derived growth factor	Age related macular degeneration
Pegnivacogin (RB006)	Coagulation factor IXa	Thrombosis
Emapticap pegol (NOX-E36)	C-C chemokine ligand 2, 8, 11 and 13	Diabetic nephropathy, chronic inflammation
Olaptesed pegol (NOX-A12)	C-X-C chemokine ligand 12	Colorectal cancer, pancreatic cancer

Table 15.1 ■ Aptamers approved or in advanced clinical studies

mals can form a recognition signal for immune activation. Specific receptors exist that recognize pathogenic DNA or RNA and subsequently activate a series of genetic programs. For example, the Toll-like receptor (TLR) family, of which TLR3 recognizes double-stranded RNA and TLR9 recognizes CpG DNA fragments, which could indicate the presence of bacterial pathogens. The broad proinflammatory activation that results of this binding, can hamper the application of oligonucleotides as therapeutics, but can also be turned around to have applications in antiviral, immune activating, vaccine adjuvant, and antitumor applications. Prokaryotic DNA contains many CpG dinucleotide sequences, while mammalian DNA has very few, which are usually methylated. Synthetic oligonucleotides containing CpG motifs can mimic prokaryotic DNA and induce immune responses (Shirota et al. 2015). The CpG sequence is a strong recognition signal for mammalian cells through interaction with Toll-like receptor 9 in the endosomes leading to B-cell proliferation and activation of cells of myeloid lineage. CpG1018 is an approved adjuvant in the marketed Heplisav® Hepatitis B vaccine. Several other CpG based oligonucleotides are currently tested in clinical trials for a variety of applications (Table 15.2), e.g. together with anthrax antigens as vaccine, together with melanoma antigens to boost cancer immune surveillance, and to limit allergic responses with house dust mite allergen. In ulcerative colitis, the somewhat counterintuitive approach to stimulate the immune system with the TLR9 agonist Kappaproct®, actually appears to support regeneration by breaking the smoldering chronic inflammation characteristic for the disease.

CpG 1018 in Heplisav®	Hepatitis B antigen	Hepatitis B vaccine
AS15 in GSK 2132231A	Melanoma-associated antigen MAGE-A3 fused to protein D of *Haemophilus influenzae*	Melanoma
CpG7909 in NuThrax™	BioThrax™, anthrax vaccine without adjuvant	Anthrax vaccine
QbG10 in virus-like particles	House dust mite allergen	Asthma
Cobitolimod or DIMS0150 (Kappaproct®)	DNA-based ImmunoModulatory sequence (DIMS)	Ulcerative colitis
Poly-ICLC (Hiltonol®)	Poly I:C mimic	Ovarian carcinoma

Table 15.2 ■ Immunostimulatory oligonucleotides approved or in advanced clinical studies

In a similar approach, ssRNA as well as dsRNA can be a predictor of viral infection and Toll-like receptors recognize ssRNA (TLR7/8) and dsRNA (TLR3) in the endosomes, respectively. In particular, synthetic dsRNA composed of polyinosinic and polycytidylic acids (poly-IC) is a strong activator (Martins et al. 2015). It is clinically tested as poly-ICLC (Hiltonol®) by Oncovir Inc., as a polylysine-complexed formulation of poly-IC, to protect the dsRNA from nuclease-mediated degradation. The system is being developed in recurrent advanced ovarian cancer together with the antibody oregovomab.

INTERFERING WITH GENE EXPRESSION

Antisense oligonucleotides (ASO), ribozymes, DNAzymes, external guide sequences, triple helix-forming oligonucleotides, siRNA, miRNA, and transcription factor decoys are all members of the class of oligonucleotides that can knock down gene expression, but they function at different stages of the gene expression process.

■ Antisense/Ribozymes/External Guide Sequences

The function of oligonucleotides to act as antisense molecules was discovered by Zamecnik and Stephenson in 1978, making it the oldest oligonucleotide-based therapeutic approach (Stephenson and Zamecnik 1978). Many of the difficulties associated with the use of oligonucleotides for medical applications have consequently been encountered for antisense molecules first, explaining why clinical progress has been difficult. Improvements in synthetic chemistry, knowledge on genome, transcriptome and proteome, and new delivery strategies have revived interest in the technology (Shen and Corey 2018). "Classical" antisense oligonucleotides are single-stranded DNA or RNA molecules that generally consist of 13–25 nucleotides. They are complementary to a sense mRNA sequence and can hybridize to it through Watson-Crick base pairing. Three classes of translation inhibiting oligonucleotides can be distinguished based on their mechanism of action (Fig. 15.3):

- mRNA-blocking oligonucleotides, which physically prevent or inhibit the progression of splicing or translation through binding of complementary mRNA sequences.
- mRNA-cleaving oligonucleotides, which induce degradation of mRNA by binding complementary mRNA sequences and recruiting the cytoplasmic nuclease RNase H.
- mRNA-cleaving oligonucleotides, which induce degradation of mRNA by recruiting nuclear RNase P via external guide sequences or by nuclease activity of the nucleic acid itself (ribozymes/DNAzymes).

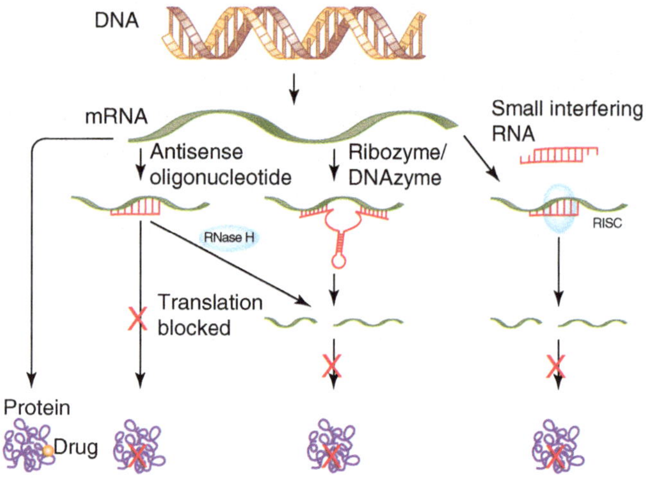

Figure 15.3 ■ Mechanism of action of oligonucleotides that act at the level of mRNA. Antisense oligonucleotides can inhibit mRNA translation by sterically blocking translation or inducing RNaseH-mediated mRNA cleavage. In the ribzoyme/DNAzyme approach, the oligonucleotide possesses mRNA degradative properties or functions as a recruiting factor (known as external guide sequences) for endogenous ribozymes (RNase P). Finally, siRNA- and miRNA-based strategies make use of short double-stranded RNA molecules which unwind and bind complementary mRNA in the RNA-induced silencing complex (RISC), which subsequently cleaves the mRNA

Formivirsen (Vitravene®)	Cytomegalovirus	Cytomegalovirus eye infection
Mipomersen (Kynamro®)	Apolipoprotein B-100	Homozygous familial hypercholesterolemia
Nusinersen (Spinraza®)	Survival motor neuron protein 2	Spinal muscular atrophy
Miravirsen	miR-122	Hepatitis C
Inotersen	Transthyretin	Familial amyloid polyneuropathy
Volanesorsen	Apolipoprotein C-III	Hypertriglyceridemia, familial chylomicronemia syndrome and familial partial lipodystrophy

Table 15.3 ■ Antisense molecules approved and in advanced clinical studies

The majority of the clinically studied antisense oligonucleotides act through RNase H. RNase H-mediated knockdown generally reaches >80% down regulation of protein and mRNA expression. In contrast to blocking oligonucleotides, RNase H-recruiting antisense oligonucleotides can inhibit protein expression without a priori restrictions to the region of the mRNA that is targeted. Most blocking oligonucleotides, however, require targeting regions within the 5′-untranslated region or AUG initiation codon region as the ribosome is apparently able to remove bound antisense molecules in the coding region.

The first antisense drug that was introduced to the market in 1998 was fomivirsen (Vitravene®), for the treatment of cytomegalovirus-induced retinitis in AIDS-patients. Due to the success of highly active antiretroviral therapy (HAART), the market for this drug has virtually disappeared, and the product has effectively been discontinued. Vitravene® was injected into the vitreous at a dose of 165 μg or 330 μg/eye in 25 μl, once weekly for 3 weeks, followed by 2-week administrations. Reported side effects are related to irritation and inflammation of the eye likely caused by the injection procedure. The oligonucleotide has a phosphorothioate (PS) backbone which limits nuclease degradation. Local injection at the pathological site improves target cell accumulation.

Over the past years, two additional antisense products received approval (Table 15.3): mipomersen and nusinersen. Mipomersen is indicated for patients with familial hypercholesterolemia. The drug targets translation of apolipoprotein B-100 in the liver, the main protein constituent in low density lipoprotein. It is administered by subcutaneous injections of 200 mg once weekly. The nucleotides are linked by phosphorothioate linkages and the distal ends are 2′-O-methyl modified. It comes with a black box warning for severe liver toxicity.

Nusinersen is administered at a dose of 12 mg intrathecally per administration. The compound is composed of nucleotides with 2′-O-(2-methoxyethyl) groups and the phosphate linkages are replaced with phosphorothioate linkages. It targets the splicing of SMN2 and converts part of it to SMN1, the protein that patients with spinal muscular atrophy lack. After four initial loading doses over a period of 30 days, the drug is injected every 4 months for maintenance. Yearly costs to treat a patient are estimated at US$ 750,000 placing it amongst the most expensive drugs in the world.

Interestingly, one antisense molecule in advanced clinical trial is designed to target an endogenous miRNA instead of a mRNA. In this particular case, the antisense miravirsen targets miR-122. This liver-specific miRNA is needed for the hepatitis C virus to replicate. Low levels of miR-122 strongly limit viral load. Miravirsen cuts HCV RNA levels 15-fold at a 3 mg/kg dose, up to ~1000-fold at 5- and 7 mg/kg dose.

Inotersen is designed to limit translation of mutated transthyretin (TTR) in patients with adult hereditary transthyretin amyloidosis. The compound is composed of phosphorothioate linked nucleotides. In clinical trials it is administered as 300 mg of inotersen via subcutaneous injection three times on alternate days for the first week, and then once weekly.

Volanesorsen is partly composed of 2′-O-(2-methoxyethyl)-modified nucleotides. It targets apolipprotein C-III translation in the liver and aims to correct the disturbed triglyceride distribution in patients with familial chylomicronemia syndrome and familial partial lipodystrophy. It is administered subcutaneously at a dosage of 300 mg once weekly.

Although sequence specificity is one of the most attractive features for antisense application, there are reports that show that knockdown of related genes with only limited sequence homology can occur.

Ribozymes and DNAzymes are molecules that combine a mRNA binding sequence with a catalytic domain and are capable of cleaving mRNA molecules (see Fig. 15.3). A single molecule is potentially capable to cleave multiple targets capable of multiple turnovers. Several different types of ribozymes are found in nature: the hammerhead, hairpin, hepatitis delta virus (HDV), Varkud satellite RNA, group I and II introns, and the RNA subunit of RNase P. Smaller ribozymes, such as hammerhead and hairpin, consist of 40–150 nucleotides. But other ribozymes can be hundreds of nucleotides long and fold into protein-like structures containing single- and double-stranded regions, base triplets, loops, bulges, and junctions, showing similarity to RNase P. Ribozymes have been applied clinically (Rossi 1999). In a study in HIV patients, hematopoietic progenitor cells were transduced ex vivo using a retroviral vector carrying an anti-HIV-1 ribozyme. Sustained output of ribozyme expressing mature myeloid and T-lymphoid cells was detected, showing that the concept may work.

DNAzymes structurally and functionally resemble ribozymes, but are made of DNA (Chan and Khachigian 2009). They are artificial molecules and have, so far, not been found in nature. The mechanism of action of DNAzymes is similar to that of ribozymes, but they offer some advantages. Because they are made of DNA rather than RNA, they are easier and less expensive to synthesize, they are much more resistant to degradation, and they possess improved catalytic efficiency. DNAzymes recently produced therapeutic effects in animal models of ischemia, inflammation, and cancer. RNase P is an endogenous nuclear ribozyme that is substantially larger (several hundred bases) than hammerhead and hairpin ribozymes, which makes it far more difficult to make and apply exogenously (Ellis and Brown 2009). However, by making use of oligonucleotides that function as so-called small external guide sequences (EGS), they can form a structure together with the mRNA that resembles the endogenous target of RNase P and thereby recruits the enzyme to digest the mRNA-oligonucleotide sequence combination. This concept has not yet been validated in vivo.

Triple Helix-Forming Oligonucleotides

Triple helix-forming oligonucleotides (Figs. 15.4 and 15.5) can bind DNA but can also act at the level of transcription of mRNA (Duca et al. 2008). They can prevent transcription initiation or elongation by binding to promoter, gene or regulatory DNA-regions. The concept has been validated in vivo but suffers some drawbacks for straightforward application. Because insertion of the third strand in the duplex requires the negatively charged backbones of the nucleic acid strands to come close, it is often difficult to find sufficiently long uninterrupted polypurine sequences in the genome that overcome the electrostatic repulsion and provide stable

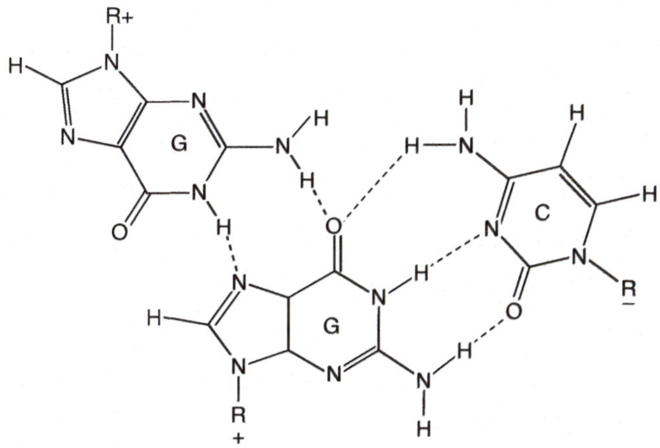

Figure 15.4 ■ Triple helices are formed through Watson-Crick-base pairing combined with Hoogsteen base pairing, here shown for guanosine = guanosine v cytosine

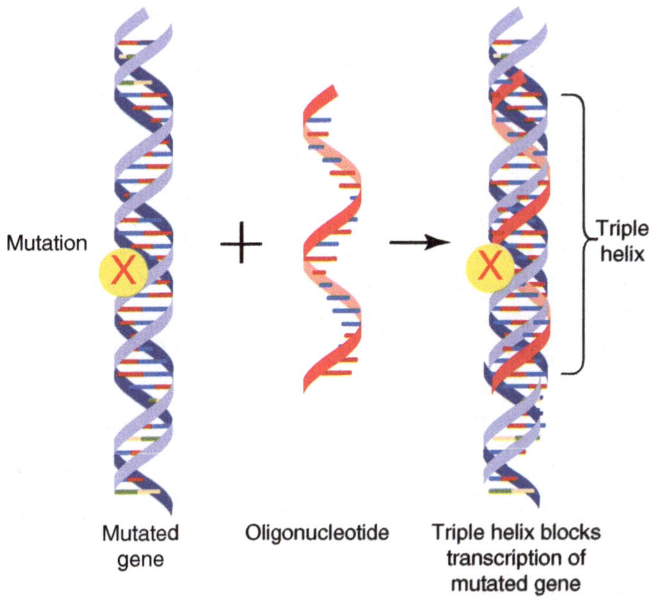

Figure 15.5 ■ Mechanism of action of triple helix-forming oligonucleotides. The oligonucleotide interacts with DNA via Hoogsteen base pairing and thereby prevents mRNA transcription. The four bases are indicated by different colors (i.e., *red/blue*, *yellow/green*). However, the region where the three strands bind should be of one type, i.e., blue-red-blue or red-blue-red (or the same with *yellow-green*) but not mixed. So only two colors for every three-base-bond-combination in the triple helix region

triplex binding. The use of chemically modified nucleic acids, such as peptide nucleic acids (PNA) (Fig. 15.1) that bear no charge in their backbone, strongly facilitates triplex formation and seems especially important for this application. The approach has not been tested clinically.

■ Transcription Factor Decoys

Transcription factors are nuclear proteins that usually stimulate and occasionally down regulate gene expression by binding to specific DNA sequences, approximately 6–10 base pairs in length, in promoter, or in enhancer regions of the genes that they influence. The corresponding decoys are oligonucleotides that match the attachment site for the transcription factor, known as consensus sequence, thus luring the transcription factor away from its natural target and thereby altering gene expression (Fig. 15.6) (Hecker and Wagner 2017).

The fact that many transcription factors are involved in regulation of a certain gene and that many genes are controlled by a single transcription factor represents important limitations to the decoy approach, especially when decoy action is only desired in the pathological tissue. Clinically, this strategy has been evaluated in patients at risk of postoperative neo-intimal hyperplasia after bypass vein grafting. The oligonucleotide, edifoligide, was delivered to grafts intraoperatively by ex vivo pressure-mediated transfection and was designed to target E2F, a transcription factor that regulates a family of genes involved in smooth muscle cell proliferation. While preclinical studies demonstrated beneficial effects, a series of clinical trials yielded mixed results. Ultimately no benefit compared to placebo was noted in 5-year graft survival (Lopes et al. 2012). The studies did indicate good safety of this local ex vivo treatment strategy.

Current clinical studies focus on topical administration of NFκB-decoys for atopic dermatitis (AMG0101) and local injection for lumbar disc degeneration (AMG0103). A decoy targeting both STAT6 and NF-κB is aiming to alleviate allergic and autoimmune diseases, such as asthma, rheumatoid arthritis, osteoarthritis, and chronic inflammatory bowel disease.

■ siRNA/miRNA

MicroRNA (miRNA) and small interfering RNA (siRNA) are double-stranded RNA oligonucleotides of 21–26 base pairs that can cause gene silencing, a process known as RNA interference (RNAi) (Fig. 15.7) (Chakraborty et al. 2017). In 1998, RNAi was first described in the nematode *Caenorhabditis elegans* (Fire et al. 1998). This silencing phenomenon also occurs in plants, protozoa, fungi, and animals and appears to be conserved in all eukaryotes and may even play a role in prokaryotic cells. It is an important process in endogenous gene expression/translation regulation and defense against pathogens.

miRNAs are endogenous oligonucleotides produced from transcripts that form stem-loop struc-

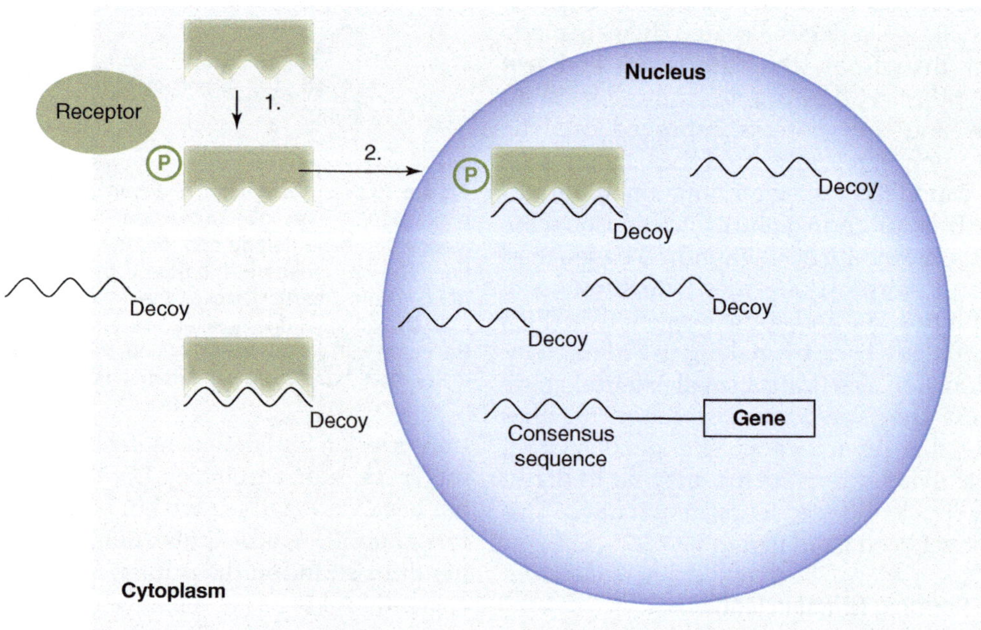

Figure 15.6 ■ Mechanism of action of transcription factor decoys. Transcription factor decoys match the consensus attachment site of the factor and thereby prevent it from binding to the DNA, inhibiting the factor's modulating activity on gene expression level

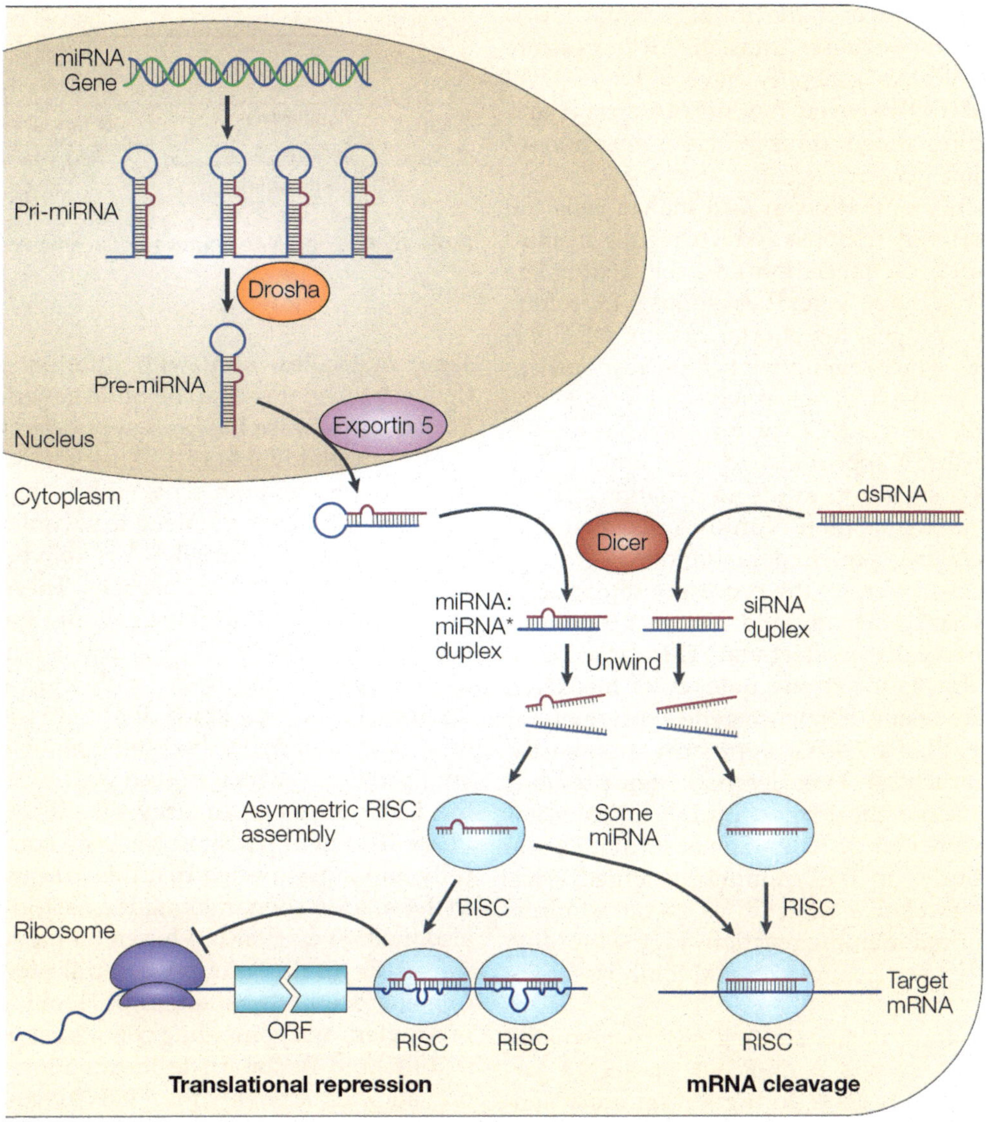

Figure 15.7 ■ Mechanism of action of RNA interference by miRNA and siRNA. RNA is transcribed from specific miRNA genes in the nucleus, which folds into characteristic hairpin loops. These are excised and processed by DROSHA in the nucleus to form pre-miRNA. These pre-miRNA fragments are transported out of the nucleus and into the cytosol. Dicer cleaves the dsRNA, cutting off the loop and separating the RNA strands with the help of Argonaute. Similarly, dicer cuts invading dsRNA coming from either viruses, or synthetic dsRNA which was introduced on purpose. The guide strand is integrated into the RNA-induced silencing complex (RISC). RISC can now regulate gene expression at the mRNA transcript level in two ways. (1) By inducing mRNA degradation. For this route a near-perfect complementary match is required between the guide strand and the target mRNA as well as a catalytically active Argonaute protein. (2) By indterfering with translation. Translational repression only requires a partial sequence match between the guide strand and the target mRNA

tures. These are processed in the nucleus into 65–75 nucleotides long pre-miRNA followed by transport to the cytoplasm. Pre-miRNA is further cleaved by an enzyme complex known as Dicer to form miRNA, which is loaded into the RNA-induced silencing complex (RISC).

siRNAs are usually exogenous double-stranded RNAs (dsRNA) of 21–26 nucleotides. They can be made from dsRNA-precursors through intracellular cleavage by Dicer. siRNAs can also be synthesized with a size that corresponds to the mature Dicer-cleavage product. siRNAs are also loaded into RISC. Subsequently one strand leaves the RISC and is degraded. By chemical modifications the preference for either strand to remain incorporated in the RISC can be influenced to reduce off-target effects. The remaining strand remains associated to the RISC. When a homologous mRNA is bound two processes can occur, depending on the level of complementarity between the mRNA and miRNA/siRNA. Complete complementarity induces

Patisiran	Transthyretin	Transthyretin amyloidosis
Inclisiran	PCSK9	Familial hypercholesterolemia
Fitusiran	Antithrombin	Hemophilia
Givosiran	Aminolevulinic acid synthase 1	Acute hepatic porphyrias

Table 15.4 ■ siRNAs approved or in advanced clinical studies

RISC-mediated cleavage of the mRNA, while lower level complementarity causes translational repression. Endogenous miRNAs generally have a lower level of complementarity between the miRNA strand and mRNA providing broad translational repression of several genes in a genetic program.

The presence of dsRNA in mammalian cells can induce an interferon response, which results in non-specific inhibition of translation and cell death. The longer the dsRNA the stronger the response. Therefore, in mammalian systems, the shorter mature siRNA is primarily used which circumvents this response to a certain degree. Next to the direct endonucleolytic cleavage of mRNAs via RISC or translational repression, miRNA/siRNA appear also to act at other levels. They have been shown to affect methylation of promoters, increase degradation of mRNA not mediated by RISC, and enhance protein degradation.

Since the discovery of the process, a remarkably rapid progress has been made, and several compounds are currently clinically investigated. This rapid progress is partly due to the strong potency of the RNAi technique which seems to silence gene expression far more efficiently than antisense approaches and partly, also, because much has been learned from previous nucleic acid-based clinical trials. Initial clinical studies focused on macular degeneration as local injection of oligonucleotides in this immunopriviliged environment allows relative high doses to be administered with minimal immune reactions (as exemplified by the clinically used pegaptanib and fomivirsen, see above).

The first study demonstrating siRNA-mediated reduction of disease was ALN-RSV01, a siRNA targeting nucleocapsid N gene during a respiratory syncytial virus infection. In the Phase II GEMINI study, a decrease in infection rate in adults experimentally infected with the virus was shown.

Calando Pharmaceuticals was the first to show RNAi-mediated knockdown of the M2 subunit of ribonucleotide reductase in melanoma patients after intravenous administration (Davis et al. 2010). The siRNA was delivered by their proprietary RONDEL technology, consisting of a targeted sterically stabilized cyclodextrin polymer. Both these projects have been abandoned since.

Alnylam is currently developing a portfolio of siRNA drugs designed to inhibit proteins in the liver. They have two technologies that ensure hepatocyte delivery based on coupling of triantennary *N*-acetylgalactosamine (GalNAc) to the siRNA or incorporating the siRNA into lipid nanoparticles. With these delivery technologies they seem to have fulfilled one of the best promises of the oligonucleotide field. Because oligonucleotides are physicochemically essentially the same molecules, only with different sequences, the delivery technology can be quite generic.

This promise has been supported by a number of clinical studies (Table 15.4). The most successful one to date is with patisiran. This siRNA targets transthyretin, a protein that is involved in several rare, but severe amyloid diseases. The siRNA is delivered to the hepatocytes by a lipid nanoparticle. These nanoparticles are composed of ionizable lipids designed to be highly potent transfectants. The particle is temporarily stabilized by PEGylated lipids with short fatty acid tails. As these PEGylated lipids dissociate from the particles in vivo, the particles become opsonized in situ with apoliprotein E, which in turn mediates recognition by the LDL receptor primarily on the hepatocytes. The Phase III trial of patisiran has been completed successfully and it is expected that this drug will be admitted to the market soon, making it a first-in-class drug, but also the first ever siRNA based therapeutic.

This marks an important milestone in the development of RNA therapeutics, but looking at the pipeline of Alnylam and competing companies, it seems that the siRNA-lipid nanoparticle formulation will be phased out and replaced by the GalNAc-conjugates. These conjugates are much smaller than the lipid nanoparticles and therefore much more straightforward to produce, as is also illustrated by the large number of late-stage clinical trials with these compounds. All the triantennary GalNAc targeted formulations in clinical studies consist of alternating 2′-O-(2-methoxyethyl) and 2′-fluoro modified nucleotides with phosphorothioate linkages on the end.

Givosiran, is a subcutaneously administered *N*-acetylgalactosamine-targeted siRNA, designed against aminolevulinic acid synthase 1 mRNA for the treatment of acute hepatic porphyrias. It has like patisiran received 'Breakthrough Designation' from the FDA as it can change the lives of patients with this orphan disease when successful. Currently, it is in a Phase III clinical trial where it is dosed at 2.5 mg/kg every month.

Fitusiran is also a subcutaneously administered *N*-acetylgalactosamine targeted siRNA against the endogenous anticoagulant antithrombin produced in the liver. It is designed to improve hemostasis in patients with hemophilia and currently progressing to Phase II clinical trials (Pasi et al. 2016). In the dose-escalation Phase I study the 80 mg dose given once monthly reduced antithrombin levels >80%. With this, the company is making steps also in a disease indication that is not designated orphan. From a commercial perspective this is very important, as these conjugates are not easy and cheap to develop, so a larger patient population would make the production more commercially feasible.

But the real key to making siRNA therapeutics a blockbuster, might be inclisiran. This is an siRNA that targets Proprotein convertase subtilisin/kexin type 9 (PCSK9) mRNA. Circulating PCSK9 causes hypercholesterolemia by reducing LDL receptors in hepatocytes. Inclisiran is delivered to the hepatocytes by *N*-acetylgalactosamine targeting. In a study with 501 patients the drug strongly lowered LDL cholesterol in patients that are refractory to other interventions (Ray et al. 2017). The dose of inclisiran in clinical trials is 300 mg given subcutaneously, once every 3 months. This is obviously a huge benefit compared to the conventional statins that are dosed multiple times per day and this patient convenience could be the critical factor for inclisiran to win a (small) part of the huge market for cholesterol lowering drugs.

Nevertheless, siRNA development for hepatic diseases is not always as straightforward as these three examples illustrate. Development of the siRNA-GalNAc conjugate revusiran for patients with transthyretin amyloidosis with cardiomyopathy was halted following a Phase III trial in which more of the revusiran-treated patients died than in the control group for as yet unknown reasons.

For these patients, the lipid-nanoparticle formulation patisiran might offer an alternative as it also targets TTR, but this setback has startled the field, because questions arose whether this may be class-specific and risks could be involved with the use of *all* GalNAc-conjugates.

Besides siRNA, miRNAs may offer some advantages with regard to their natural occurrence and ability to mediate downregulating of pathways rather than specific genes, but clinical activity with miRNAs has been limited. MRX34 reached the Phase I clinical trial stage. It is a mimic of endogenous miR-34a, which is a miRNA with tumor-suppressor activity. It was delivered in a lipid nanoparticle. This clinical study was halted in 2016 because of multiple immune-related severe adverse events. Thus, despite recent successes, the delivery challenge of RNA therapeutics is still not solved. Furthermore, the two main delivery technologies we have at hand right now, are both only suited for targeting cells in the liver. There are many diseases originating from altered protein expression in the liver, but for diseases involving other tissues, the delivery challenges remain relevant as ever.

GENE REPAIR AND CHROMOSOMAL CHANGE

Therapeutic oligonucleotides can interfere at different levels in the process of transcription and translation, for the treatment of many inherited diseases, a permanent change at the genome level is to be preferred. Actually changing the genomic DNA sequence in a straightforward manner has long been thought to be beyond the possibilities for oligonucleotides. However, several technologies have emerged that now make this possible.

■ Triplex Helix-Forming Oligonucleotides

Triple helix formation occurs when a polypurine or polypyrimidine DNA or RNA oligonucleotide binds to a polypurine/polypyrimidine region of genomic DNA. Twin helical strands form the DNA backbone. Between the strands grooves exist. These voids are unequally sized as the strands are not directly opposite each other. Triple helix-forming oligonucleotides can bind specifically in the major groove of such stretches of DNA to the polypurine strand, forming (reverse) Hoogsteen hydrogen bonds (Figs. 15.4 and 15.5). The triplex-forming oligonucleotides have been used for site-directed mutagenesis, in which a mutation is created at a specific site in the chromosomes with or without the use of coupled mutagens, as well as homologous site-specific recombination using triplex-forming oligonucleotides alone or in combination with a donor fragment to correct genetic disorders (Ricciardi et al. 2014). Although the site specificity is an important benefit for this technique, it has been overtaken by CRISPR/Cas.

■ CRISPR/Cas

Class 2 Clustered Regularly Interspaced Short Palindromic Repeat (CRISPR) systems, which form part of the adaptive immune system in bacteria, have been engineered for genome editing in human cells (Jinek et al. 2012; Cong et al. 2013). These engineered CRISPR systems contain two main components: a guide RNA (gRNA or sgRNA) and a CRISPR-associated endonuclease (Cas protein) (Fig. 15.8). The most commonly used is the CRISPR-associated protein-9 nuclease (Cas9) from *Streptococcus pyogenes*. The gRNA is a short synthetic RNA composed of a scaffold sequence that bind to the Cas protein and a 20 nucleotide spacer that binds to genomic DNA in a sequence specific manner. Thus, the gRNA guides the Cas9 protein to a specific locus in the genome, where it will introduce a double strand break. Simply changing the

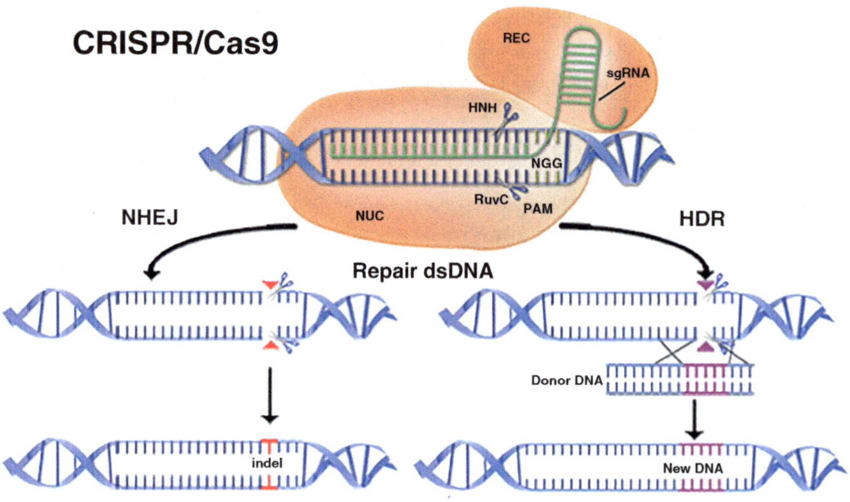

Figure 15.8 ■ RNA-guided introduction of double strand breaks by Cas9. The cas9 nuclease binds to specific sequences in the genome by virtue of an attached single guide RNA (sgRNA). This results in a double strand cut in the genome that lead to gene knock out (via NHEJ) or insertion of new DNA template (via HDR). The latter mechanism can lead to gene repair

spacer sequence of the guide RNA suffice to change the genomic target at which Cas9 will cut. Subsequently, the endogenous DNA repair system will repair the double strand breaks via a mechanism called non-homologous end-joining (NHEJ), leading to random insertions or deletions at the cut site. This will in general disrupt the open reading frame of the targeted genes and thus lead to loss of function. However, in the presence of a DNA template, the cell may choose to repair the double strand break via homology directed repair (HDR). This latter mechanism can lead to gene correction at the genomic level. The main application of this technology is in gene therapy and will therefore be further discussed in Chap. 16.

■ Antisense-Induced Ribonucleoprotein Inhibition

Ribonucleoproteins (RNP) are a complex of ribonucleic acid and RNA-binding protein. Antisense oligonucleotides can be used to inhibit or alter the functions of ribonucleoproteins by specifically binding to the RNA part of the ribonucleoprotein. For example, telomerase, the enzyme involved in preventing the shortening of telomere ends after each cell division, can be inhibited by using oligonucleotides directed against the human telomerase reverse transcriptase (hTERT) domain (i.e., RNA binding domain) (Rankin et al. 2008). Telomerase inhibition resulted in progressive shortening of telomere ends and in some cases induction of apoptosis. As telomerase activity is found in many types of cancer, inhibition of telomerase may be an effective approach for cancer treatment. The compound imetelstat is a lipid-conjugated phosphorothioate-modified DNA oligonucleotide developed by Geron corporation. Imetelstat is a competitive enzyme inhibitor that binds and blocks the active site of telomerase and is currently in Phase II clinical trials for a variety of cancers (Tefferi et al. 2016).

Eteplirsen (Exondys 51®)	Exon 51	DMD
DS-5141b	Exon 45	DMD
SRP4045/SRP4053	Exon 45/exon 53	DMD

Table 15.5 ■ Exon skipping oligonucleotides approved or in advanced clinical studies

TRANSCRIPT REPAIR

■ Antisense-Induced Exon Skipping

The detrimental effects of certain gene mutations on protein function can be alleviated by removing the faulty exon during RNA splicing, which contain the mutation that causes a frameshift or translation termination. This so-called exon-skipping technique tries to restore the reading frame by artificially removing one or more exons before or after the deletion or point mutation in the mRNA (Aartsma-Rus et al. 2017). The most popular disease target to work on is Duchenne's muscular dystrophy (DMD) which, using this technique, could be changed into the much milder Becker's dystrophy (Table 15.5).

Exons can be skipped from the mRNA with antisense oligoribonucleotides (Fig. 15.9). They attach inside the exon to be removed, or at its borders. The oligonucleotides interfere with the splicing machinery so that the targeted exons are no longer included in the mRNA. In Duchenne's disease the central region of the dystrophin protein is often not essential, and the resulting shorter protein can still perform its stabilizing role of the muscle cell membrane. The technique is currently in clinical trials for Duchenne's dystrophy, after demonstrating preclinical efficacy in mice and dogs. Sarepta Therapeutics' eteplirsen aiming at exon 51 has received accelerated approval by the FDA. This was based on an increase in dystrophin in skeletal muscle observed in some patients treated with eteplirsen. Average levels rose to 0.93% of the normal amount of dystrophin, as compared to a base-

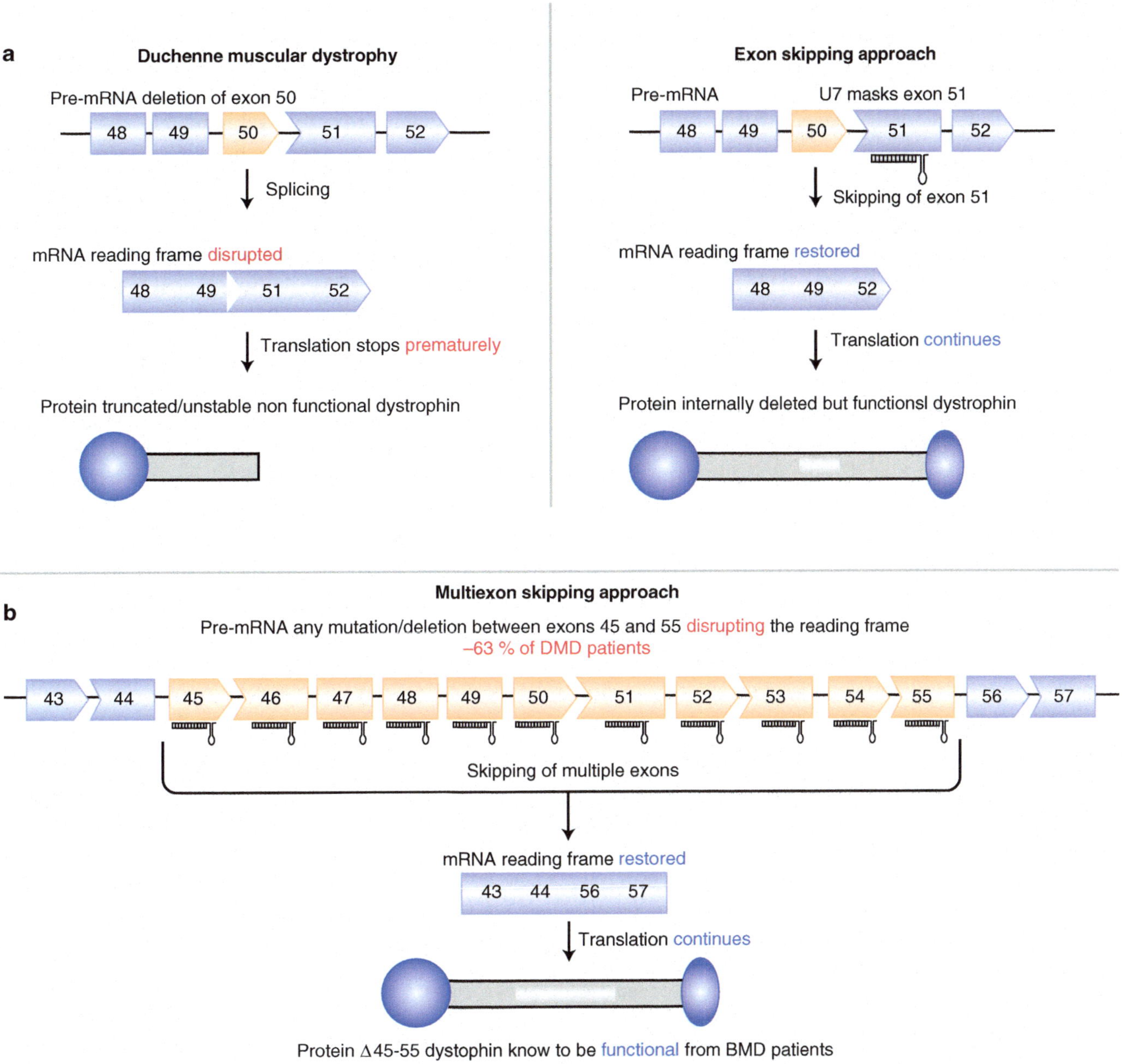

Figure 15.9 ■ Exon-skipping in Duchenne's muscular dystrophy. (**a**) Left panel. In Duchenne's muscular dystrophy the mutations in the DMD gene encoding dystrophin cause premature termination of translation. This leads to a non-functional protein that misses the second attachment point to the cytoskeleton. Right panel. By adding an oligonucleotide that preventing splicing factors from interacting with the pre-mRNA, the affected exon is skipped and the mutated region is not incorporated in the mRNA, leading to translation of a functional (albeit shorter) dystrophin molecule that contains both attachment points to the cytoskeleton. (**b**) The same strategy can also be followed to correct mutations in multiple exons, which is the case in the majority of DMD patients

line value of 0.08% in biopsies of untreated Duchenne muscles (FDA drug approval package, 2016).

The field has witnessed disappointments. Prosensa/GlaxoSmithKline/BioMarin's drisapersen, also targeting exon 51, was tested in two phase 2 and one phase 3 placebo-controlled trials in more than 300 DMD patients. The primary endpoint in these trials was a 6-min walk test but the trials failed to demonstrate significant clinical benefit. Development of this drug is currently discontinued.

PHARMACOKINETICS OF OLIGONUCLEOTIDE-BASED THERAPEUTICS

Pharmacokinetic properties and biodistribution of oligonucleotides are largely driven by the backbone chemistry and to a lesser extent to modifications on sugars or bases. Within an oligonucleotide class, the pharmacokinetic properties are largely independent of the sequence. Studies with different types of oligonucleotides (in particular phosphorothioate oligonucleotides) have demonstrated that oligo-nucleotides are rapidly absorbed from injection sites. Bioavailability of oligonucleotides can be as high as 90% after intradermal and subcutaneous injections. Oral bioavailability, however, is generally very low due to their large molecular weight, multiple charges at physiological pH, and limited stability in the gastrointestinal tract due to nuclease digestion. Oligonucleotides distribute –broadly speaking- to peripheral tissues, with highest accumulation in liver, kidney, bone marrow, skeletal muscle, and skin. Passage over the blood–brain barrier has not been reported. However, direct injection in the cerebrospinal fluid (CSF) results in broad distribution throughout the spinal cord and brain. Bolus injections are to be preferred over slow infusions for distribution to the brain. Distribution from the CSF to the tissues of the central nervous system is rapid with a distribution half-life of less than 1 h. Due to the size of oligonucleotide therapeutics (10–13 kDa), which lies below the renal clearance cut-off, they are normally rapidly cleared from the circulation by renal filtration, with plasma elimination half-lives of <10 min. However, many types of modified oligonucleotides, especially the phosphorothioate oligonucleotides, bind extensively to plasma proteins. This high plasma protein binding protects oligonucleotides from renal filtration, so that urinary excretion of intact compound is only a minor elimination pathway for highly bound oligonucleotides and plasma elimination half-lives are much longer. Plasma protein binding is also enhanced for lipid-modified oligonucleotides, such as cholesterol-oligonucleotide conjugates.

Furthermore, renal filtration can be prevented by modifying the oligonucleotides with large molecules such as polyethylene glycol as long as modification does not hamper its function. PEGylation of aptamers, for instance, results in increased blood residence times, without hampering the ability to bind protein targets. In addition to renal elimination, metabolism by exo- and endonucleases plays an important role in the elimination of oligonucleotides. Nuclease-mediated metabolism is the predominant elimination route for oligonucleotides that have been extensively distributed to peripheral tissues and/or are protected from renal elimination.

IMPROVING OLIGONUCLEOTIDE STABILITY

Nuclease resistance of oligonucleotides can be improved by modifying the backbone of the oligonucleotides. Since the early 1960s of the last century, several chemical modifications have been introduced to prevent such enzymatic degradation. The first-generation DNA analogs consisted of the phosphorothioate oligonucleotides, in which one of the non-bridging oxygen atoms in the phosphodiester bond is replaced by sulfur (Fig. 15.1). These phosphorothioate oligonucleotides are more stable in serum, but also show higher binding to proteins than those unmodified oligonucleotides, which can cause toxicity problems. However, protein binding also contributes to the increased circulation half-life seen for phosphorothioate-oligonucleotide (40–60 h).

The second-generation oligonucleotides are those containing alkyl modifications at the 2′-position of the ribose unit (Fig. 15.1). Although less toxic than the PS-oligonucleotides, they have the disadvantage to be a poor substrate for RNase H and thus can only inhibit translation by forming a steric block. However, oligonucleotides consisting of 2′-O-(2-methoxyethyl) oligonucleotides have greatly improved plasma and tissue half-lives (up to 30 days), presumably due to their ability to withstand nuclease attack.

Third generation oligonucleotides consist of a variety of different chemical modifications all aimed to improve stability, pharmacokinetics, and interaction with RNA, while reducing immunogenicity (Fig. 15.1). Examples are peptide nucleic acids (PNAs) that have a polyamide backbone rather than a deoxyribose phosphate backbone, locked nucleic acids (LNAs) that have a methylene bridge between the 2′-oxygen of the ribose and the 4′-carbon, and morpholino nucleic acids containing a nonionic morpholino subunit instead of a ribose interlinked by a phosphoroamidate bond (Fig. 15.1). These third-generation oligonucleotides all have in common the superior stability and RNA binding properties, but all lack RNase H activation. Therefore, chimeras of third generation oligonucleotides with DNA (so-called gapmers) have been made that combine good stability and effective RNase H activation. Modification of ribozymes or aptamers to obtain better stability and resistance against nucleolytic degradation is even more challenging, as such alterations most likely result in loss of enzymatic activity or binding of the complementary strand. The effect of each nucleotide modification on the stability and activity of the ribozyme or aptamer often has to be established empirically. The serum half-life of a DNA ribozyme could be tenfold increased by protecting the 3′-end with 3′-3′inverted nucleotides (Schubert et al. 2003).

The *N*-acetyl galactosamine targeted siRNAs currently in clinical studies are all consisting of alternating 2′O-(2-methoxyethyl) and 2′-fluoro modified nucleotides with phosphorothioate linkages at the end. Because of the improved protection of the lipid nanoparticle delivered siRNA by lipid complexation, patisiran can be composed of native ribose nucleotides alternating with 2′-O-(2-methoxyethyl) modified ones.

IMPROVING CELLULAR UPTAKE

Besides metabolic elimination by nucleases, the poor cellular uptake of oligonucleotides poses a problem for therapeutic application of oligonucleotides. Compared to conventional drugs, oligonucleotides are relatively large and polyanionic, making passage over cellular membranes virtually impossible (cf. Chap. 5). This is particularly true for siRNA and single stranded oligonucleotides having morpholino or peptide nucleic acid backbones as these structures poorly bind to cell membranes. However, scarce evidence exists that oligonucleotides bound to plasma proteins are taken up by endocytosis. At least the following two distinct uptake mechanisms have been identified: (1) a nonproductive uptake pathway that leads to lysosomal degradation of the plasma protein-bound oligonucleotides and which is the dominant uptake route and (2) a productive pathway that appears to be clathrin and caveolin independent and which is cell type dependent and accounts for only a minor fraction of the internalized oligonucleotides.

For PS-modified oligonucleotides the stabilin receptors on liver sinusoidal endothelial cells seem to play an important role in cellular uptake (Miller et al. 2016). Besides direct internalization via these receptors, the involvement of binding to plasma proteins, low density lipoproteins or extracellular matrix proteins as an intermediate step in cellular internalization of these PS-oligonucleotidess cannot be excluded.

Double-stranded RNA also appears to be transported into (nematode) cells by a transmembrane channel: Systemic RNA Interference Deficiency-1, SID-1. It has been suggested that the mammalian SID-1 ortholog, SIDT2, may transport internalized extracellular dsRNA from endocytic compartments into the cytoplasm (Nguyen et al. 2017).

Cellular uptake of oligonucleotides can be improved in vitro and in vivo by physical methods, chemically modifying the oligonucleotides, or by making use of specialized delivery systems. Electroporation of tissue after local injection of oligonucleotides results in improved cellular uptake.

Due to high-voltage pulses, transient perforations in the cell membrane occur that allow passage of oligonucleotides into the cytosol. This technique can of course only be applied for delivery of oligonucleotides in vitro and in vivo to tissues readily available for electroporation (e.g., skin, skeletal muscle, or superficial tumor tissue).

Grafting oligonucleotides with cationic groups in order to reduce the ionic repulsion between oligonucleotide and the negatively charged cell membrane represents an alternative strategy to enhance cellular uptake. Synthetic guanidinium-containing oligonucleotides showed improved duplex and triplex stability in addition to enhanced cellular uptake. The uptake pattern suggests that these cationic oligonucleotides are internalized by endocytosis, although cytosolic localization could also be observed.

Lipid modification of siRNA has also been proven to be beneficial for cellular uptake and subsequent gene silencing. siRNA against apolipoprotein B100 mRNA, which was modified by attaching a cholesterol group to the 3′-terminus of the sense strand, showed increased silencing of the gene encoding for apolipoprotein B100 compared to the unmodified siRNA after intravenous injection into mice. It is suggested that the siRNA is transported by lipoproteins to arrive at the liver.

Clinically, coupling of triantennary *N*-acetylgalactosamine to siRNAs has been shown to drive efficient uptake by hepatocytes. This strategy has been pursued for three products that are currently in advanced stages of clinical investigation. Due to the highly specific expression of the target receptor in the liver a low level of non-target tissue uptake is achieved.

Alternatively, cell-penetrating peptides (CPPs) can be conjugated to oligonucleotides with the purpose to enhance membrane translocation. CPPs are small basic peptides derived from protein transduction domains present in a variety of proteins which have strong membrane translocating properties (Lehto et al. 2016).

Another strategy involves the use of sophisticated delivery systems to enhance cellular uptake and to target oligonucleotides to specific tissues or cells. Most of the delivery systems for oligonucleotides are based on complexation of oligonucleotides with cationic molecules, of which cationic lipids are the most common. The progress in this field has been remarkable, where small changes in lipid structure were shown to result in dramatic changes in transfection efficiency (Tam et al. 2013).

The complexation has a dual function: it protects the oligonucleotides from nuclease attack and clearance while it enhances cellular internalization. By temporarily shielding the complexes with polyethylene glycol, gradual in situ opsonization with apoliprotein E is promoted, leading to hepatocyte uptake. This approach is taken for the patisiran product.

The fact that the triantennary *N*-acetylgalactosamine and lipid nanoparticle formulations can specifically inhibit target protein production shows that these challenging nanomedicine formulations can be developed for clinical applications. It is clear, however, that still only a fraction of the injected dose arrives at the target site and even more importantly within the target cell cytoplasm.

Recent studies attempted to quantify the cytoplasmic localization of siRNA delivered by lipid nanoparticles. The particles enter cell by clathrin-mediated endocytosis as well as macropinocytosis. Escape of siRNAs from the endosomes into the cytoplasm occurs at a low efficiency of 1–2%. Even so, the progress that has been made in improving cationic lipid structures, has now enabled the clinical feasibility of siRNA therapeutics.

A most intriguing finding is the observation that miRNA (and mRNA) can be transported between cells through endogenous carrier systems. Cellular export of miRNAs via HDL was demonstrated to be regulated by neutral sphingomyelinase. HDL-mediated delivery of both exogenous and endogenous miRNAs was shown to inhibit mRNA and dependent on cellular uptake via scavenger receptor class B type I (Vickers et al. 2011). In addition, extracellular vesicles, including exosomes and microvesicles, have been shown to contain miRNA and mRNA in their aqueous interior. The functional delivery of mRNA was recently demonstrated (Zomer et al. 2015). Mimicking these endogenous delivery systems or hybrid vesicles may enable more efficient functional RNA delivery than those based on synthetic approaches.

PERSPECTIVES

At present, a handful of oligonucleotide-based drugs are marketed. They all contain chemically modified nucleotides. In addition, they are either delivered locally (directly into the vitreous or CSF) or via the systemic route (to reach the liver). These choices reflect two of the main difficulties in applying oligonucleotides as therapeutics: (1) oligonucleotides are sensitive towards nucleases, and (2) oligonucleotides have difficulties in reaching their target site.

It is not a coincidence that most approved oligonucleotide drugs are for administration into the eye as this organ shows slow clearance rates and is immune privileged. Similarly, intrathecal delivery enables prolonged dosing intervals at relatively low concentrations. Therapeutic applications of oligonucleotides administered via the systemic route are still limited to the liver. By using triantennary *N*-acetylgalactosamine as targeting ligand conjugated to siRNAs efficient liver targeting has been achieved. Current chemical modifications offer nuclease resistance and enhanced cellular uptake that allows a subcutaneously injected oligonucleotide to reach the hepatocyte. It is expected that this strategy will be further exploited for the development of a range of therapeutics for hepatic diseases that are targeted by siRNAs.

Also, for patisiran, a nanotechnological delivery approach to the liver has been chosen. Complexing nucleic acids within nanoparticles increases their apparent molecular weight, preventing renal excretion, protects against nuclease digestion, and improves target cell recognition and uptake by in situ opsonization with apolipoprotein.

The biggest challenge for the development of oligonucleotide therapeutics in the near future is finding ways to target these molecules beyond the liver. Targeted delivery seems especially important in view of the plethora of activities nucleic acids can display. It seems virtually impossible to find nucleic acids that will not interact with any of the other pathways apart from the desired one. Limiting the number of cell types that the nucleic acids can reach and interact with will likely contribute to reduce side effects.

SELF-ASSESSMENT QUESTIONS

Questions

1. Which AS-oligonucleotide modifications are able to recruit RNase H, and which not?
2. Explain the principle of RNAi.
3. What are the major obstacles in therapeutic applications of oligonucleotides?
4. What is the difference between gene correction and gene silencing?
5. Why are the eye and liver popular target organ for oligonucleotide delivery?
6. What are the different requirements for antisense oligonucleotides that are made for exon skipping and those that are made to inhibit translation of a mutated gene?

Answers

1. Only charged antisense oligodeoxyribonucleotide phosphodiesters and phosphorothioates elicit efficient RNase H activity. Non-charged oligonucleotides, including, for example, the peptide nucleic acids, morpholino-oligos, and 2′-O-alkyloligoribon ucleotides, do not recruit RNAse H activity and act by physical mRNA-blockade.
2. RNAi is a mechanism for RNA-guided regulation of gene expression in which double-stranded ribonucleic acid inhibits the expression of genes with complementary nucleotide sequences. The RNAi pathway is initiated by the enzyme Dicer, which cleaves double-stranded RNA to short doublestranded fragments of 20–25 base pairs. One of the two strands of each fragment, known as the guide strand, is then incorporated into the RNA-induced silencing complex and base pairs with complementary sequences. The most well-studied outcome of this recognition event is a form of post-transcriptional gene silencing; however, the process also affects methylation of promoters, increases deg-

radation of mRNA (not mediated by RISC), blocks protein translation, and enhances protein degradation.
3. Poor pharmacokinetics, instability, and inability to cross membranes.
4. Gene correction makes use of a homologous recombination process to permanently correct single or multiple point mutations within a region of the gene of interest and therefore acts at the level of DNA. Gene silencing aims at reducing the level of active transcripts of the gene of interest by targeted degradation of the mRNA.
5. The eye is an immunopriviliged organ and allows local injection. The liver can be reached via N-acetylgalactosamine modification of oligonucleotides or by lipid nanoparticle encapsulation.
6. Exons can be skipped from the mRNA with antisense oligoribonucleotides. They attach inside the exon to be removed, or at its borders. The oligonucleotides interfere with the splicing machinery so that the targeted exons are no longer included in the mRNA. Classical antisense oligonucleotides are singlestranded DNA or RNA molecules that generally consist of 13–25 nucleotides. They are complementary to a sense mRNA sequence and can hybridize to it through Watson-Crick base pairing. Translation inhibition can be achieved through physical mRNA blockade, or mRNA cleavage by recruitment of RNase H.

REFERENCES

Aartsma-Rus A, Straub V, Hemmings R, Haas M, Schlosser-Weber G, Stoyanova-Beninska V, Mercuri E, Muntoni F, Sepodes B, Vroom E, Balabanov P (2017) Development of exon skipping therapies for Duchenne muscular dystrophy: a critical review and a perspective on the outstanding issues. Nucleic Acid Ther 27(5):251–259

Chakraborty C, Sharma AR, Sharma G, Doss CGP, Lee SS (2017) Therapeutic miRNA and siRNA: moving from bench to clinic as next generation medicine. Mol Ther Nucleic Acids 8:132–143

Chan CW, Khachigian LM (2009) DNAzymes and their therapeutic possibilities. Intern Med J 39(4):249–251

Cong L, Ran FA, Cox D, Lin S, Barretto R, Habib N, Hsu PD, Wu X, Jiang W, Marraffini LA, Zhang F (2013) Multiplex genome engineering using CRISPR/Cas systems. Science 339(6121):819–823

Davis ME, Zuckerman JE, Choi CH, Seligson D, Tolcher A, Alabi CA, Yen Y, Heidel JD, Ribas A (2010) Evidence of RNAi in humans from systemically administered siRNA via targeted nanoparticles. Nature 464(7291):1067–1070

Dirin M, Winkler J (2013) Influence of diverse chemical modifications on the ADME characteristics and toxicology of antisense oligonucleotides. Expert Opin Biol Ther 13(6):875–888

Duca M, Vekhoff P, Oussedik K, Halby L, Arimondo PB (2008) The triple helix: 50 years later, the outcome. Nucleic Acids Res 36(16):5123–5138

Ellis JC, Brown JW (2009) The RNase P family. RNA Biol 6(4):362–369

FDA Drug Approval Package 2016. https://www.accessdata.fda.gov/drugsatfda_docs/nda/2016/206488_TOC.cfm. Accessed 9 Jan 2019

Fire A, Xu S, Montgomery MK, Kostas SA, Driver SE, Mello CC (1998) Potent and specific genetic interference by double-stranded RNA in Caenorhabditis elegans. Nature 391(6669):806–811

Geary RS, Norris D, Yu R, Bennett CF (2015) Pharmacokinetics, biodistribution and cell uptake of antisense oligonucleotides. Adv Drug Deliv Rev 87:46–51

Hecker M, Wagner AH (2017) Transcription factor decoy technology: a therapeutic update. Biochem Pharmacol 144:29–34

Jinek M, Chylinski K, Fonfara I, Hauer M, Doudna JA, Charpentier E (2012) A programmable dual-RNA-guided DNA endonuclease in adaptive bacterial immunity. Science 337(6096):816–821

Lehto T, Ezzat K, Wood MJA, El Andaloussi S (2016) Peptides for nucleic acid delivery. Adv Drug Deliv Rev 106(Pt A):172–182

Lopes RD, Williams JB, Mehta RH, Reyes EM, Hafley GE, Allen KB, Mack MJ, Peterson ED, Harrington RA, Gibson CM, Califf RM, Kouchoukos NT, Ferguson TB, Lorenz TJ, Alexander JH (2012) Edifoligide and long-term outcomes after coronary artery bypass grafting: project of ex-vivo vein graft engineering via transfection IV (PREVENT IV) 5-year results. Am Heart J 164(3):379–386. e371

Martins KA, Bavari S, Salazar AM (2015) Vaccine adjuvant uses of poly-IC and derivatives. Expert Rev Vaccines 14(3):447–459

Miller CM, Donner AJ, Blank EE, Egger AW, Kellar BM, Ostergaard ME, Seth PP, Harris EN (2016) Stabilin-1 and Stabilin-2 are specific receptors for the cellular internalization of phosphorothioate-modified antisense oligonucleotides (ASOs) in the liver. Nucleic Acids Res 44(6):2782–2794

Moulton JD (2017) Making a morpholino experiment work: controls, favoring specificity, improving efficacy, storage, and dose. Methods Mol Biol 1565:17–29

Nguyen TA, Smith BRC, Tate MD, Belz GT, Barrios MH, Elgass KD, Weisman AS, Baker PJ, Preston SP, Whitehead L, Garnham A, Lundie RJ, Smyth GK, Pellegrini M, O'Keeffe M, Wicks IP, Masters SL, Hunter CP, Pang KC (2017) SIDT2 transports extracellular dsRNA into the cytoplasm for innate immune recognition. Immunity 47(3):498–509. e496

Nimjee SM, White RR, Becker RC, Sullenger BA (2017) Aptamers as therapeutics. Annu Rev Pharmacol Toxicol 57:61–79

Pasi KJ, Georgiev P, Mant T, Lissitchkov T, Creagh MD, Bevan D, Austin S, Hay CR, Hegemann I, Kazmi R, Chowdary P, Ragni MV, Soh CH, Akinc A, Partisano AM, Sorenson B, Rangarajan S (2016) Fitusiran, an investigational RNAi therapeutic targeting antithrombin for the treatment of hemophilia: updated results from a phase 1 and phase 1/2 extension study in patients with inhibitors. Blood 128(22):1397

Pinheiro VB, Taylor AI, Cozens C, Abramov M, Renders M, Zhang S, Chaput JC, Wengel J, Peak-Chew SY, McLaughlin SH, Herdewijn P, Holliger P (2012) Synthetic genetic polymers capable of heredity and evolution. Science 336(6079):341–344

Povsic TJ, Lawrence MG, Lincoff AM, Mehran R, Rusconi CP, Zelenkofske SL, Huang Z, Sailstad J, Armstrong PW, Steg PG, Bode C, Becker RC, Alexander JH, Adkinson NF, Levinson AI, Investigators R-P (2016) Pre-existing anti-PEG antibodies are associated with severe immediate allergic reactions to pegnivacogin, a PEGylated aptamer. J Allergy Clin Immunol 138(6):1712–1715

Rankin AM, Faller DV, Spanjaard RA (2008) Telomerase inhibitors and 'T-oligo' as cancer therapeutics: contrasting molecular mechanisms of cytotoxicity. Anti-Cancer Drugs 19(4):329–338

Ray KK, Landmesser U, Leiter LA, Kallend D, Dufour R, Karakas M, Hall T, Troquay RP, Turner T, Visseren FL, Wijngaard P, Wright RS, Kastelein JJ (2017) Inclisiran in patients at high cardiovascular risk with elevated LDL cholesterol. N Engl J Med 376(15):1430–1440

Ricciardi AS, McNeer NA, Anandalingam KK, Saltzman WM, Glazer PM (2014) Targeted genome modification via triple helix formation. Methods Mol Biol 1176:89–106

Rossi JJ (1999) The application of ribozymes to HIV infection. Curr Opin Mol Ther 1(3):316–322

Schubert S, Gul DC, Grunert HP, Zeichhardt H, Erdmann VA, Kurreck J (2003) RNA cleaving '10-23' DNAzymes with enhanced stability and activity. Nucleic Acids Res 31(20):5982–5992

Shen X, Corey DR (2018) Chemistry, mechanism and clinical status of antisense oligonucleotides and duplex RNAs. Nucleic Acids Res 46(4):1584–1600

Shirota H, Tross D, Klinman DM (2015) CpG oligonucleotides as Cancer vaccine adjuvants. Vaccines (Basel) 3(2):390–407

Stephenson ML, Zamecnik PC (1978) Inhibition of Rous sarcoma viral RNA translation by a specific oligodeoxyribonucleotide. Proc Natl Acad Sci U S A 75(1): 285–288

Stoltenburg R, Reinemann C, Strehlitz B (2007) SELEX--a (r) evolutionary method to generate high-affinity nucleic acid ligands. Biomol Eng 24(4):381–403

Tam YY, Chen S, Cullis PR (2013) Advances in lipid nanoparticles for siRNA delivery. Pharmaceutics 5(3):498–507

Tefferi A, Al-Kali A, Begna KH, Patnaik MM, Lasho TL, Rizo A, Wan Y, Hanson CA (2016) Imetelstat therapy in refractory anemia with ring sideroblasts with or without thrombocytosis. Blood Cancer J 6:e405

Vickers KC, Palmisano BT, Shoucri BM, Shamburek RD, Remaley AT (2011) MicroRNAs are transported in plasma and delivered to recipient cells by high-density lipoproteins. Nat Cell Biol 13(4):423–433

Wilusz JE (2018) A 360 degrees view of circular RNAs: from biogenesis to functions. Wiley Interdiscip Rev RNA 9(4):e1478

Zhou G, Latchoumanin O, Hebbard L, Duan W, Liddle C, George J, Qiao L (2018) Aptamers as targeting ligands and therapeutic molecules for overcoming drug resistance in cancers. Adv Drug Deliv Rev 134:107–121

Zimmermann GR, Wick CL, Shields TP, Jenison RD, Pardi A (2000) Molecular interactions and metal binding in the theophylline-binding core of an RNA aptamer. RNA 6(5):659–667

Zomer A, Maynard C, Verweij FJ, Kamermans A, Schafer R, Beerling E, Schiffelers RM, de Wit E, Berenguer J, Ellenbroek SIJ, Wurdinger T, Pegtel DM, van Rheenen J (2015) In vivo imaging reveals extracellular vesicle-mediated phenocopying of metastatic behavior. Cell 161(5):1046–1057

16 Gene Therapy

Hao Wu, Amit Kumar Chaudhary, and Ram I. Mahato

INTRODUCTION

The discovery of the DNA double-helical structure and genome sequencing has advanced the accumulation of biological insights. The genomic DNA of any organisms is constantly under the influence of various intrinsic and extrinsic agents. These agents sometimes lead to the generation of thousands of genetic mutations, resulting in nonfunctional protein production leading to genetic disorders. However, repairing, turning-off or replacing dysfunctional genes with exogenous DNA act as a novel approach to treat, cure, or ultimately prevent disease by changing (the expression) a person's genes. The insertion, alteration, or removal of genetic material to treat a disease or to improve and manage the clinical status of a patient is commonly known as gene therapy. It is a promising approach to treat diseases, where conventional drug treatments fail. Gene therapy has the potential to control a broad range of diseases, including cystic fibrosis, heart diseases, diabetes, cancer, and blood diseases. The faulty genes can be corrected either by inserting a normal gene within the genome or by correcting the faulty sequence to restore its normal function. In a strict sense, gene therapy is the use of a DNA vector as a pharmaceutical agent to treat various diseases (Fig. 16.1). The application of oligonucleic acid techniques will be discussed in Chap. 15. Gene therapy derives its name from the idea that DNA can be used to supplement or alter genes within an individual's cells as a therapy to treat disease. Unlike small molecule or protein drugs, which are usually formulated as capsule, tablet or in a parenteral dosage form, therapeutic nucleic acids are packaged within a specialized vector to enter cells within the body upon administration. Gene therapy usually targets one or more defected genes without affecting the normal genes at the site of diseases. A gene therapy target can be an abnormal oncogene whose product has the potential to cause a tumor or a defect gene whose product is critical to maintaining normal physiological functions.

The potential use of nucleic acids as therapeutics has attracted considerable attention to treat severe and debilitating genetic diseases. Gene therapy is less likely to suffer from drug resistance commonly seen in small molecular drugs after repeated treatments because gene therapy is less likely to be affected by molecular evolution, mutagenesis, and alternated pharmacokinetics. Moreover, this technique could be a permanent alternative for a patient born with a genetic disease to live a healthy life. However, there are certain limitations to gene therapy as well. The major obstacle for the successful implementation of gene therapy is that gene medicines are not easy to formulate into conventional dosage forms and delivered for routine use. Therefore, the clinical application of gene therapy so far is only conducted in hospitals with well-trained specialists. In addition, the cost of gene therapy is also much higher compared to traditional medicines.

The first approved gene therapy case in the United States took place on September 14, 1990 at the National Institute of Health (NIH). The patient was a 4-year-old girl with severe combined immunodeficiency (SCID) disease caused by a defect adenosine deaminase (ADA) gene. In the therapy procedure, the medical group isolated patient's T lymphocytes through aphaeresis, exposed these cells *ex vivo* to a genetically engineered live nonvirulent retrovirus carrying the normal ADA gene, and transfused these genetically modified T-cells back into the patient's bloodstream. The treatment was successful (Blaese et al. 1995). Ten years after treatment, lymphocytes from the patient continued to express the recombinant transgene, indicating that the effects of gene transfer can be long-lasting (Muul et al. 2003). After years of additional research, in 2016, the European Commission approved

H. Wu
WuXi Biologics, a WuXi AppTec Affiliate, Shanghai, China

A. K. Chaudhary · R. I. Mahato (✉)
Department of Pharmaceutical Sciences, College of Pharmacy, University of Nebraska Medical Center, Omaha, NE, USA
e-mail: ram.mahato@unmc.edu

D. J. A. Crommelin et al. (eds.), *Pharmaceutical Biotechnology*, https://doi.org/10.1007/978-3-030-00710-2_16

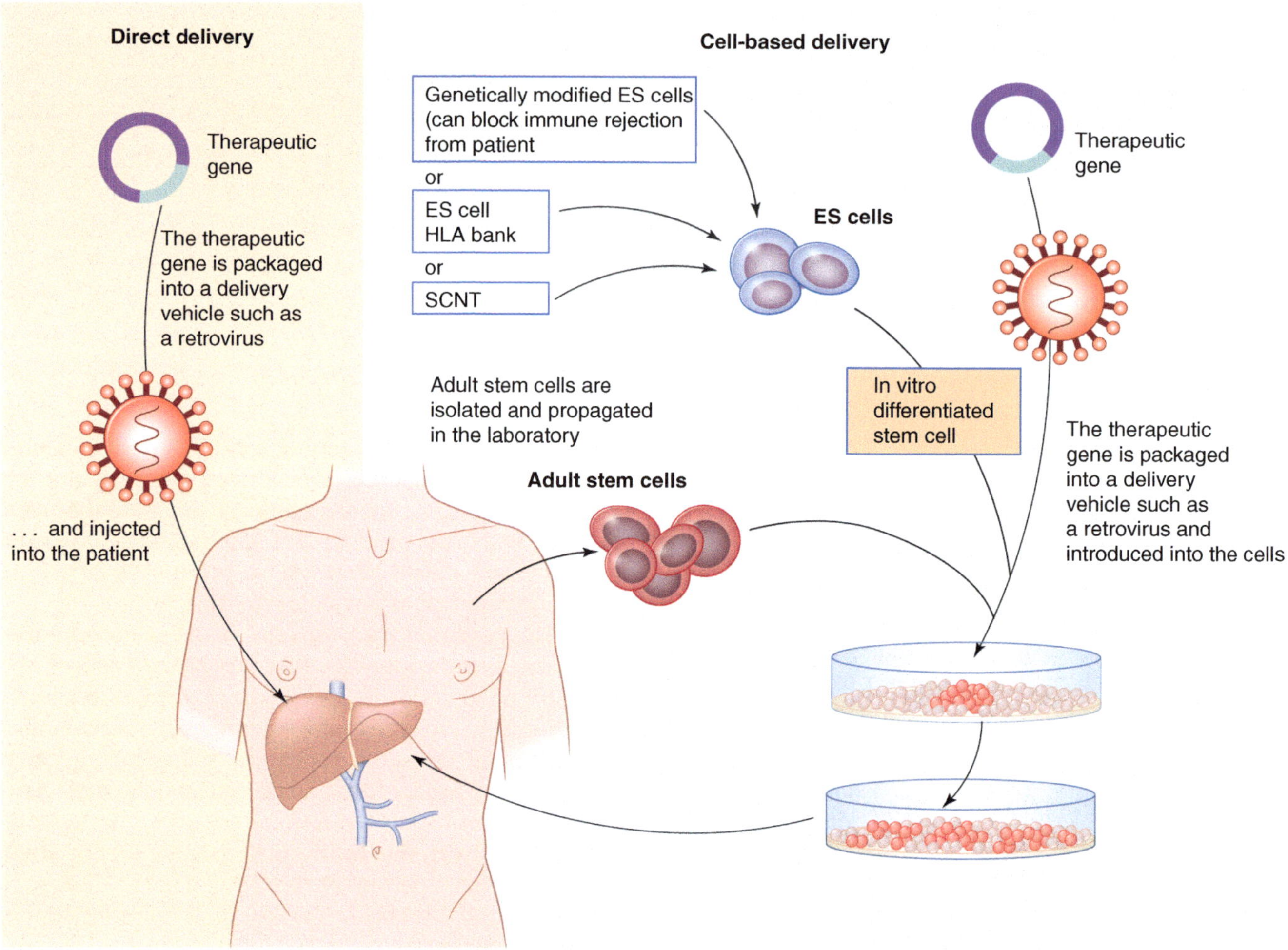

Figure 16.1 ■ Methods of administration of gene therapy vectors. In vivo gene transfer involves direct administration of the vector in the tissue of interest. Ex vivo gene transfer requires the collection of cellular targets from the patient. The cells are treated in culture with the vector. Cells expressing the therapeutic transgene are harvested and given back to the patient. *ES* Embryonic Stem Cell, *SCNT* somatic cell nuclear transfer (strategy). From Zwaka 2006; with permission to reprint (also cf. Chap. 17)

hematopoietic stem cell (HSC)-based gene therapy for ADA-SCID (Aiuti et al. 2017). This is considered *ex vivo* gene therapy. On the other hand, regarding *in vivo* gene therapy, Luxturna is an adeno-associated virus (AAV)-mediated gene therapy for the treatment of blindness caused by RPE65 gene mutations, such as in Leber's congenital amaurosis or retinitis pigmentosa. It was developed by Spark Therapeutics and first approved in 2017. Valoctocogene roxaparvovec, another AAV–mediated gene transfer of human coagulation factor VIII is currently in phase 3 clinical trial for the treatment of hemophilia A. Both *ex vivo* and *in vivo* gene therapy products are considered 'human gene therapy products' in the USA and 'advanced therapy medicinal products' (ATMPs) in the European Union (EU) (see for regulatory details Chap. 17).

In this chapter, we discuss the current state of medicinal products with a focus on *in vivo* gene transfer. The biology and utility of gene transfer systems, the diseases currently subjected to gene therapy, and the regulation of gene therapy products are touched upon. Medicinal products based on *ex vivo* genetic modification of cells are the prime topic of Chap. 17.

GENE THERAPY APPROACHES

The major objective of gene therapy is to develop good quality (i.e., stable and consistently manufactured), safe, and efficient vector systems to enable delivery of the therapeutic gene of interest to target cells to effectively treat the disease. Currently, biological (viruses and bacteria) and non-biological vectors are being explored, where both approaches have their own advantages and limitations. These delivery approaches rely on the successful construction of a gene expression plasmid and its delivery into target cells. In the following sections both approaches will be discussed.

BASIC COMPONENTS OF PLASMIDS (CF. CHAP. 1)

A plasmid is a circular, double-stranded DNA molecule, which contains a complementary DNA (cDNA) sequence coding for the therapeutic gene. In addition, it also contains several other genetic elements including bacterial elements, transcription regulatory elements, multiple cloning sites (MCS), untranslated regions (UTR), introns, polyadenylation (polyA) sequences, and fusion tags, all of which have great impact on the functioning of the final genetic products. After constructing a plasmid, certain screening methods are needed to validate the construct. For example, DNA sequencing, polymerase chain reactions (PCR), restriction digestions, agarose gel electrophoresis, Southern-Western blots and enzyme-linked immunosorbent assays (ELISA) are a few useful tools to validate the structure and function of the construct (see also Chaps. 1 and 3).

■ Bacterial Elements

Plasmids have two features that are important for their propagation in bacteria. One is the bacterial origin of replication (Ori), which is a specific DNA sequence that binds to factors that regulate replication of plasmid and control its copy number per bacterium. The second required element is a selectable marker, usually a gene that confers resistance to an antibiotic. The marker helps in the selection of bacteria that have the gene expression plasmid of interest. *Escherichia coli* (E. coli) is a commonly used bacterium for propagating plasmids. It has the property to transfer DNA either by bacterial conjugation, transduction, or transformation. The extensive knowledge about E. coli's physiology and genetics accounts for its preferential use as a host for gene expression. Human insulin was the first product to be produced using recombinant DNA technology from E. coli.

Transcription Regulatory Elements

Gene-expressing plasmids contain transcription regulatory elements to control transcription. Various transcription regulatory elements (promoters, enhancers, operators, silencers, insulators, etc.) interact with the molecular machinery (general transcription factors, activators, co-activators, and repressors) to control the patterns of gene expression.

A promoter is a DNA sequence that enables a gene to be transcribed. The promoter is recognized by RNA polymerase and transcriptional factors. Any mutation in this region will prevent the binding of RNA polymerase and the subsequent transcription and translation. The proper choice of promoter governs the strength and duration of transgene expression. Cytomegalovirus (CMV), Rous sarcoma virus (RSV), and Simian viral 40 (SV40) promoters are some of the strongest known promoters. The potency of a promoter can be cell and tissue specific. Overwhelming evidence suggests that the CMV promoter is—surprisingly—silenced in both embryonic stem cells (ES) and other adult stem cells, making such promoter unsuitable for the new evolving stem cell-based gene therapy. Other promoters such as EF-1α, chicken β-actin promoter coupled with CMV early enhancer, and SV40 are more efficient to drive the transgene expression in stem cells (Qin et al. 2010; McGinley et al. 2011). The distance between the promoter and the transgene cassette also has great impact on gene expression. Several reports have suggested that an insertion between the CMV promoter and transgene cassette surprisingly increases the transgene expression (Li and Mahato 2009).

An enhancer is a short DNA sequence that can bind transcription factors or activators to enhance transcription levels of genes in a gene cluster. While most enhancers are usually close to the promoters and genes, certain enhancers control gene expression from a far distance or even from different chromosomes (Spilianakis et al. 2005). Enhancer-promoter interaction plays a major role to drive gene expression. Enhancers do not directly act on the promoter region but elicit their effects once they are bound by activators or other transcription factors. These proteins recruit the RNA polymerase and the general transcription factors and stabilize the transcription initiation complex. Various enhancer-promoter combinations have been widely explored to improve the gene transfer efficiency in a variety of tissues and species (Hagstrom et al. 2000).

Other transcription regulatory elements include insulators, operators, and silencers. Insulators are mainly genetic boundary elements to block the enhancer-promoter interaction or more rarely barriers against condensed chromatin proteins. Operators and silencers are usually short DNA sequences close to the promoter with binding affinity to a set of proteins named repressors and inducers. Based on these interactions, an inducible or repressible system can be constructed to either increase or decrease transcription depending on the requirements. For example, the tetracycline-repressor-regulated gene expression system is a popular inducible system in constructing transcription regulatory plasmids (Fig. 16.2a). Based on this system, more advanced Tet-On and Tet-Off systems are constructed for reversible control of the transgene expression (Fig. 16.2b, c).

Multiple Cloning Site (MCS)

A multiple cloning site (MCS), also known as a polylinker, is a short DNA segment which contains many restriction endonuclease recognition sites. Restriction sites within an MCS are typically unique and occur

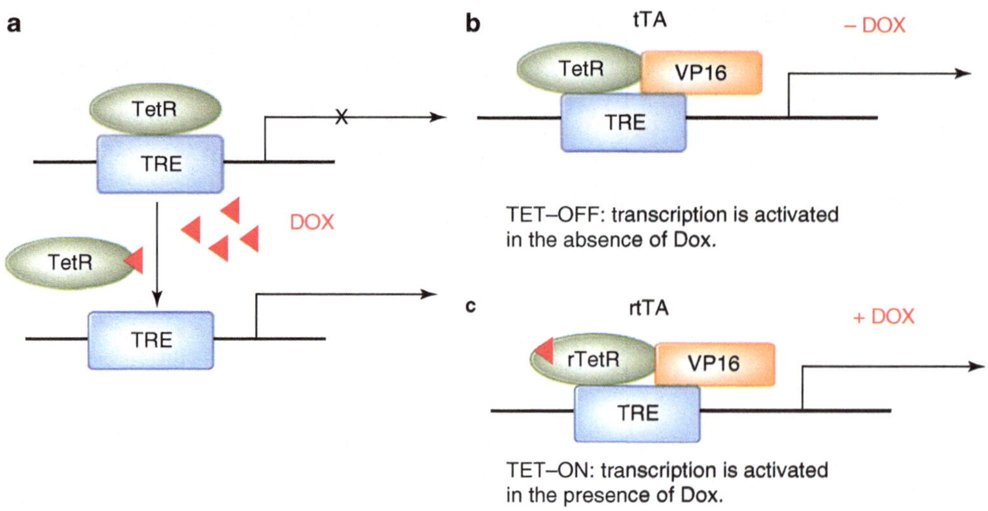

Figure 16.2 ■ Tetracycline (*Tet*)-based reversible inducible gene expression systems. (**a**) Unmodified Tet system. In the absence of the tetracycline doxycycline (*Dox*), the tetracycline repressor (*TetR*) binds to the Tet response element (*TRE*) and inhibits expression through steric hindrance; after administration of Dox, Dox binds to TetR, removes TetR from TRE, and activates expression. (**b**) Modified Tet-off system. In the Tet-off system, the chimeric tetracycline transactivator protein (*tTA*) consists of the TetR domain fused to the VP16 transactivating domain of herpes simplex virus. tTA binds to TRE to activate gene expression. (**c**) Modified Tet-On system. TetR is mutated to rTetR. Therefore, tTA is mutated to rtTA, which must have Dox present in order to bind to TRE and activate gene expression, and *r* stands for repressor

only once within a given plasmid. Within each MCS, there are usually up to 20 restriction sites which can be identified and easily cleaved with commonly used restriction endonucleases. MCS allows the insertion of single cDNA or multiple cDNA depending on the requirement of the therapeutic genes. Generally, the choice of the restriction site for cDNA cloning has no impact on the ultimate transgene expression. However, the choice of the cloning site might occasionally lead to a change in the secondary structure of mRNA and a subsequent translation inhibition. It might call for reengineering MCS for function and convenience (Crook et al. 2011).

Untranslated Regions (UTR)

To express a therapeutic protein, an mRNA must be generated from a cDNA template, which is inserted in the MCS and transported into the cytoplasm to be translated. In molecular genetics, untranslated regions (UTR) refer to two sections on each side of a coding sequence on a strand of mRNA. The 5′ UTR is the region of the mRNA transcript that is located between the capsite and the initiation codon. The 5′ UTR contains regulatory elements controlling gene expression. Such elements include the binding sites for proteins to stabilize the mRNA structure, the riboswitches to regulate mRNA's own translation activities, the binding sequence to stabilize or inhibit the translation-initiation complex, and introns to control mRNA splicing and export. The 3′ UTR is the region of the mRNA transcript following the termination codon. 3′ UTR plays an important role in mRNA stability. It contains binding sites for proteins, which may affect the mRNA's stability or location in the cell; a polyadenylation tail which is important for the nuclear export, translation, and stability of mRNA; and binding sites for microRNAs (miRNAs) which are part of the endogenous gene-silencing machinery.

Introns

The protein coding region in the eukaryotic gene is often interrupted by the stretches of noncoding DNA called introns. In any eukaryotic cells, introns are co-transcribed with protein-encoding exons into a pre-mature mRNA and removed by the mRNA splicing. There is no intron in the cDNA sequence. However, extensive studies have shown that transcripts from the intronless gene are degraded rapidly and that at least one intron should be included in the transcription unit for the optimal transgene expression (Ryu and Mertz 1989). Introns are frequently inserted into the 5′ UTR of the transcript unit (Huang and Gorman 1990).

Polyadenylation (polyA) Sequence

The polyadenylation (polyA) sequence is important for the nuclear export, translation, and stability of mRNA. At the end of transcription, the 3′ segment of the newly made RNA is first cleaved off by a set of proteins. These proteins then synthesize the polyA tail at the RNA's 3′ end. The polyA signal is a recognition site consisting of AAUAAA hexamer positioned 10–30 nucleotides upstream of the 5′ end and a GU- or U-rich element located maximally 30 nucleotides downstream of the 3′end (Mahato et al. 1999). The most important function of the polyA sequence is to prevent the mRNA from enzymatic degradation.

Fusion Tag

Fusion tag is a protein, or a peptide located either on the C- or N-terminal of the target protein to exert one or several functions such as improving expression, solubility, detection, purification, or localization. For example, (1) fusion of the N-terminus of the target protein to the C-terminus of a highly expressed fusion partner results in high-level expression of the target protein. Maltose binding protein (MBP) is frequently used to increase the solubility of recombinant proteins expressed in E. coli systems (Bedouelle and Duplay 1988). (2) Fluorescent protein tags, such as green fluorescent protein (GFP), provide information about the intracellular location of the transgene expression. (3) Fusion tags like glutathione S-transferase (GST) and MBP made the isolation of recombinant proteins easy using affinity chromatography with specific resins. (4) Other fusion tags such as several peptide sequences of the human c-myc protein were used to increase the nuclear translocation of the target protein to exert physiological functions (Dang and Lee 1988).

■ Minicircle DNA

Apart from conventional plasmid DNA consisting of bacterial elements, a novel gene delivery plasmid system has been designed called minicircles. These minicircles are supercoiled plasmids composed of eukaryotic sequences only and have a high safety profile. Due to the lack of bacterial plasmid DNA sequences including the antibiotic resistance gene, Ori, and inflammatory sequences intrinsic to bacterial DNA, the minicircles have a small size allowing them to transfect mammalian cells very efficiently with an efficient expression of transgenes and shRNAs in vitro and in vivo (Stenler et al. 2014). These minicircles are constructed by site-specific recombinases in E. coli by removing bacterial plasmid backbone elements. Several recombinases including the Cre recombinase (Bigger et al. 2001), the λ integrase (Darquet et al. 1997), PBAD/araC arabinose, and a phage phiC31 integrase (Sanei Ata-Abadi et al. 2015; Chen et al. 2003) have been employed for the construction of minicircle plasmids. In short, the overall idea behind developing minicircles is increasing both transfection efficiency and safety compared to conventional plasmids.

VIRAL VECTORS

Viruses hold the inherited advantage to bind to their hosts and introduce their genetic material into the host cell with high efficiency. To construct a viral vector, the genes responsible for the viral replication and pathogenicity are first replaced with a transgene cassette. Then the resulting recombinant viral genome is inserted into a shuttle plasmid and transduced into a packaging cell line containing the genes responsible for viral replication to generate recombinant viral vectors (Fig. 16.3). The vector construct contains the terminal sequences (ITRs or LTRs), the packaging signal (ψ), and the transgene cassette. The packaging signal (ψ) regulates the essential process of packaging the genetic materials into the viral capsid during replication. Viral vectors typically hold a high transduction efficiency and do not need additional carriers for efficient gene delivery. To date, approximately 70% of all gene therapy clinical trials employ viral vectors (Fig. 16.4). Retrovirus, lentivirus, adenovirus, and AAV are the most extensively studied and used viral vectors for human gene therapy, both ex vivo and in vivo. Their characteristics are presented and compared in Table 16.1.

■ Retrovirus

Biology

Retroviruses are enveloped RNA viruses containing two copies of a single-stranded RNA genome (Fig. 16.5). Retroviruses are 80–100 nm in diameter and have a genome of about 7–10 kb, composed of group-specific antigen (gag) gene codes for core and structural proteins of the virus; polymerase (pol) gene codes for reverse transcriptase, protease, and integrase; and envelope (env) gene codes for the retroviral coat proteins. The long terminal repeats (LTRs) control the expression of viral genes, hence act as enhancer-promoter. The final element of the genome, the packaging signal (ψ), helps in differentiating the viral RNA from the host RNA (Verma 1990).

After viral binding and introducing the viral RNA into the host cell, reverse transcriptase converts the viral RNA to linear double-stranded DNA that integrates into the host genome with the help of the viral integrase. The integrated construct, the provirus, will later undergo transcription and translation as cellular genes do to produce viral genomic RNA and mRNA encoding viral proteins. Virus particles then assemble in the cytoplasm and bud from the host cell to infect other cells.

Suitability of Retroviruses as Vectors for Gene Transfer

To generate replication-deficient retroviral vectors, the sequences encoding the virion proteins (gag, pol, and

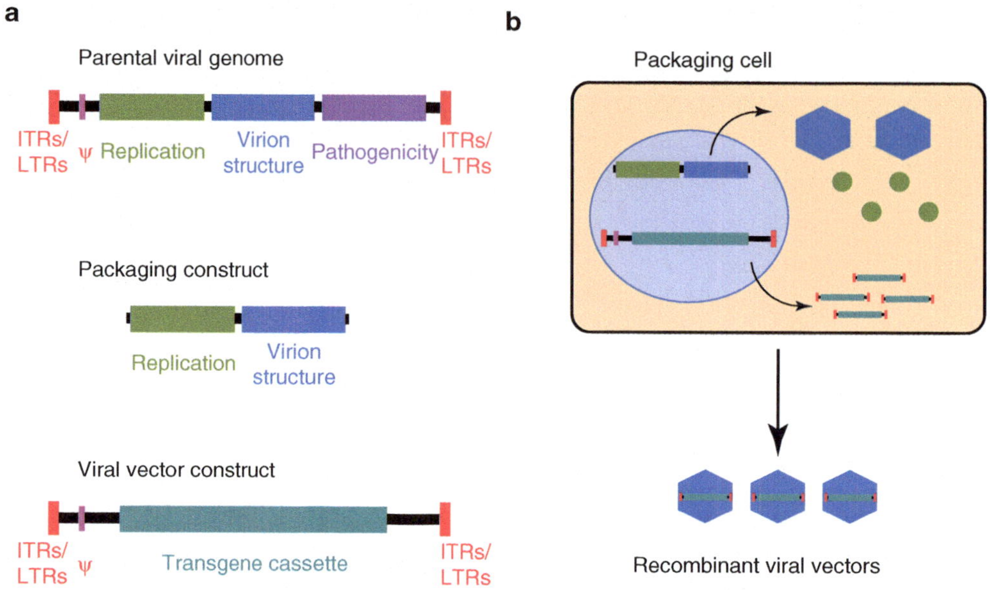

Figure 16.3 ■ General overview of constructing and maintaining a viral vector. (**a**) Schematic overview of a viral genome, the packaging construct, and the vector construct. The viral genome containing genes involved in replication, production of the virion structure, and pathogenicity of the virus is flanked by the terminal sequences (ITRs or LTRs) and the packaging signal (ψ). The packaging construct contains only genes that encode replication and structural proteins. The vector construct contains the terminal sequences (ITRs or LTRs), the packaging signal (ψ), and the transgene cassette. (**b**) The packaging and vector constructs are introduced into the packaging cell by transfection, by infection with a helper virus, or by generating stable cell lines. The packaging construct expresses replication-related proteins and viral particles. The vector constructs are replicated and encapsidated into virus particles to generate the recombinant viral vector

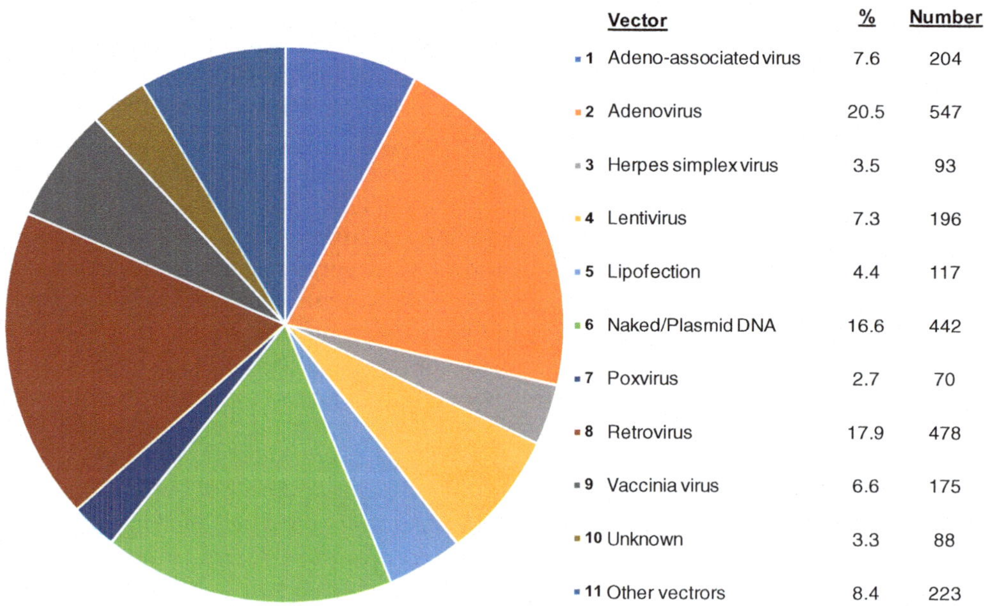

Figure 16.4 ■ Vectors used in gene therapy clinical trials (Wiley 2017, http://www.abedia.com/wiley/vectors.php). Others indicate the clinical trials in which vector used was not reported

env) responsible for the viral replication and pathogenicity are replaced by transgenes. The transgenes can be controlled by the native LTRs or exogenous enhancer-promoter sequences, which can be engineered into the genome along with the transgene. The chimeric genome is then introduced into packaging cell lines, mostly HEK293 cells to produce the retroviral vectors.

Retroviral vectors have several features for gene transfer applications (Table 16.1). They can accommodate transgene cassettes of 8 kb. They can integrate into the host genome. Therefore, retroviruses can produce stable, long-term transgene expression in dividing cells with low immunogenic potential. Retroviruses can also be used to direct the transdifferentiation of stem cells or

	Retrovirus	Lentivirus	Adenovirus	Adeno-associated virus
Genetic material	RNA	RNA	dsDNA	ssDNA
Genome size	7–11 kb	8 kb	26–45 kb	4.7 kb
Cloning capacity	8 kb	8 kb	7[b]–35[c] kb	<5 kb
Genome forms	Integrated	Integrated	Episomal	Stable/episomal
Diameter	100–145 nm	80–120 nm	80–100 nm	20–22 nm
Tropism	Dividing cells only	Broad, dividing and nondividing cells	Broad, dividing and nondividing cells	Broad, not suitable for hematopoietic cells
Virus protein expression	No	Yes/no	Yes b/no c	No
Transgene expression	Slow, constitutive	Slow, constitutive	Rapid, transient	Moderate, constitutive, transient
Delivery method	Ex vivo	Ex vivo	Ex/in vivo	Ex/in vivo
Typical yield (viral particle/ml)	$<10^8$	$<10^7$	$<10^{14}$	$<10^{13}$
Preexisting immunity	Unlikely	Perhaps, post-entry	Yes	Yes
Immunogenicity	Low	Low	High	Moderate
Potential pathogenicity	Low	High	Low	None
Safety	Insertional mutagenesis	Insertional mutagenesis	Potent inflammatory response	None to date but long term not clear
Physical stability	Poor	Poor	Fair	High

[a]Information compiled from references (Edelstein et al. 2004; Weber and Fussenegger 2006)
[b]First-generation, replication-defective adenovirus
[c]Helper-dependent adenovirus

Table 16.1 ■ Characteristics of viral vectors for gene transfer[a]

reprogram the differentiated somatic cells to have stem cell-like properties. Such features made retroviruses a valuable tool in a newly emerging area named "stem cell-based gene therapy" in the past two decades (see Chap 17). However, there are several disadvantages of these vectors. Retroviruses cannot transduce nondividing cells, which are often targets for gene transfer applications. In addition, current methods of virus production generate preparations in which the virus titer is very low (1×10^5–1×10^7 active virus particles/mL), making its clinical application difficult. Retroviruses are also inactivated by elements of the complement system and rapidly removed from the systemic circulation in response to cellular proteins incorporated in the viral envelope during the budding process. Therefore, the clinical trials with retroviral vectors are decreasing.

The major limitation of retrovirus-based gene therapy is that the retrovirus randomly inserts the genetic material into the host genome. If genetic material happens to be inserted in the middle of a gene of the host cell, this gene will be disrupted (insertional mutagenesis). If the gene happens to be one regulating cell division, uncontrolled cell division (i.e., insertional oncogenesis) can occur. Fortunately, this problem has begun to be addressed by custom-designed nucleases (cf. Chap. 9) or by genetic manipulation of the LTRs of the viral genome (Montini et al. 2009).

Clinical Use of Retrovirus

Approximately 18% of the currently active clinical trials employ retroviral vectors for gene transfer (Fig. 16.4). The Moloney murine leukemia virus (MoMLV), one of the most thoroughly characterized retroviruses, was the first viral vector to be used in the clinic for treating ADA deficiency caused by SCID, an inherited disease in which the buildup of deoxyadenosine caused by ADA deficiency prohibits the expansion of lymphocytes (Blackburn and Kellems 2005). MoMLV-expressing recombinant ADA was used for ex vivo genetic modification of autologous T lymphocytes isolated from the patient (Muul et al. 2003; Aiuti et al. 2017) (see Chap. 17).

Another successful clinical trial employing retroviruses was for treating a rare form of X-linked SCID (X-SCID) (Cavazzana-Calvo et al. 2000). MoMLV expressing the γc-interleukin receptor was used to transduce HSCs isolated from the patient ex vivo. Then, the genetically modified HSCs were transfused back to the patient to reconstitute the immune system. More than 20

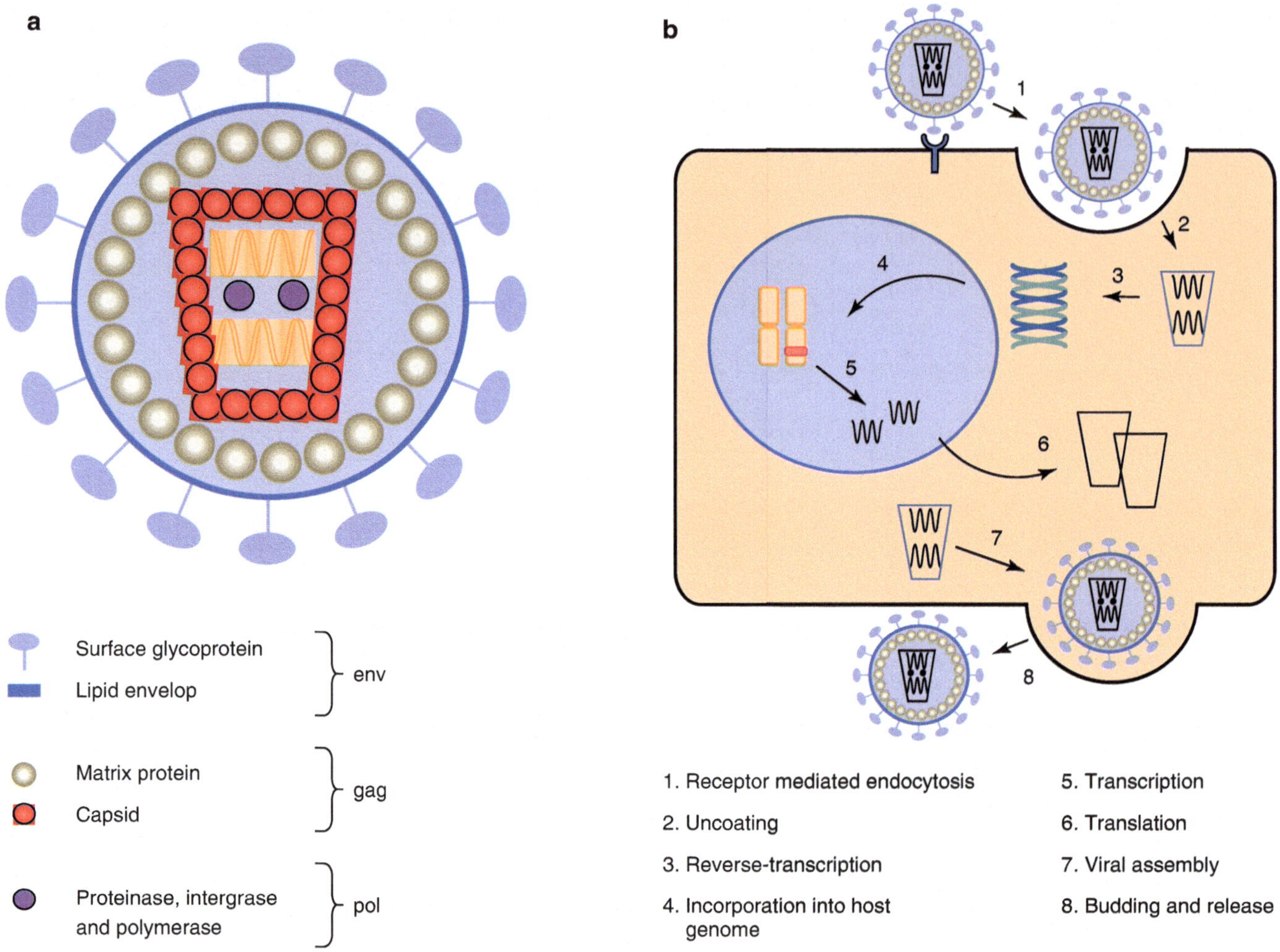

Figure 16.5 ■ The retrovirus. (**a**) Cross section of a retrovirus. (**b**) The retrovirus replication cycle. Retroviruses enter cells by receptor-mediated endocytosis. In the endosome, the lipid envelope and capsid matrix proteins are degraded. The viral RNA is reverse-transcribed into double-stranded DNA, which is then shuttled to the nucleus. In the nucleus, the double-stranded viral DNA is inserted into genomic DNA as a provirus. RNA polymerase in the cell copies the viral RNA in the nucleus. These molecules are shuttled out of the nucleus and serve as templates for making additional copies of viral RNA and mRNA that is translated into viral proteins that form the envelope. New virus particles are assembled in the cytoplasm and bud from the cell membrane

patients have been treated worldwide, with a high rate of immune system reconstitution observed. However, a leukemia syndrome was reported in several patients enrolled in the trial (Hacein-Bey-Abina et al. 2003). As a result, the US Food and Drug Administration (FDA), the Gene Therapy Advisory Committee (GTAC), and Committee of Safety of Medicine in the United Kingdom have declared that this approach should not be first-line therapy for X-SCID but should only be considered in the absence of other therapeutic options.

■ Lentivirus

Biology

Lentiviruses are unique retroviruses being able to replicate in both dividing and nondividing cells. The biology of lentiviruses resembles that of retroviruses. Apart from the genes gag, pol, and env, lentivirus has six accessory genes such as tat, rev, vpr, vpu, nef, and vif, which regulate the synthesis and processing of viral RNA and other replicative functions.

Human immunodeficiency virus (HIV) is the best-known lentivirus. HIV virus has been genetically manipulated to generate viral vectors for efficient gene transfer into human helper T cells and macrophages. Apart from the genes gag, pol, and env, the accessory genes of the lentiviral genome can also be removed to incorporate more genetic materials without affecting the production efficiency of the virus. HEK293 cells were the most frequently used packaging cell lines for lentivirus generation.

Suitability of Lentiviruses as Vectors for Gene Transfer

The significance of lentiviral vectors lies in the fact that they can efficiently transduce nondividing cells or terminally differentiated cells such as neurons, macrophages, HSCs, muscle, and liver cells as well as other cell types for which traditional retrovirus-based gene therapy methods cannot be used. Previous studies have shown that when injected into the rodent brain, liver, muscle, or pancreatic islet cells, lentivirus promoted a sustained gene expression for over 6 months (Miyoshi et al. 1997). Lentiviruses do not elicit significant immune responses and thus can be ideal for in vivo gene expression. Magnetic nanoparticles have been employed for targeted delivery of lentiviral vectors to the endothelial cells even in perfused blood vessels (Hofmann et al. 2009).

Lentiviruses only have limited integrating potential and consequently induce less risk of insertional mutagenesis. However, the generation of replication-competent lentiviruses (RCL) during the production phase or after introduction into target cells is still a primary concern for the clinical use of lentiviruses, and therefore needs to be tested for. Development of self-inactivating vectors that contain deletions within the 3′ LTR, eliminating transcription of the packaging signal to prevent virus assembly, has significantly improved the safety profile of lentiviruses (Zufferey et al. 1998). Another choice is to develop non-integrating lentiviral vectors by point mutations into the catalytic site, chromosome binding site, and viral DNA binding site of the viral integrase (Apolonia et al. 2007).

Clinical Use of Lentiviral Vectors

Because of the perceived risks associated with the use of lentiviruses, clinical trials with these vectors were not initiated until 2001. Most of lentiviral vectors are designed for treating HIV infection (MacGregor 2001). In these studies, peripheral blood mononuclear cells (PBMCs) were obtained from the patient. After selective depletion of CD8 T cells, the remaining cells, CD4 T cells were enriched, transduced with the lentiviral vector VRX496, and expanded in culture. The VRX496-transduced cells were then infused back into the patient. The VRX496 vector contains an antisense sequence targeted to the HIV env gene. Expression of the antisense env from an HIV vector transcript would target wild-type HIV env RNA and destroy it and hence, decrease the productive HIV replication from CD4 T cells. The clinical goal of this treatment approach is to decrease HIV viral loads and promote CD4 T cell survival in vivo. Results from this trial showed that although no treatment-related severe adverse events have occurred; no statistically significant anti-HIV effects could be observed in a pilot trial (Manilla et al. 2005) (cf. Chap. 17).

■ Adenovirus

Biology

Adenoviruses are non-enveloped (without an outer lipid bilayer), icosahedral, lytic DNA viruses composed of a nucleocapsid and a linear double-stranded genome (Fig. 16.6a). Adenoviruses are capable of infecting both dividing and nondividing cells. Fifty-seven serotypes of adenoviruses have been identified to date. They are grouped into 7 subgroups (A-G) based on genome size, composition, hemagglutinating properties, and oncogenicity. The adenoviruses serotype 2 and 5 are the most extensively studied and the first to be used as vectors for gene therapy. The adenoviral genome is linear, non-segmented dsDNA, between 26 and 45 kb, composed of six early (E1a, E1b, E2a, E2b, E3, and E4) and five late (L1, L2, L3, L4, L5) genes. The early genes encode proteins necessary for the viral replication, while the late genes encode proteins to assemble into viral particles.

Adenovirus infection begins with binding of the fiber knob on the surface of the viral capsid to the CAR and major histocompatibility complex (MHC) class I (Fig. 16.6c). After initial binding, the penton base interacts with integrin on the cell surface to initiate a series of cell signaling processes allowing internalization via receptor-mediated endocytosis. (Nemerow and Stewart 1999; Medina-Kauwe 2003). Adenovirus particles enter the nucleus as early as 30 min after initial cellular contact. Viral DNA replication and particle assembly in the nucleus starts 8 h after infection and culminates in the release of 10^4–10^5 mature virus particles per cell, 30–40 h post-infection by cell lysis (Majhen and Ambriovic-Ristov 2006).

Suitability of Adenoviruses as Vectors for Gene Transfer

To construct an adenoviral vector for gene therapy, the E1 region and the E3 region of the viral genome were often removed to prevent viral replication and accommodate transgene cassettes. Adenoviruses have a large genome capable of accommodating large transgene cassettes. The adenoviral genome is also easy to be manipulated to generate a vector with multiple deletions and inserts without affecting its transduction efficiency. Recently, adenoviruses with both E1 and E3 inserts to simultaneously express two therapeutic genes have been reported (Panakanti and Mahato 2009). Moreover, adenoviruses with E1, E3, and E4 deletions and even "gutless" adenovirus (adenovirus without viral coding regions) have been constructed to drive transgene expression (Armentano et al. 1995; Chen et al. 1997).

Other favorable characteristics of adenoviruses include that the biology of the virus is well understood,

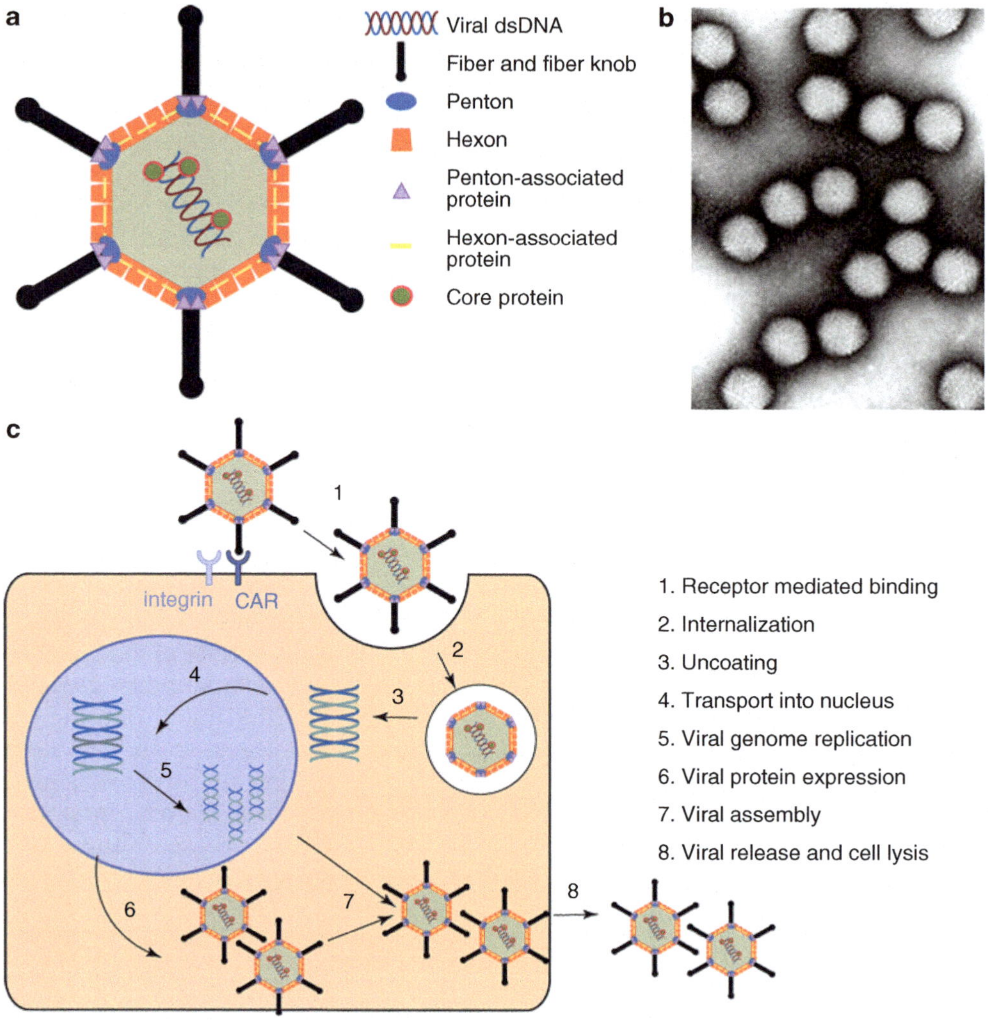

Figure 16.6 ■ The adenovirus. (**a**) Cross section of an adenovirus particle. The virus consists of a double-stranded DNA genome encased in a protein capsid. The capsid is primarily made up of hexon proteins. Penton proteins are positioned at each of the vertices of the icosahedral capsid and serve as the base for each fiber protein. Hexon-associated and penton-associated proteins are the glue that holds these proteins together within and across the facets of the capsid. Core proteins bind to penton proteins and serve as a bridge between the virus core and the capsid. (**b**) Electron micrograph of intact adenovirus serotype 5 particles. (**c**) The adenovirus replication cycle. Adenovirus infection begins with the attachment of fiber proteins to cellular receptors such as coxsackie and adenovirus receptors (CAR) and integrins. Through receptor-mediated endocytosis, the virus enters the cytoplasm. In the endosome, capsid proteins are degraded, and viral DNA is released into the cytoplasm and transported to the nucleus for replication. After assembly into new viral particles in the cytoplasm, the host cell is lysed, and viruses are released. In the case of gene therapy, recombinant replication-defective adenoviruses are used to transduce targeted cells. The inserted transgenes are transcribed to mRNA in the nucleus. Messenger RNA is then transported out of the nucleus and into the cytoplasm where it is translated to therapeutic proteins

that recombinant virus can be generated with high titer and purity, that transgene expression from adenoviruses is rapid and robust, and that adenoviruses can infect a wide range of dividing and nondividing cells. Adenoviruses do not integrate into the host genome. While this minimizes the risk of insertional mutagenesis, gene expression is transient making adenoviruses unsuitable for long-term correction of genetic defects.

A significant drawback to the use of recombinant adenoviruses is the ability of the virus to elicit a strong immune response including T lymphocyte-mediated "cellular immunity" and antibody-producing "humoral immunity." The cellular response results in the killing of adenovirus transfected cells by T lymphocytes, whereas the humoral response results in the production of antibodies to adenovirus, resulting in the clearance of the adenoviral vectors from the bloodstream. Both actions bring an end to the transgene expression (Dai et al. 1995). Moreover, the preexisting adenovirus serotype 5 immunity in human populations has been shown to significantly reduce the efficacy of these vectors in both preclinical studies and clinical trial (Ertl 2005).

The immunogenicity of recombinant adenovirus also raises a serious safety concern for its clinical applications. The massive immune responses caused by administration of adenovirus could lead to multiple organ failures and brain death. In 1999, a patient died 4 days after injection with an adenoviral vector. This was the first death of a participant in a clinical trial for gene therapy (Stolberg 1999). Another patient experienced a severe immune response syndrome characterized by multiple organ failure and sepsis and died soon after an adenoviral injection in 2003 (Raper et al. 2003). Preclinical studies also confirmed that the immune response generated by adenoviral vectors must be suppressed before a therapeutic effect can be expected. The transgene expression from adenovirus-transduced cells lasted for about 5–10 days, partially due to the clearance of the transduced cells by the host immune system (Lochmuller et al. 1996). Adenoviruses show the extended duration of expression when given to nude mice (mice with an "inhibited" immune system) or when an immunosuppressant is administered (Dai et al. 1995).

A significant effort has been put forth to address the issue of the adenovirus-induced systemic immune response. Adenoviruses with more deletions in the early genes and even "gutless" helper-dependent adenoviruses have been constructed to reduce the inflammatory response and accommodate more transgene cassettes (Chen et al. 1997). Other strategies involved the incorporation of an arginine-glycine-aspartic acid (RGD) sequence and tissue-specific ligands to the surface of the viral particles to decrease the systemic immune responses and increase the gene transfer efficiency (Stewart et al. 1997; Wu et al. 2011). However, none of these strategies provided the full elimination of the immune response. Coadministration of immunosuppressive agents such as cyclophosphamide, FK506, and cyclosporin A extended the duration of transgene expression but did not prevent the development of neutralizing antibodies (Xu et al. 2005; Lochmuller et al. 1996). "Stealth" adenoviruses coated with polyethylene glycol (PEG) or other polymers were also designed to reduce the immunogenicity, increase the blood circulation time, and prolong the transgene expression (Chillon et al. 1998). However, masking adenovirus with PEG or other polymers significantly decreased the gene transfer efficiency of adenoviruses.

Generation of replication-competent adenovirus (RCA) is another problem of using adenovirus in the human body; however, this can be tested for. Although the early genes responsible for viral replication and pathogenicity are already removed in the vector construction process, RCA can still be generated by homologous recombination if there is some overlap between sequences in the virus genome and packaging cell. The RCA mixed in the clinically used adenoviral products could be extremely dangerous for the patients. Several groups have observed the production of RCA from HEK293 cells owing to sequence overlap (Louis et al. 1997). Some new packaging cell lines with less overlap have been reported to overcome such problem.

Clinical Use of Adenoviral Vectors

Today, approximately 20.5% of all gene therapy clinical trials involve recombinant adenoviruses, making them the most widely used vector for gene transfer (Fig. 16.4). However, the safety concern regarding the immunogenicity of adenovirus is the major hurdle for its clinical application. Adenoviral gene therapy faced a major setback in 1999 when a patient died 4 days after injection with an adenoviral vector carrying a corrected gene to test the safety of the procedure (Stolberg 1999). Gendicine, adenoviral p53-based gene therapy was approved by the Chinese food and drug regulators in 2003 for treatment of head and neck cancer. Advexin, a similar gene therapy approach from Invitrogen, was turned down by the FDA in 2008. Moreover, despite over 300 clinical trials that have shown it to be well tolerated and efficient in gene transfer, the clinical efficacy of this vector has yet to be proven (Shirakawa 2009).

A number of breakthroughs in adenovirus-based gene therapy have been made. With the help of the tissue-specific targeted delivery strategies, the new generation of adenoviral vectors is less likely to induce severe systemic immunity. For example, the aerosol administration of a recombinant adenovirus expressing the cystic fibrosis transmembrane conductance regulator (CFTR) to cystic fibrosis patients demonstrated the safety and the proof of concept of adenovirus-based gene therapy (Bellon et al. 1997). In another phase I/II trial, using the gene-directed enzyme-prodrug therapy concept ("suicide gene therapy," see Figs. 16.12 and 16.13 and Disease Targets for Gene Therapy), the intratumoral administration of adenovirus encoding a suicide gene (thymidine kinase, TK) and of intravenous ganciclovir increased the median survival time of patients with malignant glioma from 37.7 to 62.4 weeks without adverse effects (Immonen et al. 2004). Cerepro, a drug composed of TK encoding recombinant adenoviruses was granted orphan drug status for the treatment of patients with high-grade operable glioma by the European Committee for Orphan Medicinal Products and the FDA Office of Orphan Products Development (OOPD). However, in 2010 Ark Therapeutics Ltd. notified the Committee for Medicinal Products for Human Use (CHMP) that it withdrew its marketing authorization application for Cerepro (see also under Disease Targets for Gene Therapy).

Adeno-Associated Virus (AAV)

Biology

The AAV genome is a 4.7 kb linear, single-stranded DNA molecule composed of two open reading frames (ORFs), rep, cap, and two inverted terminal repeats (ITRs) that define the start and end of the viral genome and packaging sequence. The rep genes encode proteins responsible for viral replication, while the cap genes encode structural capsid proteins. ITRs are required for genome replication, packaging, and integration.

The icosahedral AAV capsid is 25 nm in diameter. AAV is deficient in replication, and there are no packaging cells, which can express all the replication-related proteins of the AAV. Therefore, AAV requires coinfection with a helper virus, such as an adenovirus or a herpes simplex virus to replicate (Fig. 16.7). Eleven distinct AAV serotypes have been identified, and over 100 AAV variants have been found in human and non-human primate tissues in 2006 (Wu et al. 2006; Mori et al. 2004). The biology of AAV serotype 2 (AAV2) has been the most extensively studied, and this serotype is most often used as a vector for gene transfer.

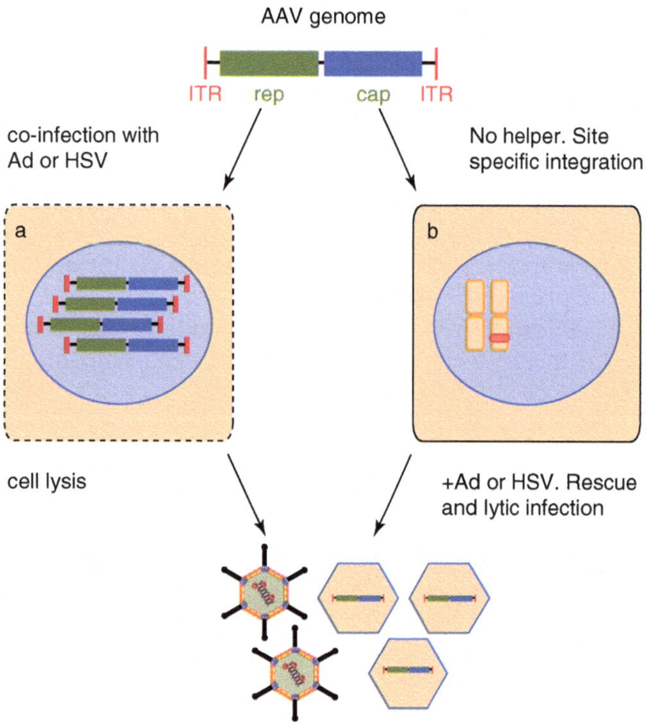

Figure 16.7 ■ Lifecycle of AAV. AAV can enter cells through receptor-mediated endocytosis. Once in the nucleus, the virus can follow one of two distinct and interchangeable pathways. (**a**) In the presence of helper virus (adenovirus or herpes simplex virus), AAV enters a lytic phase. The AAV genome undergoes DNA replication resulting in amplification of the genome and production of progeny virions. The newly formed AAV viral particles along with helper viruses are released from the cell by helper-induced lysis. (**b**) In the absence of helper virus, it enters a latent phase. During this phase, part of the AAV vectors integrates into host genomic DNA. While the majority of the AAV vector persists in an extrachromosomal latent state without integrating into the host genome. The latent AAV genome cannot undergo replication and production of progeny virions in the absence of helper virus. However, the transgenes carried in the AAV genome are transferred to the host cell and co-express using the host gene expression machinery ITRs inverted terminal repeats, rep replication

Suitability of Adeno-Associated Viruses for Gene Transfer

Recombinant AAV vectors have rapidly gained popularity for gene therapy applications within the last decade, due to their lack of pathogenicity and ability to establish long-term gene expression (Table 16.1). The viral genome is simple, making it easy to manipulate. The virus is resistant to physical and chemical challenges during purification and long-term storage (Wright et al. 2003; Croyle et al. 2001). The ability of the virus to integrate into the human chromosome was an initial concern, but eventually, it turned out that AAV only integrates into a fixed location of human chromosome and the integration frequency of recombinant AAV is quite low (Surosky et al. 1997).

The AAV vectors are produced by replacing the rep and cap genes with the transgene. Only one out of 100–1000 viral particles are infectious. Apart from the production of AAV vectors being laborious, these vectors also have the drawback of limited packaging capacity (4.7 kb) for the transgene. Large genes are therefore not suitable for use in a standard AAV vector. To overcome the limited coding capacity, the ITRs of two AAV genomes can anneal to form a head-to-tail structure through trans-splicing between two genomes, almost doubling the capacity of the vector (Yan et al. 2000).

Since recombinant AAV vectors do not contain any viral ORFs, they induce only limited immune responses in humans. Intravenous administration of AAV vectors in mice causes the transient production of pro-inflammatory cytokines and limited infiltration of neutrophils, in contrast to an innate response lasting 24 h or longer induced by aggressive viruses (Zaiss et al. 2002). However, despite the limited innate immunity elicited by AAV vectors, the humoral immunity elicited by AAV is still a common event. Up to 80% of individuals are thought to be positive for AAV2 antibodies in the human population (Erles et al. 1999). The associated neutralizing activity limits the usefulness of the most commonly used serotype AAV2 in certain applications.

Clinical Use of Adeno-Associated Virus Vectors

The first clinical use of recombinant AAV was to transfer the CFTR cDNA to the respiratory epithelium for treating cystic fibrosis (Flotte et al. 1996). This is the first trial to suggest that gene therapy could treat cystic fibrosis in a positive manner. Since then, 204 clinical trials employing recombinant AAV vectors have been initiated worldwide (Fig. 16.4). The only approved AAV gene therapy by European Commission was granted to Glybera® (alipogene tiparvovec), which encode the gene for lipoprotein lipase deficiency for the treatment of patients with familial lipoprotein lipase deficiency (LPLD, synonym: type I hyperlipidaemia) (Büning 2013; Salmon et al. 2014). Other phase I and phase II trials have shown that AAV-mediated gene transfer is safe and effective for treating Leber's congenital amaurosis (High and Aubourg 2011; Simonelli et al. 2010), hemophilia (Nathwani et al. 2011), lipoprotein lipase deficiency (Rip et al. 2005), and Parkinson's disease (LeWitt et al. 2011). There are currently several trials using AAV vectors in phase III testing for metastatic hormone-resistant prostate cancer and other diseases (Simons and Sacks 2006; Naso et al. 2017). Production and testing of these viral vector systems, both for *in vivo* and *ex vivo* gene therapy, are discussed in Chap. 17.

BACTERIAL VECTORS

Like transduction of a gene with nonvirulent viruses, the innate biological properties of bacteria allow efficient delivery of DNA to cells or tissues. Bacterial vectors maintain their integrity and biological functions, to attract antigen presenting cell (APC) and thus gene delivery. Therefore, nonpathogenic bacteria can be engineered as an efficient cell-based factory for the transfer of plasmids encoding heterologous proteins (protein antigens, hormones, toxins or enzymes) to mammalian cells by the process of bactofection. Different bacterial species including *Salmonella, Shigella, Listeria and E. coli* have been used as potent delivery vectors expressing heterologous proteins in different mammalian cells (van Pijkeren et al. 2010; Vassaux et al. 2006). However, due to side effects related to the host–bacteria interactions and the response of the immune system, the patient body might cause rapid clearance of these bacteria or even autoimmune reactions. Therefore, work is in progress to genetically modify these bacteria to reduce this clinical risk. For example, since APC can engulf particles with a size ranging from 1–10 μm based on host–bacteria interactions, a E. coli strain was engineered to express two proteins with different functions. The pore-forming toxin listeriolysin O (LLO) protein provides a pH-sensitive way to promote the internalization on its carrier into the target cells. On the other hand, the lethal lysis *gene E* (*LyE*) from bacteriophage ΦX174 induces cellular lysis. Taking these two features together, an E. coli strain was engineered to generate an E. coli bactofection vector that resulted in improved gene delivery to APC due to attenuation properties of the newly introduced lysis mechanism (Chung et al. 2015).

NON-VIRAL VECTORS

The inherent problems with recombinant viruses such as immunogenicity, a.o. reflected in the generation of neutralizing antibodies, and insertional mutagenesis have called for the design of efficient, non-biological vectors for human gene therapy. Non-viral vectors are significantly less immunogenic and are not likely to induce insertional mutagenesis and unwanted homologous recombination after uptake by the cells. They are also relatively easy to be manipulated, produced, and purified on a large scale compared with their viral counterparts. Non-viral gene therapy includes local administration of naked plasmid or using specialized carriers to deliver plasmids. However, their clinical utility is still hampered by the low transfection efficiency, which stems from the nonspecific uptake of the vector by epithelial barriers and extracellular matrix and poor delivery into the therapeutic target cells (Fig. 16.8). The intracellular gene-silencing machinery also prevents the long-term transgene expression. New emerging delivery systems and vector-constructing technologies try to address these issues.

■ Physical Methods for Gene Transfer

Physical methods involve the transfer of naked plasmid by direct disruption of (target) cell membranes. Chemical methods increase the plasmid uptake by the targeted cells using lipid-, peptide-, or polymer-based carriers.

The earliest techniques to deliver recombinant DNA to cellular targets include microinjection, particle bombardment, and electroporation (Table 16.2). Microinjection, direct injection of DNA or RNA into the cytoplasm or nucleus of a single cell, is the simplest and most effective method for physical delivery of genetic material to cells. This transfects 100% of the treated cells and minimizes waste of plasmid DNA. However, it requires highly specialized equipment and skills. Moreover, microinjection is not suitable for in vivo gene transfer or in vitro gene transfer into tissues or organs composed of many cells. Particle bombardment, or gene gun treatment, starts with coating tungsten or gold particles with plasmid DNA. The coated particles are loaded into a gene gun barrel, accelerated with gas pressure and shot into targeted cells or tissues in a petri dish. Particle bombardment can be used to introduce a variety of DNA vaccines into desirable cells in vitro. However, particle bombardment has a low penetration capacity, making it unsuitable for in vivo gene delivery apart from easily accessible tissue, e.g., the skin. Electroporation is used to generate temporary pores in the plasma membrane to transfer plasmid DNA to the cells by an externally applied high-voltage electrical field. Electroporation

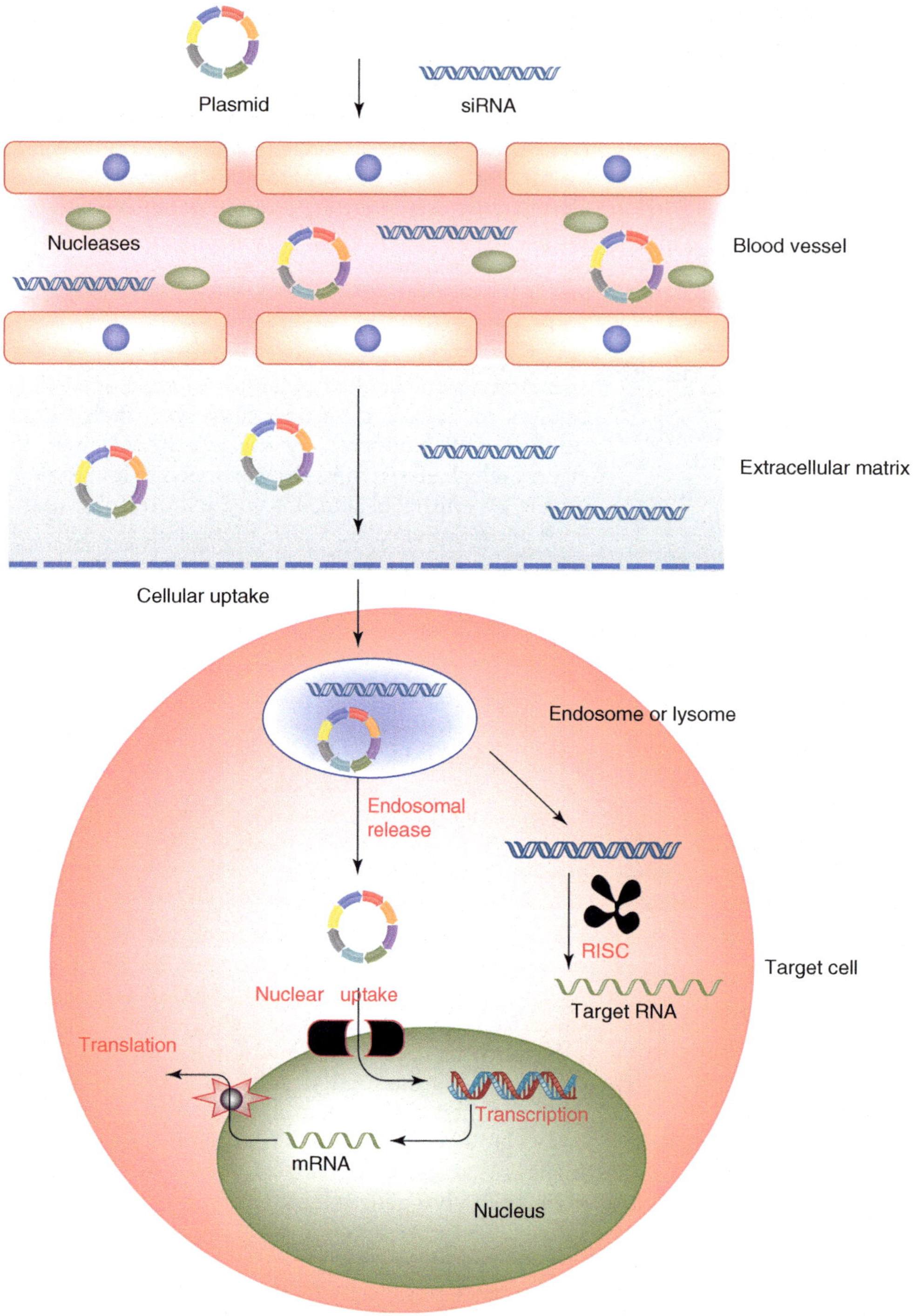

Figure 16.8 ■ Barriers for non-biological gene delivery. Following systemic administration, the gene medicine (plasmid or siRNA) meets blood nucleases. Then they may traverse the blood vessel barrier and the extracellular matrix compartment before crossing the plasma membrane barrier. Upon entering the cell via receptor-mediated endocytosis, they are trapped in endosomes and need to be released into the cytosol. Endosomal escape is a major rate-limiting step in gene delivery. From Singh et al. 2011; with permission to reprint

increases the gene transfer efficiency by 100–1000 folds compared to naked DNA solutions and has met with great success in laboratory practices and clinical trials (Wells 2004). For example, it is frequently used to produce transgenic animals, a powerful tool in preclinical studies (see Chap. 9). Electroporation-mediated gene transfer also demonstrated safety and efficacy in clinical trials to treat melanoma, prostate cancer, and HIV infection (Daud et al. 2008; Vasan et al. 2011). Other physical methods for gene transfer include sonoporation, laser irradiation, magnetofection, and hydroporation. However, because most of the physical methods induce stress and disruption of cellular structure and function, physical methods are less widely studied compared with chemical methods (see below) and are generally restricted to in vitro gene transfer of cultured cells or embryonic stem cells (Table 16.2).

	Advantages	Disadvantages
Naked DNA	No special skills needed, easy to produce	Low transduction efficiency, transient gene expression
Physical methods		
Microinjection	Up to 100% transduction efficiency (nuclear injection)	Requires highly specialized skills for delivery Limited to ex vivo delivery
Gene gun	Easy to perform Effective immunization with low amount of DNA	Poor tissue penetration
Electroporation	High transduction efficiency	Transient gene expression Toxicity, tissue damage Highly invasive
Sonoporation	Method well tolerated for other applications	Transient gene expression Toxicity not yet established
Laser irradiation	Can achieve 100% transduction efficiency	Special skills and expensive equipment necessary
Magnetofection	Safety of method established in the clinic	Poor efficiency with naked DNA
Chemical methods		
Liposomes	Easy to produce	Protein and tissue binding, transient gene expression
Micelles	Easy to produce and manipulate	Unstable Protein and tissue binding
Cationic polymers	High DNA loading Easy to produce and manipulate	Transient gene expression, toxicity
Dendrimers	High DNA loading High transduction efficiency	Extremely toxic
Solid lipid nanoparticles	Low toxicity Controlled release and targeting	NA

NA: Not Applicable

Table 16.2 ■ Summary of non-biological methods used for gene transfer

■ Cationic Lipids

Since the invention of lipofectamine in 1987, numerous cationic lipids have been synthesized and tested for gene delivery. Most cationic lipids are composed of three parts: (1) a hydrophobic lipid anchor group; (2) a linker group, such as an ester, amide, or carbamate; and (3) a positively charged head group, which interacts with the negatively charged plasmid DNA, leading to its condensation and aggregate (nanometer/micrometer range) formation (Fig. 16.9) (Mahato et al. 1997). 2,3-dioleyloxypropyl-1-trimethyl ammonium chloride (DOTMA) and 3-β[N(NV,NV-dimethylaminoethane)-carbamoyl] cholesterol (DC-Chol) are two commonly used cationic lipids with different structures. Cationic lipids are usually mixed with a neutral co-lipid such as dioleoylphosphatidylethanolamine (DOPE) at a certain molar ratio to reduce the toxicity and enhance gene delivery. PEGylation of polyplexes is frequently used to reduce the plasma binding and increase the circulation time of cationic liposomes.

Lipoplexes are taken up by cells through the endosomal route (Fig. 16.8). For endosomal escape and transport to and through the nuclear membrane, additional functional elements may be attached: for endosomal escape (pH sensitive fusogenic peptides), for transport in the cytoplasm, and nuclear membrane passage (a nuclear translocation peptide).

■ Peptides

Just like cationic lipids, cationic peptides condense DNA in a similar manner and can be used as gene delivery carriers. Poly (L-lysine) (PLL), a polydisperse, synthetic repeat of the amino acid lysine, was one of the first cationic peptides to deliver genes. However, increase in length of PLL leads to increasing cytotoxicity. Besides, PLL shows limited transfection efficiency and needs the addition of endosomolytic agents such as fusogenic peptides (see above) to facilitate plasmid release into the cytoplasm. Due to these issues, many researchers have turned to the development of PLL-containing "active" peptides and have met with some success (McKenzie et al. 1999). Such peptides offer many advantages over PLL, such as lower toxicity, precise control of synthesis, and homogeneity of peptide length.

Peptide-based gene delivery systems have the potential to overcome extracellular and intracellular barriers to gene delivery using a single peptide sequence. However, they suffer from nonspecific plasma protein binding and uptake by the reticuloendothelial system. Here again, PEGylation was demonstrated to be an effective strategy to increase the blood circulation time of the complex (Mannisto et al. 2002). Another unique challenge for peptide-based gene delivery systems is cytosolic proteasomes, which degrade unneeded or damaged proteins by proteolysis. Proteasomes destabilize and degrade the DNA/peptide condensates and prevent effective gene transfer. The involvement of proteasomes in the gene delivery process was first identified in AAV-mediated gene transfer and further confirmed in peptide-based, non-viral gene transfer strategies. In

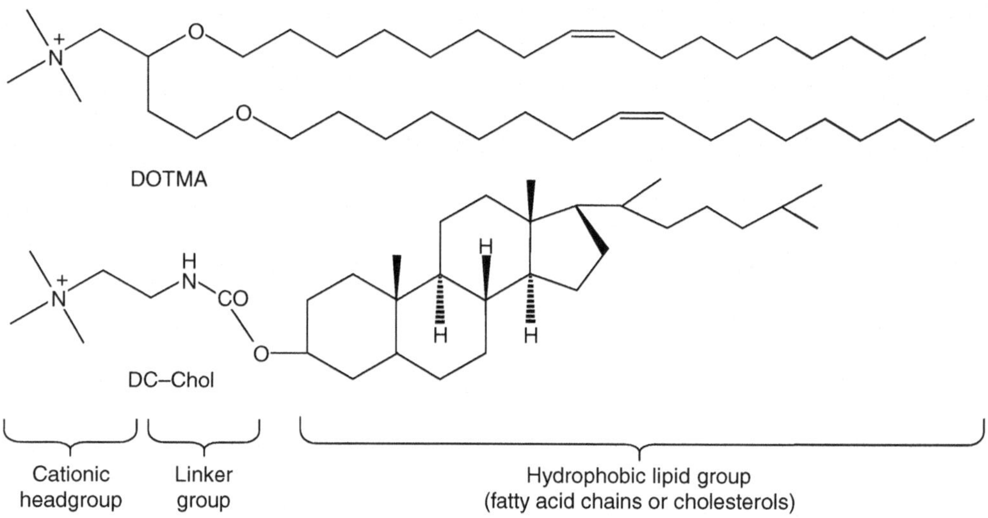

Figure 16.9 ■ Basic components of cationic lipids N-[1-(2,3-dioleyloxy)propyl]-N,N,N-trimethylammonium chloride (DOTMA) and 3-β [N(NV,NV-dimethylaminoethane)-carbamoyl] cholesterol (DC-Chol). From Mahato et al. 1997; with permission to reprint

both cases, gene transfer efficiency was significantly higher in the presence of a proteasome inhibitor (Duan et al. 2000; Kim et al. 2005). Co-administration of proteasome inhibitors is the most effective strategy to address this issue.

■ Polymers

Synthetic and naturally occurring cationic polymers constitute another category of gene carrier. Polyethyleneimine (PEI) has been the most widely used cationic polymer for gene delivery in the last two decades. Boussif et al. first reported that PEI condensed with oligonucleotides and plasmids forms colloid particles (1–1000 nm) that are a highly efficient delivery system, both in vitro and in vivo (Boussif et al. 1995). However, PEI, especially PEI with a high molecular weight (>25 kD), is extremely cytotoxic. PEI induces the disruption of the cell membrane leading to immediate necrotic cell death and disruption of the mitochondrial membrane after internalization leading to apoptosis. PEI binds to blood components, extracellular matrix, and untargeted cells after intravenous injection. Chemical modification of PEI was proposed to overcome these problems. For example, cholesteryl chloroformate readily formed micelles (10–100 nm) in aqueous solution when conjugated to branched PEI (Wang et al. 2002). This new lipopolymer showed decreased toxicity and optimal gene transfer efficiency. A simple mixing of plasmid DNA and PEG-b-PLL polymer resulted in the spontaneous formation of polyion complex (PIC) micelles characterized by small particle size, excellent colloidal stability, and optimal gene transferring ability in serum-containing media (Itaka et al. 2003). However, these micelles are thermodynamically unstable upon dilution and may disintegrate following intravenous injection, leading to inefficient gene transfer. To address this issue, cross-linked micelles were prepared using thiol-modified PEG-b-PLL through the formation of disulfide bonds in the core area (Miyata et al. 2004). These cross-linked micelles are more stable in the blood during circulation, and the disulfide bonds are assumed to be cleavable in the cytoplasm (Miyata et al. 2005). On the other hand, the connection of cyclodextrin-PEI-based polymer (PEI-β-CyD) with TAT peptide (TAT-PEI-β-CyD polymer) improve the transfection efficiency of plasmid DNA delivery to placenta mesenchymal stem cells (Lai et al. 2011).

■ Clinical Use of Non-Viral Vectors

It is not possible, with current non-viral technologies, to match the high transduction efficiencies and high levels of expression reported with certain viral methods in vivo. Nevertheless, non-viral gene therapies may provide a means for achieving short-term expression of therapeutic gene products in certain tissues with a high degree of safety. Principal approval specifications and recommended assays for assessing the final plasmid DNA preparation's purity, safety, and potency for gene therapy and DNA vaccines applications are listed in Table 16.3. There are currently 442 clinical trials using plasmid DNA to treat some diseases (Fig. 16.4). Many of these trials are still in phase I testing so far. Collectively, these clinical studies provided "proof-of-principle" for non-viral gene therapy but also highlighted the need for the development of formulations with enhanced transfection efficiency and therapeutic efficacy. It should also be mentioned that most of these trials were uncontrolled, open-label, phase I designs primarily investigating safety and feasibility. The possibility of strong placebo effects cannot be overlooked in these trials. The efficacy results from these studies should be interpreted with caution and can only be assessed by conducting further phase II/III trials.

Impurity	Recommended assay	Approval specification
Proteins	BCA protein assay	< 3 μg/mg pDNA
RNA	Analytical HPLC	<0.2 μg/mg pDNA
gDNA	Real-time PCR	<0.2 μg/mg pDNA
Endotoxins	LAL assay	< 10 E.U./mg pDNA
Plasmid isoforms (linear, relaxed, denatured)	Analytical HPLC or capillary gel electrophoresis	<3%
Bacterial and fungal	Method outlined in 21 CFR 610.12	No growth
Biological activity and identity	Restriction endonucleases	Coherent fragments with the plasmid restriction map
	Agarose gel electrophoresis	Expected migration from size and supercoiling
	Transformation efficiency	Comparable with plasmid standards

Information compiled from references (Manthorpe et al. 2005; U.S. Department of Health and Human Services 1998). *BCA* Bicinchoninic Acid, *LAL* Limulus amebocyte lysate

Table 16.3 ■ Principal approval specifications and recommended assays for assessing the final plasmid DNA preparation purity, safety, and potency for gene therapy and DNA vaccines applications

STEM CELL-BASED GENE THERAPY

Ex vivo gene therapy, which refers to the *ex vivo* genetic modification of human cells, including stem cells, is discussed in Chap. 17 'Advanced therapies: therapeutic, manufacturing and regulatory considerations'.

GENOME ENGINEERING FOR GENE THERAPY

The genome of living organisms, especially humans is mostly effected by various agents that cause double-strand breaks (DSB) into the genomic sequence. (Khanna and Jackson 2001). These DSBs are subsequently repaired by the endogenous DNA repair system that leads to targeted mutations in the genome. Since after a DSB living organisms opt for survival, they take the advantage of their own endogenous repair machinery for repairing DSB by either non-homologous end joining (NHEJ) or by homology-directed repair (HDR) (Fig. 16.10). In particular, when following the NHEJ-mediated repair routes, nucleotides are introduced or deleted generating indels. However, alternatively, HDR-mediated repair may lead to the introduction of site-specific mutations or insertion of desired sequences through recombination of exogenously supplied donor DNA template to the target locus. This alternative route evolved as a powerful approach in the life sciences, especially for genome engineering (Capecchi 2005).

Genome engineering or genome editing is a type of engineering that introduces changes (e.g. insertions, deletions or base modifications) in the genome of living organisms. Different engineered nucleases have been developed for this purpose with the common denominator that they bind to unique sequences in the genome where they introduce a DSB. The first genome engineering tools developed were zinc finger nucleases (ZFN) and transcription activator-like effector nucleases (TALEN). They have modular protein domains responsible for binding a specific DNA sequence that is fused to a FokI nuclease. The downside of having an engineered protein domain for DNA recognition is that for each genome engineering application a novel TALEN or ZFN needs to be developed, which is time consuming. For this reason, clustered regularly interspaced short palindromic repeats associated protein 9 (CRISPR-Cas9) has gained increased popularity as genome engineering tool. It is unique in the sense that DNA binding of this nuclease is mediated by an associated RNA (see section below on CRISPR-Cas9).

■ CRISPR-Cas9 System

The most widely used Type II CRISPR-Cas system for genome engineering is the CRISPR array and *Cas* genes. The basic features of this system are shown in Fig. 16.10. The *Cas* genes cluster is located adjacent to the CRISPR array having a series of repetitive sequences separated by short stretches of non-repetitive DNA sequence called spacers. These ~20 base-pair long spacers arise from invading viruses and plasmids and are stored for future encounters as an immunological memory. Preceding the *Cas* genes, the trans-activating CRISPR RNA (tracrRNA) gene is located encoding for RNA that is homologous to repeats (Jiang and Doudna 2017). At the adaptation stage, proteins Cas1, Cas2, and Csn2 identify and integrate exogenous genetic elements from viruses and plasmids into the CRISPR array forming a new spacer (Heler et al. 2015). Following integration, the CRISPR array and new spacer are co-transcribed into a long precursor RNA (pre-crRNA) containing repeats and spacers. On the other side, the tracrRNA is also transcribed and hybridized to repeats of pre-crRNA to form a short crRNA unit in the maturation stage by bacterial RNase III. Further processing of the 5′ end of crRNA results in a 20 nucleotides-long crRNA with a single spacer flanked by a part of a repeat sequence. Finally, the mature crRNA and tracrRNA form a complex with Cas-associated

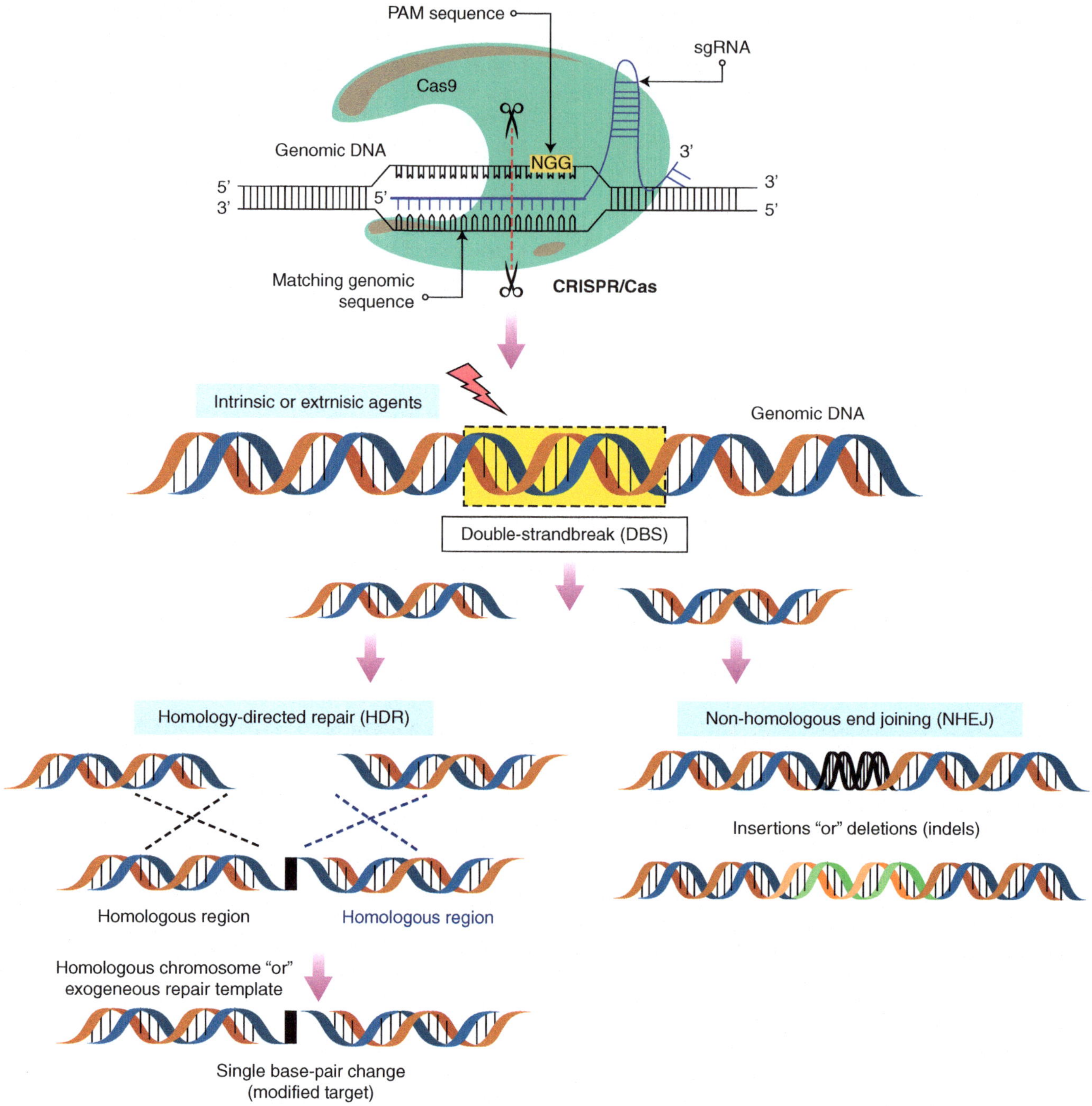

Figure 16.10 ■ The nucleases or various intrinsic and extrinsic agents mediated DNA DSBs repair mechanisms by HDR and NHEJ. A representation of the CRISPR-Cas9 system recognizing the target DNA, resulting in the formation of a DNA DSB break. The DNA DSB break is detected by the cellular DNA repair machinery and subsequently repaired via HDR and NHEJ

nuclease 9 (Cas9) and this cleaves the DNA strand complementary to the guide RNA (Kennedy and Cullen 2015). Since the protospacer is associated with a protospacer adjacent motif (PAM) within the target DNA, the crRNA-tracrRNA-Cas9 complex scans for the foreign DNA target inside the cells containing the crRNA complementary sequence preceding PAM leading to degradation of the target nucleic acid (Burnight et al. 2018).

■ Application of CRISPR-Cas9 in Gene Therapy

CRISPR/Cas9-based genome editing holds a great potential to provide an entirely new class of therapeutics. However, to achieve an effective therapeutic efficacy, the delivery of CRISPR-Cas9 components to the target cells of the patients is still a major hurdle and a prime topic for research. Several studies suggest an efficient delivery of the ~4 kb Cas9 from *Streptococcus pyogenes* into mammalian cells using adenoviral and lentiviral vectors (Eyquem et al. 2017). Non-viral approaches including cationic polymer-based vectors (Platt et al. 2014), cationic lipid-based vectors (Zuris et al. 2015), and conjugated vectors (Ramakrishna et al. 2014) are also studied as delivery vehicles. For instance, in a recent study, CRISPR-Cas9 was used to target frequently mutated oncogene KRAS alleles in cancer cells and in vivo tumors using lentivirus or AAV expressing Cas9 and single guide RNA (sgRNA) (Kim et al. 2018). Also, more than 97% reduction in serum transthyretin level was achieved in mice when the CRISPR-Cas9 system was delivered using lipid nanoparticles (Finn et al. 2018). Other, ex vivo, delivery methods such as electroporation and nucleofection, are also extensively applied for delivery of CRISPR-Cas9 components.

DISEASE TARGETS FOR GENE THERAPY

There are currently 2597 active gene therapy clinical trials worldwide (Fig. 16.11). Approximately 65% of these trials are for cancer treatment. Treatment of monogenetic diseases, cardiovascular diseases, and infectious diseases each take ~7 to 10% of the number of active clinical trials. Treatment of neurological diseases, which has expanded very fast in the last 10 years, is the goal of ~2% of active clinical trials (Fig. 16.12). Currently, gene therapy trials are primarily performed in the United States (63.3% of all trials), the United Kingdom (8.5%), and Germany (3.5%). The geographical distribution of gene therapy clinical trials is summarized in Fig. 16.13. General indications for all gene therapy trials in the clinic are summarized in Table 16.4.

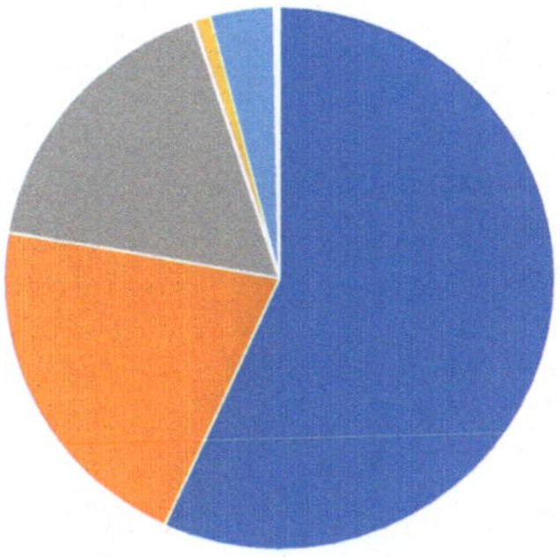

Phase	Number	%
1 Phase I	1476	56.8
2 Phase I/II	544	20.9
3 Phase II	445	17.1
4 Phase II/III	25	1
5 Phase III	98	3.8
6 Phase IV	3	0.1
7 Single subject	6	0.2

Figure 16.11 ■ Phases of gene therapy in clinical trials (Wiley 2017, http://www.abedia.com/wiley/phases.php).

CANCER GENE THERAPY

Most of today's gene therapy clinical trials are devoted to treat cancer. There are two potential benefits of using gene therapy to treat-prevent cancer: (a) gene-based treatments can attack existing cancer at the molecular level, eliminating the need for drugs, radiation, or surgery and (b) identifying and correcting cancer susceptibility genes in individuals or families that may have a significant impact in preventing the disease before it occurs.

Strategies to achieve these goals include (a) correction of genetic mutations contributing to the malignant phenotype by replacing missing genes or altered defect genes with healthy genes, (b) enhancement of a patient's immune response to cancer (immunotherapy), (c) insertion of genes into cancer cells to make them more sensitive to conventional chemotherapy and radiotherapy or other treatments, (d) introduction of "suicide genes" into a patient's cancer cells that can enzymatically activate a prodrug in these cells to destroy them, and (e) direct tumor killing through oncolytic viruses.

■ Correction of Genetic Mutations

In this approach, gene therapy is used to correct genetic mutations contributing to the malignant phenotype by replacing missing genes or removing defect genes. Understanding cancer at the molecular level is the starting point for gene correction in cancer therapy.

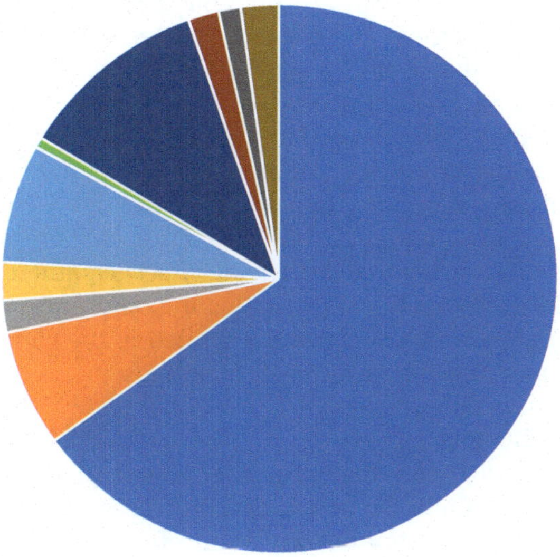

	Indications	%	Number
1	Cancer diseases	65	1688
2	Cardiovascular diseases	6.9	180
3	Gene marking	1.9	50
4	Healthy volunteers	2.2	56
5	Infectious diseases	7	182
6	Inflammatory diseases	0.6	15
7	Monogenic diseases	11.1	287
8	Neurological diseases	1.8	47
9	Ocular diseases	1.3	34
10	Others	2.2	58

Figure 16.12 ■ Disease targets of gene therapy clinical trials (Wiley 2017, http://www.abedia.com/wiley/indications.php). Other diseases include inflammatory bowel disease, rheumatoid arthritis, chronic renal disease, carpal tunnel syndrome, Alzheimer's disease, diabetic neuropathy, Parkinson's disease, erectile dysfunction, retinitis pigmentosa, and glaucoma

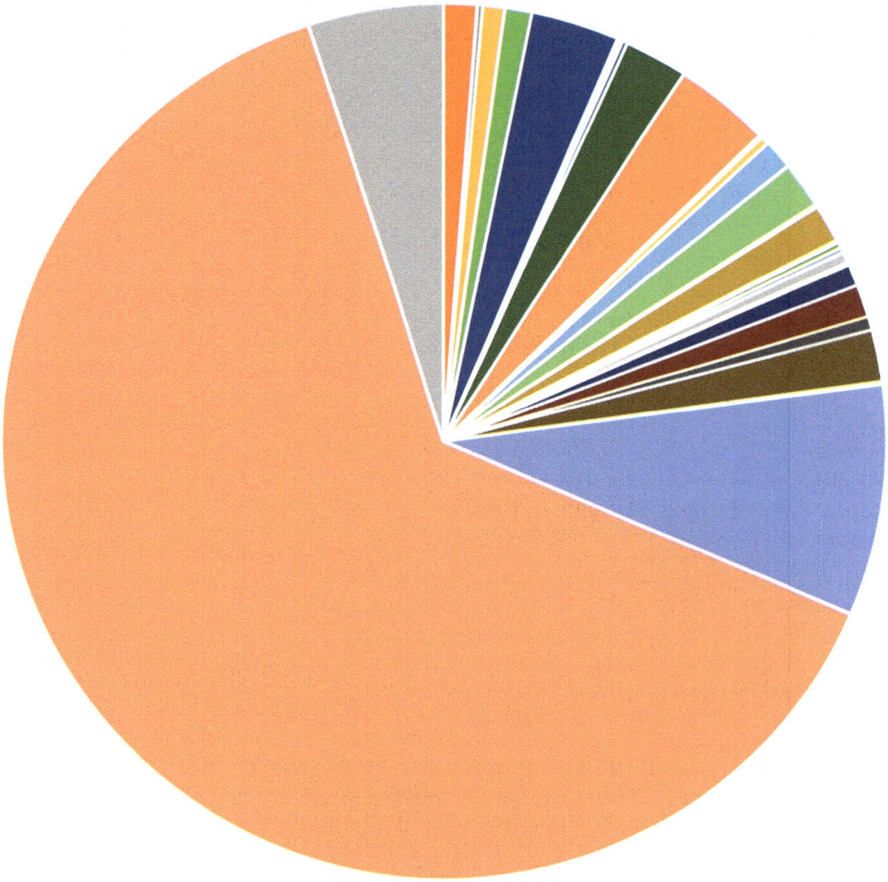

	Country	%	Number
1	Argentina	0	1
2	Australia	1.2	32
3	Austria	0.2	4
4	Belgium	0.8	22
5	Burkina Faso	0	1
6	Canada	1	27
7	China	3.2	84
8	Czech Republic	0.1	2
9	Denmark	0.1	2
10	Egypt	0	1
11	Finland	0.2	6
12	France	2.3	59
13	Gambia	0	1
14	Germany	3.5	92
15	Ireland	0.1	2
16	Israel	0.3	8
17	Italy	1.1	28
18	Japan	1.7	44
19	Kenya	0	1
20	Kuwait	0	1
21	Mexico	0.1	2
22	Netherlands	1.4	37
23	New Zealand	0.1	2
24	Norway	0.2	4
25	Poland	0.2	6
26	Romania	0	1
27	Russia	0.4	10
28	Saudi Arabia	0	1
29	Senegal	0	1
30	Singapore	0.1	3
31	South Korea	0.8	20
32	Spain	1.2	32
33	Sweden	0.5	13
34	Switzerland	1.9	50
35	Taiwan	0.1	2
36	Uganda	0	1
37	UK	8.5	221
38	USA	63.3	1643
39	Multi-country	5	130

Figure 16.13 ■ International status of gene therapy clinical trials (Wiley 2017, http://www.abedia.com/wiley/countries.php)

The inactivation or activation of certain genes may contribute to tumor growth. Although the complex process of tumor development and growth limits the utility of this strategy, approximately 12% of cancer gene therapy clinical trials involve overexpression of tumor-suppressor genes such as p53, MDA-7, and ARF (Majhen and Ambriovic-Ristov 2006). Mutations in the p53 gene are most commonly seen in a wide spectrum of tumors (Roth and Cristiano 1997). Efficient delivery and expression of the wild-type p53 tumor-suppressor gene prevents the growth of human cancer cells in culture, causes regression of established human tumors in nude mice, or sensitizes existing tumors to the therapeutic effect of conventional chemotherapy and radiotherapy (Roth and Cristiano 1997). The results from clinical trials indicated that the therapeutic effect of gendicine, the first gene therapy product was promising in patients with head and neck squamous cancers (Peng 2005). However, the results were only validated in China. Gendicine has also been used to treat various other cancers, which prolong overall survival when combined with other drugs. Although it does not show any adverse effects on the patients, vector-associated transient fever that lasts for only a few hours cannot be overcome in 50–60% of the patients (Zhang et al. 2018). Efficient delivery of tumor-suppressor genes deep within tumors is difficult, and restriction of gene expression in malignant tissue is challenging. Gene silencing by this approach has also limited success, especially when a prolonged silencing effect is required. Despite these reservations, prostate, lung, and pancreatic tumors have been successfully treated in the clinic with a variety of genes and transfer methods.

■ Immunotherapy

In this approach, gene therapy is used to stimulate the body's natural ability to attack cancer cells. One best example of gene therapy that works by stimulating the

Cancer	**Other diseases**	**Cardiovascular disease**
Gynecological	Inflammatory bowel disease	Peripheral vascular disease
Breast, ovary, cervix	Rheumatoid arthritis	Intermittent claudication
Nervous system	Chronic renal disease	Critical limb ischemia
Glioblastoma, leptomeningeal carcinomatosis, glioma, astrocytoma, neuroblastoma	Fractures	Myocardial ischemia
Gastrointestinal	Erectile dysfunction	Coronary artery stenosis
Colon, colorectal, liver metastases, post-hepatitis liver cancer, pancreas	Anemia of end stage renal disease	Stable and unstable angina
Genitourinary	Parotid salivary hypofunction	Venous ulcers
Prostate, renal	Type I diabetes	Vascular complications of diabetes
Skin	Detrusor overactivity	Pulmonary hypertension
Melanoma	Graft-versus-host disease	Heart failure
Head and neck		
Nasopharyngeal carcinoma	*Monogenic disorders*	*Infectious disease*
Lung	Cystic fibrosis	HIV/AIDS
Adenocarcinoma, small cell, non-small cell	Severe combined immunodeficiency (SCID)	Tetanus
Mesothelioma	Alpha-1 antitrypsin deficiency	Epstein-Barr virus
Hematological	Hemophilia A and B	Cytomegalovirus infection
Leukemia, lymphoma, multiple myeloma	Hurler syndrome	Adenovirus infection
Sarcoma	Hunter syndrome	Japanese encephalitis
Germ cell	Huntington's chorea	Hepatitis C
	Duchenne muscular dystrophy	Hepatitis B
Neurological diseases	Becker muscular dystrophy	Influenza
Alzheimer's disease	Canavan disease	
Carpal tunnel syndrome	Chronic granulomatous disease (CGD)	
Cubital tunnel syndrome	Familial hypercholesterolemia	
Diabetic neuropathy	Gaucher disease	
Epilepsy	Fanconi's anemia	
Multiple sclerosis	Purine nucleoside phosphorylase deficiency	
Myasthenia gravis	Ornithine transcarbamylase deficiency	
Parkinson's disease	Leukocyte adherence deficiency	
Peripheral neuropathy	Gyrate atrophy	
	Fabry disease	
Ocular diseases	Familial amyotrophic lateral sclerosis	
Age-related macular degeneration	Junctional epidermolysis bullosa	
Diabetic macular edema	Wiskott-Aldrich syndrome	
Glaucoma	Lipoprotein lipase deficiency	
Retinitis pigmentosa	Late infantile neuronal ceroid lipofuscinosis	
Superficial corneal opacity	RPE65 mutation (retinal disease)	
	Mucopolysaccharidosis	

Information obtained from reference (Ginn et al. 2018).

Table 16.4 ■ Conditions for which human gene transfer trials have been approved

immune response of patient is Imlygic® (talimogene laherparepvec). It is a genetically engineered herpex simplex virus-1, which is designed to infect and make copies of itself by replicating within the cancer cells to produce an immunostimulatory protein called GM-CSF. Imlygic® shows its anti-tumor immune response by entering the cancer cell; it uses the cell's energy to replicate, thus inducing the cancer cells to lyse-die. Once an infected cancer cell dies, the viruses are released into the bloodstream of the patient to infect other cancer cells without infecting or replicating in healthy cells. Immunotherapy through ex vivo genetic modification of patient's cells is discussed in detail in Chap 17.

■ Tumors Sensitization

In this approach, genes are inserted into cancer cells to make them more sensitive to conventional chemotherapy and radiotherapy or other treatments. We previously mentioned that transgene expression of p53 indeed sensitized the tumors to the therapeutic effect of conventional chemotherapy and radiotherapy (Lesoon-Wood et al. 1995; Chen et al. 1996). In other studies, the RNAi mechanism (see Chap. 15) was used to overcome multidrug resistance (MDR) in cancer cells. MDR, which typically represents overexpression of P-glycoprotein, a drug efflux transporter on cancer cell membranes, is a frequent impediment to successful chemotherapy. Synthetic siRNA or vector-mediated MDR1 gene silencing were widely reported to be successful to reduce the chemoresistance of certain types of cancers (Huang et al. 2008). Since, miRNAs have the ability to target multiple genes at the same time, the use of miR-205-5p, which was downregulated in gemcitabine resistant pancreatic cancer cells, resensitizes the cells to gemcitabine after its overexpression (Chaudhary et al. 2017; Mondal et al. 2017; Mittal et al. 2014; Singh et al. 2013).

■ Gene-Directed Enzyme-Prodrug Therapy

In this approach, gene therapy aims to maximize the effect of a toxic drug and to minimize its systemic effects by generating the drug *in-situ* within the tumor. In the first step of this procedure, the gene for an exogenous enzyme is delivered and expressed in the tumor cells. Subsequently, a prodrug is administered and converted to the active drug (toxic metabolites) by the foreign enzyme expressed inside or on the surface of tumor cells (Fig. 16.14). The suicide gene is usually of viral or prokaryotic origin with no human homolog. However, this is not an absolute requirement provided the prodrug is not activated to any significant degree by the native cellular enzyme. In preclinical studies, Chen et al. first reported a successful combination of a suicide gene/prodrug system and immunotherapy to treat hepatic metastases in mice (Chen et al. 1996). Uckert et al. further improved the system to a double suicide gene system as a safety mechanism for the elimination of tumor cells in a reliable fashion (Uckert et al. 1998). There are several variants of gene-directed enzyme-prodrug therapy. The herpes simplex virus-thymidine kinase (HSV-tk)/ganciclovir system, the cytosine deaminase/5-fluorocytosine system and the nitroreductase/CB1954 system, and the carboxypeptidase G2/CMDA system are the most "popular" systems (Fig. 16.13). Cerepro is a gene medicine developed by Ark Therapeutics Ltd. and has been granted orphan drug status by the European Medicines Agency and the FDA. Cerepro is an adenovirus that contain herpes simplex type-1 thymidine kinase transgene for treating malignant glioma together with ganciclovir. In a phase II clinical trial with Cerepro, the mean survival time of patients increased to 15 months as compared to 7.4 months in patients treated with retroviral therapy or 8.3 months with a noneffective adenovirus (Sandmair et al. 2000). However, Ark Therapeutics Ltd. notified the Committee for Medicinal Products for Human Use (CHMP) for withdrawing their marketing authorization application for Cerepro in 2010 (Figs. 16.15 and 16.16).

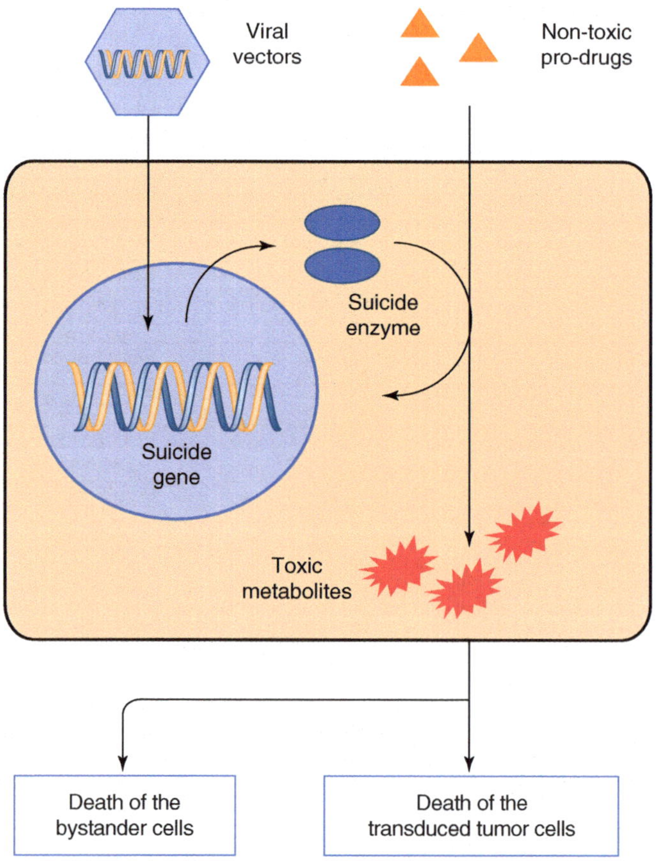

Figure 16.14 ■ A schematic illustration of gene-directed enzyme-prodrug therapy. The suicide gene for an exogenous enzyme is delivered and expressed in the tumor cells. Then a prodrug is administered and converted to the active drug by the foreign enzyme expressed inside or on the surface of tumor cells

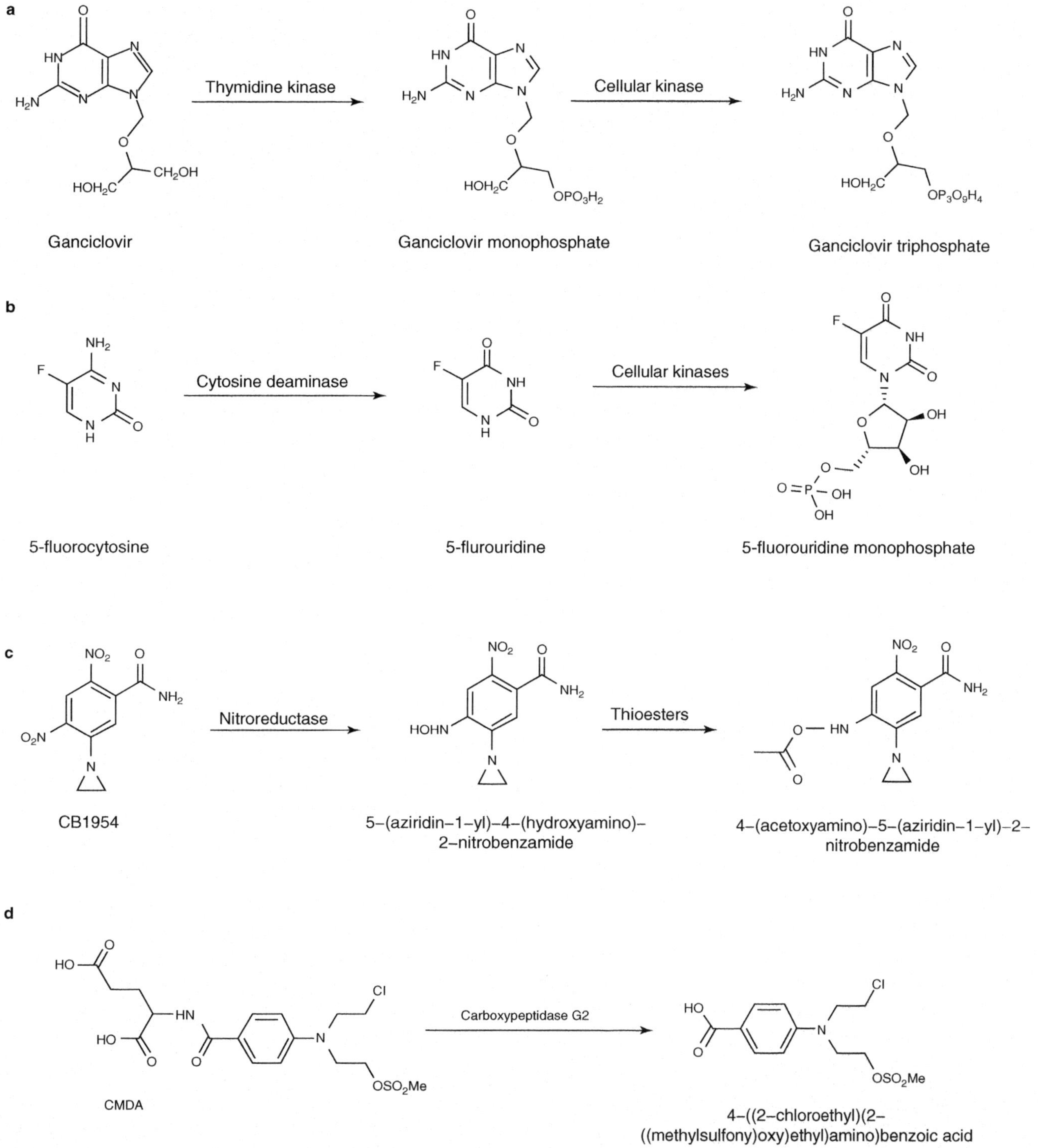

Figure 16.15 ■ Models of gene-directed enzyme-prodrug therapy. (**a**) The herpes simplex virus-thymidine kinase (HSV-tk) system. A vector expressing the gene for HSV-tk enters a cellular target. This enzyme is expressed and phosphorylates the drug ganciclovir. This is subsequently converted to the di- and triphosphate forms by guanylate kinase and other cellular kinases. The triphosphate is incorporated into cellular DNA during cell division causing single strand breaks. (**b**) The cytosine deaminase/5-fluorocytosine system. A vector expressing cytosine deaminase (CD) enters a cellular target. Overexpression of CD activates 5-fluorocytosine (5-FC) to 5-fluorouridine (5-FU). 5-FU is converted to mono-, di-, and triphosphate forms by cellular kinases. All these compounds are cytotoxic. (**c**) The nitroreductase/CB1954 system. A vector expressing E. coli nitroreductase enters a cellular target. Expression of NTR allows the cell to convert the compound CB1954 to a potent DNA-cross-linking agent. (**d**) The carboxypeptidase G2/CMDA system. The bacterial enzyme carboxypeptidase G2 (CPG2) can cleave the glutamic acid moiety from the prodrug releasing the DNA-cross-linking mustard drug 4-[(2-chloroethyl-2-mesyloxyethyl) amino] benzoic acid without further catalytic requirements

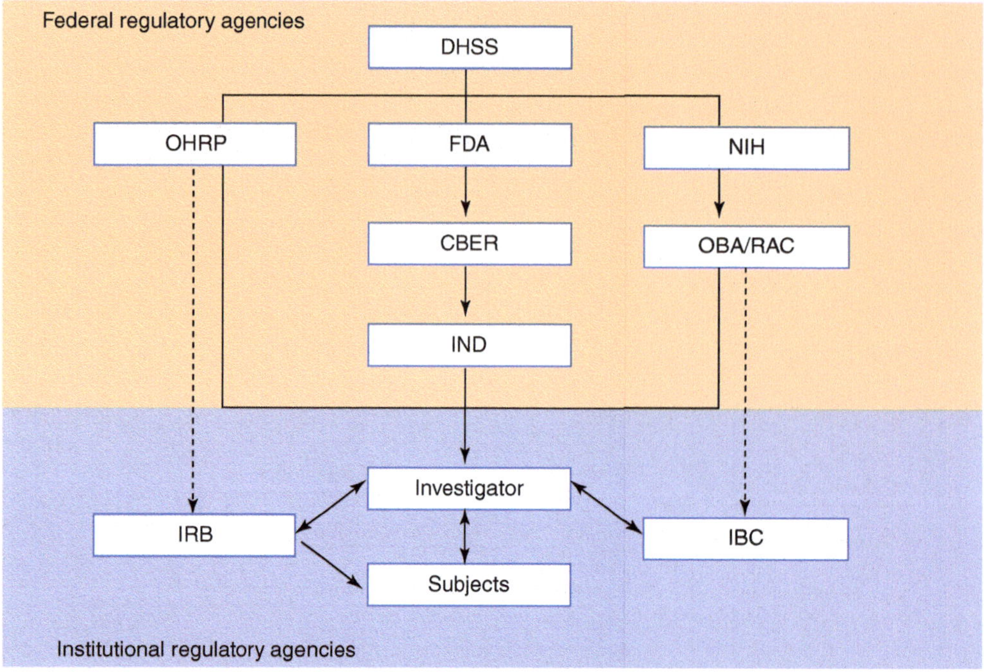

Figure 16.16 ■ The interactions of the regulatory agencies involved in the implementation of a gene therapy protocol. Abbreviations are explained in the text. From Mendell and Miller (2004) with permission to reprint

■ Oncolytic Viruses (Virotherapy)

In this approach, oncolytic viruses were directly introduced into tumors to induce cell death through viral replication, expression of cytotoxic proteins, and cell lysis. Vaccinia virus, herpes simplex type-I (HSV), reovirus, newcastle disease virus, poliovirus, and adenovirus are often selected for this application because they naturally target cancers and contain genomes that can be easily manipulated. Despite some clinical success, significant safety precautions must be taken, making clinical trials with these viruses extremely expensive and cumbersome (Markert et al. 2000; Varghese and Rabkin 2002). The clearance of the virus by cellular immunity and preexisting neutralizing antibodies in most of the population also negatively affects the efficacy of virotherapy. In 2006, Oncorine, a drug made of conditionally replicative adenoviruses by Shanghai Sunway Biotech Co., Ltd. gained marketing approval in China for treating head and neck cancer. This adenovirus contains a deletion in the E1B 55 K region and only replicates in p53-deficient cancer cells. The company has claimed significant benefits of using Oncorine in clinical trials of lung cancer, liver cancer, pancreatic cancer, and malignant effusion (Xia et al. 2004). The first oncolytic virus named ECHO-7 was approved in 2004 for the treatment of skin melanoma by a national regulatory agency. After years of long research, it was also approved in Georgia and Armenia in 2015 and 2016, respectively. Similarly, OncoVex was the first genetically modified herpes simplex virus approved in 2015 for the treatment of advanced inoperable melanoma by the FDA and European Medicines Agency (EMA).

■ Non-viral Gene Therapy

In the last three decades, gene therapy has been widely used in clinical trials for cancer treatment and the results were quite encouraging. Most of the clinical trials employed viral vector-based gene therapeutics, probably because of the high transfection efficiency of this strategy. Despite the fact that non-viral-based gene therapeutics are safer and less tumorigenic, extensive work is still needed to further optimize this strategy. For instance, by increasing transgene expression, reducing plasma protein binding, avoiding the reticuloendothelial system (RES), and escaping from the endosome, etc. non-viral-based gene therapy efficacy can be enhanced.

MONOGENETIC DISEASES

The greatest successes of gene therapy to date have been achieved in treating monogenetic diseases, which is the second largest disease group treated by gene therapy, comprising 11.1% of all the active gene therapy clinical trials in 2017 (Fig. 16.12). The ultimate therapeutic goal of gene therapy for monogenetic disorders is to permanently replace a defect gene with a 'good' copy to restore normal function and permanently reverse disease processes. To date, clinical trials have not met this objective. Of the 287 active clinical gene therapy trials for monogenetic diseases, approximately one third targeted cystic fibrosis (CF), the most common inherited genetic disease in Europe and the United States (Wiley 2017, Fig. 16.12). Until now, the group of severe combined immunodeficiency diseases (SCID), comprising 20% of the trials for inherited disorders, is the only group of diseases in which gene therapy has shown a lasting, clinically meaningful therapeutic benefit. Other monogenetic diseases currently in clinical trials are listed in Table 16.4.

Issues which have prevented successful gene transfer for monogenetic diseases are (a) lack of suitable gene delivery technologies, (b) unfavorable interactions between the host and gene transfer vector, (c) complex biology and pathology of monogenetic diseases and target organs, and (d) lack of relevant measures to assess the clinical efficacy and long-term efficacy of gene transfer. The greatest challenges that remain in treating monogenetic diseases are to induce gene expression sufficiently to correct the clinical phenotype without induction of host immune responses and minimizing the risk of insertional mutagenesis for integrating vectors in target cells. Improvements in vector technology and advancements in the understanding of cellular processes will vastly improve methods for correction of genetic diseases.

CARDIOVASCULAR DISEASES

Cardiovascular diseases are the fourth largest group of diseases actively treated by gene therapy clinical trials (Wiley 2017). The current understanding of molecular mechanisms of cardiovascular diseases has uncovered many genes that could serve as potential targets for molecular therapies. For example, overexpression of genes involved in vasodilation such as endothelial nitric oxide synthase and heme oxygenase-1 or inhibition of molecules involved in vasoconstriction (angiotensin converting enzyme, angiotensinogen) have reduced blood pressure in animal models of hypertension (Melo et al. 2006). Most clinical trials for cardiovascular diseases are designed for treating coronary and peripheral ischemia. Overexpression of pro-angiogenic factors such as vascular endothelial growth factor (VEGF), fibroblast growth factor (FGF), and hepatocyte growth factor (HGF) have been effective in myocardial and peripheral ischemia in preclinical studies (Springer 2006). Despite the lack of significant benefit in several earlier clinical trials, VEGF gene therapy did show an excellent safety profile and improvement of symptoms in patients following adenovirus or plasmid intramyocardial administration in both pilot studies and long-term follow-ups (Stewart et al. 2006; Reilly et al. 2005). However, limited success was experienced in using gene therapy to treat cardiovascular diseases compared to other areas. Larger, double-blind, randomized, placebo-controlled trials are needed to minimize the potential bias for placebo effects suspected to occur in some trials. Stringent criteria for patient selection are needed as many with cardiovascular disease often have underlying conditions that may influence the results. Endpoints for assessing efficacy and measures to assess potential short- and long-term complications must also be standardized among research groups. The efficacy of gene therapy for cardiovascular disease will most likely be enhanced by strategies that incorporate multiple gene targets with cell-based approaches. Few of the gene therapy approaches for cardiovascular diseases are in phase II or III clinical trials. These include generation of VEGF, FGF, sarcoendoplasmic reticulum calcium-ATPase 2a (SERCA2a), stromal-derived factor-1 (SDF-1) etc. (Rincon et al. 2015; Wolfram and Donahue 2013).

INFECTIOUS DISEASES

One hundred and eighty-two clinical trials for treating infectious diseases have been initiated, comprising 7% of the total number of gene therapy clinical trials (Wiley 2017). Gene transfer for acquired immunodeficiency syndrome (AIDS) is the main application in this category. Many gene therapy trials for AIDS involve ex vivo transfer of genetic material to autologous T cells using self-inactivating or conditionally replicating viral vectors to improve the immune system of the patients (Levine et al. 2006; Manilla et al. 2005). Other trials employed overexpression of HIV inhibitors such as RevM10 to increase $CD4^+$ T cell survival in HIV-infected individuals (Morgan et al. 2005; Ranga et al. 1998).

The most important achievement in the gene therapy studies to treat infectious diseases is the development of DNA vaccination. It is an approach for the treatment or prevention of diseases by producing an immunological response through injecting genetically engineered viral DNA (Cf. Chap. 14). Legally, it is not seen as gene therapy, but the techniques used are largely the same. Clinical studies using DNA vaccines for other infectious diseases caused by hepatitis B virus (HBV), influenza virus, and Ebola virus were also reported (Tacket et al. 1999). In 2010, researchers from the USA and France reported the first HIV DNA vaccine that can induce a long-lasting HIV-specific immune response in nonhuman primates, a discovery that could prove significant in the development of HIV vaccines (Arrode-Bruses et al. 2010). Currently, PENNVAX®-GP, a DNA vaccine product for HIV developed by Inovio Pharmaceuticals Inc., is in a phase I clinical study. In 2018, Inovio Pharmaceuticals Inc. announced that an HIV-vaccine maintained a robust immune response in a study in humans.

NEUROLOGICAL DISEASES

Significant progress has been made in gene therapy for neurological diseases in the last 10 years. The two most common neurological diseases targeted by gene therapy are Alzheimer's disease and Parkinson's disease. In 2005, a phase I trial of ex vivo nerve growth factor (NGF) gene delivery in eight individuals with mild Alzheimer disease was performed at the University of California in San Diego. Briefly, autologous fibroblasts obtained from small skin biopsies of the patient were genetically modified to produce and secrete human NGF using retroviral vectors and reimplanted into the forebrain. The results indicated improvement in the rate of cognitive decline, significant increases in cortical 18-fluorodeoxyglucose concentrations (by PET imaging), and robust nerve growth responses to NGF (Tuszynski et al. 2005). In 2007, the first gene therapy clinical trial was conducted at the New York Presbyterian Hospital. Briefly, serial doses of AAV encoding glutamic acid decarboxylase (GAD) were infused into the subthalamic nucleus of patients with Parkinson's disease. The results indicated that AAV-GAD gene therapy is safe and well tolerated by patients with advanced Parkinson's disease. Although this open label, non-randomized phase I study did not include a sham group and was not designed to assess the effectiveness of gene therapy, the preliminary data were encouraging, showing substantial improvements in the Unified Parkinson's Disease Rating Scale (UPDRS), beginning at 3 months after surgery and continuing until the end of the trial (12 months after surgery) (Kaplitt et al. 2007). The outcome of a phase II study with the AAV2-GAD vector supports its further development for the treatment of Parkinson's disease (LeWitt et al. 2011). Today, clinical trials for neurological diseases account for 1.8% of the total number of gene therapy-based clinical trials (Wiley 2017).

REGULATORY ISSUES OF GENE THERAPY PRODUCTS

Any studies involving humans must be carefully reviewed before permission is granted. Gene therapy presents unique safety and infection control issues. This makes it necessary for scientists to take special precautions with gene therapy. In the USA two organizations within the United States Department of Health and Human Services (DHHS), the Office for Human Research Protections (OHRP) and the FDA, have specific authority described in the Code of Federal Regulations (CFR). The OHRP mandates any gene therapy clinical trial involving human subjects to be reviewed, approved, and monitored by the Institutional Review Board (IRB) at each investigative site. The FDA's Center for Biologics Evaluation and Research (CBER) oversees human gene therapy clinical trials conducted by the manufacturers. Any gene therapy product must be tested extensively to meet the FDA requirements for safety and efficacy before approval for marketing is given. All gene therapy clinical trial protocols must be conducted under Investigational New Drug (IND) applications. Regulations pertaining to this process appear in Title 21 of the CFR, Part 312. Another DHHS organization, the NIH oversees the gene therapy studies and clinical trials conducted by federally funded investigators. The NIH monitors scientific progress in human genetics research through the Office of Biotechnology Activities (OBA). Inside OBA, the Recombinant DNA Advisory Committee (RAC) was established in 1974 in response to public concerns regarding the safety of manipulating genetic material using recombinant DNA techniques. Any human gene transfer research receiving the NIH funding must be registered with OBA and reviewed by the RAC. Another responsibility of RAC is to cooperate with the Institutional Biosafety Committees (IBC) to oversee recombinant DNA research at each investigative site. Figure 16.14 shows the interactions of these different regulatory agencies in the development process of a gene product. Other countries also have several committees that must approve gene therapy protocols and address scientific and ethical concerns associated with these clinical trials.

In Europe, and some other jurisdictions, including Canada, most Gene Therapy Medicinal Products (GTMPs) are also considered a GMO. A GMO is any organism, except for human beings, in which the genetic material has been altered in a way that does not occur naturally by mating or natural recombination. In EU a GMO approval must be obtained at a national level, in addition to ethics committee and competent authority approval, before a clinical trial can commence for such investigational GTMPs. However, the regulatory classification processes and requirements for GMO approvals are not sufficiently harmonized between EU member states, despite the EU Deliberate Release (2001/18/EC) and Contained Use (2009/41/EC) Directives, which results in significant challenges and timeline considerations.

In the USA, regulatory product development considerations for gene therapies are quite similar in their basic concepts to those in the EU. However, there are differing processes for clinical trial approval and green light to commence the study. As of April 2016, IBCs and/or IRBs are responsible for recommending protocols involving gene transfer to be submitted to the

NIH for RAC review and a public consultation meeting. Notably, RAC meetings are public discussions, so a clinical trial only can start after a RAC review is completed, when RAC recommendations have been received, and IRB and FDA approvals are available. The additional review by the RAC is often an extra, unplanned regulatory step for developers in the field (approximately an additional 4 months) compared to small molecules and less complex biologics products where a 30-day, no-objection review timeline to add a protocol to an existing IND application is all that is required.

CONCLUDING REMARKS

Within the last 30 years, the field of gene therapy has come a long way from bench to bedside. Many vectors developed for gene transfer have now been tested in the clinic. Various products (as mentioned in the text) have been given marketing approval, and several others are in late phases of testing. Although the biology of gene transfer vectors is well understood, several barriers must be overcome for turning genes into therapeutics. The immune responses and the insertional mutagenesis of viral vectors and the lack of transgene efficiency of non-viral vectors are the most significant barriers for gene therapy. Targeted delivery of gene expression systems and spatial and temporal control of transgene expression in target tissues based on the severity and the nature of the disease are also critical to the success of many gene therapy applications. Although clinical trials have shown short-term safety and efficacy, long-term surveillance over a period of decades is lacking, and the safety and efficacy of genetic medicines have so far only been validated in limited patient populations. Other factors such as the use of concurrent medications and concurrent medical conditions, objective assessment of improvements and endpoints, and the assessment of placebo effects need to be standardized to get reliable and reproducible results among different research groups. In addition, cost-effectiveness analyses must be considered as the production of gene therapy vectors itself is costly and requires specialized equipment and personnel. In the future, further development of genetic medicines that can be widely used will heavily rely on collaborations between academic institutions and commercial partners from the pharmaceutical and biotechnology industries. Further, the rapid advance in the CRISPR-Cas9-based genome engineering system has changed the picture of life science research, providing new therapeutic approaches for personalized medicine through gene therapeutics.

SELF-ASSESSMENT QUESTIONS AND ANSWERS

Questions

1. What was the disease target for the first gene therapy clinical trial? What vector was selected for gene transfer?
2. Identify and describe five transcription regulatory elements discussed in the chapter.
3. Several clinical trials involve gene transfer for treating malignant glioma. One approach involves the use of a recombinant retrovirus expressing the HSV-tk transgene. Another involves the use of a recombinant adenovirus expressing the p53 transgene.
   (a) Which of the five current strategies to treat cancer by viral gene therapy does each of these trials employ? Describe the principle behind each strategy.
   (b) List 2 advantages and 2 disadvantages associated with the vector used in each of these trials.
   (c) Outline potential drawbacks to the use of each of these strategies for cancer therapy.
   (d) What other approaches could have been selected to prevent the growth and spread of malignant tissue? Explain the principle behind each.
4. What is the purpose of the packaging cell line during the production of recombinant viral vectors for gene transfer? What is the risk associated with using packaging cell lines for vector production?
5. Provide two examples of how gene therapy is used to modulate the immune system to fight infection.
6. Describe one clinical trial for retrovirus-based gene therapy and adenovirus-based gene therapy and identify the most significant adverse effects that have been reported for each trial.
7. Identify the three marketed gene therapy products in the world and describe the mechanism of actions of each product.

Answers

1. The first gene therapy clinical trial was initiated in 1990 for treating adenosine deaminase (ADA) deficiency. In this trial, patients with ADA deficiency were given peripheral blood lymphocytes treated with a retroviral vector expressing the ADA transgene.
2. Promoter is a DNA sequence that enables a gene to be transcribed. The promoter is recognized by RNA polymerase and transcriptional factors. Enhancer is a short DNA sequence that can bind transcription factors or activators to enhance tran-

scription levels of a gene from a distance. Insulators are mainly genetic boundary elements to block the enhancer-promoter interaction or rarely as a barrier against condensed chromatin proteins. Operators and silencers are usually short DNA sequence close to the promoter with binding affinity to a set of proteins named repressors and inducers.

3. (a) Retrovirus trial

   Gene-directed enzyme-prodrug therapy. Cells transduced by the virus express an enzyme capable of converting a prodrug (in this case ganciclovir) to a cytotoxic metabolite. This conversion cannot occur in cells that do not express the transgene, limiting the cytotoxic effect to transduced cells and their neighbors through the bystander effect.

   Adenovirus trial

   Correction of genetic mutations that contribute to a malignant phenotype. Cells transduced by the virus express a gene such as p53 that is necessary for controlled cell division and development. This prevents the uncontrolled growth and division associated with malignant disease.

   (b) Retrovirus

   Advantages—(1) Retroviruses can infect dividing cells which are the therapeutic target in this trial. Despite this fact, transduction efficiency of this vector in vivo has been low. (2) Retroviruses can induce long-term gene expression which should be sufficient for effective removal of malignant tissue.

   Disadvantages—(1) Retroviruses have the potential for inducing insertional mutagenesis in normal, healthy cells. (2) Transgene expression is sometimes limited by the host immune response to cellular components acquired by the virus during large scale production.

   Adenovirus

   Advantages—(1) Adenoviruses can infect dividing cells which are the therapeutic target in this trial. (2) Adenoviruses can induce high levels of transgene expression in short periods of time. (3) Adenoviruses do not have the risk of insertional mutagenesis. (4) It is relatively easy to produce large amounts of recombinant adenovirus sufficient for clinical use.

   Disadvantages—(1) Transgene expression is transient, making readministration necessary for continued effect. (2) Adenoviral vectors can induce a potent immune response. This not only limits the success of gene transfer after a second dose of virus but also is associated with severe toxicity at certain doses. (3) Preexisting immunity to adenovirus serotype 5 is common in the general population. This may also limit gene transfer.

   (c) Drawbacks to gene-directed enzyme-prodrug therapy.

   - (1) Efficacy relies on efficient transgene expression and drug bioavailability. (2) The therapeutic effect may spread to healthy cells through the bystander effect.

   Drawbacks to gene correction therapy.

   - (1) Gene correction may stop tumor growth but not eliminate it. (2) Expression is not limited to malignant tissue.

   (d) Other approaches for cancer gene therapy

   - Immunotherapy. A vector expressing pro-inflammatory cytokines, co-stimulatory molecules, or tumor-specific antigens is injected directly into the tumor mass. This facilitates the formation of an antitumor immune response that targets and destroys malignant cells.
   - Virotherapy. A replication-competent virus that naturally targets cancers is directly injected in the tumor mass. The virus can induce cell death during replication in malignant tissue by producing cytotoxic proteins and subsequent cell lysis.

4. (1) The primary purpose of the packaging cell line is to provide genetic elements that support virus replication and assembly. These have been eliminated from the vector to prevent it from causing disease in the patient. (2) The recombinant virus can incorporate elements for replication into its genome through homologous recombination during the production process. The potential for generation of replication-competent virus (RCV) in this manner does exist for each vector but can vary due to specific features of a given packaging cell line.
5. (1) Gene transfer into autologous immunocytes to increase the immune system of a patient. (2) Overexpression of protein inhibitors that interfere with virus infection and replication. (3) Overexpression of known antigenic epitopes of the pathogen by DNA vaccination to stimulate an immune response.
6. (1) One trial employed aerosol administration of a recombinant adenovirus expressing cystic fibrosis transmembrane conductance regulator (CFTR) to treat cystic fibrosis (CF). Another trial employed a recombinant retrovirus expressing recombinant adenosine deaminase (ADA) to transduce autologous T lymphocytes isolated from patients for treating ADA deficiency-induced severe combined immunodeficiency (ADA-SCID). (2) CF trial. Massive immune response to the recombinant viral vector.

   ADA-SCID trial. Lymphoproliferative leukemia caused by insertional mutagenesis.
7. Gendicine is a recombinant adenoviral vector which expresses p53 tumor suppressor and is used to treat patients with head and neck squamous cancers.

Oncorine is a recombinant adenoviral vector which contains a deletion in the E1B 55 K region and only replicates in p53 deficient cancer cells. Oncorine kills tumor cells through viral replication, expression of cytotoxic proteins, and cell lysis. Cerepro is a recombinant adenoviral vector encoding herpes simplex type-1 thymidine kinase (TK).

Cerepro is used for treating malignant glioma together with ganciclovir through gene-directed enzyme-prodrug therapy.

Acknowledgements We would like to thank the National Institutes of Health (NIH) for the financial support (R01DK69968 and R01GM113166).

REFERENCES

Aiuti A, Roncarolo MG, Naldini L (2017) Gene therapy for ADA-SCID, the first marketing approval of an *ex vivo* gene therapy in Europe: paving the road for the next generation of advanced therapy medicinal products. EMBO Mol Med 9(6):737–740

Apolonia L, Waddington SN, Fernandes C, Ward NJ, Bouma G, Blundell MP, Thrasher AJ, Collins MK, Philpott NJ (2007) Stable gene transfer to muscle using non-integrating lentiviral vectors. Mol Ther 15(11):1947–1954

Armentano D, Sookdeo CC, Hehir KM, Gregory RJ, St George JA, Prince GA, Wadsworth SC, Smith AE (1995) Characterization of an adenovirus gene transfer vector containing an E4 deletion. Hum Gene Ther 6(10):1343–1353

Arrode-Bruses G, Sheffer D, Hegde R, Dhillon S, Liu Z, Villinger F, Narayan O, Chebloune Y (2010) Characterization of T-cell responses in macaques immunized with a single dose of HIV DNA vaccine. J Virol 84(3):1243–1253

Bedouelle H, Duplay P (1988) Production in Escherichia coli and one-step purification of bifunctional hybrid proteins which bind maltose. Export of the klenow polymerase into the periplasmic space. Eur J Biochem 171(3):541–549

Bellon G, Michel-Calemard L, Thouvenot D, Jagneaux V, Poitevin F, Malcus C, Accart N et al (1997) Aerosol administration of a recombinant adenovirus expressing CFTR to cystic fibrosis patients: a phase I clinical trial. Hum Gene Ther 8(1):15–25

Bigger BW, Tolmachov O, Collombet JM, Fragkos M, Palaszewski I, Coutelle C (2001) An araC-controlled bacterial cre expression system to produce DNA minicircle vectors for nuclear and mitochondrial gene therapy. J Biol Chem 276(25):23018–23027

Blackburn MR, Kellems RE (2005) Adenosine deaminase deficiency: metabolic basis of immune deficiency and pulmonary inflammation. Adv Immunol 86:1–41

Blaese RM, Culver KW, Miller AD, Carter CS, Fleisher T, Clerici M, Shearer G et al (1995) T lymphocyte-directed gene therapy for ADA-SCID: initial trial results after 4 years. Science 270(5235):475–480

Boussif O, Lezoualc'h F, Zanta MA, Mergny MD, Scherman D, Demeneix B, Behr P (1995) A versatile vector for gene and oligonucleotide transfer into cells in culture and in vivo: polyethylenimine. Proc Natl Acad Sci U S A 92(16):7297–7301

Burnight ER, Giacalone JC, Cooke JA, Thompson JR, Bohrer LR, Chirco KR, Drack AV, Fingert JH, Worthington KS, Wiley LA, Mullins RF, Stone EM, Tucker BA (2018) CRISPR-Cas9 genome engineering: treating inherited retinal degeneration. Prog Retin Eye Res 65:28–49 pii: S1350-9462(17)30079-4

Büning H (2013) Gene therapy enters the pharma market: the short story of a long journey. EMBO Mol Med 5(1):1–3

Capecchi MR (2005) Gene targeting in mice: functional analysis of the mammalian genome for the twenty-first century. Nat Rev Genet 6(6):507–512

Cavazzana-Calvo M, Hacein-Bey S, de Saint Basile G, Gross F, Yvon E, Nusbaum P, Selz F et al (2000) Gene therapy of human severe combined immunodeficiency (SCID)-X1 disease. Science 288(5466):669–672

Chaudhary AK, Mondal G, Kumar V, Kattel K, Mahato RI (2017) Chemosensitization and inhibition of pancreatic cancer stem cell proliferation by overexpression of microRNA-205. Cancer Lett 402:1–8

Chen HH, Mack LM, Kelly R, Ontell M, Kochanek S, Clemens PR (1997) Persistence in muscle of an adenoviral vector that lacks all viral genes. Proc Natl Acad Sci U S A 94(5):1645–1650

Chen SH, Kosai K, Xu B, Pham-Nguyen K, Contant C, Finegold MJ, Woo SL (1996) Combination suicide and cytokine gene therapy for hepatic metastases of colon carcinoma: sustained antitumor immunity prolongs animal survival. Cancer Res 56(16):3758–3762

Chen ZY, He CY, Ehrhardt A, Kay MA (2003) Minicircle DNA vectors devoid of bacterial DNA result in persistent and high-level transgene expression in vivo. Mol Ther 8(3):495–500

Chillon M, Lee JH, Fasbender A, Welsh MJ (1998) Adenovirus complexed with polyethylene glycol and cationic lipid is shielded from neutralizing antibodies in vitro. Gene Ther 5(7):995–1002

Chung TC, Jones CH, Gollakota A, Kamal Ahmadi M, Rane S, Zhang G, Pfeifer BA (2015) Improved Escherichia coli Bactofection and cytotoxicity by heterologous expression of bacteriophage ΦX174 Lysis gene E. Mol Pharm 12(5):1691–1700

Crook NC, Freeman ES, Alper HS (2011) Re-engineering multicloning sites for function and convenience. Nucleic Acids Res 39(14):e92

Croyle MA, Cheng X, Wilson JM (2001) Development of formulations that enhance the physical stability of viral vectors for human gene therapy. Gene Ther 8(17):1281–1291

Dai Y, Schwarz EM, Gu D, Zhang WW, Sarvetnick N, Verma IM (1995) Cellular and humoral immune responses to adenoviral vectors containing factor IX gene: tolerization of factor IX and vector antigens allows for long-term expression. Proc Natl Acad Sci U S A 92(5):1401–1405

Dang CV, Lee WM (1988) Identification of the human c-myc protein nuclear translocation signal. Mol Cell Biol 8(10):4048–4054

Darquet AM, Cameron B, Wils P, Scherman D, Crouzet J (1997) A new DNA vehicle for nonviral gene delivery: supercoiled minicircle. Gene Ther 4(12):1341–1349

Daud AI, Deconti RC, Andrews S, Urbas P, Riker AI, Sondak VK, Munster PN et al (2008) Phase I trial of interleukin-12 plasmid electroporation in patients with metastatic melanoma. J Clin Oncol 26(36):5896–5903

Duan D, Yue Y, Yan Z, Yang J, Engelhardt JF (2000) Endosomal processing limits gene transfer to polarized airway epithelia by adeno-associated virus. J Clin Invest 105(11):1573–1587

Edelstein ML, Abedi MR, Wixon J, Edelstein RM (2004) Gene therapy clinical trials worldwide 1989-2004-an overview. J Gene Med 6(6):597–602

Erles K, Sebokova P, Schlehofer JR (1999) Update on the prevalence of serum antibodies (IgG and IgM) to adeno-associated virus (AAV). J Med Virol 59(3):406–411

Ertl HC (2005) Challenges of immune responses in gene replacement therapy. IDrugs 8(9):736–738

Eyquem J, Mansilla-Soto J, Giavridis T, van der Stegen SJ, Hamieh M, Cunanan KM, Odak A, Gönen M, Sadelain M (2017) Targeting a CAR to the TRAC locus with CRISPR/Cas9 enhances tumor rejection. Nature 543(7643):113–117

Finn JD, Smith AR, Patel MC, Shaw L, Youniss MR, van Heteren J, Dirstine T, Ciullo C, Lescarbeau R, Seitzer J, Shah RR, Shah A, Ling D, Growe J, Pink M, Rohde E, Wood KM, Salomon WE, Harrington WF, Dombrowski C, Strapps WR, Chang Y, Morrissey DV (2018) A single administration of CRISPR/Cas9 lipid nanoparticles achieves robust and persistent in vivo genome editing. Cell Rep 22(9):2227–2235

Flotte T, Carter B, Conrad C, Guggino W, Reynolds T, Rosenstein B, Taylor G, Walden S, Wetzel R (1996) A phase I study of an adeno-associated virus-CFTR gene vector in adult CF patients with mild lung disease. Hum Gene Ther 7(9):1145–1159

Ginn SL, Amaya AK, Alexander IE, Edelstein M, Abedi MR (2018) Gene therapy clinical trials worldwide to 2017: an update. J Gene Med 25:e3015

Hacein-Bey-Abina S, von Kalle C, Schmidt M, Le Deist F, Wulffraat N, McIntyre E, Radford I, Villeval JL, Fraser CC, Cavazzana-Calvo M, Fischer A (2003) A serious adverse event after successful gene therapy for X-linked severe combined immunodeficiency. N Engl J Med 348(3):255–256

Hagstrom JN, Couto LB, Scallan C, Burton M, McCleland ML, Fields PA, Arruda VR, Herzog RW, High KA (2000) Improved muscle-derived expression of human coagulation factor IX from a skeletal actin/CMV hybrid enhancer/promoter. Blood 95(8):2536–2542

Heler R, Samai P, Modell JW, Weiner C, Goldberg GW, Bikard D, Marraffini LA (2015) Cas9 specifies functional viral targets during CRISPR-Cas adaptation. Nature 519(7542):199–202

High KA, Aubourg P (2011) RAAV human trial experience. Methods Mol Biol 807:429–457

Hofmann A, Wenzel D, Becher UM, Freitag DF, Klein AM, Eberbeck D, Schulte M et al (2009) Combined targeting of lentiviral vectors and positioning of transduced cells by magnetic nanoparticles. Proc Natl Acad Sci U S A 106(1):44–49

Huang C, Li M, Chen C, Yao Q (2008) Small interfering RNA therapy in cancer: mechanism, potential targets, and clinical applications. Expert Opin Ther Targets 12(5):637–645

Huang MT, Gorman CM (1990) The simian virus 40 small-t intron, present in many common expression vectors, leads to aberrant splicing. Mol Cell Biol 10(4):1805–1810

Immonen A, Vapalahti M, Tyynela K, Hurskainen H, Sandmair A, Vanninen R, Langford G, Murray N, Yla-Herttuala S (2004) AdvHSV-tk gene therapy with intravenous ganciclovir improves survival in human malignant glioma: a randomised, controlled study. Mol Ther 10(5):967–972

Itaka K, Yamauchi K, Harada A, Nakamura K, Kawaguchi H, Kataoka K (2003) Polyion complex micelles from plasmid DNA and poly(ethylene glycol)-poly(L-lysine) block copolymer as serum-tolerable polyplex system: physicochemical properties of micelles relevant to gene transfection efficiency. Biomaterials 24(24):4495–4506

Jiang F, Doudna JA (2017) CRISPR-Cas9 structures and mechanisms. Annu Rev Biophys 46:505–529

Kaplitt MG, Feigin A, Tang C, Fitzsimons HL, Mattis P, Lawlor PA, Bland RJ et al (2007) Safety and tolerability of gene therapy with an adeno-associated virus (AAV) borne GAD gene for Parkinson's disease: an open label, phase I trial. Lancet 369(9579):2097–2105

Kennedy EM, Cullen BR (2015) Bacterial CRISPR/Cas DNA endonucleases: a revolutionary technology that could dramatically impact viral research and treatment. Virology 479-480:213–220

Khanna KK, Jackson SP (2001) DNA double-strand breaks: signaling, repair and the cancer connection. Nat Genet 27(3):247–254

Kim J, Chen CP, Rice KG (2005) The proteasome metabolizes peptide-mediated nonviral gene delivery systems. Gene Ther 12(21):1581–1590

Kim W, Lee S, Kim HS, Song M, Cha YH, Kim YH, Shin J, Lee ES, Joo Y, Song JJ, Choi EJ, Choi JW, Lee J, Kang M, Yook JI, Lee MG, Kim YS, Paik S, Kim HH (2018) Targeting mutant KRAS with CRISPR-Cas9 controls tumor growth. Genome Res 28(3):374–382. https://doi.org/10.1101/gr.223891.117

Lai WF, Tang GP, Wang X, Li G, Yao H, Shen Z, Lu G, Poon WS, Kung HF, Lin MC (2011) Cyclodextrin-PEI-tat polymer as a vector for plasmid DNA delivery to placenta mesenchymal stem cells. Bionanoscience 1(3):89–96

Lesoon-Wood LA, Kim WH, Kleinman HK, Weintraub BD, Mixson AJ (1995) Systemic gene therapy with p53 reduces growth and metastases of a malignant human breast cancer in nude mice. Hum Gene Ther 6(4):395–405

Levine BL, Humeau LM, Boyer J, Macgregor RR, Rebello T, Lu X, Binder GK, Slepushkin V, Lemiale F, Mascola JR, Bushman FD, Dropulic B, June CH (2006) Gene transfer in humans using a conditionally replicating lentiviral vector. Proc Natl Acad Sci U S A 103(46):17372–17377

Lewitt PA, Rezai AR, Leehey MA, Ojemann SG, Flaherty AW, Eskandar EN, Kostyk SK et al (2011) AAV2-GAD gene therapy for advanced Parkinson's disease: a double-blind, sham-surgery controlled, randomised trial. Lancet Neurol 10(4):309–319

Li F, Mahato RI (2009) Bipartite vectors for co-expression of a growth factor cDNA and short hairpin RNA against an apoptotic gene. J Gene Med 11(9):764–771

Lochmuller H, Petrof BJ, Pari G, Larochelle N, Dodelet V, Wang Q, Allen C et al (1996) Transient immunosuppression by FK506 permits a sustained high-level dystrophin expression after adenovirus-mediated dystrophin minigene transfer to skeletal muscles of adult dystrophic (mdx) mice. Gene Ther 3(8):706–716

Louis N, Evelegh C, Graham FL (1997) Cloning and sequencing of the cellular-viral junctions from the human adenovirus type 5 transformed 293 cell line. Virology 233:423–429

MacGregor RR (2001) Clinical protocol. A phase 1 open-label clinical trial of the safety and tolerability of single escalating doses of autologous CD4 T cells transduced with VRX496 in HIV-positive subjects. Hum Gene Ther 12(16):2028–2029

Mahato RI, Rolland A, Tomlinson E (1997) Cationic lipid-based gene delivery systems: pharmaceutical perspectives. Pharm Res 14(7):853–859

Mahato RI, Smith LC, Rolland A (1999) Pharmaceutical perspectives of nonviral gene therapy. Adv Genet 41:95–156

Majhen D, Ambriovic-Ristov A (2006) Adenoviral vectors–how to use them in cancer gene therapy? Virus Res 119(2):121–133

Manilla P, Rebello T, Afable C, Lu X, Slepushkin V, Humeau LM, Schonely K et al (2005) Regulatory considerations for novel gene therapy products: a review of the process leading to the first clinical lentiviral vector. Hum Gene Ther 16(1):17–25

Mannisto M, Vanderkerken S, Toncheva V, Elomaa M, Ruponen M, Schacht E, Urtti A (2002) Structure-activity relationships of poly(L-lysines): effects of pegylation and molecular shape on physicochemical and biological properties in gene delivery. J Control Release 83(1):169–182

Manthorpe M, Hobart P, Hermanson G, Ferrari M, Geall A, Goff B, Rolland A (2005) Plasmid vaccines and therapeutics: from design to applications. Adv Biochem Eng Biotechnol 99:41–92

Markert JM, Medlock MD, Rabkin SD, Gillespie GY, Todo T, Hunter WD, Palmer CA, Feigenbaum F, Tornatore C, Tufaro F, Martuza RL (2000) Conditionally replicating herpes simplex virus mutant, G207 for the treatment of malignant glioma: results of a phase I trial. Gene Ther 7(10):867–874

McGinley L, McMahon J, Strappe P, Barry F, Murphy M, O'Toole D, O'Brien T (2011) Lentiviral vector mediated modification of mesenchymal stem cells & enhanced survival in an in vitro model of ischaemia. Stem Cell Res Ther 2(2):12

McKenzie DL, Collard WT, Rice KG (1999) Comparative gene transfer efficiency of low molecular weight polylysine DNA-condensing peptides. J Pept Res 54(4):311–318

Medina-Kauwe LK (2003) Endocytosis of adenovirus and adenovirus capsid proteins. Adv Drug Deliv Rev 55(11):1485–1496

Melo LG, Pachori AS, Gnecchi M, Dzau VJ (2006) Genetic therapies for cardiovascular diseases. Trends Mol Med 11(5):240–250

Mendell JR, Miller A (2004) Gene transfer for neurologic disease: agencies, policies, and process. Neurology 63(12):2225–2232

Mittal A, Chitkara D, Behrman SW, Mahato RI (2014) Efficacy of gemcitabine conjugated and miRNA-205 complexed micelles for treatment of advanced pancreatic cancer. Biomaterials 35(25):7077–7087

Miyata K, Kakizawa Y, Nishiyama N, Harada A, Yamasaki Y, Koyama H, Kataoka K (2004) Block catiomer polyplexes with regulated densities of charge and disulfide cross-linking directed to enhance gene expression. J Am Chem Soc 126(8):2355–2361

Miyata K, Kakizawa Y, Nishiyama N, Yamasaki Y, Watanabe T, Kohara M, Kataoka K (2005) Freeze-dried formulations for in vivo gene delivery of PEGylated polyplex micelles with disulfide crosslinked cores to the liver. J Control Release 109(1–3):15–23

Miyoshi H, Takahashi M, Gage FH, Verma IM (1997) Stable and efficient gene transfer into the retina using an HIV-based lentiviral vector. Proc Natl Acad Sci U S A 94(19):10319–10323

Mondal G, Almawash S, Chaudhary AK, Mahato RI (2017) EGFR-targeted cCationic polymeric mixed micelles for codelivery of gemcitabine and miR-205 for treating advanced pancreatic cancer. Mol Pharm 14(9):3121–3133

Montini E, Cesana D, Schmidt M, Sanvito F, Bartholomae CC, Ranzani M, Benedicenti F et al (2009) The genotoxic potential of retroviral vectors is strongly modulated by vector design and integration site selection in a mouse model of HSC gene therapy. J Clin Invest 119(4):964–975

Morgan RA, Walker R, Carter CS, Natarajan V, Tavel JA, Bechtel C, Herpin B, Muul L, Zheng Z, Jagannatha S, Bunnell BA, Fellowes V, Metcalf JA, Stevens R, Baseler M, Leitman SF, Read EJ, Blaese RM, Lane HC (2005) Preferential survival of CD4+ T lymphocytes engineered with anti-human immunodeficiency virus (HIV) genes in HIV-infected individuals. Hum Gene Ther 16(9):1065–1074

Mori S, Wang L, Takeuchi T, Kanda T (2004) Two novel adeno-associated viruses from cynomolgus monkey: pseudotyping characterization of capsid protein. Virology 330(2):375–383

Muul LM, Tuschong LM, Soenen SL, Jagadeesh GJ, Ramsey WJ, Long Z, Carter CS, Garabedian EK, Alleyne M, Brown M, Bernstein W, Schurman SH, Fleisher TA, Leitman SF, Dunbar CE, Blaese RM, Candotti F (2003) Persistence and expression of the adenosine deaminase gene for 12 years and immune reaction to gene transfer components: long-term results of the first clinical gene therapy trial. Blood 101(7):2563–2569

Naso MF, Tomkowicz B, Perry WL 3rd, Strohl WR (2017) Adeno-associated virus (AAV) as a vector for gene therapy. BioDrugs 31(4):317–334

Nathwani AC, Tuddenham EG, Rangarajan S, Rosales C, McIntosh J, Linch DC, Chowdary P et al (2011) Adenovirus-associated virus vector-mediated gene transfer in hemophilia B. N Engl J Med 365(25):2357–2365

Nemerow GR, Stewart PL (1999) Role of a_v integrins in adenovirus cell entry and gene delivery. Microbiol Mol Biol Rev 63(3):725–734

Panakanti R, Mahato RI (2009) Bipartite adenoviral vector encoding hHGF and hIL-1Ra for improved human islet transplantation. Pharm Res 26(3):587–596

Peng Z (2005) Current status of gendicine in China: recombinant human ad-p53 agent for treatment of cancers. Hum Gene Ther 16(9):1016–1027

Platt RJ, Chen S, Zhou Y, Yim MJ, Swiech L, Kempton HR, Dahlman JE, Parnas O, Eisenhaure TM, Jovanovic M, Graham DB, Jhunjhunwala S, Heidenreich M, Xavier RJ, Langer R, Anderson DG, Hacohen N, Regev A, Feng G, Sharp PA, Zhang F (2014) CRISPR-Cas9 knockin mice for genome editing and cancer modeling. Cell 159(2):440–455

Qin JY, Zhang L, Clift KL, Hulur I, Xiang AP, Ren BZ, Lahn BT (2010) Systematic comparison of constitutive promoters and the doxycycline-inducible promoter. PLoS One 5(5):e10611

Ramakrishna S, Kwaku Dad AB, Beloor J, Gopalappa R, Lee SK, Kim H (2014) Gene disruption by cell-penetrating peptide-mediated delivery of Cas9 protein and guide RNA. Genome Res 24(6):1020–1027

Ranga U, Woffendin C, Verma S, Xu L, June CH, Bishop DK, Nabel GJ (1998) Enhanced T cell engraftment after retroviral delivery of an antiviral gene in HIV-infected individuals. Proc Natl Acad Sci U S A 95(3):1201–1206

Raper SE, Chirmule N, Lee FS, Wivel NA, Bagg A, Gao GP, Wilson JM, Batshaw ML (2003) Fatal systemic inflammatory response syndrome in a ornithine transcarbamylase deficient patient following adenoviral gene transfer. Mol Genet Metab 80(1–2):148–158

Reilly JP, Grise MA, Fortuin FD, Vale PR, Schaer GL, Lopez J, Van Camp JR et al (2005) Long-term (2-year) clinical events following transthoracic intramyocardial gene transfer of VEGF-2 in no-option patients. J Interv Cardiol 18(1):27–31

Rincon MY, Vandendriessche T, Chuah MK (2015) Gene therapy for cardiovascular disease: advances in vector development, targeting, and delivery for clinical translation. Cardiovasc Res 108(1):4–20

Rip J, Nierman MC, Sierts JA, Petersen W, Van den Oever K, Van Raalte D, Ross CJ et al (2005) Gene therapy for lipoprotein lipase deficiency: working toward clinical application. Hum Gene Ther 16(11):1276–1286

Roth JA, Cristiano RJ (1997) Gene therapy for cancer: what have we done and where are we going? J Natl Cancer Inst 89(1):21–39

Ryu WS, Mertz JE (1989) Simian virus 40 late transcripts lacking excisable intervening sequences are defective in both stability in the nucleus and transport to the cytoplasm. J Virol 63(10):4386–4394

Salmon F, Grosios K, Petry H (2014) Safety profile of recombinant adeno-associated viral vectors: focus on alipogene tiparvovec (Glybera®). Expert Rev Clin Pharmacol 7(1):53–65

Sandmair AM, Loimas S, Puranen P, Immonen A, Kossila M, Puranen M, Hurskainen H et al (2000) Thymidine kinase gene therapy for human malignant glioma, using replication-deficient retroviruses or adenoviruses. Hum Gene Ther 11(16):2197–2205

Sanei Ata-Abadi N, Dormiani K, Khazaie Y, Ghaedi K, Forouzanfar M, Lachinani L, Rezaei N, Kiani-Esfahani A, Nasr-Esfahani MH (2015) Construction of a new minicircle DNA carrying an enhanced green florescent protein reporter gene for efficient expression into mammalian cell lines. Mol Biol Rep 42(7):1175–1185

Shirakawa T (2009) Clinical trial design for adenoviral gene therapy products. Drug News Perspect 22(3): 140–145

Simonelli F, Maguire AM, Testa F, Pierce EA, Mingozzi F, Bennicelli JL, Rossi S et al (2010) Gene therapy for Leber's congenital amaurosis is safe and effective through 1.5 years after vector administration. Mol Ther 18(3):643–650

Simons JW, Sacks N (2006) Granulocyte-macrophage colony-stimulating factor-transduced allogeneic cancer cellular immunotherapy: the GVAX vaccine for prostate cancer. Urol Oncol 24(5):419–424

Singh S, Chitkara D, Kumar V, Behrman SW, Mahato RI (2013) miRNA profiling in pancreatic cancer and restoration of chemosensitivity. Cancer Lett 334(2): 211–220

Singh S, Narang AS, Mahato RI (2011) Subcellular fate and off-target effects of siRNA, shRNA, and miRNA. Pharm Res 28(12):2996–3015

Spilianakis CG, Lalioti MD, Town T, Lee GR, Flavell RA (2005) Interchromosomal associations between alternatively expressed loci. Nature 435(7042):637–645

Springer ML (2006) A balancing act: therapeutic approaches for the modulation of angiogenesis. Curr Opin Investig Drugs 7(3):243–250

Stenler S, Wiklander OP, Badal-Tejedor M, Turunen J, Nordin JZ, Hallengärd D, Wahren B, Andaloussi SE, Rutland MW, Smith CI, Lundin KE, Blomberg P (2014) Micro-minicircle gene therapy: implications of size on fermentation, Complexation, shearing resistance, and expression. Mol Ther Nucleic Acids 2:e140

Stewart DJ, Hilton JD, Arnold JM, Gregoire J, Rivard A, Archer SL, Charbonneau F et al (2006) Angiogenic gene therapy in patients with nonrevascularizable ischemic heart disease: a phase 2 randomized, controlled trial of AdVEGF(121) (AdVEGF121) versus maximum medical treatment. Gene Ther 13(21):1503–1511

Stewart PL, Chiu CY, Huang S, Muir T, Zhao Y, Chait B, Mathias P, Nemerow GR (1997) Cryo-EM visualization of an exposed RGD epitope on adenovirus that escapes antibody neutralization. EMBO J 16(6):1189–1198

Stolberg SG (1999) The biotech death of Jesse Gelsinger. N Y Times Mag 136–140:149–150

Surosky RT, Urabe M, Godwin SG, McQuiston SA, Kurtzman GJ, Ozawa K, Natsoulis G (1997) Adeno-associated virus rep proteins target DNA sequences to a unique locus in the human genome. J Virol 71(10):7951–7959

Tacket CO, Roy MJ, Widera G, Swain WF, Broome S, Edelman R (1999) Phase 1 safety and immune response studies of a DNA vaccine encoding hepatitis B surface antigen delivered by a gene delivery device. Vaccine 17(22):2826–2829

Tuszynski MH, Thal L, Pay M, Salmon DP, Hs U, Patel P et al (2005) A phase 1 clinical trial of nerve growth factor gene therapy for Alzheimer disease. Nat Med 11(5):551–555

U.S. Department of Health and Human Services (1998) Guidance for industry: guidance for human somatic cell therapy and gene therapy. Center for Biologics Evaluation and Research. United States Food and Drug Administration, Rockville

Uckert W, Kammertons T, Haack K, Qin Z, Gebert J, Schendel DJ, Blankenstein T (1998) Double suicide gene (cytosine deaminase and herpes simplex virus thymidine kinase) but not single gene transfer allows reliable elimination of tumor cells in vivo. Hum Gene Ther 9(6):855–865

van Pijkeren JP, Morrissey D, Monk IR, Cronin M, Rajendran S, O'Sullivan GC, Gahan CG, Tangney M (2010) A novel Listeria monocytogenes-based DNA delivery system for cancer gene therapy. Hum Gene Ther 21(4):405–416

Varghese S, Rabkin SD (2002) Oncolytic herpes simplex virus vectors for cancer virotherapy. Cancer Gene Ther 9(12):967–978

Verma IM (1990) Gene therapy. Sci Am 263(5):68–72 81–64

Vasan S, Hurley A, Schlesinger SJ, Hannaman D, Gardiner DF, Dugin DP, Boente-Carrera M et al (2011) In vivo electroporation enhances the immunogenicity of an HIV-1 DNA vaccine candidate in healthy volunteers. PLoS One 6(5):e19252

Vassaux G, Nitcheu J, Jezzard S, Lemoine NR (2006) Bacterial gene therapy strategies. J Pathol 208(2):290–298

Wang DA, Narang AS, Kotb M, Gaber AO, Miller DD, Kim SW, Mahato RI (2002) Novel branched poly(ethylenimine)-cholesterol water-soluble lipopolymers for gene delivery. Biomacromolecules 3(6):1197–1207

Weber W, Fussenegger M (2006) Pharmacologic transgene control systems for gene therapy. J Gene Med 8(5):535–556

Wells DJ (2004) Gene therapy progress and prospects: electroporation and other physical methods. Gene Ther 11(18):1363–1369

Wiley (2017) The Journal of Gene Medicine Clinical Trials Worldwide Database. http://www.abedia.com/wiley/index.html

Wolfram JA, Donahue JK (2013) Gene therapy to treat cardiovascular disease. J Am Heart Assoc 2(4):e000119

Wright JF, Qu G, Tang C, Sommer JM (2003) Recombinant adeno-associated virus: formulation challenges and strategies for a gene therapy vector. Curr Opin Drug Discov Devel 6(2):174–178

Wu H, Yoon AR, Li F, Yun CO, Mahato RI (2011) RGD peptide-modified adenovirus expressing HGF and XIAP improves islet transplantation. J Gene Med 13(12):658–669

Wu Z, Asokan A, Samulski RJ (2006) Adeno-associated virus serotypes: vector toolkit for human gene therapy. Mol Ther 14(3):316–327

Xia ZJ, Chang JH, Zhang L, Jiang WQ, Guan ZZ, Liu JW, Zhang Y et al (2004) Phase III randomized clinical trial of intratumoral injection of E1B gene-deleted adenovirus (H101) combined with cisplatin-based chemotherapy in treating squamous cell cancer of head and neck or esophagus. Ai Zheng 23(12):1666–1670

Xu ZL, Mizuguchi H, Sakurai F, Koizumi N, Hosono T, Kawabata K, Watanabe Y, Yamaguchi T, Hayakawa T (2005) Approaches to improving the kinetics of adenovirus-delivered genes and gene products. Adv Drug Deliv Rev 57(5):781–802

Yan Z, Zhang Y, Duan D, Engelhardt JF (2000) Trans-splicing vectors expand the utility of adeno-associated virus for gene therapy. Proc Natl Acad Sci U S A 97(12):6716–6721

Zaiss AK, Liu Q, Bowen GP, Wong NC, Bartlett JS, Muruve DA (2002) Differential activation of innate immune responses by adenovirus and adeno-associated virus vectors. J Virol 76(9):4580–4590

Zhang WW, Li L, Li D, Liu J, Li X, Li W, Xu X, Zhang MJ, Chandler LA, Lin H, Hu A, Xu W, Lam DM (2018) The first approved gene therapy product for Cancer ad-p53 (Gendicine): 12 years in the clinic. Hum Gene Ther 29(2):160–179

Zufferey R, Dull T, Mandel RJ, Bukovsky A, Quiroz D, Naldini L, Trono D (1998) Self-inactivating lentivirus vector for safe and efficient in vivo gene delivery. J Virol 72(12):9873–9880

Zuris JA, Thompson DB, Shu Y, Guilinger JP, Bessen JL, Hu JH, Maeder ML, Joung JK, Chen ZY, Liu DR (2015) Cationic lipid-mediated delivery of proteins enables efficient protein-based genome editing in vitro and in vivo. Nat Biotechnol 33(1):73–80

Zwaka T (2006) Use of genetically modified stem cells in experimental gene therapies. In: Regenerative medicine. National Institutes of Health, Bethesda

SUGGESTED READING

Narang A, Mahato RI (2010) Targeted delivery of small and macromolecular drugs. CRC Press, Boca Raton

National Institutes of Health (2006) Regenerative medicine. National Institutes of Health, Bethesda

Schleef M et al (2001) Plasmids for therapy cbrsand vaccination. Wiley-VCH, New York

Schleef M (2005) DNA pharmaceuticals: formulation and delivery in gene therapy, DNA vaccination and immunotherapy. John Wiley & Sons, Hoboken

17 Advanced Therapies: Clinical, Non-clinical and Quality Considerations

Karin H. Hoogendoorn

INTRODUCTION

Cell therapy, tissue engineering, and gene therapy, together called "regenerative medicine" or "advanced therapies" or "advanced therapy medicinal products" ((ATMPs), European union (EU) legal term), represent the most recent branch of the biotechnology revolution in medicine. These therapies constitute an innovative group of heterogeneous, research driven biopharmaceuticals, based on cells, tissues, and/or nucleic acids packaged within a viral or non-viral vector. As with many medicinal products, advanced therapies are based on ground-breaking scientific discoveries and technological advancement. With increasing knowledge of the human body's cell and tissue architecture in a healthy and in a diseased state, medical therapy became targeted. This refers not only to the metabolic, immunological, and/or pharmacological interaction but also to the more complex regeneration, repair, and replacement of human diseased tissues.

The use of advanced therapies based on live cells in medical practice is not a new concept. The first successful human hematopoietic stem cell transplantation from a healthy donor to a cancer patient took place in 1968 and is now a routine clinical procedure for bone-marrow regeneration. The true value of (stem) cell therapies was not further explored until the early 1990s when the therapeutic relevance of mesenchymal stromal cells (MSCs) was considered for the regeneration of skeletal tissue and later for broader therapeutic use. Since the turn of the millennium there has been a steady increase in the number of advanced therapy clinical trials, with a growing number of target indications. Particularly for the treatment of diseases and tissue/organ defects for which traditional therapies and medicinal products have not always provided high benefit/risk outcomes, such as Alzheimer's disease, Parkinson's disease, cancer, and muscular dystrophy, advanced therapies hold high expectations.

Currently, worldwide there are over 700 advanced therapy companies and more than 1000 active clinical trials are ongoing. However, only eight advanced therapies have been approved by the Unites States (US) Food and Drug Administration (FDA) and ten by the European Commission (EC) (December 2017; see Table 17.1) and less than a handful by other jurisdictions (e.g., Canada and Japan). The inherent complexity of these products poses unique challenges compared to other therapeutics. The manufacture of "living" materials (i.e., cells and tissues) carries great challenges in terms of consistency and process and product characterization, the latter due to the lack of (sensitive) analytical techniques. Such challenges are analogous, in many ways, to those faced in the past when the first recombinant protein biopharmaceutical products were being developed and regulated. Bringing advanced therapies to market at an acceptable cost, benefit/risk ratio, and quality has proven extremely difficult for certain products.

In this chapter we discuss the current status and unique aspects of cell therapy medicinal products, tissue engineered products, and medicinal products based on the *ex-vivo* genetic modification of cells. The latter fall legally in the category of gene therapy medicinal products. Gene therapy products involving *in-vivo* gene transfer are discussed in Chap. 16.

(DIS)SIMILARITIES WITH RECOMBINANT THERAPEUTIC PROTEINS AND OTHER BIOPHARMACEUTICALS

Although advanced therapies fall within the group of biopharmaceuticals, there are substantial differences in the area of quality/chemical, manufacturing, and controls (CMC), non-clinical, clinical, regulatory, and

Parts of this chapter were taken from the fourth edition chapter 25 authored by Colin W. Pouton.

K. H. Hoogendoorn (✉)
Leiden University Medical Center, Hospital Pharmacy, Interdivisional GMP Facility, Leiden, The Netherlands
e-mail: k.h.hoogendoorn@lumc.nl

D. J. A. Crommelin et al. (eds.), *Pharmaceutical Biotechnology*, https://doi.org/10.1007/978-3-030-00710-2_17

Product and classification	INN/description	Indication	Company	Approval month
Europe (EMA)				
ChondroCelect® (TEP)	Characterized viable autologous cartilage cells expanded *ex-vivo* expressing specific marker proteins	Cartilage defects of the femoral condyle of the knee	Tigenix NV	10/2009 (withdrawn 08/2016)
Glybera® (*in-vivo* GTMP)	Alipogene tiparvovec (AAV1 vector)	Hyperlipoproteinemia Type I	uniQure biopharma BV	10/2012 (withdrawn 10/2017)
MACI® (TEP)	Autologous cultured chondrocytes	Fractures, cartilage	Genzyme Europe BV	06/2013 (withdrawn 10/2014)
Provenge® (SCTMP)	Sipuleucel-T; autologous peripheral blood mononuclear cells activated with PAP-GM-CSF	Prostatic neoplasms	Dendreon UK Ltd.	09/2013 (withdrawn 05/2015)
Imlygic® (*in-vivo* GTMP)	Talimogene laherparepvec	Treatment of adults with melanoma that is regionally or distantly metastatic	Amgen Europe BV	12/2015
Holoclar® (TEP)	*Ex-vivo* autologous corneal epithelial cells including stem cells	Corneal diseases stem cell transplantation	Chiesi farmaceutici SpA.	02/2015
Strimvelis® (*ex-vivo* GTMP)	Autologous $CD34^+$ cells transduced with retroviral vector containing the adenosine deaminase gene	Treatment of severe combined immunodeficiency due to adenosine deaminase deficiency (ADA-SCID)	GlaxoSmithKline Trading Services Ltd.	05/2016
Zalmoxis® (*ex-vivo* GTMP)	Allogeneic T cells genetically modified with a retroviral vector encoding for a truncated form of the human low affinity nerve growth factor receptor (ΔLNGFR) and the herpes simplex I virus thymidine kinase (HSV-TK Mut2)	Treatment in haploidentical haematopoeitic stem cell transplantation	MolMed SpA	08/2016
Spherox® (TEP)	Spheroids of human autologous matrix associated chondrocytes	Cartilage defects of the femoral condyle of the knee	Co.don AG.	07/2017
Alofisel® (SCTMP)	Darvadstroce; contains allogeneic expanded adipose stem cells	Treatment of complex perianal fistulas in adult patients with non-active/mildly active luminal Crohn's disease	Tigenix NV	12/2017
USA (FDA)				
Provenge® (SCTMP)	Sipuleucel-T; autologous cellular immunotherapy	Treatment of asymptomatic or minimally symptomatic metastatic castrate resistant (hormone refractory) prostate cancer	Dendreon Corporation	04/2010
LaViv® (SCTMP)	Azficel-T	Autologous cellular product indicated for improvement of the appearance of moderate to severe nasolabial fold wrinkles in adults	Fibrocell Technologies, Inc.	06/2011
Gintuit® (SCTMP)	Allogeneic cultured keratinocytes and fibroblasts in bovine collagen	Allogeneic cellularized scaffold product indicated for topical (non-submerged) application to a surgically created vascular wound bed in the treatment of mucogingival conditions in adults	Organogenesis Inc.	03/2012
Imlygic® (*in-vivo* GTMP)	Talimogene laherparepvec	Local treatment of unresectable cutaneous, subcutaneous, and nodal lesions in patients with melanoma recurrent after initial surgery	Amgen Inc.	10/2015

Table 17.1 ■ ATMPs approved in Europe and the USA (2008–2017)

Product and classification	INN/description	Indication	Company	Approval month
MACI® (SCTMP)	Autologous cultured chondrocytes on a porcine collagen membrane	Autologous cellularized scaffold product indicated for the repair of symptomatic, single or multiple full-thickness cartilage defects of the knee with or without bone involvement in adults	Vericel Corp.	12/2016
Kymriah® (*ex-vivo* GTMP)	Tisagenlecleucel	Treatment of patients up to 25 years of age with B-cell precursor acute lymphoblastic leukemia (ALL) that is refractory or in second or later relapse	Novartis Pharmaceuticals Corporation	08/2017
Yescarta® (*ex-vivo* GTMP)	Axicabtagene ciloleucel	A CD19-directed genetically modified autologous T cell immunotherapy indicated for the treatment of adult patients with relapsed or refractory large B-cell lymphoma after two or more lines of systemic therapy, including diffuse large B-cell lymphoma (DLBCL) not otherwise specified, primary mediastinal large B-cell lymphoma, high grade B-cell lymphoma, and DLBCL arising from follicular lymphoma	Kite Pharma Inc.	10/2017
Luxturna® (*in-vivo* GTMP)	Voretigene neparvovec-rzyl (AAV2 vector)	Inherited retinal disease in patients who have a biallelic mutation of the RPE65 gene	Spark Therapeutics	12/2017

Table 17.1 ■ (continued)

costs/reimbursement structure compared to recombinant proteins and other biopharmaceuticals. This is summarized in Table 17.2 and further discussed in this chapter. Therefore, the format of this chapter has a different set up as the other product group related chapters in this book.

CLASSIFICATION OF ADVANCED THERAPIES

Advanced therapies can be classified in many ways, e.g., by:

1. The therapeutic indication they aim to address, e.g., neurological, cardiovascular, ophthalmological.
2. Whether they comprise cells and/or tissues (see Fig. 17.1):
   (a) derived from and administered to the same human individual (autologous = autogeneic), hence the donor = the recipient (patient);
   (b) derived from a human (healthy) donor, who is different to the patient (allogeneic);
   (c) derived from an animal (xenogeneic; see Chap. 9); e.g., porcine islets to treat diabetes mellitus (DM)
3. The potency of the cells (i.e., omnipotent, pluripotent, multipotent, oligopotent, unipotent (see Table 17.6).
4. The *in-vivo* mode of action (i.e., pharmacological, immunological, metabolic or regenerative (i.e., regenerate, repair or replace a human tissue); see Fig. 17.2 below).
5. Their underlying technology, as described in this chapter (Mount et al. 2015):
   (a) somatic cell technologies;
   (b) cell immortalization technologies;
   (c) *ex-vivo* gene modification of cells using viral vector technologies;
   (d) *in-vivo* gene modification of cells using viral vector technologies (see Chap. 16);
   (e) genome editing technologies;
   (f) cell plasticity technologies;
   (g) three-dimensional technologies;
   (h) combinations of the above technologies.
6. The cell types (e.g., MSCs, dendritic cells (DCs), T-cells).
7. The regulatory/legislative regime applied, as briefly discussed below.

■ Advanced Therapies: Medicinal Products for Human Use Versus "Cell and Tissue Transplantations"

Advanced therapies often are considered biological medicinal products, a category of medicinal products for human use, meaning they are typically subject to two regulatory regimes: public health legislation and pharmaceutical legislation (see British standards institution publicly available specification (BSI PAS) 83:2012). However, some clinical interventions for cell- and tissue-based advanced therapies (*gene therapies are excluded*) are not considered being medicinal and these

Category	Characteristic	Advanced therapies	Other biopharmaceuticals
Non-clinical	Animal models	Often no relevant animal models to predict safety and particularly efficacy in humans available	Relevant animal models to predict safety/efficacy often available
	Safety testing	Tumorigenicity testing may be needed (stem cell derived products)	N.A.[a]
	ADME[b]/ pharmacodynamic studies	Often not possible/relevant	Generally performed
Clinical	Disease pathway(s) and mode of action	Often not well understood	Well understood
	First in human trials	Always in patients	Often in healthy volunteers
	PK[c]/PD[d] studies	Often not feasible/relevant	Performed
	Route of administration	Often IV[e]infusion, some times local injection, e.g., intotumor, subretinal space of eye; spinal cord; brain; intra-dermal	IV injection or infusion, SC[f], intradermal, IM[g]
	Patient monitoring	Often long-term follow-up (10-20 years)	Short term follow-up
	Track & traceability	From donor start material (tissue/cell) through manufacturing process to patient and vice versa	From starting material through manufacturing process to patient
Quality/CMC[h]	Product group	Heterogeneous	Less heterogeneous
	Type of formulation	Often a dispersion /suspension of cells	Often a solution (liquid or reconstituted lyophilizate); sometimes emulsion or suspension (vaccines)
	Dose	Mostly number of (viable) cells/kg body weight or cm^2 tissue	Usually milligram range for proteins; microgram range for vaccines; or defined as units activity/mg
	Manufacturing process	Often continuous process, no designated drug substance	Often discontinuous process, designated drug substance and drug product
		Often open and manual process steps; no platform technologies yet, automation in its infancy	Closed and mostly automated process steps; platform technologies

Table 17.2 ■ Examples of differences between advanced therapies and other biopharmaceuticals

Category	Characteristic	Advanced therapies	Other biopharmaceuticals
		Often aseptic manufacture, no sterilization possible (no viral removal and/or inactivation steps) due to viability of cell/tissue	Viral removal and/or inactivation steps; sterilization (mostly through ≤ 0.2 micron filtration)
	Batch definition	Often one batch for one to few patients; off-the-shelf products less common	Off-the-shelf (one batch for multiple patients)
	Safety	Risk for transmission of human viral infections from donor to patient; animal and human derived raw materials and excipients	Risk extremely low due to viral removal/inactivation steps; chemically defined raw materials and excipients
	Product storage and supply	Sometimes 2-8°C or room temperature - short shelf - life; often vapor phase of liquid nitrogen (at < -150°C) - longer shelf -l ife(months - years)	Mostly 2-8°C and longer shelf-life (years)
Regulatory	Landscape	Evolving regulatory landscape	Established regulatory landscape
	Guidances	Specific “advanced therapy” guidances	Guidances for biologicals and vaccines
	Classification	Product classification and product terminology not harmonized globally	Product classification and product terminology mostly harmonized globally
Ethics	Uncontrolled access to non-approved product	Stem cell tourism	Illicit use of biopharmaceuticals
	Acceptability starting material (tissue/cells)	Use of human embryos to manufacture human embryonic stem cell based product not allowed in some countries	N.A.
Reimbursement	Costs	Very high (20,000-1,000.000 Euros) per treatment	Medium-high (500-5,000 Euros)per injection

[a]N.A. = not applicable
[b]ADME = absorption, distribution, metabolism, elimination
[c]PK = pharmacokinetics
[d]PD = pharmacodynamics
[e]IV = intravenous
[f]SC = subcutaneous
[g]IM = intramuscular
[h]CMC = chemical, manufacturing, and controls

Table 17.2 ■ (continued)

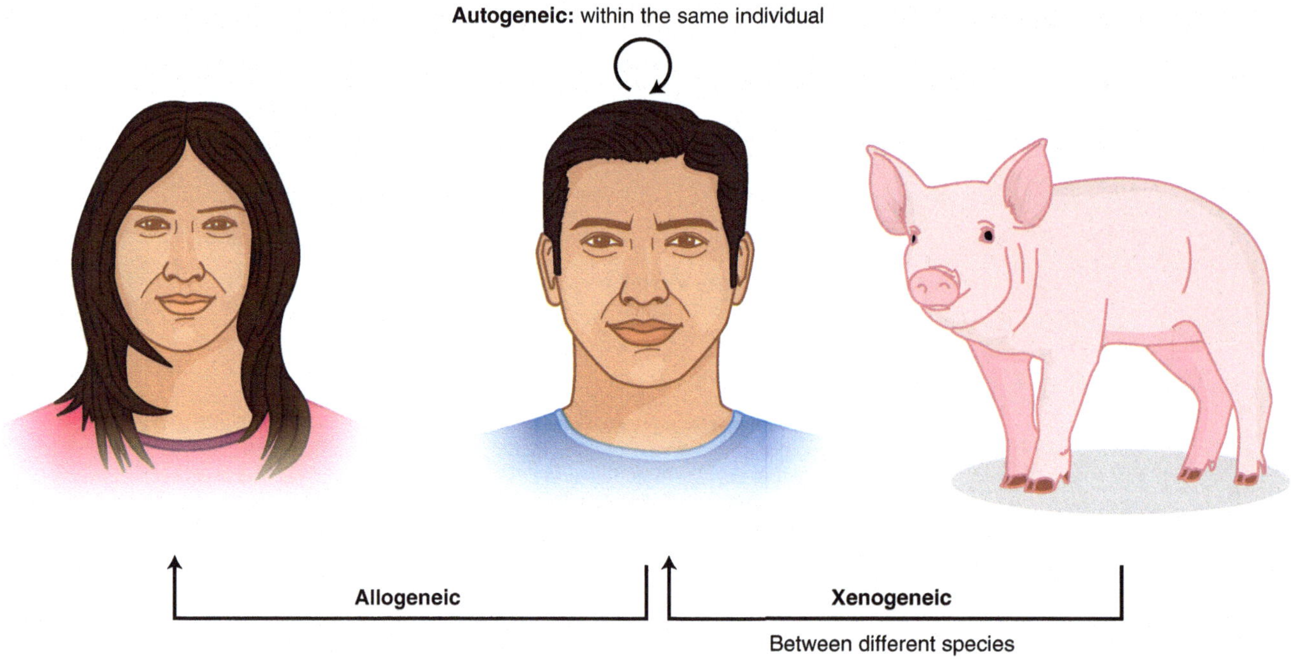

Figure 17.1 ■ Types of transplants/advanced therapy cell source

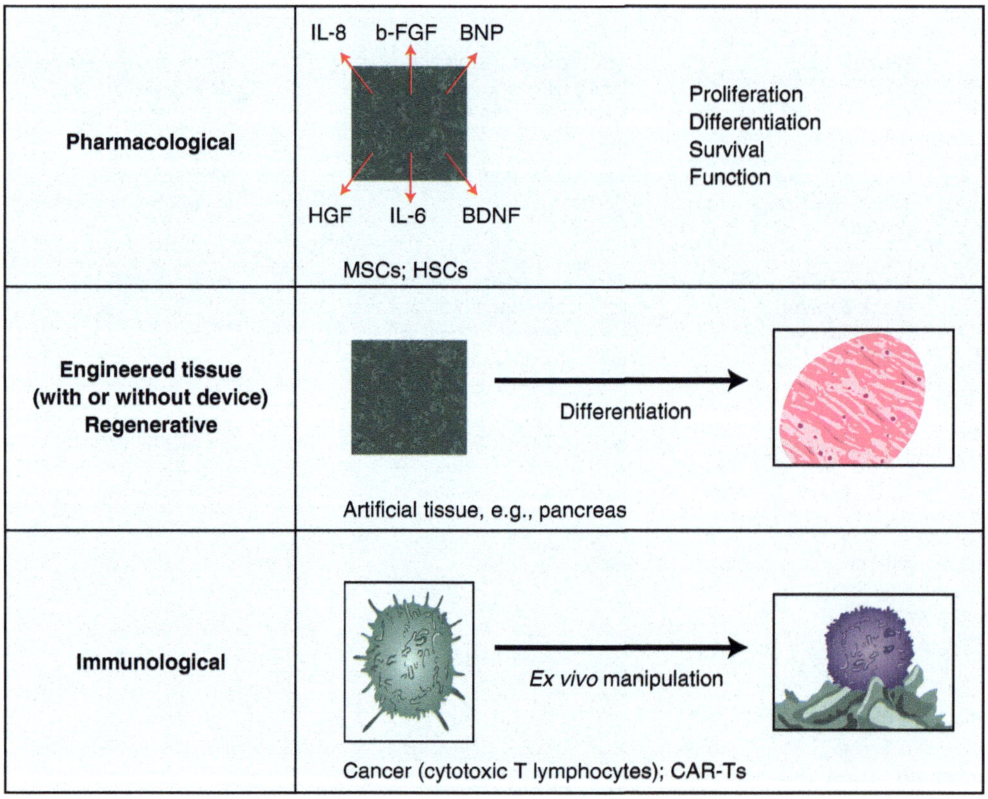

Figure 17.2 ■ Possible MoAs of advanced therapies

Substantial manipulation	Non-substantial manipulation
Specific manipulations considered substantial are: 1. Cell expansion (culture; *ex-vivo*) 2. Differentiation and/or activation with growth factors 3. *Ex-vivo* genetic modifications of cells (e.g., with viral vector)	Specific manipulations *not* considered substantial: 1. Cutting 2. Grinding 3. Shaping 4. Centrifugation 5. Soaking in antibiotic or antimicrobial solutions 6. Sterilization 7. Irradiation 8. Cell separation, concentration or purification 9. Filtering 10. Lyophilization 11. Freezing 12. Cryopreservation 13. Vitrification

Table 17.3 ■ Substantial and non-substantial manipulations; see for details PAS83:2012

therapies are subject to public health legislation only. These therapies are often called "cell and tissue transplant products" or "cell and tissue transplantations" and have to meet all of the following criteria:

1. A cell or tissue, which is *not* substantially manipulated. Table 17.3, below, provides guidance on the definition of substantial and non-substantial manipulations;
2. Cells/tissues are used for the *same* essential function in the donor and recipients (sometimes called "homologous use");
3. It is not combined with a medical device or active implantable medical device.

These criteria are elaborated in the EU and the US legislation (see for references to the legislation BSI PAS83:2012). Whether an advanced therapy meets these three criteria is important because, if so, no clinical trials and no marketing authorization (MA) prior to commercial availability are required. If the product falls into the 'non-substantial manipulation' category only public health legislation applies. An example of such a transplantation product is a hematopoietic stem cell (HSC) transplantation which is already a well-established treatment for blood disorders since the late 1960s (see Fig. 17.5).

Advanced Therapy Classification in the EU and USA

Globally, slightly different definitions for an "advanced therapy, which is a medicinal product" are being used by regulatory bodies. In the EU, such a product is called an ATMP, which is defined as being a Somatic Cell Therapy Medicinal Product (SCTMP), a Tissue Engineered Product (TEP), a Gene Therapy Medicinal Product (GTMP) or a combined ATMP. The four subtypes of ATMPs are further defined in the following ways:

1. SCTMPs contain cells or tissues that have been manipulated to change their biological characteristics or cells or tissues not intended to be used for the same essential functions of the body. They can be used to cure, diagnose or prevent disease.
2. TEPs contain cells or tissues that have been modified so they can be used to repair, regenerate or replace human tissue.
3. GTMPs contain genes that lead to a therapeutic, prophylactic or diagnostic effect. They work by inserting recombinant genes into the body to treat cancer, genetic disorders or long-term diseases (see also Chap. 16).
4. Combined ATMPs contain one or more medical devices as an integral part of the medicine, such as cells embedded in a biodegradable matrix or scaffold (not further discussed here).

Hence, products used for HSC transplantation don't fall under the European Medicines Agency (EMA) "ATMP" definition.

See for details on these four ATMP classes Table 17.4 below.

By contrast, the US FDA's definition for ATMPs is broader than the EU's description (i.e., ATMPs + transplant products). FDA defines ATMPs as:

1. Human cells, tissues, and cellular and tissue-based products (HCT/Ps). HCT/Ps consist of human cells or tissues intended for implantation, transplantation, infusion or transfer into a human recipient and include cellular immunotherapies, cancer vaccines, and other types of both autologous and allogeneic cells for certain therapeutic indications, including HSCs and adult and embryonic stem cells (ESCs). This category covers both the transplant products and the medicinal products.
2. Human gene therapy products, which refers to medicinal products that are aimed to introduce genetic material into a person's deoxyribonucleic acid (DNA) to replace faulty or missing genetic material, thus treating a disease or abnormal medical condition.
3. Unlike the EU it is possible for human cells and tissues to be regulated as devices, however, this possibility is outside of the scope of this chapter and will not be discussed in detail (similarly to the combined ATMPs in Europe).

Hence, products used for HSC transplantation fall under the FDA "ATMP" definition.

■ What Is a Stem Cell?

The fundamental property of a stem cell is the capability to multiply i.e., it has self-renewal capacity, which is the ability to go through numerous cycles of cell division (through mitosis) while maintaining the undifferentiated state and to give rise to a variety of differentiated cells. But the general term "stem cell" is used in several contexts, each important for different reasons, as shown in Table 17.5. Adult (or somatic) stem cells, e.g., MSCs, ESCs, and induced pluripotent stem cells (iPSCs) are currently the subject of intense non-clinical and clinical investigation. Stem cells differ in the breadth of mature,

ATMP classification	Definition	Examples
Gene therapy medical product (GTMP)	A GTMP is a biological medicinal product (*excluding vaccines*) that: (a) Contains an active substance which contains or consists of a recombinant nucleic acid used in or administered to human beings with a view to regulating, repairing, replacing, adding or deleting a genetic sequence and; (b) Its therapeutic, prophylactic or diagnostic effect relates *directly* to the recombinant nucleic acid sequence it contains, or to the product of genetic expression of this sequence Gene therapy medicinal products shall not include *vaccines against infectious diseases* (see Chap. 14), which have their own set of vaccine specific guidances	Glybera® (see Chap. 16); Kymriah® (autologous $CD19^+$ CAR-T cells)[a]; Strimvelis® (genetically modified autologous $CD34^+$ cells)
Somatic cell therapy medicinal product (SCTMP)	A SCTMP is a biological medicinal product which fulfils the following two characteristics: (a) Contains or consists of cells or tissues that have been subject to substantial manipulation so that biological characteristics, physiological functions or structural properties relevant for the intended clinical use have been altered or of cells or tissues that are not intended to be used for the same essential function(s) in the recipient and the donor (b) Is presented as having properties for or is used in or administered to human beings with a view to treating, preventing or diagnosing a disease through the pharmacological, immunological or metabolic action of its cells or tissues	Alofisel® (allogeneic MSCs); irradiated plasmacytoid dendritic cell line (allogeneic) loaded with peptides from tumor antigens
Tissue engineered product (TEP)	A TEP is a biological medicinal product that meets the following two characteristics: (a) Contains or consists of engineered cells or tissues, and (b) Is presented as having properties for, or is used in or administered to human beings with a view to regenerating, repairing or replacing a human tissue A TEP may contain cells or tissues of human or animal origin, or both. The cells or tissues may be viable or non-viable. It may also contain additional substances, such as cellular products, bio-molecules, biomaterials, chemical substances, scaffolds or matrices. Products containing or consisting exclusively of non-viable human or animal cells and/or tissues, which do not contain any viable cells or tissues and which do not act principally by pharmacological, immunological or metabolic action, are excluded from this definition. Cells or tissues shall be considered "engineered" if they fulfill at least one of the following conditions: (a) The cells or tissues have been subject to substantial manipulation, so that biological characteristics, physiological functions or structural properties relevant for the intended regeneration, repair or replacement are achieved (b) The cells or tissues are not intended to be used for the same essential function or functions in the recipient as in the donor	Spherox® (autologous chondrocytes); Holoclar® (autologous corneal epithelial cells, which contain stem cells)
Combined ATMP	A combined ATMP fulfills the following conditions: (a) It must incorporate, as an integral part of the product, one or more medical devices or one or more active implantable devices, and (b) Its cellular or tissue part must contain viable cells or tissues, or (c) Its cellular or tissue part containing non-viable cells or tissues must be liable to act upon the human body with action that can be considered primary to that of the devices referred to	Allogenic adipose derived regenerative cells encapsulated in hyaluronic acid (TEP + device)[b]; encapsulated allogeneic cells secreting GM-CSF[c] + irradiated autologous tumor cells (GTMP + device)

[a]*$CD19^+$ (CAR-T cells)* = cluster of differentiation (CD) 19 'chimeric antigen receptor T cells,' CAR-T cells
[b]Hassan et al. (2013)
[c]*GM-CSF* = Granulocyte-macrophage colony-stimulating factor

Table 17.4 ■ EU-ATMP classification definitions according to the EU pharmaceutical legislation, adapted from Smith et al. (2015)

Type of stem cell	Origin	Characteristic potential (see also Table 17.6)	Application
Adult (= somatic) stem cells	Exist in small number in many tissues, often in a well-defined and supportive niche	Multipotent: Give rise to cells of the relevant tissue or local environment	Neural stem cells & limbal stem cells in pre-clinical and clinical development
MSCs (a group of adult stem cells)	A collective term for cells from mesodermal lineage, sourced from stromal or connective tissue (e.g., bone marrow, adipose tissue, and umbilical cord tissue)	Multipotent: A heterogeneous pool of cells. They have a "stem cell-like" character and can differentiate into cells of connective tissues, e.g., chondrocytes, osteoblasts, and adipocytes, but they have also been reported to give rise to many other unrelated cell types	Pre-clinical development & clinical PI-III trials; commercial (Prochymal® and Alofisel®)
Cord blood-derived MSCs (primitive stem cells, somewhere between ESCs and mature adult stem cells)	A specific source of MSCs. Extracted at birth from umbilical cord blood	Multipotent: Yet to be fully determined. Potentially they could be a source of many cell types for individual patients	Private cell banks are established for cryopreservation of cord blood samples; pre-clinical development and clinical phase I/II trials
ESC (no adult stem cells)	Result from *ex-vivo* culture of the inner cell mass of a blastocyst (embryoblast = 5–9 days old embryo)	Pluripotent	Vital source of differentiated cells for different research applications and clinical first in human (FIH) trials ongoing
iPSC (no adult stem cells	Derived by reprogramming of somatic cells (often skin fibroblasts) taken from an adult biopsy	Pluripotent, although methods for full reprogramming are still in development	From autologous source for disease modelling, drug screening including toxicity testing, and FIH trial; pre-clinical development and plans for human leukocyte antigens (HLA)-matched allogeneic iPSCs for FIH trial; research is ongoing with allogeneic iPSCs eliminating HLA-class I expression using genome editing technologies to generate universal cell lines

Table 17.5 ■ Origin, characteristics, and uses of "stem" cells

non-stem cell phenotypes to which they can give rise. These non-stem cells cannot differentiate anymore and are not capable of self-renewal (e.g., DCs, pre-ß-cells). However, some stem cells, such as skin and muscle stem cells, do only multiply and do not differentiate (i.e., unipotent stem cells). Stem cells can be characterized by their potency as defined in Table 17.6.

Before the practical applications of stem cells can be fully realized, in both the research laboratory and clinic, it will be necessary to understand in detail how to control stem cell differentiation towards mature post-mitotic phenotypes.

ESCs and iPSCs are capable of unlimited *ex-vivo* (in culture) growth. In contrast, MCSs and oligo- and unipotent stem cells cannot be grown in culture indefinitely, i.e., they grow to senescence.

■ Advanced Therapy Possible Mode of Action(s)

The *in-vivo* mode of action(s) (MoA(s)) of an advanced therapy depends on the type of cell/tissue, the *ex-vivo* manipulations performed on the cells/tissue in the manufacturing facility (e.g., genetic modification), the route of administration, and the *in-vivo* environment the cells/tissue occur. Fig. 17.2 provides an overview of the possible MoAs:

1. Pharmacological: cells/tissue release molecules such as cytokines and growth factors upon interaction with their/its environment. An example is the immunoregulatory effect of MSCs. E.g., Alofisel contains expanded adipose derived MSCs which, once activated, impair proliferation of lymphocytes and reduce the release of pro-inflammatory cytokines at inflammation sites in patients with luminal

Stem cell potency	Explanation and examples
Totipotent (or omnipotent) stem cell	Can differentiate into all embryonic and extraembryonic cell types (i.e., in humans they give rise to the foetus, umbilical cord, and the placenta: morula's cells (0–5 days old embryo)
Pluripotent stem cell	Can differentiate into all three germ cell types (endoderm, mesoderm, or ectoderm lineage) but not the placenta and umbilical cord, and subsequently into all embryonic cell types: ESCs, iPSCs
Multipotent stem cell	Can differentiate into closely related cells, such as all cells in a particular organ: MSCs, other adult (=somatic) stem cells
Oligopotent stem cell	Can differentiate into a restricted closely related group, such as a hematopoietic progenitor cell that can produce a subset of blood cell types, such as B and T cells; vascular stem cell that has the capacity to become both endothelial or smooth muscle cells
Unipotent stem cells (or precursor cell)	Have the property of self-renewal but can only give rise to cells of their own lineage, such as muscle or skin stem cells. This distinguishes these cells from real stem cells as they do not differentiate into other cell phenotypes

Table 17.6 ■ Categorization of stem cells on their potency

Crohn's disease. This immunoregulatory activity reduces inflammation and may allow the tissues around the fistula tract to heal;

2. Regenerative: *ex-vivo* manipulated cells/tissue regenerate, repair or replace a diseased or damaged human tissue. E.g., human (h)ESCs are *ex-vivo* differentiated into pre-ß cells, loaded into a device, and administered under the skin to replace damaged ß-cells of a patient suffering from DM type I.
3. Immunological: cells of the immune system are *ex-vivo* activated. E.g., cytotoxic T lymphocytes (CTL) or genetically modified (e.g., CAR-T cells) cells activate the patient's own immune system upon administration, e.g., to treat cancer.

TECHNOLOGIES

Although advanced therapies can be classified by the regulatory regime to be applied (see above), the diversity of this new group of biopharmaceuticals may be better illustrated by the underlying technology and the therapeutic use (Mount et al. 2015). Below, these technologies are briefly discussed with examples of products currently in clinical development or approved for commercial use.

■ Somatic Cell Technologies

This technology involves adult (somatic) stem cells which are isolated from a donor and subsequently *ex-vivo* manipulated using purification, propagation and/or differentiation steps to manufacture a specific cell- or tissue-based product. Thereafter, the product is administered to a patient for a therapeutic indication.

Examples of such cells are chondrocytes, HSCs, MSCs, skin stem cells, and immune cells (see Table 17.5 above). The challenge is that in each tissue a very small number of stem/progenitor cells reside and, once removed from the body, these cells grow to senescence; hence obtaining large quantities of stem cells is difficult. Also the separation of stem cells from other (unwanted) cell populations may be difficult. For some products master and working cell bank (MCB and WCB) strategies are applied, but potential changes to the genetic information and the phenotypic stability (i.e., markers present on the cell surface as measured by flow cytometry techniques) of the cells during culture over time have to be carefully assessed.

What Are Adult Stem Cells and Where Are They Found in the Body?

Adult stem cells are known to be present in many if not all individual organs in adults and are generally thought to be "multipotent," meaning they can give rise to the cells found in their organ of origin, but not in other organs (Fig. 17.3). The identification of adult stem cells in human tissues has necessitated a repositioning of basic tenets of some biological sciences, most notably in neuroscience, where the prevailing view was that no new neurons were born in humans after birth (Zhao et al. 2008). Adult stem cells are rare and they cannot always be isolated and grown in culture. Even when they can be grown in culture, usually they grow to senescence. In tissues, they exist in a defined, organized environment of supporting cells that define the architecture of the "stem cell niche" (Scadden 2006). For example, in the bone marrow there are many hematopoietic stem cell niches, each of which contain MSCs to support the function of HSCs. Each HSC is capable of producing the progenitors of all types of blood cells (Taichman 2005). Differentiation of HSCs has been studied extensively and is now well understood (Fig. 17.4), but at present conditions that allow HSCs to be maintained and expanded *ex-vivo* have not been established. A hallmark of adult stem cells is their ability to "self-renew" both *in-vivo* and *ex-vivo* and they undergo asymmetric cell division. This means that when they divide they usually give rise to two different cells, one an identical stem cell and the other a partly differentiated progenitor cell (Fig. 17.4), a process that occurs in a polarized manner controlled by the niche. The common pattern in adult tissues is that the resulting progenitor cells, sometimes referred to as "transit amplifying" cells, are capable of expansion by symmetric division and can subsequently differentiate to form the various cell types needed for repair or replenishment of the relevant tissue. Such mechanisms

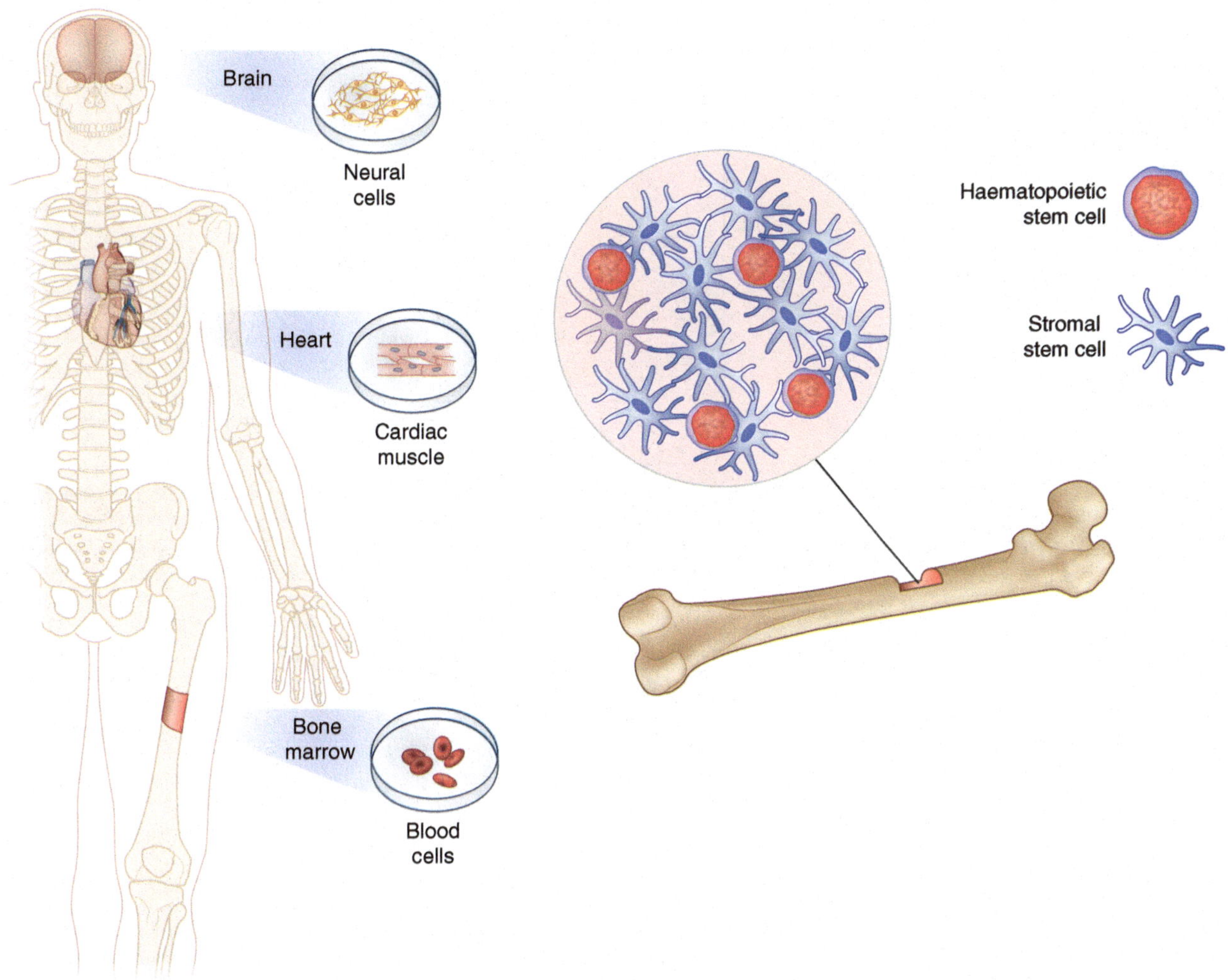

Figure 17.3 ■ Adult stem cells are present in many tissues in specific stem cell niches, giving rise to a specific group of cells found in the relevant tissue. The examples shown have been studied in detail but adult stem cells, yet to be defined, may be present in many other tissues

are well documented in tissues that are regenerated continuously in the adult, such as the epithelia of the skin, intestine and other mucosal tissues, and the bone marrow (Lander et al. 2012). Similar processes are also found in organs that are not continuously replenished, such as the brain. The realization that adult stem cells are present in many organs offers the possibility that repair and regeneration could be stimulated and controlled in degenerative diseases by drug therapy, but whether this will be possible remains to be seen. In the brain, neural stem cells have been identified in the subventricular zone and in the dentate gyrus (part of the hippocampus) (Alvarez-Buylla et al. 2001; Landgren and Curtis 2010).

Adult Stem Cells Used as Transplant Product

Adult stem cells have been used since the 1950s to treat cancers of blood cells, as one of the components of bone marrow transplants (Santos 1983). This procedure involves whole body irradiation to kill malignant cells in multiple myelomas and leukemia. The patient then receives a bone marrow transplant, not in itself a stem cell product, but the transplant contains a few HSCs which subsequently home to the bone marrow stem cell niches and begin to replenish the blood (Fig. 17.5). Rejection and graft-versus-host disease (GvHD) are still threatening complications of this form of therapy, but its practice can now be considered to be routine. These products are not medicinal products, but transplant products and fall under a different legislative regime worldwide, as discussed above.

Adult Stem Cells for Clinical Application: Immune Cells

Immune cell types currently investigated for their therapeutic value, mostly in the field of cancer, are DCs (see also Chap. 14), tumor infiltrating lymphocytes (TILs), γδ T cells, regulatory T cells (Tregs), macrophages, and viral reconstitution T cells. Both autologous and allogeneic cells are used as cell source. These immune cells have a highly specific mode of

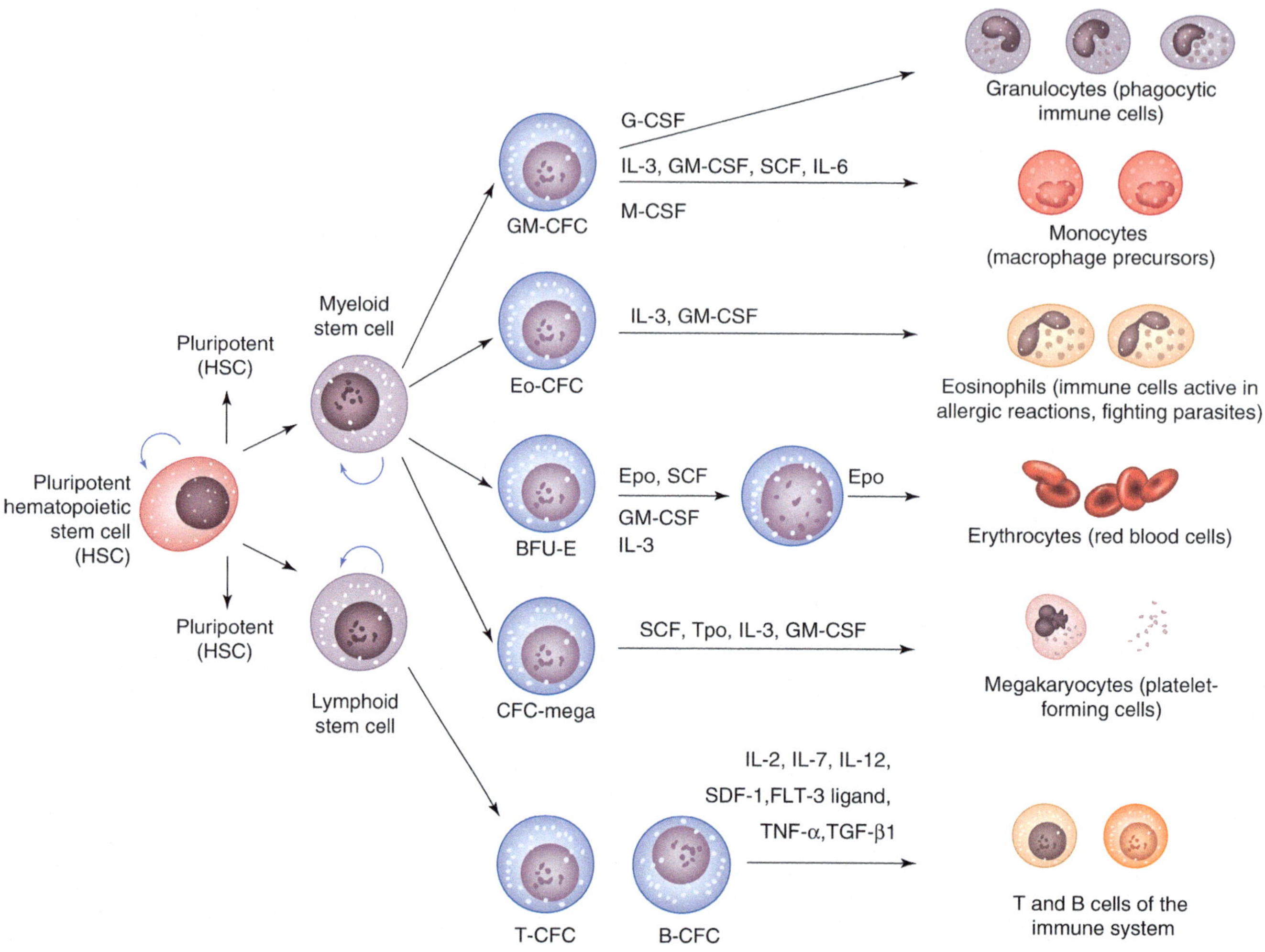

Figure 17.4 ■ Asymmetric division of adult HSCs, to produce myeloid or lymphoid stem cells, further differentiation to form mitotic progenitors, and subsequently under the control of specific growth factors and cytokines, to form fully differentiated blood cells. The differentiation pathways of the hematopoietic system are better characterized than those of other tissues, but the pattern of differentiation is typical of other tissues. *GM-CSF* = Granulocyte-macrophage colony-stimulating factor, *Eo-CFC* = Eosinophil-leukocyte Colony Forming Cell, *BFU-E* = Bone marrow erythroid progenitor cells, *IL* = interleukin, *SCF* = stem cell factor, *SDF* = stromal cell-derived factor, *TNF* = tumor necrosis factor, *TGF* = transforming growth factor

action and are in different stages of clinical development. T cells which are genetically modified using a viral vector, e.g., CAR-T cells, are much more complex to manufacture due to the modification step and fall within a different technology class, i.e., *ex-vivo* gene modification of cells using viral vector technologies (see below).

Adult Stem Cells for Clinical Application: MSCs

MSCs, sometimes called multipotent stromal cells or mesenchymal stem cells, have generated considerable interest in recent years for cell therapy applications (Bianco et al. 2008). However, the description of the cells, their source, and manufacturing processes are quite heterogeneous. MSCs can e.g., be isolated from bone marrow, adipose tissue, and umbilical cord tissue (from the particularly rich source of Wharton's jelly and also from umbilical cord blood). Because cord blood can be sampled, frozen, and banked at birth, this source of MSCs has been identified as a potential source of cells for use in a regenerative capacity in later life. There are now several private companies that offer personal cell banking services, and public cord blood banks that supply pooled cord blood samples for clinical use. Whether cord blood banking will prove to be useful remains to be seen. However, this cell source has already been tested clinically in Phase I/II trials. MSCs have been reported to differentiate into various phenotypes (including chondrocytes, osteoblasts, and adipocytes) as well as other phenotypes. Due to their pleiotropic properties, e.g., growth factors and chemokines producing, anti-apoptotic, angiogenetic, anti-fibrotic, and neuroprotective, they have been extensively tested in pre-clinical models. Hundreds of Phase I-III clinical trials have been performed and are ongoing globally in a wide variety of indications: bone/cartilage repair, heart, lung, liver, gastrointestinal, neurological diseases, and rheuma-

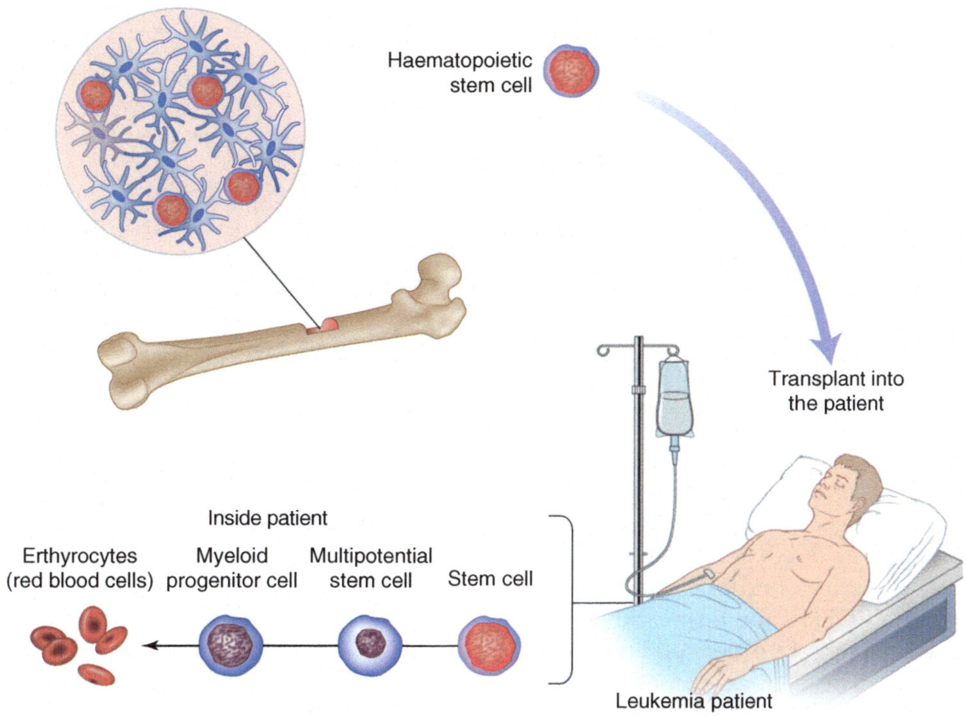

Figure 17.5 ■ Schematic representation of bone marrow transplantation, a form of stem cell therapy that was first used over 50 years ago. The transplant contains hematopoietic stem cells from the donor. These cells repopulate niches in the recipient bone marrow

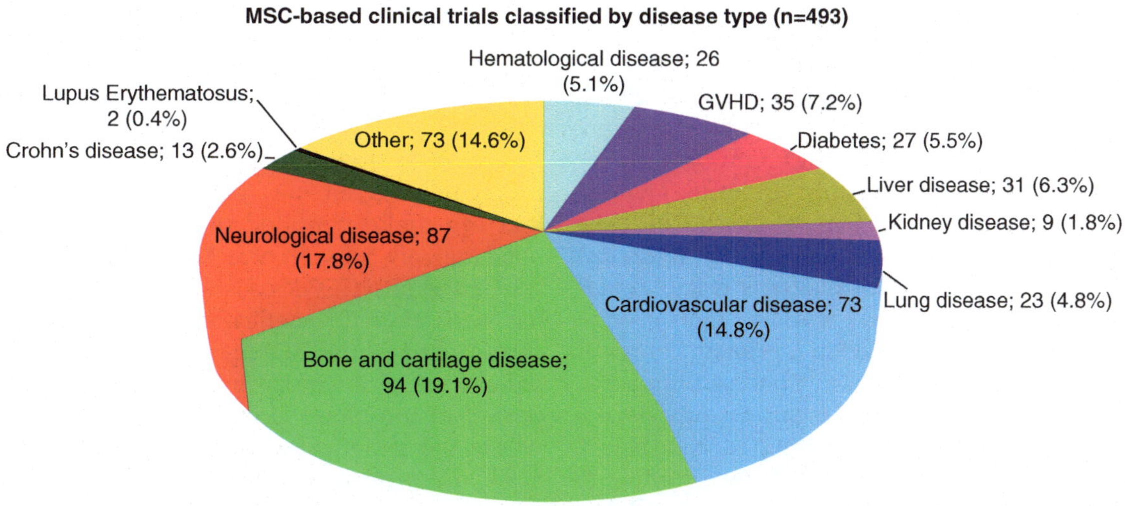

Figure 17.6 ■ Clinical trials with MSC-derived products and their indication (in percentages), adapted from Squillaro et al. (2016)

tology, Crohn's, and other autoimmune diseases, GvHD after organ transplantation, DM and kidney diseases (Trounson and McDonald 2015; Heathman et al. 2015), see Fig. 17.6.

MSC can be administered locally (e.g. intralesionally or subcutaneously) and intravascularly. While local administration has been found effective in case of local injury e.g. to treat bone and joint diseases, heart disease, for repair of muscle and ligament damage, Crohn's fistulas and even for repair of ischemic brain tissue, systemic infusion is preferable in the case of systemic diseases such as GvHD (Kean et al. 2013). Both autologous and allogeneic cell sources have been studied. To date only three MSC products have been approved globally: Alofisel in the EU for the treatment of Crohn's fistulas and Prochymal in Canada and New Zealand and Temcell HS in Japan for the treatment of pediatric acute GvHD. This is due to amongst others the lack of understanding of the therapeutic MoA, limited evidence for the preferred route of administration, lack of delivery systems and analytical tools to characterize the cells (especially their potency), as well as limited experience on optimal manufacturing technologies to support late phase clinical trial and commercial production.

Other adult stem cell sources tested in the clinic, less frequently though, are limbal stem cells, neural stem/progenitor cells, and endothelial stem/progenitor cells (Trounson and McDonald 2015).

■ Cell Immortalization Technologies

Another technology makes use of immortalized cell lines as starting material for the manufacture of cell-based products. An example of such a cell line is the neural stem cell line CTX0E03, derived from human fetal cortical brain and genetically modified with a retroviral vector encoding the immortalizing gene, c-mycER^{TAM} (Pollock et al. 2006; Stevanato et al. 2009). This gene enables, under the conditional regulation by 4-hydroxytamoxifen (4-OHT), the large-scale production of the CTX cells using a two-tier cell banking system (MCB and WCB). The CTX cell-based product is currently in a clinical Phase II program for stroke. Although cell immortalization technologies have been in development for quite some time now, this is not a mainstream technology yet in the pharmaceutical world.

■ *Ex-vivo* Gene Modification of Cells Using Viral Vector Technologies

Ex-vivo genetic modifications using viral vector technology are used for several cell types; the most common are T cells, HSCs, and MSCs. The viral vector systems for transfer of genetic information into the cells are e.g., adeno associated virus (AAV), herpes virus (HPV), adenovirus (Ad), lentivirus (LV), and gamma-retrovirus (γ-RV). Cells are of autologous or allogeneic origin, *ex-vivo* purified, activated, modified with a viral vector, expanded, formulated, and filled in a primary container for direct infusion or stored frozen prior to administration. More details of the manufacturing process are described in the manufacturing and testing section below.

Gene modifications of HSCs show promise to treat diseases such as adenosine deaminase severe combined immunodeficiency disease (ADA SCID) and genetically modified MSCs are entering the FIH trials for indications such as advanced adenocarcinoma. In the case of T cells, which are currently the dominating cell type in this technology area, the approach is to genetically modify the isolated T cells in various ways to target and activate them to selectively destruct different types of systemic and solid malignancies.

HSCs Ex-vivo Genetically Modified

Since the 1990s, genetically modified HSCs have been viewed as a promising cell type for gene therapy for several reasons. Not only are HSCs readily accessible and easily separated from the bone marrow or peripheral blood; they also have the potential to expand into differentiated, long-living cell types that can carry a therapeutic gene to different sites of the patient's body, which are accessible to blood cells. Diseases of the blood and immune system, where one gene (monogenic) is involved, are now fairly well characterized and good candidates for treatment with genetically modified HSCs, as shown in Table 17.7.

Disease category	Examples
Primary immune deficiencies	ADA-SCID, Wiskott-Aldrich syndrome, granulomatous disease, X-linked syndrome
Hemoglobulin pathologies and red blood cell disorders	Sickle cell disease, thalassemia
Lysosomal storage diseases and metabolic disorders	Gaucher, mucopolysaccharidosis

Table 17.7 ■ Candidates for *ex-vivo* HSC therapy, adapted from Scott and DeFrancesco (2016)

One of the most successful genetically modified HSC products is Strimvelis against ADA-SCID. This is the second gene therapy approved in the EU after Glybera (withdrawn shortly after approval) and it represents a historic first for *ex-vivo* gene therapy. Children with ADA-SCID are vulnerable to life-threatening infections, a result of defects in the housekeeping enzyme adenosine deaminase (ADA), which causes metabolites of adenosine to accumulate to toxic levels. To manufacture Strimvelis, patient cells are collected from the bone marrow. Then, CD34$^+$ cells (i.e., HSCs that can make lymphocytes) are extracted from the bone marrow cells. A correct copy of the gene for ADA is inserted into CD34$^+$ cells using a γ-RV vector, which has been altered genetically so that it can transfer a correct copy of the ADA gene. Once given back to the patient via intravenous infusion, Strimvelis is transported in the blood circulation to the bone marrow, where the genetically modified CD34$^+$ cells start to grow and produce healthy B- and T-lymphocytes that can produce ADA. These lymphocytes improve the patient's ability to fight infections, and so overcome the symptoms of the condition related to the immune deficiency. The effects are expected to last for the patient's lifetime, but this still has to be proven.

T-cells Ex-vivo Genetically Modified

The immune system comprises the innate and adaptive immune systems (see Chap. 14 and handbooks on immunology for explanation). Through immune surveillance, any molecules that are identified as non-self are eliminated. Targets include not only virally infected cells, as discussed in Chap. 14, but also transformed (tumor) cells, which can become immunogenic through the expression of neo-antigens that can be recognized as non-self and can interact with an immunologically specific antibody or T cell receptor (Sharpe and Mount 2015). However, cancer cells have developed strategies to escape the immune system, which results in a failure to initiate and maintain adequate anti-tumor immunity, and consequently facilitates tumor survival and progression.

Over the last 20 years, genetically modified T cell immunotherapies have been widely tested in clinical trials, mostly in the oncology field. These cells play a key role in cell-mediated immunity. The genetic modification of the T cells occurs either through altering the specificity of the T-cell receptor (TCR) or through introducing antibody-like recognition in CARs. Both approaches enhance tumor specificities.

The potential of these T cell therapies has been demonstrated, particularly in the treatment of B cell hematological malignancies, for the following reasons: (1) B cell malignancies are relatively common; (2) B cells express several conserved cell surface markers; (3) the i.v. route provides an easy route of administration to interact with circulating B cell tumors. The product cells don't have to traffic to the tumor-site, which would be the case for a solid tumor (Fesnak et al. 2016). Most malignant B cells as well as healthy B cells express the extracellular glycoprotein CD19 antigen on their cell surface. As there is extremely limited non-B cell expression of CD19, it is an attractive therapeutic target for cell therapy (anti-CD19 CAR-Ts), see Fig. 17.7. The greatest clinical success in terms of response rates to CAR-T19 cells has been reported for patients with B cell acute lymphoblastic leukaemia (B-ALL), with one product being approved by the FDA for commercial use (Kymriah®). Yescarta® is a CAR-T19 immunotherapy commercially available in the US for the treatment of diffuse large B-cell lymphoma (DLBCL). Other cell surface markers used as a target (antigen) are e.g., CD20, CD22, and CD30. Currently, both CAR-T and engineered TCR cell therapies are also under investigation for the treatment of solid tumors, e.g., neuroblastoma, prostate cancer, breast cancer, and glioblastoma. Although successful in treatment of hematologic malignancies, the effectiveness of genetically modified T cells in the treatment of solid tumors remains modest. Table 17.8 provides an overview of genetically modified T cell clinical trials.

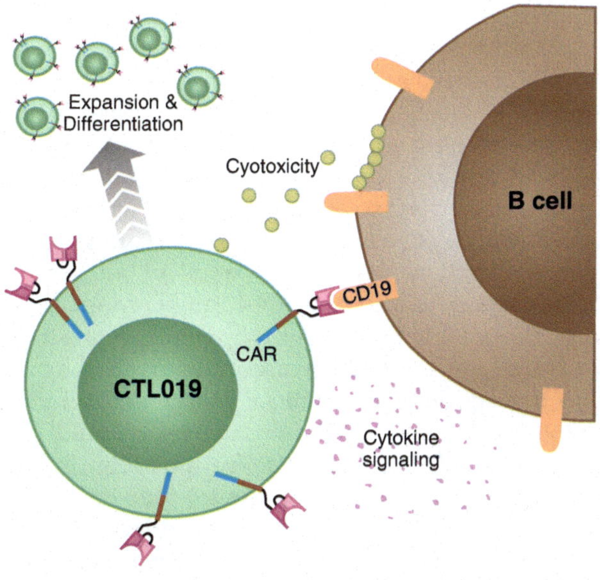

Figure 17.7 ■ Schematic presentation of Kymriah's MoA, adapted from https://www.fda.gov/downloads/AdvisoryCommittees/CommitteesMeetingMaterials/Drugs/OncologicDrugsAdvisoryCommittee/UCM566166.pdf

Factors That Can Affect Efficacy

A number of factors may contribute to the variability observed in (long term) efficacy of genetically modified T cell therapies (Sharpe and Mount 2015). These include e.g.:

- Persistence and survival of the engineered T cells in the body.
- Patients who have shown disappearance of all signs of cancer in response to the engineered T cell treatment (complete responders), have shown greater cell persistence and survival. This may be impacted by a preparative conditioning regime (e.g., fludarabine) to reduce the number of circulating patient T cells (lymphodepletion) prior to administration of the genetically modified T cells.
- Cell dose.
- T cell therapies are normally dosed on the basis of a defined number of cells per kilogram of body weight. However, because T cells will replicate and expand after administration, which may vary among patients, there may not be a direct correlation between cell dose and efficacy. It is suggested that the ability of cells to proliferate and persist may be more important than the initial cell dose.
- Cancer cells may down-regulate or lose expression of the targeted (e.g., CD19) antigens. This may impact long-term maintenance of efficacy.
- Many factors present in the tumor microenvironment, which is composed of tumor cells, vasculature, and immune cells.
- Tumors propagate conditions that favor immune tolerance and this might impact the effectiveness of the genetically modified T cell therapy.

Factors That Can Affect Safety

A number of factors may affect safety of genetically modified T-cell therapies (Sharpe and Mount 2015). These include:

- Cytokine-release syndrome.
- Genetically modified T cells can be very effective against target tumor cells by inducing tumor cell lysis and potential tumor cell removal at a fast rate. This can result in high levels of cytokine (e.g., interferon-gamma and interleukin-6 (IL-6)) release and macrophage activation syndrome, leading to

Genetically modified T-cell therapy	Target (antigen on the cell surface of cancer cell)	Indication
Hematological tumor		
CAR-T cell	CD19 or CD20	(ALL)
		Chronic lymphocytic leukemia (CLL)
		DLBCL
		Multiple Myeloma
	CD22	B cell malignancy
	CD30	Lymphoma
	CD138	Multiple myeloma
	CD33	Myeloid malignancies
	Receptor tyrosine kinase-like orphan receptor (ROR1)	Leukaemia
Engineered TCR	Cancer-testis antigen NY-ESO-1 with/without additional antigens	Multiple myeloma
Solid tumor		
CAR-T cell	Epidermal growth factor receptor variant III (EGFRvIII)	Glioblastoma
	Mesothelin	Mesothelioma, pancreatic cancer, ovarian cancer
	Prostate-specific membrane antigen (PSMA)	Prostate cancer
	Hepatocyte growth factor receptor, a protein tyrosine kinase (c-met)	Breast cancer
	Lewis-Y	Solid tumors and myeloid malignancies
Engineered TCR	Cancer-testis antigen NY-ESO-1 with/without additional antigens	Various solid tumors
	Wilms tumor protein 1 (WT1)	Myeloid malignancy; mesothelioma and non-small cell lung cancer (NSCL)

Table 17.8 ■ Overview of CAR-T and engineered TCR cell-based clinical trials, adapted from Fesnak et al. (2016), Sharpe and Mount (2015)

high fevers, rigors, nausea, and diarrhea. Anti-IL-6 receptor antibody administration can inhibit these side effects.

– On-target off-tumor activity.

This phenomenon occurs when the antigen target of the T cell therapy is expressed on normal cells as well, even at low levels. An example of this side effect is depletion of normal B cells, which also express CD19. Since B cells play an important role in the humoral immunity component of the adaptive immune system by secreting antibodies (see Chap. 14), a lack of these cells may cause infectious diseases. This side effect can be managed by the administration of antibodies. Strategies are being explored to engineer T-cells with higher selectivity for tumor than for normal cells. E.g., dual-CAR-T cells, in which T cells are genetically modified to express simultaneously two CARs with different antigen specificities (e.g., CD19 and CD123).

– Off-target reactivity.

This side effect can occur as cross-reactivity and is particularly a risk for TCR T cells, which could react against peptides and proteins other than the target ones.

■ *In-vivo* Gene Modification of Cells Using Viral or Non-viral Vector Technologies

In-vivo gene therapy refers to the direct introduction of genetic material into the human body. This technology is discussed in Chap. 16.

■ Genome Editing Technologies

The emerge of genome editing tools, such as zinc finger nucleases (ZNFs), meganucleases, transcription activator-like effector nucleases (TALENs), and lately the cluster regularly interspaced short palindrome repeat (CRISPR)-CRISPR-associated protein 9 (Cas9) has further advanced the application of advanced therapies. Especially CRISPR-Cas9 systems are gaining interest because of signs of efficacy.

With these genetic engineering techniques, as discussed in detail in Chap. 16, it is now possible to generate human cellular disease models in a precise and predicable manner These techniques can be used to make changes in the genome which results into the formation of cells/tissues/organs identical to those of a person with a specific disease. Genome editing has been applied to introduce genetic alterations to create cardiac disease models or correct genetic mutations in e.g., iPSC- cardiac myocytes to model cardiac diseases, such as long QT- (Sayed et al. 2016; see Chap. 9), e.g., cardiomyocytes. Single genetic mutations responsible for cardiomyopathies, such as Barth syndrome and Duchenne muscular dystrophy have been corrected by use of these genome-editing tools. However, these engineered nucleases could introduce unintended genomic alterations (e.g., in addition to cleaving the on-target site, they might have off-target effects). Similarly, other challenges, such as methods for local delivery and efficiency, still need to be sorted out.

Targeted gene editing is still considered an early stage technology from a translational point of view. However, the first applications have reached the first-in-human trial phase: Human Immuno-deficiency

Virus (HIV) treatment by gene editing of autologous CD4+ T cells (CCR5 gene dysfunction) using the ZFN technology (Tebas et al. 2014).

■ Cell Plasticity Technologies

The cell plasticity technology area takes advantage of discoveries during the last 50 years that certain cells have the ability to evolve to cell types formerly considered outside their normal differentiation repertoire, i.e., hESCs and iPSCs. This technology has an extensive clinical potential due to the high probability of an almost unlimited supply of cells (MCB and WCB approach) and also for the possibility to HLA-match the resulting cell-based product (partly) with the recipient patient. The application of pluripotent stem cells, such as ESCs and iPSCs, goes beyond the administration of cell-based medicinal products and are investigated as a source for tissue engineering and organogenesis (see below three dimensional technologies). In addition, autologous and allogeneic iPSCs are currently extensively used for disease modeling (i.e., patient specific iPSC derived cardiomyocytes, cultured *in-vitro*, can be used to identify the genetic basis of a cardiac disease, leading to the identification of pharmacogenetic biomarkers that support effective and personalized drug therapy) and drug discovery including toxicity screening (Sayed et al. 2016).

Embryonic Stem Cells

During the earliest stages of mammalian development, soon after egg and sperm combine, the resulting diploid cells are said to be "totipotent," i.e., they can give rise to both the embryo and placental tissue. At the blastocyst stage of embryogenesis (day 5 in humans), the "inner cell mass" or "embryoblast" is compacted and separated from the surrounding "trophoblast." The latter combines with the maternal endometrium to form the placenta. The inner cell mass can be extracted and grown *ex-vivo* as ESCs, which can give rise to all three germ cell types (mesoderm, endoderm, and ectoderm), and therefore potentially any cell type found in the adult (Fig. 17.8). Mouse ESCs were first isolated in 1981 (Evans and Kaufman 1981; Martin 1981), but it took until 1998 for a similar procedure to be described allowing hESCs to be grown in culture (Thomson et al. 1998). ESCs can now be grown for many cell divisions, limited only by genetic damage that occurs by mutation after extensive culturing. The pluripotency of ESCs can be demonstrated in mice by injecting cells into a fertilized egg, resulting in the production of chimeric mice (i.e., mice made up of cells derived from both the donor and the injected ESCs). This process has been used routinely over the past 20 years to produce transgenic mice for research purposes. HESCs are currently investigated by a set of cell surface markers (CD markers) and their capacity to differentiate. The criteria for this assessment include the expression of surface markers and transcription factors associated with an undifferentiated state. In addition, extended proliferative capacity, pluripotency and an euploid karyotype are important characteristics of these cells. Recent evidence suggests that the epigenetic status of the cells is also a relevant criterion for hESCs. Examination of

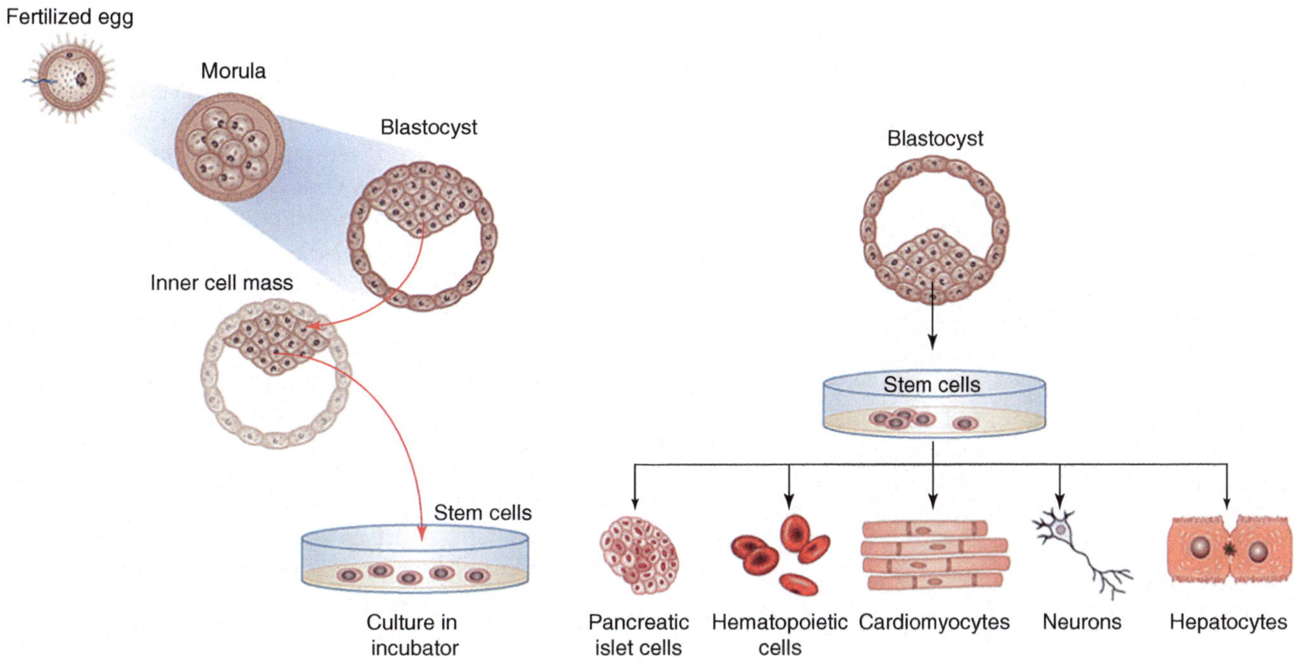

Figure 17.8 ■ Extraction of the inner cell mass of the blastocyst gives rise to ESCs, which have the capacity to differentiate into all 200+ somatic cell types found in the adult human

hESCs over extended periods *ex-vivo* should also be considered as critical parameter, to demonstrate that hESC characteristics do not change over time, and that the lines are stable in their expression of markers, expression of telomerase, ability to differentiate into the three germlines ecto- meso- and endoderm, and maintenance of a normal karyotype (i.e., number and appearance of the 46 chromosomes).

Maintenance and Differentiation of ESCs in Culture

Mouse ESCs were first grown as compact colonies on a feeder layer of mouse embryonic fibroblasts, in media containing leukemia inhibitory factor (LIF) and fetal bovine serum (FBS). Efforts to simplify culture methods soon established that the feeders could be substituted with gelatin-coated culture plates, though differentiation occurs to some extent in the absence of the feeder layer. The vital component in serum was found to be bone morphogenetic protein (BMP). Thus, mouse ESCs can be grown in chemically defined medium with LIF and BMP4 (Ying et al. 2003). HESCs are grown in the presence of high concentrations of basic fibroblast growth factor-2 (FGF2) and are unresponsive to LIF (Levenstein et al. 2006). The difference in responsiveness between mouse and human ESCs has been extensively studied and debated. The two methods of derivation may result in isolation of cells from slightly different stages of development. HESCs are thought to resemble cells from the later epiblast stage. More recently, it has been demonstrated that mouse ESCs can be maintained and grown very efficiently in the presence of small molecule inhibitors of mitogen-activated protein kinase (MEK1/2) and glycogen synthase kinase-3β (GSK-3β). This medium changes their phenotype slightly to what may be represent a "ground state" for mouse ESCs (Ying et al. 2008). A better understanding of the ground state and how this relates to hESCs will be an important step forward and will allow human ES-technology to be reproduced more effectively.

The technical challenge, now that hESCs can be maintained and expanded, is to develop robust methods to control and direct ESC differentiation, so that human cells of any desired phenotype can be obtained (Keller 2005; Murry and Keller 2008). In the context of cell based therapies, it is also important to ensure that no undesired cells are present in a product for clinical use, such as undifferentiated cells, or cells that are capable of de-differentiation (into undifferentiated cells or into cells of a different lineage), either of which could cause tumor formation after implantation, both at the site of administration or elsewhere in the body after cell migration. This science is not mature at present and will remain a priority for investigation for several years. Thus far, attention has focused on the differentiation of human ESCs towards products that could be of obvious use for clinical administration, e.g., midbrain dopaminergic neurons for Parkinson's disease, cardiomyocytes for reinforcement of damaged heart tissue, and pancreatic pre-β-islet cells for implantation in Type I DM.

At present, fine tuning of differentiation programs is still a challenge. Differentiation usually results in mixed populations of cells. For example, neural differentiation can be induced quite effectively, but the result of further differentiation is a mixed population of cells that often include both neurons and glia, and the neurons are comprised of a variety of neuronal subtypes. Timing, duration, and concentration of exposure to specific morphogenic compounds are of critical importance to the outcome and will need to be optimized in each case.

Since they were isolated for the first time, the use of hESC remains controversial. Whereas researchers clearly have experienced and experience their therapeutic potential, both pre-clinically as well as clinically, the regulators and public became widely divided, from being very supportive to seeking a regulatory ban on hESC research for ethical/religious reasons. Ocular diseases dominate these FIH trials, and these trials are showing promising safety data as well as signs of efficacy, as shown in Table 17.9.

ESC Somatic Cell Nuclear Transfer (Therapeutic Cloning)

An alternative, particularly when an HLA-donor match cannot be found, is to produce ESCs for individual patients, by somatic cell nuclear transfer (SCNT) (Wilmut et al. 2002). This process, also known as "therapeutic cloning," involves implantation of a cell nucleus from the patient (i.e., genomic DNA extracted from a skin biopsy) into a human egg, which has undergone removal of its own DNA. The environment in the enucleated egg is able to reprogram the DNA from the patient, removing epigenetic marks and restoring the DNA to an embryonic state. The development of an inner cell mass in the egg, after a period of incubation, allows extraction of ESCs that have the patient's exact genotype. These cells could be used subsequently for production of implants for cell therapy (Fig. 17.9). SCNT is also the first step in the process by which animals are cloned by "reproductive cloning," which involves implantation of the engineered egg into a surrogate mother (Fig. 17.10) (Campbell et al. 1996). Reproductive cloning of humans is illegal but is also likely to be impractical. It is known from experience with animal cloning that SCNT is an inefficient process. Most eggs that have undergone SCNT are unable to completely reprogram the donor DNA and as a result the surrogate pregnancy is usually unproductive. Even when the pregnancy comes to term, the cloned offspring is known to carry many epigenetic marks that may compromise normal development, and the famous sheep, "Dolly," the first large animal to be cloned by way of SCNT,

Indication	Active substance	Trial sponsor (country)
AMD[a]	hESC derived RPEs[b]	Chabiotech (South Korea)
Dry AMD; myopic AMD; Stargardt's macular dystrophy	hESC derived RPEs	Ocata therapeutics (USA)
Wet AMD	hESC derived RPEs	Pfizer (UK)
Dry AMD	hESC derived RPEs	Cell cure neurosciences (Israel)
Type I DM	hESC derived pancreatic endoderm cell	Viacyte/Johnson& Johnson
Heart failure	hESC derived CD^{15+} $Isl\text{-}^{1+}$ progenitors	Assistance Publique-Hopitaux de Paris (France)
Parkinson's disease	Human parthenogenic-derived neural stem cells	International stem cell Corp. (Australia)
Spinal cord injury	hESC derived oligodendrocyte precursors	Asterias Biotherapeuticcs (USA)
Wet AMD	hESC derived RPEs	The London project to cure blindness (UK)
Wet AMD	iPSC-derived RPEs (autologous)	Riken institute (Japan)

[a]*AMD* = age related macular degeneration
[b]*RPEs* = retinal pigmented epithelial cells

Table 17.9 ■ Example of clinical trials with pluripotent stem cells (hESCs and iPSC), adapted from Trounson and McDonald 2015 and Ilic et al. (2015)

had several developmental defects (Wilmut et al. 2009). Second-generation animals, produced by mating a clone with another parent, are usually unaffected by such defects, indicating that SCNT is much less efficient than the natural process of reprogramming of DNA in a fertilized egg. Given that defects are known to occur after SCNT, the subsequent derivation of cells for clinical uses might also be prone to failure due to defects in ESC differentiation. There is insufficient data available at this stage to judge whether this will be a limitation in practice. There are significant ethical concerns that have limited the practice of SCNT. A human egg donor is required, and unless the process becomes more efficient, women who are prepared to donate eggs would need to provide several eggs to produce a single ESC line. There is concern that women could be exploited, particularly women from low economic backgrounds, and as a result SCNT is not supported by government funding at present in most countries. A restricted number of ESC lines have been produced using spare eggs from *in-vitro* fertilization programs, but the status of SCNT remains a controversial topic and is subject to legal constraints that vary from country to country. An alternative source of cells for clinical application are umbilical cord blood stem cells, which are now being banked at childbirth (i.e., biobank), at least in private practice and the first clinical trials have been initiated. Whether cord blood cells can be harnessed to produce all cell phenotypes is not clear at present (see also above "cord blood derived MSCs"). However, many of the ethical issues surrounding SCNT, and uncertainty of cord blood stem cell potency (*in-vivo* activity), may become irrelevant if the promise of iPSCs can be realized.

IPS Cell Technology

Initially, work on pluripotent stem cells (PSCs) was conducted using hESCs; however, the requirement to destroy early-stage embryos in the process of ESC derivation makes their use ethically controversial. In addition, practical considerations hinders their medical applications, because any cells or tissues generated from hESCs by definition would be allotransplants into the recipient patient (see above). The discovery by Takahashi et al. (that mouse skin fibroblasts could be reprogrammed to produce pluripotent cells by forcing expression of just four genes (*Sox2*, *Oct4*, *Klf4*, and *cMyc*) using LV vectors (Takahashi and Yamanaka 2006) became a landmark in regenerative medicine. A year later similar methods were published for production of iPSCs from human fibroblasts (Takahashi et al. 2007; Yu et al. 2007). This indicated that patient-specific (i.e., autologous) pluripotent stem cells could be produced without the need for human eggs, using cells extracted from a simple skin biopsy. These cells retain similar properties as hESCs, such as indefinite growth and pluripotency. The significance of this discovery to regenerative medicine cannot be overestimated. Over the last 15 years, the iPSC field has exploded with activity, and the technology is now in use in hundreds of stem cell biology laboratories around the world. The four genes initially identified can be partly substituted by alternatives, and several experiments have shown that integrated lentiviral constructs can be avoided to reduce safety concerns, by using non-viral plasmids (Jia et al. 2010), micro ribonucleic acids (RNAs) (Yang et al. 2011), protein transduction, and even by substituting some of the factors with small molecules (Yuan et al. 2011). Often the safer alternative methods work with reduced efficiency, but nevertheless produce the same result. The technology is still in its infancy, but if it delivers its potential, iPSC technology will have profound effects on the understanding of disease by disease modeling, drug discovery and toxicity screening, correction of genetic defects, and cell-and tissue-based medici-

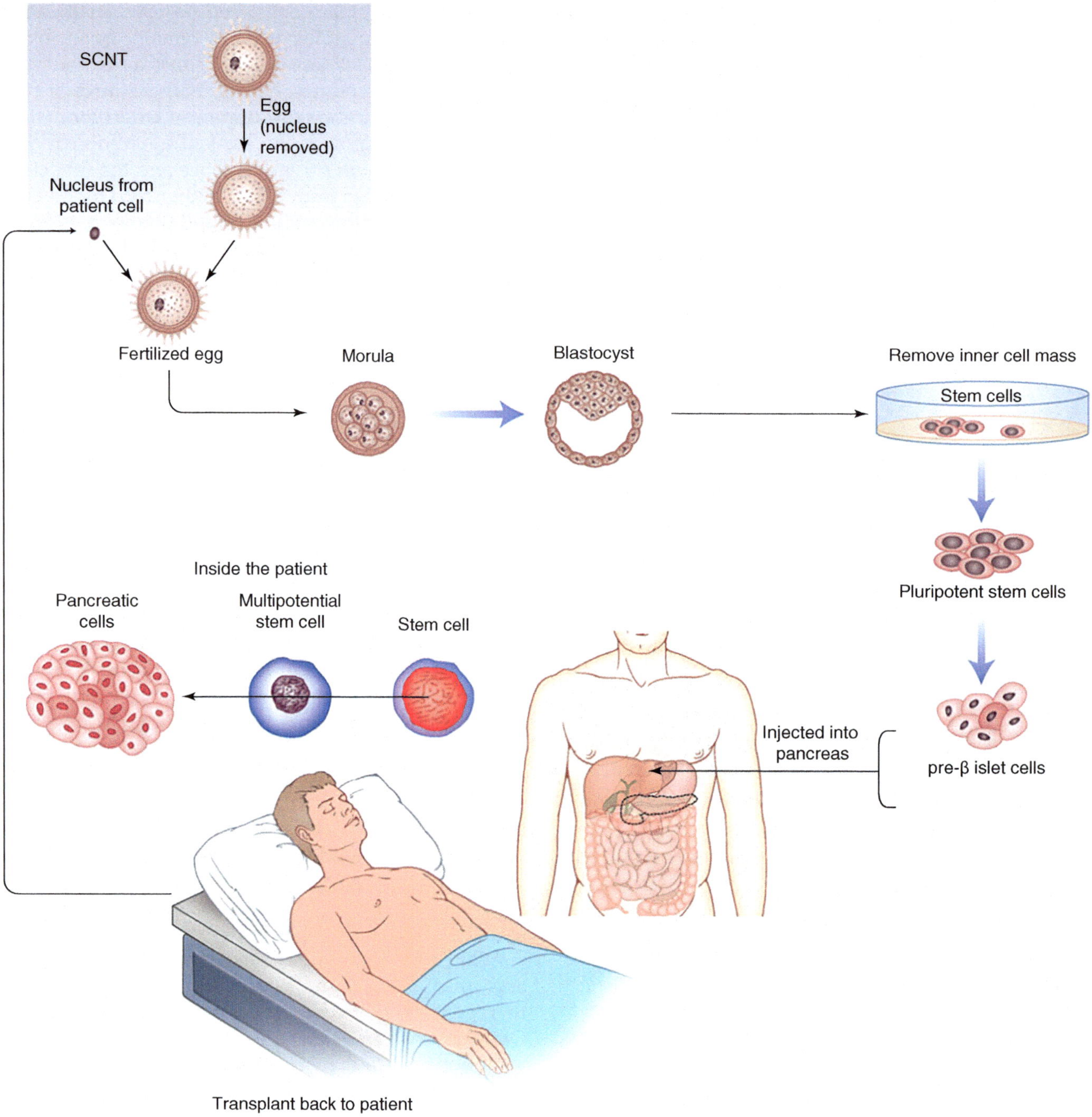

Figure 17.9 ■ Schematic diagram of the production and clinical use of cell therapies derived using somatic cell nuclear transfer (therapeutic cloning). The example given is for possible treatment of Type I insulin-dependent DM. The final maturation of the pre-β islet cells occur in the patient's body

nal products (Sayed et al. 2016). Already iPSCs have been used to correct defects in mouse models of Parkinson's disease (Hargus et al. 2010), to cure a model of sickle cell anemia in mice (Hanna et al. 2007), and other diseases (Kimbrel and Lanza 2015).

Considerable effort has been directed at investigating how iPSCs differ from ESCs and whether reprogramming is complete enough to produce truly pluripotent cells. True pluripotency is difficult to demonstrate unequivocally in human iPSCs so the development of methods to measure the extent of reprogramming will be important for practical applications. There are indications that iPSCs can have chromosomal defects and are not fully reprogrammed (Chin et al. 2010). Female human iPSCs appear to maintain the inactivated X chromosome that was present in the skin fibroblasts, though this has not been a problem with mouse iPSCs (Tchieu et al. 2010).

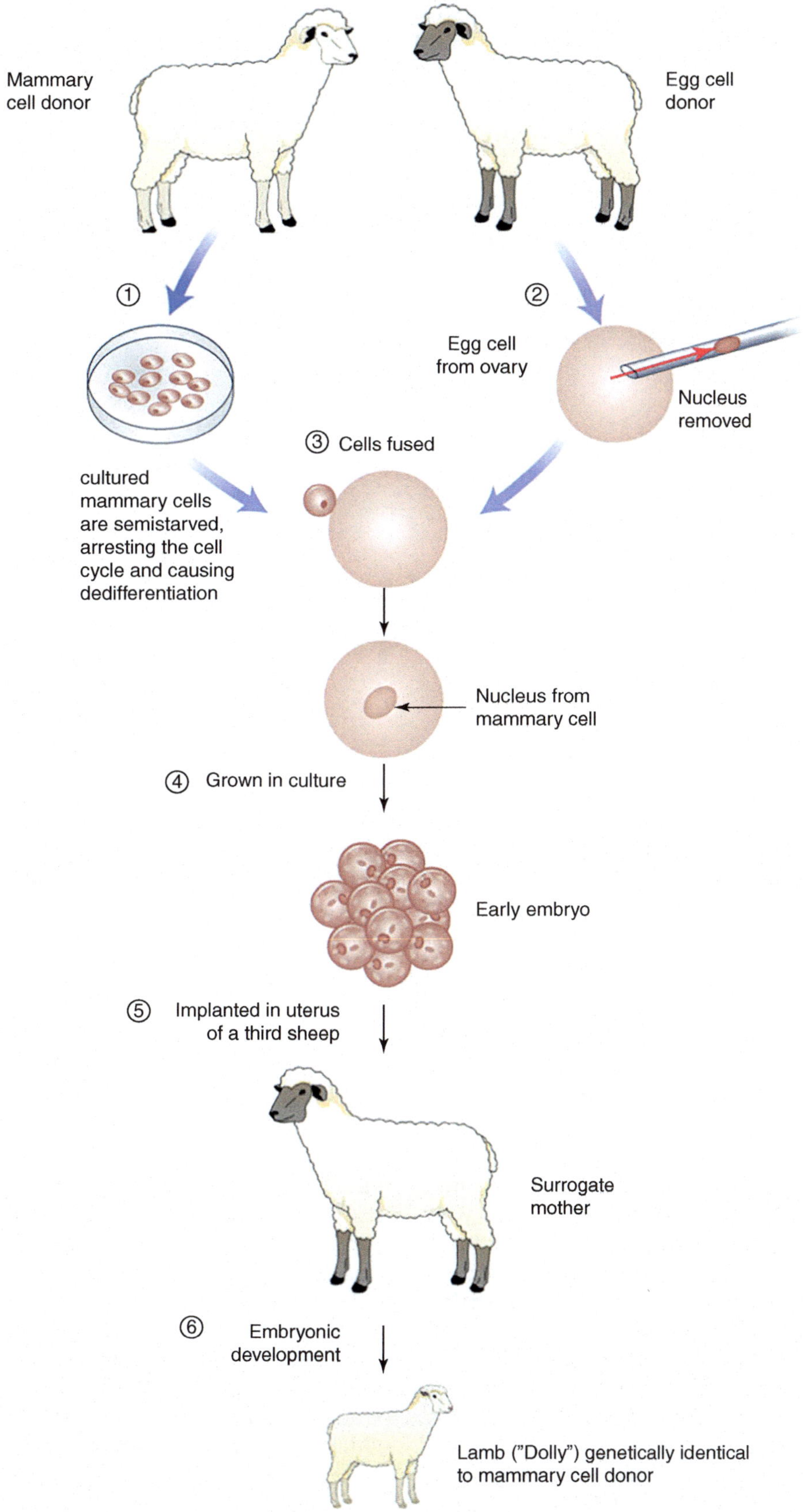

Figure 17.10 ■ Schematic diagram of the concept of reproductive cloning, as used to produce the cloned sheep "Dolly"

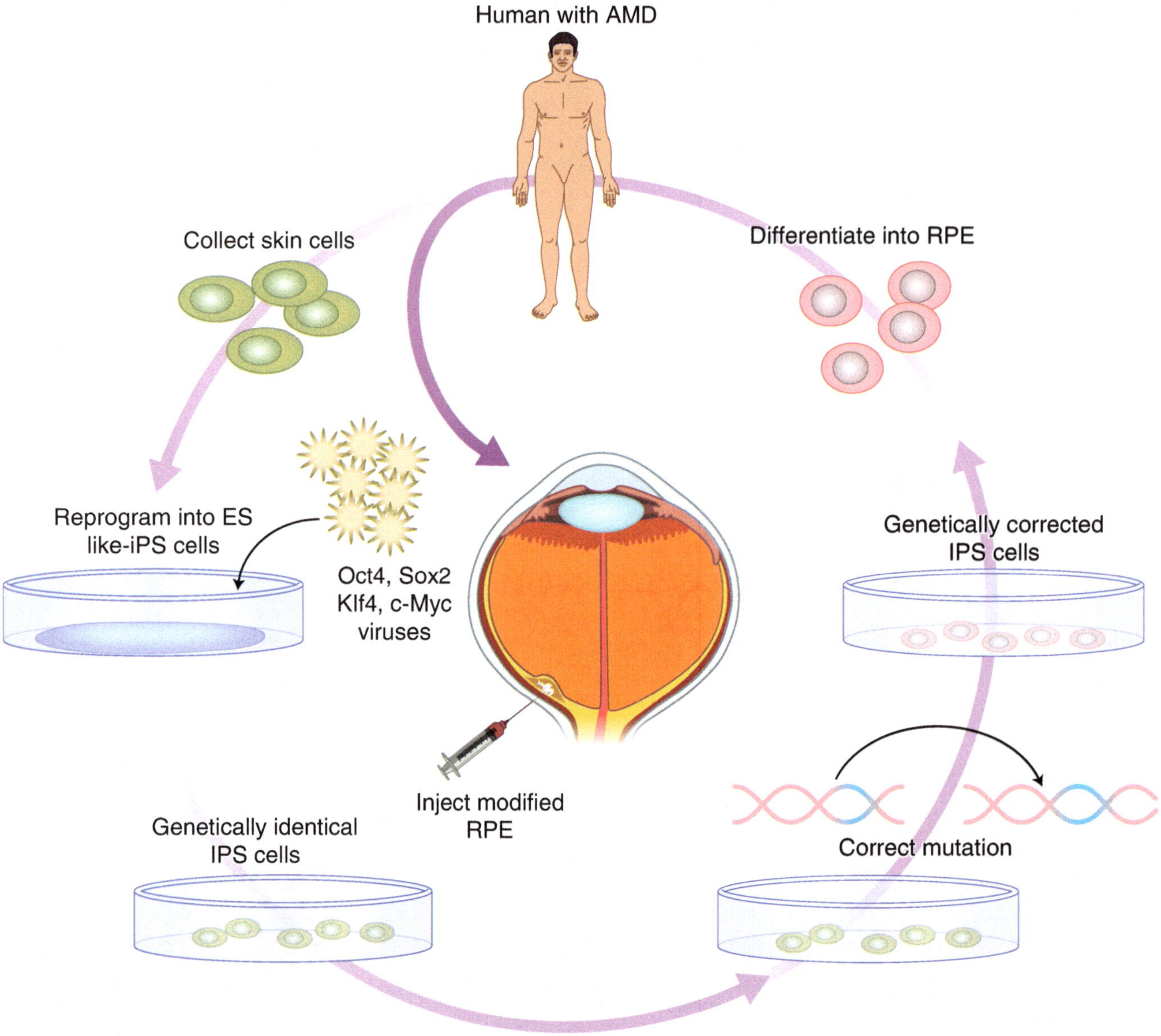

Figure 17.11 ■ Method used to produce iPS cells, correct a genetic defect responsible for AMD, and implant the corrected stem cells into humans to cure AMD

In mice iPSCs induced an immune response in a genetically identical host from which the cells were derived (Zhao et al. 2011). The mechanisms causing this immunogenicity need to be studied in more detail to investigate whether this is a widespread problem. The above unfavorable reports may be the result of inadequate control over reprogramming. In recent years, progress has been made with improved culture techniques and differentiation protocols, which resulted in safer and clinically relevant cells with lower tumorigenic risk. So far, one clinical trial has been initiated by the Riken Institute in Japan (Table 17.9; Fig. 17.11), using autologous iPSC derived RPE to treat wet AMD (Sayed et al. 2016). After the second patient was dosed, the study was temporarily put on hold due to genetic mutations found in the iPSC-RPEs (Ilic et al. 2015). The switch to allogeneic iPSC sources, both HLA-matched and HLA-inactivated, to manufacture cell based medicinal products, has the potential to broaden the accessibility of stem cell therapies to a wider population. In addition, the ability to use 'off-the-shelf' cell products makes them available for use immediately and decreases the cost of treatment compared to using the patient's own cells to generate autologous therapies, which can be time consuming and costly. Still, there is debate in the scientific community over using iPSCs derived from an allogeneic donor because of the potential immune rejection as is the case for many other allogeneic cell types. Progress has been made to address this concern through identification of HLA superdonors, individuals whose HLA profiles make their cells widely compatible for donation to unrelated patients. Companies worldwide are generating and banking HLA superdonor iPSC lines (see above ESC lines). In Japan the first AMD patient has been treated with allogeneic skin cell derived iPSCs which were differentiated into retinal cells and transplanted onto the retina of the patient. Since the eye is an immune-privileged site, the risk for rejection of the transplant is considered low.

Direct Reprogramming/Transdifferentiation

Forced expression of genes has been used to convert fibroblasts directly into unrelated differentiated cells, including neurons (Ambasudhan et al. 2011; Wernig et al. 2008), hepatocytes (Huang et al. 2011), endothelial cells (Sayed et al. 2015) and cardiomyocytes (Burridge et al. 2012) by skipping the iPSC stage. The technique used is analogous to that used to derive iPSCs, except that genes associated with the desired somatic cell are expressed instead of pluripotency genes. The realization that cellular phenotypes can be transformed in this way has been met with astonishment and is certainly breakthrough technology. It raises the possibility that interconversion could be performed *in-vivo*, though it does not allow for expansion of cells in preparation for an implant. However, direct reprogramming of fibroblasts to neural stem cells, as reported in 2012 (Han et al. 2012; Thier et al. 2012), may be a short cut to neurons. This approach may offer some advantages over production of neurons by way of iPSCs.

Three-Dimensional Technologies

Another technology, tissue engineering, is combining somatic cell technologies or cell-therapy technologies described above, with various types of biocompatible materials to solve structural challenges that are often surgical or immunological in nature. Three-dimensional (3D) technologies, including biomaterial scaffolds, can have many purposes, such as supporting cell viability, induction of cell differentiation, provision of a substrate for cell growth and support of tissue regeneration, provision of the shape, scale, and volume of a desired tissue, provision of growth factors, and encapsulation of cell-based products to protect the product from the host immune system to avoid rejection. This is schematically presented in Fig. 17.12 (Smith and Grande 2015). 3D technologies can be divided into four subtypes of technologies as shown in Table 17.10. For further reading see Murphy and Atala (2014); Wegst et al. (2015); Smith and Grande (2015); Pedersen et al. (2012); Kim and Matsunaga (2017).

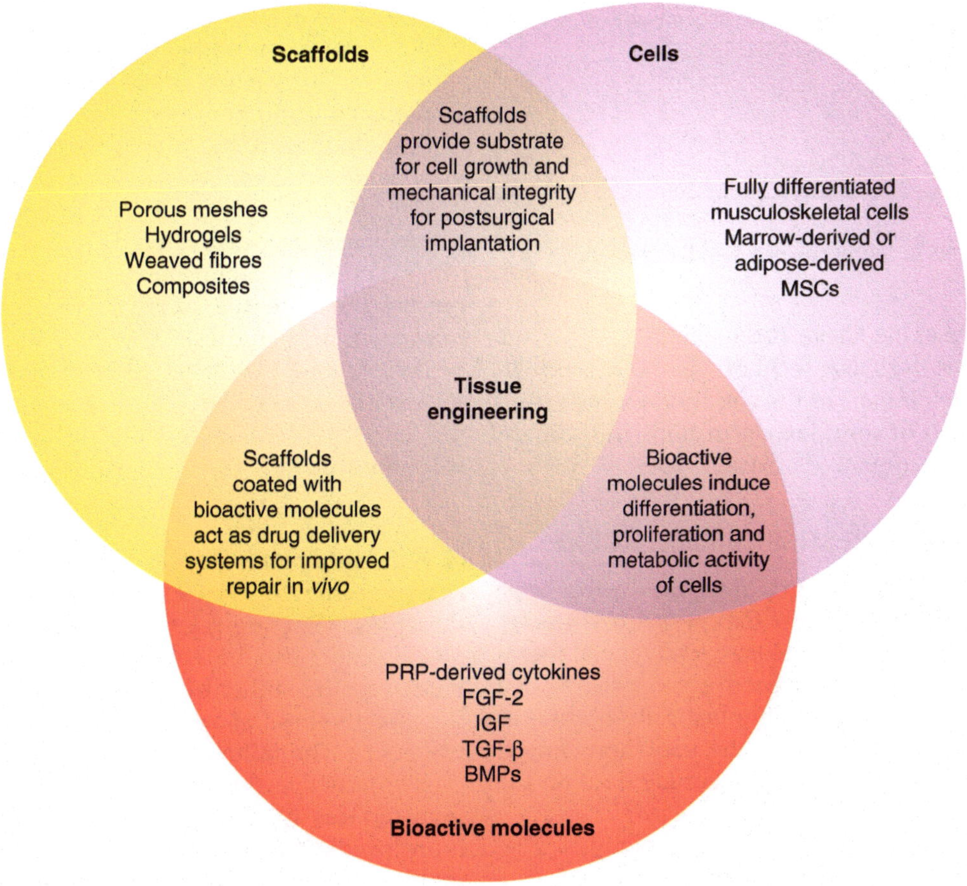

Figure 17.12 ■ The role of scaffolds in tissue engineering strategies. Scaffolds are an important component of the tissue engineering triad. *BMP* = bone morphogenetic protein, *FGF-2* = fibroblast growth factor 2, *IGF* = insulin-like growth factor, *MSC* = mesenchymal stromal cells, *PRP* = platelet-rich plasma, *TGF-β* = transforming growth factor β. adapted from Smith and Grande (2015)

Subtype of 3D technologies	Examples of products/organs in pre-clinical or clinical development or commercially used
Simple biomaterials e.g., hyaluronic acid, bone substitutes, alginate-encapsulated islets	Allogenic adipose derived regenerative cells (keratinocytes) encapsulated in hyaluronic acid to regenerate extracellular matrix–like material to treat corneal blindness; transplantation of pancreatic islets in immune protective alginate capsules to treat DM Type I; MACI® for repair of cartilage defects of the knee (see Figure 17.13)
3D/shaped scaffolds that provide organ shape and bio-resorbable substrate for cell growth	Bladder; trachea; 3D-printing technologies
Tissue-derived (decellularized) scaffolds that are 3D but with added benefits of native biomechanical strengths and matrix factors	Esophagus; trachea
Smart (second generation) biomaterials that may have thixotropic, thermo-responsive, growth-factor-encapsulating or *in-situ* self-assembly properties	Chitosan and hyaluronic acid are typically used as excipients for thermoset injectable hydrogels encapsulating cells

Table 17.10 ■ 3D technologies and examples

■ Combinations of the Above Technologies

A combination of the above technologies is currently in pre-clinical development in the cell therapy area, e.g., the self-formation of complex organ buds into organ-like structures, i.e., organoids (Sasai 2013).

NON-CLINICAL ANIMAL TESTING CONSIDERATIONS

A full pre-/non-clinical testing program during drug development as presented in Chap. 8 for mAbs, may not always be feasible or necessary for advanced therapies due to the nature of these products, consisting of a heterogeneous population of human cells or tissues (see also Table 17.2). Generally, the pre-/non-clinical testing package entails studies to provide data on the following:

(a) safety (toxicity, including immunogenicity);
(b) tolerance (local, systemic);
(c) biodistribution;
(d) persistence (duration of exposure);
(e) *in-vivo* proliferation, maturation, and/or differentiation into an unwanted lineage of stem cells (ESCs, iPSCs);
(f) tumorigenicity;
(g) reproducibility;
(h) biological activity (potency) *in-vivo* and/or *in-vitro*; *in-vivo* mechanism of action
(i) *in-vitro* and *in-vivo* efficacy studies to understand which cells/cell-sub-populations and cell characteristics have therapeutic value;
(j) PK/PD to serve dose definition, e.g., number of (viable) cells;
(k) PK/PD to serve route of administration and schedule;
(l) study duration to monitor for toxicity;
(m) safety of surgical procedure for local delivery of cells/tissues.

Non-clinical animal safety (toxicology) and efficacy (pharmacology) studies pose significant challenges when applied to advanced therapies, e.g., for the following reasons:

1. Molecular incompatibility and immune rejection in xenogeneic human-animal combinations (i.e., human tissues/cells tested in animal models). This is also true for genetically transduced cells, where the genetic modification leads to the expression of human protein(s), e.g., CAR-T cells.
2. A cellular immunotherapy to treat cancer (e.g., TILs) relies on interaction of the cellular product with the patient's immune system for its effect. The *in-vivo* immunological effect will very likely be different between species.
3. Cells do not undergo ADME in a way conventional medicinal products often do.

Without non-clinical data it may be difficult to predict the potential safety of the proposed first-in-human clinical studies. Therefore, alternatives should be investigated that could yield evidence of safety and, for late stage clinical trials, evidence of efficacy, including the use of models explained in Table 17.11 (adapted from BSI PAS83:2012).

■ Relevant Animal Models

Mice are often the species of choice to study advanced therapies. They are relatively inexpensive, reproduce quickly, and can be easily manipulated genetically. However, the ability of mouse experiments to predict the effectiveness of advanced therapies remains controversial. The failure of many mouse models to precisely predict particular human diseases has compelled investigators to examine animal species that may be more predictive of humans. Larger animals, such as rabbits, dogs, pigs, goats, sheep, and non-human primates, are potentially better models than mice for this

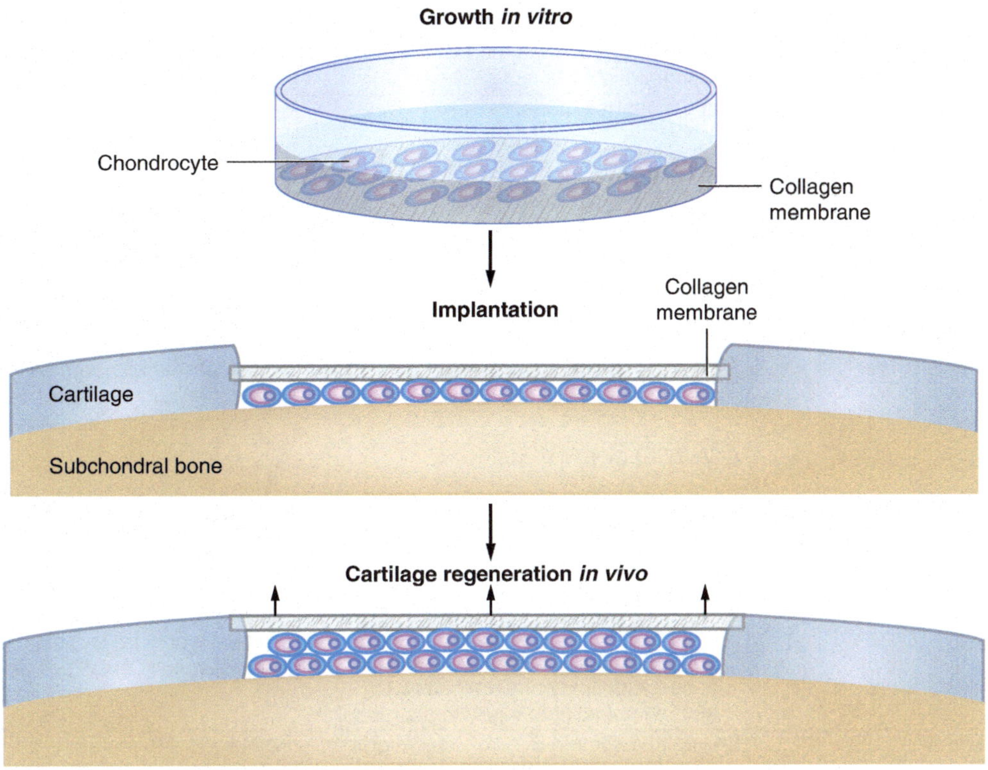

Figure 17.13 ■ Matrix-assisted chondrocyte implantation (MACI) in cartilage repair. MACI uses chondrocytes that have been seeded into a collagen scaffold and cultured for a period of time prior to surgical implantation, adapted from Smith and Grande (2015)

purpose. They have a longer life span, which facilitates long-term (e.g., years) studies that are critical for some advanced therapy products with a life-long effect. Many physiological parameters (e.g., immune system properties that play an important role in the reaction of the host animal to advanced therapies) are much closer to humans than are those of rodents. Large animals also have significant advantages regarding the number and types of cells or amounts of tissues that can be reproducibly isolated from a single donor animal and *ex-vivo* manipulated in sufficient quantity for analysis and for various non-clinical applications.

In case animal safety data do not provide meaningful information based on which an extrapolation can be made to potential risks posed to humans, those studies may be (partially) waived by regulatory authorities. Study set-up and duration for evaluation of the toxicity and/or biodistribution have to be determined on a case-by-case basis and depend on, e.g.:

- product half-life which may vary between hours–days and months–years, the latter for cells which engraft in a specific niche in the human body;
- potential alterations of cells over time upon administration;
- dose regime of single or repeat dosing over a period of weeks–months–years;
- chance for migration of the cells in the body to unwanted sites upon administration (e.g., local administration of an adult stem cell in the sub-retinal space of the eye may be safer than the systemic administration of an ESC/iPSC derived product);
- type and number of *ex-vivo* cell manipulations performed during manufacture (i.e., in case cells are expanded for multiple passages close to the point where these cells senesce, animal studies should be performed with cells beyond the cell passage used to manufacture the advanced therapy).

Generally, genotoxicity and specific safety pharmacology studies are not conducted for cell and tissue based products, unless there is a reason for concern (e.g., novel excipient or novel route of administration for an approved excipient). Reproductive toxicity studies are only required when there is a potential risk for exposure to the reproductive organs.

And finally, literature data may be used to support the (lack of) animal data. See Herberts et al. (2011) and Vestergaard et al. (2013) for further reading.

CLINICAL CONSIDERATIONS

For investigating the safety and efficacy in humans, generally the same principles apply to advanced therapies as to other medicinal products (see Table 17.2). However,

Animal and other model options	Example	Comment
Immunodeficient or immunosuppressed animal	NOD.SCID-rd1 mouse model of retinitis pigmentosa	See Chap. 9 for details on transgenic animal models
Animal disease model	Diabetic mouse model	Not always possible especially in case of immune based disease
Homologous animal model	AMD mouse model	Copy of human condition regarding pathology, symptoms and prognosis of disease. Use species specific autologous or allogeneic cells instead of human cells and apply the same manufacturing process to produce the animal cell based product; characterize the product to the extent possible; mimic the clinical setting in terms of route of administration, surgical procedure, and dose regime, to the extent possible
Homologous animal model plus use of a vector	ADA-SCID mouse model	See above plus vector encoding the animal homologue for animal cell transduction
Non-invasive whole animal modeling system	Magnetic resonance imaging (MRI) or computed tomography imaging (CTI) techniques	Cell fate/biodistribution studies in animals
Large animal model	Delivery of cells in the sub-retinal space of a pig's eye to train surgeons to safely administer cells in the eye of AMD patients; delivery of stem cells for treating spinal cord injury in pig model	Development of complex surgical procedures which would be technically difficult or impossible in small species
In-vitro assay system	Cell culture system to mimic cell migration upon immune stimulus	Potency test to characterize an advanced therapy

Table 17.11 ■ Examples of animal and other pre-clinical models applied for assessment of safety, efficacy, and product potency testing

considering the nature and complexity of the products and potential risks and benefits, there are some unique aspects to the clinical programs (see Mount et al. 2015):

1. Different set-up of trials compared to most conventional medicinal products:
   (a) First-in-human trials are always in patients and never in healthy volunteers;
   (b) A seamless development path rather than the traditional route of separate formal phase I (safety), phase II (hint of efficacy), and phase III (safety confirmation and efficacy) studies.
2. Traditional PK (ADME)/PD studies may not be feasible.
   (a) Dose (defined as number of cells/mL; number of cells/kg body weight) escalation studies may not be feasible as there may not be clear dose-response correlations. Often, a low-, medium-, and high-dose are selected, based on literature data concerning the number of cells that have historically been administered to humans.
   (b) Advanced therapies are frequently administered via the intravenous route and rapidly cleared via the lungs, spleen and liver (Leibacher and Henschler 2016). Other possible routes are intranodal (DCs to treat rheumatoid arthritis) or local administration via a surgical procedure, e.g., into the eye, brain, spinal cord or knee.
3. For safety evaluation, the following risks may need to be taken into account, depending on many factors, including type of product, cell differentiation status upon administration, cell proliferation capacity, cell source being autologous, allogeneic or xenogeneic, half-life of the cells in the body/lifelong persistence, site and method of administration/implantation, quality of the starting material (derived from healthy donor or very sick patient), and disease environment(s) which cells may encounter in the patient's body:
   (a) Tumor formation (tumorigenicity) e.g., in case of ESC- and iPSC-derived products which are *ex-vivo* expanded and differentiated;
   (b) Potential adverse reactions at the site of administration e.g., dimethyl sulfoxide (DMSO) related side effects upon i.v. administration;
   (c) Cells, being sub-visible particles, make it difficult to assess sub-visible particles potentially present in the product. These foreign particles may damage the tissue upon administration e.g., in the sub-retinal space of the eye;
   (d) Inflammatory responses and infections (e.g., side effect of CAR-T cells);
   (e) Implantation procedure for cells or 3-D tissue replacement therapies using a complex surgical

procedure (e.g., to administer cells in the subretinal space of the eye, in the spinal cord or in the brain; 3-D cultured trachea placed in the throat);
(f) Immuno-mediated side effects (CAR-T cells may cause cytokine release syndrome);
(g) Immunogenicity, which may depend on:
- Relative immune privilege of the administration site (e.g., eye);
- Allelic differences between product and patient cells (e.g., allogeneic dendritic cells);
- Immune competence of the patient;
- Need for repeat dosing (more doses may increase the chance of immune rejection of the advanced therapy);
- Maturation status of the cells (e.g., ESCs).

Often, advanced therapies derived from an allogeneic cell source require immune-suppressant medicines to be administered together with the cell-/tissue-based product. However, some allogeneic cell-/tissue-based products, such as MSCs, have shown relatively low immunogenicity profiles, in part due to the short half-life of the cells in the body. See for more details below.

4. Selecting the right patient population for the initial clinical program is challenging as there is a tension between choosing the patients most likely to benefit from an efficacious advanced therapy (e.g., early stage cancer patients) and limiting the risk to which patients are exposed with the unlicensed therapy (late stage cancer patients who may not benefit from the therapy at all due to their severe illness).
5. Establishment of surrogate biomarkers for efficacy assessment may be needed to predict long-term clinical outcome of cells that may persist in the body for years, e.g. CAR-T cells which engraft in the peripheral blood and bone marrow and transduced $CD34^+$ cells, which engraft in the bone marrow.
6. Particularly for genetically modified cells, which may persist in the body for many years or lifelong, long-term (10–20 years) patient follow-up for safety, efficacy, and durability monitoring may be necessary.

Immunological Considerations in Advanced Therapy

The potential application of adult stem cell based medicinal products derived from allogeneic source as well as hESC based therapies is limited by risks for graft-host rejection issues, as with all therapeutic strategies based on cell, tissue and organ transplantation, unless the transplant is derived from an autologous source. A way to overcome this challenge is the use of a device to protect the allogeneic cellular product from the host immune system. An example of this strategy is Viacyte's cell-based combination product, where the hESC derived β-islet progenitors are contained in the Encaptra® cell delivery system, which is placed subcutaneously (see Table 17.9 and Fig. 17.19). The additional advantage of this system is that cells cannot migrate in the body to unwanted sites and the device can be taken out in case of e.g., tumor formation. The disadvantages of such an immune-protective device are fibrosis and the lack of vascularisation around the device, required for cell viability and insulin production. Certain sites of the human body have immune privilege, i.e., they tolerate the introduction of non-self-antigens without eliciting an inflammatory immune response. These sites include the eyes, the testicles, the fetus and certain tumors. There is debate in the cell therapy world regarding the immunogenicity of allogeneic MSCs (Consentius et al. 2015; Ankrum et al. 2014). Clinical trials with standardized immune monitoring programs and a better understanding of the *in-vivo* mode of action of allogeneic MSCs may provide answers.

Administration of drugs to suppress the immune response is standard practice for patients undergoing transplantation, but with immunosuppression come side effects and uncertainty. The hope is that iPSC technology (see above) may overcome rejection problems but it is too early to be sure at this stage as there is only one product tested clinically in one subject and this is from an autologous cell source (Table 17.9). Another approach is to bank a collection of ESC lines that allows selection of a matched ABO and HLA haplotype or a close match (Lui et al. 2009). It has been estimated that with a bank of 70–100 ESC lines, a partially matched ESC line can be chosen that is adequate for each recipient. The downside of this approach is that at the time the cell lines are banked, it may not be clear yet for which diseases they will be used in the future, hence what the critical parameters are to characterize the banks for (e.g., purity of the cells, stability, potency, viral safety), see Bravery (2015). Preparing cell banks, extensive testing, and long term storage under frozen conditions are very expensive undertakings.

MANUFACTURING AND TESTING CONSIDERATIONS

Manufacturing

Cell and tissue based products are distinct from traditional biopharmaceuticals in that the modified cell/tissue itself is the active ingredient in the medicinal product rather than "simply" the means by which the cells produce an active ingredient (e.g., a recombinant protein; a viral vector). However, many of the production platforms, cell culture media, storage and transport bags, and product excipients and primary containers, which have been established for traditional cell-based recombinant protein manufacturing processes (see other chapters), can be readily applied to these innovative products.

Manipulation step	Equipment used (examples)
Collection or generation of autologous or allogeneic donor cells; collection of tissue biopsy (i.e., starting material). This step is not considered a GMP manufacturing step and takes place outside the GMP facility at a clinical site	Bone marrow aspiration system, surgical procedure, apheresis/leukopheresis system (Fig. 17.14)
Isolation of specific cell population(s). This is usually where the GMP manufacturing process starts	Knife; fluorescence-activated cell sorting (FACS) (see below); positive/negative selection by e.g., magnetic-activated cell sorting (MACS®) technology (microbeads and column); Elutra®; LOVO spinning membrane filtration device
Cultivation, expansion, and/or (genetic) modification of cells; tissue culture	Cell culture systems (see Chap. 4)
Cell differentiation	Specific raw materials, such as growth factors, are added to the culture medium manually or automatically
Purification of desired cell population(s); purification of tissue	Counter-flow centrifugal elutriation (Ficoll). This technique separates cells by size and density while maintaining cell viability. Cell enrichment kit for the magnetic separation of the desired cells by negative selection. It utilizes antibody magnetic bead complexes. Undesired cells are bound by the antibody and then magnetic beads that, when placed in a magnetic field, leave the desired cells untouched and free in the medium. The same principles and systems can be applied as for isolation of specific cell population(s) (see above)
Cell harvest and cell wash/cell concentration; tissue harvest and wash	Centrifuge; fluidized bed + elutriation-closed system (K-Sep); tangential flow filtration (TFF) technology; spinning-membrane filtration;
Formulation of the harvested cells in excipient mixture; formulation of tissue	Manually; mixing station with disposable bag set-closed system (Invetech)
Filling in the primary container of cell suspension; transfer of tissue to primary container (this is considered the drug product (DP)	Manual vial filling, stopping, and capping (Flexicon pump); manual bag filling and sealing; (semi) automated vial filling (FPC50, Flexicon system)
Labelling of the primary container	Manually; automatically with labelling machine
Short/long term storage of the DP	Refrigerator; controlled rate freezer; freezer, cryopreservation tank
Shipment of the DP to the clinical site	Temperature controlled shipment in cool box, on dry ice, in cryogenic Dewar
Handlings of the DP at the clinical site to allow for administration of the DP to the patient (e.g., thawing, washing, mixing with other ingredient)	Plasmatherm controlled temperature rate dry thawing instrument; centrifuge, mostly manual handlings

Table 17.12 ■ Typical advanced therapy manipulation steps and equipment used for each step

Since the fast majority of advanced therapies contain viable cells/tissue that can be easily destroyed through sterilization procedures and cannot be sterile filtered (≤0.2 μm filter pore size), as cells have a size of 10–30 μm on average and tissues are even bigger, the manufacturing of these products must take place under aseptic conditions. For non-sterile raw and starting materials as well as excipients, additional steps may need to be taken to ensure subsequent aseptic manufacturing (e.g., heat inactivation, gamma-irradiation or sterile filtration of the material). The facilities, equipment, raw materials, viral vectors, and cells/tissues used must be of suitable quality to allow for good manufacturing practice (GMP) production of the drug product for human application. At every stage of production, materials and final product should be protected from microbial, viral, and other contamination.

The manufacturing of advanced therapies typically requires many or all of the following "manipulation" steps, see Table 17.12.

Control of Manufacturing Process

As for any biopharmaceutical manufacturing process, process variables need to be chosen carefully and monitored to allow for adjustments to the process and to ensure a product of high quality is consistently produced. Process variables assessed are e.g., medium perfusion or exchange rate, feeding regime, biomass, stirring speed, pH, dissolved oxygen (DO), and lactate production. Particularly in the case of open and manual culture steps, this is challenging because any handling of the cells/tissue may impact the quality of the viable material and could potentially contaminate the culture system. Examples of fully-closed production

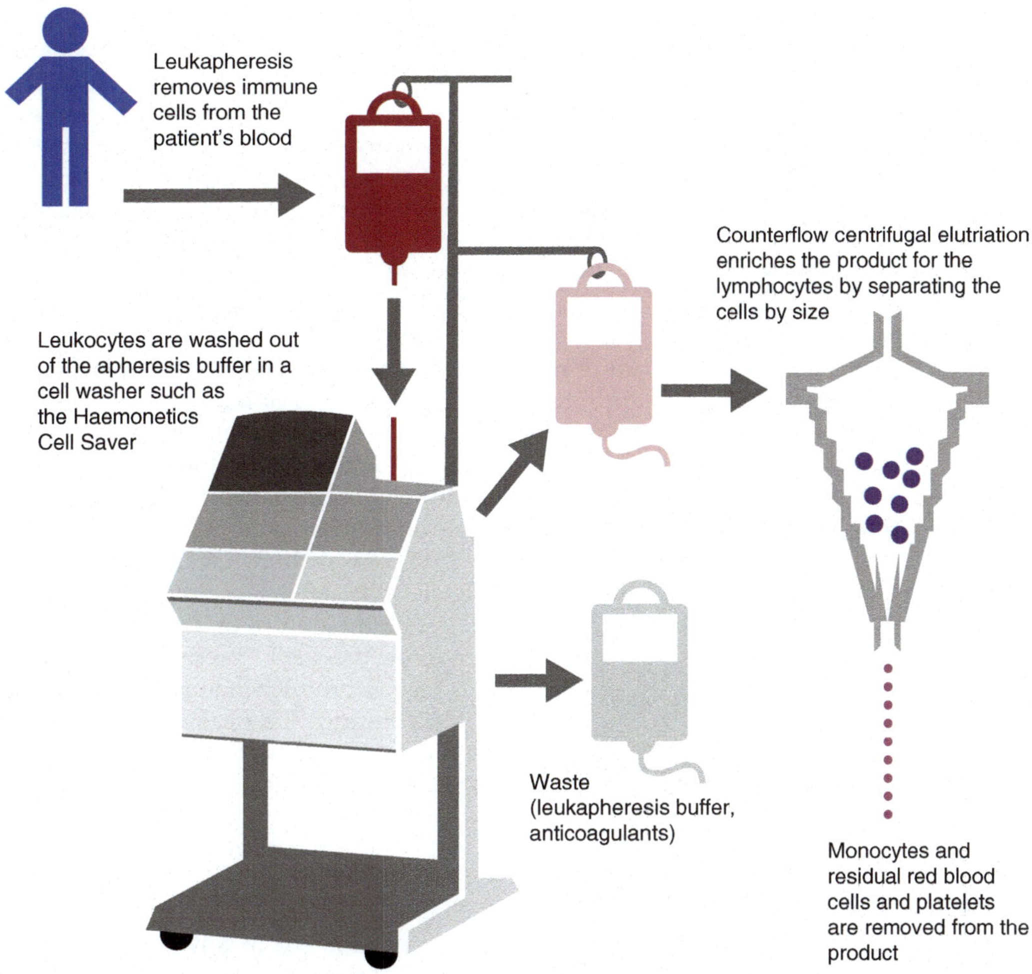

Figure 17.14 ■ Example of a leukapheresis system, which collects lymphocytes from the donor's peripheral blood, reprinted with permission (Levine et al. 2017)

systems enabling different manipulation steps in one system are the CliniMACs Prodigy® and the Octane Technology (see Figs. 17.15 and 17.16, respectively).

A fully closed processing system is the CliniMACS Prodigy. This is a single-use device that performs all manufacturing steps (i.e., cell wash, enrichment, activation, genetic modification, expansion, final formulation, and sampling). This contrasts with other manufacturing approaches, which use separate machines for the cell culture, cell washing, and other steps in the production chain.

The manufacturing process for advanced therapies show parallels with the processes for E.coli/mammalian production cells described in Chap. 4 for therapeutic proteins. But they differ considerably from those processes at a number of critical points. On top of that, the various types of cell therapy products vary widely between each other. Below follow examples of manufacturing process flow-charts for three different types of advanced therapy medicinal products:

1. *Off-the shelf* or *non-off-the-shelf* MSC production process, as described below and presented in (Fig. 17.17);
2. *Non-off-the-shelf* CAR T production process, as this procedure is a prime example of "personalized medicine" (see Chap. 9) the complexity is caught both in the text below and shown in Fig. 17.18;
3. *Off-the-shelf* human ESC derived pre-beta cell production process, as described below and presented in Fig. 17.19.

Manufacturing of MSC Product

The manufacturing of an off the-shelf (allogeneic) or non-off-the-shelf (autologous or allogeneic) cell based product, e.g., MSC-derived product, is a multi-step process with slight modifications for each specific product (see Fig. 17.17):

- Step 1: Starting material procurement via bone marrow (BM) aspiration (1a) or adipose tissue biopsy (1b) from a healthy donor (allogeneic cell source) or patient (autologous cell source). Other sources of

MSCs are not discussed here. The donor (healthy person or patient) is tested for specific human viruses prior to donation of the starting material.

- Step 2: Mononuclear cell separation from BM (2a) using separation techniques; adipose tissue digestion using enzymes, such as collagenase (2b).
- Step 3: Mononuclear cell separation from digested adipose tissue.
- Step 4: MSC expansion: MSCs are adherent cells and can therefore either be cultured in a culture flask (2D culture) or on micro-carriers in suspension culture (3D culture). Cells grow and multiply via mitosis and meiosis. By selecting the appropriate surface and culture medium, and culture conditions, unwanted cell populations do not adhere and are separated from the wanted cell populations.

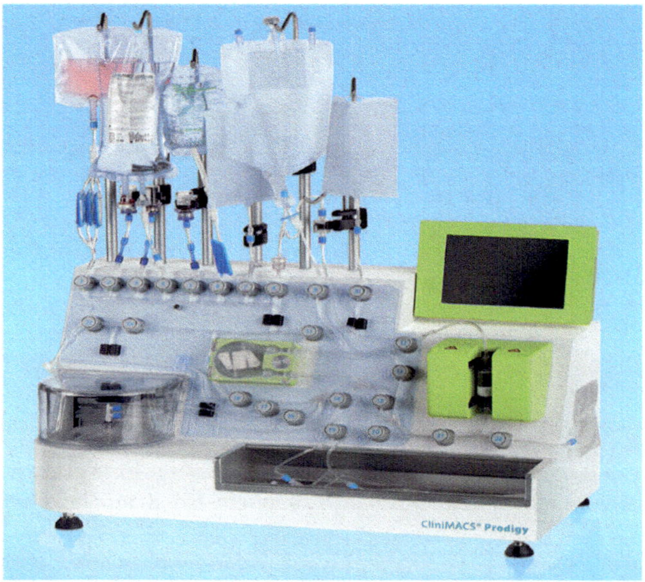

Figure 17.15 ■ Miltenyi's CliniMACs Prodigy closed processing system for cells grown in suspension (DCs, T cells)

- Step 5: Cell detachment from the surface via trypsinization. Cells are washed to remove dead cells, unwanted cell populations, and trypsine. Steps 4 & 5 are repeated as many times as needed for the targeted dose or to freeze-down a cell bank (MCB/WCB strategy; which is an off-the-shelf product approach).
- Step 6: Cell concentration.
- Step 7: Resuspension of the cells in formulation buffer.
- Step 8: Filling of the cell suspension in the primary container (vial or bag) and labelling of the primary container. This is considered the drug product (DP).
- Step 9: For some products, the cells are immediately shipped by a qualified courier to the side of administration after step 8. In such cases, the hospital should be at short distance, as the product cells are generally stable for hours to a couple of days at room temperature or at 2–8 °C (short term storage; non-off-the-shelf product). To allow for time between product manufacture plus quality control (QC) testing plus release of the DP and administration, and to allow for easy shipment to distant hospitals, the product is stored and shipped frozen, often in the vapor phase of liquid nitrogen at <–120 °C (long term storage).
- Step 10: Shipment of the DP to the clinical site.
- Step 11: Administration to the patient systemically (IV infusion) or locally with/without the use of a surgical procedure.

Manufacturing of CAR-T Product

The manufacturing of genetically modified T cells is a multi-step process with slight modifications for each specific product (Fig. 17.18):

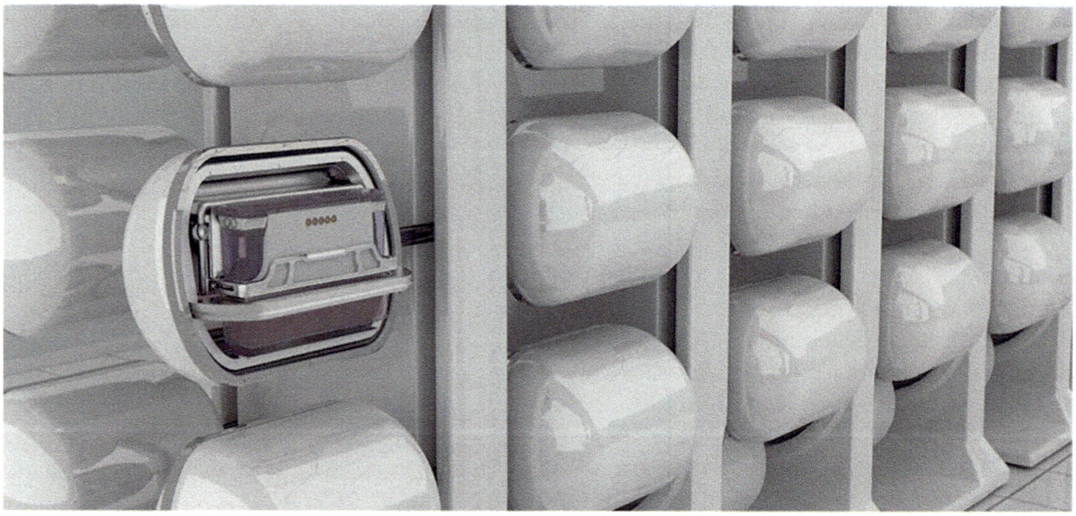

Figure 17.16 ■ Octane Technology, a fully closed production system for scale-out of autologous or allogeneic tissue- and cell-based products

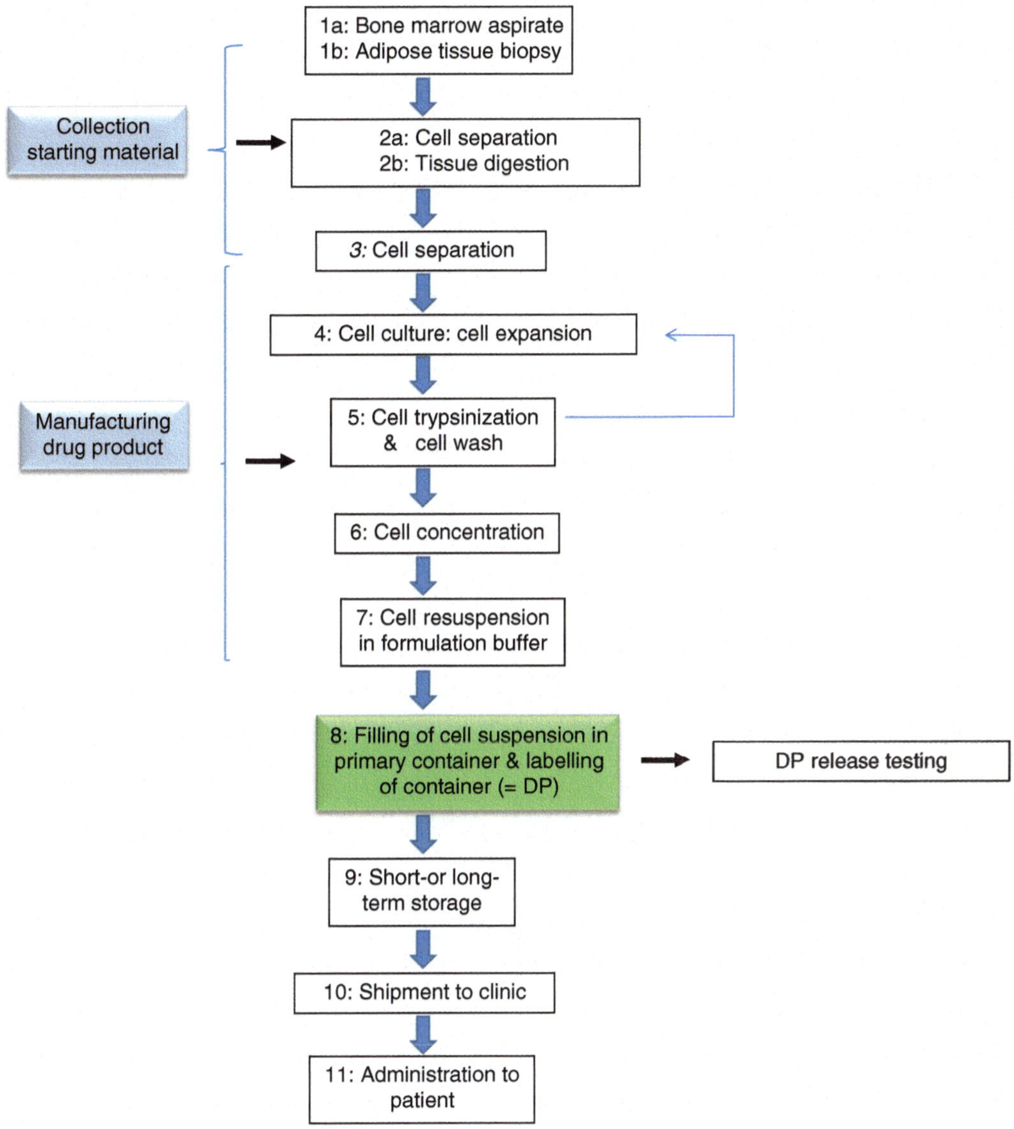

Figure 17.17 ■ Flow diagram of a manufacturing process for an off-the-shelf (allogeneic) or non-off-the-shelf (autologous or allogeneic) cell-based product based on adherent cells which do expand *ex-vivo*, such as MSCs

- Step 1: Harvest of blood cells by apheresis (whole blood collection) or leukapheresis (collection of leukocytes) from the patient (autologous cell source). The so called "starting material" is shipped either "fresh" (i.e., at room temperature or at 2–8 °C) or "frozen" (≤−80 °C) to the GMP manufacturing site. The patient is tested for specific human viruses prior to donation of the starting material.
- Step 2: From this starting material lymphocytes can be enriched either by counter-flow centrifugal elutriation or by subset selection according to the cellular phenotype.
- Step 3: The enriched lymphocyte population is placed in culture and stimulated with bead-based artificial antigen presenting cells (e.g., magnetic beads, coupled with mAbs).
- Step 4: The viral vector is added to transduce the genetic insert (CAR) into the T cells.
- Step 5: The cell culture is expanded in a bioreactor for several days until sufficient numbers of CAR-T cells are obtained for dosing and QC testing. The beads from step 3 are removed by a magnet as they are considered a process impurity.
- Step 6: The T cells are harvested, washed, and concentrated.
- Step 7: The cells are resuspended in the final product formulation buffer (7a) and filled in the primary container (infusion bag or vial). This is the so called "DP" (7b). Samples are taken for quality control testing.
- Step 8: For some products, the cells are immediately shipped by a qualified courier to the side of administration after step 7. In such cases, the hospital should be at short distance, as the product cells are

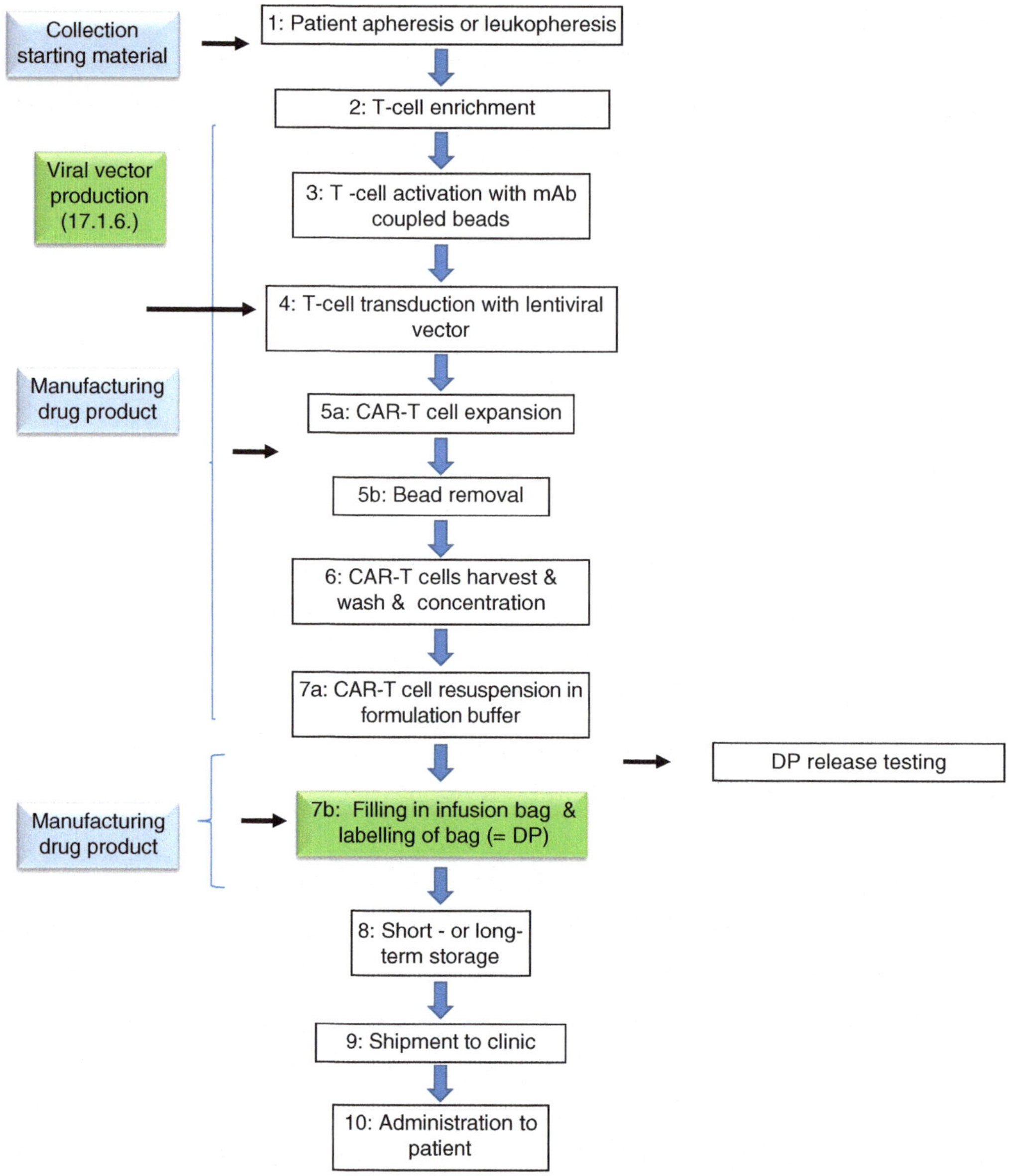

Figure 17.18 ■ Flow diagram of a CAR-T cell product manufacturing process. At the hospital white blood cells are harvested by leukapheresis (1). The starting material is shipped to the manufacturing facility for enrichment of the wanted T-cell populations (2); T-cell activation (3); transduction (genetic modification) of the T-cells with the lentiviral vector encoding the CAR genetic information (4). Thereafter, transduced cells (CAR-T cells) are *ex-vivo* expanded (5a) and purified via bead removal (5b). Cells are harvested, washed, and concentrated (6); cells are resuspended in formulation buffer (7a) and filled in the primary container (7b), which is labelled. This is considered the drug product. The product is stored (8) and thereafter shipped to the clinic (9). Prior to administration via IV infusion of the CAR-T cells at the hospital (10), the patient is pre-conditioned with chemotherapeutic medicines. Except steps 1 and 10, which take place at the hospital, all other steps take place at a manufacturing facility under GMP conditions. QC testing occurs between steps 1–2 (control of the starting material), in-process (steps 2–7a), and on the final drug product (step 7b)

generally stable for hours to a couple of days at room temperature or at 2–8 °C (short term storage). To allow for time between product manufacture plus QC testing plus release of the DP and administration, and to allow for easy shipment to distant hospitals, the product is stored and shipped frozen, often in the vapor phase of liquid nitrogen at < −120 °C (long term storage).

- Step 9: See step 10 manufacturing of MSC product.
- Step 10: At the site of administration the product is either administered directly to the patient or first thawed and sometimes washed to remove certain excipients such as dimethyl sulfoxide (DMSO) and then administered, often via IV infusion.

The chain-of identity of the entire process from leukapheresis to infusion and throughout all manufacturing steps vice versa (i.e., from donor to recipient and from recipient to donor) is controlled by a computer based system to ensure the product's identity and product traceability.

Manufacturing of hESC Product

The manufacturing of a hESC derived combination product (cells in device) to treat DM type I is a multi-step process with expansion and complex differentiation steps, with slight modifications for each specific product (Fig. 17.19):

- Step 1: Isolation of the starting material (hESCs) via extraction of the inner cell mass from a 5-days old embryo (= blastocyte). This procedure can only take place after informed consent from the parent(s) and testing of the mother's blood for specific human viruses. This step does not take place at a manufacturing facility under GMP, but at an accredited tissue establishment, which is often a hospital.
- Step 2: Production of the pre-MCB by hESC culture initiation, cell expansion, cell wash, cell harvest, formulation of the cells in cryogenic medium, fill in a vial, and storage under cryogenic conditions in the vapor phase of liquid nitrogen.
- Step 3: Production of the MCB from a pre-MCB. A pre-MCB vial is thawed and cells are cultured expanded as described under "step 2" and followed by release testing of the MCB.
- Step 4: Production of a WCB from the MCB (see step 3) and release testing of the WCB.
- Step 5: A WCB vial is thawed and cells are expanded to obtain the required cell number for cell differentiation. Steps 2 through 5 take a couple of weeks.
- Step 6: Differentiation of undifferentiated hESCs into anterior definitive endoderm cells by adding specific growth factors and other factors to the culture medium. This step takes about 2 days.
- Step 7: Differentiation of anterior definitive endoderm cells into foregut endoderm cells by adding specific growth factors and other factors to the culture medium. This step takes about 3 days.
- Step 8: Differentiation of foregut endoderm cells into posterior foregut cells by adding specific growth factors and other factors to the culture medium. This step takes about 3 days.
- Step 9: Differentiation of posterior foregut cells into pancreatic endoderm cells by adding specific growth factors and other factors to the culture medium. This step takes about 4 days.
- Step 10: Pancreatic endoderm cells are harvested, washed, resuspended in cryo-preservation medium, and filled in cryovials. The cryovials are labelled. This is considered the "intermediate DP".
- Step 11: The intermediate DP is cryopreserved in the vapor phase of liquid nitrogen at < −120 °C (long term storage) and extensively QC tested prior to release of the intermediate DP.
- Step 12: Intermediate DP cryovials are thawed. In case steps 2 through 11 take place at a GMP facility on long distance from the clinical site where the drug product will be administered to the patient, the cryopreserved intermediate DP is shipped frozen to a GMP facility, often the hospital pharmacy, for preparation of the final drug product.
- Step 13: Intermediate DP cells are recovered from the freezing and thawing steps by placing them in culture for another 3–4 days.
- Step 14: The recovered cells are harvested and washed to remove dead cells and culture medium.
- Step 15: Cells are concentrated and formulated in a buffer.
- Step 16: Cells are uploaded into the immune-protective device using a loading device. The pancreatic pre-beta cells in the device is considered the DP. Limited QC release testing is performed on the DP.
- Step 17: The device is administered to the patient via a surgical procedure.

Key Factors for a Successful Manufacturing Process

To consistently manufacture advanced therapies at a large scale, automated manufacturing processes as well as the implementation of functionally closed systems are key success factors for the following reasons: (1) lower the risk of viral and bacterial contamination during manual and open process steps; (2) decrease costs associated with manual handlings; (3) improve product consistency; (4) shorten production times. Other key factors for success are: logistics around the manufacturing, supply chain of the product, and cost of goods. Particularly animal and human derived raw materials (for example growth factors, FBS), antibody coupled beads, and viral vectors are very expensive. Considering the high cost and increased risk of validating sterilization cycles of multiple-use bioreactors, these closed-processes for advanced therapies utilize single use, disposable bioreactors, mimicking current recombinant protein platform approaches (see Chap. 4). Despite some progress made in this field, there remains a requirement for better understanding of potential manufacturing platforms and how they can be best utilized for advanced therapies, taking the variety of cell and tissue types and clinical application into account.

Viral Vector Production for Ex-vivo Gene Modification of Cells

Recombinant viral vectors, e.g., retroviruses like lentiviruses, are produced by transfecting packaging cells, cultured with 3–4 plasmids that encode viral structural proteins (e.g., GAG, POL, Vesicular stomatitis virus (VSV)-G, and REV; the so called packaging plasmids) and the plasmid encoding the therapeutic gene of interest (e.g., CAR, ADA-SCID; the so called transfer plasmid). The transfer plasmid encoding the

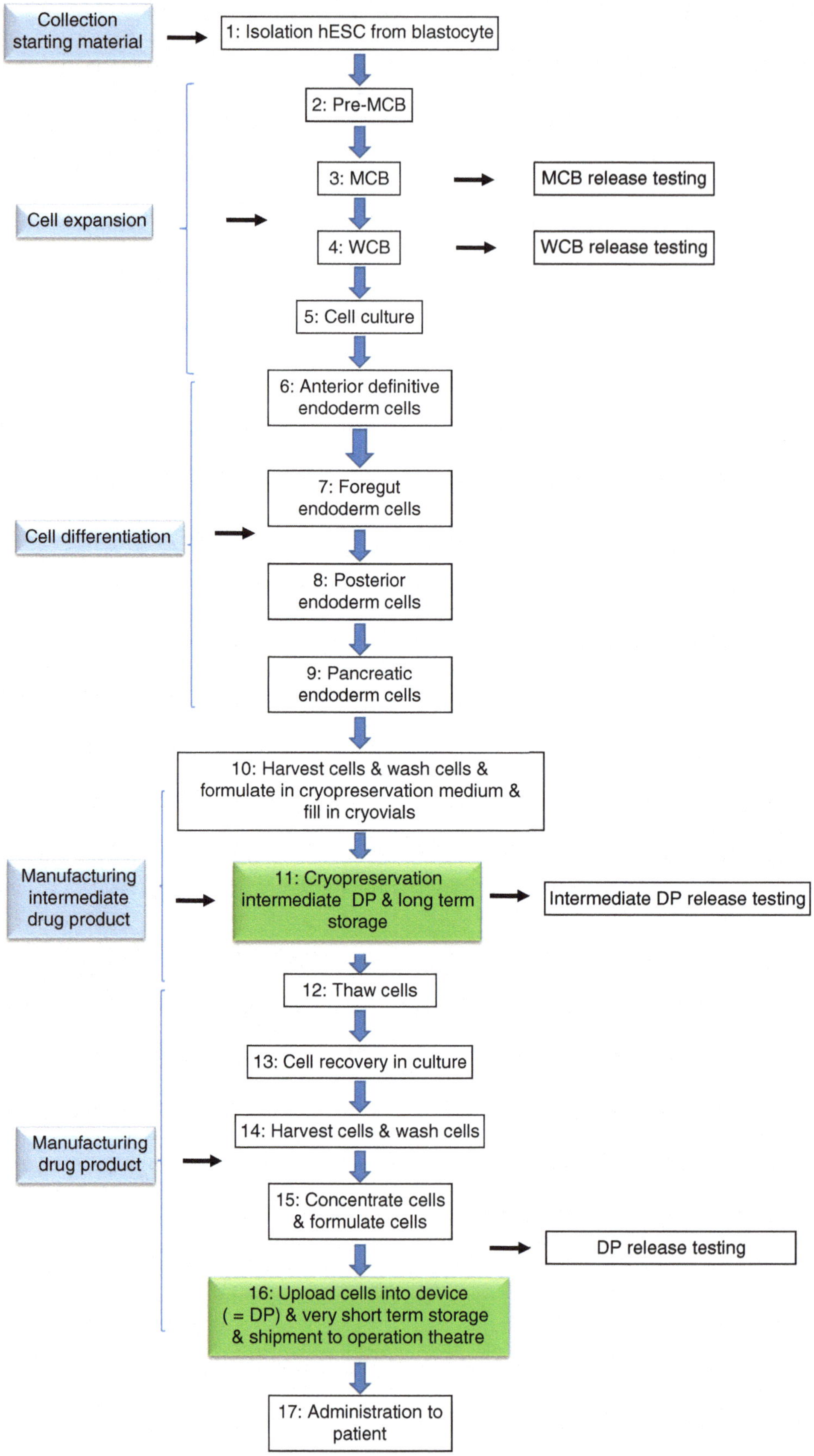

Figure 17.19 ■ Flow diagram of a hESC-derived combination product manufacturing process to treat DM type I

therapeutic gene contains the regulatory sequences that control its expression and a packaging sequence that enables its recognition. Within the packaging cell (e.g., the human embryonic kidney (HEK) 293 cell line), the RNA transcribed from the plasmid encoding the therapeutic gene is recognized by the viral proteins that assemble around it. The recombinant virus is then transported to the plasma membrane of the packaging cell that expresses viral envelope proteins (VSV-G). During budding the virus acquires the lipid bilayer from the packaging cell surface and incorporates the envelope proteins. The viral vector particles are released from the cells, which are cultured as adherent cells in culture flasks, into the cell culture medium. The above described steps are considered the upstream processing (USP) steps. From the medium the virus particles are subsequently harvested, formulated in a buffer and filled in the primary container. These production steps are considered the downstream processing (DSP) steps (Morenweiser 2005). DSP steps applied for viral vector production are steps traditionally used in the biotechnology industry for the manufacture of recombinant proteins. These are membrane-based (filt ration/clarification, concentration/diafiltration using tangential flow filtration, membrane-based chromatography) and chromatography based (ion-exchange chromatography, affinity chromatography, and size exclusion chromatography) process steps. The combination of these different process steps is variable and in some cases, different purification principles are used for the same purpose. Furthermore, a benzonase/DNase treatment for the degradation of contaminating DNA from the packaging cells is either part of the USP or DSP part of the manufacturing process. Subsequently, the purified virus particles are formulated in a buffer, filled in the primary container, stored frozen, and tested until further use for transduction of the cells to make a genetically modified cell therapy product (see Wright 2018). Figure 17.20 provides a schematic overview of the entire viral vector material manufacturing process used in the production of a genetically modified cell therapy product. For production of a viral vector product for *in-vivo* gene therapy (see Chap. 16), the production process is identical.

■ Excipients

Common excipients used in the formulation of advanced therapies are presented in Table 17.13. Most of these excipients overlap with those used in therapeutic protein products. However, KCl, $MgCl_2$, nucleosides, FBS, and DMSO are not found in therapeutic protein drug products.

Table 17.14 provides an overview of a few commercially available advanced therapies with their formulation and shelf-life.

■ Primary Container

Generally, two types of containers are used for cell-based products: vials (small volume, low dose), and infusion bags (higher volume and dose), as shown in Fig. 17.21. Tissue-based products often have a non-standard container for storage and shipment.

■ Storage and Shipment

Stability of the starting material (cells or tissue and viral vector) and DP are an important element for successful production, storage, shipment, and administration of advanced therapies. Starting materials and DPs either have a very short shelf-life of hours–days and are stored and transported at 2–8 °C or at room temperature or have a longer shelf-life (months–years) and are stored and shipped frozen (cryopreserved in the vapor phase of liquid nitrogen at <−120 °C or in a −80 °C or −150 °C freezer).

■ Manufacturing Model: Scale–Up Versus Scale–Out

Broadly speaking, there are two paradigms in advanced therapy manufacture: off-the-shelf (always allogeneic source of cells/tissue) and patient specific (commonly autologous source of starting materials, but sometimes allogeneic) DPs. Off-the-shelf products represent a business model akin to current biopharmaceuticals, where one batch can be manufactured to treat multiple patients. This allows for increasing economies of scale, which drives down the per-dose cost of the final product. This means that there is a wealth of engineering and process knowledge and technologies that can be leveraged to support the manufacture of off-the-shelf advanced therapies at increasing scale.

However, scale-up is not just about making the reactor growing the cells bigger. Conventional scale-up bioprocesses typically use cells to produce therapeutic agents (e.g., mAbs), which can then be isolated and purified without the need to recover the cell. For the manufacture of advanced therapies, where the cells/tissue culture is the product of interest, retention of cell viability, phenotype, and function to assure quality, is of primary importance in order to preserve product safety and efficacy. As the number of cells increase during expansion this can become increasingly challenging, as the greater cell numbers lead to an increased chance of inhomogeneity of culture and hence of cellular performance being altered. This means that the desired quality of the cells/tissue must be maintained through the entire manufacturing process, including the harvest and DSP, storage, shipment, and delivery to the patient. This will require the development of scalable harvesting, DSP, and formulation technologies to cope with the large batch size produced.

Patient-specific advanced therapies offer a new challenge for process scalability, where the manufacturing process must be scaled-out, in order to pro-

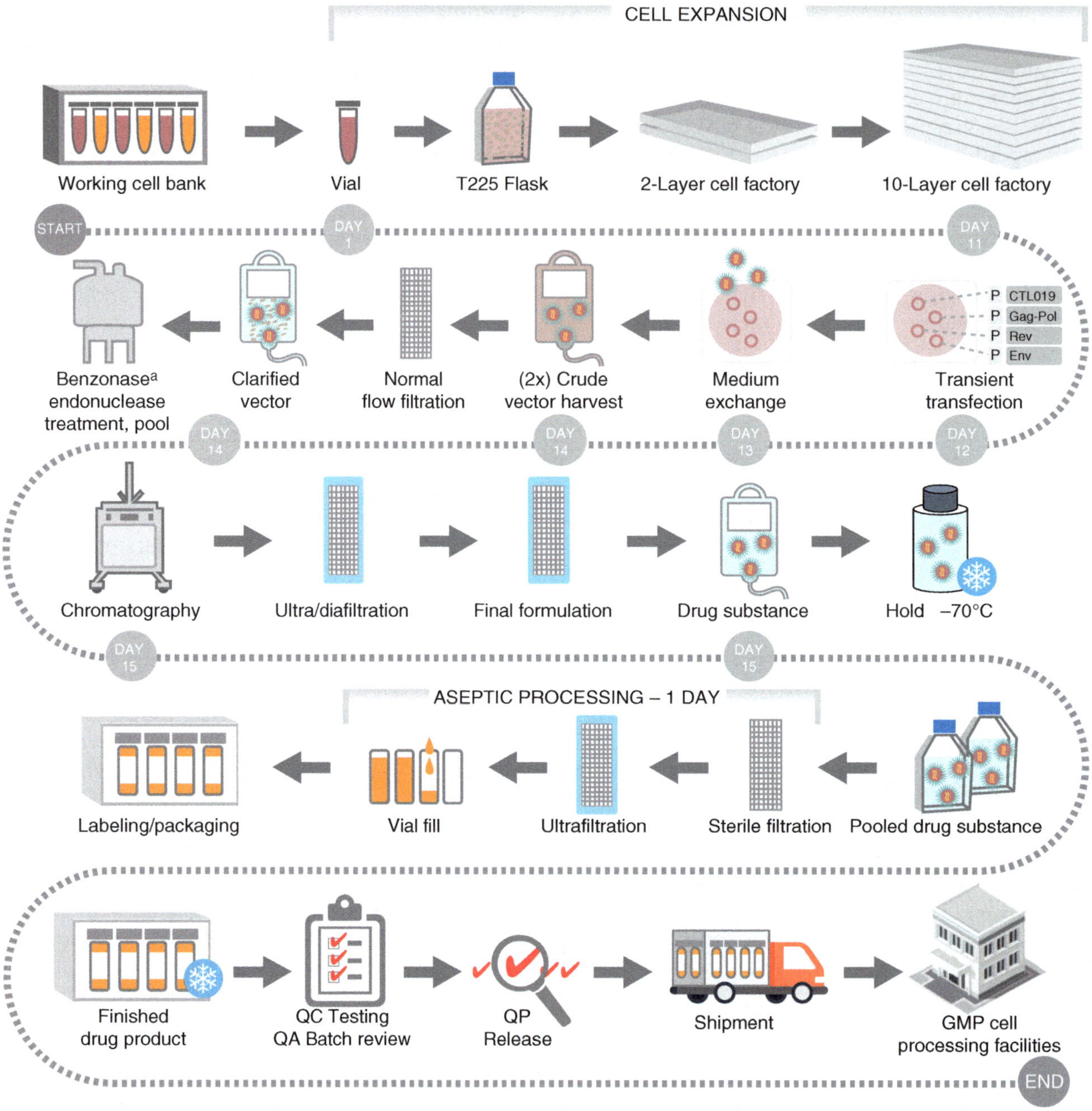

Figure 17.20 ■ Schematic overview of a lentiviral vector manufacturing process. The produced viral vector is used as starting material for the genetic modification of T-cells in the manufacture of a CAR-T product, reprinted with permission (Levine et al. 2017). A similar production approach is taken for other *ex-vivo* gene therapy as well as *in-vivo* gene therapy products (cf. Chap. 16). *QC* = quality control, *QP* = qualified person, *QA* = quality assurance

duce one batch for each patient (Fig. 17.22). This introduces the concept of "personalized medicine" (see Chap. 9), where the cost of production per batch cannot be reduced by exploiting an increasing economy of scale by simply producing a larger batch. Reducing the cost of these patient-specific cell- and tissue-based products must therefore be achieved by advances in engineering and manufacturing technology, reducing the number of complex, labor-intensive, and open-process steps that are commonplace in manufacture of these products at research labs. The developments of closed and automated processes as well as process simplification are key factors for commercial success as this will allow multiple batches to be produced in parallel (scale-out), with reduced burden of oversight by highly-trained scientists. These new processes must be GMP-compliant and closed for sterility.

■ Testing

As for any DP, cell- and tissue-based therapies are subject to detailed characterization. This involves assessment of quality attributes (i.e., identity, purity and impurities, viability (Cadena-Herrera et al. 2015), bioactivity (potency; Bravery et al. 2013), safety, quantity, and general attributes, such as appearance, pH, morphology) both of the cellular/tissue/vector starting material and the final DP, see Table 17.15. The latter includes QC testing to allow release of the DP for administration. In addition, at different stages of the production, in-process controls are performed to assess the quality and stability of the cells/tissue during manufacture. A sub-set of characterization tools is used for assessment of stability of the starting material(s) and DP.

Excipients class	Function	Example
Buffer	pH stabilizer	TRIS, histidine, Na-acetate
Salt	Stabilizer	NaCl, KCl, $MgCl_2$
Antioxidant	Prevent oxidation	Methionine
Sugar	Stabilizer, cryoprotectant, tonicity modifier	Mannitol, trehalose, sucrose, glucose
Polyol	Collapse temperature modifier	Dextran (low and high molecular weight)
Nucleoside	Stabilizer	Adenosine, guanosine
Protein	Stabilizer, preservative	Fetal bovine serum, human serum albumin
Organic solvent	Stabilizer, cryoprotectant, solvent	Glycerol, ethylene glycol, DMSO

Table 17.13 ■ Examples of excipients used in the formulation of advanced therapy products

However, for a lot of autologous and some allogeneic DPs that are not "off-the-shelf", performing QC tests may be challenging due to the time constraints between manufacture and administration, i.e., the shelf-life of the drug product is hours–days. Moreover, for some autologous products all the available cell/tissue material is needed for the dose. In such cases, product release may be justified by extensive process validation; in-process control testing and/or QC testing data becoming available after product administration. These approaches require a paradigm shift in the pharma world, where traditionally products are only administered after extensive testing and batch release.

Adequate QC of starting materials such as cells/tissue biopsy and viral vectors is crucial as poor quality starting material will affect the quality of the final product. Autologous or allogeneic cells/tissue can be very heterogeneous due to the inherent donor variability (age, sex, health status, medication), the variable amount of cells other than the intended cells, and because the collected cells are not in a synchronized cell cycle. In addition, the origin of the cells (e.g., MSCs of bone marrow, adipose, and cord blood origin) may have significant impact on the activity and phenotype of the cells after manufacture.

The challenge is that a lot of the techniques used for the characterization of this heterogeneous group of products are not sensitive methods, hence they are not able to pick-up subtle changes to the process and/or to the product.

For further reading on characterization of cell- and tissue-based products, see BSI PAS 93:2011.

Product	Shelf-life and storage condition	Composition (active substance)	Excipients/mixtures
Provenge® Suspension of cells for IV infusion	18 h at 2–8 °C	≥50 × 10^6 autologous $CD54^+$ cells/250 mL activated with PAP-GM-CSF[a]	Lactated Ringer's solution (NaCl, $NaC_3H_5O_3$, KCl, $CaCl_2$)
ChondroCelect® Suspension of cells for implantation	48 h at 15–25 °C	4 × 10^6 autologous human cartilage cells/ 0.4 ml	DMEM[b]
MACI® Implantation matrix plus cells in solution for implantation	6 days at ≤37 °C and keep out of fridge	0.5 × 10^6 to 1 × 10^6 autologous cultured chondrocytes/cm^2 porcine derived type I/III collagen membrane	DMEM, HEPES[c] adjusted for pH with HCl or NaOH and osmality with NaCl
Kymriah® Suspension of cells for IV infusion	9 months at ≤−120 °C in the vapor phase of liquid nitrogen	2 × 10^6–2.5 × 10^8 autologous CAR-positive viable T cells	Plasmalyte-A[d], glucose/NaCl, human serum albumin, dextran 40-low molecular weight/glucose, DMSO

[a]Prostatic acid phosphatase granulocyte-macrophage colony-stimulating factor

[b]Calcium Chloride anhydrous, Ferric Nitrate.$9H_2O$, Potassium Chloride, Magnesium Sulphate anhydrous, Sodium Chloride, Sodium Bicarbonate, Potassium Phosphate Monobasic.H_2O, D-Glucose, L-Arginine.HCl, L-Cystine.2HCl, L-Glutamine, Glycine, L-Histidine.HCl.H_2O, L-Isoleucine, L-Leucine, L-Lysine.HCl, L-Methionine, L-Phenylalanine, L-Serine, L-Threonine, L-Tryptophan, L-Tyrosine.2Na.$2H_2O$, L-Valine, D-Calcium Pantothenate, Choline Chloride, Folic Acid, i-Inositol, Niacinamide, Riboflavin, Thiamine.HCl, Pyridoxine.HCl

[c]4-(2-Hydroxyethyl)piperazine-1-ethanesulfonic acid sodium

[d]Plasmalyte-A sodium chloride: 5.26 g/l potassium chloride: 0.37 g/l magnesium chloride hexahydrate: 0.30 g/l sodium acetate trihydrate

Table 17.14 ■ Examples of approved advanced therapies, their formulation, and shelf-lives

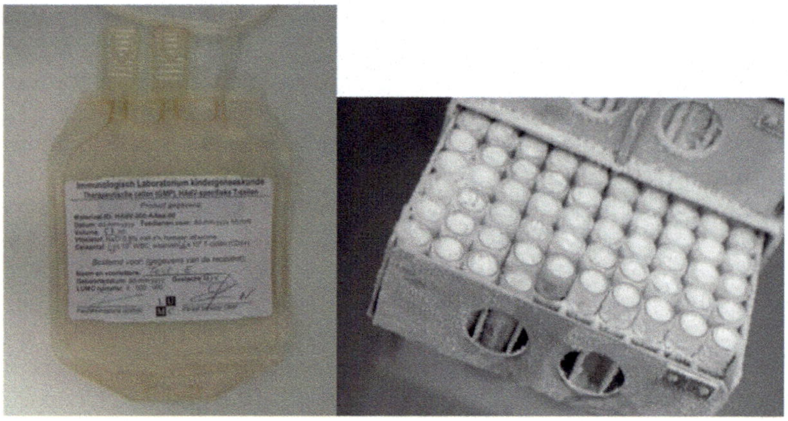

Figure 17.21 ■ Examples of primary containers for the storage and transport of advanced therapies. Left photo: infusion bag; right photo: cryovials in box to allow for storage in the vapor phase of liquid nitrogen (courtesy of M. de Haan)

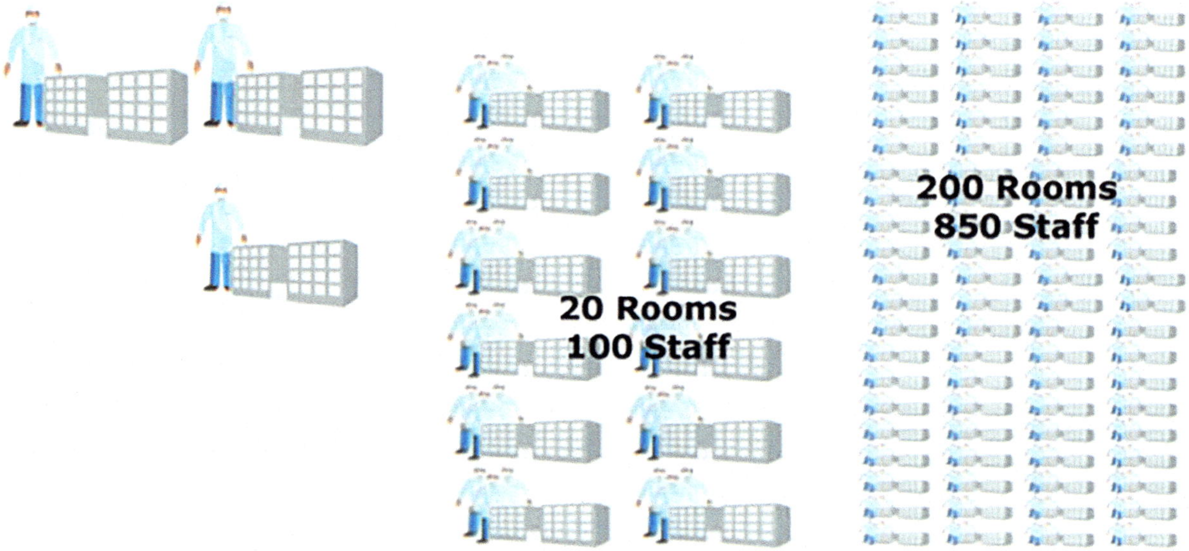

Figure 17.22 ■ Scale-out of a labor intensive manual process

For details on testing (lot release and additional characterization) of viral vectors for *ex-vivo* and *in-vivo* gene therapy products, see Gombold (Gombold et al. 2006a, b); Wright (2018).

Table 17.16 provides an overview of the QC testing panel for an MSC–derived and a CAR-T product.

Flow Cytometry

One of the key technologies in advanced therapy manufacturing is flow cytometry. It can be operated in a QC test environment and in production of advanced therapies products (see next section). As this technique is not used regularly to characterize therapeutic proteins, it is not discussed in Chap. 3. We pay attention to it in this chapter.

Flow cytometry assays may be used to assess cell- and tissue-based product identity, active substance purity, cellular impurity, viability, and potency testing. It is a powerful technique, which allows for specific measurement of cellular components on the cell surface (e.g., CD73, CD90, and CD105 to characterize MSCs) and intracellular components. It is also amenable to the measurement of soluble analyte(s) such as cytokines, released by the cells in the extracellular environment, e.g., upon cell activation.

Flow cytometry is a technology that simultaneously measures and then analyzes multiple physical characteristics of single particles, usually cells, as they flow in a fluid stream through a beam of light. The properties measured include a particle's relative size, relative granularity or internal complexity, and relative fluorescence intensity. These characteristics are determined using an optical-to-electronic coupling system that records how the cell or particle scatters incident laser light and emits fluorescence. A flow cytometer is made up of three main systems: fluidics, optics, and electronics.

- The fluidics system transports single particles (cells) in a stream to the laser beam for interrogation.
- The optics system consists of a light source, mostly lasers, to illuminate the particles in the sample stream and optical filters to direct the resulting light signals to the appropriate detectors. Light scattering or fluorescence emission from auto-fluorescence of the particle or from fluorophores, which are fluorescence labels (e.g., bound to specific anti-

Quality attribute	Explanation	Possible techniques applied
Identity	Distinguish the cellular active substance (s)/tissue from unwanted cell population(s); donor specific test; sometimes a combination of tests	Flow cytometry[g]; karyology, STR[a], FISH[b], CGH[c], microscopy, immunocytochemistry, electrochemiluminescence, protein array, microarray
Active substance purity	Number of viable cells with specific cell surface markers present/absent, unique for the active substance. Closely related to identity	Flow cytometry; ELISA[d]; immunocytochemistry; electrochemiluminescence; protein ligation assay
Cellular (product) impurities	Dead cells (based on total and viable cell numbers); unwanted cell populations. Closely related to identity and purity	Flow cytometry; ELISA; electrochemiluminescence; MS[e]
Process impurities	Depends on process and raw materials used, e.g. antibiotics, cytokines, growth factors, FBS, beads, viral vector starting material	– Cytokines, growth factors, FBS, TryPLESelect: ELISA – Beads: microscopic evaluation; – Antibiotics: LC-MS[f]; – Viral vector: qPCR[h]
Potency/ bioactivity	Quantitative measure of relevant biologic function(s) based on the attributes that are linked to relevant *in-vivo* biologic properties; often a combination of assays. Receptors, cellular metabolism, secreted proteins, migration of cells, (lack of) proliferation, differentiation potential, mRNA expression	ELISA; qPCR; flow cytometry; cell migration in Dunn or Boyden chamber; protein array; LC; MS; animal model (not quantitative), microarray
Viability and total cell count	Viability is a critical parameter and related to dose, purity and cellular impurities	Colorimetric assay (spectrophotometer), fluorescent assay (including flow cytometry), membrane integrity assay (e.g., trypan blue), microscope. Manual, semi-automated or automated equipment
Dose	Often number of total or viable cells per unit (mL, kg body weight); cm^2 of tissue	Total cell count and viability techniques
Safety	Sterility, endotoxin, mycoplasma, human and animal viruses derived from starting material or raw materials, replication competent viral vector, chromosomal aberrations	Pharmacopoeial tests for sterility, mycoplasma, endotoxin-standard or rapid tests; chromosomal aberrations by karyology, FISH, CGH
General attribute	Appearance, pH, osmolality, particles, cell/tissue morphology	Pharmacopoeial tests, microscope for morphology assessment

[a]*STR* = short tandem repeat
[b]*FISH* = Fluorescence in situ hybridization
[c]*CGH* = comparative genomic hybridization
[d]*ELISA* = Enzyme-Linked Immuno Sorbent Assay; see Chap. 3 for details on this technique
[e]*MS* = mass spectrometry
[f]*LC-MS* = liquid chromatography-mass spectrometry; see Chap. 3 for details on this technique
[g]Flow cytometry technique is explained below; it can be used for intracellular and cell surface markers
[h]*qPCR* = quantitative polymerase chain reaction; see Chap. 1 for details on PCR

Table 17.15 ■ Examples of techniques applied for the analysis of different quality attributes of cell- and tissue based therapies. Some techniques are also used for starting material characterization

bodies) used to detect the expression of cellular molecules such as specific proteins or nucleic acids) provides information about the particle's properties. (1) Light that is scattered in the forward direction after interacting with a particle, typically up to 20° offset from the laser beam's axis, is collected by a photomultiplier tube or photodiode and is known as the forward scatter (FSC) channel. This FSC measurement can give an estimation of a particle's size with larger particles refracting more light than smaller particles. (2) Light measured at a 90° angle to the excitation line is called side scatter (SSC). The SSC can provide information about the relative complexity (e.g., granularity and internal structures) of a cell or particle; however, as with forward scatter this can depend on various factors. Both FSC and SSC are unique for every particle and a combination of the two can be used to roughly differentiate cell types in a heterogeneous population such as blood or bone marrow aspirate. However, this scatter information and cell typing depends on the sample type and the quality of sample preparation, so fluorescent labelling is generally required to obtain more detailed information.

– The electronics system converts the detected light signals into electronic signals that can be processed by the computer.
– In the flow cytometer, particles are carried to the laser intercept in a fluid stream. Any suspended particle or cell from 0.2–150 µm in size is suitable for

Quality attribute	MSC derived cell based product; allogeneic off-the-shelf (1 batch of multiple vials/bags for multiple patients)	CAR-T *ex-vivo* gene therapy product; autologous (1 batch of 1 infusion bag for 1 patient)
Identity	$CD73^+$, $CD90^+$, $CD105^+$, HLA-DR^-, $CD3^-$, $CD45^-$ cells by flow cytometry	CAR expression by qPCR
Viability by manual or automated cell count	Number of total cells	Number of total cells
	Number of viable cells	Number of viable cells
	Percentage of viable cells	Percentage of viable cells
Purity by flow cytometry (% of viable cells with a certain CD-marker profile)	Percentage of $CD73^+$, $CD90^+$, $CD105^+$, 7-AAD^- cells by flow cytometry	Percentage of viable T cells
		Transduction efficiency by CAR q-PCR
Product = cellular impurities (dead cells and unwanted cell populations) by flow cytometry	Percentages of 7-AAD^+ (dead cells), $CD3^+$ (T cells), $CD45^+$ (lymphocytes), $CD34^+$ (HSCs and endothelial cells), $CD14^+$ (monocytes), $CD19^+$ (B cells)	Percentages of red blood cells, granulocytes, dead cells, $CD19^+$ B cells
Process impurities	Residual bovine serum albumin (BSA) by ELISA	Residual antibody conjugated beads (CD3/CD28)
	Residual TryPLESelect by ELISA	BSA by ELISA
	Residual antibiotic by liquid chromatography-mass spectrometry	Residual VSV-G DNA by qPCR-derived from viral vector
Potency	CD marker expression (e.g., adhesion molecules) upon immune activation by flow cytometry	Determination of CAR expression by flow cytometry
		Release of interferon-gamma in response to CD19-expressing target cells
Safety	Sterility	Sterility
	Bacterial endotoxins	Endotoxin
	Mycoplasma	Mycoplasma
	Karyology	PCR-based replication competent lentivirus assay
	Human viral testing; test for the presence of inapparent virus; *in-vitro* assay for the presence of viral contaminants	N.A.
Dose (calculated)	a–b × 10^6 viable $CD73^+$, $CD90^+$, $CD105^+$, 7-AAD^- cells/ml	a–b × 10^6 $CD19^+$ T cells/kg body weight
General attribute	pH	pH
	Osmolality	Osmolality
	Appearance of primary container and content	Appearance of primary container and content
	Content uniformity	N.A.
	Extractable volume from the vial	N.A.

Table 17.16 ■ Example of QC testing panel for an MSC-derived cell based product and a CAR-T *ex-vivo* gene therapy product

analysis. Cells from solid tissue must be desegregated into single cells before analysis. The portion of the fluid stream where particles are located is called the sample core. When particles pass through the laser intercept, they scatter laser light. Any fluorescent molecules present on the particle fluoresce. The scattered and fluorescent light is collected by appropriately positioned lenses. A combination of beam splitters and filters steers the scattered and fluorescent light to the appropriate detectors. The detectors produce electronic signals proportional to the optical signals striking them. Read outs are collected on each particle or single event. The characteristics or parameters of each event are based on its light scattering and fluorescent properties. The data are collected and stored in the computer. This data can be analyzed to provide information about sub-populations of cells within the sample (see Fig. 17.23).

Figure 17.24 provides representative flow cytometry histograms for an MSC product.

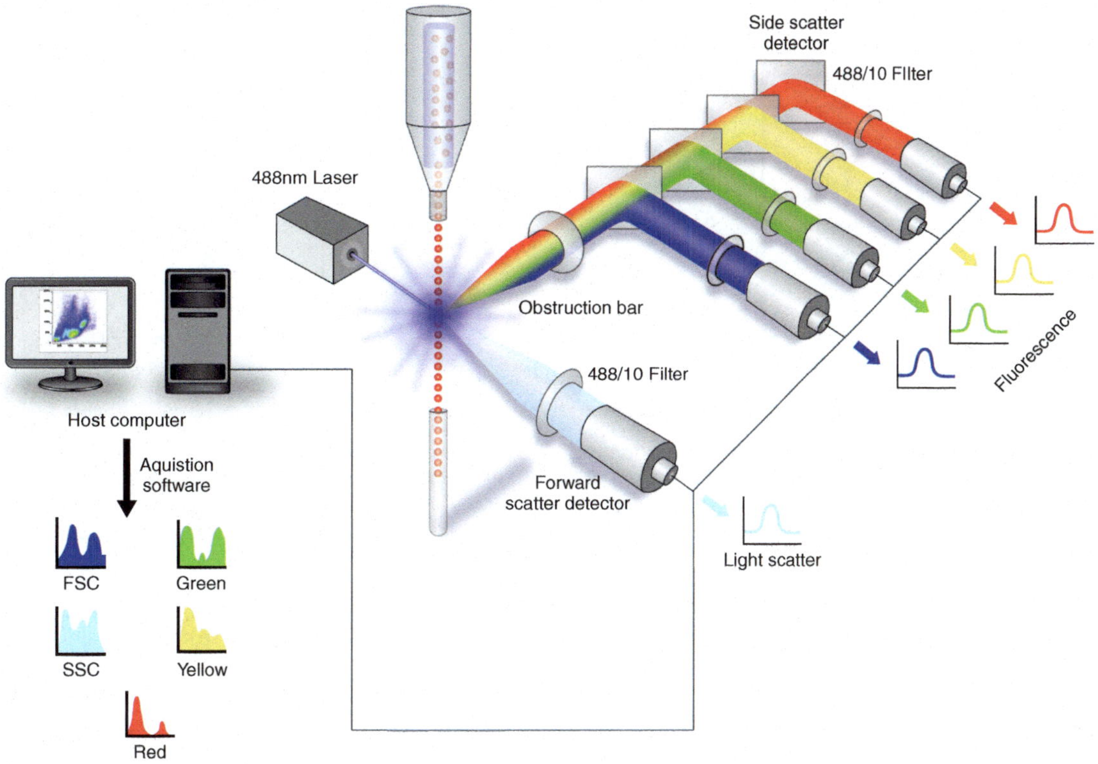

Figure 17.23 Schematic view of a flow cytometer. Scattered and emitted light signals are converted to electronic pulses, adapted from ThermoFisher Scientific. http://www.thermofisher.com/nl/en/home/life-science/cell-analysis/cell-analysis-learning-center/molecular-probes-school-of-fluorescence/flow-cytometry-basics/flow-cytometry-fundamentals/how-flow-cytometer-works.html#overview

Fluorescence-Activated Cell Sorting (FACS)

Flow cytometry techniques can also be used for sorting of specific cell (sub) populations, e.g., to increase product yield and/or to reduce the amount of unwanted cell populations, which are considered impurities. A FACS machine provides the ability to separate cells identified by flow cytometry. Droplet based cell sorters first analyze the particles but also have hardware that can generate droplets and a means of deflecting or directing wanted particles into a collection tube. Cell dispersions are often purified based on surface markers such as CD34+ in HSCs or on their viability. Common uses of cell sorting include identifying and isolating cell populations or single cells followed by subsequent downstream applications where DNA, protein or cellular function is investigated.

Improvements of Testing Strategies Needed

Developing robust, sensitive, rapid, and in-line analytical testing and characterization tools will be required as cell/tissue and viral vector processing platvforms continue to evolve. Significant improvements are needed to establish next-generation analytics for (in-process) QC, stability, and additional characterization testing to assess the quality attributes of starting materials, intermediates, and advanced therapy products. Improvements are also to be made in the field of in-line and on-line testing of cell culture conditions (e.g., pH, morphology and viability). Reducing the sampling frequency, technical complexity, amount of sample needed, and labor intensiveness of testing is especially critical for a non-off-the-shelf autologous *ex-vivo* gene therapy product. This contrasts with traditional biopharmaceuticals where a single batch of QC tested product may treat hundreds or thousands of patients. Cell processing automation will also be enabled through the development of high throughput in-process and release assays providing results in a very short timeframe (minutes–hours). Advanced cell/tissue characterization techniques based on nanofluidics, transcriptomics, and proteomics, and next generation sequencing techniques may allow better understanding of what happens to desired cell population(s)/tissue once they are processed and before patient administration (see Chap. 9 for more details on "-omics"), both in the cytosol as well as in the extracellular environment. Examples are changes in intracellular genetic profiles and patterns within the micro RNA and exosome pools secreted into the culture medium by the cells.

Different advanced therapy technologies are currently at different stages in translation and do have their particular manufacturing and testing challenges, as summarized in Table 17.17.

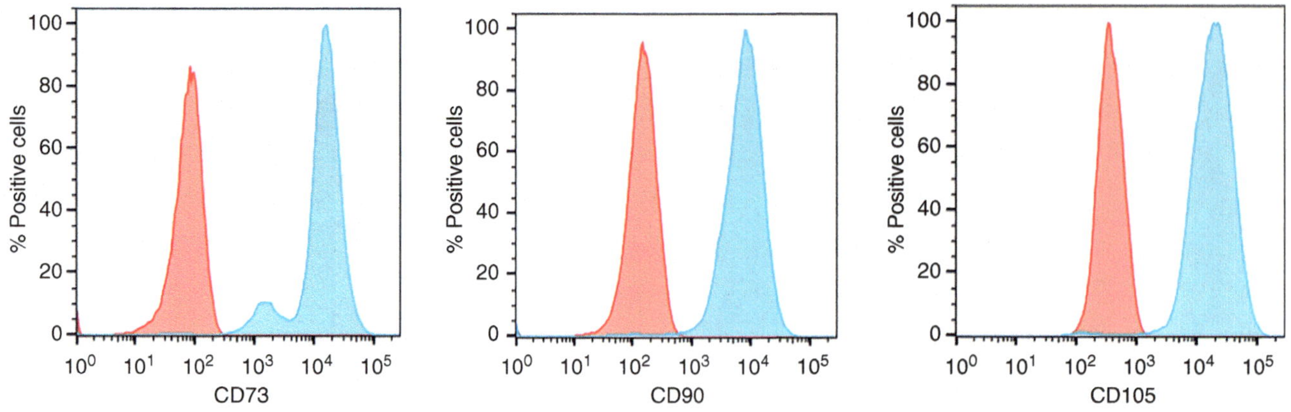

Figure 17.24 Flow cytometry histograms of MSC product cells. Flow cytometric analysis of MSC product cells against three defined MSC markers (CD73, CD90, and CD105) show that these cells are of mesenchymal cell phenotype. On the X-axis the density of the respective cell surface marker molecule is shown. A single peak is observed for each of the markers tested (blue peak at the right side of each histogram), indicating a single population of cells. The red peak at the left side of each histogram represents the isotype control staining. Courtesy of M. van Pel

OTHER ASPECTS OF ADVANCED THERAPIES

Regulatory Bodies Involved in Regulating Advanced Therapies in Europe

In Europe, the responsibility for regulating transplant products according to the public health legislation lies with the national Competent Authority for tissues and cells in each member state. ATMPs in contrast are regulated by the pharmaceutical legislation, hence a marketing approval must be obtained prior to the marketing of an ATMP through the centralized procedure, like for any other biological medicinal product. The scientific evaluation of these products is led by a specialized committee within the EMA (the Committee for Advanced Therapies—"CAT"). The CAT drafts an opinion for the Committee for Medicinal Products for Human Use (CHMP), which is responsible for providing a second scientific opinion. Based on a positive CHMP opinion, the approval of a marketing authorization application (MAA) is granted by the EC. Clinical trials involving ATMPs are regulated and authorized in the same manner as other medicinal products, i.e., on a national level by the appropriate national competent authority (NCA).

Regulatory Bodies Involved in Regulating Advanced Therapies in the USA

The situation in the US is simpler in that the FDA is responsible for both aspects of the legislation: the public health and the pharmaceutical legislation. Within the FDA, the responsibility for the regulation of HCT/Ps and human gene therapy products lies with the Center for Biologics Evaluation and Research (CBER), both for clinical trials and marketing authorization. As of 2016, the CBER structure includes the Office of Blood Research and Review (OBRR), the Office of Vaccines Research and Review (OVRR), and the Office of Tissues and Advanced Therapies (OTAT), which was formerly known as the Office of Cellular, Tissue and Gene Therapies (OCTGT). To monitor activity, review data, and anticipate future needs, the FDA operates the Cellular, Tissue and Gene Therapies Advisory Committee.

Regulatory Guidances

Links to the relevant regulatory bodies involved in advanced therapies in the EU and US as well as applicable guidances can be found in Table 17.18.

Stem Cell Tourism

The general interest in advanced therapies around the world has allowed unregulated practice particularly of cell-based products to develop in some countries, i.e., "stem cell tourism". This is a major concern for many stakeholders in the field of ATMPs, because treatments are being offered in the absence of a strong safety data package and any proven efficacy. In addition, there is suspicion that the products in use have been manufactured with insufficient attention to GMP including quality control. It is very important that patients are warned of the dangers of falling prey to unethical operations. An up-to-date source of information on private clinics and stem cell tourism is available at the website of the International Society for Stem Cell Research (www.isscr.org).

CONCLUDING REMARKS

Although progress has been made in the area of ATMPs, with about 30 products approved globally and 20 in the EU&US (see Table 17.1) for commercial use and many products in clinical development, this field is currently struggling with similar problems as the first recombinant proteins 20 years ago. Appropriate manufacturing platforms, supply chain models, healthcare systems, reimbursement models, and regulatory frameworks for these medicinal products need to be established by developers and other key stakeholders, while specific knowledge about quality (production and testing), safety, and efficacy of advanced therapies is steadily growing.

Technologies	Development stage of the field	Current manufacturing technologies	Manufacturing and testing challenges
(a) Somatic cell technologies	Many products in early clinical development phase; few products approved, e.g., Alofisel	Manual process with open handling steps; automated multi-planar flasks and stack systems; micro-carriers in disposable stirred tank systems; hollow fiber growth systems; membrane and contraflow centrifugation systems	Scale-up and control of large scale batches. Recovery of cells from micro-carriers. DSP: Large volume handling, primary container filling at scale using enclosed technologies. Relevant potency assays lacking
(b) Cell immortalization technologies	One product in early clinical development	CompacT SelecT[a] fully automated and programmable scalable cell culture platform consisting of a robot arm that can access T175 flask or multi-well plate incubator. Standard cell culture activities, such as passage or media change, are conducted and controlled with no manual intervention	Similar to protein manufacturing platform technologies
(c) *Ex-vivo* gene modification of cells using viral vector technologies	Mainly small trials in early and late clinical development phase (gene modified autologous T-cells and HSCs); few products approved, e.g., Strimvelis and Kymriah	Manual processes often not fully enclosed using static bags, gas-permeable pots + lateral movement bioreactors (wave bags) for higher cell yield. Positive or negative cell selection process steps often used. High cell purity becoming possible with sterile cell sorter	Adapting systems to deal with variation in quality and amount of incoming starting material. Lack of product stability pressuring manufacturing and distribution model. Lack of fast QC assays. Low transduction efficiency with non-replicating viral vectors. Enclosed and automated manufacturing systems are becoming available for the entire process (e.g., prodigy)
(d) Cell plasticity technologies	Mainly pre-clinical phase with few ESC and iPSC-derived FIH trials	Current processes are extremely 'manual' and rely on small scale cell culture and harvest technologies. High risk processes with extensive process and product characterization testing to assess product quality, safety, and efficacy	A two-tier banking strategy (MCB/WCB) scale-up process of pluripotent cells prior to differentiation steps needed. Dynamic cell culture systems to expand PSC numbers. Robotic scale-out of current plate-based iPSC technology is also being explored
(e) 3D-technologies	Mainly pre-clinical phase with few FIH trials	A complex manufacturing interplay between (bio)materials, scaffolds, cells, and biological coatings. Incorporates decellularization/recellularization tissue-based products such as trachea, esophagus, and veins	Enclosed bioreactors to control cell and material interface. Improved stability and delivery systems. Robust product quality to ensure large clinical application

[a]Thomas et al. (2009)

Table 17.17 ■ Development stage manufacturing and testing challenges for different advanced therapy technologies, adapted from Mount et al. (2015)

Regulatory agency/institute	Link
EMA	http://www.ema.europa.eu/ema/index.jsp?curl=pages/regulation/general/general_content_000294.jsp&mid=WC0b01ac05800241e0
FDA	https://www.fda.gov/BiologicsBloodVaccines/default.htm
International Conference on Harmonisation (ICH)	http://www.ich.org/home.html
British Standards Institution (BSI)	BSI PAS 83:2012, BSI PAS 84:2012, and BSI PAS 93:2011

Table 17.18 ■ Regulatory agencies and applicable guidances for advanced therapies in the US and EU

This rapidly evolving field does require highly trained practitioners, both at the technical level and with regard to advising and counseling patients. Pharmaceutical scientists and pharmacists are important members of the teams of professionals that deliver these changes in healthcare to seriously ill patients. Much can be learned from the research & development (R&D) processes used by traditional biotech (e.g., during development of recombinant proteins and vaccines). Pharmaceutical scientists and pharmacists can play a key role in development of advanced therapies, as many applications are conceived by academic groups and small spin-off companies, who do not necessarily know how to translate a research concept into a medicinal product for human use. Pharmacy professionals can provide valuable experience in relation to the application of the principles of GMP, GLP, GCP, GDP (good distribution practice), and other available guidances.

SELF-ASSESSMENT QUESTIONS

■ Questions

1. What is the difference between embryonic and adult stem cells?
2. How is somatic cell nuclear transfer carried out and what are the problems with this technique?
3. What are iPSCs and why are they important?
4. What is the difference between *in-vivo* gene therapy and *ex-vivo* gene therapy?
5. Which disease areas are predominantly investigated clinically with ATMPs?
6. What problems could arise in use of stem cell-derived products for clinical application?

■ Answers

1. Embryonic stem cells are grown *ex-vivo* after extraction of the inner cell mass from a blastocyst. Adult stem cells are found *in-vivo* in many tissues, usually in the specialized environment of a stem cell niche, that supports their asymmetric cell division.
2. Somatic cell nuclear transfer (SCNT) involves the injection of a donor genome into an enucleated egg, such that the embryo develops as a clone of the donor genome. This allows the generation of embryonic stem cells using the donor genome and, in principle, allows implantation into the uterus of a recipient female leading to pregnancy. There are ethical problems concerned with supply of fertilized human eggs and also technical problems caused by incomplete reprogramming of the donor nucleus.
3. iPSCs are produced by transient expression of pluripotency genes in somatic cells, leading to reprogramming to form pluripotent cells resembling embryonic stem cells. The production of iPSCs allows pluripotent cells to be obtained from a patient without the need for SCNT. iPSCs can be used to derive differentiated cells for the production of ATMPs for clinical application or for disease modeling purposes.
4. *In-vivo* gene therapy refers to the direct introduction of genetic material into the human body, whereas *ex-vivo* gene therapy refers to the use of cells, which are genetically modified outside the body (i.e., *ex-vivo*) prior to administration of these genetically modified cells into the human body. In the latter case, the genetic material is introduced into the human body using cells as "delivery system". See also Chap. 16 for details on gene therapy.
5. Various cancers, autoimmune disorders, such as DM type I and Crohn's disease, neurological disorders, such as Parkinson's disease and Alzheimer's disease, myocardial infarction, and macular degeneration.
6. One of the concerns with stem cell derived ATMPs is the possibility that rare pluripotent or multipotent cells in the product could give rise to tumors after administration to humans (i.e., tumorigenicity risk). Thus, the quality control of the medicinal product is of paramount importance. Often, in particular in treatment of neurological diseases, it is not clear whether a progenitor, precursor, or fully mature cell should be administered. Careful preclinical work is required in each clinical indication to establish the most effective approach. Where the strategy is designed to replace a cell that is lost in a particular disease, the environment into which the cell-based medicinal product is placed may not be supportive of cell survival and integration/persistence. In general, one needs to pay attention to provide a protective environment for the medicinal product.

REFERENCES

Alvarez-Buylla A, Garcia-Verdugo JM, Tramontin AD (2001) A unified hypothesis on the lineage of neural stem cells. Nat Rev Neurosci 2:287–293

Ambasudhan R, Talantova M, Coleman R, Yuan X, Zhu S, Lipton SA, Ding S (2011) Direct reprogramming of adult human fibroblasts to functional neurons under defined conditions. Cell Stem Cell 9:113–118

Ankrum JA, Ong JF, Karp JM (2014) Mesenchymal stem cells: immune evasive, not immune privileged. Nat Biotechnol 32(3):252–260

Bianco P, Robey PG, Simmons PJ (2008) Mesenchymal stem cells: revisiting history, concepts, and assays. Cell Stem Cell 2:313–319

Bravery CA (2015) Do human leukocyte antigen-typed cellular therapeutics based on induced pluripotent stem cells make commercial sense? Stem Cells Dev 24(1):1–10

Bravery CA, Carmen J, Fong T, Oprea W, Hoogendoorn KH, Woda J, Burger SR, Rowley JA, Bonyhadi ML, van't Hof W (2013) Potency assay development for cellular therapy products: an ISCT review of the requirements and experiences in the industry. Cytotherapy 15:9–19

Burridge PW, Keller G, Gold JD, Wu JC (2012) Production of de novo cardiomyocytes: human pluripotent stem cell differentiation and direct reprogramming. Cell Stem Cell 10:16–28

Cadena-Herrera D, Esparza-De Lara JE, Ramírez-Ibañez ND, López-Morales CA, Pérez NO, Flores-Ortiz LF, Medina-Rivero E (2015) Validation of three viable-cell counting methods: manual, semi-automated, and automated. Biotechnol Rep 7:9–16

Campbell KH, McWhir J, Ritchie WA, Wilmut I (1996) Sheep cloned by nuclear transfer from a cultured cell line. Nature 380:64–66

Chin MH, Pellegrini M, Plath K, Lowry WE (2010) Molecular analyses of human induced pluripotent stem cells and embryonic stem cells. Cell Stem Cell 7:263–269

Consentius C, Reinke P, Volk H-D (2015) Immunogenicity of allogeneic mesenchymal stromal cells: what has been seen in vitro and *in vivo*? Regen Med 10(3):305–315

Evans MJ, Kaufman MH (1981) Establishment in culture of pluripotential cells from mouse embryos. Nature 292:154–156

Fesnak AD, June CH, Levine BL (2016) Engineered T cells: the promise and challenges of cancer immunotherapy. Nature 16:566–581

Gombold J, Peden K, Gavin D, Wei Z, Baradaran K, Mire-Sluis A, Schenerman M (2006a) Lot release and characterization testing of live-virus-based vaccines and gene therapy products, part 1: factors influencing assay choices - WCBP CMC Forum. Bioprocess Int 46–54, April 2006

Gombold J, Peden K, Gavin D, Wei Z, Baradaran K, Mire-Sluis A, Schenerman M (2006b) Lot release and characterization testing of live-virus-based vaccines and gene therapy products, part 2: case studies and discussion - WCBP CMC Forum Bioprocess Int 56–65, May 2006

Han DW, Tapia N, Hermann A, Hemmer K, Hoing S, Arauzo-Bravo MJ, Zaehres H, Wu G, Frank S, Moritz S, Greber B, Yang JH, Lee HT, Schwamborn JC, Storch A, Scholer HR (2012) Direct reprogramming of fibroblasts into neural stem cells by defined factors. Cell Stem Cell 10:465–472

Hanna J, Wernig M, Markoulaki S, Sun CW, Meissner A, Cassady JP, Beard C, Brambrink T, Wu LC, Townes TM, Jaenisch R (2007) Treatment of sickle cell anemia mouse model with iPS cells generated from autologous skin. Science 318:1920–1923

Hargus G, Cooper O, Deleidi M, Levy A, Lee K, Marlow E, Yow A, Soldner F, Hockemeyer D, Hallett PJ, Osborn T, Jaenisch R, Isacson O (2010) Differentiated Parkinson patient-derived induced pluripotent stem cells grow in the adult rodent brain and reduce motor asymmetry in Parkinsonian rats. Proc Natl Acad Sci U S A 107:15921–15926

Hassan W, Dong Y, Wang W (2013) Encapsulation and 3D culture of human adipose-derived stem cells in an in-situ crosslinked hybrid hydrogel composed of PEG-based hyperbranched copolymer and hyaluronic acid. Stem Cell Res Ther 4(32):1–11

Heathman T, Nienow AW, McCall MJ, Coppman K, Kara B, Hewitt CJ (2015) The translation of cell-based therapies: clinical landscape and manufacturing challenges. Regen Med 10(1):49–64

Herberts CA, Kwa MS, Hermsen HP (2011) Risk factors in the development of stem cell therapy. J Transl Med 9:29

Huang P, Zhang L, Gao Y, He Z, Yao D, Wu Z, Cen J, Chen X, Liu C, Hu Y, Lai D, Hu Z, Chen L, Zhang Y, Cheng X, Ma X, Pan G, Wang X, Hui L (2011) Direct reprogramming of human fibroblasts to functional and expandable hepatocytes. Cell Stem Cell 14:370–384

Ilic D, Devito L, Miere C, Codognotto S (2015) Human embryonic and induced pluripotent stem cells in clinical trials. Br Med Bull 116:19–27

Jia F, Wilson KD, Sun N, Gupta DM, Huang M, Li Z, Panetta NJ, Chen ZY, Robbins RC, Kay MA, Longaker MT, Wu JC (2010) A nonviral minicircle vector for deriving human iPS cells. Nat Methods 7:197–199

Kean TJ, Lin P, Caplan AI, Dennis JE (2013) MSCs: delivery routes and engraftment, cell-targeting strategies, and immune modulation. Stem Cells Int 2013:732742

Keller G (2005) Embryonic stem cell differentiation: emergence of a new era in biology and medicine. Genes Dev 19:1129–1155

Kim YJ, Matsunaga YT (2017) Thermo-responsive polymers and their application as smart biomaterials. J Mater Chem B 5:4307–4321

Kimbrel EA, Lanza R (2015) Current status of pluripotent stem cells: moving the first therapies to the clinic. Nat Rev Drug Discov 14:681–692

Lander AD, Kimble J, Clevers H, Fuchs E, Montarras D, Buckingham M, Calof AL, Trumpp A, Oskarsson T (2012) What does the concept of the stem cell niche really mean today? BMC Biol 10:19

Landgren H, Curtis MA (2010) Locating and labeling neural stem cells in the brain. J Cell Physiol 226:1–7

Leibacher J, Henschler R (2016) Biodistribution, migration and homing of systematically applied mesenchymal stem/stromal cells. Stem Cell Res Ther 7:7:1–12

Levenstein ME, Ludwig TE, Xu RH, Llanas RA, VanDenHeuvel-Kramer K, Manning D, Thomson JA (2006) Basic fibroblast growth factor support of human embryonic stem cell self-renewal. Stem Cells 24:568–574

Levine BL, Miskin J, Wonnacott K, Keir C (2017) Global manufacturing of CAR T cell therapy. Mol Ther Methods Clin Dev 4:92–101

Lui KO, Waldmann H, Fairchild PJ (2009) Embryonic stem cells: overcoming the immunological barriers to cell replacement therapy. Curr Stem Cell Res Ther 4:70–80

Martin GR (1981) Isolation of a pluripotent ell line from early mouse embryos cultured in medium conditioned by teratocarcinoma stem cells. Proc Natl Acad SCi USA 78:7634–7638

Morenweiser R (2005) Downstream processing of viral vectors and vaccines. Gene Ther 12:S103–S110

Mount NM, Ward SJ, Kefalas P, Hyllner J (2015) Cell-based therapy technology classifications and translational challenges. Philos Trans R Soc Lond B Biol Sci 370:1–16

Murphy SV, Atala A (2014) 3D bioprinting of tissues and organs. Nat Biotechnol 32(8):773–785

Murry CE, Keller G (2008) Differentiation of embryonic stem cells to clinically relevant populations: lessons from embryonic development. Cell 132:661–680

Pedersen RA, Macetti V, Mendjan S (2012) Synthetic organs for regenerative medicine. Cell Stem Cell 10:646–647

Pollock K, Stroemer P, Patel S, Stevanato L, Hope A, Miljan E, Dong Z, Hodges H, Price J, Sinden JD (2006) A conditionally immortal clonal stem cell line from human cortical neuroepithelium for the treatment of ischemic stroke. Exp Neurol 199:143–155

Santos GW (1983) History of bone marrow transplantation. Clin Haematol 12:611–639
Sasai Y (2013) Next-generation regenerative medicine: organogenesis from stem cells in 3D culture. Cell Stem Cell 12:520–530
Sayed N, Liu C, Wu JC (2016) Translation of human-induced pluripotent stem cells. J Am Coll Cardiol 67(18):2161–2176
Sayed N, Wong WT, Ospino F, Meng S, Lee J, Jha A, Dexheimer P, Aronow BJ, Cooke JP (2015) Transdifferentiation of human fibroblasts to endothelial cells: role of innate immunity. Circulation 131:300–9
Scadden DT (2006) The stem-cell niche as an entity of action. Nature 441:1075–1079
Scott CT, DeFrancesco L (2016) Gene therapy's out-of-body experience. Nat Biotechnol 34(6):600–607
Sharpe M, Mount N (2015) genetically modified T cells in cancer therapy: opportunities and challenges. Dis Model Mech 8:337–350
Smith BD, Grande DA (2015) The current state of scaffolds for musculoskeletal regenerative applications. Nat Rev Rheumatol 11:213–222
Smith JA, Bravery CA, Hollander G, Brindley DA (2015) Regenerative medicine regulation: cell therapy, gene therapy and tissue engineering. In: Fundamentals of EU regulatory affairs, 7th edn. RAPS, Rockville
Squillaro T, Peluso G, Galderisi U (2016) Clinical trials with mesenchymal stem cells: an update. Cell Transplant 25:829–848
Stevanato L, Corteling RL, Stroemer P, Hope A, Heward J, Miljan EA, Sinden JD (2009) c-MycERTAM transgene silencing in a genetically modified human neural stem cell line implanted into MCAo rodent brain. BMC Neurosci 10:86
Taichman RS (2005) Blood and bone: two tissues whose fates are intertwined to create the hematopoietic stem-cell niche. Blood 105:2631–2639
Takahashi K, Yamanaka S (2006) Induction of pluripotent stem cells from mouse embryonic and adult fibroblast cultures by defined factors. Cell 126:663–676
Takahashi K, Tanabe K, Ohnuki M, Narita M, Ichisaka T, Tomoda K, Yamanaka S (2007) Induction of pluripotent stem cells from adult human fibroblasts by defined factors. Cell 131:861–872
Tchieu J, Kuoy E, Chin MH, Trinh H, Patterson M, Sherman SP, Aimiuwu O, Lindgren A, Hakimian S, Zack JA, Clark AT, Pyle AD, Lowry WE, Plath K (2010) Female human iPSCs retain an inactive X chromosome. Cell Stem Cell 7:329–342
Tebas P, Stein D, Tang WW, Frank I, Wang SQ, Lee G, Spratt SK, Surosky RT, Giedlin MA, Nichol G, Holmes MC, Gregory P et al (2014) Gene editing of CCR5 in autologous CD4 T cells of persons infected with HIV. N Engl J Med 370:901–910
Thier M, Worsdorfer P, Lakes YB, Gorris R, Herms S, Opitz T, Seiferling D, Quandel T, Hoffmann P, Nothen MM, Brustle O, Edenhofer F (2012) Direct conversion of fibroblasts into stably expandable neural stem cells. Cell Stem Cell 10:473–479
Thomas RJ, Anderson D, Chandra A, Smith NM, Young LE, Williams D, Denning C (2009) Automated, scalable culture of human embryonic stem cells in feeder-free conditions. Biotechnol Bioeng 102:1636–1644
Thomson JA, Itskovitz-Eldor J, Shapiro SS, Waknitz MA, Swiergiel JJ, Marshall VS, Jones JM (1998) Embryonic stem cell lines derived from human blastocysts. Science 282:1145–1147
Trounson A, McDonald C (2015) Stem cell therapies in clinical trials: progress and challenges. Cell Stem Cell 17:11–22
Vestergaard HT, D'Apote L, Schneider CK, Herberts C (2013) The evolution of nonclinical regulatory science: advanced therapy medicinal products as a paradigm. Mol Ther 21(9):644–1647
Wegst UGK, Bai H, Saiz E, Tomsia AP, Richie RO (2015) Bioinspired structural materials. Nat Mater 14:23–36
Wernig M, Zhao JP, Pruszak J, Hedlund E, Fu D, Soldner F, Broccoli V, Constantine-Paton M, Isacson O, Jaenisch R (2008) Neurons derived from reprogrammed fibroblasts functionally integrate into the fetal brain and improve symptoms of rats with Parkinson's disease. Proc Natl Acad Sci U S A 105:5856–5861
Wilmut I, Beaujean N, de Sousa PA, Dinnyes A, King TJ, Paterson LA, Wells DN, Young LE (2002) Somatic cell nuclear transfer. Nature 419:583–586
Wilmut I, Sullivan G, Taylor J (2009) A decade of progress since the birth of Dolly. Reprod Fertil Dev 21:95–100
Wright JF (2018) Manufacturing and characterization of AAV-based vectors for use in clinical studies. Gene Ther 15:840–848
Yang CS, Li Z, Rana TM (2011) microRNAs modulate iPS cell generation. RNA 17:1451–1460
Ying QL, Nichols J, Chambers I, Smith A (2003) BMP induction of Id proteins suppresses differentiation and sustains embryonic stem cell self-renewal in collaboration with STAT3. Cell 115:281–292
Ying QL, Wray J, Nichols J, Batlle-Morera L, Doble B, Woodgett J, Cohen P, Smith A (2008) The ground state of embryonic stem cell self-renewal. Nature 453:519–523
Yu J, Vodyanik MA, Smuga-Otto K, Antosiewicz-Bourget J, Frane JL, Tian S, Nie J, Jonsdottir GA, Ruotti V, Stewart R, Slukvin II, Thomson JA (2007) Induced pluripotent stem cell lines derived from human somatic cells. Science 318:1917–1920
Yuan X, Wan H, Zhao X, Zhu S, Zhou Q, Ding S (2011) Brief report: combined chemical treatment enables Oct4-induced reprogramming from mouse embryonic fibroblasts. Stem Cells 29:549–553
Zhao C, Deng W, Gage FH (2008) Mechanisms and functional implications of adult neurogenesis. Cell 132:645–660
Zhao T, Zhang ZN, Rong Z, Xu Y (2011) Immunogenicity of induced pluripotent stem cells. Nature 474:212–215

SUGGESTED READING

BSI PAS 83:2012 (2012) Developing human cells for clinical applications in the Euopean Union and the United States of America – guide. Publicly Available Specification PAS83:2012, The British Standards Institution, ISBN 978 0 580 71052 0
BSI PAS 84:2012 (2012) Cell therapy and regenerative medicine – glossary. Publicly Available Specification PAS84:2012, The British Standards Institution, ISBN 978 0 580 74904 9
BSI PAS 93:2011 (2011) Characterization of human cells for clinical applications – guide. Publicly Available Specification PAS93:2011, The British Standards Institution, ISBN 978 0 580 69850 7

18 Insulin

John M. Beals, Michael R. DeFelippis, Chad D. Paavola, David P. Allen, Ashish Garg, and D. Bruce Baldwin

INTRODUCTION

Insulin was discovered by Banting and Best in 1921 (Bliss 1982). Soon afterwards, manufacturing processes were developed to extract the insulin from porcine and bovine pancreata. From 1921 to 1980, efforts were directed at increasing the purity of the insulin and providing different formulations for enhanced glucose control by altering time action (Brange 1987a, b; Galloway 1988). Purification was improved by optimizing extraction and processing conditions and by implementing chromatographic processes (size exclusion, ion exchange, and reversed-phase (Kroeff et al. 1989)). These improvements reduce the levels of both general protein impurities and insulin-related proteins such as proinsulin and insulin polymers. Formulation development focused on improving chemical stability by moving from acidic to neutral formulations and by modifying the time-action profile through the use of various levels of zinc and protamine. The evolution of recombinant DNA technology led to the widespread availability of human insulin, which has eliminated issues with sourcing constraints while providing the patient with an exogenous source of native insulin. Combining the improved purification methodologies and recombinant DNA (rDNA) technology, manufacturers of insulin are now able to provide the purest human insulin ever made available, >98% pure. Further advances in rDNA technology, coupled with a detailed understanding of the molecular properties of insulin and knowledge of its endogenous secretion profile, enabled the development of insulin analogs with improved pharmacology relative to existing human insulin products.

CHEMICAL DESCRIPTION

Insulin, a 51-amino acid protein, is a hormone that is synthesized as a single-chain proinsulin precursor, containing a leader sequence, the B-chain, a connecting peptide (C-peptide), and an A-chain, in the β-cells of the pancreas. The proinsulin precursor is converted to insulin by enzymatic cleavage. Current manufacturing strategies mimic this enzymatic approach. The resulting insulin molecule is composed of two polypeptide chains that are connected by two inter-chain disulfide bonds (Fig. 18.1) (Baker et al. 1988). The A-chain is composed of 21 amino acids, and the B-chain is composed of 30 amino acids. The inter-chain disulfide linkages occur between A^7–B^7 and A^{20}–B^{19}, respectively. A third intra-chain disulfide bond is located in the A-chain, between residues A^6 and A^{11}.

Bovine and porcine insulin preparations were the first commercially available insulin-therapies. However, all major manufacturers of insulin have discontinued production of these products, marking an end to future supply of animal-sourced insulin products. Difficulties obtaining sufficient supplies of bovine or porcine pancreata and recent concerns over transmissible spongiform encephalopathies associated with the use of animal-derived materials were major reasons for the product deletions.

Recombinant DNA technology enabled the production of human insulin from microorganisms, such as bacteria or yeast. In most cases, a precursor proinsulin is produced by the introduction of an exogenous gene into the microorganism. This proinsulin contains a leader sequence on the N-terminus of the B-chain and a connecting peptide between the A- and B-chain. The connecting peptide enables proper folding of the

J. M. Beals (✉) · C. D. Paavola
Lilly Research Laboratories, Biotechnology Discovery Research, Eli Lilly and Company, Indianapolis, IN, USA
e-mail: beals_john_m@lilly.com

M. R. DeFelippis · D. P. Allen · A. Garg
Lilly Research Laboratories, Bioproduct Research and Development, Eli Lilly and Company, Indianapolis, IN, USA

D. Bruce Baldwin
Lilly Research Laboratories, Technical Services and Manufacturing Sciences, Eli Lilly and Company, Indianapolis, IN, USA
e-mail: baldwin_bruce@lilly.com

D. J. A. Crommelin et al. (eds.), *Pharmaceutical Biotechnology*, https://doi.org/10.1007/978-3-030-00710-2_18

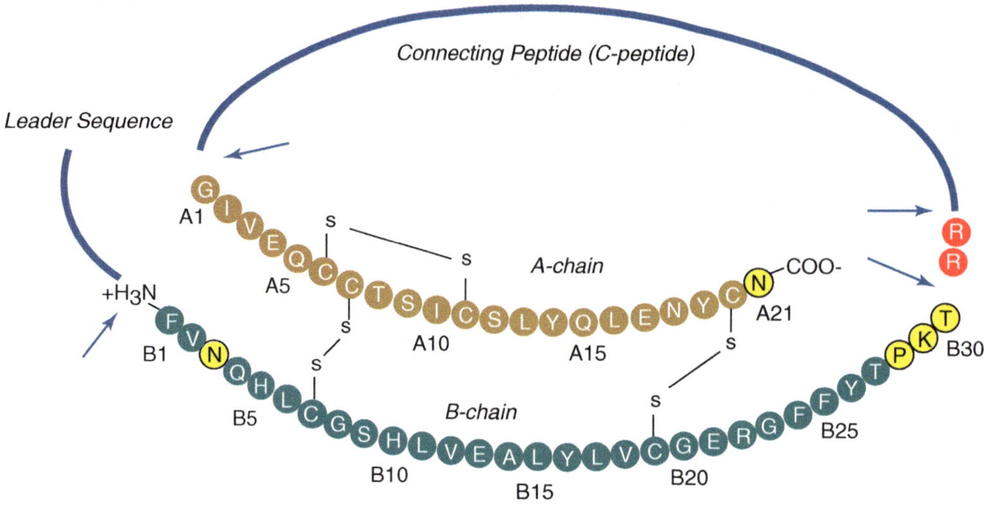

Figure. 18.1 ■ Primary sequence of insulin. The A-chain is displayed in tan. The B-chain is displayed in teal. The yellow-highlighted amino acids represent sites of sequence alterations denoted in Table 18.1. The arrows indicate sites of enzymatic processing that remove the leader sequence and connecting peptide from the expressed proinsulin. The sequences of the leader and connecting peptide are not shown, with the exception of the two arginine residues (red) that are retained in an analog to alter their time action (e.g., insulin glargine)

Species	A^{21}	B^{3}	B^{28}	B^{29}	B^{30}	B^{31}	B^{32}
human insulin (Humulin®, Novolin®, Afrezza®)	Asn	Asn	Pro	Lys	Thr	–	–
insulin lispro (Humalog®, Liprolog®, Admelog®)	Asn	Asn	Lys	Pro	Thr	–	–
insulin aspart (NovoRapid®, NovoLog®)	Asn	Asn	Asp	Lys	Thr	–	–
insulin glulisine (Apidra®)	Asn	Lys	Pro	Glu	Thr	–	–
insulin glargine (Lantus®, Basaglar®, Toujeo®)	Gly	Asn	Pro	Lys	Thr	Arg	Arg
insulin detemir (Levemir®)	Asn	Asn	Pro	Lys-(*N*-tetradecanoyl)	–	–	–
insulin degludec (Tresiba®)	Asn	Asn	Pro	Lys-(N^{ε}-hexadecandioyl-γ-Glu)	–	–	–

Table 18.1 ■ Amino acid substitutions in insulin analogs compared to human insulin

proinsulin in the cells or during in vitro processing. The leader sequence and connecting peptide can vary in their amino acid composition and size, dependent on the expression system being used. In most cases, the leader sequence and connecting peptide are removed by enzymatic cleavage during the purification process. After processing and final purification, the two-chain insulin is delivered with sufficient purity.

The establishment of these biotechnological processes for generating insulin, coupled with understanding of its chemical and physical properties, enabled the engineering of new analogs of insulin. These new analogs (listed with human insulin in Table 18.1) contain various mutations and/or chemical modifications of the human insulin protein that enable differing in vivo time action profiles and stability within their commercial drug product formulations.

Follow-on biologic versions of already-approved insulin analogs are beginning to enter the market (see, Basaglar® and Admelog® in Table 18.1). A follow-on biologic version of insulin is a marketed insulin that exhibits no clinically meaningful difference from the existing approved insulin product. Regulatory agencies compare the characteristics of the follow-on biologic version of insulin to an already-approved originator product. To warrant approval, the follow-on biologic version insulin must demonstrate comparable purity, chemical identity, bioactivity, and safety through preclinical and clinical evaluation (Peters et al. 2015).

The net charge on human insulin is produced from the ionization potential of four glutamic acid residues, four tyrosine residues, two histidine residues, a lysine residue, and an arginine residue, in conjunction with two α-carboxyl and two α-amino groups. Human insulin has an isoelectric point (pI) of 5.3 in the denatured state; thus, the insulin molecule is negatively charged at neutral pH (Kaarsholm et al. 1990). This net

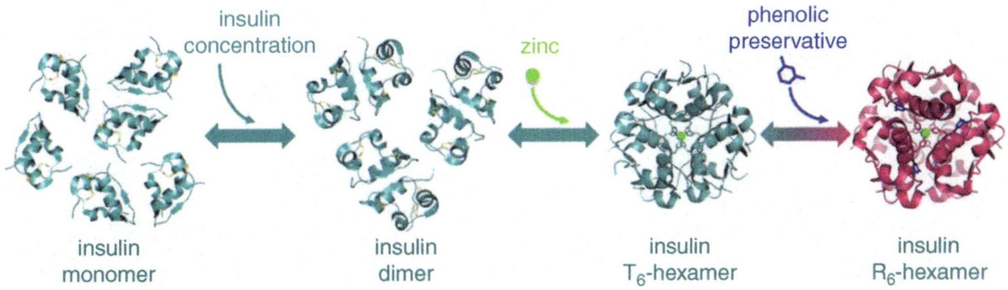

Figure. 18.2 ■ Schematic representation of insulin association in the presence and absence of zinc and phenolic preservatives, e.g., phenol or m-cresol

negative charge state of insulin has been used in formulation development, as will be discussed later.

In addition to the net charge on insulin, another important intrinsic property of the molecule is its ability to readily associate into dimers and higher-order associated states (Figs. 18.2 and 18.3) (Pekar and Frank 1972). The driving force for dimerization appears to be the formation of favorable hydrophobic interactions at the C-terminus of the B-chain (Ciszak et al. 1995). Insulin can associate into discrete hexameric complexes in the presence of various divalent metal ions, such as zinc at 0.33 g-atom/monomer (Goldman and Carpenter 1974), where each zinc ion (a total of two) is coordinated by a His^{B10} residue from three adjacent monomers. Physiologically, insulin is stored as a zinc-containing hexamer in the β-cells of the pancreas. As will be discussed later, the ability to form discrete hexamers in the presence of zinc has been used to develop therapeutically useful formulations of insulin.

Commercial insulin formulations contain phenolic excipients (e.g., phenol and m-cresol) as antimicrobial agents. As represented in Figs. 18.2 and 18.3d, these phenolic species also bind to specific sites on insulin hexamers, causing a conformational change that increases the chemical stability of insulin in commercial preparations (Brange and Langkjaer 1992). X-ray crystallographic studies have identified the location of six phenolic ligand binding sites on the insulin hexamer and the nature of the conformational change induced by the binding of these ligands (Derewenda et al. 1989). The phenolic ligands occupy a binding pocket between monomers of adjacent dimers by hydrogen bonds with the carbonyl oxygen of Cys^{A6} and the amide proton of Cys^{A11} as well as numerous van der Waals contacts. The binding of these ligands stabilizes a conformational change that occurs at the N-terminus of the B-chain in each insulin monomer, shifting the conformational equilibrium of residues B1 to B8 from an extended structure (T-state) to an α-helical structure (R-state). This conformational change is referred to as the T↔R transition (Brader and Dunn 1991) and is illustrated in Fig. 18.3c, d.

In addition to the presence of zinc and phenolic preservatives, modern insulin formulations may contain a tonicity agent (e.g., glycerol or NaCl), a buffer (e.g., sodium phosphate or TRIS listed as trometamol or tromethamine), and surfactants (e.g., polysorbate 20 or polysorbate 80). The tonicity agent is used to minimize subcutaneous tissue damage and pain upon injection. The buffer is present to minimize pH drift in some pH-sensitive formulations. The surfactant is present to increase physical stability of the formulation. Afrezza® is a dry powder inhalation product, so it differs from the solution forumlations described above. This pulmonary insulin formulation contains fumaryl diketopiperazine to create technospheres on which human insulin is coated.

PHARMACOLOGY AND FORMULATIONS

Normal insulin secretion in the nondiabetic person falls into two categories: (1) insulin that is secreted in response to a meal and (2) the background or basal insulin that is continually secreted between meals and during the nighttime hours (Fig. 18.4). The pancreatic response to a meal typically results in peak serum insulin levels of 50–80 μU/mL, whereas basal serum insulin levels fall within the 5–15 μU/mL range (Galloway and Chance 1994). Because of these vastly different insulin demands, considerable effort has been expended to develop insulin formulations that meet the pharmacokinetic (PK) and pharmacodynamic (PD) requirements of each condition. More recently, insulin analogs and insulin analog formulations have been developed to improve PK and PD properties.

■ Regular and Rapid-Acting Soluble Preparations

Initial soluble insulin formulations were prepared under acidic conditions and were chemically unstable. In these early formulations, considerable deamidation was identified at Asn^{A21}, significant potency loss was observed during prolonged storage under acidic conditions, and time action was impaired due to the pH transition across the pI of the insulin molecule,

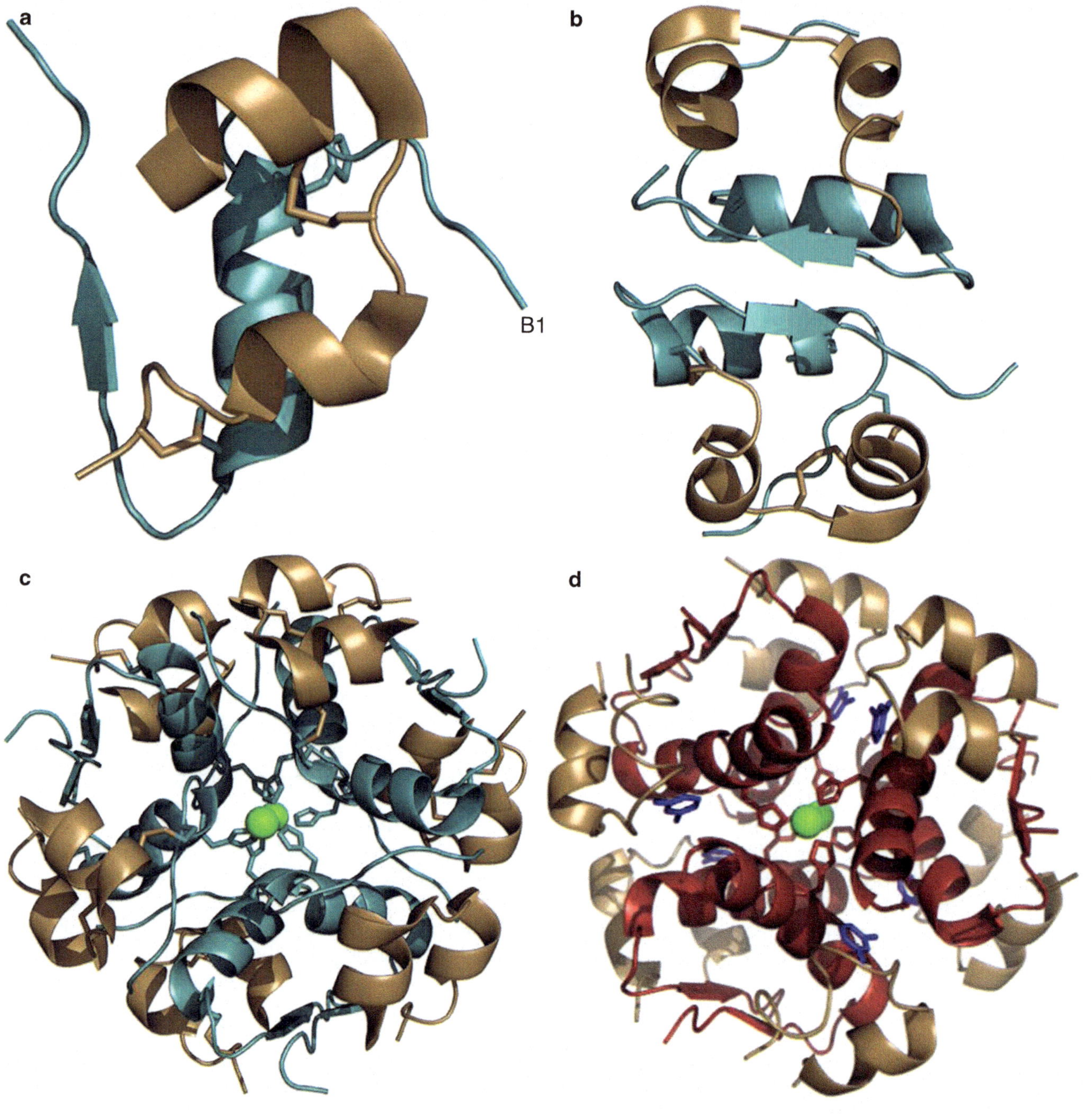

Figure. 18.3 (**a**) A cartoon representation of the secondary and tertiary structures of an insulin monomer, with the B1–B8 region in an extended conformation (T-state). The A-chain is colored tan and the B-chain is colored teal. The α-helices are depicted as coils and the β-sheet formed during dimerization is depicted as arrow. (**b**) A cartoon representation of the secondary and tertiary structures of a insulin dimer, with the B1–B8 regions in an extended conformation (T-state). The A-chains are colored tan and the B-chains are colored teal. (**c**) A cartoon representation of the secondary and tertiary structures of a zinc-induced T_6-state insulin hexamer, with the B1–B8 regions in an extended conformation (T-state). The A-chains are colored tan, the B-chains are colored teal, and zinc is colored green. (**d**) A cartoon representation of the secondary and tertiary structures of the zinc- and phenolic preservative-induced R_6-state insulin hexamer, wherein the B1-B8 regions are locked in the α-helical conformation (R-state). The A-chains are colored tan, the B-chains are colored red, zinc is colored green, and preservative is colored purple

which resulted in protein precipitation at the site of injection. Efforts to improve the chemical stability of these soluble formulations led to the development of neutral, zinc-stabilized solutions.

The insulin in these neutral pH, regular formulations is chemically stabilized by the addition of zinc (~0.4% (w/w) relative to the insulin concentration) and phenolic preservatives. As mentioned above, the

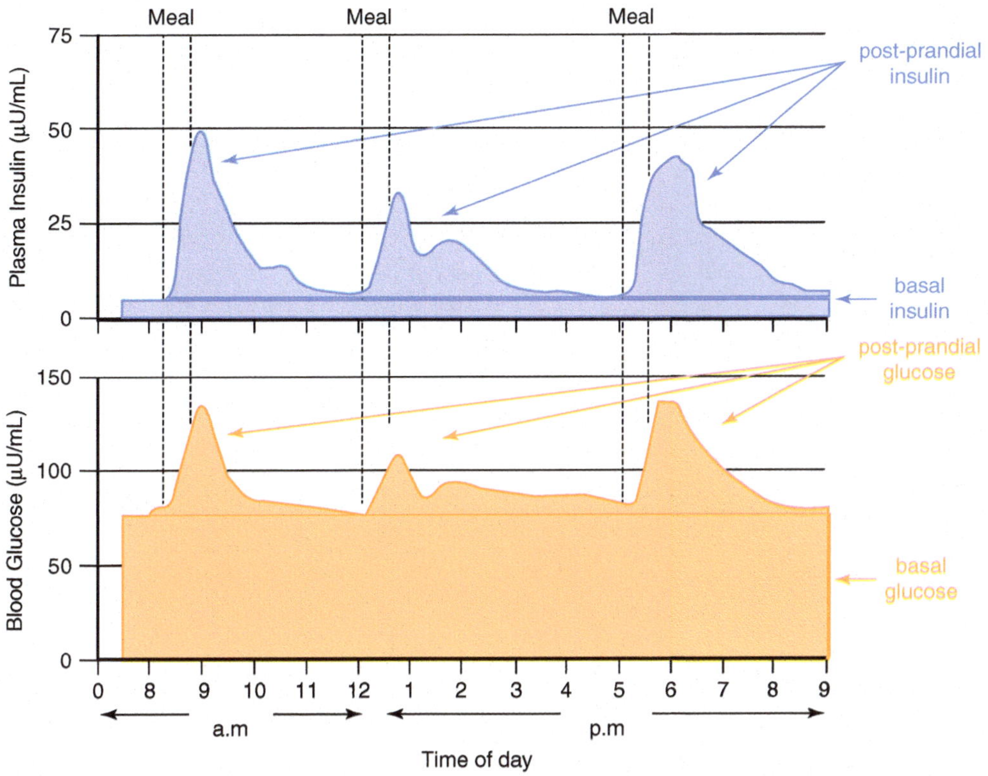

Figure. 18.4 ■ A schematic representation of glucose and insulin profiles during the day in nondiabetic individuals (Adapted and reprinted from Schade et al. 1983)

addition of zinc leads to the formation of discrete T_6 hexameric structures (containing 2 Zn^{+2} atoms per hexamer) that can bind six molecules of phenolic preservatives, e.g., m-cresol to form R_6 hexamers (Figs. 18.2 and 18.3c). This in turn decreases the availability of residues involved in deamidation and high molecular weight polymer formation (Brange et al. 1992a, b).

The pharmacodynamic profile of these soluble formulations (marketed in the U.S. under the designation type R) is listed in Table 18.2. The neutral pH, regular formulations show peak insulin activity between 2 and 3 h with a maximum duration of 5–8 h. As with other formulations, the variations in time action can be attributed to factors such as dose, site of injection, temperature, and the patient's physical activity. Despite the soluble state of insulin in these formulations, a delay in activity is still observed. This delay has been attributed to the time required for the hexamer to dissociate into the dimeric and/or monomeric substituents prior to absorption from the interstitium. This dissociation requires time-dependent diffusion of the preservative, zinc, and insulin from the site of injection, effectively diluting the protein and shifting the equilibrium from hexamers to dimers and monomers (Fig. 18.5a) (Brange et al. 1990). Studies exploring the relationship of molecular weight and cumulative dose recovery of various compounds in the popliteal lymph following subcutaneous injection suggest that lymphatic transport may account for approximately 20% of the absorption of insulin from the interstitium (Supersaxo et al. 1990; Porter and Charman 2000; Charman et al. 2001). The remaining balance of insulin is predominately absorbed through the microvascular endothelium.

Insulin analogs with monomerizing mutations were designed to weaken the dimerization interface and achieve a faster response to prandial glucose increases, while providing dosing convenience to the patient. The pharmacological properties of these soluble formulations are listed in Table 18.3. The development of monomeric analogs of insulin for the treatment of insulin-dependent diabetes mellitus has focused on shifting the self-association properties of insulin to favor the monomeric species and consequently minimizing the delay in time action (Brange et al. 1988, 1990; Brems et al. 1992). One such monomeric analog, $Lys^{B28}Pro^{B29}$-human insulin (insulin lispro; CAS Number 133107-64-9; Humalog®, Liprolog®, Admelog®) has demonstrated a more rapid time-action profile, with a peak activity of approximately 1 h (Howey et al. 1994). The sequence inversion of amino acids at positions B28 and B29 yields an analog with reduced self-association behavior compared to human insulin (Fig. 18.1; Table 18.1); yet, insulin lispro can be stabilized in a preservative- and zinc-dependent hexameric complex that provides the necessary chemical and vphysical stability required for

Type[a]	Description	Appearance	Components	Action (h)[b]		
				Onset	Peak	Duration
R[c]	Regular soluble insulin human injection	Clear solution	Metal ion: zinc (10–40 μg/mL) Buffer: none Preservative: m-cresol (2.5 mg/mL) Tonicity agent: glycerin (16 mg/mL) pH: 7.2–7.6 Dosages: U100	0.5–1	2–4	5–8
Afrezza®	Insulin human inhalation powder	Dry powder	Metal ion: none Buffer: none Preservative: none Tonicity agent: none pH: N/A Carrier Particles: fumaryl diketopiperazine and polysorbate 80 Dosages: 4 U and 8 U	0.1–0.2	0.5–0.9	2.5–3.0
N	NPH insulin human isophane suspension	Turbid or cloudy suspension	Metal ion: zinc (21–40 μg/mL) Buffer: dibasic sodium phosphate (3.78 mg/mL) Preservatives: m-cresol (1.6 mg/mL), phenol (0.73 mg/mL) Tonicity agent: glycerin (16 mg/mL) Modifying protein: protamine (~0.35 mg/mL) pH: 7.0–7.5 Dosages: U100	1–2	2–8	14–24
70/30	70% insulin human isophane suspension, 30% regular insulin human injection	Turbid or cloudy suspension	Metal ion: zinc (21–35 μg/mL) Buffer: dibasic sodium phosphate (3.78 mg/mL) Preservatives: m-cresol (1.6 mg/mL), phenol (0.73 mg/mL) Tonicity agent: glycerin (16 mg/mL) Modifying protein: protamine (~0.241 mg/mL) pH: 7.0–7.8 Dosages: U100	0.5	2–4	14–24

[a]US designation
[b]The time-action profiles of Lilly insulins are the average onset, peak action, and duration of action that are taken from a composite of studies. The onset, peak, and duration of insulin action depend on numerous factors, such as dose, injection site, presence of insulin antibodies, and physical activity. The action times listed represent the generally accepted values in the medical community
[c]Another notable designation is S (Britain). Other soluble formulations have been designed for pump use and include Velosulin® and HOE 21PH®

Table 18.2 ■ A list of human insulin formulations

insulin preparations. Despite the hexameric complexation of this analog, insulin lispro retains its rapid time action. Based on the crystal structure of the insulin lispro hexameric complex (Ciszak et al. 1995) and the self-association behavior in solution (Bakaysa et al. 1996), it is hypothesized that the reduced dimerization properties of the analog, coupled with the zinc- and preservative-dependent hexamerization requirements, yield a hexameric complex that readily dissociates into monomers after rapid diffusion of the phenolic preservative into the subcutaneous tissue at the site of injection (Fig. 18.5b). Consequently, the time-dependent diffusion, dilution, and dissociation of the zinc hexamers is not necessary for the analog to generate monomers/dimers, which are required for adsorption across the microvascular endothelium.

It is important to highlight that the properties engineered into insulin lispro not only provide the patient with a more convenient therapy, but also improve control of postprandial hyperglycemia and reduce the frequency of non-severe hypoglycemic events (Holleman et al. 1997; Anderson et al. 1997).

Since the introduction of insulin lispro, two additional rapid-acting insulin analogs have been introduced to the market. The amino acid modifications made to the human insulin sequence to produce these analogs are depicted in Table 18.1. Like insulin lispro, both analogs are supplied as neutral pH solutions containing phenolic preservative. The design strategy for Asp^{B28}-human insulin (insulin aspart; CAS Number 116094-23-6; NovoRapid® or NovoLog®) (Brange et al. 1988, 1990) involves the replacement of Pro^{B28} with a

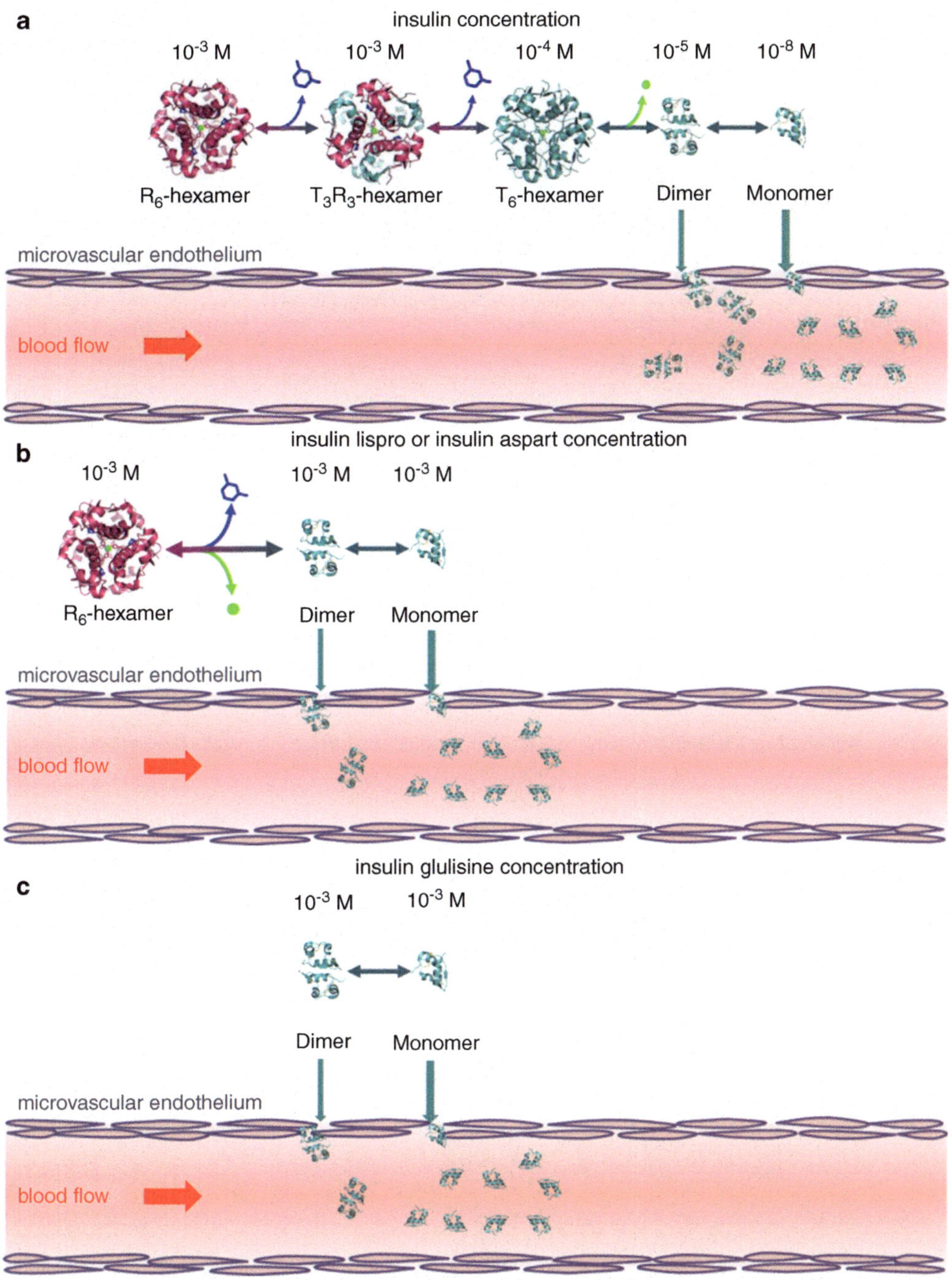

Figure. 18.5 ■ A schematic representation of Regular (R, see Table 18.2) or rapid-acting (see Table 18.3) insulin dissociation and absorption after subcutaneous administration; (**a**) insulin, (**b**) insulin lispro or insulin aspart, and (**c**) insulin glulisine

negatively charged aspartic acid residue. Like $Lys^{B28}Pro^{B29}$-human insulin, Asp^{B28}-human insulin has a more rapid time action following subcutaneous injection (Fig. 18.5b) (Heinemann et al. 1997). This rapid action is also achieved through a reduction in the self-association behavior compared to human insulin (Brange et al. 1990; Whittingham et al. 1998). The other rapid-acting analog, Lys^{B3}-Glu^{B29}-human insulin (insulin glulisine; CAS Number 160337-95-1; Apidra®), involves a substitution of the lysine residue at position 29 of the B-chain with a negatively charged glutamic acid. Additionally, this analog replaces the Asn^{B3} with a positively charged lysine. Scientific reports describing the impact of these changes on the molecular properties of this analog are lacking. However, the glutamic acid substitution occurs at a position known to be involved in dimer formation (Brange et al. 1990) and may result in disruption of key interactions at the monomer-mono-

Type[a]	Description	Appearance	Components	Action (h)[b] Onset	Peak	Duration
Humalog®, Admelog®, Liprolog®	Rapid-acting soluble insulin analog for injection	Aqueous, clear, and colorless solution	Metal ion: zinc (19.7 μg/mL U100; 46 μg/mL U200) Buffer: dibasic sodium phosphate (1.88 mg/mL U100) tromethamine (5 mg/mL U200) Preservatives: m-cresol (3.15 mg/mL), phenol (trace) Tonicity agent: glycerin (16 mg/mL) pH: 7.0–7.8 Dosage: Humalog® U100 and U200: Admelog® U100	0.25–0.5	0.5–2.5	≤5[c]
Humalog® Mix75/25™	75% insulin lispro protamine suspension and 25% insulin lispro for injection	Turbid or cloudy suspension	Metal ion: zinc (25 μg/mL) Buffer: dibasic sodium phosphate (3.78 mg/mL) Preservative: m-cresol (1.76 mg/mL), phenol (0.715 mg/mL) Tonicity agent: glycerin (16 mg/mL) Modifying protein: protamine sulfate (0.28 mg/mL) pH: 7.0–7.8 Dosage: U100	0.25–0.5	2–3	14–24[d]
Humalog® Mix50/50™	50% insulin lispro protamine suspension and 50% insulin lispro for injection	Turbid or cloudy suspension	Metal ion: zinc (30.5 μg/mL) Buffer: dibasic sodium phosphate (3.78 mg/mL) Preservative: m-cresol (2.20 mg/mL), phenol (0.89 mg/mL) Tonicity agent: glycerin (16 mg/mL) Modifying protein: protamine sulfate (0.19 mg/mL) pH: 7.0–7.8 Dosage: U100	0.25–0.5	2–3	14-20[d]
NovoLog®	Rapid-acting soluble insulin analog for injection	Aqueous, clear, and colorless solution	Metal ion: zinc (19.6 μg/mL) Buffer: disodium hydrogen phosphate dihydrate (1.25 mg/mL) Preservative: m-cresol (1.72 mg/mL), phenol (1.50 mg/mL) Tonicity agents: glycerin (16 mg/mL), sodium chloride (0.58 mg/mL) pH: 7.2–7.6 Dosage: U100	0.25[c]	1–3[c]	3–5[c]
Fiasp®	Rapid-acting soluble insulin analog for injection	Aqueous, clear, and colorless solution	Metal ion: zinc Buffer: disodium hydrogen phosphate dihydrate Preservative: m-cresol, phenol Tonicity agents: glycerol Other: arginine hydrochloride, niacinamide (vitamin B3), pH: 7.1 Dosage: U100	0.26–0.33	1.5–2.2	5–7[d]

Table 18.3 ■ A list of insulin analog formulations

Type[a]	Description	Appearance	Components	Action (h)[b]		
				Onset	Peak	Duration
Novolog® Mix 70/30	70% insulin aspart protamine suspension and 30% insulin aspart for injection	Turbid or cloudy suspension	Metal ion: zinc (19.6 μg/mL) Buffer: dibasic sodium phosphate (1.25 mg/mL) Preservatives: m-cresol (1.72 mg/mL), phenol (1.50 mg/mL) Tonicity agents: sodium chloride (0.58 mg/mL), mannitol (36.4 mg/mL) Modifying protein: protamine (0.33 mg/mL) pH: 7.2–7.4 Dosage: U100	<0.5[e]	1–4[e]	≤24[e]
Apidra®	Rapid-acting soluble insulin analog for injection	Aqueous, clear, and colorless solution	Metal ion: none Buffer: tromethamine (6 mg/mL) Preservative: m-cresol (3.15 mg/mL) Tonicity agent: sodium chloride (5 mg/mL) Stabilizing agent: polysorbate 20, (0.01 mg/mL in vials) pH: ~7.3 Dosage: U100	~0.3[c]	0.5–1.5[c]	~5.3[c]
Lantus®, Basaglar®	Long-acting soluble insulin analog for injection	Aqueous, clear, and colorless solution	Metal ion: zinc (30 μg/mL) Buffer: none Preservative: m-cresol (2.7 mg/mL) Tonicity agent: glycerin (20 mg 8%/mL) Modifying protein: none Stabilizing agent: polysorbate 20 (20 μg/mL – Vials only) pH: ~ 4 Dosage: U100		Constant release with no pronounced peak[c]	10.8 to >24.0[e]
Toujeo®	Long-acting soluble insulin analog for injection	Aqueous, clear, and colorless solution	Metal ion: zinc (90 μg/mL) Buffer: none Preservative: m-cresol (2.7 mg/mL) Tonicity agent: glycerin (20 mg 85%/mL) Modifying protein: none pH: ~4 Dosage: U300	0–6[e]	Steady state after 5 days[e]	24 at steady state[e]
Levemir®	Long-acting soluble insulin analog for injection	Aqueous, clear, and colorless solution	Metal ion: zinc (65.4 μg/mL) Buffer: dibasic sodium phosphate (0.89 mg/mL) Preservatives: m-cresol (2.06 mg/mL), phenol (1.8 mg/mL) Tonicity agents: sodium chloride (1.17 mg/mL) Modifying protein: none pH: 7.4 Dosage: U100		3–14[c]	5.7–23.2[c]

Table 18.3 ■ (continued)

Type[a]	Description	Appearance	Components	Action (h)[b]		
				Onset	Peak	Duration
Tresiba®	Long-acting soluble insulin analog for injection	Aqueous, clear, and colorless solution	Metal ion: zinc (32.7 μg/mL U100; 71.9 μg/mL U200) Buffer: none Preservatives: m-cresol (1.72 mg/mL), phenol (1.50 mg/mL) Tonicity agents: none Modifying protein: none pH: 7.6 Dosage: U100 and U200		9[c]	24 at steady state
Ryzodeg® 70/30	70% long-acting soluble insulin degludec and 30% rapid-acting insulin aspart for injection	Aqueous, clear, and colorless solution	Metal ion: zinc (27.4 μg/mL) Buffer: none Preservatives: m-cresol (1.72 mg/mL), phenol (1.50 mg/mL) Tonicity agents: glycerol (19 mg/mL), sodium chloride (0.58 mg/mL) Modifying protein: none pH: 7.4		2.3	24 after attaining steady state after 3–4 days)[d]

[a]US designation
[b]The time-action profiles of Lilly insulins are the average onset, peak action, and duration of action taken from a composite of studies. The onset, peak, and duration of insulin action depend on numerous factors, such as dose, injection site, presence of insulin antibodies, and physical activity. The action times listed represent the generally accepted values in the medical community
[c]DRUGDEX® System [Internet database]. Greenwood Village, Colo: Thomson Micromedex. Updated periodically
[d]Prescribing Information insert
[e]PDR® Electronic Library™ [Internet database]. Greenwood Village, Colo: Thomson Micromedex. Updated periodically

Table 18.3 ■ (continued)

mer interface. The Asn residue at position 3 of the B-chain plays no direct role in insulin self-association (Brange et al. 1990), but it is flanked by two amino acids involved in the assembly of the insulin hexamer. Despite the limited physicochemical information on insulin glulisine, studies conducted in persons with either type 1 (T1DM) or type 2 diabetes (T2DM) (Dreyer et al. 2005; Dailey et al. 2004) confirm that the analog displays similar pharmacological properties as insulin lispro. Interestingly, insulin glulisine is not formulated in the presence of zinc as are the other rapid-acting analogs. Instead, insulin glulisine is, in vials, formulated in the presence of a stabilizing agent (polysorbate 20) (Table 18.3). The surfactant in the vial formulation presumably minimizes aggregation. Apidra®, which is a non-hexameric formulation, demonstrates small but statistically significant faster onset and time to maximum insulin concentration (Heise et al. 2007; Arnolds et al. 2010) with small but statistically significant differences in PD properties from Novolog® (insulin aspart) and Humalog® (insulin lispro). The clinical significants of these differences have yet to be demonstrated clinically (Dreyer et al. 2005). Consequently, the hexameric breakdown of the two latter formulations must be rapid relative to the rate-limiting step, subcutaneous absorption (Fig. 18.5c) (Home 2012).

The aforementioned commercially available rapid-acting insulin analogs are approved for use in external infusion pumps. Buffer, and surfactant in the case of Apidra®, are included in these formulations to minimize the physical aggregation of insulin that can lead to clogging of the infusion sets. In early pump systems, gas-permeable infusion tubing was used with the external pumps. Consequently, a buffer was added to the formulation in order to minimize pH changes due to dissolved carbon dioxide. With continued improvements in external pumping systems, tubing composed of materials having greater resistance to carbon dioxide diffusion has been introduced and the potential for pH-induced precipitation of insulin is greatly reduced.

■ Ultra-Rapid Initiatives

Products with increasingly fast time action represent the most recent development in prandial insulins. These will likely have greatest impact in artificial pancreas systems that are under development. These systems are comprised of an external insulin pump controlled by an algorithm that uses data from a continuous glucose monitor to determine how much insulin to automatically administer for optimal blood glucose control. Reductions in the time to onset and the overall duration of an insulin product are likely to result in better glycemic control for these automated systems. The first product in the ultra-rapid space is a reformulation of insulin aspart marketed as Fiasp® (insulin aspart; CAS Number 116094-23-6). The formulation differs from NovoLog® primarily in the addition of nicotinamide and arginine. In a study with T1DM patients, onset of action across a range of doses was reduced relative to NovoLog® by 5–6 min with 95% confidence intervals of 0–10 min, while time to peak action was reduced by 10% (Heise et al. 2015). No change in duration of action was reported (Heise et al. 2017). Two other approaches are currently under active clinical development. One employs "biochaperones" to assist transport of insulin across the capillary membrane via a mechanism of action that is not fully-defined (Soula et al. 2014; Hardy et al. 2017), while the other takes advantage of excipients to increase vascular permeability and blood flow in the site of injection (Kazda et al. 2017; Kapitza et al. 2017). In the context of ultra-rapid insulin it is worth taking note of the fact that, while not compatible with artificial pancreas systems, an inhaled insulin, Afrezza® (human insulin; CAS Number 11061-68-0), achieves peak action faster than any currently marketed subcutaneously-injected insulin, with a mean of 0.9 ± 1.2 h and a duration of action of about 2.7 h.

■ Basal Insulin Suspension Preparations

The normal human pancreas secretes approximately 1 unit of insulin (0.035 mg) per hour to maintain basal glycemic control (Waldhäusl et al. 1979). Adequate basal insulin levels are a critical component of diabetes therapy because they regulate hepatic glucose output, which is essential for proper maintenance of glucose homeostasis during the diurnal cycling of the body. Consequently, basal insulin formulations must provide a very different PK profile than "mealtime" insulin formulations.

This detailed understanding of specific insulin requirements was unknown at the time the original NPH suspension product was introduced. This first commercially-available basal insulin preparation is known as Neutral Protamine Hagedorn (NPH) and is named after its inventor H. C. Hagedorn (1936). This preparation is a neutral microcrystalline suspension that is prepared by the cocrystallization of insulin with protamine. Originally produced using animal-derived insulins, the currently marked products are exclusively manufactured using human insulin. The cocrystallizing agent, protamine, consists of a closely related group of very basic peptides that are isolated from fish sperm. Protamine is heterogeneous in composition; however, four primary components have been identified and each show a high degree of sequence homology (Hoffmann et al. 1990). In general, protamine is ~30 amino acids in length and has an amino acid composition that is primarily composed of arginine, 65–70%. Using crystallization conditions later identified by Krayenbuhl and Rosenberg (1946), oblong tetragonal NPH insulin crystals with volumes between 1 and 20 μm^3 can be consistently prepared from protamine and insulin (Deckert 1980). These formulations, by design, have very minimal levels of soluble insulin in solution. The condition at which no measurable protamine or insulin exists in solution after crystallization is referred to as the isophane point of insulin. Crystal dissolution is presumed to be the rate-limiting step in the absorption of NPH insulin. Consequently, the time action of the formulation is prolonged by further delaying the dissociation of the hexamer into dimers and monomers (Fig. 18.6a).

NPH has an onset of action from 1 to 2 h, peak activity from 6 to 12 h, and duration of activity from 18 to 24 h (Table 18.2). As with other formulations, the variations in time action are due to factors such as dose, site of injection, temperature, and the patient's physical activity. In T2DM patients, NPH can be used as either once-daily or twice-daily therapy; however, in T1DM patients, NPH is predominately used as a twice-daily therapy.

NPH can be readily mixed with regular insulin either extemporaneously by the patient or as obtained from the manufacturer in a premixed formulation (Table 18.2). Premixed insulin, e.g., Humulin® 70/30 or Humulin® 50/50 (NPH/regular), has been shown to provide the patient with improved dose accuracy and consequently improved glycemic control (Bell et al. 1991). In these preparations, a portion of the soluble regular insulin will reversibly adsorb to the surface of the NPH crystals through an electrostatically mediated interaction under formulation conditions (Dodd et al. 1995); however, this adsorption is reversible under physiological conditions and consequently has no clinical significance (Galloway et al. 1982; Hamaguchi et al. 1990; Davis et al. 1991). Due, in part, to the reversibility of the adsorption process, NPH/regular mixtures are uniquely stable and have a 3-year shelf life.

The rapid-acting insulin analog, insulin lispro, can be extemporaneously mixed with NPH; however, such mixtures must be injected immediately after the two insulins are combined due to the potential for exchange between the soluble and suspension components upon long-term storage. Exchange refers to the release of human insulin from the NPH crystals into the solution phase and concomitant loss of the analog into the crystalline phase. The presence of human insulin in solution could diminish the rapid time-action effect of the rapid-acting analog. One way to overcome the problem of exchange is to prepare mixtures

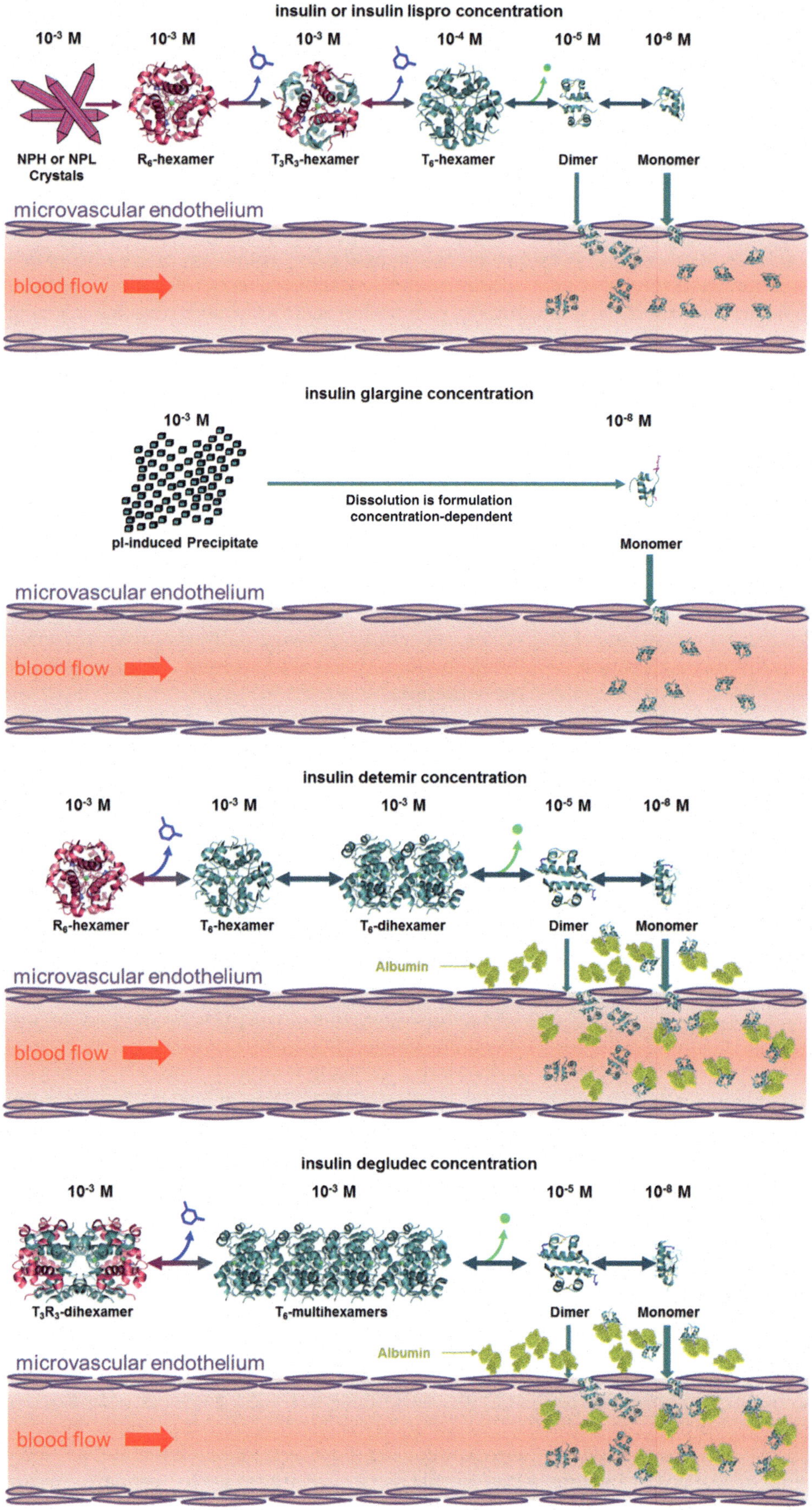

Figure. 18.6 ■ A schematic representation of basal insulin dissociation and absorption after subcutaneous administration; (**a**) NPH or NPL, (**b**) insulin glargine, (**c**) insulin detemir, and (**d**) insulin degludec (see Tables 18.1 and 18.3 for analogs descriptions)

containing the same insulin species in both the suspension and the solution phases, analogous to human insulin regular/NPH preparations. However, this approach requires an NPH-like preparation of the rapid-acting analog.

An NPH-like suspension of insulin lispro, referred to as neutral protamine lispro (NPL), and its physicochemical properties relative to human insulin NPH have been described (DeFelippis et al. 1998). In order to prepare the appropriate crystalline form of the analog, significant modifications to the NPH crystallization procedure are required. The differences between the crystallization conditions have been proposed to result from the reduced self-association properties of insulin lispro.

Pharmacological studies reported for NPL (DeFelippis et al. 1998; Janssen et al. 1997), indicate that the PK and PD properties of this analog suspension are analogous to human insulin NPH (Table 18.3). Clinical trials of insulin lispro protamine suspension alone in T2DM and in combination with insulin lispro in T1DM have been reported (Strojek et al. 2010; Fogelfeld et al. 2010; Chacra et al. 2010). In T2DM patients, the PK/PD profile of NPL can support a once-daily therapy regimen (Hompesch et al. 2009).

Homogeneous, biphasic, premixture preparations containing NPL and rapid-acting insulin lispro, Humalog® Mix 75/25 and Humalog® Mix 50/50, are marketed (Table 18.3). As with insulin lispro, premixed preparations containing insulin aspart combined with a protamine-containing microcrystalline suspension of insulin aspart (Balschmidt 1996) are commercially available (Novolog® 70/30). Clinical data on insulin lispro mixtures and those composed of insulin aspart have been reported in the literature (Weyer et al. 1997; Heise et al. 1998). The pharmacological properties of the rapid-acting analogs are preserved in these stable mixtures (Table 18.3).

Immunogenicity issues with protamine have been documented in a small percentage of diabetic patients (Kurtz et al. 1983; Nell and Thomas 1988). Individuals who show sensitivity to the protamine in NPH formulations (or premixed formulations of insulins lispro and aspart) are routinely switched to other long-acting insulin formulations (e.g., Lantus®, Toujeo®, Levemir®, Tresiba®, Basaglar®) to control their basal glucose levels.

Basal Insulin Solution Preparations

While the NPH and NPH-like analog preparations are still widely used in diabetes treatment regimens, research and development efforts continuing into present time remain focused on strategies to design improved basal insulin products. Advancements in basal insulin therapy have concentrated on developing solution formulations that exhibit flatter and peakless PK profiles and a longer duration of action. The result of this work has produced three commercially available basal insulin analog products that address hypoglycemia risk and decrease the number of injections needed on a daily basis to achieve glycemic control.

Lantus® (insulin glargine) and Levemir® (insulin detemir) were the first of these new basal insulin analog preparations to be approved for diabetes treatement (Table 18.1; Fig. 18.1). Lantus® derives its protracted time-action profile from the slow and relatively constant dissolution of solid particles that form as result of a pH shift of the acidic formulation to neutral pH in the subcutaneous tissue. This slow dissolution precedes the dissociation of insulin into absorbable units, and thus, the rate of absorption (units per hour) into the bloodstream is significantly decreased in comparison to that of prandial or bolus (mealtime) formulations. Levemir®, on the other hand, achieves its protracted effect by a combination of structural interactions and physiological binding events (Havelund et al. 2004).

The active ingredient in Lantus® and Basaglar® is the insulin analog, insulin glargine (Gly^{A21}, Arg^{B31}, Arg^{B32}-human insulin; CAS Number 160337-95-1), whose amino acid sequence modifications are highlighted in Table 18.1 and Fig. 18.1. This analog differs from human insulin in that the amino acid asparagine is replaced with glycine at position Asn^{A21} and two arginine residues have been added to the C-terminus of the B-chain. The additional arginine residues shift the isoelectric point from ~5.7 to ~6.9, thereby producing an insulin analog that is soluble at acidic pH values, but is less soluble at the neutral pH environment within subcutaneous tissue. As a result of this property, Lantus® is a solution formulation of insulin glargine prepared at pH 4.0. The introduction of glycine at position Asn^{A21} yields a protein with acceptable chemical stability since the asparagine side chain of human insulin is susceptible to acid-mediated degradation (deamidation and increased high-molecular weight proteins) and reduced potency. Thus, the changes to the molecular sequence of insulin have been made to improve chemical stability and to modulate absorption from the subcutaneous tissue, resulting in an analog that has approximately the same potency as human insulin. The Lantus® formulation is a clear solution that incorporates zinc and m-cresol (anti-microbial preservative). Consequently, Lantus® does not need to be resuspended prior to dosing like the protamine-containing insulin suspension products. Immediately following injection into the subcutaneous tissue, the insulin glargine precipitates due to the shift to neutral pH conditions. The slowly dissolving precipitate results in a relatively constant rate of absorption over

24 h with no pronounced peak (Fig. 18.6b; Table 18.3). This profile allows once-daily dosing and can satisfy basal insulin requirements of persons with diabetes. As with all insulin preparations, the time course of Lantus® may vary in different individuals or at different times in the same individual, and the rate of absorption is dependent on blood supply, temperature, and the patient's physical activity. Lantus® should not be diluted or mixed with any other solution or insulin, as will be discussed below.

A follow-on biologic version of Lantus® is approved for use in patients with type 1 or 2 diabetes, Basaglar® (Abasaglar® in Europe). This product has comparable physiochemical and pharmacological properties to the reference compound, Lantus®. For Basaglar®, comparability was demonstrated in clinical studies, where it exhibited similar pharmacodynamic and pharmacokinetic parameters to reference product in healthy volunteers, and provides effective glycemic control equivalent to that of reference Lantus® (Lamb and Syed 2018).

Insulin detemir (Lys^{B29}(*N*-tetradecanoyl)des(B30) human insulin; CAS Number 169148-63-4) is the active ingredient in Levemir® and the analog strategy employs acylation of insulin with a fatty acid moiety as a means to achieve a protracted pharmacological effect. As shown in Table 18.1 and Fig. 18.1, the B30 threonine residue of human insulin is eliminated in insulin detemir, and a 14-carbon, myristoyl fatty acid is covalently attached to the ε-amino group of Lys^{B29}. The analog forms a zinc hexamer at neutral pH in a preserved solution. Clinical studies have reported that insulin detemir displays lower PK and PD variability than NPH and/or insulin glargine (Hermansen et al. 2001; Vague et al. 2003; Heise et al. 2004; Porcellati et al. 2011). An approximate description of the PD profile of Levemir® is listed in Table 18.3. This analog appears to display a slower onset of action than NPH without a pronounced peak (Heinemann et al. 1999). Binding of the tetradecanoyl-acylated insulin to albumin was originally proposed as the underlying mechanism behind the observed prolonged effect for insulin detemir analog; however, investigations on insulin detemir have determined that the mechanism is more complex (Havelund et al. 2004). It has been proposed that subcutaneous absorption is initially delayed as a result of hexamer stability and dihexamerization (Fig. 18.6c). Such interactions between hexamers are likely a consequence of the symmetrical arrangement of fatty acid moieties around the outside of the hexamers as shown by X-ray crystallographic studies (Whittingham et al. 2004). These associated forms further bind to albumin within the injection site depot, and further prolongation may result due to this binding.

Although Lantus® and Levemir® have improved basal insulin therapy, these insulin formulations may not achieve full 24 h coverage in all patients. Moreover, the desire to eliminate or minimize nocturnal hypoglycemia has driven the exploration of improved basal insulin therapies. Two commercial products have emerged from research efforts in this area. Tresiba® builds upon the the design strategy of Levemir® by incorporating an acylated insulin analog as its active ingredient. The second product, Toujeo®, represents a departure from a molecular engineering approach and utilizes changes in precipitation behavior at higher formulation concentrations of insulin glargine.

The active ingredient in Tresiba® is insulin degludec (LysB29(Nε-hexadecandioyl-γ-Glu) des(B30) human insulin; CAS Number 844439-96-9). As shown in Table 18.1, it differs from human insulin in that the amino acid threonine in position B30 has been omitted and the ε-amino group of Lys^{B29} is covalently modified with a γ-L-glutamic acid linker containing a bound C16 fatty acid with a terminal carboxylic acid. Tresiba® is a clear, colorless solution that contains either insulin degludec 100 units/mL (U100) or 200 units/mL (U200). In the presence of the phenolic preservatives and zinc, insulin degludec forms a soluble and stable dihexamer described as a closed configuration that results from an interaction between one of the fatty diacid side chains of one hexamer and the zinc atom of the adjacent hexamer. After injection, as the bound preservative molecules diffuse away, the dihexamers adopt an open configuration and interact with each other to form multihexamer units facilitated by the interaction of fatty diacid chains and zinc atoms between adjacent hexamers (Fig. 18.6d). Subsequent diffusion of zinc from each end of the chain results in terminal hexamers breaking apart into dimers, which then dissociate into monomers. This process enables gradual release of monomers that are absorbed into the systemic circulation. The complex self-association and dissociation characteristics result in insulin degludec exhibiting the longest duration of action at the injection depot compared to all other basal insulins (Jonassen et al. 2012; Steensgaard et al. 2013).

Tresiba® U100 and U200 have shown to be bioequivalent and exhibit a mean half-life of 25 h and at least a 42-h duration of action at steady state using once-daily administration. Tresiba® achieves steady state in 3–5 days with serum insulin concentration increasing slowly until a very flat profile is achieved. This results in a reduced risk of nocturnal hypoglycaemia versus Lantus® for both T1DM patients (Birkeland et al. 2011). Because of its slow accumulation, long duration of action and flat, and predictable PD profile, Tresiba® can be dosed any time of the day versus Lantus® which has to be dosed at the same time everyday (Heise and Mathieu 2017).

Toujeo® is a higher concentration preparation of insulin glargine formulated at 300 U/mL and is thus, three times more concentrated than the 100 U/mL Lantus® product. The amino acid composition of the active ingredient, insulin glargine, is the same in Toujeo® and Lantus® and maintains the same physical and chemical properties. However, the higher concentration allows a dose to be administered in a third of the injection volume of Lantus®. It is believed that this lower volume produces a subcutaneous precipitate with reduced surface area, resulting in more prolonged and constant release of insulin into the bloodstream (Fig. 18.6b) (Ritzel et al. 2015). PK and PD studies have shown that Toujeo® exhibits a flatter profile and more prolonged glucose-lowering activity over ≥24 h compared to Lantus®. Toujeo® achived steady state in 3–4 days and exhibits a half-life of 19 h versus Lantus®, which achieves steady state in 2–4 days with a half-life of 12 h. In addition, lower within day and day-to-day glycemic variability is also observed at clinically relevant basal insulin doses. It is important to note that Lantus® U100 and Toujeo® U300 are *not bioequivalent*, since the time actions are different and 12% more U300 is needed for a similar glycemic effect (Ritzel et al. 2015). This effect possibly results from increased enzymatic inactivation of the drug by tissue peptidases in the subcutaneous tissue due to longer residence time of Toujeo®. Toujeo® offers comparable glycemic control to Lantus® in both T1DM and T2DM but the main clinically relevant benefit of Toujeo® is that it provides lower nocturnal hypoglycemia risk (Lau et al. 2017).

Basal Insulin Preparations Co-formulated with Rapid-Acting Insulin Analog or GLP-1R Agonists

Following the successful commercialization of Tresiba® and Lantus®, premixture preparations incorporating their respective basal insulin analog active ingredients with either a rapid-acting insulin analog or a human incretin analog of glucagon-like peptide-1 (GLP-1) were introduced. A stable premixture of insulin degludec and insulin aspart is marketed as Ryzodeg® 70/30. The rationale for combining a basal insulin with a rapid-acting insulin in a single product is similar to the biphasic solution/suspension products discussed earlier. However, Ryzodeg® is a stable solution composed of 70% insulin degludec and 30% insulin aspart. (Havelund et al. 2015). Clinical studies have shown that Ryzodeg® 70/30 can be effectively used in patients with T1DM in combination with Novolog® (Hirsch et al. 2017) and patients with T2DM (Park et al. 2017). However it should be noted that the Ryzodeg® label states that the administration of insulin formulation should be subcutaneously once or twice daily with any main meal(s); thus, requiring administration of a rapid- or short-acting insulin at other meals, if needed.

Two basal insulin analog/GLP-1 incretin premixture preparations are commercially available for use in patients with T2DM, Xultophy® and Soliqua®. Both the basal insulin analog and incretin components lower blood glucose, but do so in different ways. GLP-1 facilitates a glucose-dependent increase in insulin secretion by β-cells and decreased glucagon secretion by α-cells with a lower risk of hypoglycemia. Additionally, GLP-1 can reduce body weight, but may not cause sufficient insulin secretion to achieve desired glycemic control. Basal insulin therapy increases circulating insulin in a non-glucose-dependent manner, improves β-cell function, and plays a role in regulation and production of glucose, but may cause weight gain and carries the risk of hypoglycemia. Therefore, a combination of the two therapies compliments their respective therapeutic benefits while compensating for undesired effects (Gough et al. 2016; Rodbard et al. (2016).

A premixture preparation of 100 units/mL insulin degludec and 3.6 mg/mL of the GLP-1 analog liraglutide is marketed as Xultophy®. This product is supplied as a prefilled, single-patient multi-use disposable pen. The formulation contains 19.7 mg/mL glycerol, 5.70 mg/mL phenol and 55 μg/mL zinc, and has a pH of approximately 8.15. The product is considered an alternative to basal–bolus therapy in the treatment of Type 2 Diabetes (Hughes 2016; Rodbard et al. 2016).

The other commercial premixture preparation marketed is Soliqua® 100/33, which combines insulin glargine with the GLP-1 analog lixisenatide for the treatment of patients with T2DM (Goldman and Trujillo 2017). This product is supplied as a prefilled, single-patient multi-use disposable pen. The solution formulation contains 100 units insulin glargine, 33 μg/mL lixisenatide, 3 mg/mL methionine, 2.7 mg/mL metacresol, 20 mg/mL glycerol and 30 μg/mL of zinc. The pH of the formulation is not clearly stated in the prescribing information.

Concentrated Human Insulin Formulations

Most insulin and insulin analog formulations are manufactured at a concentration of 100 insulin units/mL, referred to as U100; however, with the advent of delivery device systems, manufacturers have steadily introduced more concentrated insulin formulations (U200, U300, and U500). These more concentrated formulations enable clinicians to tailor insulin therapy for the needs of their patients; particularly those with obesity and/or severely insulin resistant patients. However with some knowledge of the PK/PD profiles, the usage of concentrated formulations can benefit a wide range of patients allowing for reduced injection volume or for modifying the time action profile; consequently some educational information is required for both the clinician and the patient. As discussed above, many human insulin and insulin analog preparations are now marketed in dedicated devices at concentrations >U100 (Johnson et al. 2017; Reid et al. 2017; Ovalle et al. 2018); however, it cannot be assumed that all concentrated insulins have PK and PD properties equivalent to their U100 counterparts. Humalog® U200 and Tresiba® U200 have been shown to be bioequivalent to their U100 counterparts (Korsatko et al. 2013; de la Pena et al. 2016). Conversely, Humulin® R U500 and Toujeo® (U300) are not bioequivalent (de la Pena et al. 2011; Becker et al. 2015). Thus, safety concerns can be addressed with patient education and the use of precise and accurate, dedicated insulin delivery devices. However, Humulin® R U500 human insulin formulations warrant separate discussion, as it is used in patients that exhibit insulin resistance and possess a different time action profile. This higher concentration insulin provides a preferential treatment option for those needing higher doses.

Early pharmacological studies demonstrated reduced absorption associated with increasing concentrations of insulin (Binder 1969; Binder et al. 1984). Galloway et al. (1981) showed no statistically significant differences in PK serum insulin levels with increasing concentrations of pork regular insulin (at 0.25 U/kg) from U40 to U500; however, time to peak glucose responses were mildly delayed, and peak effect was variably reduced as concentration increased. The first PK/PD study of human U500 vs. U100 regular insulin in healthy obese subjects was recently published (de la Peña et al. 2011). Overall insulin exposure and overall effect were similar at both 50 U and 100 U doses (0.5 and 1.0 U/kg) with both formulations. However, the two formulations were not bioequivalent: peak insulin concentration (C_{max}) and effect (R_{max}) were significantly reduced for U500 vs. U100 for both doses. Time to peak concentration (t_{max}) and time to maximal effect (tR_{max}) were significantly longer for U500 vs. U100 only at the U100 dose. Duration of action (tR_{last}) was prolonged for U500 at both doses vs. U100 (50 U: 19.7 vs. 18.3 h; U100: 21.5 vs. 18.3 h; $p < 0.05$ for both). The onset of action (t_{onset}) was within 20 min for both formulations and supports the clinical use of human U500 regular 30 min before meals to leverage the prandial effect. Basal insulin between-meal requirements are expected to be covered by the long "tail" of action of the U500 formulation (de la Peña et al. 2011); futher work is needed to assess if overnight coverage in T2D patients is possible.

A randomized controlled trial comparing twice-daily and thrice-daily U500 in insulin-resistant T2DM demonstrated that both dosing regimes were efficacious and safe, although higher hypoglycemia rates were observed in higher-dose groups (Wysham et al. 2016). Moreoover a series of other studies have demonstrated reductions in HbA1c (glycated hemoglobin) of 1.0–1.7% over 3–98 months of use (Lane et al. 2009; Ziesmer et al. 2012; Boldo and Comi 2012). Paradoxically, insulin dose generally did not statistically increase after conversion to human U500 regular insulin, although one large case series did report an increase in total daily dose by 0.44 U/kg (Boldo and Comi 2012). Weight gain with treatment was variable, up to 4.2–6.8 kg (Lane et al. 2009; Boldo and Comi 2012). Reports of severe hypoglycemia have been infrequent, although an increase in non-severe hypoglycemia was reported in one large study (Boldo and Comi 2012). Most studies have used twice-daily or thrice-daily regimens (Lane et al. 2009; Ziesmer et al. 2012; Boldo and Comi 2012). A simplified dosing algorithm was published by Segal et al. (2010).

In the past, safety concerns with concentrated insulin therapy in diabetes patients, besides hypoglycemia and weight gain, mainly relate to the risk of dose confusion due to lack of a dedicated injection device for U500 insulin. In November of 2016, Becton, Dickinson and Company in collaboration with Eli Lilly and Company launched the first insulin syringe specifically developed for patients prescribed Humulin® R U500, thus eliminating complex dosing conversion tables and formulas required when having to use the standard U100 insulin syringes. Also early in 2016 Eli Lilly and Company launched a Humulin® R U500 single-patient multiple-use disposable pen. For product differentiation the Humulin® R U500 single-patient multiple-use disposable pen has a distinctive aqua color. The U500 insulin vial and labeling of vial and box are distinctive from U100 insulins, with black and white-colored and green-colored lettering, aqua-colored labeling and a larger box size (20 mL containing 10,000 U) with the green coloring matching the secondary packaging and needle shield color for the U500 syringe. The aqua-color labeling was selected to align with the distinctive aqua-colored use for the Humulin® R U500 single-patient multiple-use disposable pen.

PHARMACEUTICAL CONCERNS

Chemical Stability of Insulin Formulations

The purity of insulin formulations is typically assessed by high-performance liquid chromatography using reversed-phase and size exclusion separation modes (USP Monographs: Insulin 2013). Insulin has two primary routes of chemical degradation upon storage and use: hydrolytic transformation of amide to acid groups and formation of covalent dimers and higher-order polymers. Primarily the pH, the storage temperature, and the components of the specific formulation influence the rate of formation of these degradation products. In acidic solution, the main degradation reaction is the transformation of asparagine (Asn) at the terminal 21 position of the A-chain to aspartic acid. This reaction is relatively facile at low pH, but is extremely slow at neutral pH (Brange et al. 1992b). This was the primary degradation route in early soluble (acidic) insulin formulations. However, the development of neutral solutions and suspensions has diminished the importance of this degradation route. Stability studies of neutral solutions indicate that the amount of A21 desamido insulin does not change upon storage. Thus, the relatively small amounts of this bioactive material present in the formulation arise either from the source of insulin or from pharmaceutical process operations.

The deamidation of the AsnB3 of the B-chain is the primary degradation mechanism at neutral pH. The reaction proceeds through the formation of a cyclic imide that results in two products, aspartic acid (Asp) and iso-aspartic acid (iso-Asp) (Brennan and Clarke 1994). This reaction occurs relatively slowly in neutral solution (approximately 1/12 the rate of A21 desamido formation in acid solution) (Brange et al. 1992b). The relative amounts of these products are influenced by the flexibility of the B-chain, with approximate ratios of Asp:iso-Asp of 1:2 and 2:1 for solution and crystalline formulations, respectively. As noted earlier, the use of phenolic preservatives provides a stabilizing effect on the insulin hexamer that reduces the formation of the cyclic imide, as evidenced by reduced deamidation. The rate of formation also depends on temperature; typical rates of formation are approximately 2% per year at 5 °C. Studies have shown B3 deamidated insulin to be essentially fully potent (R.E. Chance, personal communication).

High molecular weight protein (HMWP) products form at both refrigerated and room temperature storage conditions. Accelerated conditions (37 °C for 1 year) were used to enrich and then characterize the HMWP species from a neutral pH insulin formulations (Hjorth et al. 2015). The primary species identified were covalent dimers of insulin linked at the A21Asn and B29Lys positions originating from the attack of the B29Lys on the anhydride intermediate of A21Asn. These purified covalent dimers were then further characterized for biological activity, conformational structure including self-association and fibrillation properties (Hjorth et al. 2016). The covalent dimer showed little to no biological activity and the covalent dimer tertiary structure was identical to the non-covalent dimer such that in the presence of Zn it participated in hexamer assembly. In studies aimed at evaluating physical attributes like self-association and fibrillation, the non-covalent dimer reduced the propensity for self-association and delayed onset of fibril formation. There is evidence that insulin-protamine heterodimers also form in NPH suspensions (Brange et al. 1992a). At higher temperatures, the probability of forming higher-order insulin oligomers increases. The rate of formation of HMWP is less than that of hydrolytic reactions; typical rates are less than 0.5% per year for soluble neutral regular insulin formulations at 5 °C. The rate of formation can be affected by the strength of the insulin formulation or by the addition of glycerol as a tonicity agent. The latter increases the rate of HMWP formation presumably by introducing impurities such as glyceraldehyde. HMWP formation is believed to also occur as a result of a reaction between the N-terminal B1 phenylalanine amino group and the C-terminal A21 asparagine of a second insulin molecule via a cyclic anhydride (or succinimide, based on unpublished results of the authors) intermediate (Darrington and Anderson 1995). Reaction with the intermediate may also occur via the N-terminus of the A-chain. Disulfide exchange leading to polymer formation is also possible at basic pH; however, the rate for these reactions is very slow under neutral pH formulation conditions. The quality of excipients such as glycerol is also critical because small amounts of aldehyde and other glycerol-related chemical impurities can accelerate the formation of HMWP. The biopotency of HMWP is significantly less (1/12–1/5 of insulin) than monomeric species (Brange 1987c).

Only limited chemical stability data has been published in the scientific literature for the insulin analog formulations containing insulin lispro, insulin aspart, insulin glulisine, insulin glargine, insulin detemir, or insulin degludec; however, it is reasonable to presume that similar chemical degradation pathways are present to varying extents in these compounds. Nevertheless, since some analogs are formulated under acidic conditions, e.g., Lantus®, Basaglar®, and Toujeo®, or have been modified with hydrophobic moieties, e.g., Levemir® or Tresiba®, it is reasonable to presume that alternate chemical degradation pathways may be possible. It should be noted that the amino acid substitution of glycine for asparagine at position 21 of the insulin glargine A-chain effectively eliminates the potential for deamidation that would occur under the acidic pH conditions used in the Lantus®, Basaglar®, and Toujeo® formulations. This glycine substitution may also result in lower covalent dimer formation.

Physical Stability of Insulin Formulations

The physical stability of insulin formulations is mediated by noncovalent aggregation of insulin. Hydrophobic forces typically drive the aggregation, although electrostatics plays a subtle but important role. Aggregation typically leads to a loss in potency of the formulation, and therefore conditions promoting this type of physical degradation (i.e., extreme mechanical agitation or exposure to air-liquid interfaces often in combination with elevated temperatures) should be avoided for all insulin products. A particularly severe type of nonreversible aggregation results in the formation of insulin fibrils. The mechanism of insulin fibrillation is widely believed to result from destabilization of hexamers (i.e., the predominant self-associated form of most insulin solution preparations) causing an increase in the population of monomers that can partially unfold and initiate the aggregation process (Jansen et al. 2005). Physical attributes of insulin formulations are readily assessed by visual observation for macroscopic characteristics as well as by instrumental methods such as light and differential phase contrast microscopy. Insulin fibrillation can be confirmed using atomic force microscopy (Jansen et al. 2005). Various particle-sizing techniques also may be used to characterize physical degradation phenomena. Fluorescence spectroscopy using specific dyes has proven useful in monitoring the time course of insulin fibrillation process (Nielsen et al. 2001).

In general, insulin solutions have good physical stability. Physical changes in soluble formulations may be manifested as color or clarity change or, in extreme situations, increases in solution viscosity, a phenomenon referred to as gelation, or the formation of a precipitate that could be an indication of fibrillation. Insulin suspensions, such as NPH, are the most susceptible to changes in physical stability. Such physical instability typically occurs as a result of both elevated temperature and mechanical stress to the insulin preparation. The increase in temperature favors hydrophobic interactions, while mechanical agitation serves to provide mixing and stress across interfacial boundaries. Nucleation and higher-order forms of aggregation in suspensions can lead to conditions described as visible clumping of the insulin microcrystalline particles or adherence of the aggregates to the inner wall of the glass storage container. The latter phenomenon is referred to as frosting. In severe cases, resuspension may be nearly impossible because of caking of the suspension in the vial. Temperatures above ambient (>25 °C) can accelerate the aggregation process, especially those at or above body temperature (37 °C). Normal mechanical mixing of suspensions to achieve dispersion of the microcrystalline insulin particles prior to administration is not deleterious to physical stability. However, vigorous shaking or mixing should be avoided. Consequently, this latter constraint has, in part, led to the observation that patients do not place enough effort into resuspension. Thus, proper emphasis must be placed on training the patient in resuspension of crystalline, amorphous, and premixed suspension formulations of insulin and insulin analogs. The necessity of rigorous resuspension may be the first sign of aggregation and should prompt a careful examination of the formulation to verify its suitability for use.

As with the chemical stability data, published information regarding the physical stability of the newer insulin analog formulations containing insulin lispro, insulin aspart, insulin glulisine, insulin glargine, or insulin detemir is limited. However, it is reasonable to assume that similar controls are practiced for preventing exposures to extreme agitation and thermal excursions to minimize undesirable physical transformations such as precipitation, aggregation, gelation, or fibrillation.

CLINICAL AND PRACTICE ASPECTS

Vial Presentations

Insulin is available in 10-mL vials. In the United States, a strength of U100 (100 U/mL) is the standard, whereas outside the USA both U100 and U40 (40 U/mL) are commonly used. Recent introduction of U100 insulins (Humalog®, Humulin® N, R, and 70/30) in 5-mL vials (filled to 3 mL: 300 U) has met a need for smaller volumes and less waste in hospital usage. The result is a combined economic impact of reduced acquisition cost and purchased volume (Edmondson et al. 2014, Eby et al. 2014).

It is essential to obtain the proper strength and formulation of insulin in order to maintain glycemic control. In addition, brand/method of manufacture is important. Any change in insulin should be made cautiously and only under medical supervision (Galloway 1988; Brackenridge 1994). Common formulations, such as regular and NPH, are listed in Table 18.2, and the newer insulin analog formulations are listed in Table 18.3. Mixtures of rapid- or fast-acting with intermediate-acting insulin formulations are popular choices for glycemic control. The ratio is defined as ratio of protamine-containing fraction/rapid- or fast-acting fraction, e.g., Humalog® Mix 75/25 where 75% of a dose is available as insulin lispro protamine suspension and 25% as insulin lispro for injection. With regard to NPH regular mixtures, caution must be used in the nomenclature because it may vary depending on the country of sale and the governing regulatory body. In the USA, for example, the predominant species is listed first as in N/R 70/30, but in Europe the same formulation is described as R/N 30/70 (Soluble/Isophane) where the base ("normal") ingredient is listed first. Currently, an effort is being made to standardize worldwide to the European nomenclature. The predominant human insulin mixture formulations sold globally are N/R 70/30; however, the number of suppliers may vary from country to country.

■ Injection Devices

Insulin syringes should be purchased to match the strength of the insulin that is to be administered (e.g., for U100 strength use 30-, 50-, or 100-unit syringes designated for U100 and for U500 strength use the syringe designated for U500). The gauge of needles available for insulin administration has been reduced to very fine gauges (30–32 G) in order to minimize pain during injection. In addition to finer gauge needles, the length of needles has shortened to a minimum of 5 mm, in part, to prevent unintended IM injection. Recently, studies have shown that skin thickness is rarely >3 mm and that needles of 4–5 mm consistently deliver insulin into the subcutaneous adipose tissue (Gibney et al. 2010). The use of a new needle for each dose maintains the sharp point of the needle and ensures a sterile needle for the injection.

The availability of insulin pen devices has made dosing and compliance easier for the patient with diabetes as well as allowing manufacturers to introduce higher concentration formulations in dedicated, disposable pens. Moreover advances in engineering are enabling pen devices with ½ unit dosing as well as increasing capacity for maximum single injection dose of 80 units/injection from a U100 formulation, 160 units/injection for U200 formulation, and 300 units/injection for U500 formulations.

The first pen injector used a 1.5-mL cartridge of U100 insulin (NovoPen® by Novo Nordisk in 1985). A needle was attached to the end of the pen, and the proper dose was selected and then injected by the patient. The cartridge was replaced when the content was exhausted, typically 3–7 days. Currently, 3.0-mL cartridges in U100 strength for regular, NPH, and the range of R/N mixtures, as well as the various rapid- and long-acting insulin analogs, have become the market standard, particularly in disposable pen devices with prefilled insulin reservoirs, that vary with regard to size and strength. The advantages of the pen devices are primarily better compliance for the patient through a variety of factors including more accurate and reproducible dose control, easier transport of the drug, more discrete dose administration, timelier dose administration, and greater convenience.

■ Continuous Subcutaneous Insulin Infusion: External Pumps

As previously mentioned, solution formulations of human insulin specifically designed for continuous subcutaneous insulin infusion (CSII) are commercially available. CSII systems were traditionally used by a small population of patients with diabetes but have become more popular with the recent introduction of rapid-acting insulin analogs. Currently, all three rapid-acting insulin analog formulations have received regulatory approval for this mode of delivery. Specific in vitro data demonstrating physicochemical stability for CSII has been reported for Humalog® (DeFelippis et al. 2006; Sharrow et al. 2012), Novolog®, and Apidra® (Senstius et al. 2007a, b). Early pump devices contained glass or plastic reservoirs that must be hand filled from vial presentations by the patient. Some newer pumps have been specifically designed to accept the same glass 3-mL cartridges used in pen injector systems. Due to concerns over the impact of elevated temperature exposure and mechanical stress on the integrity of the insulin molecule along with the potential increased risk of microbial contamination, the patient information leaflets for the rapid-acting insulin analog products specify time intervals for changing the CSII infusion set as well as the infusion site. The package information leaflets should be consulted for the maximum duration each product may remain in the CSII reservoir. This time period of use varies with 7, 6, or 2 days listed for Humalog®, Novolog®, and Apidra®, respectively, due to formulation stability. As always, the patient information leaflets supplied with these products should be consulted for the most current information related to in-use periods.

A number of systems have been developed or are under development to automatically dose insulin in response to continuous glucose monitoring data. The first step in this direction is a relatively simple system to turn off basal insulin delivery when glucose drops below a predetermined threshold (low glucose suspend), as is implemented in the Medtronic 530G pump. The Medtronic 640G and t:slim X2 pumps incorporate an algorithm to predict future glucose levels and prospectively reduce or stop insulin delivery (predictive low glucose suspend). Numerous systems are under development to more completely automate insulin delivery decisions. Some of these include delivery of both insulin at high glucose and glucagon at low glucose, while others depend only on modulation of insulin dosing; however, the bihomonal system requires a stable formulation of glucagon, which is not yet commercially available. The latter, which are broadly described as "closed-loop insulin pumps," are being advanced by several companies, including Medtronic, which has launched the first pump widely recognized as closed-loop in the 670G. Clinical studies are currently underway to better understand the extent to which systems employing both glucagon and insulin may or may not deliver better outcomes than those that deliver only insulin. Patients impatient with the pace of commercial development and regulatory approval have also developed open-source closed-loop insulin delivery systems based on commodity electronics and medical devices. The best known of these is the Open Artificial Pancreas System (https://openaps.org/). While assembling the OpenAPS system requires a high degree of technical sophistication, users report a lower daily burden in managing their diabetes and their experience is potentially valuable in speeding the development of commercial systems.

Noninvasive Delivery

Since the discovery of insulin, there has been a strong desire to overcome the need for injection-based therapy (cf. Chap. 5). Progress has been made in the form of needle-free injector systems (Robertson et al. 2000), but these devices have not gained widespread acceptance presumably because administration is not entirely pain-free, device costs are high, and other factors make it less desirable than traditional injection. Extensive research efforts have also focused on noninvasive routes of administration with attempts made to demonstrate the feasibility of transdermal, nasal, buccal, ocular, pulmonary, oral, and even rectal delivery of insulin (Heinemann et al. 2001). Unfortunately, most attempts failed to progress beyond the proof of concept stage because low bioavailability, dose–response variability, and other adverse factors seriously called into question commercial viability. This situation has changed to some extent for pulmonary and buccal delivery of insulin.

As noted above, Afrezza® is an approved pulmonary insulin product for the treatment of post-prandial hyperglycemia. The formulation uses the dry powder Technosphere® technology wherein, particles composed of fumaryl diketopiperazine and polysorbate 80 are coated with human insulin. The delivery system utilizes single-use plastic cartridges containing 4 U, 8 U, or 12 U of the formulated insulin powder. The powder is aerosolized and delivered to the lung via oral inhalation using an inhaler.

Oralin®, a buccal product, consists of a solution formulation of insulin containing various absorption enhancers needed to achieve mucosal absorption (Modi et al. 2002), and a metered-dose inhaler is used to administer a fine mist into the oral cavity. Clinical studies evaluating this buccal delivery system in healthy subjects as well as patients with T1DM and T2DM have been reported (Modi et al. 2002; Cernea et al. 2004). The availability of Oralin® is limited to only a few countries.

Storage

Insulin solution formulations should be stored in a cool place that avoids sunlight. Vials or cartridges that are not in active use should be stored under refrigerated (2–8 °C) conditions. Vials or cartridges in active use may be stored at ambient temperature. The in-use period for insulin formulations ranges from 28 to 56 days depending upon the product and its chemical, physical, and microbiological stability during use. High temperatures, such as those found in non-air-conditioned vehicles in the summer or other non-climate-controlled conditions, should be avoided due to the potential for chemical and/or physical changes to the formulation properties. Insulin formulations should not be frozen; if this occurs, the product should be disposed of immediately, since either the formulation or the container-closure integrity may be compromised. Insulin formulations should never be purchased or used past the expiration date on the package. Further information on storage and use of specific insulin products are contained in their respective patient information leaflets.

USAGE

Resuspension

Insulin suspensions (e.g., NPH, NPL, premixtures) should be resuspended by gentle back-and-forth mixing and rolling of the vial between the palms to obtain a uniform, milky suspension. The patient should be advised of the resuspension technique for specific insoluble insulin and insulin analog formulations, which is detailed in the package insert. The homogeneity of suspensions is critical to obtaining an accurate dose. Any suspension that fails to provide a homogeneous dispersion of particles should not be used. Insulin formulations contained in cartridges in pen injectors may be suspended in a similar manner; however, the smaller size of the container and shape of the pen injector may require slight modification of the resuspension method to ensure complete resuspension. A bead (glass or metal) is typically added to cartridges to aid in the resuspension of suspension formulations.

Dosing

Dose withdrawal should immediately follow the resuspension of any insulin suspension. The patient should be instructed by their doctor, pharmacist, or nurse educator in proper procedures for dose administration. Of particular importance are procedures for disinfecting the container top and injection site. The patient is also advised to use a new needle and syringe for each injection. Reuse of these components, even after cleaning, may lead to contamination of the insulin formulation by microorganisms or by other materials, such as cleaning agents.

Extemporaneous Mixing

As discussed above in the section on "Basal Insulin Suspension Preparations," regular insulin can be mixed in the syringe with NPH and is stable enough to be stored for extended periods of time.

With regard to extemporaneous mixing of the newer insulin analogs, caution must be used. Lantus®, due to its acidic pH, should not be mixed with other fast- or rapid-acting insulin formulations which are formulated at neutral pH. If Lantus® is mixed with other insulin formulations, the solution may become cloudy due to isoelectric point (pI) precipitation of both the insulin glargine and the fast- or rapid-acting insulin resulting from pH changes. Consequently, the PK/PD profile, e.g., onset of action and time to peak effect, of insulin glargine and/or the mixed insulin may be altered in an unpredictable manner. With regard to rapid-acting insulin analogs, extemporaneous mixing with human insulin NPH formulations is acceptable if used immediately. Under no circumstances should these formulations be stored as mixtures, as human insulin and insulin analog exchange can occur between solution and the crystalline matter, thereby potentially altering time-action profiles of the solution insulin analog. With regard to Levemir®, the human prescription drug label states that the product should not be diluted or mixed with any other insulin or solution to avoid altered and unpredictable changes in PK or PD profile (e.g., onset of action, time to peak effect).

SELF-ASSESSMENT QUESTIONS

Questions

1. Which insulin analog formulations cannot be mixed and stored? Why?
2. What are the primary chemical and physical stability issues with human insulin formulations?
3. What are some benefits and concerns around higher concentration insulin formulations?

Answers

1. Lantus® and Basaglar® are long-acting insulin formulations which are formulated at pH 4.0, which should not be mixed with rapid- or fast-acting insulin formulated under neutral pH. If Lantus® or Basaglar® is mixed with other insulin formulations, the solution may become cloudy due to pI precipitation of both the insulin glargine and the fast- or rapid-acting insulin resulting from pH changes. Consequently, the PK/PD profile, e.g., onset of action and time to peak effect, of insulin glargine and/or the mixed insulin may be altered in an unpredictable manner.
2. The two primary modes of chemical degradation are deamidation and HMWP formation. These routes of chemical degradation occur in all formulations. However, they are generally slower in suspension formulations. Physical instability is most often observed in insulin suspension formulations and pump formulations. In suspension formulations, particle agglomeration can occur resulting in the visible clumping of the crystalline and/or amorphous insulin. The soluble insulin in pump formulations can also precipitate or aggregate.
3. The main benefit of higher insulin concentration is the ability for insulin resistant patients to deliver larger doses of insulin with lower injection volumes, potentially reducing patient discomfort and number of injections, thus enhancing patient compliance. Major concerns with higher concentration insulin formulations relate to the potential for dose confusion that could lead to hypoglycemic events. The coordination of insulin packaging with specialized syringes is an attempt to reduce this risk.

REFERENCES

Anderson JH Jr, Brunelle RL, Keohane P, Koivisto VA, Trautmann ME, Vignati L, DiMarchi R (1997) Mealtime treatment with insulin analog improves postprandial hyperglycemia and hypoglycemia in patients with non-insulin-dependent diabetes mellitus. Multicenter Insulin Lispro Study Group. Arch Intern Med 157:1249–1255

Arnolds S, Rave K, Hövelmann U, Fischer A, Sert-Langeron C, Heise T (2010) Insulin glulisine has a faster onset of action compared with insulin aspart in healthy volunteers. Exp Clin Endocrinol Diabetes 118(9):662–664

Bakaysa DL, Radziuk J, Havel HA, Brader ML, Li S, Dodd SW, Beals JM, Pekar AH, Brems DN (1996) Physicochemical basis for the rapid time-action of $Lys^{B28}Pro^{B29}$-insulin: dissociation of a protein-ligand complex. Protein Sci 5(12):2521–2531

Baker EN, Blundell TL, Cutfield JF, Cutfield SM, Dodson EJ, Dodson GG, Hodgkin DM, Hubbard RE, Isaacs NW, Reynolds CD, Sakabe K, Sakabe N, Vijayan NM (1988) The structure of 2Zn pig insulin crystals at 1.5 Å resolution. Philos Trans R Soc Lond Ser B Biol Sci 319:369–456

Balschmidt P (1996) AspB28 insulin crystals. US Patent 5,547,930

Becker RH, Dahmen R, Bergmann K, Lehmann A, Jax T, Heise T (2015) New insulin glargine 300 units mL^{-1} provides a more even activity profile and prolonged glycemic control at steady state compared with insulin glargine 100 units mL^{-1}. Diabetes Care 38:637–643

Bell DS, Clements RS Jr, Perentesis G, Roddam R, Wagenknecht L (1991) Dosage accuracy of self-mixed vs premixed insulin. Arch Intern Med 151:2265–2269

Binder C (1969) Absorption of injected insulin. a clinical-pharmacologic study. Acta Pharmacol Toxicol (Copenh) 27(Suppl 2):1–84

Binder C, Lauritzen T, Faber O, Pramming S (1984) Insulin pharmacokinetics. Diabetes Care 7:188–199

Birkeland KI, Home PD, Wendisch U, Ratner RE, Johansen T, Endahl LA, Lyby K, Jendle JH, Roberts AP, DeVries JH, Meneghini LF (2011) Insulin degludec in type 1 diabetes: a randomized controlled trial of a new-generation ultra-long-acting insulin compared with insulin glargine. Diabetes Care 34:661–665

Bliss M (1982) Who discovered insulin. In: The discovery of insulin. McClelland and Stewart Limited, Toronto, pp 189–211

Boldo A, Comi RJ (2012) Clinical experience with U500 insulin: risks and benefits. Endocr Pract 18:56–61

Brackenridge B (1994) Diabetes medicines: insulin. In: Brackenridge B (ed) Managing your diabetes. Eli Lilly and Company, Indianapolis, pp 36–50

Brader ML, Dunn MF (1991) Insulin hexamers: new conformations and applications. Trends Biochem Sci 16:341–345

Brange J (1987a) Insulin preparations. In: Galenics of insulin. Springer, Berlin, pp 17–39

Brange J (1987b) Production of bovine and porcine insulin. In: Galenics of insulin. Springer, Berlin, pp 1–5

Brange J (1987c) Insulin preparations. In: Galenics of insulin. Springer, Berlin, pp 58–60

Brange J, Langkjaer L (1992) Chemical stability of insulin. 3. Influence of excipients, formulation, and pH. Acta Pharm Nord 4:149–158

Brange J, Ribel U, Hansen JF, Dodson G, Hansen MT, Havelund S, Melberg SG, Norris F, Norris K, Snel L et al (1988) Monomeric insulins obtained by protein engineering and their medical implications. Nature 333:679–682

Brange J, Owens DR, Kang S, Vølund A (1990) Monomeric insulins and their experimental and clinical applications. Diabetes Care 13:923–954

Brange J, Havelund S, Hougaard P (1992a) Chemical stability of insulin. 2. Formation of higher molecular weight transformation products during storage of pharmaceutical preparations. Pharm Res 9:727–734

Brange J, Langkjaer L, Havelund S, Vølund A (1992b) Chemical stability of insulin. 1. Hydrolytic degradation during storage of pharmaceutical preparations. Pharm Res 9:715–726

Brems DN, Alter LA, Beckage MJ, Chance RE, DiMarchi RD, Green LK, Long HB, Pekar AH, Shields JE, Frank BH (1992) Altering the association properties of insulin by amino acid replacement. Protein Eng 6:527–533

Brennan TV, Clarke S (1994) Deamidation and isoasparate formation in model synthetic peptides. In: Aswad DW (ed) Deamidation and isoaspartate formation in peptides and proteins. CRC Press, Boca Raton, pp 65–90

Cernea S, Kidron M, Wohlgelernter J, Modi P, Raz I (2004) Comparison of pharmacokinetic and pharmacodynamic properties of single-dose oral insulin spray and subcutaneous insulin injection in healthy subjects using the euglycemic clamp technique. Clin Ther 26:2084–2091

Chacra AR, Kipnes M, Ilag LL, Sarwat S, Giaconia J, Chan J (2010) Comparison of insulin lispro protamine suspension and insulin detemir in basal-bolus therapy in patients with type 1 diabetes. Diabet Med 27:563–569

Charman SA, McLennan DN, Edwards GA, Porter CJH (2001) Lymphatic absorption is a significant contributor to the subcutaneous bioavailability of insulin in a sheep model. Pharm Res 18:1620–1626

Ciszak E, Beals JM, Frank BH, Baker JC, Carter ND, Smith GD (1995) Role of the C-terminal B-chain residues in insulin assembly: the structure of hexameric LysB28ProB29-human insulin. Structure 3:615–622

Dailey G, Rosenstock J, Moses RG, Ways K (2004) Insulin glulisine provides improved glycemic control in patients with type 2 diabetes. Diabetes Care 27:2363–2368

Darrington RT, Anderson BD (1995) Effects of insulin concentration and self-association on the partitioning of its A-21 cyclic anhydride intermediate to desamido insulin and covalent dimer. Pharm Res 12:1077–1084

Davis SN, Thompson CJ, Brown MD, Home PD, Alberti KG (1991) A comparison of the pharmacokinetics and metabolic effects of human regular and NPH mixtures. Diabetes Res Clin Pract 13:107–117

de la Peña A, Riddle M, Morrow LA, Jiang HH, Linnebjerg H, Scott A, Win KM, Hompesch M, Mace KF, Jacobson JG, Jackson JA (2011) Pharmacokinetics and pharmacodynamics of high-dose human regular U-500 insulin versus human regular U-100 insulin in healthy obese subjects. Diabetes Care 34:2496–2501

de la Pena A, Seger M, Soon D, Scott AJ, Reddy SR, Dobbins MA et al (2016) Bioequivalence and comparative pharmacodynamics of insulin lispro 200 U/mL relative to insulin lispro (Humalog (R)) 100 U/mL. Clin Pharmacol Drug Dev 5:69–75

Deckert T (1980) Intermediate-acting insulin preparations: NPH and lente. Diabetes Care 3:623–626

DeFelippis MR, Bakaysa DL, Bell MA, Heady MA, Li S, Pye S, Youngman KM, Radziuk J, Frank BH (1998) Preparation and characterization of a cocrystalline suspension of [LysB28, ProB29]-human insulin analogue. J Pharm Sci 87:170–176

DeFelippis MR, Bell MA, Heyob JA, Storms SM (2006) In vitro stability of insulin lispro in continuous subcutaneous insulin infusion. Diabetes Technol Ther 8:358–368

Derewenda U, Derewenda Z, Dodson EJ, Dodson GG, Reynolds CD, Smith GD, Sparks C, Swenson D (1989) Phenol stabilizes more helix in a new symmetrical zinc insulin hexamer. Nature 338:594–596

Dodd SW, Havel HA, Kovach PM, Lakshminarayan C, Redmon MP, Sargeant CM, Sullivan GR, Beals JM (1995) Reversible adsorption of soluble hexameric insulin onto the surface of insulin crystals cocrystallized with protamine: an electrostatic interaction. Pharm Res 12:60–68

Dreyer M, Prager R, Robinson A, Busch K, Ellis G, Souhami E, Van Leendert R (2005) Efficacy and safety of insulin glulisine in patients with type 1 diabetes. Horm Metab Res 37:702–707

Eby E, Smolen L, Pitts A, Krueger LA, Grimm D (2014) Economic impact of converting from pen and 10-mL vial to 3-mL vial for insulin delivery in a hospital setting. Hosp Pharm 49(11):1033–1038

Edmondson G, Criswell J, Krueger L, Eby EL (2014) Economic impact of converting from 10-mL insulin vials to 3-mL vials and pens in a hospital setting. Am J Health-Syst Pharm 70:1485–1489

Fogelfeld L, Dharmalingam M, Robling K, Jones C, Swanson D, Jacober SJ (2010) A randomized, treat-to-target trial comparing insulin lispro protamine suspension and insulin detemir in insulin-naive patients with type 2 diabetes. Diabet Med 27:181–188

Galloway JA (1988) Chemistry and clinical use of insulin. In: Galloway JA, Potvin JH, Shuman CR (eds) Diabetes mellitus, 9th edn. Lilly Research Laboratories, Indianapolis, pp 105–133

Galloway JA, Chance RE (1994) Improving insulin therapy: achievements and challenges. Horm Metab Res 26:591–598

Galloway JA, Spradlin CT, Nelson RL, Wentworth SM, Davidson JA, Swarner JL (1981) Factors influencing the absorption, serum insulin concentration, and blood glucose responses after injections of regular insulin and various insulin mixtures. Diabetes Care 4:366–376

Galloway JA, Spradlin CT, Jackson RL, Otto DC, Bechtel LD (1982) Mixtures of intermediate-acting insulin (NPH and Lente) with regular insulin: an update. In: Skyler JS (ed) Insulin update: 1982. Exerpta Medica, Princeton, pp 111–119

Gibney MA, Arce CH, Byron KJ, Hirsch LJ (2010) Skin and subcutaneous adipose layer thickness in adults with diabetes at sites used for insulin injections: implications for needle length recommendations. Curr Med Res Opin 26:1519–1530

Goldman J, Carpenter FH (1974) Zinc binding, circular dichroism, and equilibrium sedimentation studies on insulin (bovine) and several of its derivatives. Biochemistry 13:4566–4574

Goldman J, Trujillo JM (2017) iGlarLixi: a fixed-ratio combination of insulin glargine 100 U/mL and lixisenatide for the treatment of type 2 diabetes. Ann Pharmacother 51(11):990–999

Gough SC, Jain R, Woo VC (2016) Insulin degludec/liraglutide (IDegLira) for the treatment of type 2 diabetes. Expert Rev Endocrinol Metab 11(1):7–19

Hagedorn HC, Jensen BN, Krarup NB, Wodstrup I (1936) Protamine insulinate. JAMA 106:177–180

Hamaguchi T, Hashimoto Y, Miyata T, Kishikawa H, Yano T, Fukushima H, Shichiri M (1990) Effect of mixing short and intermediate NPH insulin or Zn insulin suspension acting human insulin on plasma free insulin levels and action profiles. J Jpn Diabet Soc 33:223–229

Hardy TA, Andersen G, Meiffren G, Lamers D, Ranson A, Alluis B, Gaudier M, Soula O, Kazda C, Heise T, Bruce S (2017) Ultra-rapid BioChaperone Lispro (BCLIS) improves postprandial blood glucose (PPG) excursions vs. insulin Lispro (LIS) in a 14-day treatment study in subjects with type 1 diabetes (T1DM). Diabetes A249:964

Havelund S, Plum A, Ribel U, Jonassen I, Vølund A, Markussen J, Kurtzhals P (2004) The mechanism of protraction of insulin detemir, a long-acting, acylated analog of human insulin. Pharm Res 21:1498–1504

Havelund S, Ribel U, Hubálek F, Hoeg-Jensen T, Wahlund PO, Jonassen I (2015) Investigation of the Physico-chemical properties that enable co-formulation of basal insulin degludec with fast-acting insulin Aspart. Pharm Res 32(7):2250–2258

Heinemann L, Weyer C, Rave K, Stiefelhagen O, Rauhaus M, Heise T (1997) Comparison of the time-action profiles of U40- and U100-regular human insulin and the rapid-acting insulin analogue B28 Asp. Exp Clin Endocrinol Diabetes 105:140–144

Heinemann L, Sinha K, Weyer C, Loftager M, Hirschberger S, Heise T (1999) Time-action profile of the soluble, fatty acid acylated, long-acting insulin analogue NN304. Diabet Med 16:332–338

Heinemann L, Pfützner A, Heise T (2001) Alternative routes of administration as an approach to improve insulin therapy: update on dermal, oral, nasal and pulmonary insulin delivery. Curr Pharm Des 7:1327–1351

Heise T, Weyer C, Serwas A, Heinrichs S, Osinga J, Roach P, Woodworth J, Gudat W, Heinemann L (1998) Time-action profiles of novel premixed preparations of insulin lispro and NPL insulin. Diabetes Care 21:800–803

Heise T, Nosek L, Rønn BB, Endahl L, Heinemann L, Kapitza C, Draeger E (2004) Lower within-subject variability of insulin detemir in comparison to NPH insulin and insulin glargine in people with type 1 diabetes. Diabetes 53:1614–1620

Heise T, Nosek L, Spitzer H, Heinemann L, Niemöller E, Frick AD, Becker RH (2007) Insulin glulisine: a faster onset of action compared with insulin lispro. Diabetes Obes Metab 9(5):746–753

Heise T, Hövelmann U, Brøndsted L, Adrian CL, Nosek L, Haahr H (2015) Faster-acting insulin aspart: earlier onset of appearance and greater early pharmacokinetic and pharmacodynamic effects than insulin aspart. Diabetes Obes Metab 17(7):682–688

Heise T, Mathieu C (2017) Impact of the mode of protraction of basal insulin therapies on their pharmacokinetic and pharmacodynamic properties and resulting clinical outcomes. Diabetes Obes Metab 19(1):3–12

Heise T, Stender-Petersen K, Hövelmann U, Jacobsen JB, Nosek L, Zijlstra E, Haahr H (2017) Pharmacokinetic and Pharmacodynamic properties of faster-acting insulin Aspart versus insulin Aspart across a clinically relevant dose range in subjects with type 1 diabetes mellitus. Clin Pharmacokinet 56(6):649–660

Hermansen K, Madsbad S, Perrild H, Kristensen A, Axelsen M (2001) Comparison of the soluble basal insulin analog insulin detemir with NPH insulin: a randomized open crossover trial in type 1 diabetic subjects on basal-bolus therapy. Diabetes Care 24:296–301

Hirsch IB, Franek E, Mersebach H, Bardtrum L, Hermansen K (2017) Safety and efficacy of insulin degludec/insulin aspart with bolus mealtime insulin aspart compared with standard basal-bolus treatment in people with type 1 diabetes: 1-year results from a randomized clinical trial (BOOST® T1). Diabet Med 34(2):167–173

Hjorth CF, Hubalek F, Andersson J, Poulsen C, Otzen D, Naver H (2015) Purification and identification of high molecular weight products formed during storage of neutral formulation of human insulin. Pharm Res 32:2072–2085

Hjorth CF, Norrman M, Wahlund P, Benie AJ, Petersen BO, Jessen CM, Pedersen TA, Vestergaard K, Steensgaard DB, Pedersen JS, Naver H, Hubalek F, Poulsen C, Otsen D (2016) Structure, aggregation, and activity of a covalent insulin dimer formed during storage of neutral formulation of human insulin. J Pharm Sci 105:1376–1386

Hoffmann JA, Chance RE, Johnson MG (1990) Purification and analysis of the major components of chum salmon protamine contained in insulin formulations using high-performance liquid chromatography. Protein Expr Purif 1:127–133

Holleman F, Schmitt H, Rottiers R, Rees A, Symanowski S, Anderson JH (1997) Reduced frequency of severe hypoglycemia and coma in well-controlled IDDM patients treated with insulin lispro. The Benelux-UK Insulin Lispro Study Group. Diabetes Care 20:1827–1832

Home PD (2012) The pharmacokinetics and pharmacodynamics of rapid-acting insulin analogues and their clinical consequences. Diabetes Obes Metab 14:780–788

Hompesch M, Ocheltree SM, Wondmagegnehu ET, Morrow LA, Kollmeier AP, Campaigne BN, Jacober SJ (2009) Pharmacokinetics and pharmacodynamics of insulin lispro protamine suspension compared with insulin glargine and insulin detemir in type 2 diabetes. Curr Med Res Opin 25:2679–2687

Howey DC, Bowsher RR, Brunelle RL, Woodworth JR (1994) [Lys(B28), Pro(B29)]-human insulin: a rapidly-absorbed analogue of human insulin. Diabetes 43:396–402

Hughes E (2016) IDegLira: Redefining insulin optimisation using a single injection in patients with type 2 diabetes. Primary Care Diabetes 10(3):202–209

Jansen R, Dzwolak W, Winter R (2005) Amyloidogenic self-assembly of insulin aggregates probed by high resolution atomic force microscopy. Biophys J 88:1344–1353

Janssen MM, Casteleijn S, Devillé W, Popp-Snijders C, Roach P, Heine RJ (1997) Nighttime insulin kinetics and glycemic control in type 1 diabetic patients following administration of an intermediate-acting lispro preparation. Diabetes Care 20:1870–1873

Johnson JL, Downes JM, Obi CK, Asante NB (2017) Novel concentrated insulin delivery devices: developments for safe and simple dose conversions. J Diabetes Sci Technol 11(3):618–622

Jonassen I, Havelund S, Hoeg-Jensen T, Steensgaard DB, Wahlund PO, Ribel U (2012) Design of the novel protraction mechanism of insulin degludec, an ultra-long-acting basal insulin. Pharm Res 29(8):2104–2114

Kaarsholm NC, Havelund S, Hougaard P (1990) Ionization behavior of native and mutant insulins: pK perturbation of B13-Glu in aggregated species. Arch Biochem Biophys 283:496–502

Kapitza C, Leohr J, Liu R, Reddy S, Dellva MA, Matzopoulos M, Knadler MP, Loh MT, Hardy T, Kazda C (2017) A novel formulation of insulin Lispro containing citrate and Treprostinil shows significantly faster absorption and an improvement in postprandial glucose excursions vs. Humalog® in patients with T2DM. Diabetes 66(suppl 1). 978-P, A253

Kazda C, Leohr J, Liu R, Dellva MA, Lim ST, Loh MT, Knadler MP, Hardy T, Plum-Moerschel L (2017) A novel formulation of insulin Lispro containing citrate and Treprostinil shows faster absorption and improved postprandial glucose excursions vs. Humalog® in patients with T1DM. Diabetes 66(suppl 1). 959-P, A247

Korsatko S, Deller S, Koehler G, Mader JK, Neubauer K, Adrian CL et al (2013) A comparison of the steady-state pharmacokinetic and pharmacodynamic profiles of 100 and 200 U/mL formulations of ultra-long-acting insulin degludec. Clin Drug Investig 33:515–521

Krayenbuhl C, Rosenberg T (1946) Crystalline protamine insulin. Rep Steno Hosp (Kbh) 1:60–73

Kroeff EP, Owen RA, Campbell EL, Johnson RD, Marks HI (1989) Production scale purification of biosynthetic human insulin by reversed-phase high-performance liquid chromatography. J Chromatogr 461:45–61

Kurtz AB, Gray RS, Markanday S, Nabarro JD (1983) Circulating IgG antibody to protamine in patients treated with protamine-insulins. Diabetologia 25:322–324

Lamb YN, Syed YY (2018) LY2963016 insulin glargine: a review in type 1 and 2 diabetes. BioDrugs 32(1): 91–98

Lane WS, Cochran EK, Jackson JA, Scism-Bacon JL, Corey IB, Hirsch IB, Skyler JS (2009) High-dose insulin therapy: is it time for U-500 insulin? Endocr Pract 15:71–79

Lau IT, Lee KF, So WY, Tan K, Yeung VTF (2017) Insulin glargine 300 U/mL for basal insulin therapy in type 1 and type 2 diabetes mellitus. Diabetes Metab Syndr Obes 30(10):273–284

Modi P, Mihic M, Lewin A (2002) The evolving role of oral insulin in the treatment of diabetes using a novel RapidMistSystem. Diabetes Metab Res Rev 18(Suppl 1):S38–S42

Nell LJ, Thomas JW (1988) Frequency and specificity of protamine antibodies in diabetic and control subjects. Diabetes 37:172–176

Nielsen L, Khurana R, Coats A, Frokjaer S, Brange J, Vyas S, Uversky VN, Fink AL (2001) Effect of environmental factors on the kinetics of insulin fibril formation: elucidation of the molecular mechanism. Biochemistry 40:6036–6046

Ovalle F, Segal AR, Anderson JE, Cohen MR, Morwick TM, Jackson JA (2018) Understanding concentrated insulins: a systematic review of randomized controlled trials. Curr Med Res Opin 10:1–15

Park SW, Bebakar WM, Hernandez PG, Macura S, Hersløv ML, de la Rosa R (2017) Insulin degludec/insulin aspart once daily in type 2 diabetes: a comparison of simple or stepwise titration algorithms (BOOST® : SIMPLE USE). Diabet Med 34(2):174–179

Pekar AH, Frank BH (1972) Conformation of proinsulin. A comparison of insulin and proinsulin self-association at neutral pH. Biochemistry 11:4013–4016

Peters AL, Pollom RD, Zielonka JS, Carey MA, Edelman SV (2015) Biosimilar and new versions. Endocr Pract 21(12):1387–1394

Porcellati F, Bolli GB, Fanelli CG (2011) Pharmacokinetics and pharmacodynamics of basal insulins. Diabetes Technol Ther 13(Suppl 1):S15–S24

Porter CJ, Charman SA (2000) Lymphatic transport of proteins after subcutaneous administration. J Pharm Sci 89:297–310

Reid TS, Schafer F, Brusko C (2017) Higher concentration insulins: an overview of clinical considerations. Postgrad Med 129(5):554–562

Ritzel R, Roussel R, Bolli GB, Vinet L, Brulle-Wohlhueter C, Glezer S, Yki-Järvinen H (2015) Patient-level meta-analysis of the EDITION 1, 2 and 3 studies: glycaemic control and hypoglycaemia with new insulin glargine 300 U/ml versus glargine 100 U/ml in people with type 2 diabetes. Diabetes Obes Metab 17(9): 859–867

Robertson KE, Glazer NB, Campbell RK (2000) The latest developments in insulin injection devices. Diabetes Educ 26:135–152

Rodbard HW, Buse JB, Woo V, Vilsbøll T, Langbakke IH, Kvist K, Gough SC (2016) Benefits of combination of insulin degludec and liraglutide are independent of baseline glycated haemoglobin level and duration of type 2 diabetes. Diabetes Obes Metab 18(1):40–48

Schade DS, Santiago JV, Skyler JS, Rizza RA (1983) Intensive insulin therapy. Medical Examination Publishing, Princeton, p 24

Segal AR, Brunner JE, Burch FT, Jackson JA (2010) Use of concentrated insulin human regular (U-500) for patients with diabetes. Am J Health Syst Pharm 67:1526–1535

Senstius J, Harboe E, Westermann H (2007a) In vitro stability of insulin aspart in simulated continuous subcutaneous insulin infusion using a MiniMed 508 pump. Diabetes Technol Ther 9:75–79

Senstius J, Poulsen C, Hvass A (2007b) Comparison of in vitro stability for insulin aspart and insulin glulisine during simulated use in infusion pumps. Diabetes Technol Ther 9:517–521

Sharrow SD, Glass LC, Dobbins MA (2012) 14-day in vitro chemical stability of insulin lispro in the MiniMed paradigm pump. Diabetes Technol Ther 14:264–270

Soula O, Soula R, Soula G (2014) Fast-acting insulin formulations, US8669227

Steensgaard DB, Schluckebier G, Strauss HM, Norrman M, Thomsen JK, Friderichsen AV, Havelund S, Jonassen I (2013) Ligand-controlled assembly of hexamers, dihexamers, and linear multihexamer structures by the engineered acylated insulin degludec. Biochemistry 52(2):295–309

Strojek K, Shi C, Carey MA, Jacober SJ (2010) Addition of insulin lispro protamine suspension or insulin glargine to oral type 2 diabetes regimens: a randomized trial. Diabetes Obes Metab 12:916–922

Supersaxo A, Hein WR, Steffen H (1990) Effect of molecular weight on the lymphatic absorption of water-soluble compounds following subcutaneous administration. Pharm Res 7:167–169

USP Monographs: Insulin (2013) USP36-NF31: 3911–3913

Vague P, Selam JL, Skeie S, De Leeuw I, Elte JW, Haahr H, Kristensen A, Draeger E (2003) Insulin detemir is associated with more predictable glycemic control and reduced risk of hypoglycemia than NPH insulin in patients with type 1 diabetes on a basal-bolus regimen with premeal insulin aspart. Diabetes Care 26:590–596

Waldhäusl W, Bratusch-Marrain P, Gasic S, Kom A, Nowotny P (1979) Insulin production rate following glucose ingestion estimated by splanchnic C-peptide output in normal man. Diabetologia 17:221–227

Weyer C, Heise T, Heinemann L (1997) Insulin aspart in a 30/70 premixed formulation. Pharmacodynamic properties of a rapid-acting insulin analog in stable mixture. Diabetes Care 20:1612–1614

Whittingham JL, Edwards DJ, Antson AA, Clarkson JM, Dodson GG (1998) Interactions of phenol and m-cresol in the insulin hexamer, and their effect on the association properties of B28 pro → Asp insulin analogues. Biochemistry 37:11516–11523

Whittingham JL, Jonassen I, Havelund S, Roberts SM, Dodson EJ, Verma CS, Wilkinson AJ, Dodson GG (2004) Crystallographic and solution studies of N-lithocholyl insulin: a new generation of prolonged-acting human insulins. Biochemistry 43:5987–5995

Wysham C, Hood RC, Warren ML, Wang T, Morwick TM, Jackson JA (2016) Endocr Pract 22(6):653–665

Ziesmer AE, Kelly KC, Guerra PA, George KG, Dunn KL (2012) U500 regular insulin use in insulin-resistant type 2 diabetic veteran patients. Endocr Pract 18:34–38

SUGGESTED READING

American Diabetes Association (2011) Practical insulin: a handbook for prescribing providers, 3rd edn. American Diabetes Association, New York

Beals JM (2015) Insulin analogs—"improving the therapy of diabetes". In: Fischer J, Rotella DP (eds) Successful drug discovery, vol 1. Wiley, Hoboken

Bliss M (1982) The discovery of insulin. McClelland and Stewart Limited, Toronto

Brange J (1987) Galenics of insulin. Springer, Berlin

Burant C (ed) (2008) Medical management of type 2 diabetes, 6th edn. American Diabetes Association, New York

Cooper T, Ainsburg A (2010) Breakthrough: Elizabeth Hughes, the discovery of insulin, and the making of a medical miracle. St. Martin's Press, New York

Galloway JA, Potvin JH, Shuman CR (1988) Diabetes mellitus, 9th edn. Lilly Research Laboratories, Indianapolis

Wolfsdorf JI (2009) Intensive diabetes management, 4th edn. American Diabetes Association, New York

Zaykov AN, Mayer JP, DiMarchi RD (2016) Pursuit of a perfect insulin. Nat Rev Drug Discov 15(6):425–439

19 Follicle-Stimulating Hormone

Tom Sam and Renato de Leeuw

INTRODUCTION

About 15% of all couples experience infertility at some time during their reproductive lives. Nowadays, infertility can be treated by the use of assisted reproductive technologies (ART), such as in vitro fertilization (IVF) and intracytoplasmic sperm injection (ICSI). A common element of these programs is the treatment with Follicle Stimulating Hormone (FSH) to increase the number of oocytes retrievable for the IVF or ICSI procedure (multifollicular development). Patients suffering from female infertility because of chronic anovulation may also be treated with FSH, then with the aim to achieve monofollicular development.

Natural FSH is produced and secreted by the anterior lobe of the pituitary, a gland at the base of the brain. Its target is the FSH receptor at the surface of the granulosa cells that surround the oocyte. FSH acts synergistically with oestrogens and Luteinizing Hormone (LH) to stimulate proliferation of these granulosa cells, which leads to follicular growth. As the primary function of FSH in the female is the regulation of follicle growth and development, this process explains why deficient endogenous production of FSH may cause infertility. In males, FSH plays a pivotal role in spermatogenesis.

FSH preparations for infertility treatment are traditionally derived from urine from (post) menopausal women. As over 100,000 L of urine may be required for a single batch, many thousands of donors are needed. Hence, the source of urinary FSH is heterogeneous and the sourcing cumbersome. Moreover, in addition to FSH, these urinary preparations contain impurities including pharmaceutically active proteins such as LH. Recombinant DNA technology allows the reproducible manufacturing of FSH preparations of high purity and specific activity, devoid of urinary contaminants. Recombinant FSH is produced using a Chinese Hamster Ovary (CHO) cell line, transfected with the genes encoding for the two human FSH subunits (van Wezenbeek et al. 1990; Howles 1996). The isolation procedures render a product of high purity (at least 99%), devoid of LH activity and very similar to natural FSH. Recently, a novel recombinant FSH derived from a cell line of human fetal retinal origin (follitropin delta) was introduced (Olson et al. 2014).

Currently, there are several clinically approved recombinant FSH-containing drug products on the various markets. The most widely approved products are Gonal-F®, manufactured by Merck Serono S.A., and Puregon®, with the brand name of Follistim® in the USA and Japan, manufactured by N.V. Organon, now part of Merck Sharp and Dohme. Regulatory authorities have issued two distinct International Non-proprietary Names (INN) for the three corresponding recombinant FSH drug substances, i.e. follitropin alfa (Gonal-F®), follitropin beta (Puregon®/Follistim®) and follitropin delta (Rekovelle®). In addition, a few other recombinant-FSH preparations, 'biosimilar' to follitropin alfa, were developed and are available under the names: Bemfola®, Ovaleap® (Rettenbacher et al. 2015).

FSH IS A GLYCOPROTEIN HORMONE

Follicle-stimulating hormone belongs to a family of structurally related glycoproteins which also includes luteinizing hormone (LH), chorionic gonadotropin (CG), collectively called the gonadotropins and thyroid-stimulating hormone (TSH, also named thyrotropin). These hormones belong to the 'cystine-knot protein family'. FSH is a hetero-dimeric protein consisting of two non-covalently associated glycoprotein

T. Sam
GlobalPharmCMC, Heesch, The Netherlands

R. de Leeuw (✉)
DeLeeuw Consultancy, Heesch, The Netherlands
e-mail: renato@deleeuwconsultancy.nl

D. J. A. Crommelin et al. (eds.), *Pharmaceutical Biotechnology*, https://doi.org/10.1007/978-3-030-00710-2_19

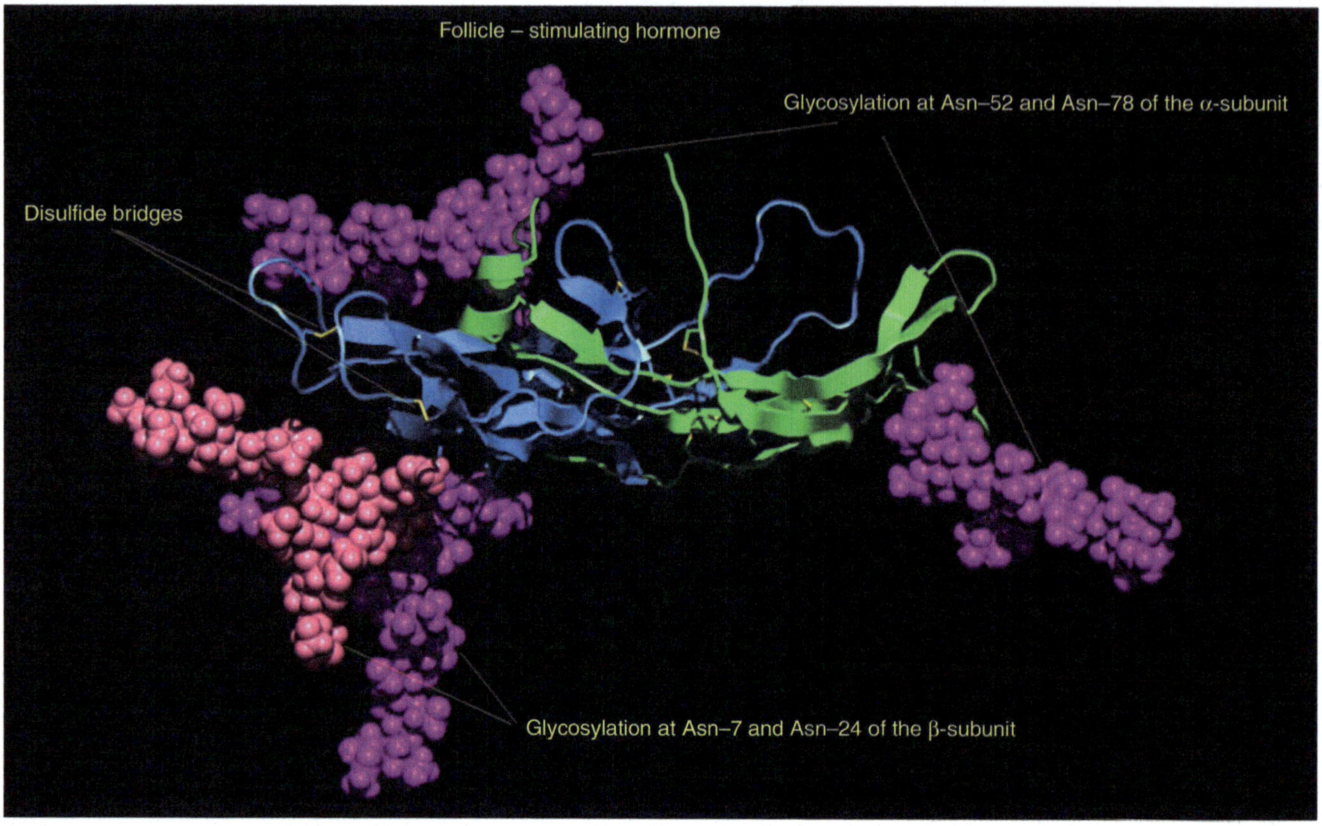

Figure 19.1 ■ A three-dimensional model of FSH. The ribbons represent the polypeptide backbones of the α-subunit (green ribbon) and the β-subunit (blue ribbon). The carbohydrate side chains (violet and pink space filled globules) cover large areas of the surface of the polypeptide subunits

subunits, denoted α and β. The α-subunit contains five intra-subunit disulfide bonds and is identical for all these glycoproteins, and it is the β-subunit (having six intra-subunit disulfide bonds) that provides each hormone with its specific biological function.

The glycoprotein subunits of FSH consist of two polypeptide backbones with carbohydrate side chains attached to the two asparagine (Asn) amino acid residues on each subunit. The oligosaccharides are attached to Asn-52 and Asn-78 on the α-subunit (92 amino acids), and to Asn-7 and Asn-24 on the β-subunit (111 amino acids). The glycoprotein FSH has a molecular mass of approximately 35 kDa. For the FSH preparation to be biologically active, the two subunits must be correctly assembled into their three-dimensional hetero-dimeric protein structure and post-translationally modified (Fig. 19.1).

Assembly and glycosylation are intracellular processes that take place in the endoplasmatic reticulum and in the Golgi apparatus. This glycosylation process leads to the formation of a population of hormone isoforms differing in their carbohydrate side-chain composition. The carbohydrate side-chains of FSH are essential for its biological activity since they (1) influence FSH receptor binding, (2) play an important role in the signal transduction into the FSH target cell, and (3) affect the plasma residence time of the hormone.

Recombinant FSH contains approximately one third carbohydrate on a mass per mass basis. The carbohydrate side chains are composed of mannose, fucose, *N*-acetyl-glucosamine, galactose and sialic acid. Structure analysis by ^{1}H-NMR-spectroscopy on oligosaccharides enzymatically cleaved from follitropin beta, reveals minor differences with natural FSH. For instance, the bisecting GlcNAc residues are lacking in the recombinant molecule, simply because the FSH-producing CHO cells do not possess the enzymes to incorporate these residues. Furthermore, the carbohydrate side-chains of recombinant FSH exclusively contain α2–3 linked sialic acid, whereas in the natural hormone α1–6 linked sialic acid occurs, as well. However, all carbohydrate side-chains identified in recombinant FSH are moieties normally found in other natural human glycoproteins. The amino acid sequences of the α-subunit and the β-subunit of the recombinant FSH derived from human fetal retina, are identical to the sequence of natural human FSH and CHO-derived FSH products in clinical use, while the sialic acid content is higher (Olson et al. 2014).

Whereas FSH only contains N-linked carbohydrates, human chorionic gonadotropin (hCG) also carries 4 O-linked (at serine or threonine residues) carbohydrates, all located at the Carboxy Terminal Peptide (CTP) of its beta subunit. This glycosylated CTP is the major difference with the beta subunit of LH and is demonstrated to be responsible for the much longer plasma residence time of hCG compared to natural LH. (Matzuk et al. 1990).

PRODUCTION OF RECOMBINANT FSH

The genes coding for the human FSH α-subunit and β-subunit were inserted in cloning vectors (plasmids) to enable efficient transfer into recipient cells. These vectors also contained promoters that could direct transcription of foreign genes in recipient cells. CHO cells were selected as recipient cells since they were easily transfected with foreign DNA, and are capable of synthesizing complex glycoproteins. Furthermore they could be grown in cell cultures on a large scale. To construct a FSH-producing cell line, N.V. Organon, the manufacturer of Puregon®/Follistim®, used one single vector containing the coding sequences for both subunit genes (Olijve et al. 1996). Merck Serono S.A., the manufacturer of Gonal-F®, used two separate vectors, one for each subunit gene (Howles 1996). Following transfection, a genetically stable transformant producing biologically active recombinant FSH was isolated. For the CHO cell line used for manufacturing Puregon®/Follistim® it was shown that approximately 150–450 gene copies were present.

To establish a master cell bank (MCB) identical homogeneous cell preparations of the selected clone are stored in individual vials and cryopreserved until needed. Subsequently a working cell bank (WCB) is established by the expansion of cells derived from a single vial of the MCB and aliquots are put in vials and cryopreserved, as well. Each time a production run is started cells from one or more vials of the WCB are cultured.

Both recombinant FSH products are isolated from cell culture supernatants. These supernatants are collected from a perfusion-type bioreactor containing recombinant FSH-producing CHO cells grown on microcarriers. This is because the CHO cell lines used are anchorage-dependent cells, which implies that a proper surface must be provided for cell growth. The reactor is perfused with growth-promoting medium during a period that may continue for up to 3 months (see also Chap. 4). The down-stream purification processes for the isolation of the two recombinant FSH products are different. For Puregon®/Follistim® a series of chromatographic steps, including anion and cation exchange chromatography, hydrophobic chromatography and size-exclusion chromatography is used. Recombinant FSH in Gonal-F® is obtained by a similar process of five chromatographic steps, but also includes an immunoaffinity step using a murine FSH-specific monoclonal antibody (from European Public Assessment Report, EPAR Gonal-F 2011). In both production processes, each purification step is rigorously controlled in order to ensure the batch-to-batch consistency of the purified product.

DESCRIPTION OF RECOMBINANT FSH

■ Structural Characteristics

Like urinary sourced (natural) FSH, the recombinant versions exist in several distinct molecular forms (isohormones), with identical polypeptide backbones but with differences in oligosaccharide structure, in particular in the degree of terminal sialylation. These isohormones can be separated by chromatofocusing or isoelectric focusing on the basis of their different isoelectric points (pI, as has been demonstrated for follitropin beta (De Leeuw et al. 1996), Fig. 19.2). The typical pattern for FSH indicates an isohormone distribution between pI values of 6 and 4. To obtain structural information at the subunit level, the two subunits were separated by RP-HPLC and treated to release the N-linked carbohydrate side-chains. Fractions with low pI values (acidic fractions) displayed a high content of tri- and tetrasialo oligosaccharides and a low content of neutral and monosialo oligosaccharides. For fractions with a high pI (basic fractions) value the reverse was found. The β-subunit carbohydrate side chains appeared to be more heavily sialylated and branched than the

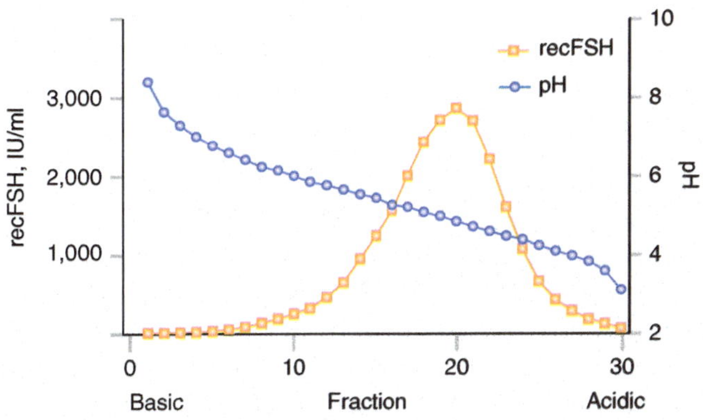

Figure 19.2 ■ Isohormone profile of recombinant follicle stimulating hormone (follitropin β beta) after preparative free flow focusing (De Leeuw et al. 1996). The FSH concentration was determined by a two-site immunoassay that is capable of quantifying the various isohormones equally well

α-subunit carbohydrate side chains. The low pI value isohormones of follitropin beta have a high sialic acid/galactose ratio and are rich in tri- and tetra-antennary N-linked carbohydrate side chains, as compared with the side chains of the high pI value isohormones.

One of the tools for further characterization is the immunoassay. Due to the specific recognition characteristics of the antibodies used, this assay determines FSH-specific structural features and provides a relative measure for the quantity of FSH, as it is not sensitive to the differences in glycosylation.

Biological Properties of Recombinant FSH Isohormones

A FSH preparation can be biologically characterized with several essentially different assays, each having its own specific merits (Mannaerts et al. 1992). The receptor binding assay provides information on the proper conformation for interaction with the FSH receptor. Receptor binding studies with calf testis membranes have shown that FSH isoform activity in follitropin beta decreases when going from high to low pI isoforms. The in vitro bioassay measures the capability of FSH to transduce signals into target cells (the intrinsic bioactivity). The in vitro bioactivity, assessed in the rat Sertoli cell bioassay, also decreases when going from high to low pI isoforms. The in vivo bioassay provides the overall bioactivity of an FSH preparation. It is determined by the number of molecules, the plasma residence time, the receptor binding activity and the signal transduction. Interestingly, in contrast to the receptor binding and in vitro bioassays, the in vivo biological activity determined in rats shows an approximate 20-fold increase between isoforms with a pI value of 5.49, as compared to those with a pI of 4.27. These results indicate that the basic isohormones exhibit the highest receptor binding and signal transduction activity, whereas the acidic isohormones are the more active forms under in vivo conditions. This notion also warrants pharmacokinetic studies to further characterize the biological properties of FSH preparations.

Pharmacokinetic Behavior of Recombinant FSH Isohormones

The pharmacokinetic behavior of follitropin beta and its isohormones was investigated in beagle dogs that were given an intramuscular bolus injection of a number of FSH isohormone fractions, each with a specific pI value. With a decrease in pI value from 5.49 (basic) to 4.27 (acidic), the AUC increased and the clearance decreased, each more than tenfold (Fig. 19.3). A more than twofold difference in elimination half-life between the most acidic and the most basic FSH isohormone fraction was calculated. The absorption rate of the two most acidic

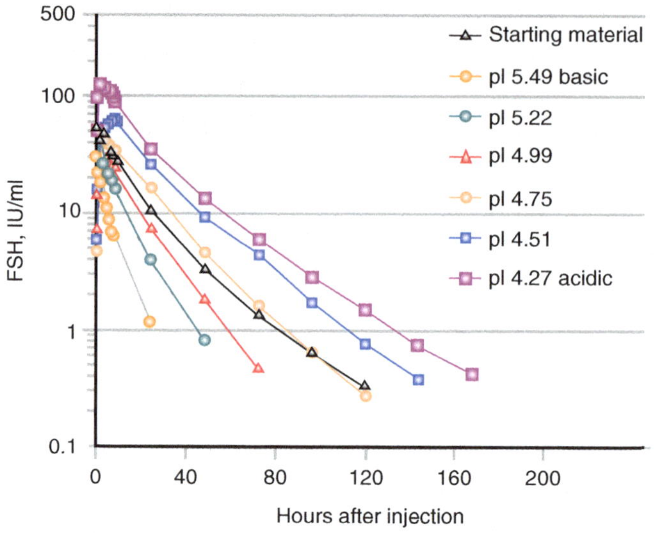

Figure 19.3 ■ Kinetic behavior of FSH isoforms after a single intramuscular injection (20 IU/kg) in beagle dogs

isoforms was higher than the absorption rates of all other isoforms. The AUC and the clearance for the follitropin beta preparation, being a mixture of all isohormone fractions, corresponded with the centre of the isohormone profile (Fig. 19.3). In contrast, the elimination of the follitropin beta preparation occurred at a rate similar to that of the most acidic fractions, indicating that the elimination rate is largely determined by the removal of the most acidic isoforms from the plasma.

Thus, for follitropin beta isohormone fractions, a clear correlation exists between pI value and pharmacokinetic behavior. Increasing acidity leads to an increase in the extent of absorption and elimination half-life and to a decrease in clearance.

PHARMACEUTICAL FORMULATIONS

Recombinant FSH preparations distinguish themselves from the earlier urinary FSH preparations by their high purity (at least 99%). However, pure proteins are relatively unstable and are therefore often lyophilized, unless some specific stabilizing measures can be taken. FSH preparations are available in different strengths and presentation forms, both as freeze-dried products (powder, cake) and as solution for injection. Follitropin alfa was originally formulated with sucrose (bulking agent, lyoprotectant), sodium dihydrogen phosphate/disodium hydrogen phosphate, phosphoric acid and sodium hydroxide (for pH adjustment). In 2002, L-methionine (antioxidant) and polysorbate 20 (to prevent adsorption losses) were added to the single dose formulation. Follitropin beta is formulated with sucrose, sodium citrate (stabilizer), polysorbate 20 (lyoprotectant and agent to prevent adsorption losses), and hydrochloride/sodium hydroxide (for pH adjustment). The lyophilized preparations are to be reconstituted before use to obtain a ready-for-use solution for injection. In addition to the freeze-dried presentation form, a solution for injection with several strengths of follitropin beta could be developed. To stabilize the solutions 0.25 mg of L-methionine had to be added. Furthermore, the solution in the cartridge contains benzyl alcohol as preservative. For follitropin alfa a multidose solution for injection in a pre-filled pen became available in 2004. This solution contains poloxamer 188 instead of polysorbate 20 and m-cresol has been added as preservative.

The Puregon®/Follistim® solution for injection is available in vials and is very suitable for titration because of the large range of available strengths as expressed in IU's. Pen injectors have been developed with multidose cartridges containing solution for injection, giving the patient improved convenience.

The solutions for injection should be stored in the refrigerator for a maximum of 3 years with the container kept in the outer carton to protect the solution from light. The patient can keep the solutions at room temperature for a maximum of 3 months. The multidose solution of follitropin α has a shelf-life of 2 years and can be stored for 1 month at room temperature.

CLINICAL ASPECTS

Recombinant FSH products on the market have been approved for two female indications. The first indication is anovulation (including polycystic ovarian disease) in women who are unresponsive to clomiphene citrate (an estrogen receptor modulator). The second indication is controlled ovarian hyperstimulation to induce the development of multiple follicles in medically assisted reproduction programs, such as in vitro fertilization (IVF) and intracytoplasmatic sperm injection (ICSI). In addition, recombinant FSH may be used in men with congenital or required hypogonadotropic hypogonadism to stimulate spermatogenesis.

For the treatment of anovulatory patients (aiming at monofollicular growth) it is recommended to start Puregon®/Follistim® treatment with 50 IU per day for 7–14 days and gradually increase dosing with steps of 50 IU if no sufficient response is seen. This gradual dose-increasing schedule is followed in order to prevent multifollicular development and the induction of ovarian hyperstimulation syndrome (a serious condition of unwanted hyperstimulation). In the most commonly applied treatment regimens in IVF, endogenous gonadotropin levels are suppressed by a GnRH agonist or by the more recently approved GnRH antagonists (Cetrotide® and Orgalutran®/ganirelix acetate injection). It is recommended to start Puregon® treatment with 100–200 IU of recombinant FSH followed by maintenance doses of 50–350 IU. The availability of a surplus of collected oocytes allows the vitrification of embryos for replacement in frozen-thawn embryo transfer (FTET) cycles. Similar treatment regimens are recommended for Gonal-F®.

After subcutaneous administration, follitropin beta has an elimination half-life of approximately 33 h (Voortman et al. 1999). Steady-state levels of follitropin beta are therefore obtained after four to five daily doses reaching therapeutically effective plasma concentrations of FSH. Follitropin β is administered via the subcutaneous route with good local tolerance. Bioavailability is approximately 77%. In a large fraction of patients treated with follitropin β, no formation of antibodies against recombinant FSH or CHO-cell derived proteins was observed. Injections of the follitropin β preparations can be given by the patient herself or her partner.

A NEWLY DEVELOPED FSH ANALOG

The need for daily injections of FSH, especially in combination with GnRH agonists, is a burden for the women treated in an ART regimen. Therefore, several different approaches have been undertaken to arrive at FSH preparations that need fewer injections, such as slow release formulations, addition of N-linked carbohydrates and other chemical modifications including pegylation (Fauser et al. 2009). An elegant approach pioneered by Irving Boime and collaborators (Fares et al. 1992; LaPolt et al. 1992), is based on the longer in vivo half-life of hCG compared to LH. Using genetic engineering, the beta subunit of FSH was extended by one or two CTPs of hCG. It was demonstrated that fewer injections with preparations containing such molecules were needed to induce similar pharmacodynamic effects in laboratory animals. Subsequently, a new cell line was generated by Organon (now part of Merck Sharp & Dohme) that produced corifollitropin alfa (the INN of this molecule), an FSH analog in which the beta subunit was extended by a single CTP (28 amino acids). Thorough biochemical analysis demonstrated the expected amino acid sequence of the alpha subunit and the extended beta subunit, but revealed two additional O-linked glycosylation sites in corifollitropin alfa (Henno van den Hooven, Ton Swolfs, personal communication) compared to the 4–5 sites reported in hCG (Fig. 19.4). Nonclinical evaluation demonstrated that the receptor binding and transactivation profile of this new molecular entity was specific and comparable to that of rec-FSH without intrinsic TSH-receptor or LH-receptor activation. However, the in vivo half-life was increased 1.5- to 2-fold in the species tested and a 2-fold to 4-fold

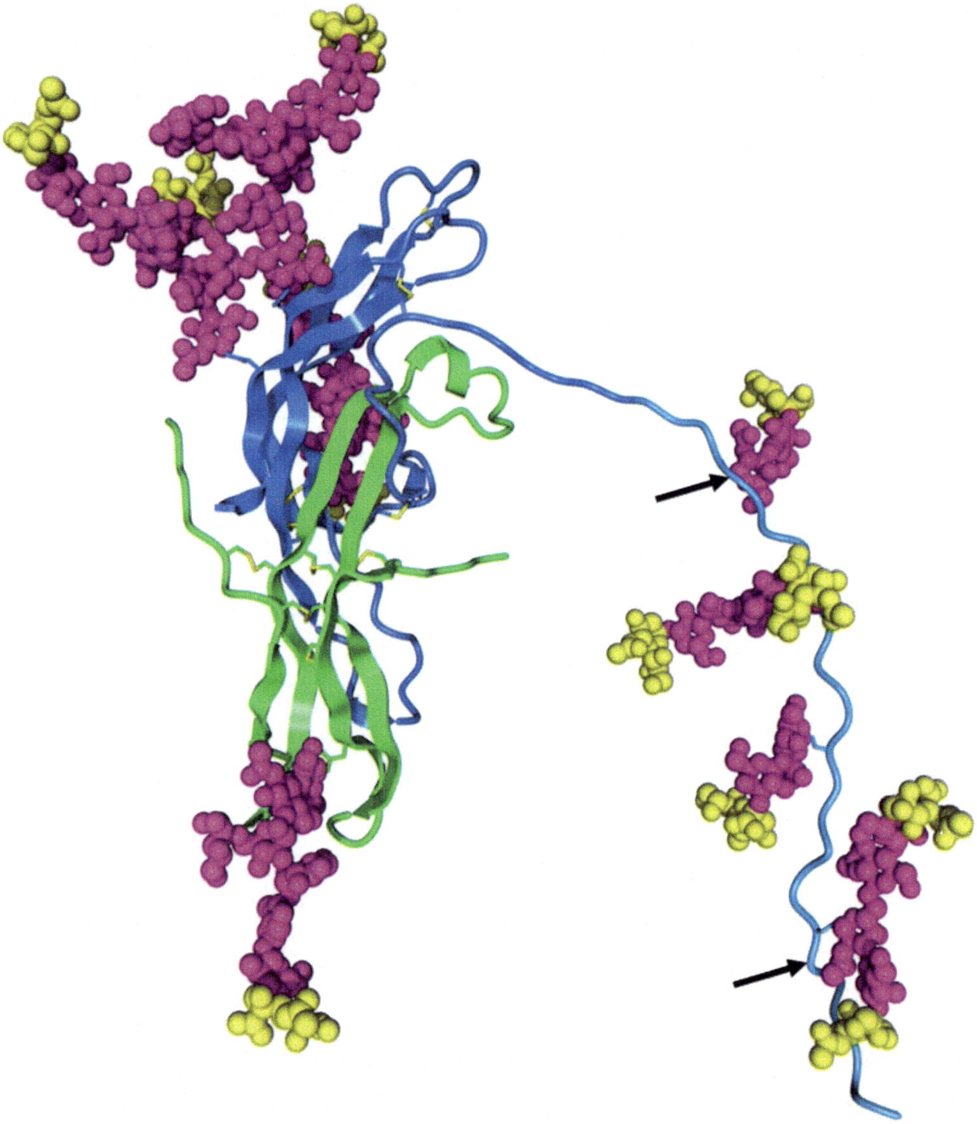

Figure 19.4 ■ A three-dimensional model of corifollitropin alfa. The ribbons represent the polypeptide backbones of the α-subunit (green ribbon) and the β-subunit (blue ribbon). The carbohydrate side chains (pink and yellow space filled globules) represent N-linked and O-linked carbohydrates. The sialic acid carbohydrates are depicted in yellow. The arrows indicate additional O-linked carbohydrate sites. Courtesy MLCE Kouwijzer and R Bosch

increase of bioactivity was found across all in vivo pharmacodynamic parameters tested (Verbost et al. 2011). These observations were corroborated by a very extensive data set obtained in a broad panel of clinical trials (phase I, II and III), including the largest comparator controlled trial of its kind in fertility (the comparator being recFSH) (Devroey et al. 2009; Fauser et al. 2010). A single subcutaneous dose of corifollitropin alfa (Elonva®) can be used to initiate and sustain multifollicular growth for 7 days while the efficacy and safety of this novel biopharmaceutical were similar to that of daily injections with recombinant FSH. Whereas normally more than 7 days of FSH treatment has to be given after the first injection, in about one third of the women treated with FSH-CTP no additional FSH treatment was needed.

Dedicated clinical research revealed no clinically relevant immunogenicity against the FSH analog (Norman et al. 2011), despite being a fusion protein. Hence, by virtue of its ~twofold increased in vivo half-life, corifollitropin alfa has demonstrated to provide a valuable alternative for FSH by acting as a sustained follicle stimulant. Elonva® is approved (EU) for Controlled Ovarian Stimulation (COS) in combination with a GnRH antagonist for the development of multiple follicles in women participating in an assisted Reproductive Technology (ART) program. It is supplied in pre-filled syringes equipped with an automatic safety system to prevent needle stick injuries after use and is packed together with a sterile injection needle. Each prefilled syringe contains 0.5 mL solution for injection (Fig. 19.5).

FSH provides a great example of the evolution of biopharmaceuticals, starting from the natural form (urine-derived), via close imitations thereof (recombinant FSH) towards further improved biopharmaceuti-

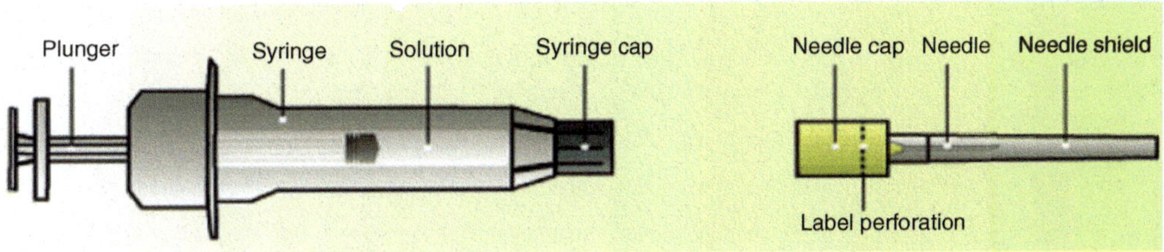

Figure 19.5 ■ Pre-filled syringe with corifollitropin alfa solution to be assembled with a needle assembly. The syringe is equipped with an automatic safety system to prevent needle sticking

cals (FSH analogs, corifollitropin alfa being the only CTP form that made it to the market). Such developments in pharmaceutical biotechnology are clearly to the benefit of the patients in need for effective, safe, and convenient treatment options.

REFERENCES

De Leeuw R, Mulders J, Voortman G, Rombout F, Damm J, Kloosterboer L (1996) Structure-function relationship of recombinant follicle stimulating hormone (Puregon®). Mol Hum Reprod 2:361–369

Devroey P, Boostanfar R, Koper NP, Ijzerman P, Mannaerts BMJL, Fauser BC, ENGAGE Investigators (2009) A double-blind, non-inferiority RCT comparing corifollitropin alfa and recombinant FSH during the first seven days of ovarian stimulation using a GnRH antagonist protocol. Hum Reprod 24:3063–3072

European public assessment report Gonal-F (Follitropin alfa), CPMP/415/95. Revision 18, 11 Apr 2011. European Agency for the Evaluation of Medicinal Products

Fares FA, Suganuma N, Nishimori K, LaPolt PS, Hsueh AJ, Boime I (1992) Design of a long-acting follitropin agnosit by fusinh the C-terminal sequence of the beta chorionic gonadotropin subunit. Proc Natl Acad Sci USA 89:4304–4308

Fauser BCJM, Mannaerts BMJL, Devroey P, Leader A, Boime I, Baird DT (2009) Advances in recombinant DNA technology: corifollitropin alfa, a hybrid molecule with sustained follicle-stimulating activity and reduced injection frequency. Hum Reprod Update 15:309–321

Fauser BCJM, Alper MM, Ledger W, Schoolcraft WB, Zandvliet A, Mannaerts BMJL (2010) Pharmacokinetics and follicular dynamics of corifollitropin alfa versus recombinant FSH during controlled ovarian stimulation for in vitro fertilisation. Reprod Biomed Online 21:593–601

Howles CM (1996) Genetic engineering of human FSH (Gonal-F®). Hum Reprod Update 2:172–191

LaPolt PS, Nishimori K, Fares FA, Perlas E, Boime I, Hsueh AJ (1992) Enhanced stimulation of follicle stimulating and ovulatory potential by long acting follicle stimulating hormone agonist with extended carboxy-termial peptide. Endocrinology 131:2514–2520

Mannaerts BMJL, De Leeuw R, Geelen J, Van Ravenstein A, Van Wezenbeek P, Schuurs A, Kloosterboer L (1992) Comparative in vitro and in vivo studies on the biological properties of recombinant human follicle stimulating hormone. Endocrinology 129:2623–2630

Matzuk MM, Hsueh AJ, Lapolt P, Tsafriri A, Keene JL, Boime I (1990) The biological role of the carboxy-terminal extension of human chorionic gonadotropin (corrected) beta-subunit. Endocrinology 126:376–383

Norman RJ, Zegers-Hochschild F, Salle BS, Elbers J, Heijnen E, Marintcheva-Petrova M, Mannaerts B (2011) Repeated ovarian stimulation with corifollitropin alfa in patients in a GnRH antagonist protocol: no concern for immunogenicity. Hum Reprod 26(8):2200–2208

Olijve W, de Boer W, Mulders JWM, van Wezenbeek PMGF (1996) Molecular biology and biochemistry of human recombinant follicle stimulating hormone (Puregon®). Mol Hum Reprod 2:371–382

Olson H, Standström R, Grundemar L (2014) Different pharmacokinetic and pharmodynamic properties of recombinant follicle-stimulating hormone (rFSH) derived from a human cell line compared with rFSH from a non-human cell line. J Clin Pharmacol 54:1299–1307

Rettenbacher M, Andersen AN, Garcia-Velasco JA, Sator M, Barri P, Lindenberg S, van der Veen K, Khalaf Y, Bentin-Ley U, Obruca A, Tews G, Schenk M, Stowitzki T, Narvekar N, Sator K, Inthurn B (2015) A multicenter phase 3 study comparing efficacy and safety of Bemfola versus Gonal-F in women undergoing ovarian stimulation for ivf. Reprod Biomed Online 30: 504–513

van Wezenbeek P, Draaier J, van Meel F, Olijve W (1990) Recombinant follicle stimulating hormone. I. Construction, selection and characterization of a cell line. In: Crommelin DJA, Schellekens H (eds) From clone to clinic, Developments in biotherapy, vol 1. Kluwer, Dordrecht, pp 245–251

Verbost P, Sloot WN, Rose UM, de Leeuw R, Hanssen RGJM, Verheijden GFM (2011) Pharmacologic profiling of corifollitropin alfa, the first developed sustained follicle stimulant. Eur J Pharmacol 651:227–233

Voortman G, van de Post J, Schoemaker RC, Gerwen J v (1999) Bioequivalence of subcutaneous injections of recombinant human follicle stimulating hormone (Puregon®) by Pen-injector and syringe. Hum Reprod 14:1698–1702

SUGGESTED READING

Seyhan A, Ata B (2011) The role of corifollitropin alfa in controlled ovarian stimulation for IVF in combination with GnRH antagonist. Int J Women's Health 3:243–255

20 Human Growth Hormone

Le N. Dao, Barbara Lippe, Michael Laird, and Ingrid Beierle

INTRODUCTION

Human growth hormone (hGH) is a protein hormone essential for normal growth and development in humans. hGH affects many aspects of human metabolism, including lipolysis, the stimulation of protein synthesis, and the inhibition of glucose metabolism. Human growth hormone was first isolated and identified in the late 1950s from extracts of pituitary glands obtained from cadavers and from patients undergoing hypophysectomy. The first clinical use of these pituitary-extracted hGHs for stimulation of growth in hypopituitary children occurred in 1957 and 1958 (Raben 1958). From 1958 to 1985 the primary material used for clinical studies was pituitary-derived growth hormone (pit-hGH). Human growth hormone was first cloned in 1979 (Goeddel et al. 1979; Martial et al. 1979). The first use in humans of recombinant human growth hormone (rhGH) was reported in the literature in 1982 (Hintz et al. 1982). The introduction of rhGH coincided with reports of a number of cases of Creutzfeldt-Jakob disease, a fatal degenerative neurological disorder, in patients receiving pituitary-derived hGH. Concern over possible contamination of the pituitary-derived hGH preparations by the prion responsible for Creutzfeldt-Jakob disease led to the removal of pit-hGH products from the market in the US in 1985 followed by the FDA approval of rhGH later in the year. The initial rhGH preparations were produced in bacteria (*E. coli*) but, unlike endogenous hGH, contained an N-terminal methionine group (met-rhGH). Natural sequence recombinant hGH products have subsequently been produced in bacteria, yeast, and mammalian cells.

HGH STRUCTURE AND ISOHORMONES

The major, circulating form of hGH is a non-glycosylated, 22 kDa protein composed of 191 amino acid residues linked by disulfide bridges in two peptide loops (Fig. 20.1). The three dimensional structure of hGH includes four antiparallel alpha-helical regions (Fig. 20.2) and three mini-helices. Helix 4 and Helix 1 have been determined to contain the primary sites for binding to the growth hormone receptor. In addition, two of the three mini-helices located within the connecting link between Helix 1 and 2 have been shown to play an important role in the binding of growth hormone to its receptor (Root et al. 2002; Wells et al. 1993). Endogenous growth hormone contains a variety of other isoforms including a 20 kDa monomer, disulfide-linked dimers, oligomers, proteolytic fragments, and other modified forms (Boguszewski 2003; Lewis et al. 2000). The 20 kDa monomer, dimers, oligomers, and other modified forms occur as a result of different gene products, different splicing of hGH mRNA, and post-translational modifications. These isoforms are generally expressed at lower amounts compared to the 22 kDa protein (Baumann 2009).

There are two hGH genes in humans, the "normal" hGH-N gene and the "variant" hGH-V gene. The hGH-N gene is expressed in the pituitary gland. The hGH-V gene is expressed in the placenta and is responsible for the production of several variant forms of hGH found in pregnant women. Non-glycosylated and glycosylated isoforms of hGH-V have been identified (Ray et al. 1989; Baumann 1991).

L. N. Dao
Clinical Pharmacology, Genentech Inc., South San Francisco, CA, USA

B. Lippe
Endocrine Care, Genentech Inc, South San Francisco, CA, USA

M. Laird
Division of Medical Affairs, Department of Bioprocess Development, Genentech Inc, South San Francisco, CA, USA

I. Beierle (✉)
Germantown, TN, USA

D. J. A. Crommelin et al. (eds.), *Pharmaceutical Biotechnology*, https://doi.org/10.1007/978-3-030-00710-2_20

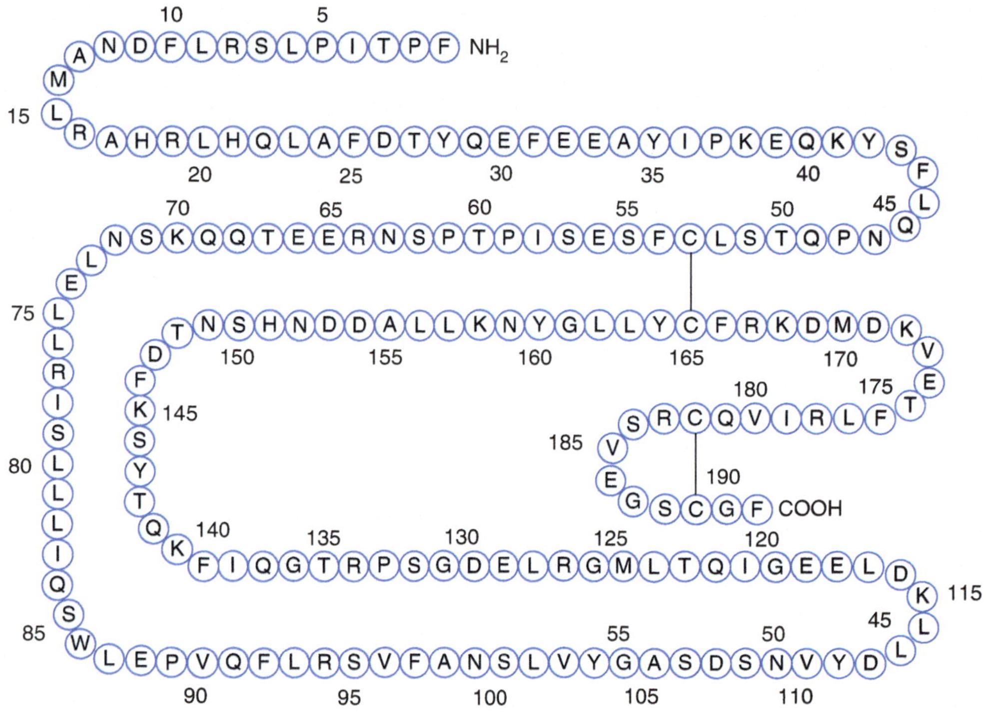

Figure 20.1 ■ Primary structure of recombinant human growth hormone

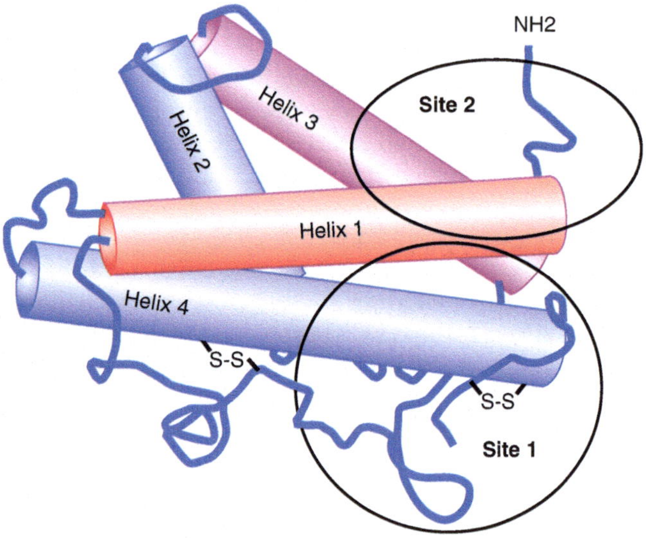

Figure 20.2 ■ Schematic 3-D structure of hGH showing four antiparallel α-helices and receptor binding sites 1 and 2. Approximate positions of the two disulfide bridges (*S-S*) are also indicated (Modified from Wells et al. (1993))

PHARMACOLOGY

■ Growth Hormone Secretion and Regulation

Growth hormone is secreted in a pulsatile manner from somatotrophs in the anterior pituitary. Multiple feedback loops are present in normal regulation of hGH secretion (Casanueva 1992; Giustina and Veldhuis 1998) (Fig. 20.3). Growth hormone release from the pituitary is regulated by a "short loop" of two-coupled hypothalamic peptides—a stimulatory peptide, growth hormone releasing hormone (GHRH), and an inhibitory peptide, somatostatin (also known as somatotropin release-inhibitory factor (SRIF)). GHRH and somatostatin are, in turn, regulated by neuronal input to the hypothalamus and the GH secretagogue, ghrelin (Kojima et al. 2001). There is possibly also an "ultra-short loop" in which hGH release is feedback regulated by growth hormone receptors present on the somatotrophs of the pituitary themselves. Growth hormone secretion is also regulated by a "long loop" of indirect peripheral signals including negative feedback via insulin-like growth factor (IGF-1) and positive feedback via ghrelin. Growth hormone-induced peripheral IGF-1 inhibits somatotroph release of hGH and stimulates somatostatin release.

Growth hormone secretion changes during human development, with the highest production rates observed during gestation and puberty (Giustina and Veldhuis 1998; Brook and Hindmarsh 1992). Growth hormone production declines approximately 10–15% each decade from age 20 to 70. Endogenous hGH secretion also varies with sex, age, nutritional status, obesity, physical activity, and in a variety of disease states. Endogenous hGH is secreted in periodic bursts over a 24-h period with great variability in burst frequency, amplitude, and duration. There is little detectable hGH released from the pituitary between

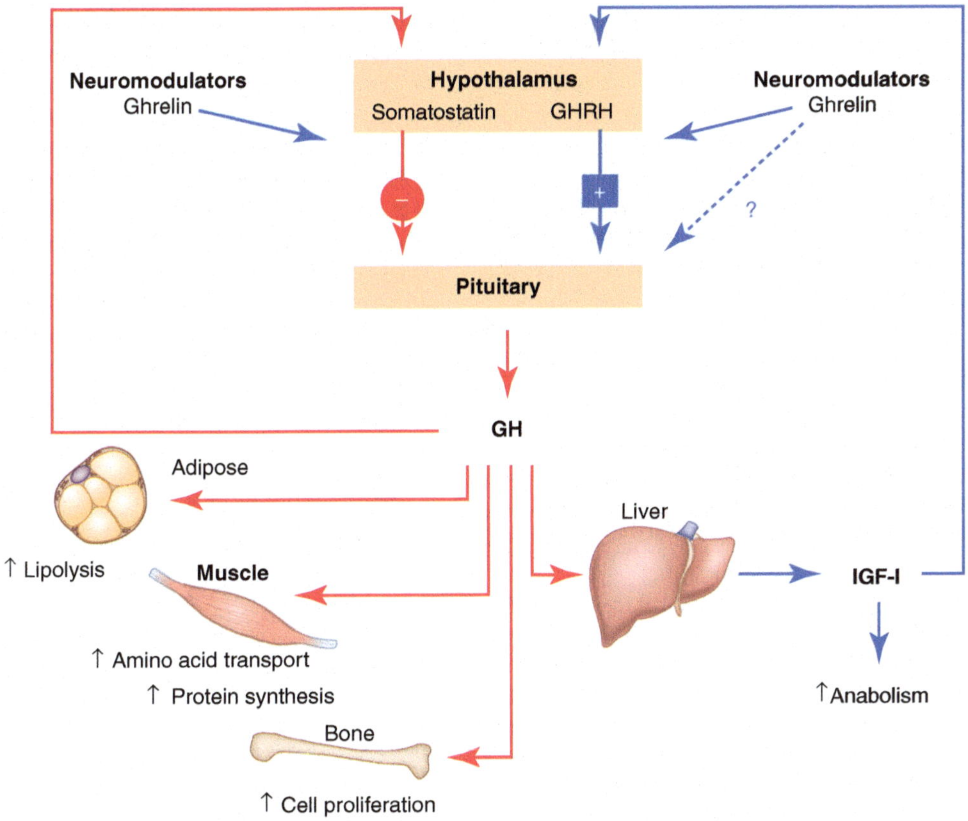

Figure 20.3 ■ Schematic representation of hGH regulation and biologic actions in man. "Short loop" regulation of hGH secretion occurs between the hypothalamus and pituitary. GHRH stimulates GH release. Somatostatin inhibits GH release. "Long loop" regulation of hGH secretion occurs through peripheral feedback signals, primarily negative feedback from insulin-like growth factor 1 (IGF-1). hGH acts directly on muscle, bone, and adipose tissue. Other anabolic actions are generally mediated through IGF-1

bursts. The highest endogenous hGH serum concentrations of 10–30 ng/mL usually occur at night when the secretory bursts are largest and most frequent.

■ Growth Hormone Biologic Actions

hGH has well-defined growth-promoting and metabolic actions. hGH stimulates the growth of cartilage and bone directly, through hGH receptors in those tissues, and indirectly, via local increases in IGF-1 (Isaksson et al. 2000; Bouillon 1991). Metabolic actions, which may be directly controlled by hGH, include the elevation of circulating glucose levels (diabetogenic effect) and acute increases in circulating concentrations of free fatty acids (lipolytic effect). Other hGH anabolic and metabolic actions believed to be mediated through increases in local or systemic IGF-1 concentrations include the following: increases in net muscle protein synthesis (anabolic effect), skeletal muscle growth, chondroblasts and osteoblasts proliferation, and linear growth; modulation of reproduction in both males and females; maintenance, control, and modulation of lymphocyte functions; increases in glomerular filtration rate and renal plasma flow rate (osmoregulation); influences on the release and metabolism of insulin, glucagon, and thyroid hormones (T3, T4); and possible direct effects on pituitary function and neural tissue development (Casanueva 1992; Strobl and Thomas 1994; Le Roith et al. 1991).

■ hGH Receptor and Binding Proteins

The hGH receptor (GHR) is a member of the hematopoietic cytokine receptor family. It has an extracellular domain consisting of 246 amino acids, a single 24-amino-acid transmembrane domain, and a 350-amino-acid intracellular domain (Fisker 2006). The extracellular domain has at least six potential N-glycosylation sites and is usually extensively glycosylated. GHRs are found in most tissues in humans. However, the greatest concentration of receptors in humans and other mammals occurs in the liver (Mertani et al. 1995).

As much as 40–45% of monomeric hGH circulating in plasma is bound to one of two growth hormone binding proteins (GHBP) (Fisker 2006). Binding proteins decrease the clearance of hGH from the circulation (Baumann 1991) and may also serve to dampen the biological effects of hGH by competing with cell receptors for circulating free hGH. The major form of GHBP in humans is a high-affinity (Ka = 10^{-9} to 10^{-8} M), low-capacity form which preferentially binds the 22 kDa form of hGH (Baumann 1991; Herington et al. 1986). Another low-affinity (Ka = 10^{-5} M), high-capacity

GHBP is also present which binds the 20 kDa form with equal or slightly greater affinity than the 22 kDa form. In humans, the high-affinity GHBP is identical to the extracellular domain of the hGH receptor and arises by proteolytic cleavage of hGH receptors by a process called ecto-domain shedding. Since the high-affinity binding protein is derived from hGH receptors, circulating levels of GHBP generally reflect hGH receptor status in many tissues (Fisker 2006; Hansen 2002).

Molecular Endocrinology and Signal Transduction

X-ray crystallographic studies and functional studies of the extracellular domain of the hGH receptor suggest that two receptor molecules form a dimer with a single growth hormone molecule by sequentially binding to Site 1 on Helix 4 of hGH and then to Site 2 on Helix 3 (Fig. 20.4) (Wells et al. 1993). Signal transduction may occur by activation/phosphorylation of JAK-2 tyrosine kinase followed by activation/

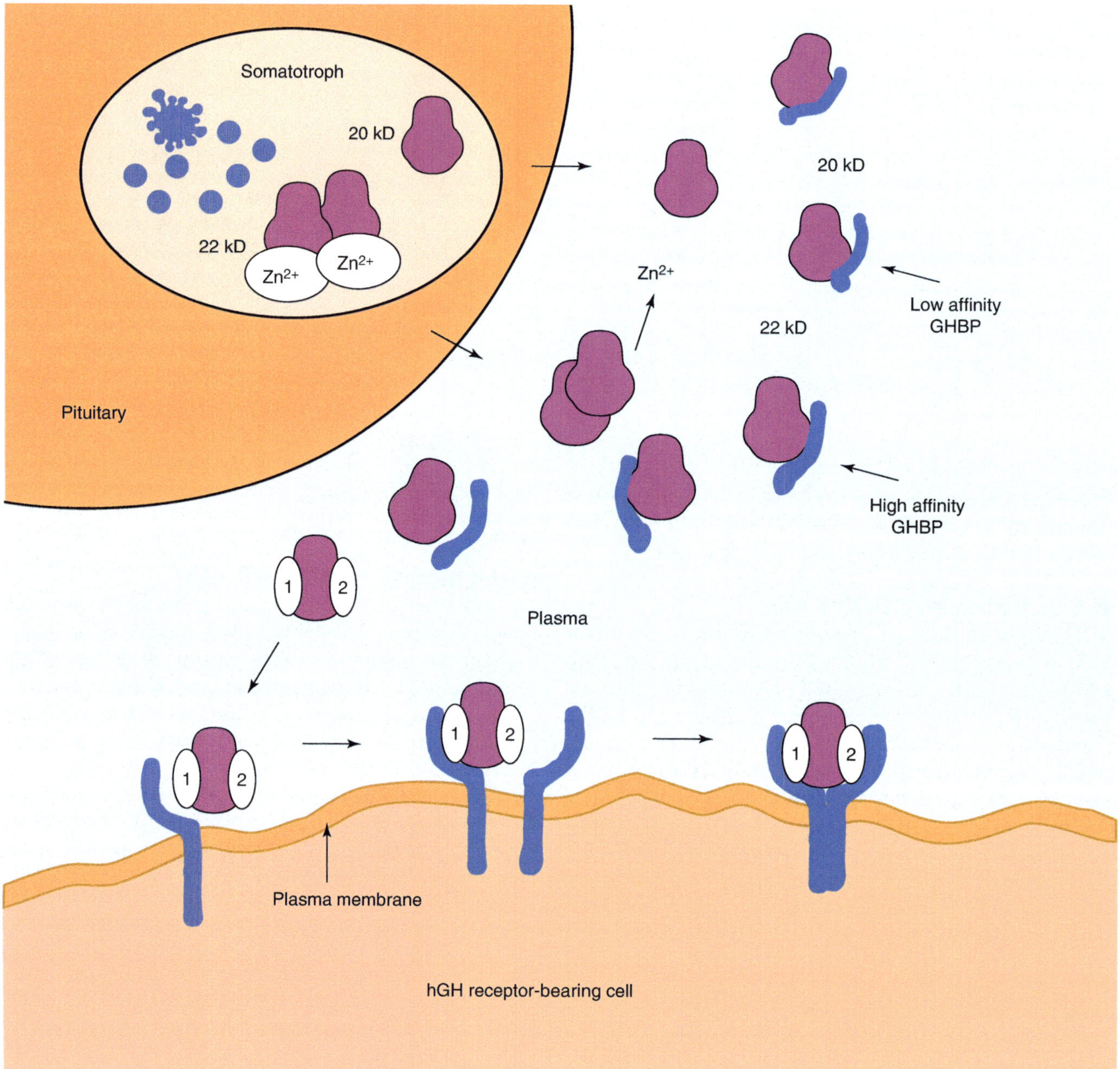

Figure 20.4 ■ Growth hormone secreted isoforms, binding proteins, and receptor interactions. Both 22 and 20 kDa forms are secreted by the pituitary. Pituitary hGH is stored bound to zinc (*Zn^{2+}*) which is released upon secretion from the pituitary. Secreted hGH is free or bound to either the low- or high-affinity GHBP in plasma. Receptor activation involves dimerization of two receptor molecules with 1 molecule of hGH (Modified from Wells et al. (1993))

phosphorylation of multiple signaling cascades (Herrington and Carter-Su 2001; Piwien-Pilipuk et al. 2002; Brooks and Waters 2010).

Dosing Schedules and Routes

The dosing levels and routes for exogenously administered growth hormone were first established for pit-hGH in growth hormone deficient (GHD) patients (Laursen 2004; Jorgensen 1991). The initial pit-hGH regimen, three times weekly by intramuscular (IM) injection, was based on a number of factors including patient compliance and limited availability of hGH derived from cadaver pituitaries and the assumption that intramuscular injections would be less immunogenic. Subsequent clinical evaluations found a very strong patient preference for subcutaneous (SC) administration and data supporting no increased immunogenicity. Furthermore, increased growth rates were observed with daily SC injections compared to the three times weekly injection schedules (MacGillivray et al. 1996). The abdomen, deltoid area, and thigh are commonly used subcutaneous injection sites. Current dosing schedules are usually daily SC injections, often self-administered with a variety of injection devices.

Pharmacokinetics and Metabolism

The earliest pharmacokinetic studies were conducted with pituitary-derived hGH (pit-hGH). The pharmacokinetic profiles of pit-hGH, met-rhGH, and rhGH have been compared (Hansen 2002; Laursen 2004) and shown to be very similar. The pharmacokinetics of hGH have been studied in normal, healthy children and adults and a variety of patient populations (Hansen 2002; Laursen 2004; Jorgensen 1991).

Exogenously administered pit-hGH, met-rhGH, and rhGH are rapidly cleared following intravenous (IV) injection with terminal half-lives of approximately 15–20 min (Hansen 2002; Laursen 2004). Distribution volumes usually approximate the plasma volume. hGH clearance in normal subjects ranges from 2.2 to 3.0 mL/kg/min. hGH clearance decreases with increasing serum GH concentrations, most likely due to saturation of hGH receptors at concentrations >10–15 μg/L (Hansen 2002). Comparative analyses of total hGH clearance have not shown consistent population differences based on age, sex, or body composition. However, hGH clearance is controlled by a complex interaction between free hGH, GHBP-bound hGH, and GH receptor status (Hansen 2002). Individual subject variations in GHBP or GH receptor levels may result in substantial differences in hGH clearance.

Human growth hormone is slowly, but relatively completely, absorbed after either IM or SC injection. Time to peak concentration ranges from 2 to 4 h following IM bolus administration and 4 to 6 h following SC bolus administration (Laursen 2004; Jorgensen 1991). Subcutaneously administered rhGH is approximately 50–80% bioavailable (Laursen 2004). The rate of absorption of hGH is slightly faster after injection in the abdomen compared with the thigh (Laursen 2004), but the extent of absorption is comparable. Elimination half-lives following extravascular administration (2–5 h) are usually longer than the IV terminal half-lives indicating absorption rate-limited kinetics.

hGH pharmacokinetics in the presence of growth hormone deficiency, diabetes, obesity, and critical illness or diseases of the thyroid, liver, and kidney have been evaluated. Results suggest disposition is not significantly altered compared with normal subjects except in severe liver or kidney dysfunction (Hansen 2002; Haffner et al. 1994; Owens et al. 1973; Cameron et al. 1972). The reduction in clearance observed in severe liver (30%) or kidney dysfunction (40–75%) is consistent with the role of the liver and kidney as major organs of hGH elimination.

Both the kidney and the liver have been shown to be important in the clearance of hGH in humans (Hansen 2002). The relative contribution of each organ has not been rigorously quantified in humans, but the preponderance of studies in laboratory animals and in isolated perfused organ systems suggests a dominant role for the kidney at pharmacologic levels of hGH. Receptor-mediated uptake of hGH by the liver is the major extrarenal clearance mechanism (Harvey 1995).

PROTEIN MANUFACTURE, FORMULATION, AND STABILITY

Commercially available hGH preparations are summarized in Table 20.1. All recombinant growth hormones except Serostim®/Saizen®/Zorbtive® are produced in bacteria (*E. coli*). Serostim®/Saizen®/Zorbtive® are produced in mammalian cells (C127 mouse cells). Growth hormone produced in the cytoplasm of *E. coli* may contain an N-terminal methionine residue. Natural sequence rhGH is produced either by enzymatic cleavage of the methionine residue during the purification process or by secreting the rhGH into the periplasmic space where the signal peptide is removed by the cell and the native N-terminus of rhGH is revealed. rhGH can be produced in the periplasm in a soluble, properly folded form (Chang et al. 1989) or as refractile/inclusion bodies which require the insoluble rhGH to be extracted, denatured, and refolded (Shin et al. 1998) (cf. Chap. 4). The rhGH is released from the cells by osmotic shock (periplasm) or mechanical lysis (cytoplasm & periplasm), and the protein is recovered and purified. rhGH synthesized in mammalian cells is transported across the endoplasmic reticulum and secreted directly

Source	Brand names	Product	Container	Injection device	Manufacturer
Recombinant protein produced in bacteria (*E. coli*)	Genotropin®	Lyophilized powder	Two-chamber cartridge	Genotropin Pen®	Pfizer
		Multiple-dose cartridge: 5 and 12 mg		Genotropin Miniquick®	
		Single-dose Miniquick cartridge: 0.2–2 mg		Genotropin Mixer®	
	Norditropin®	Liquid 5 mg/1.5 mL, 10 mg/1.5 mL, 15 mg/1.5 mL, 30 mg/3 mL	Prefilled, preloaded pen device	Norditropin FlexPro®	Novo Nordisk
	Nutropin AQ®	Liquid 5 mg/2 mL, 10 mg/2 mL, 20 mg/2 mL	Prefilled, preloaded pen device	Nutropin AQ® NuSpin	Genentech, Inc
	Humatrope®	Lyophilized powder Vial: 5 mg/5 mL Cartridge: 6 mg/3 mL, 12 mg/3 mL, 24 mg/3 mL	Vial and cartridge	Single-use syringe HumatroPen™	Eli Lilly & Co.
	Zomacton®	Lyophilized powder 5 mg/5 mL, 10 mg/1 mL	Vial	Single-use syringe	Ferring
				Needle-free device: Zoma-Jet™ 5/10	
	Omnitrope®	Lyophilized powder Vial: 5.8 mg/1.14 mL	Vial	Single use syringe	Sandoz
		Liquid Cartridge: 5 mg/1.5 mL, 10 mg/1.5 mL	Cartridge	Omnitrope® pen	
Recombinant protein produced in mammalian cells (C127 mouse cell line-derived)	Serostim® (AIDS wasting)	Lyophilized powder Single dose vial: 5 mg, 6 mg; diluent: sterile water for injection Multi dose vial: 4 mg; diluent: bacteriostatic water for injection	Vial	Syringe Needle free devive: SeroJet™	Serono
	Saizen® (growth inadequacy)	Lyophilized powder Vial: 5 mg, 8.8 mg; diluent: bateriostatic water for injection	Vial	Single-use syringe	
		Saizenprep® single use reconstituition mixing device with Saizen 8.8 mg vial and bateriostatic water for injection catridge		one.click® pen	
				easypod® drug delivery device	
	Zorbtive® (short bowel syndrome)	Lyophilized powder Multi Dose Vial: 8.8 mg; diluent: bateriostatic water for injection	Vial	Single-use syringe	

Note: This table represents rhGH products currently availalble in the US and is not meant to be an exhaustive list of globally available marketed hGH products

Table 20.1 ■ Recombinant hGH products

into the culture medium from which it is recovered and purified (Catzel et al. 2003).

Historically, the potency of hGH products was expressed in International Units per mg (IU/mg). The initial standard, established in 1982 for pit-hGH preparations, was 2 IU/mg. The standard for rhGH products was 2.6 IU/mg until September 1994. The current WHO standard, established in September 1994, is 3.0 IU/mg. Dosages are usually expressed as IU/kg or IU/m^2 in Europe and Japan and as mg/kg in the USA. However, the use of IU dosages is no longer necessary due to the high level of purity and consistent potency of recombinant hGH products.

All current rhGH products are available as lyophilized or liquid preparations. Lyophilized formulations usually include 5 or 10 mg of protein in a glycine and mannitol or sucrose-containing phosphate buffer excipient. The materials are usually reconstituted with sterile water for injection for single use or with bacteriostatic water or bacteriostatic saline for multiple injection use. Liquid formulations of rhGH (Norditropin®, Nutropin AQ®, Omnitrope®) contain excipients such as mannitol or sodium chloride, histidine or citrate buffer, poloxamer 188 or polysorbate 20, and phenol or benzyl alcohol. Product stability has been very good with shelf lives of approximately 2 years at 2–8 °C. The lyophilized rhGH preparation of Omnitrope® was approved for marketing as the first "biosimilar" rhGH product in the EU and the US in 2006. Two strengths of Omnitrope® (5 and 10 mg cartridges) were approved for marketing in 2008 for use in pen devices (Omnitrope Pen®).

CLINICAL USAGE

Clinical usage of rhGH has been reviewed for pediatric and adult indications (Franklin and Geffner 2011). Investigations of clinical usage of hGH have focused, generally, on two major areas of hGH biologic action: (1) linear growth promotion and (2) modulation of metabolism. Growth-promoting indications in children which have been approved for the market include growth hormone deficiency, idiopathic short stature, growth failure associated with chronic renal insufficiency, growth failure in children born small for gestational age, and short stature in Prader-Willi syndrome, Turner's syndrome, Noonan syndrome, and short stature homeobox-containing gene deficiency on the X chromosome (SHOX). Modulation of metabolism is the primary biologic action in long-term replacement therapy in adults with GH deficiency of either childhood or adult onset or for GH supplementation in AIDS wasting or cachexia and in short bowel syndrome. Contraindications to rhGH use include use in patients with active malignancy, active proliferative or severe nonproliferative retinopathy, acute critical illness, children with Prader-Willi syndrome (PWS) who are severely obese or have severe respiratory impairment, children with closed epiphyses, and hypersensitivity to somatropin or excipients.

■ Growth Hormone Deficiency (GHD)

The major indication for therapeutic use of hGH is the long-term replacement treatment for children with classic growth hormone deficiency in whom growth failure is due to a lack of adequate endogenous hGH secretion. Children with GHD fall into a variety of etiologic categories including genetic defects in the hypothalamic pituitary axis, developmental anomalies of the brain with or without identifiable syndromes, acquired events such as CNS lesions (craniopharyngioma most commonly) or from the treatment of CNS tumors (medulloblastoma, gliobastoma, etc.), trauma, or other events requiring CNS irradiation. When diagnosed in otherwise healthy children, it is called idiopathic. In patients suspected of having GHD, the diagnosis is usually defined based on an inadequate response to two hGH provocation tests implying a functional deficiency in the production or secretion of hGH from the pituitary gland. In patients with documented organic causes, especially if panhypopituitarism is present, two stimulation tests may not be required. Usual doses range from 0.24 to 0.30 mg/kg/week administered as daily SC injections in prepubertal children. Doses up to 0.7 mg/kg/week have been approved for GHD adolescent subjects to improve final height based on a clinical trial (Mauras et al. 2000) showing hGH treatment results in increased growth velocity and enhancement in final adult height. For most GHD children the growth response is greatest in the first year of treatment and correlates positively with hGH dose, degree of short stature, and frequency of injections and negatively with chronological age at onset of treatment. hGH therapy in children is usually continued until growth has been completed, as evidenced by epiphyseal fusion. rhGH treatment of idiopathic GH-deficient children has a positive overall safety profile documented in long-term clinical registries (Bell et al. 2010; Darendeliler et al. 2007). However, in those with organic causes, the safety profile may be dependent on the underlying medical condition and its prior treatment. In childhood cancer survivors, an increased risk of a second neoplasm has been reported in patients treated with somatropin after their first neoplasm (Sklar et al. 2002), and this information is communicated under warnings and precautions in the product labels.

■ Idiopathic Short Stature (ISS)

Idiopathic short stature (ISS) comprises a heterogeneous group of growth failure states for which the proximate cause remains unknown. Postulated defects include impaired spontaneous hGH secretion, hGH resistance due to low levels of hGH receptors, or other defects in either secreted hGH, hGH receptors or post-receptor events, or other genetic defects yet to be elucidated. Nevertheless, studies have documented that many patients in the "idiopathic" group respond to exogenous growth hormone treatment with acceleration of growth and improvement in final height. As a consequence of several long-term multicenter trials to final height, rhGH was approved for the treatment of ISS in the United States (Hintz et al. 1999; Leschek et al. 2004). The risk benefit assessment of improved growth in what is generally considered to be a population of "healthy" children continues to be debated, and while short-term safety has been documented (Bell et al.

2010), long-term safety is still a question that is being addressed by a multi-country study in Europe looking at adult patients treated with rhGH as children. Based on preliminary data and published reports (Carel et al. 2012; Savendahl et al. 2012), the FDA and the EMA preliminary assessments are that there should be no change in prescribing information with emphasis on adherence to approved dosages.

■ Turner Syndrome (TS)

Turner syndrome is a disease of females caused by partial or total loss of one sex chromosome and is characterized by decreased intrauterine and postnatal growth, short final adult height, incomplete development of the ovaries and secondary sexual characteristics, and other physical abnormalities. Although serum levels of hGH and IGF-1 are not consistently low in this population, hGH treatment (0.375 mg/kg/week), alone or in combination with oxandrolone, significantly improves growth rate and final adult height in this patient group, and its use in Turner syndrome is now an accepted indication (Rosenfeld et al. 1998; Kappelgaard and Laursen 2011).

■ Prader-Willi Syndrome (PWS)

Prader-Willi syndrome is a genetic disease usually caused by the functional deletion of a gene on the paternal allele of chromosome 15. Clinical manifestations in childhood include lack of satiety, obesity, hypotonia, short stature, hypogonadism, and behavioral abnormalities. PWS children have especially high rates of morbidity due to obesity-related illnesses. Growth hormone treatment (0.24–0.48 mg/kg/week) has been shown to improve height and, perhaps more importantly, improve body composition, physical strength, and agility in PWS children (Allen and Carrel 2004). However, growth hormone treatment is contraindicated in the face of severe obesity or severe respiratory impairment since sudden deaths in this group of patients, when treated with growth hormone, have been reported.

■ Small for Gestational Age (SGA)

Growth hormone is approved for use in long-term treatment of growth failure in children born small for gestational age who fail to manifest catch-up growth. Children born at birth weights and birth lengths more than two standard deviations below the mean are considered small for gestational age. Children who fail to catch up by age two to three are at risk for growing into adults with substantial height deficits (Rappaport 2004). Growth hormone treatment at doses of 0.24–0.48 mg/kg/week can induce catch-up growth, with the potential to normalize height at an earlier age and the potential to improve adult height.

■ Chronic Renal Insufficiency (CRI)/Chronic Kidney Disease (CKD)

Children with renal insufficiency, which is termed chronic kidney disease (CKD), grow slowly, possibly related to defects in metabolism, nutrition, metabolic bone disease, and/or defects in the IGF-1/hGH axis. Basal serum hGH concentrations may be normal or high, and IGF-1 responses to hGH stimulation is usually normal. However, there are reported abnormalities in the IGF-binding protein levels in CKD patients suggesting possible problems with GH/IGF-1 action. Growth hormone therapy (0.35 mg/kg/week) in children with chronic renal insufficiency results in significant increases in height velocity (Greenbaum et al. 2004). Increases are best during the first year of treatment for younger children with stable renal disease. Responses are less for children on dialysis. Growth hormone has not been approved for children posttransplant.

■ Noonan Syndrome

First called male Turner syndrome due to similar phenotypic characteristics, Noonan syndrome, an autosomal dominant disorder, was later recognized as a separate condition. It occurs in both males and females. Its key features are short stature (although some patients will achieve normal adult height), congenital heart disease, most commonly pulmonic stenosis or hypertrophic cardiomyopathy, a short and often webbed neck, ptosis, and chest/sternum deformities. While the GH/IGF axis is intact in Noonan syndrome, and the mechanisms through which the mutations cause short stature are unknown, clinical trials with rhGH demonstrated significant increases in growth rate and modest increases in final height (Osio et al. 2005), resulting in FDA approval of this indication in 2007. Pediatric patients with short stature associated with Noonan syndrome are given up to a rhGH dose of 0.066 mg/kg/day. Safety concerns in treatment with rhGH have been raised with respect to progression of cardiomyopathy although data to date do not support this clinical concern.

■ Short Stature Homeobox-Containing Gene (SHOX)

The SHOX gene is located on the pseudoautosomal region of the X chromosome and the homologous distal region on the Y chromosome. Healthy males and females express two active copies of the SHOX gene, one from each of the sex chromosomes. Females with TS missing an X chromosome or part of an X chromosome have one copy of the SHOX gene. A significant percentage of the growth failure in TS females is secondary to this gene loss. The variably expressed SHOX gene in long bones tends to be in the mesomelic segments. Mutations resulting in haploinsufficiency of SHOX are also responsible for the short stature in some patients with a pseudoautosomal dominant condition of mesomelic dyschondrosteosis called Leri-Weill syndrome. In addition, sporadic mutations are also responsible for short stature in a small percentage of patients who would otherwise be characterized as idiopathic short stature (Rao et al. 1997). A multicenter study of a heterogeneous group of patients with SHOX haploinsufficiency demonstrated a clinically significant effect of rhGH on growth in children with SHOX mutations compared to the untreated control group. In addition, the efficacy of rhGH treatment was similar to that seen in a comparable group of girls with TS, leading to approval of the SHOX indication (Blum et al. 2007). The FDA-approved rhGH dose for SHOX deficiency is 0.35 mg/kg/week. To date no specific safety signals attributable to rhGH treatment have emerged in these children.

■ Growth Hormone Deficient Adults

Early limitations in hGH supply severely limited treatment of adults with GHD. With the increased supply of recombinant rhGH products, replacement therapy for adults was evaluated and, ultimately, approved as a clinical indication. Growth hormone has been approved for two growth hormone deficient adult populations: (a) adults with childhood-onset GHD and (b) adults with adult-onset GHD usually due to pituitary tumors, CNS irradiation, or head trauma. Growth hormone treatment (starting dose of 0.006 mg/kg/day, increased according to individual requirements to a maximum of 0.025 mg/kg/day in patients under 35 years old and 0.0125 mg/kg/day in patients over 35 years old, or a starting dose of 0.2 mg/day and progressing based on IGF and clinical symptoms) reduces body fat, increases lean body mass, and increases exercise capacity. Increases in bone density have been observed in some bone types although treatment duration greater than 1 year may be necessary to see significant effects. hGH treatment consistently elevates both serum IGF-1 and insulin levels. Women have also been shown to require higher doses to normalize IGF-1 levels than men, especially women taking oral estrogens.

■ Clinical Malnutrition and Wasting Syndromes

Growth hormone is approved for treatment of short bowel syndrome (SBS) in adults, a congenital or acquired condition in which less than ~200 cm of small intestine is present. Short bowel syndrome patients have severe fluid and nutrient malabsorption and are often dependent upon intravenous parenteral nutrition (IPN). Administration of growth hormone, 0.1 mg/kg/day to a maximum of 8 mg for 4 weeks, alone or in combination with glutamine, reduces the volume and frequency of required IPN (Keating and Wellington 2004). Growth hormone is indicated for use in adult patients who are also receiving specialized nutritional support. Usage for periods >4 weeks, or in children, has not been investigated. Usage of growth hormone for SBS remains controversial due to potential risks associated with IGF-1-related fibrosis and cancer (Theiss et al. 2004).

Growth hormone is also approved for use in wasting associated with AIDS. Growth hormone treatment (~0.1 mg/kg daily, max. 6 mg/day), when used with controlled diets, increases body weight and nitrogen retention. rhGH treatment is also under investigation for HIV-associated lipodystrophy, a syndrome of fat redistribution and metabolic complications resulting from the highly active antiretroviral therapy commonly used in HIV infection (Burgess and Wanke 2005).

■ Other Conditions Under Investigation

Growth hormone levels and IGF decline with age, prompting the initiation of multiple clinical trials for use in adults over age 60 (Di Somma et al. 2011). However, clear long-term efficacy in muscle strength or improvements in activities of daily life have not been sufficiently demonstrated to gain regulatory approval for this indication. The use of hGH therapy to ameliorate the negative nitrogen balance seen in patients following surgery, injury, or infections has been investigated in a number of studies (Takala et al. 1999; Jeevanandam et al. 1995; Ponting et al. 1988; Voerman et al. 1995). However, due to the increased mortality found in a study of severe critical illness (Takala et al. 1999) and the subsequent contraindication for use in acute critical illness, very few registration trials examining the use of hGH for these conditions have been initiated. Studies of hGH effects in burns have shown significant effectiveness in acceleration of healing in skin graft donor sites and improvements in growth in burned children (Herndon and Tompkins 2004). Growth hormone has been shown to significantly reduce multiple disease symptoms and improve well-being and growth in children and adults with Crohn's disease, a chronic inflammatory disorder of the bowel (Theiss et al. 2004; Slonim et al. 2000; Denson et al. 2010). Growth hormone has also shown benefit in cardiovascular recovery and function in congestive heart failure (Colao et al. 2004). Recent studies indicate that growth hormone treatment improves growth, pulmonary function, and clinical status in children with cystic fibrosis (Stalvey et al. 2012).

■ Safety Concerns

hGH has been widely used for many years and has been proven to have a positive safety profile for most pediatric indications (Growth Hormone Research Society 2001). However, sudden death in some patients with PWS and severe obesity associated with rhGH treatment resulted in a contraindication to its use in severely obese or respiratory compromised PWS children (Eiholzer 2005). Adverse events have been reported in a small number of children and include benign intracranial hypertension, glucose intolerance, and the rare development of anti-hGH antibodies. In most cases, the formation of anti-hGH antibodies following rhGH treatment has not been positively correlated with a loss in efficacy.

Growth hormone therapy is also not associated with increased risk of primary malignancies or tumor recurrence (Growth Hormone Research Society 2001; Sklar et al. 2002). However, an increase in secondary malignancies in childhood cancer survivors, especially those treated with CNS irradiation, has been described (Sklar et al. 2002).

Growth hormone inhibits 11β-hydroxysteroid dehydrogenase type 1 (11βHSD-1) activity in adipose/hepatic tissue and may impact the metabolism of cortisol and cortisone (Gelding et al. 1998). Treatment with rhGH could potentially unmask undiagnosed central adrenal insufficiency (secondary hypoadrenalism) or increase the requirement for maintenance or stress doses of replacement corticosteroid in those already diagnosed with adrenal insufficiency.

Growth hormone has caused significant, dose-limiting fluid retention in adult populations resulting in increased body weight, swollen joints and arthralgias, and carpal tunnel syndrome (Carroll and van den Berghe 2001). Symptoms were usually transient and resolved upon reduction of hGH dosage or upon discontinuation of the hGH treatment. Growth hormone administration has been associated with increased mortality in clinical trials in critically ill, intensive-care patients with acute catabolism (Takala et al. 1999) and is, therefore, contraindicated for use in critically ill patients.

Growth hormone's anabolic and lipolytic effects have made it attractive as a performance enhancement drug among athletes. Illicit hGH usage has been anecdotally reported for the last 20 years. Detection of rhGH abuse proximate to the time of testing is now possible due to the development of assays which rely on detecting changed ratios of exogenous rhGH (22 kDa only) and endogenous hGH (22 kDa, 20 kDa and other forms). Screening for proximate rhGH abuse, based on the new ratio assays, was included in the 2006 Olympic Games for the first time (McHugh et al. 2005).

CONCLUDING REMARKS

The abundant supply of rhGH, made possible by recombinant DNA technology, has allowed enormous advances to be made in understanding the basic structure, function, and physiology of hGH over the past 20 years. As a result of those advances, recombinant hGH has been developed into a safe and efficacious therapy for a variety of growth and metabolic disorders in children and adults. Continuing basic research in GH and IGF-1 biology, genomics, and GH-related diseases and continuing clinical investigation into additional uses in pediatric growth disorders or disorders of metabolism may yield as yet new indications for treatment.

SELF-ASSESSMENT QUESTIONS

Questions

1. One molecule of hGH is required to sequentially bind to two receptor molecules for receptor activation. What consequences might the requirement for sequential dimerization have on observed dose–response relationships?
2. Growth hormone is known or presumed to act directly upon which tissues?
3. You are investigating the use of hGH as an adjunct therapy for malnutrition/wasting in a clinical population which also has severe liver disease. What effects would you expect the liver disease to have on the observed plasma levels of hGH after dosing and on possible efficacy (improvement in nitrogen retention, prevention of hypoglycemia, etc.)?

Answers

1. Sequential dimerization will potentially result in a "bell-shaped" dose–response curve, i.e., response is stimulated at low concentrations and inhibited at high concentrations. The inhibition of responses at high concentrations is due to blocking of dimerization caused by the excess hGH saturating all the available receptors. Inhibition of in vitro hGH binding is observed at high hGH (mM) concentrations. Reductions in biological responses (total IGF-1 increase and weight gain) have also been seen with increasing hGH doses in animal studies. However, inhibitory effects of high concentrations of hGH are not seen in treatment of human patients since hGH dose levels are maintained within normal physiological ranges and never approach inhibitory levels.
2. Growth hormone is known to act directly on both bone and cartilage and possibly also on muscle and adipose tissue. Growth hormone effects on other tissues appear to be mediated through the IGF-1 axis or other effectors.
3. Severe liver disease may reduce the clearance of the exogenously administered hGH, and observed plasma levels may be higher and persist longer compared to patients without liver disease. However, the increased drug exposure may not

result in increased anabolic effects. The desired anabolic effects require the production/release of IGF-1 from the liver. Both IGF-1 production and the number of hGH receptors may be reduced due to the liver disease. To understand the results (or lack of results) from the treatment, it is important to monitor effect parameters (i.e., IGF-1 and possibly IGF-1 binding protein levels, liver function enzymes) in addition to hGH levels.

REFERENCES

Allen DB, Carrel AL (2004) Growth hormone therapy for Prader-Willi syndrome: a critical appraisal. J Pediatr Endocrinol Metab 17:1297–1306

Baumann G (1991) Growth hormone heterogeneity: genes, isohormones, variants and binding proteins. Endocr Rev 12:424–449

Baumann GP (2009) Growth hormone isoforms. Growth Horm IGF Res 19:333–340

Bell J, Parker KL, Swinford RD, Hoffman AR, Maneatis T, Lippe B (2010) Long-term safety of recombinant human growth hormone in children. J Clin Endocrinol Metab 95:167–177

Blum WF, Crowe BJ, Quigley CA, Jung H, Cao D, Ross JL, Braun L, Rappold G, Shox Study Group (2007) Growth hormone is effective in treatment of short stature associated with short stature homeobox-containing gene deficiency: two-year results of a randomized, controlled, multicenter trial. J Clin Endocrinol Metab 92:219–228

Boguszewski CL (2003) Molecular heterogeneity of human GH: from basic research to clinical implications. J Endocrinol Invest 26:274–288

Bouillon R (1991) Growth hormone and bone. Horm Res 36(Suppl 1):49–55

Brook CGD, Hindmarsh PC (1992) The somatotropic axis in puberty. Endocrinol Metab Clin North Am 21:767–782

Brooks AJ, Waters MJ (2010) The growth hormone receptor: mechanism of activation and clinical implications. Nat Rev Endocrinol 6(9):515–525

Burgess E, Wanke C (2005) Use of recombinant human growth hormone in HIV-associated lipodystrophy. Curr Opin Infect Dis 18:17–24

Cameron DP, Burger HG, Catt KJ et al (1972) Metabolic clearance of human growth hormone in patients with hepatic and renal failure, and in the isolated perfused pig liver. Metabolism 21:895–904

Carel J-C, Ecosse E, Landier F, Meguellati-Hakkas D, Kaguelidou F, Rey G, Coste J (2012) Long-term mortality after recombinant growth hormone treatment for isolated growth hormone deficiency or childhood short stature: preliminary report of the French SAGhE study. J Clin Endocrinol Metab 97:416–425. https://doi.org/10.1210/jc.2011-1995

Carroll PV, van den Berghe G (2001) Safety aspects of pharmacological GH therapy in adults. Growth Horm IGF Res 11:166–172

Casanueva F (1992) Physiology of growth hormone secretion and action. Endocrinol Metab Clin North Am 21:483–517

Catzel D, Lalevski H, Marquis CP, Gray PP, Van Dyk D, Mahler SM (2003) Purification of recombinant human growth hormone from CHO cell culture supernatant by Gradiflow preparative electrophoresis technology. Protein Expr Purif 32(1):126–234

Chang JY, Pai RC, Bennett WF, Bochner BR (1989) Periplasmic secretion of human growth hormone by Escherichia coli. Biochem Soc Trans 17(2):335–337

Colao A, Vitale G, Pivonello R et al (2004) The heart: an end-organ of GH action. Eur J Endocrinol 151:S93–S101

Darendeliler F, Karagiannis G, Wilton P (2007) Headache, idiopathic intracranial hypertension and slipped capital femoral epiphysis during growth hormone treatment: a safety update from KIGS. Horm Res 68(Suppl 5):41–47

Denson LA, Kim MO, Bezold R et al (2010) A randomized controlled trial of growth hormone in active pediatric Crohn disease. J Pediatr Gastroenterol Nutr 51:130–139

Di Somma C, Brunelli V, Savanelli MC et al (2011) Somatopause: state of the art. Minerva Endocrinol 36:243–255

Eiholzer U (2005) Deaths in children with Prader-Willi syndrome: a contribution to the debate about the safety of growth hormone treatment in children with PWS. Horm Res 63(1):33–39

Fisker S (2006) Physiology and pathophysiology of growth hormone binding protein: methodological and clinical aspects. Growth Horm IGF Res 16:1–28

Franklin SL, Geffner ME (2011) Growth hormone: the expansion of available products and indications. Endocrinol Metab Clin North Am 38:587–611

Gelding SV, Taylor NF, Wood PJ, Noonan K, Weaver JU, Wood DF, Monson JP (1998) The effect of growth hormone replacement therapy on cortisol-cortisone interconversion in hypopituitary adults: evidence for growth hormone modulation of extrarenal 11 beta-hydroxysteroid dehydrogenase activity. Clin Endocrinol (Oxf) 48(2):153–162

Giustina A, Veldhuis JD (1998) Pathophysiology of the neuroregulation of growth hormone secretion in experimental animals and in the human. Endocr Rev 19(6):717–797

Goeddel DV, Heyreker HL, Hozumi T et al (1979) Direct expression in Escherichia coli of a DNA sequence coding for human growth hormone. Nature 281:544–548

Greenbaum LA, Del Rio M, Bamgbola F et al (2004) Rationale for growth hormone therapy in children with chronic kidney disease. Adv Chronic Kidney Dis 11(4):377–386

Growth Hormone Research Society (2001) Critical evaluation of the safety of recombinant human growth hormone administration: statement from the Growth Hormone Research Society. J Clin Endocrinol Metab 86(5):1868–1870

Haffner D, Schaefer F, Girard J et al (1994) Metabolic clearance of recombinant human growth hormone in health and chronic renal failure. J Clin Invest 93:1163–1171

Hansen TK (2002) Pharmacokinetics and acute lipolytic actions of growth hormone: impact of age, body

composition, binding proteins and other hormones. Growth Horm IGF Res 12:342–358
Harvey S (1995) Growth hormone metabolism. In: Harvey S, Scanes CG, Daughaday WH (eds) Growth hormone. CRC Press, Inc, Boca Raton, pp 285–301
Herington AC, Ymer S, Stevenson J (1986) Identification and characterization of specific binding proteins for growth hormone in normal human sera. J Clin Invest 77:1817–1823
Herndon DN, Tompkins RG (2004) Support of the metabolic response to burn injury. Lancet 363:1895–1902
Herrington J, Carter-Su C (2001) Signaling pathways activated by the growth hormone receptor. Trends Endocrinol Metab 12(6):252–257
Hintz RL, Rosenfeld RG, Wilson DM et al (1982) Biosynthetic methionyl human growth hormone is biologically active in adult man. Lancet 1:1276–1279
Hintz RL, Attie KM, Baptista J, Roche A (1999) Effect of growth hormone treatment on adult height of children with idiopathic short stature. N Engl J Med 340:502–507
Isaksson OG, Ohlsson C, Bengtsson B et al (2000) GH and bone-experimental and clinical studies. Endocr J 47(Suppl):S9–S16
Jeevanandam M, Ali MR, Holaday NJ et al (1995) Adjuvant recombinant human hormone normalizes plasma amino acids in parenterally fed trauma patients. J Parenter Enteral Nutr 19:137–144
Jorgensen JOL (1991) Human growth hormone replacement therapy: pharmacological and clinical aspects. Endocr Rev 12:189–207
Kappelgaard AM, Laursen T (2011) The benefits of growth hormone therapy in patients with Turner syndrome, Noonan syndrome, and children born small for gestational age. Growth Horm IGF Res 21(6):305–313
Keating GM, Wellington K (2004) Somatropin (zorbtive™) in short bowel syndrome. Drugs 64(12):1375–1381
Kojima M, Hosoda H, Matsuo H et al (2001) Ghrelin: discovery of the natural endogenous ligand for the growth hormone secretagogue receptor. Trends Endocrinol Metab 12(3):118–126
Laursen T (2004) Clinical pharmacological aspects of growth hormone administration. Growth Horm IGF Res 14:16–44
Le Roith D, Adamo M, Werner H, Roberts CT Jr (1991) Insulin-like growth factors and their receptors as growth regulators in normal physiology and pathologic states. Trends Endocrinol Metab 2:134–139
Leschek EW, Ross SR, Yanovski JA, Troendle JF, Quigley CA, Chipman JJ, Crowe BJ et al (2004) Effect of growth hormone treatment on adult height in peripubertal children with idiopathic short stature: a randomized, double blind, placebo-controlled trial. J Clin Endocrinol Metab 89:3140–3148
Lewis UJ, Sinhda YN, Lewis GP (2000) Structure and properties of members of the hGH family: a review. Endocr J 47:S1–S8
MacGillivray MH, Baptista J, Johanson A (1996) Outcome of a four-year randomized study of daily versus three times weekly somatropin treatment in prepubertal naïve growth hormone deficient children. J Clin Endocrinol Metab 81:1806–1809
Martial JA, Hallewell RA, Baxter JD (1979) Human growth hormone: complementary DNA cloning and expression in bacteria. Science 205:602–607
Mauras N, Attie KM, Reiter EO et al (2000) High dose recombinant human growth hormone (GH) treatment of GH-deficient patients in puberty increases near-final height: a randomized, multicenter trial. J Clin Endocrinol Metab 85:3653–3660
McHugh CM, Park RT, Sonksen PH et al (2005) Challenges in detecting the abuse of growth hormone in sport. Clin Chem 51(9):1587–1593
Mertani HC, Delehaye-Zervas MC, Martini JF et al (1995) Localization of growth hormone receptor messenger RNA in human tissues. Endocrine 3:135–142
Osio D, Dahlgren J, Wikland KA, Westphal O (2005) Improved final height with long-term growth hormone treatment in Noonan syndrome. Acta Paediatr 94(9):1232–1237
Owens D, Srivastava MC, Tompkins CV et al (1973) Studies on the metabolic clearance rate, apparent distribution space and plasma half-disappearance time of unlabelled human growth hormone in normal subjects and in patients with liver disease, renal disease, thyroid disease and diabetes mellitus. Eur J Clin Invest 3:284–294
Piwien-Pilipuk G, Huo JS, Schwartz J (2002) Growth hormone signal transduction. J Pediatr Endocrinol Metab 15:771–786
Ponting GA, Halliday D, Teale JD et al (1988) Postoperative positive nitrogen balance with intravenous hyponutrition and growth hormone. Lancet 1:438–440
Raben MS (1958) Treatment of a pituitary dwarf with human growth hormone. J Clin Endocrinol Metab 18:901–903
Rao E, Weiss B, Fukami M et al (1997) Pseudoautosomal deletions encompassing a novel homeobox gene cause growth failure in idiopathic short stature and Turner syndrome. Nat Genet 16:54–63
Rappaport R (2004) Growth and growth hormone in children born small for gestational age. Growth Horm IGF Res 14:S3–S6
Ray J, Jones BK, Liebhaber SA, Cooke NE (1989) Glycosylated human growth hormone variant. Endocrinology 125(1):566–568
Root AW, Root MJ et al (2002) Clinical pharmacology of human growth hormone and its secretagogues. Curr Drug Targets Immune Endocr Metabol Disord 2:27–52
Rosenfeld RG, Attie KM, Frane J et al (1998) Growth hormone therapy of Turner's syndrome: beneficial effect on adult height. J Pediatr 132:319–324
Savendahl L, Maes M, Albersson K, Borgstrom B, Carel J-C, Henrad S, Speybroeck N, Thomas M, Xandwijken G, Hokken-Koelega A (2012) Long-term mortality and causes of death in isolated GHD, ISS and SGA patients treated with recombinant growth hormone during childhood in Belgium, the Netherlands, and Sweden: preliminary report of a 3 countries participating in the EU SAGhE study. J Clin Endocrinol Metab 97:E213–E217. https://doi.org/10.1210/jc.2011-2882

Shin NK, Kim DY, Shin CS, Hong MS, Lee J, Shin HC (1998) High-level production of human growth hormone in Escherichia coli by a simple recombinant process. J Biotechnol 62(2):143–151

Sklar CA, Mertens AC, Mitby P et al (2002) Risk of disease recurrence and second neoplasms in survivors of children cancer treated with growth hormone: a report from the Childhood Cancer Survivor Study. J Clin Endocrinol Metab 87(7):3136–3141

Slonim AE, Bulone L, Damore MB et al (2000) A preliminary study of growth hormone therapy for Crohn's disease. N Engl J Med 342:1633–1637

Stalvey MS, Anbar RD, Konstan MVV, Jacobs JR, Bakker B, Lippe B, Geller DE (2012) A multi-center controlled trial of growth hormone treatment in children with cystic fibrosis. Pediatr Pulmonol 47:252–263. https://doi.org/10.1002/ppul.21546

Strobl JS, Thomas MJ (1994) Human growth hormone. Pharm Rev 46:1–34

Takala J, Ruokonen E, Webster NR et al (1999) Increased mortality associated with growth hormone treatment in critically ill adults. N Engl J Med 341(11):785–792

Theiss AL, Fruchtman S, Lund PK (2004) Growth factors in inflammatory bowel disease. The actions and interactions of growth hormone and insulin-like growth factor-I. Inflamm Bowel Dis 10(6):871–880

Voerman BJ, van Schijndel RJMS, Goreneveld ABJ et al (1995) Effects of human growth hormone in critically ill nonseptic patients: results from a prospective, randomized, placebo-controlled trial. Crit Care Med 23:665–673

Wells JA, Cunningham BC, Fuh G et al (1993) The molecular basis for growth hormone-receptor interactions. Recent Prog Horm Res 48:253–275

SUGGESTED READING

Boguszewski CL (2003) Molecular heterogeneity of human GH: from basic research to clinical implications. J Endocrinol Invest 26:274–288

Brooks AJ, Waters MJ (2010) The growth hormone receptor: mechanism of activation and clinical implications. Nat Rev Endocrinol 6(9):515–525

Fisker S (2006) Physiology and pathophysiology of growth hormone binding protein: methodological and clinical aspects. Growth Horm IGF Res 16:1–28

Giustina A, Veldhuis JD (1998) Pathophysiology of the neuroregulation of growth hormone secretion in experimental animals and in the human. Endocr Rev 19(6):717–797

Harvey S, Scanes CG, Daughaday WH (eds) (1995) Growth hormone. CRC Press, Inc, Boca Raton

Harris M, Hofman PL, Cutfield WS (2004) Growth hormone treatment in children. Pediatr Drugs 6(2):93–106

Laursen T (2004) Clinical pharmacological aspects of growth hormone administration. Growth Horm IGF Res 14:16–44

Simpson H, Savine R, Sonksen P et al (2002) Growth hormone replacement therapy for adults: into the new millennium. Growth Horm IGF Res 12:1–33

21 Recombinant Coagulation Factors and Thrombolytic Agents

Koen Mertens and Alexander B. Meijer

INTRODUCTION

Blood coagulation and fibrinolysis are two sides of the same coin: the hemostatic system. Hemostasis involves the interplay of the coagulation cascade with activated blood platelets and the vessel wall. This results in the formation of a thrombus, which comprises activated platelets and cross-linked fibrin. Thrombus formation is counterbalanced by coagulation inhibitors on the one hand, and the fibrinolytic system on the other hand. Upon vascular injury, coagulation *(thrombus formation)* serves to achieve local bleeding arrest, while fibrinolysis *(thrombus dissolution)* prevents obstruction of blood flow elsewhere in the circulation. Disruption of the balance between these mechanisms can cause malfunction of the hemostatic system, and becomes manifest as bleeding or thrombosis. Bleeding disorders are usually due to a defect or deficiency in one of the constituents of the coagulation cascade, and can be treated by substitution therapy to compensate for the missing component. Thrombotic disorders comprise two distinct forms: venous and arterial thrombosis. Venous thrombosis results from excessive coagulation and can ultimately lead to pulmonary embolism, while arterial thrombosis is associated with atherosclerosis, stroke and acute coronary syndrome, the major indication for thrombolytic therapy. This chapter focuses on the recombinant biopharmaceuticals that are currently available for the treatment of bleeding and thrombosis.

The Essentials of Blood Coagulation and Fibrinolysis

Formation and Dissolution of the Hemostatic Plug

While the network of hemostasis and thrombosis is generally perceived as being a complex issue in physiology, understanding the essentials thereof will greatly facilitate appreciation of the biopharmaceuticals used in this area, and in particular of the pharmacodynamics thereof. As schematically depicted in Fig. 21.1, the system can be divided into three distinct sections. The left part (panel a) comprises the coagulation cascade. This is an ordered conversion of proenzymes into active enzymes that leads to the activation of prothrombin into thrombin. Once the initial amounts of thrombin are formed, it catalyzes a variety of enzymatic conversions. These include a self-amplifying loop by feedback activation of several other components upstream in the cascade, and self-dampening of its own formation by activating an enzyme that specifically inactivates essential cofactors in the cascade. The central part (panel b) summarizes how thrombin drives the formation of the hemostatic plug, initially by activating platelets and by converting fibrinogen into fibrin polymers, and subsequently by activating factor XIII, which then cross-links fibrin into a stable network. The right section (panel c) represents the fibrinolytic system, in which activators like tissue-type plasminogen activator (t-PA) convert plasminogen into the enzyme plasmin that degrades cross-linked fibrin into soluble fragments, resulting in lysis of the hemostatic plug.

The Network of Coagulation Factors

Why do we need so many coagulation factors? The answer lies in the various regulatory steps, which allow the mechanism to act as a biological amplifier that rapidly responds to injury, while at the same time the process should remain restricted to the site of injury. The apparent complexity of the coagulation scheme in Fig. 21.1 (panel a) merits some further explanation. Apart from a few exceptions, the proteins in this system ('factors') are indicated by roman numerals, with the suffix 'a' referring to their activated form. This nomenclature dates from 1959, and has been implemented to resolve confusion by the coexistence of multiple names for the same component. For some factors, however, the old names have remained in use, such as fibrinogen (factor I), prothrombin (factor II) and Tissue Factor (factor III). The terms factor IV and factor VI are

K. Mertens (✉) · A. B. Meijer
Department of Pharmaceutical Sciences, Utrecht Institute for Pharmaceutical Sciences, Utrecht University, Utrecht, The Netherlands
e-mail: k.mertens@uu.nl

D. J. A. Crommelin et al. (eds.), *Pharmaceutical Biotechnology*, https://doi.org/10.1007/978-3-030-00710-2_21

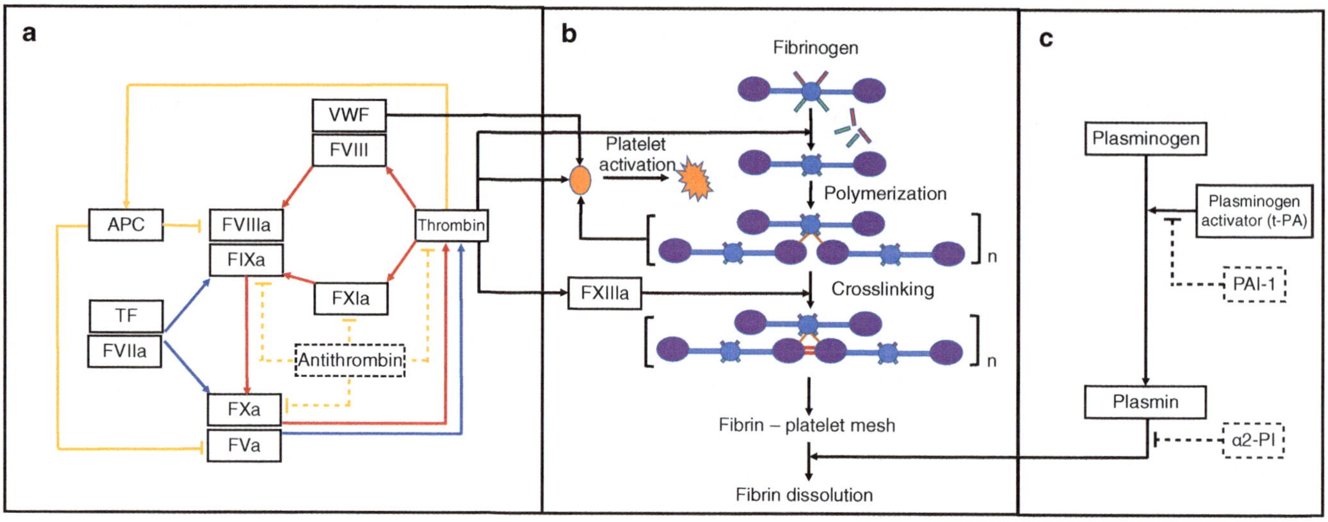

Figure 21.1 Schematic representation of hemostasis. Panel (**a**) the coagulation cascade; Panel (**b**) the hemostatic plug; Panel (**c**) the fibrinolytic system. The various pathways and constituents thereof are described in the text. Roman numerals refer to the individual coagulation factors. Von Willebrand factor is abbreviated as *VWF*, *APC* activated protein C, *TF* tissue factor, *PAI-1* plasminogen activator inhibitor-1, *α2-PI* α2-plasmin inhibitor

obsolete, as they have never been assigned to a specific protein. Of the other coagulation factors, numbers V and VIII are cofactors, while the remaining numbers VII and IX to XII are proenzymes of serine proteases that catalyze the sequential steps in the cascade (Furie and Furie 1988).

The concept of an ordered sequence of reactions as a cascade or waterfall has first been described in 1964 (Davie and Ratnoff 1964; Macfarlane 1964) and has remained essentially unaltered since then. What did change, however, is the insight into the various feed-back effects of thrombin upstream in the cascade. This introduced a distinction between successive stages in thrombin formation, which are often referred to as *initiation*, *propagation* and *termination* (Mann et al. 2009). In each of these phases, different sections of the cascade predominate. These can be summarized as follows:

1. In the *initiation phase*, indicated by *blue arrows* in Fig. 21.1a, vascular injury leads to the exposure of tissue factor (TF). The cascade then runs from FVIIa/TF to FXa/FVa complex to the conversion of prothrombin into thrombin. The initially formed thrombin starts activating platelets and cleaving fibrinogen into fibrin (Fig. 21.1b), and at the same time initiates the self-amplifying propagation loop.
2. This *propagation phase*, indicated by *red arrows*, involves the activation of factor XI (FXI) and the cofactors factor VIII (FVIII) and factor V (FV). The cascade then runs from FXIa (or FVIIa) to FIXa/FVIIIa complex, and further from FXa/FVa complex to generate large amounts of thrombin. The main difference between the initiation and the propagation phase is that the latter comprises an additional amplifying step, which involves FVIII and FIX.
3. Finally, in the *termination phase*, indicated by the *yellow arrows*, thrombin binds to an endothelial receptor (thrombomodulin), and activates Protein C. Once activated, this inactivates the cofactors FVIIIa and FVa and thereby causes thrombin formation to shut-down. The activated coagulation enzymes are neutralized by antithrombin (*yellow dashed lines*)

Local Control Mechanisms

How do the various mechanisms indicated in Fig. 21.1 remain localized to the site of injury? One reason is that assembly of enzyme-cofactor complexes in coagulation cascade requires membranes containing acidic phospholipids, which are exposed on perturbed cells such as activated platelets, but not on resting cells. Moreover, any excess of activated factors is neutralized by protease inhibitors that occur in plasma. These include tissue factor pathway inhibitor, which inhibits at the level of factor VIIa, and antithrombin, an inhibitor of most of the other enzymes from the cascade. Similar considerations apply to the fibrinolytic system (Fig. 21.1c). First, most t-PA is stored in vascular cells and released upon perturbation, while levels of t-PA in the circulation are low. Second, plasmin needs its substrate, fibrin, to express full fibrinolytic activity. Finally, the circulating inhibitors plasminogen activator inhibitor-1 (PAI-1) and α2-plasmin inhibitor (α2-PI) neutralize excess of their target proteases (indicated by dashed lines in Fig. 21.1c).

■ Hemostatic Disorders

There is little or no redundancy within the intricate protein network involved in the formation and dissolution of the hemostatic plug. Therefore, deficiency or dysfunction of a single component may have a severe impact. The consequences thereof can include both bleeding and thrombosis. Deficiency of most of the coagulation factors results in a bleeding tendency, while a shortage of coagulation inhibitors such as antithrombin or protein C predisposes for thrombosis. Likewise, thrombosis may also result from a defect in the fibrinolytic pathway, while bleeding has been associated with a deficiency in α2-plasmin inhibitor. The incidence of deficiencies in hemostatic proteins is summarized in Table 21.1 (adapted from Bishop and Lawson 2004 and Palla et al. 2015). In affected patients, bleeding can be treated by administering the missing plasma protein. This may be of human origin, as a concentrate derived from human plasma, or a biopharmaceutical from recombinant sources. Table 21.1 lists the availability of such protein therapeutics. It is evident that, with a few exceptions, recombinant products have been clustering around the field of hemophilia, which due to its relatively high incidence represents the most significant market.

Hemophilia and Other Bleeding Disorders

Hemophilia is the best-known bleeding disorder, as it occurred in several European royal families, including the Romanov dynasty in Russia. These descendants of the British Queen Victoria had a defect in the gene encoding in factor IX, and thus suffered from hemophilia B (Rogaev et al. 2009). The more frequent disorder, however, is hemophilia A, or factor VIII deficiency. Hemophilia A and B are clinically indistinguishable, which may be expected from their place in the coagulation cascade: whether the enzyme or the cofactor moiety in the FVIIIa/FIXa complex is missing, it disrupts the biological amplifier that drives the propagation phase in thrombin generation (see Fig. 21.1). Hemophilia differs from the other inherited bleeding disorders in that the genes encoding factor VIII and factor IX are located on the X-chromosome. The inheritance pattern is X-linked recessive, and mutation in the single X-chromosome in males is sufficient to cause the deficiency. In females, however, the same mutation in one X-chromosome results in heterozygosity, and in factor levels which, although reduced, still are sufficient to support normal hemostasis.

The other coagulation factor deficiencies do not display this sex-linked pattern, and a complete deficiency thereof will need a defect in both chromosomes (homozygous or compound heterozygous). For most of these deficiencies, often referred to as the Rare Bleeding Disorders, substitution therapy is available, albeit to a limited extent, in the form of concentrates from human blood (see Table 21.1).

The most common bleeding disorder is von Willebrand's disease. This is caused by a deficiency or dysfunction of von Willebrand factor, a large multimeric adhesion protein that mediates the interaction between activated platelets and the perturbed vessel wall at the site of injury. As such, von Willebrand factor is an essential constituent of the hemostatic plug (see Fig. 21.1b). Besides its role as adhesion protein, von Willebrand factor serves as carrier of factor VIII in the circulation, and protects factor VIII from degradation and premature clearance. Within von Willebrand's

Deficiency	Incidence	Bleeding phenotype	Availability of products for substitution therapy	
			Human plasma-derived	Recombinant
Fibrinogen (factor I)	1 in 1 million	None to severe	Few	None
Prothrombin (factor II)	1 in 2 million	Mild to moderate	Common	None
Factor V	1 in 1 million	Moderate	One (under evaluation)	None
Factor VII	1 in 500,000	Mild to severe	Few	Factor VIIa only
Factor VIII (hemophilia A)	1 in 5000 males	Moderate to severe	Common	Several (see Table 15.2)
Factor IX (hemophilia B)	1 in 25,000 males	Moderate to severe	Common	Several (see Table 15.3)
Factor X	1 in 1 million	Mild to severe	Common	None
Factor XI	1 in 1 million	Mild to moderate	Few	None
Factor XIII	1 in 2 million	Moderate to severe	Few	One
von Willebrand factor	~1 in 1000	Mild to severe	Common	One
α2-plasmin inhibitor	very rare	Mild to severe	None	None
Antithrombin	~1 in 5000	Thrombotic phenotype	Common	One

Table 21.1 ■ Incidence of coagulation factor deficiencies

disease, a variety of subtypes can be distinguished, with partial quantitative deficiency and different molecular defects (for review see Castaman and Linari 2017). Only the most severe deficiency (type III, 1–2% of all cases) requires substitution therapy with von Willebrand factor-containing therapeutics.

Thrombosis

While protein substitution therapy is a straightforward approach for stopping or preventing bleeding, management of thrombosis is more complex. Partial deficiencies of antitrombin or protein C are risk factors that predispose for venous thrombosis, but usually multiple, often acquired risk factors, are involved. The mechanisms involved in thrombosis are beyond the scope of the present chapter, and have been reviewed elsewhere (Mackman 2008). Treatment involves dampening the coagulation cascade, or inhibiting platelet activation, usually by small molecules rather than by protein therapeutics. Protein substitution therapy remains limited to some specific cases of antithrombin deficiency.

As for arterial thrombosis, this is associated with atherosclerosis. After rupture of an atherosclerotic plaque, a platelet-rich thrombus may lead to arterial occlusion, which then may result in ischemia, myocardial infarction or stroke (Lusis 2000; Mackman 2008). In such situations, lysis of the occluding thrombus is the immediate target. This can be accomplished by infusing large amounts of plasminogen activator. The medical need for such thrombolytic therapy is high. This explains why tissue-type plasminogen activator, after human insulin and human growth hormone, was among the first recombinant protein therapeutics that reached the market.

RECOMBINANT FACTOR VIII

In the early 1980s, the factor VIII cDNA has been cloned by two independent groups, one collaborating with Genentech (Vehar et al. 1984), and another with Genetics Institute (Toole et al. 1984). This provided access to the biotechnological development of recombinant factor VIII. Factor VIII was among the largest proteins characterized at that time. The factor VIII gene spans 180 kb, and comprises 26 exons that together encode a polypeptide of 2351 amino acids. This includes a signal peptide of 19 amino acids and a mature protein of 2332 amino acids. As reviewed in detail elsewhere (Lenting et al. 1998; Fay 2004), factor VIII displays the ordered domain structure A1-*a1*-A2-*a2*-B-*a3*-A3-C1-C2 (see Fig. 21.2a). The triplicated A-domains share homology with the copper-binding protein ceruloplasmin, while the two C-domains are structurally related to lipid-binding proteins such as lactadherin. The A-domains are bordered by short

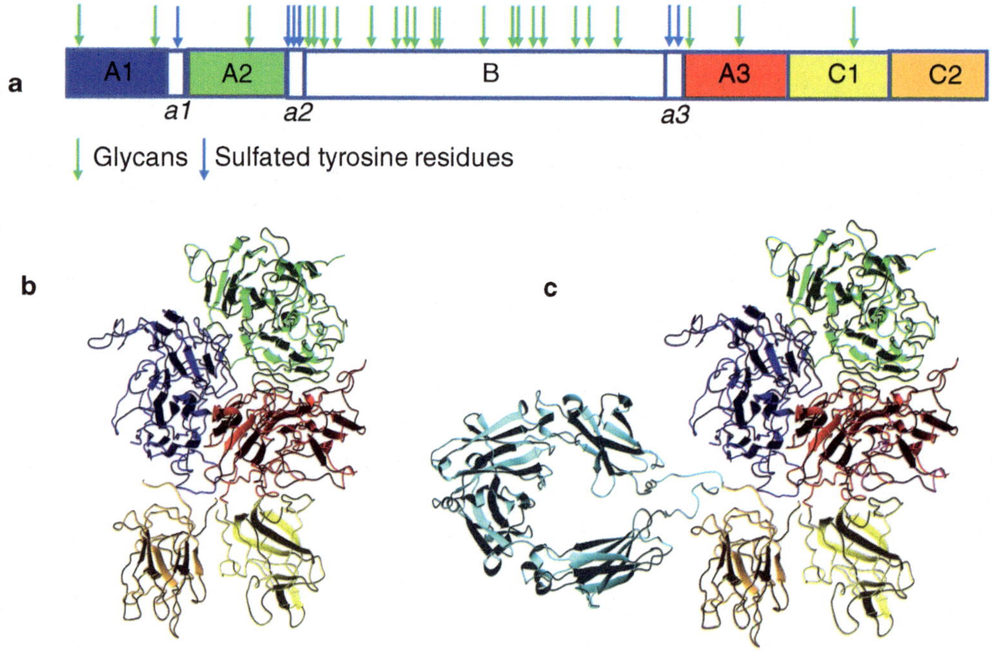

Figure 21.2 ■ Structure of factor VIII. Panel (**a**) displays the domain structure of full-length factor VIII. Panel (**b**) represents the 3D-structure of B-domain-deleted factor VIII (derived from pdb 2R7E), and panel (**c**) is the same structure with the Fc fragment of IgG1 (from pdb 1HZA) fused to the C-terminus of the C2-domain

spacers (*a1*, *a2*, and *a3*) that are also known as acidic regions. These spacers contain sulfated tyrosine residues that are needed for full biological activity.

The central B-domain carries the vast majority of the glycosylation sites in factor VIII. Due to processing at the junction B-*a3*, mature factor VIII is secreted as a heterodimer of heavy chain (A1-*a1*-A2-*a2*-B), and light chain (*a3*-A3-C1-C2). In the circulation, the B-domain is subject to cleavage at multiple sites, resulting in size heterogeneity without apparent consequence for biological activity (Andersson et al. 1986). Thus, about one third of the factor VIII protein seems dispensable for biological activity. Indeed, recombinant expression of a factor VIII variant lacking a major part of the B-domain proved functionally normal (Toole et al. 1986). For B-domain deleted factor VIII, several crystal structures are available. These reveal a compact cluster of the three A-domains, supported by a tandem of the two C-domains, in a side-by-side orientation (Fig. 21.2b). This structure represents the inactive factor VIII, and conversion into factor VIIIa involves cleavage at the *a1*-A2, *a2*-B and *a3*-A3 junctions. The resulting heterotrimer is the molecular form that participates in the coagulation cascade.

Factor VIII Products

Due the size and complexity of the factor VIII protein, mammalian cells need to be used as expression system. Commonly used cells are CHO (chinese hamster ovary), BHK (baby hamster kidney) and HEK (human embryonic kidney) or engineered derivatives thereof. Post-translational modifications (see Fig. 21.2a) include glysosylation, and the sulfation of specific tyrosine residues in the *a1*, *a2* and *a3* segments. One particular challenge is its low expression, as factor VIII tends to accumulate intracellularly, which is cytotoxic for the host cells. Another challenge is the instability of the factor VIII once secreted. Over the past 30 years, these issues have been resolved by a limited number of manufacturers only. An overview of the various products is given in Table 21.2.

Full–Length Factor VIII

The first generation of recombinant factor VIII was intended to provide exact copies of the natural protein from human plasma, which had been established as being effective in the treatment of hemophilia A since the 1960s. The first products, Kogenate (developed at Genentech and Bayer) and Recombinate (developed at Genetics Institute and Baxter) were licensed in 1992. In order to enhance secretion and stability, Recombinate was produced by co-expression with von Willebrand factor, which was removed during downstream processing. The simultaneous expression of these two exceptionally large polypeptides was a remarkable achievement in the early years of biopharmaceuticals.

Both Kogenate and Recombinate were produced using human albumin-containing culture medium, and employed an albumin-containing formulation for the final product. As such, these initial products were actually plasma-derived, except that the active ingredient was produced through recombinant technology. In 2000, Kogenate has been replaced by Kogenate-FS, with an albumin-free formulation. In 2016, this was followed by Kovaltry, which employs co-expression with heat shock protein-70 to facilitate factor VIII expression in protein-free medium (Table 21.2). As for Recombinate, a protein-free equivalent (Advate) became available in 2003. A PEGylated variant thereof, Adynovate, was licensed in 2015 (see below, section extended half-life factor VIII).

B-Domain Deleted (BDD) Factor VIII

The finding that the central B-domain is dispensable for in vitro activity (Toole et al. 1986) formed the basis for the design of a variety of deletion mutants. An advantage of B-domain deletion is that this greatly improves factor VIII expression. The first BDD-factor VIII was ReFacto (developed at Pharmacia/Pfizer), which was followed in 2009 by the protein-free equivalent ReFacto-AF/Xyntha. Other BDD-factor VIII products have slightly different deletions (see Table 21.2). All of them have conserved a small N-terminal part of the B-domain, in order to maintain the thrombin cleavage site at the *a2*-B junction (position 740–741). Moreover, most constructs have retained the processing site at the B-*a3* junction (position 1648–1649) and consequently are, like wild-type factor VIII, heterodimeric molecules (NovoEight, Nuwiq). An exception is Afstyla, which is a single-chain molecule because the deletion extends into the *a3* segment. Despite the differences between the individual constructs, these BDD-factor VIII products, once activated, are fully indistinguishable from wild-type factor VIIIa, because the B-domain remnant and the *a3*-section are released upon activation. Other BDD factor VIII products, in particular those that have been engineered to extend half-life (see in Table 21.2), may still contain the introduced modification within their activated form (see following section).

Extended Half-Life Factor VIII

One limitation of factor VIII replacement therapy is the relatively short half-life, which may vary between 10 and 17 h (see Table 21.2). Half-life extension would provide an obvious therapeutic advancement. Over the past few years several products have been developed to pursue this goal. Thus, the original paradigm that recombinant factor VIII should be identical to the natural protein has started shifting towards engineering to improve on nature.

Adynovate is a PEG (polyethylene glycol)-ylated full-length factor VIII, based on Advate. It contains on

Product type	INN name	(*Investigational*) product name(s)	First approval (USA/EU)	Half-life (mean, h)	Production technology	Reference
Full-length FVIII	Octocog alfa	Recombinate	1992	12	CHO cells, co-expression with VWF, albumin in culture and formulation	
		Advate	2003	10–14	as Recombinate, but without protein in culture, albumin-free formulation	
		Kogenate Helixate	1992	14–17	BHK cells, albumin in culture and formulation	
		Kogenate-FS	2000	14–17	as Kogenate, but with albumin-free formulation	
		Kovaltry, Iblias (*BAY 81–8973)*	2016	13	BHK, co-expression with HSP-70, protein-free culture and formulation,	Maas Enriquez et al. (2016)
	Rurioctocog alfa pegol	Adynovate (*BAX 855)*	2015	14–16	as Advate, 20 kDa pegylation to extend half-life	Turecek et al. (2012)
B-domain deleted FVIII	Moroctocog alfa	ReFacto	1999	14	CHO cells, deletion of amino acids 744–1637, albumin in culture, not in formulation	
		ReFacto-AF Xyntha	2008	13	as ReFacto, albumin-free culture and formulation	
	Turoctogoc alfa	NovoEight (*N8)*	2013	11	CHO cells, deletion of amino acids 751–1637, albumin-free culture and formulation	Thim et al. (2010)
	Simoctocog alfa	Nuwiq	2014	17	HEK cells, B-domain replaced by 16 amino acid linker, protein-free culture and formulation	Sandberg et al. (2012)
	Lonoctocog alfa	Afstyla (*rVIII-SingleChain)*	2016	14	CHO cells, deletion of amino acids 765–1652, single-chain molecule, albumin-free	Schmidbauer et al. (2015)
	Efmoroctocog alfa	Eloctate, Elocta (*rFVIIIFc)*	2014	20	HEK cells, deletion of amino acids 744–1637, dimeric IgG1-Fc fused to FVIII C2-domain	Leksa et al. (2017)
	Damoctocog alfa pegol	Jivi (*BAY 94–9027)*	2018	~19	HEK-hybrid cells, deletion of amino acids 743–1636, Lys-1804 substituted by Cys for site-specific 40 kDa pegylation in the A3-domain	Mei et al. (2010)
	Turoctocog alfa pegol	*N8GP*	pending	~19	as NovoEight, with site-specific glycopegylation in residual B-domain segment	Stennicke et al. (2013)

Table 21.2 ■ Recombinant factor VIII products

average two moles of branched 20 kDa PEG per factor VIII molecule. Approximately 60% of the PEG chains are located in the B-domain, and thus are lost upon activation. The remaining modifications are randomly dispersed over the rest of the protein, and, by virtue of the low extent of PEGylation, do not interfere in any known functional interaction (Turecek et al. 2012).

Eloctate is a fusion between BDD-factor VIII and the Fc fragment of IgG. This serves to target factor VIII to the FcRn receptor recycling pathway that endows IgG and albumin with their long half-life (see Chaps. 6 and 8). The fusion of the Fc fragment to the factor VIII C-terminus yields a derivative in which the activated form is non-natural in that it still carries the Fc moiety. Surprisingly, this C-terminal extension conserves factor VIII's potency, presumably because the Fc portion is loosely attached and, besides the linker sequence, has no specific interaction with the factor VIII surface (Leksa et al. 2017). On the other hand, the fusion protein displays aberrant response in some activity assays used for therapy monitoring (see section Clinical considerations).

One additional product in this category is currently under consideration by EMA and FDA, and may become licensed shortly. This is a PEGylated version of NovoEight (N8-GP, see Table 21.2). This is modified with a branched 40 kDa PEG using enzymatic glycoconjugation, which is targeted to the single O-linked glycan in the short B-domain remnant. Because the PEG moiety is released upon activation, the active form is the natural, unmodified factor VIIIa. Another strategy has been used for the recently approved Jivi (BAY 94–9027, see Table 21.2), developed by Bayer. This employs cysteine-targeted PEGylation with a branched 60 kDa PEG. This cysteine is introduced by mutagenesis in the factor VIII A3-domain. The PEG moiety remains conserved after activation, and thus the active species in this product is non-natural. This has some impact on activity assays used for monitoring (see section Clinical considerations).

The benefit of these half-life extensions seems limited (Table 21.2). For the current four products, cross-over studies reported a 1.5 to 1.7-fold half-life prolongation over an unmodified comparator (Peyvandi et al. 2013). So far, this seems to be the maximum achievable prolongation by such modification strategies. This apparent limitation is because factor VIII, whether or not modified to extend its half-life, circulates in complex with the recipient's endogenous von Willebrand factor. Therefore, the clearance of von Willebrand factor remains the major driver of factor VIII's half-life (Pipe et al. 2016).

■ Pharmacology

The term factor VIII, or Anti-Hemophilic Factor in the early US literature, has been introduced before the protein had been identified. Factor VIII was defined by its function, as the activity that corrects the clotting defect of hemophilic plasma. This functional definition has remained the basis for the quantification of factor VIII since then, and factor VIII concentrations are expressed in units, where one unit represents the amount of factor VIII activity in 1 ml of normal human plasma. Besides in units/ml, factor VIII levels in plasma are often also expressed as % of normal. Thus, assessment of product potency, dosing and pharmacokinetics is based on bioassays, with their inherent variability.

Pharmacokinetics

The pharmacokinetics of factor VIII is largely dependent on the plasma level of von Willebrand factor, which stabilizes factor VIII and protects against premature clearance. As reviewed in detail elsewhere (Björkman and Berntorp 2001), systemic clearance in patients with normal von Willebrand factor levels is typically 3 ml/h/kg, with an apparent distribution volume that slightly exceeds the patient's plasma volume, and an average elimination half-life of approximately 14 hours. While assessment of pharmacokinetics is mandatory for all individual factor VIII products, there is quite some variability between data reported (see Iorio 2017 and Table 21.2). Apart from variation between patients, also technical issues contribute to this variation, such as the sampling time points, and the dependence on bioassays for the determination of the administered dose and of plasma levels post-infusion. Given this variability, the pharmacokinetics of the various recombinant factor VIII products can be considered as being essentially similar, with the exception of those products that have been engineered to extend half-life.

Pharmacodynamics

Hemophilia A is a congenital deficiency or dysfunction of factor VIII which, dependent on the residual level of factor VIII activity, is categorized as mild (6–40%), moderate (1–5%) or severe (<1% of normal) (for review see Franchini and Mannucci 2013). Administration of factor VIII serves as substitution therapy, with the objective to restore the defect in thrombin generation. Normalization of factor VIII levels in the circulation requires administration by the intravenous route. The therapeutic range is rather narrow, because supra-normal factor VIII levels increase the risk of thrombosis, while the risk of bleeding tends to increase when levels drop below 40%. A usual strategy is to maintain a dosing schedule that ensures that factor VIII trough levels remain at least at 1–4% of normal, to avoid the bleeding risk of the severe form of hemophilia A.

For all licensed factor VIII products, efficacy has been established for both on-demand and prophylactic treatment. Dosing is generally based on the empirical finding that one unit factor VIII per kg body weight raises the plasma factor VIII activity by 2%, which implies the simple formula (Björkman and Berntorp 2001):

$$\text{dose}(\text{units/kg}) = 50 \times (\text{required rise in units/ml factor VIII}).$$

On-demand treatment involves factor VIII administration once bleeding occurs. Dependent on the type of bleeding, this requires administration of 20–100 units/kg, which can be repeated every 8–24 h if needed (Franchini and Mannucci 2013). In the developed countries, the general treatment has the objective not to treat, but rather to prevent bleeding episodes. This can be short-term prophylaxis to provide protection during surgical or invasive procedures, or long-term prophylaxis to prevent spontaneous bleeding. The latter involves regular treatment at a dose of 20–40 units/kg, which needs to be repeated 2–3 times per week in order to maintain the factor VIII level above 1% of normal. For extended half-life products, a recommended regimen is 50 units/kg every 4–5 days (Cafuir and Kempton 2017).

For all factor VIII products, the main side effect is the formation of antibodies against factor VIII (inhibitors) once replacement therapy is started. This involves 30–40% of all severe patients. In the majority of cases, these antibodies are transient, and can be eliminated by immuno-tolerance therapy with high doses of factor VIII. In a significant proportion of the patient population, however, the antibodies remain persistent, and thereby preclude further treatment with factor VIII (Franchini and Mannucci 2013).

Pharmaceutical Considerations

While the factor VIII concentration in human plasma is approximately 0.1 μg/ml, the potency of factor VIII products is expressed in International Units (IU). This is an activity unit relative to a reference preparation that is established from time to time by the World Health Organization. Products are available in fillings ranging between 250 and 2000 (or 3000) IU, in order to provide convenient dosing for children and adults using a single vial. Current products are freeze dried, and need to be reconstituted before infusion. Most products are stabilized in a sucrose-containing formulation, and have a shelf life of 24–36 months upon storage at 2–8 °C. For most products, data are available that establish stability at room temperature for 6–12 months, thus facilitating patients to travel while maintaining their prophylactic treatment.

As for impurities, most products may contain low amounts of residual proteins from the host expression system. With the exception of Nuwiq, which is expressed in a human cell line, these products may cause side effects in patients with hypersensitivity against rodent proteins. This adverse event, however, remains rare. To further enhance safety, the downstream processing of most recombinant factor VIII products includes virus-eliminating steps that have been previously established for plasma-derived factor VIII products, such as immuno-affinity chromatography, solvent/detergent treatment, ultrafiltration, and combinations thereof (Franchini and Mannucci 2013).

Clinical Considerations

The sole indication for recombinant factor VIII is congenital hemophilia A that is not complicated by factor VIII inhibitors. Similarly, acquired hemophilia A, which is due to the spontaneous formation of anti-factor VIII antibodies should be treated using alternative therapies such as factor VIII bypassing agents.

For all recombinant factor VIII products, appropriate treatment protocols have been established as part of the licensing procedure. Nevertheless, there is an increasing trend towards personalized prophylactic treatment, based on the pharmacokinetic profile of individual patient/product combinations. The advantage of this policy is that it allows the precise prediction of trough values and adaptation of dosing schedules accordingly. As for the extended half-life products, these tend to be used not to increase the dosing intervals, but rather to maintain higher trough levels and thus to offer better protection against spontaneous bleeding (Iorio 2017). A crucial requirement for this approach to be allowable is the availability of robust methods for monitoring post-infusion factor VIII levels. While this is feasible for full-length products, this remains a problematic issue for many of the engineered factor VIII products, including some products with B-domain deletions, the single-chain factor VIII product, some of the PEGylated products, and the Fc-fusion protein. While some manufacturers recommend the use of specific assay reagents, or reagent-dependent conversion factors, it seems evident that this approach lacks robustness, and as such is currently limiting the personalized use of these products (Kitchen et al. 2017).

RECOMBINANT FACTOR IX

While the cDNA encoding factor IX has been cloned in 1982 (Choo et al. 1982; Kurachi and Davie 1982), it took until 1997 before the first recombinant factor IX was licensed. Expressing the protein proved challenging in that factor IX requires excessive post-translational modification for full biological activity. These include 12 glutamine residues in the N-terminal section of the mature protein, which need to be modified into γ-carboxyglutamic acid (conversion of Glu into Gla) by a vitamin K-dependent carboxylase. The modification involves interaction between the carboxylase and the 46 amino acid long propeptide of factor IX, which is cleaved off by a furin-like processing enzyme prior to secretion (Jorgensen et al. 1987; Wasley et al. 1993). This results in a mature protein of 416 amino acids with the Gla-rich segment (the Gla-domain) at its N-terminus. Factor IX further comprises two epidermal growth factor-like (EGF) domains, an activation peptide (AP), and the catalytic domain (see Fig. 21.3a). Cleavage at both sides of the activation peptide yields a two-chain protein, consisting of a heavy chain (the catalytic domain) and a light chain (the Gla-EGF1-EGF2 section). Structural data indicate that factor IX is a stretched molecule, with the catalytic domain on one end, and the Gla-domain, with its Gla-residues protruding, at the opposite end (Perera et al. 2001, see Fig. 21.3b).

Why are these Gla-residues so important? Like in other vitamin K-dependent coagulation factors, such as factor VII, factor X, protein C and prothrombin, they provide high-affinity binding sites for Ca^{2+}-ions, and thereby mediate the interaction with negatively-charged lipid membranes. Thus, the appropriate assembly of coagulation factors at the site of injury is fully dependent on the presence of these clustered Ca^{2+}-binding sites (Furie and Furie 1988). Therefore, full carboxylation is a major requirement in the production of recombinant factor IX.

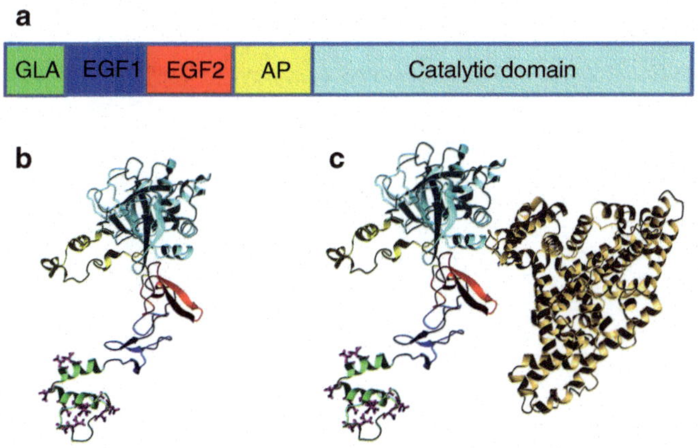

Figure 21.3 ■ Structure of factor IX. Panel (**a**) displays the domain structure. The colors of the individual domains correspond to those in panel (**b**), which provides a 3D structure of factor IX (Peirera 2001). In the Gla-domain, the γ-carboxylated residues are indicated in purple. Panel (**c**) provides the same structure with human albumin (from pdb 1AO6) fused to the C-terminus of the catalytic domain. *EGF* epidermal growth factor, *AP* activation peptide

■ Factor IX Products

The complexity of the post-translational modifications remains a major challenge in the production of recombinant factor IX. Mammalian cells need to be used as expression system, because these contain the necessary carboxylase enzyme complex. However, the capacity of host cells to perform this post-translational modification tends to be limiting, leading to under-carboxylated forms that lack full activity. Biological activity further requires removal of the propeptide, which usually implies the need for co-expression with a furin-like processing enzyme (Harrison et al. 1998). Most other post-translation modifications are located in the activation peptide, and include two N-linked glycosylation sites, tyrosine sulfation, and serine phosphorylation. With respect to these modifications, recombinant factor IX remains non-identical to its plasma-derived counterpart (Peters et al. 2010; Monroe et al. 2016).

Wild–Type Factor IX

Normal human plasma factor IX exists in two allelic forms, with alanine or threonine in position 148 in the activation peptide. This dimorphism, however, is without any known functional implication. Some recombinant factor IX products provide the Ala-148 variant, while others have Thr in position 148 (see Table 21.3). The first recombinant factor IX was BeneFIX, developed at Genetics Institute. More than 15 years later, two other products have been licensed, Rixubis and IXinity, developed at Baxter and Inspiration Biopharmaceuticals, respectively. All three products are produced in CHO cells under serum-free conditions, and undergo extensive downstream processing to remove impurities, including at least one virus eliminating step. For IXinity, the purification process includes one polishing step to specifically remove CHO-derived proteins (Monroe et al. 2016). Despite the differences in production and purification methods, the final products of these wild-type recombinant factor IX products are similar in terms of efficacy and pharmacokinetics.

Extended Half-Life Factor IX

Like factor VIII, also factor IX replacement therapy is limited by its relatively short half-life of about 24 h (see Table 21.3). For factor IX, engineering has proven more rewarding than for factor VIII. Currently, three products have been licensed that offer three to fourfold extended half-life (see Table 21.3 and references therein).

Alprolix has been developed by Biogen Idec, and is a fusion between factor IX and the Fc fragment of IgG. The targeting of factor IX to the FcRn receptor prolongs the half-life to approximately 82 h. The fusion of the Fc fragment to the factor IX C-terminus yields a derivative in which the activated form still carries the Fc-moiety. The downside thereof is that the activity of this fusion protein is considerably lower than that of 'wild-type' Factor IX.

Idelvion has been developed by CSL Behring, and is a fusion between factor IX and human albumin (Fig. 21.3c). The presence of the relatively large albumin at the C-terminus of the catalytic domain is incompatible with biological activity. This has been partially resolved by using a linker sequence that comprises the sequence of one of the two natural cleavage sites in factor IX (Metzner et al. 2009). Thus, proteolytic activation of this fusion protein involves three cleavages, the extra one serving to release the albumin moiety. Nevertheless, this fusion protein displays reduced in vitro activity, possibly because albumin release is relatively slow or incomplete. Its reported half-life is ~92 h (Iorio 2017).

Rebinyne/Refixia has been developed by Novo Nordisk. In this products, recombinant factor IX is modified with a branched 40 kDa PEG. This modification is targeted to the native N-glycans in the activation peptide by enzymatic glycoconjugation. Because the PEG moiety is released with the activation peptide upon activation, the active form is the natural, unmodified factor IXa. The in vitro activity of this factor IX derivative seems normal, although this remains dependent of assay reagents used.

■ Pharmacology

Like factor VIII, the term factor IX has been used before the protein had been identified. Factor IX was defined by its function to correct the clotting defect of plasma

Product type	INN name	*(Investigational)* product name(s)	First approval (USA/EU)	Half-life (mean, h)	Production technology	Reference
Wild-type FIX	nonacog alfa	BeneFIX	1997	17–36	CHO cells, co-expression with furin, Ala-148 polymorphic variant	Harrison et al. (1998)
	nonacog gamma	Rixubis *(Bax326)*	2013	27	CHO cells, co-expression with furin, Ala-148 polymorphic variant	Dietrich et al. (2013)
	trenonacog alfa	IXinity *(IB1001)*	2015	24	CHO cells, Thr-148 polymorphic variant	Monroe et al. (2016)
Engineered FIX	eftrenonacog alfa	Alprolix *(FIX-Fc)*	2014	82	HEK cells, Thr-148 variant, Fc fused to FIX C-terminus, co-expression with Fc alone and with processing enzyme PC5	Peters et al. (2010)
	albutrepenonacog alfa	Idelvion *(F9-fusion protein)*	2016	92	CHO cells, Thr-148 variant, albumin fused to FIX C-terminus by cleavable linker	Metzner et al. (2009)
	nonacog beta pegol	Rebinyn, Refixia *(N9-GP)*	2017	96	CHO cells, Ala-148 variant, glycoPEGylation in activation peptide region	Østergaard et al. (2011)

Table 21.3 ■ Recombinant factor IX products

of patients suffering from hemophilia B. Biological activity has remained the basis for the quantification of factor IX, and concentrations are expressed in units, where one unit represents the amount of factor IX activity in 1 ml of normal human plasma. Plasma factor IX levels can also be expressed as % of normal. Thus, assessment of product potency, dosing and pharmacokinetics are based on bioassays, and not on factor IX protein concentrations. Dosing is generally based on the empirical finding that one unit factor IX per kg body weight raises the plasma factor IX activity by 1% (or 0.01 unit/ml), according to the formula (Björkman and Berntorp 2001):

$$\text{dose}\left(\text{units/kg}\right) = 100 \times \left(\text{required rise in units/ml factor IX}\right).$$

Pharmacokinetics

The pharmacokinetics of factor IX have been reviewed in detail elsewhere (Björkman and Berntorp 2001; Iorio 2017). Systemic clearance is around 5 ml/h/kg for plasma-derived factor IX, and somewhat higher for recombinant wild-type factor IX. The distribution volume considerably exceeds the plasma volume, presumably because factor IX rapidly binds to the vascular surface. Elimination generally follows a bi-exponential pattern, with a terminal half-life of 20–34 h. Assessment of pharmacokinetics is mandatory for all individual factor IX products, and seems more consistent than that of factor VIII (see Iorio 2017 and Table 21.3). Similar to factor VIII, also factor IX pharmacokinetic data remain dependent on technical issues such as sampling time points, and the bioassays for the determination of the dose and post-infusion plasma levels. Despite this variability, it is evident that the engineered factor IX products do display a substantial half-life extension.

Pharmacodynamics

Hemophilia B is a congenital deficiency or dysfunction of factor IX which, dependent on the residual level of factor IX activity, is categorized as mild, moderate or severe (Björkman and Berntorp 2001). Like factor VIII, normalization of factor IX levels in the circulation requires intravenous administration. The therapeutic range is narrow, and similar to that of factor VIII.

For all licensed factor IX products, efficacy has been established for both on-demand and prophylactic treatment. On-demand treatment generally involves administration of 20–100 units/kg, depending on the bleeding type. Long-term prophylaxis involves regular treatment at a dose of 20–40 units/kg, with intervals of 3–4 days. For extended half-life products various regimens have been assessed, varying between 10 units/kg every 7 days for one product, to 75 units/kg every 14 days or 100 units/kg every 10 days for other products (Young and Mahlangu 2016). Thus, no general recommendation can be given so far. For the time being, dosing should strictly adhere to the product-specific recommendations for the individual products given in the Summary of Product Characteristics as issued by regulatory authorities such as EMA.

Unlike factor VIII, an immune response against factor IX is rare. Hypersensitivity and allergic reactions have been reported, and factor IX inhibitory antibodies may occur in a very small proportion of patients (1% or less). Antibodies against hamster proteins have been reported for one particular product (IXinity), but this has been resolved by introducing an additional step to further reduce these impurities (Monroe et al. 2016).

Pharmaceutical Considerations

The factor IX concentration in human plasma is approximately 4 µg/ml. However, like factor VIII, activity units are used for factor IX. The potency of factor IX products is expressed in International Units (IU) relative to an international standard established by the World Health Organization. Most products are available in fillings ranging between 250 and 3000 IU in order to provide appropriate, body-weight guided, dosing for children and adults. Current products are freeze dried, and need to be reconstituted before infusion. Most products are stabilized in a sucrose-containing formulation, and have a shelf life of 24–36 months upon storage at 2–8 °C. For most products, data are available that establish stability at room temperature for 6–24 months.

As for impurities, most products may contain low amounts of residual proteins from the host expression system. With the exception of Alprolix, which is expressed in a human cell line, these products may cause side effects in patients which hypersensitivity against rodent proteins. To enhance safety further, the downstream processing of most recombinant factor IX products includes one or more virus-eliminating steps, usually including nanofiltration.

Clinical Considerations

The sole indication for recombinant factor IX is congenital hemophilia B. For all factor IX products, appropriate treatment protocols have been established as part of the licensing procedure. Like for hemophilia A, there is an increasing interest in personalized prophylactic treatment, based on the pharmacokinetic profile of individual patient/product combinations (Iorio 2017). This remains challenging for the extended half-life products, because of the lack of uniform, robust assays for monitoring these engineered factor IX variants (Kitchen et al. 2017).

An additional complication is that the Fc- and albumin fusion proteins display reduced activity, indicating that patients are treated with factor IX that is partially inactive. This might seem irrelevant because dosing is based on activity (Peters et al. 2010). On the other hand, this introduces an extra, assay-dependent variable in personalized, pharmacokinetics-based dosing. One important implication is that patients cannot be switched from one extended half-life product to another, while maintaining the same dosing schedule.

OTHER HEMOSTATIC PROTEINS

While a variety of recombinant factor VIII and IX products is available from multiple biotechnology companies, other hemostatic proteins have received limited attention. For some proteins, a single product has been licensed so far. These are reviewed in the present section.

Recombinant Factor VIIa

Factor VIIa is the enzyme that triggers the initiation phase of thrombin generation, and acts directly upstream of factor X in the cascade. Based on theoretical considerations, it has been proposed that the presence of high concentrations of factor VIIa should have the potential of activating factor X to a sufficient extent to bypass the need for factor VIII or factor IX in the coagulation cascade (see Fig. 21.1). Once this concept had been verified (Hedner and Kisiel 1983), the use of factor VIIa became an option for treatment of bleeding in patients with inhibitory antibodies against factor VIII or IX, and a few other bleeding disorders (see Clinical Considerations).

The factor VII concentration in human plasma is low (0.5 µg/ml), and as such is insufficient to provide a source for large amounts of factor VIIa. This made factor VIIa an attractive target for production by recombinant technology. Factor VII is a glycoprotein of approximately 57 kDa, which has the same domain structure as factor IX (Fig. 21.3). It shares the same requirement for γ-carboxylation in its Gla-domain at the N-terminus of the mature protein. Recombinant factor VII has been developed at Novo Nordisk, and is produced in BHK cells under serum-free conditions. During downstream processing, single-chain factor VII is converted into two-chain factor VIIa by autoactivation (Hedner 2006). Recombinant factor VIIa (INN name eptacog alfa) has been licensed since 1996 under the product name NovoSeven. Two biosimilars have been developed, one by Baxter (investigational name BAX 817), and another (AryoSeven) by AryoGen Biopharma. The production of the former has been discontinued, and the latter has only been licensed in Iran so far. An engineered variant of factor VIIa (vatreptacog alfa) has been developed, but phase III trials have been terminated because of immunogenicity due to the amino acid substitutions made to enhance biological activity (Mahlangu et al. 2015). Consequently, NovoSeven remains the sole widely available recombinant factor VIIa so far.

Pharmacology

Factor VIIa normally activates factor X when bound to tissue factor at the site of vascular injury. NovoSeven dosing, however, is in large excess over physiological concentrations. Under such conditions, factor VIIa is believed to activate factor X on the surface of activated platelets in a tissue factor-independent manner (Hedner 2006). Factor VIIa potency and dosing is based on bioassays but, unlike factor VIII and IX, is expressed in terms of protein concentration, and not in units. Like other coagulation factors, Factor VIIa therapy requires intravenous administration. The pharmacokinetics of recombinant factor VIIa has been assessed in various patient groups. In non-bleeding patients, the overall mean clearance is approximately 30 ml/h/kg, and the half-life is around 2–3 h (Björkman and Berntorp 2001). For hemophilia A or B patients with inhibitory antibodies, the recommended dosage is 90 µg/kg every 2 h until hemostasis is achieved. Dosage is slightly different for other indications (see Clinical Considerations).

Pharmaceutical Considerations

Recombinant factor VIIa is available in fillings of 1–8 mg per vial. The product is freeze-dried, and needs to be reconstituted in a specific histidine-containing diluent before use. The product is stable for 3 years at room temperature. As for impurities, downstream processing includes a virus inactivating solvent/detergent step.

Clinical Considerations

Apart from treatment of hemophilia A and B with inhibitory antibodies, recombinant factor VIIa is also indicated for treatment of acquired hemophilia due to antibodies in non-hemophilic patients. Another indication is congenital factor VII deficiency. The recommended dosage then is 15–30 µg/kg every 4–6 h. NovoSeven is also indicated for the platelet-based bleeding disorder Glanzmann Thrombasthenia. The recommended dosage then is 90 µg/kg every 2–6 h, until hemostasis has been achieved (Hedner and Ezban 2008). The most common and serious adverse reactions are thrombotic events.

Recombinant von Willebrand Factor

Von Willebrand factor is one of the largest proteins in the circulation. Monomeric von Willebrand factor is synthesized as a preproprotein, with a signal peptide of 22 amino acids, a propeptide that is unusually large (741 amino acids) and a mature subunit of 2015 amino acids (for review see Castaman and Linari 2017). Monomers form tail-to-tail dimers via a cysteine-rich region at the C-terminus. These dimers can multimerize by the formation of cysteine bridges at the N-terminus of the mature subunit, in a process that requires the presence of the propeptide. The molecular size of von Willebrand factor thus can vary between a dimer of 500 kDa and multimers of up to 20,000 kDa. The primary function of von Willebrand factor is to promote platelet aggregation and adhesion, which is essential for appropriate thrombus formation (Fig. 21.1b). The secondary function is to carry factor VIII in the circulation and thereby to prevent its premature clearance (Pipe et al. 2016; Castaman and Linari 2017).

It seems evident that the size of this protein and the complexity of its processing into dimers and multimers make production of recombinant von Willebrand factor to a challenge. Nevertheless this has already been achieved in the 1980s at Genetics Institute, by the co-expression of von Willebrand factor and factor VIII. While the factor VIII products resulting from co-expression (Recombinate and Advate, see Table 21.2) were depleted of von Willebrand factor, this byproduct has subsequently been developed into a separate product. Downstream processing includes in vitro processing with recombinant processing enzyme (furin) to remove the propeptide and expose optimal factor VIII binding (Turecek et al. 2009). This recombinant product (INN name vonicog alfa) has first been licensed as Vonvendi in the US in 2015, and is called Veyvondi in the EU. It is the first recombinant von Willebrand factor available as an alternative for the current plasma-derived counterparts (Francini and Mannucci 2016).

Pharmacology and Pharmaceutical Considerations

Recombinant von Willebrand factor serves to control bleeding episodes in patients with severe, type-III deficiency. The deficiency of von Willebrand factor in these patients implies not only a defective platelet aggregation and adhesion, but also abnormally fast clearance of their endogenous factor VIII. Therefore, factor VIII needs to be supplemented too, usually to a level of 35–50% of normal, in order to achieve hemostasis (Mannucci 2004).

The concentration of recombinant von Willebrand factor is expressed in terms of biological activity, by its effect on platelet aggregation in the presence of ristocetin (so-called 'ristocetin cofactor activity'). Potency is expressed in International Units (IU), and is based on the International Standard for von Willebrand factor concentrate. Vonvendi is available as lyophilized powder for reconstitution in fillings of 650 and 1300 IU, and needs to be administered intravenously. Its shelf-life is 36 months at 3–5 °C, or 12 months at room temperature. Being derived from CHO cells under serum- and protein free conditions, the most relevant impurities may represent residual hamster protein, which might cause hypersensitivity reactions in some recipients. The pharmacokinetics have been studied extensively (Gill et al. 2015), both for recombinant von Willebrand factor alone, and in combination with recombinant factor VIII (see under Clinical Considerations). The overall clearance was 3 ml/h/kg, and half-life approximately 22 h. In the phase III study, the initial dosage was 40–80 IU/kg, followed by 40–60 kg every 8–24 h if clinically required.

Clinical Considerations

The vast experience with treatment of severe von Willebrand's disease is based on the use of plasma-derived products, in particular concentrates that contain both von Willebrand factor and factor VIII. The recommended regimen is 30–50 IU/kg von Willebrand factor, while keeping the trough factor VIII level >30–50% of normal (Mannucci 2004). In Vonvendi, the sole active component is recombinant von Willebrand factor. To control bleeding, the first dosage should therefore be combined with recombinant factor VIII. Because recombinant von Willebrand factor sustains the stability of the patient's endogenous factor VIII, co-administration with factor VIII for subsequent infusions might prove unnecessary (Gill et al. 2015). For the moment, the burden of co-administration and dual monitoring seems to be prohibitive for general use in less specialized centers. Ongoing post-marketing trials will help to further clarify the exact place of recombinant von Willebrand factor in the management of this complex bleeding disorder (Franchini and Mannucci 2016).

Recombinant Factor XIII

Factor XIII is the pro-enzyme of a transglutaminase that, after activation by thrombin, reinforces fibrin polymers by the formation of γ-glutamyl-ε-lysyl amide cross-links. A congenital deficiency of factor XIII is associated with severe bleeding due to impaired thrombus stability (see Fig. 21.1b). Factor XIII is a hetero-tetramer comprising two catalytic A-subunits of 82 kDa and two carrier B-subunits of 73 kDa, which are linked by noncovalent interactions (Komaromi et al. 2011). The A-and B-subunits are encoded by different genes, and in plasma the B-chain circulates in excess over the A-chain. An intracellular form of factor XIII is present in platelets, macrophages and other cells, and is a homodimer of two A-subunits only. Most patients with factor XIII deficiency have a defect in the A-subunit, which makes this a suitable target for recombinant factor XIII substitution therapy (Inbal et al. 2012).

Pharmacology and Pharmaceutical Considerations

Recombinant factor XIII A-subunit has been developed at ZymoGenetics and Novo Nordisk, and is expressed in *Saccharomyces cerevisiae* under protein-free conditions. The purified yeast-derived protein is a dimer of two non-glycosylated factor XIII A-subunits (Lovejoy et al. 2006), which upon infusion spontaneously associates with B-subunits to form the factor XIII hetero-tetramer in the circulation. The product (INN name catridecacog) has been licensed in 2012, and is available under the product name Tretten in the US, and as NovoThirteen elsewhere.

The potency of recombinant factor XIII is expressed in International Units (IU), and is based on the International Standard for factor XIII concentrate. NovoThirteen is available as lyophilized powder for reconstitution in vials of 2500 IU, to be reconstituted in physiological saline for intravenous administration. The shelf-life is 24 month at 2–8 °C. Pharmacokinetic studies have shown that the half-life varies between 6 and 9 days (Lovejoy et al. 2006). Prophylactic treatment has proven efficacious and safe using a regimen of 35 IU/kg once monthly (Inbal et al. 2012).

Clinical Considerations

Recombinant factor XIII is the first recombinant product for a rare bleeding disorder. So far, plasma-derived, hetero-tetrameric factor XIII has been used for treatment of congenital factor XIII deficiency. Due to the lack of post-translation glycosylation, the yeast protein is non-identical to the natural A-subunit homodimer. Nevertheless, this has not resulted in any detectable immunogenicity so far. For a majority of patients, therefore, recombinant A-subunit dimer proves a viable alternative for plasma-derived factor XIII.

Recombinant Antithrombin

Antithrombin belongs to the class of serine protease inhibitors ('serpins'), and as such might be considered as not being a coagulation factor in the strict sense. However, antithrombin is the major inhibitor of factor IXa, factor Xa, factor XIa and thrombin, and thereby plays a regulatory role at multiple levels in the coagulation cascade. Antithrombin is a single-chain glycoprotein, and has a molecular mass of 58 kDa. Its inhibitory potential is greatly enhanced by binding to heparin or other glycosaminoglycans. This drives antithrombin, like other serpins, into a conformation that favors the interaction with its target proteases (Huntington 2003). A partial deficiency of antithrombin reduces the down-regulation of the coagulation cascade, and thereby enhances the risk of thrombosis. In antithrombin deficiency, prophylaxis usually consists of standard anti-thrombotic therapy using heparin or small molecules that inhibit coagulation (Mackman 2008). However, the inherent bleeding risk thereof makes such therapy undesirable for use in high-risk situations such as surgery or delivery. Suppletion of antithrombin then provides an alternative treatment.

Recombinant antithrombin is licensed in the EU and US since 2006 and 2009, respectively. The product has been developed by Genzyme Transgenics (GTC Biotherapeutics), and is available as ATryn (INN name antithrombin alfa). ATryn is particularly remarkable from a biotechnological point of view, because it is harvested from the milk of transgenic goats (Edmunds et al. 1998). This technology, which is introduced in Chap. 9, has proven feasible for the expression of a wide range of therapeutic proteins in milk or other body fluids (Lubon et al. 1996, see also Table 9.4). During further development, however, transgenic technology had to deal with numerous issues, including stability of transgenic inheritance, appropriate post-translational modification and stability of heterologous proteins in milk, and regulatory affairs (Lubon et al. 1996). Upon its approval by EMA and FDA, ATryn became the first biopharmaceutical that took all hurdles of production in transgenic animals.

Pharmacology and Pharmaceutical Considerations

The potency of ATryn is expressed in International Units, which relate to the International Standard for antithrombin in concentrate as established by WHO. The unitage is based on in vitro inhibitory activity in the presence of heparin. ATryn is available as lyophilized powder for reconstitution and infusion, in fillings of 1750 IU per vial. When stored at 2–8 °C, the shelf-life is 4 years. The transgenic antithrombin in ATryn is identical to plasma-derived antithrombin, with the exception of its glycosylation, which is less complex and comprises fewer sialic acid moieties (Edmunds et al. 1998). Rigorous pharmacokinetic studies have not been reported, but the estimated mean elimination half-life is 10 h, which is sixfold shorter than that of the fully glycosylated antithrombin from human plasma. Therefore, dosing recommendations of plasma-derived and transgenic antithrombin are different. Dosing aims to maintain plasma levels between 80 and 120% of normal. For ATryn, the recommended dosing is (Tiede et al. 2008):

$$\text{Loading dose}\left(\text{IU/kg}\right) = \left(100 - \text{pretreatment antithrombin level in}\,\%\right)/\,2.28$$

$$\text{Maintenance}\left(\text{IU/kg/h}\right) = \left(100 - \text{pretreatment antithrombin level in}\,\%\right)/\,10.22$$

The loading dose can be administered as a bolus, while maintenance requires continuous infusion.

Clinical Considerations

ATryn is indicated for the prophylaxis of venous thrombosis in surgery in adult patients with congenital antithrombin deficiency. In absence of sufficient data, ATryn initially has not been recommended for use during pregnancy. More recent studies have generated additional support for using ATryn in both perioperative and peripartum settings (Paidas et al. 2014). One concern could be the potential immunogenicity of the transgenic protein, due to the glycosylation differences between transgenic and native human antithrombin. However, antibodies to neither the transgenic protein, nor to any other goat protein, have been reported (Paidas et al. 2014).

RECOMBINANT THROMBOLYTIC AGENTS

The need for thrombolytic agents dates from the 1970s, when myocardial infarction was recognized as being caused by the rupture of an atherosclerotic plaque in a coronary artery, followed by the formation of an occluding thrombus (Lusis 2000). Recanalization of the occluded vessel requires thrombus dissolution, which can be achieved by activating the fibrinolytic system (see Fig. 21.1c). The first thrombolytic agent used was streptokinase, a bacterial plasminogen activator isolated from *Streptococcus haemolyticus*. This agent has been widely used in the treatment of myocardial infarction, and as such has developed into a worldwide blockbuster. However, the use of a bacterial protein implies the risk of immunogenicity, and this may hamper repeated dosing. The search for a human plasminogen activator has resulted in the identification of tissue-type plasminogen activator (t-PA). Its low concentration in tissues and in blood is prohibitive for obtaining natural t-PA in substantial amounts. This made t-PA to an obvious candidate for production by recombinant technology (for review see Collen and Lijnen 2005).

■ Recombinant Tissue–Type Plasminogen Activator (t–PA)

The primary structure of human t-PA has been established since the cloning and expression of its cDNA (Pennica et al. 1983). The mature protein comprises an N-terminal region that is called the finger domain, followed by a single EGF-like domain, two so-called kringle domains, and the catalytic domain (see Fig. 21.4a). There are four sites for N-linked glycosylation, one in kringle-1, two in kringle-2, and one in the protease domain. Human t-PA is a single-chain protein with a molecular mass of about 70 kDa. It is converted into a two-chain form by plasmin, by cleavage at the junction between the kringle-2 and the catalytic domain. While the two-chain form represents the fully activated enzyme, the single-chain form displays very similar fibrinolytic activity. Both forms of t-PA share high-affinity interaction with fibrin and inhibition by plasminogen activator inhibitor-1 (PAI-1) (Rijken et al. 1982).

Wild-Type Recombinant t-PA (Alteplase)

Wild-type t-PA has initially been expressed in *Escherichia coli* (Pennica et al. 1983). However, the numerous (17)

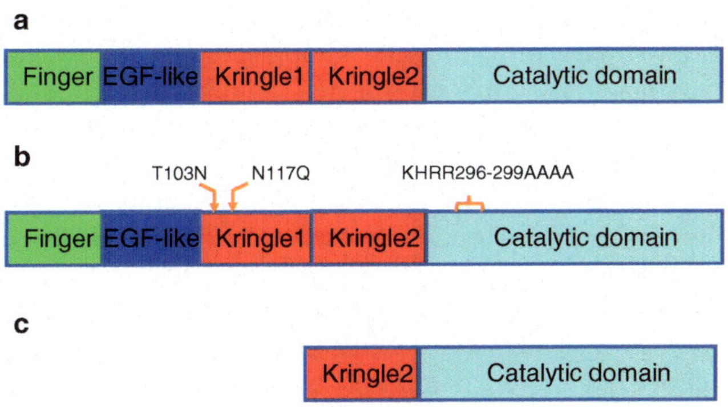

Figure 21.4 ■ Structure of recombinant tissue-type plasminogen activator. Panel (**a**) represents the domain structure of full-length t-PA (alteplase). Panel (**b**) displays the variant tenecteplase, and panel (**c**) the truncated variant reteplase. Further details are given in the text. *EGF* epidermal growth factor

internal disulfide bridges and multiple glycosylation sites make production in mammalian cells more efficient. Recombinant t-PA, (INN name alteplase), has been developed at Genentech, and is produced in CHO cells. Alteplase displays the fibrin-specificity of natural t-PA, which is mediated by the finger and kringle-2 domain. The biological half-life is only 5–6 min. Half-life is limited by the rapid inhibition by PAI-1, and by the interaction of the finger and/or EGF-like domains with clearance receptors (Collen and Lijnen 2005). Alteplase has first been licensed in 1987, and is available under multiple product names, including Activase (Genentech) and Actilyse (Boehringer Ingelheim).

Engineered Recombinant t-PA

Tenecteplase is the INN name of a t-PA variant that has been engineered at Genentech, with the aim to prolong half-life, while maintaining the fibrin specificity of natural t-PA. This has been accomplished by a few substitutions in the full-length protein (see Fig. 21.4b). The Thr103 to Asn (T103 N) substitution creates a new N-linked glycosylation site, and the Asn117 to Gln (N117Q) eliminates a high-mannose glycosylation site in the kringle-1 domain. In addition, the amino acids Lys295-His-Arg-Arg299 have been replaced by four Ala residues. The modified glycosylation in the kringle-1 domain serves to reduce clearance, while the KHRR296-299AAAA substitutions confer increased resistance against inhibition by PAI-1 (Keyt et al. 1994). Tenecteplase is produced in CHO cells, and has first been licensed in the US in 2000. It is available under the product names TNKase and Metalyse.

Reteplase is the INN name for a truncated variant of t-PA which consists of only the kringle-2 and the catalytic domain (see Fig. 21.4c). This variant was developed at Boehringer Mannheim, with the objective to eliminate the domains that drive clearance, while conserving the kringle-2 domain for fibrin-specificity. This major truncation allows for production in *Escherichia coli*. Reteplase is a single-chain, non-glycosylated protein with a molecular mass of 39 kDa. Its downstream processing includes extraction from inclusion bodies, and in vitro renaturation and refolding (Moser et al. 1998; Simpson et al. 2006). Reteplase was first licensed in 1996, and is available under the product names Rapsilysin and Retevase.

A variety of other t-PA variants has been designed, including lanoteplase. Lanoteplase has been developed at Genetics Institute. It lacks the finger and EFG-like domains, as well as the glycosylation in position Asn117 (Collen and Lijnen 2005). Like other, more recently engineered t-PA variants, lanoteplase has not been licensed, and therefore remains beyond the scope of this chapter.

■ Pharmacology

Multiple methods are being used for the quantification of t-PA. First, potency is expressed in terms of International Units (IU), which reflects biological activity against the International Standard as established by WHO. Alternatively, t-PA concentration can be defined by protein content, and expressed in mg. Which method is used for potency labelling varies between products. For reteplase, potency is expressed in units (U) using a product-specific reference. For patient monitoring or for pharmacokinetic studies, t-PA concentrations are usually based on immunological assays.

Pharmacokinetics

Assessment of the pharmacokinetics of t-PA is complex. It is reflecting a combination of 'regular' plasma elimination of free t-PA, the adsorption of t-PA to insoluble fibrin, the neutralization by PAI-1, and the elimination of t-PA/PAI-1 complexes. The reader is referred to the Summary of Product Characteristics of the individual products for details as issued by EMA. As a general parameter, most studies just use the biological half-life as estimated from levels of circulating t-PA. In these terms, the half-life of alteplase is 5–6 min, whereas the half-life of tenecteplase and reteplase is 17–20 min and 14–18 min, respectively (Collen and Lijnen 2005).

Pharmacodynamics

The recombinant plasminogen activators differ from streptokinase in that they are fibrin-specific. Fibrin has high affinity for both t-PA and plasminogen, and serves as a surface for local plasminogen activation. In contrast to free plasmin, fibrin-bound plasmin is relatively insensitive to inactivation by α2-plasmin inhibitor. These interactions make fibrin the central regulator of its own degradation (Collen and Lijnen 2005). Normally, this subtle mechanism is triggered adequately by the small amounts of t-PA in plasma (5–10 ng/ml).

Numerous clinical studies have addressed recombinant t-PA in acute myocardial infarction, usually in comparison with a standard streptokinase regimen. Due to the difference in pharmacokinetics, dosage regimens are product-specific. For alteplase, a typical regimen is a total of 100 mg, of which 60 mg during the first hour, and 20 mg over the second hour and 20 mg over the third hour. An alternative is 100 mg divided over a bolus of 15 mg, followed by 0.75 mg/kg over 30 min, and 0.5 mg/kg over 60 min (Collen and Lijnen 2004).

In contrast, tenecteplase usually is administered as a single intravenous bolus of 30–50 mg (6000–10,000 IU), dependent on body weight (Guillermin et al. 2016). For reteplase, a recommended regimen is a double bolus (10 U + 10 U, 30 min apart), independent of body weight (Simpson et al. 2006). Apparently, the engineering to extend half-life of tenecteplase and reteplase indeed resulted in the intended dosing advantage.

In thrombolytic therapy, t-PA levels are achieved that are in large excess (up to 500-fold) over the physiological concentration. This carries the inherent risk that t-PA also acts in a fibrin-independent manner, and degrades fibrinogen (fibrinogenolysis). This may lead to systemic fibrinogen shortage and a concomitant bleeding risk. Bleeding is the most common complication of thrombolysis, also because it is usually combined with anticoagulant therapy to prevent re-occlusion. This may vary between superficial bleeding at the site of injection and more severe episodes, including intracranial bleeding.

Pharmaceutical Considerations

Alteplase, tenecteplase and reteplase are lyophilized products that need to be reconstituted for intravenous infusion. Shelf-life is at least 2 years at temperatures not exceeding 25 °C. Once reconstituted, alteplase can be further diluted with a physiological saline solution to facilitate continuous infusion. Usually, thrombolytic therapy is combined with continuous infusion of heparin. This should not be co-administered through the same cannula, because of solubility issues, in particular for reteplase.

As for impurities, alteplase and tenecteplase are produced in CHO cells, and may include residual hamster protein. Reteplase is produced in *Escherichia coli,* and is subjected to a validated process of denaturation and refolding to produce the active fibrinolytic enzyme. Reteplase has a lower affinity for fibrin than alteplase and tenecteplase. It also displays lower in vitro fibrinolytic activity than alteplase (Simpson et al. 2006). Because of its different unitage used for potency labeling, the content of active agent in reteplase cannot be directly related to that of alteplase or tenecteplase.

Clinical Considerations

The primary indication for alteplase, tenecteplase and reteplase is acute myocardial infarction. Alteplase has further been licensed for use in acute pulmonary embolism and acute ischaemic stroke. For tenecteplase and reteplase, studies are addressing the extension into these indications too. For treatment of stroke, it is essential to start therapy only after prior exclusion of intracranial bleeding by appropriate imaging techniques.

In the majority of clinical trials, the recombinant agents have been compared with standard streptokinase therapy, often in combination with heparin or other anticoagulants to prevent re-occlusion (Collins et al. 1997). Overall, all agents seem to offer adequate thrombolytic therapy of acute myocardial infarction, with comparable survival rates and bleeding complications. In the absence of a direct comparison between recombinant thrombolytic agents, it remains difficult to conclude that one agent would be preferable over another. A meta-analysis suggests that tenecteplase and alteplase are equally effective in acute coronary syndrome, with a slightly lower bleeding risk for tenecteplase (Guillermin et al. 2016). It should be noted, however, that clinical studies are complex and require the inclusion of large numbers of patients to reach satisfying conclusions for all individual indications. Therefore, the current thrombolytic agents will continue to be subject of clinical studies to further explore their therapeutic potential in life-threatening thrombotic complications.

CONCLUDING REMARKS

In the early 1980s, the advent of biotechnology provided the perspective of unlimited access to recombinant coagulation factors and thrombolytic agents. This was particularly promising for low abundance proteins such as t-PA, and factors VII and VIII, for which the medical need was by far exceeding the availability for pharmaceutical production from human sources. Now, three decades later, one may wonder whether biotechnology actually has fulfilled its initial promise in this field. It remains difficult to give a fully unequivocal answer at this point.

On the positive side, there are some major achievements. The most prominent example is t-PA. Its cDNA was cloned in 1983, and recombinant t-PA became available as a life-saving product already 4 years later. It is further remarkable that for recombinant factor VIII, being a much more complex protein than t-PA, the gap between cloning and licensing could be closed in only 8 years. Another success is activated factor VII. Recombinant technology has been instrumental for obtaining this trace protein in sufficient amounts to meet the clinical need. More recently, we have seen examples of how protein engineering may generate biopharmaceuticals that display more favorable pharmacokinetics than their natural counterparts.

At the same time, however, some limitations remain apparent. For instance, recombinant t-PA now is the generally established agent for thrombolytic therapy in the US and EU, but not in territories where t-PA is not affordable, and streptokinase is still being used. Another example is factor VIII. Since the introduction of recombinant factor VIII supplies have been a limiting factor, and prices have remained prohibitive for many countries. While factor VIII is included in WHO's List of Essential Medicines, the majority (~75%) of the world's patients still have little or no access to hemophilia care, despite intense efforts to maximize the production of conventional factor VIII from human plasma. Apparently, recombinant factor VIII did not meet the full medical need. In this regard, one may question why so many new recombinant factor VIII products have been recently developed without taking the affordability issue into account. Moreover, with the exception of factor XIII deficiency, the rare bleeding disorders have remained dependent on blood-derived products, with their inherent limited supply. The initial expectation was that plasma-derived coagulation factors may soon become obsolete. It is evident that this optimism has been premature.

The next few decades offer excellent perspectives on fulfilling the initial promise of biotechnology. It may become possible to replace costly mammalian cell expression by cheaper technology. For relatively simple proteins such as t-PA, expression in transgenic plants has already proven feasible. Production in transgenic animals has, after many hurdles, resulted in the first tangible products on the market. Moreover, for most of the hemostatic proteins the dominant patents have expired, thus opening the way towards more affordable biosimilars (cf. Chap. 12). Finally, protein engineering may continue to generate therapeutics that display improved biological activity at much lower dosage. It remains an attractive challenge to a new generation of researchers to accomplish these goals in the near future.

SELF-ASSESSMENT QUESTIONS

Questions

1. Proteolytic processing

   Furin-like enzymes play a role in the post-translational modification of a several hemostatic proteins.

   (a) Give three examples and describe the relevance of processing in these proteins.

   (b) How is this modification accomplished in biotechnological production?

2. Transgenic animal bioreactors

   A variety of transgenic animals has been used to express hemostatic proteins in their milk, including rabbits, goats, sheep, pigs and cows. Recombinant antithrombin (ATryn) is produced in goats.

   (a) ATryn differs from plasma-derived antithrombin. What is the major difference? How could this be caused?

   (b) Would you consider using goats as bioreactor for producing transgenic factor VIII or IX, or would you prefer an alternative? Why?

3. Extended half-life factor IX

   The factor IX-albumin fusion protein is one of the three available products with extended half-life.

   (a) What is the mechanism underlying the half-life prolongation?

   (b) Are there particular disadvantages or limitations of this particular fusion strategy?

   (c) What are the implications for patients switching from normal factor IX to this fusion product?

4. Thrombolytic agents

   (a) Describe the mechanism by which fibrinolysis is under local control

   (b) What is the main adverse effect of thrombolysis, and how is this caused

   (c) Reteplase differs from other thrombolytic agents in that it is produced in E. coli. What are the potential advantages or disadvantages of this approach?

Answers

1. Proteolytic processing

   (a) Three examples are: (1) factor IX, wherein the propeptide that is needed for appropriate γ-carboxylation, needs to be cleaved off in order to generate the Gla-domain as the natural N-terminus of the mature factor IX, (2) von Willebrand factor, wherein the propeptide is important for the formation of multimers, but is removed prior to secretion in order to facilitate its function as carrier of factor VIII in the circulation, and (3) factor VIII, which is processed into a two chain heterodimer as in plasma-derived, natural factor VIII; the role of this cleavage is unclear, and one recombinant product is deliberately constructed to be single-chain (see Table 21.2).

   (b) If cleavage by endogenous processing proteases is limiting (as for instance in CHO cells), the usual approach is to co-express furin (or a related protease) in the same cells, or to perform in vitro maturation using a recombinant processing protease (as in recombinant von Willebrand factor).

2. Transgenic animal bioreactors
   (a) The major difference between ATryn and plasma-derived antithrombin is the glycosylation, with less complicated glycans that carry fewer end-standing sialic acid moieties. This suggests that glycosylation in goat mammary gland cells is incomplete. Apparently, this translates into a shorter half-life.
   (b) Half-life of factor VIII or IX is a key issue because these proteins are predominantly used for long-term prophylaxis. The use of transgenic goats would imply a risk of undesirably short half-life. Factor VIII and IX have been expressed in pigs, and glycosylation patterns seem less aberrant than in goats. Establishing correct glycosylation is a crucial element in assessing the potential benefit of transgenic technology for proteins that are to be used in non-acute situations.
3. Extended half-life factor IX
   (a) The factor IX-albumin fusion binds to the FcRn receptor via its albumin moiety. Due to the binding to this recycling receptor, the fusion protein escapes endosomal degradation after endocytosis and recycles back to the circulation.
   (b) The disadvantage is that factor IX is inactive as long as albumin remains fused to its catalytic domain. This has been solved by creating a cleavable linker. However, partial cleavage of the linker at the site of injury will reduce biological activity.
   (c) For the patient, dosing intervals will be significantly longer. Alternatively, trough levels of factor IX will be higher, which adds protection against spontaneous bleeding. However, because monitoring is more complex than for other factor IX products, it will be more difficult to develop an individualized dosing regimen.
4. Thrombolytic agents
   (a) Fibrinolysis is controlled by fibrin, which binds t-PA and plasminogen (see text), and thereby limits plasmin formation to the site of the occluding thrombus.
   (b) The main adverse effect of thrombolysis is bleeding. This is largely due to insufficient fibrin-specificity, leading to the degradation and consumption of fibrinogen (fibrinogenolysis).
   (c) The advantage of production in E. coli is the lower production cost. The disadvantage is the need for denaturation and refolding. Reteplase lacks a few domains of normal t-PA, including the fibrin-binding finger domain. Therefore, its affinity for fibrin is lower, which theoretically reduces its fibrin-specificity.

REFERENCES

Andersson LO, Forsman N, Huang K, Larsen K, Lundin A, Pavlu B, Sandberg H, Sewerin K, Smart J (1986) Isolation and characterization of human factor VIII: molecular forms in commercial factor VIII concentrate, cryoprecipitate and plasma. Proc Natl Acad Sci U S A 83:2979–2983

Björkman S, Berntorp E (2001) Pharmacokinetics of coagulation factors: clinical relevance for patients with haemophilia. Clin Pharmacokinet 40:815–832

Cafuir LA, Kempton CL (2017) Current and emerging factor VIII replacement products for hemophilia A. Ther Adv Hematol 8:303–313

Castaman G, Linari S (2017) Diagnosis and treatment of von Willebrand disease and rare bleeding disorders. J Clin Med 6:E45

Choo KH, Gould KG, Rees DL, Brownlee GG (1982) Molecular cloning of the gene for human anti-haemophilic factor IX. Nature 299:178–180

Collen D, Lijnen HR (2004) Tissue-type plasminogen activator: a historical perspective and personal account. J Thromb Haemost 2:541–546

Collen D, Lijnen HR (2005) Thrombolytic agents. Thromb Haemost 93:627–630

Collins R, Peto R, Baigent C, Sleight P (1997) Aspirin, heparin, and fibrinolytic therapy in suspected acute myocardial infarction. N Engl J Med 336:847–860

Davie EW, Ratnoff OD (1964) Waterfall sequence for intrinsic blood clotting. Science 145:1310–1312

Dietrich B, Schiviz A, Hoellriegl W, Horling F, Benamara K, Rottensteiner H, Turecek PL, Schwarz HP, Scheiflinger F, Muchitsch EM (2013) Preclinical safety and efficacy of a new recombinant FIX drug product for treatment of hemophilia B. Int J Hematol 98:525–532

Edmunds T, Van Patten SM, Pollock J, Hanson E, Bernasconi R, Higgins E, Manvalan P, Ziomek C, Meade H, McPherson JM, Cole ES (1998) Transgenically produced human antithrombin: structural and functional comparison to human plasma-derived antithrombin. Blood 91:4561–4571

Fay PJ (2004) Activation of factor VIII and mechanisms of cofactor action. Blood Rev 18:1–15

Franchini M, Mannucci PM (2013) Hemophilia A in the third millennium. Blood Rev 27:179–184

Franchini M, Mannucci PM (2016) Von Willebrand factor (Vonvendi®): the first recombinant product licensed for the treatment of von Willebrand disease. Expert Rev Hematol 9:825–830

Furie B, Furie BC (1988) The molecular basis of blood coagulation. Cell 53:505–518

Gill JC, Castaman G, Windyga J, Kouides P, Ragni M, Leebeek FWG, Obermann-Slupetzky O, Chapman M, Fritsch S, Pavlova BG, Presch I, Ewenstein B (2015) Hemostatic efficacy, safety, and pharmacokinetics of a recombinant von Willebrand factor in severe von Willebrand disease. Blood 126:2038–2046

Guillermin A, Yan DJ, Perrier A, Marti C (2016) Safety and efficacy of tenecteplase versus alteplase in acute coronary syndrome: a systematic review and meta-analysis of randomized trials. Arch Med Sci 12:1181–1187

Harrison S, Adamson S, Bonam D, Brodeur S, Charlebois T, Clancy B, Costigan R, Drapeau D, Hamilton M, Hanley K, Kelley B, Knight A, Leonard M, McCarthy M, Oakes P, Sterl K, Switzer M, Walsh R, Foster W (1998) The manufacturing process for recombinant factor IX. Sem Hematol 35(Suppl 2):4–10

Hedner U (2006) Mechanism of action, development and clinical experience of recombinant FVIIa. J Biotechnol 124:747–757

Hedner U, Ezban M (2008) Tissue factor and factor VIIa as therapeutic targets in disorders of hemostasis. Annu Rev Med 59:29–41

Hedner U, Kisiel W (1983) Use of human factor VIIa in the treatment of two hemophilia A patients with high-titer inhibitors. J Clin Invest 71:1836–1841

Huntington JA (2003) Mechanisms of glycosaminoglycan activation of the serpins in hemostasis. J Thromb Haemost 1:1535–1549

Inbal A, Oldenburg J, Carcao M, Rosholm A, Tehranchi R, Nugent D (2012) Recombinant factor XIII: a safe and novel treatment for congenital factor XIII deficiency. Blood 119:5111–5117

Iorio A (2017) Using pharmacokinetics to individualize hemophilia therapy. Hematology Am Soc Hematol Educ Program 2017:595–604

Jorgensen MJ, Cantor AB, Furie BC, Brown CL, Shoemaker CB, Furie B (1987) Recognition site directing vitamin K-dependent γ-carboxylation resides on the propeptide of factor IX. Cell 48:185–191

Keyt BA, Paoni NF, Refino CJ, Berleau L, Nguyen H, Chow A, Lai J, Pena L, Pater C, Ogez J, Etscheverry T, Botstein D, Bennett WF (1994) A faster-acting and more potent form of tissue plasminogen activator. Proc Natl Acad Sci U S A 91:3670–3674

Kitchen S, Tiefenbacher S, Gosselin R (2017) Factor activity assays for monitoring extended half-life FVIII and factor IX replacement therapies. Sem Thromb Hemost 43:331–337

Komaromi I, Bagoly Z, Muszbek L (2011) factor XIII: novel structural and functional aspects. J Thromb Haemost 9:9–20

Kurachi K, Davie EW (1982) Isolation and characterization of a cDNA coding for human factor IX. Proc Natl Acad Sci U S A 79:6461–6464

Leksa NC, Chiu PL, Bou-Assaf GM, Quan C, Liu Z, Goodman AB, Chambers MG, Tsutakawa SE, Hammel M, Peters RT, Waltz T, Kulman JD (2017) The structural basis for the functional comparability of factor VIII and the long-acting variant factor VIII Fc fusion protein. J Thromb Haemost 15:1167–1179

Lenting PJ, van Mourik JA, Mertens K (1998) The life cycle of coagulation factor VIII in view of its structure and function. Blood 92:3983–3996

Lovejoy AE, Reynolds TC, Visich JE, Butine MD, Young G, Belvedere MA, Blain RC, Pederson SM, Ishak LM, Nugent DJ (2006) Safety and pharmacokinetics of recombinant factor XIII-A_2 administration in patients with congenital factor XIII deficiency. Blood 108:57–62

Lusis AJ (2000) Atherosclerosis. Nature 407:233–241

Maas Enriquez M, Thrift J, Garger S, Katterle Y (2016) Bay 81-8973, a full-length recombinant factor VIII: human heat shock protein 70 improves the manufacturing process without affecting clinical safety. Prot Expr Purif 127:111–115

Macfarlane RG (1964) An enzyme cascade in the blood clotting mechanism, and its function as a biochemical amplifier. Nature 202:498–499

Mahlangu JN, Weldingh KN, Lentz SR, Kaicker S, Karim FA, Matsushita T, Recht M, Tomczak W, Windyga J, Ehrenfort S, Knobe K (2015) Changes in the amino acid sequence of the recombinant human factor VIIa analog, vatreptacog alfa, are associated with clinical immunogenicity. J Thromb Haemost 13:1989–1998

Mann KG, Orfeo T, Butenas S, Undas A, Brummel-Ziedins K (2009) Blood coagulation dynamics in haemostasis. Hämostaseologie 29:7–16

Mannucci PM (2004) Treatment of von Willebrand's disease. N Engl J Med 531:683–694

Mei B, Pan C, Jiang H, Tjandra H, Strauss J, Chen Y, Liu T, Zhang X, Severs J, Newgren J, Chen J, Gu J-M, Subramanyam B, Fournel MA, Pierce GF (2010) Rational design of a fully active, long-acting PEGylated factor VIII for hemophilia A treatment. Blood 116:270–279

Metzner HJ, Weimer T, Kronthaler U, Lang W, Schulte S (2009) Genetic fusion to albumin improves the pharmacokinetic properties of factor IX. Thromb Haemost 102:634–644

Monroe DM, Jenny RJ, Van Cott KE, Buhay S, Saward LL (2016) Characterization of IXINITY (trenonacog alfa), a recombinant factor IX with primary sequence coresponding to the threonine-148 polymorph. Adv Hematol 2016:7678901

Moser M, Kohler B, Schmittner M, Bode C (1998) Recombinant plasminogen activators: a comparative review of the clinical pharmacology and therapeutic use of alteplase and reteplase. BioDrugs 9:455–463

Østergaard H, Bjelke JR, Hansen L, Petersen LC, Pedersen AA, Elm T, Møller F, Hermit MB, Holm PK, Krogh TN, Petersen LM, Ezban M, Sørensen BB, Andersen MD, Agersø H, Ahmandian H, Balling KW, Christiansen MLS, Knobe K, Nichols TC, Bjørn SE, Tranholm M (2011) Prolonged half-life and preserved enzymatic properties of factor IX selectively PEGylated on native N-glycans in the activation peptide. Blood 118:2333–2341

Paidas MJ, Forsyth C, Quéré I, Rodger M, Frieling JTM, Tait RC (2014) Perioperative and peripartum prevention of venous thromboembolism in patients with hereditary antithrombin deficiency using recombinant antithrombin therapy. Blood Coagul Fibrinolysis 25:444–450

Palla R, Peyvandi F, Shapiro A (2015) Rare bleeding disorders: diagnosis and treatment. Blood 125:2052–2061

Pennica D, Holmes WE, Kohr WJ, Harkins RN, Vehar GA, Ward CA, Bennett WF, Yelverton E, Seeburg PH,

Heyneker HL, Goeddel DV, Collen D (1983) Cloning and expression of human tissue-type plasminogen activator cDNA in E. coli. Nature 301:214–221

Perera L, Darden T, Pedersen LG (2001) Modeling human zymogen factor IX. Thromb Haemost 85:596–603

Peters RT, Low SC, Kamphaus GD, Dumont JA, Amari JV, Lu Q, Zarbis-Papastoitsis G, Reidy TJ, Merricks EP, Nichols TC, Bitonti AJ (2010) Prolonged activity of factor IX as a monomeric Fc fusion protein. Blood 115:2057–2064

Pipe SW, Montgomery RR, Pratt KP, Lenting PJ, Lillicrap D (2016) Life in the shadow of a dominant partner: the FVIII-VWF association and its clinical implications for hemophilia A. Blood 128:2007–2016

Rijken DC, Hoylaerts M, Collen D (1982) Fibrinolytic properties of one-chain and two-chain human extrinsic (tissue-type) plasminogen activator. J Biol Chem 257:2920–2925

Rogaev EI, Grigorenko AP, Faskhutdinova G, Kittler ELW, Moliaka YK (2009) Science 326:817

Sandberg H, Kannicht C, Stenlund P, Dadaian M, Oswaldsson U, Cordula C, Walter O (2012) Functional characteristics of the novel, human-derived recombinant FVIII protein product, human-cl rhFVIII. Thromb Res 130:808–817

Schmidbauer S, Witzel R, Robbel L, Sebastian P, Grammel N, Metzner HJ, Schulte S (2015) Physicochemical characterisation of rVIII-SingleChain, a novel recombinant single-chain factor VIII. Thromb Res 136:388–395

Simpson D, Siddiqui MAA, Scott LJ, Hilleman DE (2006) Reteplase: a review of its use in the management of thrombotic occlusive disorders. Am J Cardiovasc Drugs 6:265–285

Stennicke HR, Kjalke M, Karpf DM, Baling KW, Johansen PB, Elm T, Øvlisen K, Möller F, Holmberg HL, Gudme CN, Persson E, Hilden I, Pelzer H, Rahbeck-Nielsen H, Jespersgaard C, Bogsnes A, Pedersen AA, Kristensen AK, Peschke B, Kappers W, Rode F, Thim L, Tranholm M, Ezban M, Olsen EHN, Bjørn SE (2013) A novel B-domain O-glycoPEGylated FVIII (N8-GP) demonstrates full efficacy and prolonged effect in hemophilic mice models. Blood 121:2108–2116

Thim L, Vandahl B, Karlsson J, Klausen NK, Pedersen J, Krogh TN, Kjalke M, Petersen JM, Johnsen LB, Bolt G, Nørby PL, Steenstrup TD (2010) Purification and characterization of a new recombinant factor VIII (N8). Haemophilia 16:349–359

Tiede A, Tait RC, Shaffer DW, Baudo F, Boneu B, Dempfle CE, Horrelou MH, Klamroth R, Lazarchick J, Mumford AD, Schulman S, Shiach C, Bonfiglio LJ, Frieling JTM, Conard J, von Depka M (2008) Antithrombin alfa in hereditary antithrombin deficient patients: a phase 3 study of prophylactic intravenous administration in high risk situations. Thromb Haemost 99:616–622

Toole JJ, Knopf JL, Wozney JM, Sultzman LA, Bueker JL, Pittman DD, Kaufman RJ, Brown E, Shoemaker C, Orr EC, Amphlett GW, Foster WB, Coe ML, Knutson GJ, Fass DN, Hewick RM (1984) Molecular cloning of a cDNA encoding human antihaemophilic factor. Nature 312:342–347

Toole JJ, Pittman DD, Orr EC, Murtha P, Wasley LC, Kaufman RJ (1986) A large region (approximately equal to 95 kDa) of human factor VIII is dispensable for in vitro procoagulant activity. Proc Natl Acad Sci U S A 83:5939–5942

Turecek PL, Bossard M, Graniger M, Gritsch H, Höllriegl W, Kaliwoda M, Matthiessen P, Mitterer A, Muchitsch E-M, Purtscher M, Rottensteiner H, Schiviz A, Schrenk G, Siekmann J, Varadi K, Riley T, Ehrlich HJ, Schwarz HP, Scheiflinger F (2012) BAX 855, a PEGylated rFVIII product with prolonged half-life: development, functional and structural characterisation. Hämostaseologie 32(Suppl 1):S29–S38

Turecek PL, Mitterer A, Matthiessen HP, Gritsch H, Varadi K, Siekmann J, Schnecker K, Plaimauer B, Kaliwoda M, Purtscher M, Woehrer W, Mundt W, Muchitsch E-M, Suiter T, Ewenstein BM, Ehrlich HJ, Schwarz HP (2009) Development of a plasma- and albumin-free recombinant von Willebrand factor. Hämostaseologie 29(Suppl 1):S32–S38

Vehar GA, Keyt B, Eaton D, Rodriguez H, O'Brien DP, Rotblatt F, Oppermann H, Keck R, Wood WI, Harkins RN, Tuddenham EGD, Lawn RM, Capon DJ (1984) Structure of human factor VIII. Nature 312:337–342

Wasley LC, Rehemtulla A, Bristol JA, Kaufman RJ (1993) PACE/furin can process the vitamin K-dependent pro-factor IX precursor within the secretory pathway. J Biol Chem 268:8458–8465

Young G, Mahlangu JN (2016) Extended half-life clotting factor concentrates: results from published clinical trials. Haemophilia 22(Suppl 5):25–30

SUGGESTED READING

Bishop P, Lawson J (2004) Recombinant biologics for treatment of bleeding disorders. Nat Rev Drug Disc 3:684–694

Lubon H, Paleyanda RK, Velander WH, Drohan WN (1996) Blood proteins from transgenic animal bioreactors. Transf Med Rev 10(2):131–143

Mackman N (2008) Triggers, targets and treatments for thrombosis. Nature 451:914–918

Peyvandi F, Garagiola I, Seregni S (2013) Future of coagulation factor replacement therapy. J Thromb Haemost 11(Suppl 1):84–98

22 Recombinant Human Deoxyribonuclease I

Robert A. Lazarus and Jeffrey S. Wagener†

INTRODUCTION

Human deoxyribonuclease I (DNase I) is an endonuclease that catalyzes the hydrolysis of extracellular DNA and is just one of the numerous types of nucleases found in nature (Horton 2008; Yang 2011). It is the most extensively studied member in the family of DNase I-like nucleases (Keyel 2017; Lazarus 2002; Baranovskii et al. 2004; Shiokawa and Tanuma 2001); the homologous bovine DNase I has received even greater attention historically (Laskowski 1971; Moore 1981; Chen and Liao 2006). Mammalian DNases have been broadly divided into several families initially based upon their products, pH optima, and divalent metal ion requirements. These include the neutral DNase I family (EC 3.1.21.1), the acidic DNase II family (EC 3.1.22.1), as well as apoptotic nucleases such as DFF40/CAD and endonuclease G (Keyel 2017; Lazarus 2002; Evans and Aguilera 2003; Widlak and Garrard 2005). The human DNase I gene resides on chromosome 16p13.3 and contains 10 exons and 9 introns, which span 15 kb of genomic DNA (Kominato et al. 2006). DNase I is synthesized as a precursor and contains a 22-residue signal sequence that is cleaved upon secretion, resulting in the 260-residue mature enzyme. It is secreted by the pancreas and parotid glands, consistent with its proposed primary role of digesting nucleic acids in the gastrointestinal tract. However, it is also present in blood and urine as well as other tissues, suggesting additional functions.

Recombinant human DNase I (rhDNase I, rhDNase, Pulmozyme®, dornase alfa) has been developed clinically where it is aerosolized into the airways for treatment of pulmonary disease in patients with cystic fibrosis (CF) (Suri 2005; Wagener and Kupfer 2012). Cystic fibrosis is an autosomal recessive disease caused by mutations in the CF transmembrane conductance regulator (CFTR) gene (Kerem et al. 1989; Riordan et al. 1989). Mutations of this gene result in both abnormal quantity and function of an apical membrane protein responsible for chloride ion transfer. The CFTR protein is a member of the ATP-binding cassette transporter superfamily (member ABCC7) and in addition to transporting chloride has many other functions including the regulation of epithelial sodium channels, ATP-release mechanisms, anion exchangers, sodium bicarbonate transporters, and aquaporin water channels found in airways, intestine, pancreas, sweat duct, and other fluid-transporting tissues (Guggino and Stanton 2006). Clinical manifestations of the disease include chronic obstructive airway disease, increased sweat electrolyte excretion, male infertility due to obstruction of the vas deferens, and exocrine pancreatic insufficiency.

In the airways, abnormal CFTR results in altered secretions and mucociliary clearance, leading to a cycle of obstruction, chronic bacterial infection, and neutrophil-dominated inflammation. This bacterial infection and neutrophil-dominated airway inflammation begins early in the patient's life and, while initially it helps to control infection, the degree of inflammation remains excessive to the degree of infection. Poorly regulated neutrophil-dominated inflammation damages the airways over time due to the release of potent oxidants and proteases. Additionally, necrosis of neutrophils leads to the accumulation of extracellular DNA and actin, increasing the viscosity of mucous and creating further obstruction, and a downward spiral of lung damage, loss of lung function, and ultimately premature death (Fig. 22.1).

rhDNase I has also been studied in a variety of other diseases where extracellular DNA has been postulated to play a pathological role, including prolonged mechanical ventilation due to persistent airway obstruction (Riethmueller et al. 2006),

†This chapter is dedicated in honor of a lifetime of scientific and clinical contributions by Jeffrey S. Wagener, deceased October 24, 2018.

R. A. Lazarus (✉)
Department of Early Discovery Biochemistry, Genentech Inc., South San Francisco, CA, USA
e-mail: lazarus.bob@gene.com

J. S. Wagener
Department of Pediatrics, University of Colorado School of Medicine, Aurora, CO, USA

D. J. A. Crommelin et al. (eds.), *Pharmaceutical Biotechnology*, https://doi.org/10.1007/978-3-030-00710-2_22

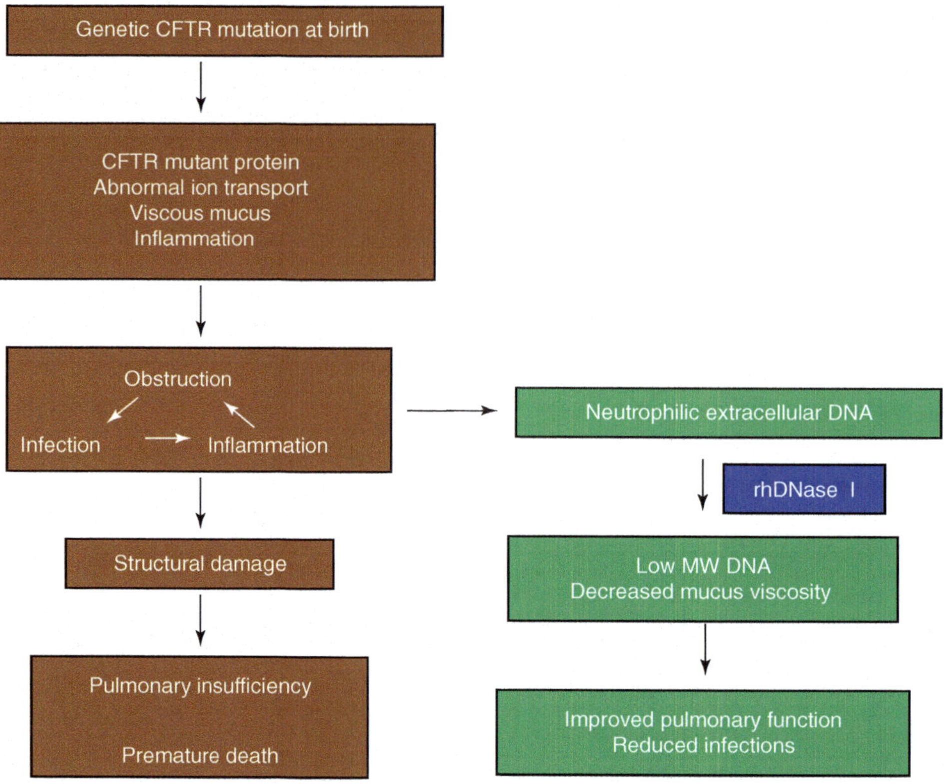

Figure 22.1 ■ Cystic fibrosis and rhDNase I. CFTR genetic mutation at birth leads to either reduced or improperly folded CFTR protein, which results in altered ion transport, viscous mucus, and inflammation in the airways. Eventually, this leads to obstruction of the airways, bacterial infection, and further inflammation. After neutrophils arrive to fight the infection, they die and release cellular contents, one of which is DNA. Persistent obstruction, infection, and inflammation leads to structural damage and eventually pulmonary insufficiency and premature death. rhDNase I is aerosolized into the airways where it degrades DNA to lower molecular weight fragments, thus reducing CF mucus viscosity and allowing expectoration, which improves lung function and reduces bacterial infections

ventilator-associated pneumonia in infants (Scala et al. 2017), atelectasis (Hendriks et al. 2005), chronic sinusitis (Cimmino et al. 2005), primary ciliary dyskinesia (Desai et al. 1995; ten Berge et al. 1999; El Abiad et al. 2007), other non-CF lung diseases in children (Boogaard et al. 2007a), and empyema (Simpson et al. 2003; Rahman et al. 2011). rhDNase I has also been studied to examine its effectiveness in the presence or absence of antibiotics against biofilm producing strains of *Staphylococcus aureus* and *Staphylococcus epidermidis* (Kaplan et al. 2012). rhDNase I exhibits potent antibiofilm and antimicrobial-sensitizing activities at clinically achievable concentrations.

Finally, the use of rhDNase I has been investigated in systemic lupus erythematosus (SLE) where degradation or prevention of immune complexes containing anti-DNA antigens may have therapeutic benefit (Lachmann 2003; Davis et al. 1999).

■ Historical Perspective and Rationale

Macromolecules that contribute to the physical properties of lung secretions include mucus glycoproteins, filamentous actin, and DNA. Experiments in the 1950s and 1960s revealed that DNA is present in very high concentrations (3–14 mg/mL) only in infected lung secretions (Matthews et al. 1963). This implied that the DNA that contributes to the high viscoelastic nature of CF sputum is derived from neutrophils responding to chronic infections (Potter et al. 1969). These DNA-rich secretions also bind aminoglycoside antibiotics commonly used for treatment of pulmonary infections and thus may reduce their efficacy (Ramphal et al. 1988; Bataillon et al. 1992).

Early in vitro studies in which lung secretions were incubated for several hours with partially purified bovine pancreatic DNase I showed a large reduction in viscosity (Armstrong and White 1950; Chernick et al. 1961). Based on these observations, bovine pancreatic DNase I (dornavac or pancreatic dornase) was approved in the United States for human use in 1958. Numerous uncontrolled clinical studies in patients with pneumonia and one study in patients with CF suggested that bovine pancreatic DNase I was effective in reducing the viscosity of lung secretions (Lieberman 1968). However, severe adverse reactions occurred occasionally, perhaps due to allergic reactions to a foreign protein or from contaminating proteases, since up to 2% of trypsin and chymotrypsin were present in the final product (Raskin 1968; Lieberman 1962). Both bovine DNase I products were eventually withdrawn from the market.

In the late 1980s, human deoxyribonuclease I was cloned from a human pancreatic cDNA library, sequenced and expressed recombinantly using mammalian cell culture in Chinese hamster ovary (CHO) cells to reevaluate the potential of DNase I as a therapeutic for cystic fibrosis (Shak et al. 1990). In vitro incubation of purulent sputum from CF patients with catalytic concentrations of rhDNase I reduced its viscoelasticity (Shak et al. 1990). The reduction in viscoelasticity was directly related to both rhDNase I concentration and reduction in the size of the DNA in the samples. Therefore, reduction of high molecular weight DNA into smaller fragments by treatment with aerosolized rhDNase I was proposed as a mechanism to reduce the mucus viscosity and improve mucus clearability from obstructed airways in patients. It was hoped that improved clearance of the purulent mucus would enhance pulmonary function and reduce recurrent exacerbations of respiratory symptoms requiring parenteral antibiotics. This proved to be the case and rhDNase I was approved by the Food and Drug Administration in 1993. Since that time the clinical use of rhDNase I has continued to increase with over 67% of CF patients receiving chronic therapy (Konstan et al. 2010).

PROTEIN CHEMISTRY, ENZYMOLOGY, AND STRUCTURE

The protein chemistry of human DNases including DNase I has been reviewed (Lazarus 2002; Baranovskii et al. 2004). Recombinant human DNase I is a monomeric, 260-amino acid glycoprotein (Fig. 22.2) produced by mammalian CHO cells (Shak et al. 1990). The protein has four cysteines, which are oxidized into two disulfides between Cys101–Cys104 and Cys173–Cys209 as well as two potential N-linked glycosylation sites at Asn18 and Asn106 (Fig. 22.2). rhDNase I is glycosylated at both sites and migrates as a broad band on polyacrylamide gel electrophoresis gels with an approximate molecular weight of 37 kDa, which is significantly higher than the predicted molecular mass from the amino acid sequence of 29.3 kDa. rhDNase I is an acidic protein and has a calculated pI of 4.58. The primary amino acid sequence is identical to that of the native human enzyme purified from urine.

DNase I cleaves double-stranded DNA, and to a much lesser degree single-stranded DNA, nonspecifically by nicking phosphodiester linkages in one of the strands between the 3′-oxygen atom and the phosphorus to yield 3′-hydroxyl and 5′-phosphoryl oligonucleotides with inversion of configuration at the phosphorus. rhDNase I enzymatic activity is dependent upon the presence of divalent metal ions for structure, as there are two tightly bound Ca^{2+} atoms and catalysis, which requires either Mg^{2+} or Mn^{2+} (Pan and Lazarus 1999). The active site includes two histidine

```
                   10                  20                  30
L K I A A F N I Q T F G E T K M S N A T L V S Y I V Q I L S
                   40                  50                  60
R Y D I A L V Q E V R D S H L T A V G K L L D N L N Q D A P
                   70                  80                  90
D T Y H Y V V S E P L G R N S Y K E R Y L F V Y R P D Q V S
                  100                 110                 120
A V D S Y Y Y D D G C E P C G N D T F N R E P A I V R F F S
                  130                 140                 150
R F T E V R E F A I V P L H A A P G D A V A E I D A L Y D V
                  160                 170                 180
Y L D V Q E K W G L E D V M L M G D F N A G C S Y V R P S Q
                  190                 200                 210
W S S I R L W T S P T F Q W L I P D S A D T T A T P T H C A
                  220                 230                 240
Y D R I V V A G M L L R G A V V P D S A L P F N F Q A A Y G
                  250                 260
L S D Q L A Q A I S D H Y P V E V M L K
```

Figure 22.2 ■ Primary amino acid sequence of rhDNase I. Active site residues are highlighted in *blue*, cysteine residues that form disulfide bonds are shown in *yellow*, N-linked glycosylation sites are highlighted in *pink*, and residues involved in Ca^{2+} coordination are shown in *beige*. The 22-residue signal sequence that is cleaved prior to secretion is not shown

residues (His134 and His252) and two acidic residues (Glu78 and Asp 212), all of which are critical for the general acid–base catalysis of phosphodiester bonds since alanine substitution of any of these results in a total loss of activity (Ulmer et al. 1996). Other residues involved in the coordination of divalent metal ions at the active site and DNA contact residues have also been identified by mutational analysis and include Asn7, Glu39, Asp168, Asn170, and Asp251 (Pan et al. 1998a; Parsiegla et al. 2012). The two Ca^{2+} binding sites require acidic or polar residues for coordination of Ca^{2+}; for site 1 these include Asp201 and Thr203 and for site 2 these include Asp99, Asp107, and Glu112 (Pan and Lazarus 1999). DNase I is a relatively stable enzyme and shows optimal activity at pH 5.5–7.5. It is inactivated by heat and is potently inhibited by EDTA and G-actin. Surprisingly, DNase I is also inhibited by NaCl and has only ca. 30% of the maximal activity in physiological saline.

rhDNase I belongs to the DNase I-like structural superfamily according to SCOP and is also related to the endonuclease-exonuclease-phosphatase family (Andreeva et al. 2008; Dlakic 2000; Wang et al. 2010). The X-ray crystal structure of rhDNase I was initially solved at 2.2 Å resolution and superimposes with the biochemically more widely studied bovine DNase I, which shares 78% sequence identity, with an rms deviation for main chain atoms of 0.56 Å (Wolf et al. 1995). DNase I is a compact α/β protein having a core of two tightly packed six-stranded β-sheets surrounded by eight α-helices and several loop regions (Fig. 22.3). Bovine DNase I has also been crystallized in complex with G-actin (Kabsch et al. 1990) as well as with several short oligonucleotides, revealing key features of DNA recognition in the minor groove and catalytic hydrolysis (Suck 1994).

More recently, the structure of rhDNase I containing a divalent Mg^{2+} and a phosphate in the active site has been solved at 1.95 Å resolution (Parsiegla et al. 2012). The combined structural and mutagenesis data suggest a Mg^{2+}-assisted pentavalent phosphate transition state during catalysis of rhDNase I, where Asp168 may play a key role as a catalytic general base. Asn170 is also in close proximity to both the attacking water molecule and the phosphoryl oxygen. His134 and His252 appear to act as general acids in stabilizing the pentavalent transition state. There is also a critical catalytic role for rhDNase I Asn7, a residue that is highly conserved among mammalian DNase I enzymes and members of the DNase I-like superfamily. The Mg^{2+} cation resides at the computationally predicted site IVb (Gueroult et al. 2010) and interacts with Asn7, Glu39, and Asp251 via a complex set of water-mediated hydrogen bond interactions. A comprehensive analysis of the rhDNase I

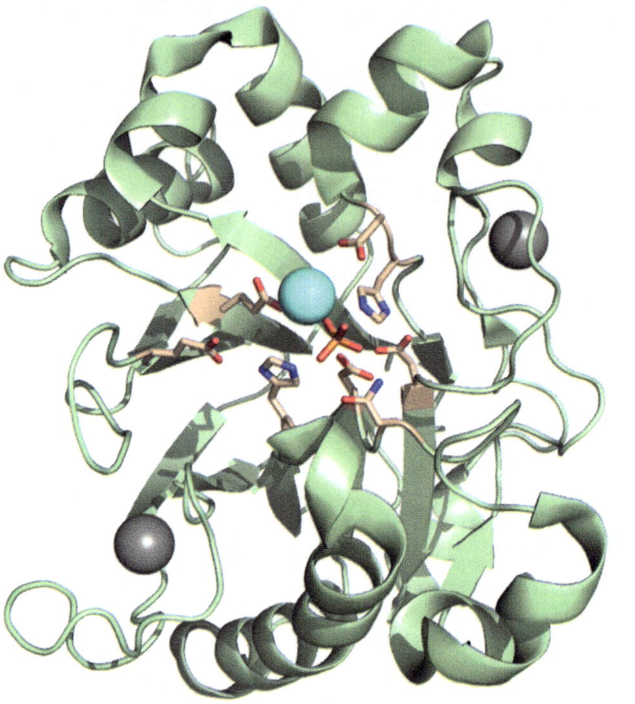

Figure 22.3 ■ Cartoon representation of rhDNase I depicting the active site of the enzyme. The active site residues are shown as *beige sticks* where oxygen and nitrogen atoms are in *red* and *blue*, respectively. The Mg^{2+} ion is shown as a *cyan sphere* and Ca^{2+} ions are shown as *grey* spheres. The phosphate ion is shown in sticks with the phosphorus atom in *orange*. The figure was made using PyMOL (www.pymol.org) using accession code 4AWN for rhDNase I (Parsiegla et al. 2012)

with members of the DNase I-like structural superfamily (Andreeva et al. 2008; Dlakic 2000) such as the apurinic/apyrimidinic endonucleases from human (APE1) (Mol et al. 2000) and *Neisseria meningitidis* (Nape) (Carpenter et al. 2007), sphingomyelin phosphodiesterase (SMase) from *Bacillus cereus* (Ago et al. 2006), or the C-terminal domain of human CNOT6L nuclease (Wang et al. 2010) solved in complex with cations or DNA have revealed new insights into the catalytic mechanism of DNA hydrolysis.

Several variants of rhDNase I with greatly improved enzymatic properties have been engineered by site-directed mutagenesis (Pan and Lazarus 1997; Pan et al. 1998a). The methods for production of the variants and the assays to characterize them have been reviewed recently (Pan et al. 2001; Sinicropi and Lazarus 2001). The rationale for improving activity was to increase binding affinity to DNA by introducing positively charged residues (Arg or Lys) on rhDNase I loops at the DNA binding interface to form a salt bridge with phosphates on the DNA backbone. These so-called "hyperactive" rhDNase I variants are substantially more active than wild-type rhDNase I and are no longer inhibited by physiological saline. The greater catalytic activity of the hyperactive variants is due to a change in the catalytic mechanism from a "single nicking" activity in the case of wild-type rhDNase I to a "processive nicking" activity in the hyperactive rhDNase I variants (Pan and Lazarus 1997), where gaps rather than nicks result in a higher frequency of double strand cleavages.

It is interesting to note that significantly greater activity can result from just a few mutations on the surface that are not important for structural integrity. For whatever reason DNase I is not as efficient an enzyme as it could be for degrading DNA into small fragments. Furthermore the inhibition by G-actin can be eliminated by a single amino acid substitution (see below). Thus, DNase I is under some degree of regulation in vivo. One can only speculate that nature may have wanted to avoid an enzyme with too much DNA degrading activity that could result in undesired mutations in the genome.

EMERGING BIOLOGY

Neutrophil Extracellular Traps

Neutrophils are important effector cells that play a key role in innate immunity. They have well documented 'first-line defense' roles in phagocytosis of foreign organisms such as bacteria and fungi. NETosis, the formation and release of neutrophil extracellular traps (NETs) is another defense mechanism that has emerged more recently (Brinkmann et al. 2004). Neutrophils can degranulate, releasing NETs, which are structures of DNA filaments coated with toxic histones, proteases, oxidative enzymes and other proteins that can immobilize and neutralize bacteria in the extracellular environment. NETosis can lead to a cell death process that is distinct from both apoptosis and necrosis, but it can also be independent of cell death (Jorch and Kubes 2017; Honda and Kubes 2018). NETs and NETosis have been broadly studied in biology and their role in a wide variety of diseases is of great interest (Jorch and Kubes 2017; Brinkmann 2018). These have included autoimmune, inflammatory, thrombotic, cancer and other diseases such as SLE, vasculitis, acute pancreatitus, rheumatoid arthritis, Type 1 diabetes mellitus and wound healing, gout, inflammatory bowel disease; vascular occlusion, sepsis, ARDS, metastasis and others (Cools-Lartigue et al. 2014; Martinod and Wagner 2014; Merza et al. 2015; Wong et al. 2015; Lood et al. 2016; Park et al. 2016; Gupta and Kaplan 2016; Jiménez-Alcázar et al. 2017b; Apel et al. 2018; Honda and Kubes 2018). It is particularly significant that DNase I or rhDNase I was almost always used in the biological studies on the above mentioned disease areas to show the effect of NET degradation, most often resulting in beneficial effects. Notably, serum DNase I had been shown to be essential for degradation of NETs (Hakkim et al. 2010); however, other DNase I like nucleases like DNase 1L3 can also degrade NETs (Jiménez-Alcázar et al. 2017b).

While it is clear that NETs and NETosis plays an important role in biology, that role is quite complex. In many cases they likely play a beneficial role, however in others they may play a pathological role. Like many areas of biology and disease, it is likely the right balance as well as the their locality that makes the difference. Furthermore, it is not always clear if they are the cause or result of a given pathology; there is evidence supporting both in thrombosis (Jiménez-Alcázar et al. 2017a). There is much evidence showing that diseases involve a multitude of pathways. For example, there are strong connections between coagulation, inflammation and cancer pathways. It is not surprising that NETs also have connections with these pathways. NETosis is a factor in tumor progression as well as cancer associated thrombosis (Demers and Wagner 2014). Both neutrophils and circulating extracellular DNA have been suggested to play an important role in cancer (Hawes et al. 2015).

With respect to rhDNase I, it is especially noteworthy that NETs play a significant role in CF (Gray et al. 2015; Law and Gray 2017), since this is the major use of rhDNase I clinically. While rhDNase I has a rheological effect in reducing the viscoelasticity in CF sputum, it also has biological effects related to releasing various enzymes and proteins from the NETs upon hydrolysis of the DNA. In the CF lung, NETs may play less of a role as an antibacterial and more of a role in fostering inflammation. rhDNase I likely exerts its anti-inflammatory function due to degradation of NETs.

PHARMACOLOGY

In Vitro Activity in CF Sputum

In vitro, rhDNase I hydrolyzes the DNA in sputum of CF patients and reduces sputum viscoelasticity (Shak et al. 1990). Effects of rhDNase I were initially examined using a relatively crude "pourability" assay. Pourability was assessed qualitatively by inverting a tube of sputum and observing the movement of sputum after a tap on the side of the tube. Catalytic amounts of rhDNase I (50 μg/mL) greatly reduced the viscosity of the sputum, rapidly transforming it from a viscous gel to a flowing liquid. More than 50% of the sputum moved down the tube within 15 min of incubation, and all the sputum moved freely down the tube within 30 min. The qualitative results of the pourability assay were confirmed by quantitative measurement of viscosity using a Brookfield Cone-Plate viscometer (Fig. 22.4). The reduction of viscosity by rhDNase I is rhDNase I concentration-dependent and is associated with reduction in size of sputum DNA as measured by agarose gel electrophoresis (Fig. 22.5).

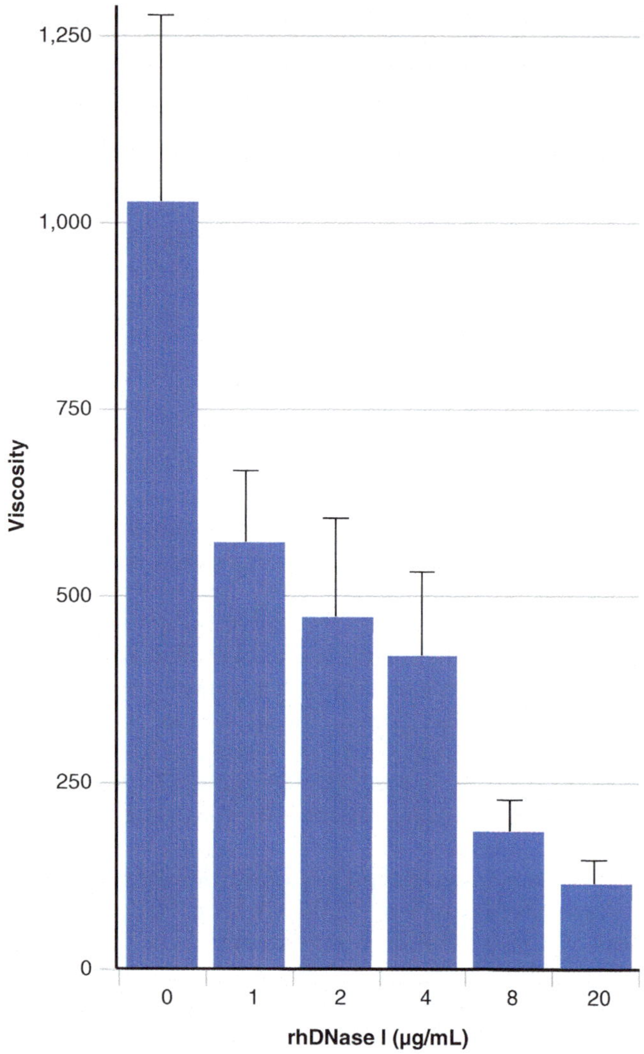

Figure 22.4 ■ In vitro reduction in viscosity (in centipoise) of cystic fibrosis sputum by cone-plate viscometry. Cystic fibrosis sputum was incubated with various concentrations of rhDNase I of 15 min at 37 °C

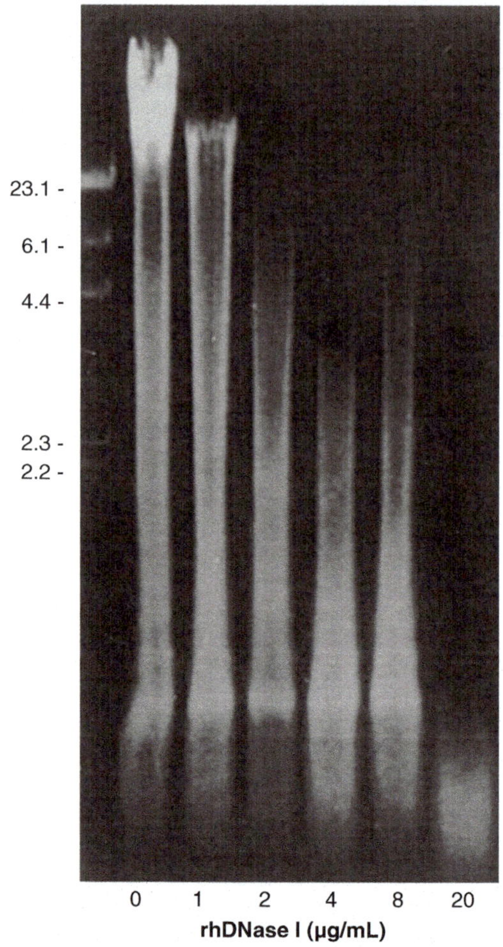

Figure 22.5 ■ In vitro reduction in sputum DNA size as measured by agarose gel electrophoresis. Cystic fibrosis sputum was incubated with increasing concentrations (0–20 µg/mL) of rhDNase I for 150 min at 37 °C. Molecular weight standards for DNA in kb are indicated

Additional in vitro studies of CF mucus samples treated with rhDNase I demonstrated a dose-dependent improvement in cough transport and mucociliary transport of CF mucus using a frog palate model and a reduction in adhesiveness as measured by mucus contact angle (Zahm et al. 1995). The improvements in mucus transport properties and adhesiveness were associated with a decrease in mucus viscosity and mucus surface tension, suggesting rhDNase I treatment may improve the clearance of mucus from airways. The in vitro viscoelastic properties of rhDNase I have also been studied in combination with normal saline, 3% hypertonic saline, or nacystelyn, the L-lysine salt of N-acetyl cysteine (King et al. 1997; Dasgupta and King 1996). The major impact of rhDNase I on CF sputum is to decrease spinnability, which is the thread forming ability of mucus under the influence of low amplitude stretching. CF sputum spinnability decreases 25% after 30 min incubation with rhDNase I (King et al. 1997). rhDNase I in normal saline and saline alone both increased the cough clearability index. With the combination of rhDNase I and 3% hypertonic saline, there was minimal effect on spinnability however mucus rigidity and cough clearability improved greater than with either agent alone. The predicted mucociliary clearance did not significantly increase with 3% saline either alone or in combination with rhDNase I. Combining rhDNase I with nacystelyn has an additive benefit on spinnability, but no effect on mucus rigidity or cough clearability (Dasgupta and King 1996). These effects of rhDNase I can be variable in vivo and do not necessarily correlate with the level of DNA in sputum. For example, sputum from CF patients that clinically responded to rhDNase I contains significantly higher levels of magnesium ions compared with sputum from patients who do not have a clear response (Sanders et al. 2006). Although this response is consistent with the requirement for divalent cations and their mode of action on DNase I (Campbell and Jackson 1980), the mechanism of increased rhDNase I activity by magnesium ions has been attributed to altering the polymerization state of actin such that equilibrium favors increased F-actin and decreased G-actin (see below).

The mechanism of action of rhDNase I to reduce CF sputum viscosity has been ascribed to DNA hydrolysis (Shak et al. 1990). However, an alternative mechanism involving depolymerization of filamentous actin (F-actin) has been suggested since F-actin contributes to the viscoelastic properties of CF sputum and the actin-depolymerizing protein gelsolin also reduces sputum viscoelasticity (Vasconcellos et al. 1994). F-actin is in equilibrium with its monomeric form (G-actin), which binds to rhDNase I with high affinity and is also a potent inhibitor of DNase I activity (Lazarides and Lindberg 1974). DNase I is known to depolymerize F-actin by binding to G-actin with high affinity, shifting the equilibrium in favor of rhDNase I/G-actin complexes (Hitchcock et al. 1976). To elucidate the mechanism of rhDNase I in CF sputum, the activity of two types of rhDNase I variants were compared in CF sputum (Ulmer et al. 1996). Active site variants were engineered that were unable to catalyze DNA hydrolysis but retained wild-type G-actin binding. Actin-resistant variants that no longer bound G-actin but retained wild-type DNA hydrolytic activity were also characterized. The active site variants did not degrade DNA in CF sputum and did not decrease sputum viscoelasticity (Fig. 22.6). Since the active site variants retained the ability to bind G-actin, these results argue against depolymerization of F-actin as the mechanism of action. In contrast, the actin-resistant variants were more potent than wild-type DNase I in their ability to degrade DNA and reduce sputum viscoelasticity (Fig. 22.6). The increased potency of the actin-resistant variants indicated that G-actin was a significant inhibitor of wild-type DNase I in CF sputum and confirmed that hydrolysis of DNA was the mechanism by which rhDNase I decreases sputum viscoelasticity. The mechanism for reduction of sputum viscosity by gelsolin was subsequently determined to result from an unexpected second binding site on actin that competes with DNase I, thus relieving the inhibition by G-actin (Davoodian et al. 1997). Additional in vitro studies characterizing the relative potency of actin-resistant

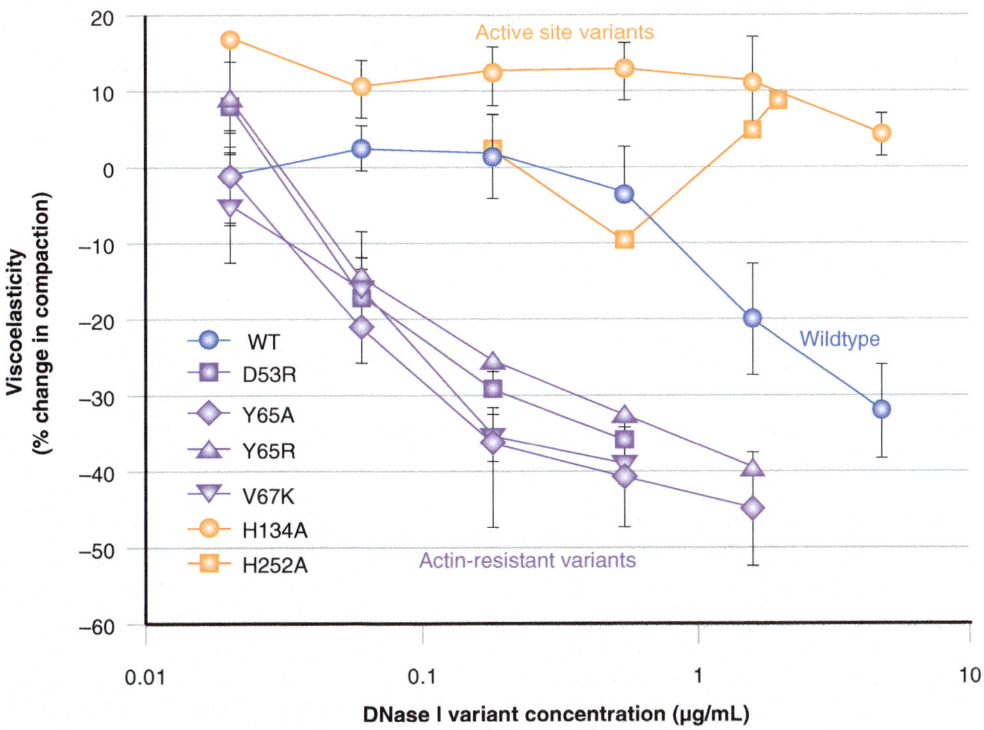

Figure 22.6 ■ Mechanism of action in CF mucus for rhDNase I. The change in viscoelasticity in CF mucus as a function of DNase I concentration was determined for wild-type rhDNase I, two active site variants that no longer catalyze DNA hydrolysis and four variants that are no longer inhibited by G-actin (Ulmer et al. 1996)

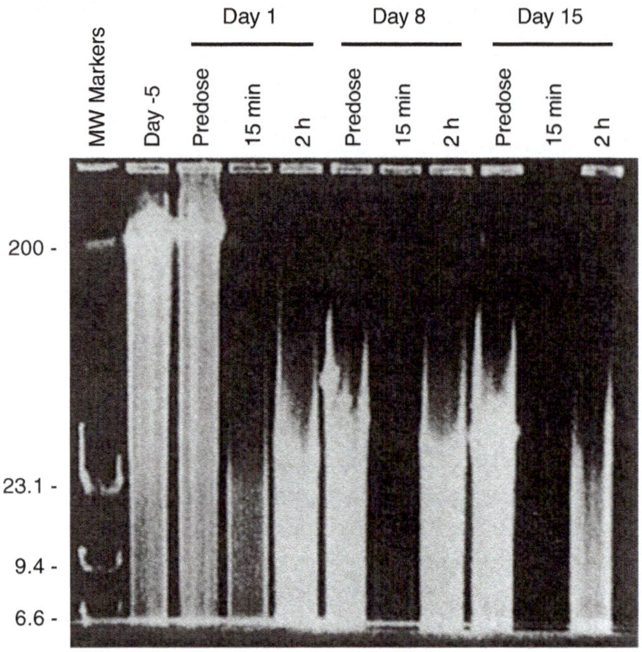

Figure 22.7 ■ Sustained reduction in DNA length in sputum recovered from a CF patient treated with 2.5 mg rhDNase I BID for up to 15 days. Samples were analyzed by pulsed field agarose gel electrophoresis. Molecular weight standards for DNA in kb are indicated

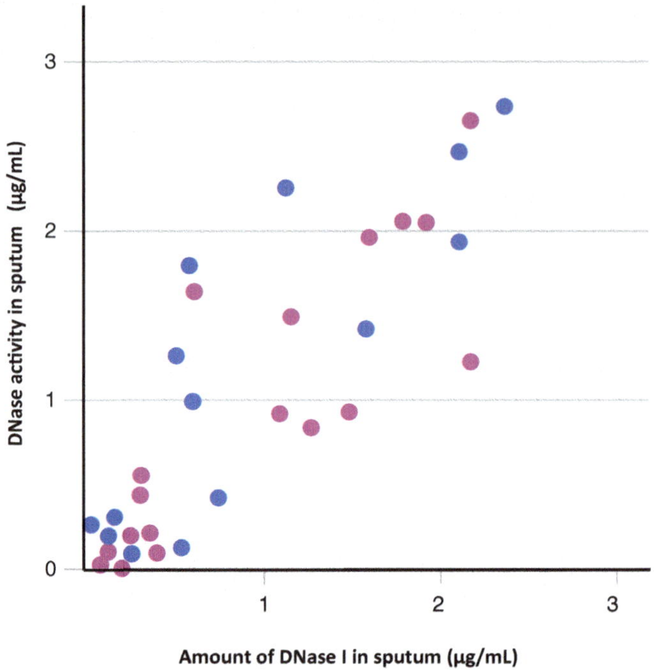

Figure 22.8 ■ Immunoreactive concentrations and enzymatic activity of rhDNase I in sputum following aerosol administration of either 10 mg (purple filled circle) or 20 mg (blue filled circle) rhDNase I to patients with cystic fibrosis. Each data point is a separate sample measured in duplicate

and hyperactive rhDNase I variants in serum and CF sputum have been reported (Pan et al. 1998b).

■ In Vivo Activity in CF Sputum

In vivo confirmation of the proposed mechanism of action for rhDNase I has been obtained from direct characterization of apparent DNA size (Fig. 22.7) and measurements of enzymatic and immunoreactive (ELISA) activity of rhDNase I (Fig. 22.8) in sputum from cystic fibrosis patients (Sinicropi et al. 1994a). Sputum samples were obtained 1–6 h post-dose from adult cystic fibrosis patients after inhalation of 5–20 mg of rhDNase I. rhDNase I therapy produced a sustained reduction in DNA size in recovered sputum (Fig. 22.7), in good agreement with the in vitro data.

Inhalation of the therapeutic dose of rhDNase I produced sputum levels of rhDNase I which have been shown to be effective in vitro (Fig. 22.8) (Shak 1995). Similarly, delivery to CF patients as young as 3 months can produce bronchoalveolar lavage fluid levels similar to that of older patients (Wagener et al. 1998). The recovered rhDNase I was also enzymatically active. Enzymatic activity was directly correlated with rhDNase I concentrations in the sputum. Viscoelasticity was reduced in the recovered sputum, as well. Furthermore, results from scintigraphic studies in using twice daily 2.5 mg of rhDNase I in CF patients suggested possible reductions in pulmonary obstruction and increased rates of mucociliary sputum clearance from the inner zone of the lung compared to controls (Laube et al. 1996). This finding was not confirmed in a crossover design study using once-daily dosing, suggesting that improvement of mucociliary clearance may require higher doses (Robinson et al. 2000). Epidemiologic evaluation of patients changing from once-daily dosing to twice-daily and vice versa has also shown improvement in lung function and fewer pulmonary exacerbations on higher doses, although the clinical indication for a dose change is not clear (VanDevanter et al. 2018).

■ Pharmacokinetics and Metabolism

Nonclinical pharmacokinetic data in rats and monkeys suggest minimal systemic absorption of rhDNase I following aerosol inhalation of clinically equivalent doses. rhDNase I is cleared from the systemic circulation without any accumulation in tissues following acute exposure (Green 1994). Additionally, nonclinical metabolism studies suggest that the low rhDNase I concentrations present in serum following inhalation will be bound to binding proteins (Green 1994; Mohler et al. 1993). The low concentrations of endogenous DNase I normally present in serum and the low concentrations of rhDNase I in serum following inhalation are inactive due to the ionic com-

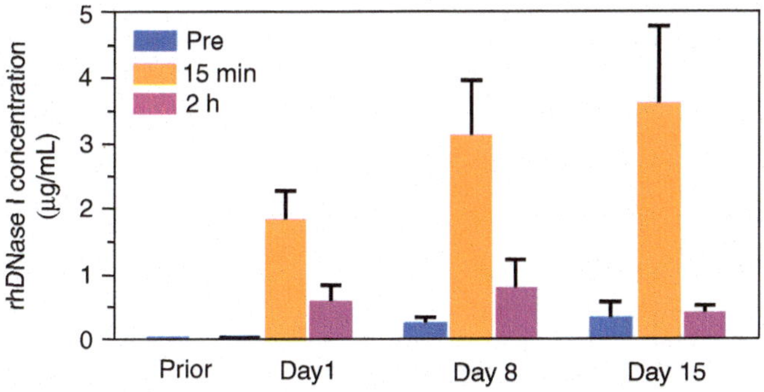

Figure 22.9 ■ rhDNase I concentration in sputum following administration of 2.5 mg of rhDNase I twice daily by inhalation to CF patients. The blue, orange, and purple bars represent concentrations at pre-dose, 15 min post-dose, and 2 h post-dose, respectively. The mean ± SD is shown with $N = 18$

position and presence of binding proteins in serum (Prince et al. 1998).

When 2.5 mg of rhDNase I was administered twice daily by inhalation to 18 CF patients, mean sputum concentrations of 2 μg/mL DNase I were measurable within 15 min after the first dose on Day 1 (Fig. 22.9). Mean sputum concentrations declined to an average of 0.6 μg/mL 2 h following inhalation. The peak rhDNase I concentration measured 2 h after inhalation on Days 8 and 15 increased to 3.0 and 3.6 μg/mL, respectively. Sputum rhDNase I concentrations measured 6 h after inhalation on Days 8 and 15 were similar to Day 1. Predose trough concentrations of 0.3–0.4 μg/mL rhDNase I measured on Day 8 and Day 15 (sample taken approximately 12 h after the previous dose) were, however, higher than Day 1, suggesting possible modest accumulation of rhDNase I with repeated dosing. Inhalation of up to 10 mg three times daily of rhDNase I by 4 CF patients for 6 consecutive days did not result in significant elevation of serum concentrations of DNase above normal endogenous levels (Aitken et al. 1992; Hubbard et al. 1992). After administration of up to 2.5 mg of rhDNase I twice daily for 6 months to 321 CF patients, no accumulation of serum DNase was noted (assay limit of detection is approximately 0.5 ng DNase/mL serum).

PROTEIN MANUFACTURING AND FORMULATION

rhDNase I is expressed in mammalian cell culture and purified to homogeneity using a variety of chromatographic steps. The development of the formulation of rhDNase I is especially important in that a suitable formulation is required to take into account protein stability, aerosolization properties, tonicity, and the sealed container for storage (Shire 1996). rhDNase I (Pulmozyme®, dornase alfa) is manufactured by Genentech, Inc. and formulated as a sterile, clear, and colorless aqueous solution containing 1.0 mg/mL dornase alfa, 0.15 mg/mL calcium chloride dihydrate, and 8.77 mg/mL sodium chloride. The solution contains no preservative and has a nominal pH of 6.3. Pulmozyme® is administered by the inhalation of an aerosol mist produced by a compressed air-driven nebulizer system. Pulmozyme® is supplied as single-use ampoules, which deliver 2.5 mL of solution to the nebulizer.

The choice of formulation components was determined by a need to provide 1–2 years of stability and to meet additional requirements unique to aerosol delivery (Shire 1996). A simple colorimetric assay for rhDNase I activity was used to evaluate the stability of rhDNase I in various formulations (Sinicropi et al. 1994b). In order to avoid adverse pulmonary reactions, such as cough or bronchoconstriction, aerosols for local pulmonary delivery should be formulated as isotonic solutions with minimal or no buffer components and should maintain pH >5.0. rhDNase I has an additional requirement for calcium to be present for optimal enzymatic activity. Limiting formulation components raised concerns about pH control, since protein stability and solubility can be highly pH-dependent. Fortunately, the protein itself provided sufficient buffering capacity at 1 mg/mL to maintain pH stability over the storage life of the product.

DRUG DELIVERY

The droplet or particle size of an aerosol is a critical factor in defining the site of deposition of the drug in the patient's airways (Gonda 1990). A distribution of particle or droplet size of 1–6 μm is optimal for the uniform deposition of rhDNase I in the airways (Cipolla et al. 1994). Jet nebulizers are the simplest method of producing aerosols in the desired respirable range. However, recirculation of protein solutions under high shear rates in the nebulizer bowl can present risks to the integrity of the protein molecule. rhDNase I survived recirculation and high shear rates during the nebulization process with no apparent degradation in protein quality or enzymatic activity (Cipolla et al. 1994). Ultrasonic nebulizers produce greater heat than jet nebulizers and protein breakdown prevents their use with rhDNase I. Significant advances in nebulizer technology have occurred since the original approval of rhDNase I. Newer nebulizers using a vibrating, perforated membrane do not produce protein breakdown and provide more rapid and efficient delivery of particles in the respirable range (Scherer et al. 2011).

Approved jet nebulizers produce aerosol droplets in the respirable range (1–6 μm) with a mass median aerodynamic diameter (MMAD) of 4–6 μm. The delivery of rhDNase I with a device that produces smaller droplets leads to more peripheral deposition in the smaller airways and thereby improves efficacy (Geller et al. 1998). Results obtained in 749 CF patients with mild disease confirmed that patients randomized to the Sidestream nebulizer powered by the Mobil Aire Compressor (MMAD = 2.1 μm) tended to have greater improvement in pulmonary function than patients using the Hudson T nebulizer with Pulmo-Aide Compressor (MMAD = 4.9 μm). These results indicate that the efficacy of rhDNase I is dependent, in part, on the physical properties of the aerosol produced by the delivery system. Nebulizers with vibrating mesh technology (Pari eFlow®) produce similarly small particles, suggesting these may result in further improved efficacy of rhDNase I. Furthermore, "smart" nebulizers are now available that coach the patient on taking a proper breath to improve delivery to the lower airways. Delivery of rhDNase I improves and lung function improves more when these nebulizers are used (Bakker et al. 2011). A randomized trial of efficacy and safety of dornase alfa delivered by the eRapid® nebulizer in CF patients showed comparable efficacy and safety, shorter nebulization times, and higher patient preference when compared to standard jet nebulizer systems such as the LC Plus (Sawicki et al. 2015).

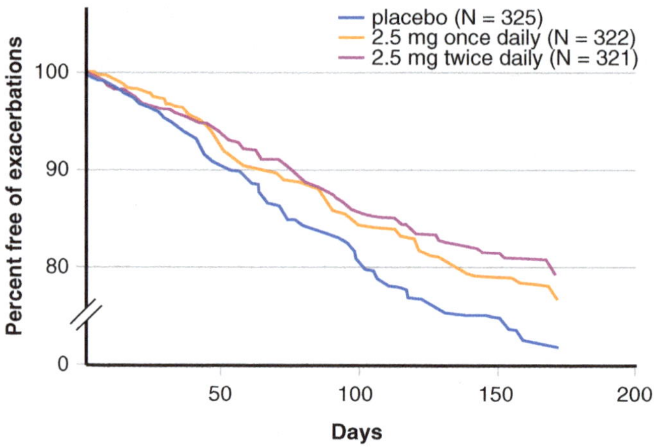

Figure 22.10 ■ Proportion of patients free of exacerbations of respiratory symptoms requiring parenteral antibiotic therapy from a 24-week study

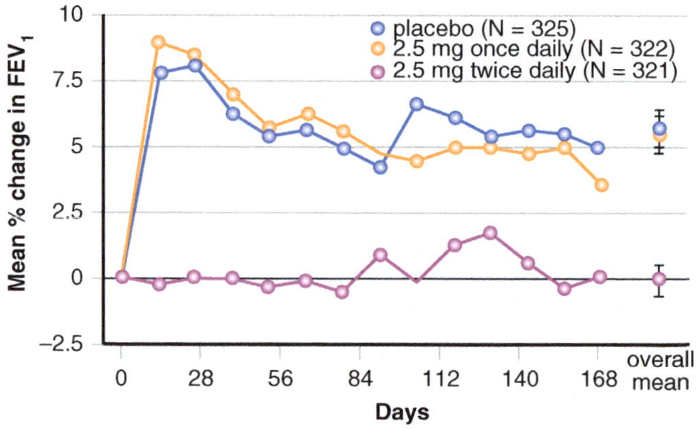

Figure 22.11 ■ Mean percent change in FEV_1 from baseline through a 24-week study

CLINICAL USE

■ Indication and Clinical Dosage

rhDNase I (Pulmozyme®, dornase alfa) is currently approved for use in CF patients, in conjunction with standard therapies, to reduce the frequency of respiratory infections requiring parenteral antibiotics and to improve pulmonary function (Fig. 22.1). The recommended dose for use in most CF patients is one 2.5 mg dose inhaled daily.

■ Cystic Fibrosis

rhDNase I was evaluated in a large, randomized, and placebo-controlled trial of clinically stable CF patients, 5 years of age or older, with baseline forced vital capacity (FVC) greater than or equal to 40% of predicted (Fuchs et al. 1994). All patients received additional standard therapies for CF. Patients were treated with placebo or 2.5 mg of rhDNase I once or twice a day for 6 months. When compared to placebo, both once daily and twice daily doses of rhDNase I resulted in a 28–37% reduction in respiratory tract infections requiring use of parenteral antibiotics (Fig. 22.10). Within 8 days of the start of treatment with rhDNase I, mean forced expiratory volume in 1 s (FEV_1) increased 7.9% in patients treated once a day and 9.0% in those treated twice a day compared to the baseline values. The mean FEV_1 observed during long-term therapy increased 5.8% from baseline at the 2.5 mg daily dose level and 5.6% from baseline at the 2.5 mg twice daily dose level (Fig. 22.11). The risk of respiratory tract infection was reduced even in patients whose pulmonary function (FEV_1) did not improve. This finding may be due to improved clearance of mucus from the small airways in the lung, which will have little effect on FEV_1 (Shak 1995). Supporting this concept is the finding that rhDNase I improves the lung clearance index in 6–18-year-old CF patients with normal lung function (Amin et al. 2011). Alternatively, use of rhDNase I may be altering the neutrophilic inflammatory response that occurs early in the course of CF lung disease, similar to the use of other anti-inflammatory therapies (Konstan and Ratjen 2012). The administration of rhDNase I also lessened shortness of breath, increased the general perception of well-being, and reduced the severity of other cystic fibrosis-related symptoms. Based on these findings, the US Cystic Fibrosis Foundation, in their chronic therapy pulmonary guidelines, strongly recommends the use of rhDNase I in patients 6 years old and older with moderate to severe lung disease and recommends its use in patients with mild lung disease (Flume et al. 2007).

The safety and deposition, but not efficacy, of rhDNase I has been studied in CF patients <5 years old (3 months to 5 years) since therapy may provide clinical benefit for young CF patients with mild disease (Wagener et al. 1998). After 2 weeks of daily administration of 2.5 mg rhDNase I, levels of rhDNase I deposited in the lower airways were similar for children <5 years compared to a group of 5–10-year-olds. Moreover, rhDNase I was well tolerated in the younger age group with an adverse event frequency similar to that in the older age group. To further understand how rhDNase I might alter the progression of lung disease, children with mild CF related lung disease were treated for 2 years in a randomized controlled trial (Quan et al. 2001). Children with a mean age of 8.4 years and an FVC greater than 85% of predicted were treated once daily with either placebo or 2.5 mg rhDNase I. After 96 weeks, lung function was significantly better in the treated group compared with placebo, particularly for tests measuring function of smaller airways. Respiratory exacerbations were also reduced in the treated group.

Clinical trials have indicated that rhDNase I therapy can be continued or initiated during an acute respiratory exacerbation (Wilmott et al. 1996). rhDNase I however does not produce a pulmonary function benefit when used short-term in the most severely ill CF patients (FVC less than 40% of predicted) (Shah et al. 1995; McCoy et al. 1996). Short-term dose ranging studies demonstrated that doses in excess of 2.5 mg twice daily did not provide further significant improvement in FEV_1 (Aitken et al. 1992; Hubbard et al. 1992; Ramsey et al. 1993). Patients who have received drug on a cyclical regimen (i.e., administration of rhDNase I 10 mg twice daily for 14 days, followed by a 14-day washout period) showed rapid improvement in FEV_1 with the initiation of rhDNase I and a return to baseline following withdrawal (Eisenberg et al. 1997). rhDNase I use improves quality of life as measured by the validated CFQ-R questionnaire (Rozov et al. 2010).

Concomitant therapy with rhDNase I and other standard CF therapies often show additive effects. The intermittent administration of aerosolized tobramycin was approved for use in CF patients with or without concomitant use of rhDNase I (Ramsey et al. 1999). Aerosolized tobramycin was well tolerated, enhanced pulmonary function, and decreased the density of *P. aeruginosa* in sputum. In combination with rhDNase I a larger treatment effect was noted but did not reach statistical significance. No differences in safety profile were observed following aerosolized tobramycin in patients that did or did not use rhDNase I. Chronic use of azithromycin has also been studied in CF patients chronically infected with *P. aeruginosa* (Saiman et al. 2005). Similar improvement in lung function and reduction in respiratory exacerbations was seen in patients receiving rhDNase I as those not, suggesting an additive, but not synergistic benefit of the two therapies used together. The combination of hypertonic saline therapy with chronic use of rhDNase I has similar additive benefits (Elkins et al. 2006), in agreement with the previously mentioned in vitro studies. Finally, combining ivacaftor, which potentiates chloride transport in CF patients with the G551D gene mutation, with chronic rhDNase I use produces an additive benefit in both improved lung function and reduced respiratory exacerbations (Ramsey et al. 2011). Notably, there was no evidence of a change in adverse events related to combination therapy in any of these studies.

Following FDA approval of rhDNase I in 1993, a large epidemiologic study of CF patients was initiated (the Epidemiologic Study of Cystic Fibrosis or ESCF), which continued until 2005 (Morgan et al. 1999). This study was designed to evaluate practice patterns in CF patients and has included data from over 24,000 patients. Recent analysis of ESCF data showed that chronic use of rhDNase I is associated with a decreased rate of decline in lung function overtime (Konstan et al. 2011). This reduced rate of decline in lung function is similar to findings with oral ibuprofen (Konstan et al. 1995, 2007) and inhaled corticosteroids (Ren et al. 2008), suggesting that there may be a long-term anti-inflammatory benefit with the use of rhDNase I. This potential anti-inflammatory effect is supported by a randomized trial in 105 CF patients with mild lung disease (FEV_1 >80% predicted) (Paul et al. 2004). Based on an initial bronchoscopy and alveolar lavage, patients were divided into two groups, those without airway inflammation ($n = 20$) and those with. The patients with inflammation were then randomized to treatment with rhDNase I ($n = 46$) or not ($n = 39$). Follow-up bronchoscopy and lavage was performed at 18 and 36 months. In the patients treated with rhDNase I, there was no change in inflammation as measured by elastase and IL-8 levels and neutrophil number. Patients not treated with rhDNase I and patients who did not have inflammation at baseline all had worsening neutrophilic inflammation on follow-up. Although this study was not designed to evaluate the rate of lung function decline, treated patients dropped FEV_1 by 1.99% predicted per year compared to a 3.26% predicted drop per year in the untreated subjects. Finally, rhDNase I is associated with a 15% reduction in the odds of subsequent year mortality in patients with CF (Sawicki et al. 2012).

Non-cystic Fibrosis Respiratory Disease

Although originally considered beneficial for the treatment of non-CF related bronchiectasis (Wills et al. 1996), rhDNase I had no effect on pulmonary function or the frequency of respiratory exacerbations in a randomized controlled trial (O'Donnell et al. 1998).

In another randomized controlled trial of rhDNase I, young children had shorter periods of ventilatory support following cardiac surgery when rhDNase I was instilled twice daily into the endotracheal tube (Riethmueller et al. 2006). Complicating atelectasis was less frequent in the treated group, consistent with numerous case reports suggesting that rhDNase I decreases, and can be used to treat, atelectasis when directly instilled into the airway (Hendriks et al. 2005). This effectiveness in treating atelectasis seems particularly true for newborns with lung disease requiring mechanical ventilation (MacKinnon et al. 2011; Dilmen et al. 2011; Fedakar et al. 2012; Altunhan et al. 2012). Limited benefit has been seen in children with asthma (Puterman and Weinberg 1997) although no benefit has been seen in adults (Silverman et al. 2012), consistent with the lack of neutrophil dominated inflammation in asthma. Finally, while there is increased free DNA in the secretions of infants with respiratory syncytial virus caused bronchiolitis, early suggestions of benefit (Nasr et al. 2001) have not translated into reduced hospitalization or the need for supplemental oxygen (Boogaard et al. 2007b).

Empyema and Para-Pneumonic Effusion

In principle rhDNase I may be useful for treating any condition where high levels of extracellular DNA and associated viscoelastic properties are pathological. Pulmonary empyema involves the collection of purulent material in the pleural space and the use of rhDNase I instilled into the pleural space has been reviewed (Simpson et al. 2003; Corcoran et al. 2015). In one large, multicenter clinical trial for the treatment of empyema in adults, twice daily intrapleural administration over 3 days was evaluated in four groups: 5 mg rhDNase, 10 mg tissue plasminogen activator (t-PA), with the combination of both, and a double placebo. Patients receiving the combination therapy had improved fluid drainage and a reduced frequency of surgical referral (Rahman et al. 2011). Additional studies using similar doses have demonstrated similar clinical benefits in children, although determining when and if to perform surgery remains unclear (Piccolo et al. 2015; Gilbert and Gorden 2017). Importantly, it appears that using either t-PA or rhDNase 1 alone does not produce the benefit of combined therapy.

Other Medical Conditions

rhDNase I has also been instilled into the nasal sinuses after surgery for chronic infections (Cimmino et al. 2005; Raynor et al. 2000). While daily use over 28 days of nasal nebulized rhDNase I in patients with CF did not produce a significant change in the sinuses on MRI, there was a significant clinical improvement as measured by quality of life questionnaire (Mainz et al. 2011, 2014).

Children with otitis media develop chronic neutrophil inflammation and an associated increase in NETs. rhDNase I has been proposed for the management of chronic otitis disease in patients not responding well to antibiotics, although no significant clinical trials have been conducted (Thornton et al. 2013).

The effect of rhDNase I has been studied in a small group of advanced head and neck cancer patients with thick, tenacious upper airway secretions while receiving chemoradiationtherapy (Mittal et al. 2013). Preliminary results did not show a significant difference versus placebo in quality of life measures, but did show improvement in secondary endpoints of oropharyngeal secretions and DNA concentrations.

Safety

The administration of rhDNase I has not been associated with an increase in any major adverse events. Most adverse events were not more common with rhDNase I than with placebo treatment and probably reflect complications related to the underlying lung disease. Most events associated with dosing were mild, transient in nature, and did not require alterations in dosing. Observed symptoms included hoarseness, pharyngitis, laryngitis, rash, chest pain, and conjunctivitis. Within all the studies a small percentage (average 2–4%) of patients treated with rhDNase I developed serum antibodies to rhDNase I. None of these patients developed anaphylaxis and the clinical significance of serum antibodies to rhDNase I is unknown. rhDNase I has also been associated with a slight increased risk of allergic bronchopulmonary aspergillosis in CF patients, although this most likely represents the chronic use of a wet nebulizer and not a complication of rhDNase I (Jubin et al. 2010).

SUMMARY

DNase I, a secreted human enzyme whose normal function is thought to be for digestion of extracellular DNA, has been developed as a safe and effective adjunctive agent in the treatment of pulmonary disease in cystic fibrosis patients. rhDNase I reduces the viscoelasticity and improves the transport properties of viscous mucus both in vitro and in vivo. Inhalation of aerosolized rhDNase I reduces the risk of infections requiring antibiotics and improves pulmonary function and the well-being of CF patients with mild to moderate disease. Studies also suggest that rhDNase I has benefit in infants and young children with CF and in patients with early disease who may have "normal" lung function. Additional studies may assess the usefulness of rhDNase I in early-stage CF pulmonary disease and other diseases where extracellular DNA and NETs may play a pathological role.

SELF-ASSESSMENT QUESTIONS

Questions

1. Mutations of the CF gene result in abnormalities of the CF transmembrane conductance regulator protein. How do abnormalities of this protein lead to eventual lung damage?
2. How does rhDNase I result in improved pulmonary function in patients with cystic fibrosis?
3. rhDNase I is strongly recommended by the US Cystic Fibrosis Foundation for use in CF patients with moderate and severe lung disease. What other CF patients may benefit from using this therapy?
4. In addition to improving lung function in CF patients, what benefits have been demonstrated in clinical trials of rhDNase I?
5. What other medical conditions may benefit from treatment with rhDNase I?
6. Why should ultrasonic nebulizers not be used to administer rhDNase I? What other types of nebulizers might be effective for delivering rhDNase I?

Answers

1. Abnormal CFTR protein results in abnormal airway surface liquid, which leads to a vicious cycle of airway obstruction, infection, and inflammation. The chronic, excessive neutrophilic inflammation in the airway results in release of neutrophil elastase, oxidants, and extracellular DNA. These substances result in worsening obstruction and progressive airway damage.
2. rhDNase I cleaves extracellular DNA in the airway of CF patients, resulting in improved airway clearance of secretions. Additionally, rhDNase I may have anti-inflammatory properties, resulting in a slower progression of lung damage and reduced rate of decline in lung function. This anti-inflammatory benefit is more likely present in patients with earlier, less severe lung disease.
3. rhDNase I is also recommended in CF patients over age 6 with mild lung disease. It has also been demonstrated as safe in younger patients, although efficacy has not been studied.
4. rhDNase I use decreases the frequency of respiratory exacerbations. rhDNase I also lessened shortness of breath, increased the general perception of well-being, and reduced the severity of other cystic fibrosis-related symptoms.
5. Although only approved by the FDA for treatment of lung disease in patients with CF, controlled trials have also shown efficacy for treating empyema (in combination with t-PA) and sinus disease in patients with CF.
6. Ultrasonic nebulizers generate heat, which breaks down the protein in rhDNase I. Vibrating permeable membrane nebulizers and "smart" nebulizers do not damage the drug and may improve the effectiveness of rhDNase I.

REFERENCES

Ago H, Oda M, Takahashi M, Tsuge H, Ochi S, Katunuma N, Miyano M, Sakurai J (2006) Structural basis of the sphingomyelin phosphodiesterase activity in neutral sphingomyelinase from *Bacillus cereus*. J Biol Chem 281:16157–16167

Aitken ML, Burke W, McDonald G, Shak S, Montgomery AB, Smith A (1992) Recombinant human DNase inhalation in normal subjects and patients with cystic fibrosis. A phase 1 study. JAMA 267:1947–1951

Altunhan H, Annagür A, Pekcan S, Ors R, Koç H (2012) Comparing the efficacy of nebulizer recombinant human DNase and hypertonic saline as monotherapy and combined treatment in the treatment of persistent atelectasis in mechanically ventilated newborns. Pediatr Int 54:131–136

Amin R, Subbarao P, Lou W, Jabar A, Balkovec S, Jensen R, Kerrigan S, Gustafsson P, Ratjen F (2011) The effect of dornase alfa on ventilation in homogeneity in patients with cystic fibrosis. Eur Respir J 37:806–812

Andreeva A, Howorth D, Chandonia JM, Brenner SE, Hubbard TJ, Chothia C, Murzin AG (2008) Data growth and its impact on the SCOP database: new developments. Nucleic Acids Res 36:D419–D425

Apel F, Zychlinsky A, Kenny EF (2018) The role of neutrophil extracellular traps in rheumatic diseases. Nat Rev Rheumatol 14:467–475

Armstrong JB, White JC (1950) Liquefaction of viscous purulent exudates by deoxyribonuclease. Lancet 2:739–742

Bakker EM, Volpi S, Salonini E, van der Wiel-Kooij EC, Sintnicolaas CJJCM, Hop WCJ, Assael BM, Merkus PJFM, Tiddens HAWM (2011) Improved treatment response to dornase alfa in cystic fibrosis patients using controlled inhalation. Eur Respir J 38:1328–1335

Baranovskii AG, Buneva VN, Nevinsky GA (2004) Human deoxyribonucleases. Biochemistry (Mosc) 69:587–601

Bataillon V, Lhermitte M, Lafitte JJ, Pommery J, Roussel P (1992) The binding of amikacin to macromolecules from the sputum of patients suffering from respiratory diseases. J Antimicrob Chemother 29:499–508

Boogaard R, de Jongste JC, Merkus PJ (2007a) Pharmacotherapy of impaired mucociliary clearance in non-CF pediatric lung disease. A review of the literature. Pediatr Pulmonol 42:989–1001

Boogaard R, Hulsmann AR, van Veen L, Vaessen-Verberne AA, Yap YN, Sprij AJ, Brinkhorst G, Sibbles B, Hendriks T, Feith SW, Lincke CR, Brandsma AE, Brand PL, Hop WC, de Hoog M, Merkus PJ (2007b) Recombinant human deoxyribonuclease in infants with respiratory syncytial virus bronchiolitis. Chest 131:788–795

Brinkmann V (2018) Neutrophil extracellular traps in the second decade. J Innate Immun 10:414–421

Brinkmann V, Reichard U, Goosmann C, Fauler B, Uhlemann Y, Weiss DS, Weinrauch Y, Zychlinsky A (2004) Neutrophil extracellular traps kill bacteria. Science 303:1532–1535

Campbell VW, Jackson DA (1980) The effect of divalent cations on the mode of action of DNase I. The initial reaction products produced from covalently closed circular DNA. J Biol Chem 255:3726–3735

Carpenter EP, Corbett A, Thomson H, Adacha J, Jensen K, Bergeron J, Kasampalidis I, Exley R, Winterbotham M, Tang C, Baldwin GS, Freemont P (2007) AP endonuclease paralogues with distinct activities in DNA repair and bacterial pathogenesis. EMBO J 26:1363–1372

Chen WJ, Liao TH (2006) Structure and function of bovine pancreatic deoxyribonuclease I. Protein Pept Lett 13:447–453

Chernick WS, Barbero GJ, Eichel HJ (1961) In vitro evaluation of effect of enzymes on tracheobronchial secretions from patients with cystic fibrosis. Pediatrics 27:589–596

Cimmino M, Nardone M, Cavaliere M, Plantulli A, Sepe A, Esposito V, Mazzarella G, Raia V (2005) Dornase alfa as postoperative therapy in cystic fibrosis sinonasal disease. Arch Otolaryngol Head Neck Surg 131:1097–1101

Cipolla D, Gonda I, Shire SJ (1994) Characterization of aerosols of human recombinant deoxyribonuclease I (rhDNase) generated by jet nebulizers. Pharm Res 11:491–498

Cools-Lartigue J, Spicer J, Najmeh S, Ferri L (2014) Neutrophil extracellular traps in cancer progression. Cell Mol Life Sci 71:4179–4194

Corcoran JP, Wrightson JM, Belcher E, DeCamp MM, Feller-Kopman D, Rahman NM (2015) Pleural infection: past, present, and future directions. Lancet Respir Med 3:563–577

Dasgupta B, King M (1996) Reduction in viscoelasticity in cystic fibrosis sputum in vitro using combined treatment with nacystelyn and rhDNase. Pediatr Pulmonol 22:161–166

Davis JC Jr, Manzi S, Yarboro C, Rairie J, McInnes I, Averthelyi D, Sinicropi D, Hale VG, Balow J, Austin H, Boumpas DT, Klippel JH (1999) Recombinant human DNase I (rhDNase) in patients with lupus nephritis. Lupus 8:68–76

Davoodian K, Ritchings BW, Ramphal R, Bubb MR (1997) Gelsolin activates DNase I in vitro and cystic fibrosis sputum. Biochemistry 36:9637–9641

Demers M, Wagner DD (2014) NETosis: a new factor in tumor progression and cancer-associated thrombosis. Semin Thromb Hemost 40:277–283

Desai M, Weller PH, Spencer DA (1995) Clinical benefit from nebulized human recombinant DNase in Kartagener's syndrome. Pediatr Pulmonol 20:307–308

Dilmen U, Karagol BS, Oguz SS (2011) Nebulized hypertonic saline and recombinant human DNase in the treatment of pulmonary atelectasis in newborns. Pediatr Int 53:328–331

Dlakic M (2000) Functionally unrelated signalling proteins contain a fold similar to Mg^{2+}-dependent endonucleases. Trends Biochem Sci 25:272–273

Eisenberg JD, Aitken ML, Dorkin HL, Harwood IR, Ramsey BW, Schidlow DV, Wilmott RW, Wohl ME, Fuchs HJ, Christiansen DH, Smith AL (1997) Safety of repeated intermittent courses of aerosolized recombinant human deoxyribonuclease in patients with cystic fibrosis. J Pediatr 131:118–124

El Abiad NM, Clifton S, Nasr SZ (2007) Long-term use of nebulized human recombinant DNase I in two siblings with primary ciliary dyskinesia. Respir Med 101:2224–2226

Elkins MR, Robinson M, Rose BR, Harbour C, Moriarty CP, Marks GB, Belousova EG, Xuan W, Bye PT (2006) A controlled trial of long-term inhaled hypertonic saline in patients with cystic fibrosis. N Engl J Med 354: 229–240

Evans CJ, Aguilera RJ (2003) DNase II: genes, enzymes and function. Gene 322:1–15

Fedakar A, Aydogdu C, Fedakar A, Ugurlucan M, Bolu S, Iskender M (2012) Safety of recombinant human deoxyribonuclease as a rescue treatment for persistent atelectasis in newborns. Ann Saudi Med 32:131–136

Flume PA, O'Sullivan BP, Robinson KA, Goss CH, Mogayzel PJ Jr, Willey-Courand DB, Bujan J, Finder J, Lester M, Quittell L, Rosenblatt R, Vender RL, Hazle L, Sabadosa K, Marshall B (2007) Cystic fibrosis pulmonary guidelines: chronic medications for maintenance of lung health. Am J Respir Crit Care Med 176:957–969

Fuchs HJ, Borowitz DS, Christiansen DH, Morris EM, Nash ML, Ramsey BW, Rosenstein BJ, Smith AL, Wohl ME (1994) Effect of aerosolized recombinant human DNase on exacerbations of respiratory symptoms and on pulmonary function in patients with cystic fibrosis. N Engl J Med 331:637–642

Geller DE, Eigen H, Fiel SB, Clark A, Lamarre AP, Johnson CA, Konstan MW (1998) Effect of smaller droplet size of dornase alfa on lung function in mild cystic fibrosis. Pediatr Pulmonol 25:83–87

Gilbert CR, Gorden JA (2017) Use of intrapleural tissue plasminogen activator and deoxyribonuclease in pleural space infections: an update on alternative regimens. Curr Opin Pulm Med 23:371–375

Gonda I (1990) Aerosols for delivery of therapeutic and diagnostic agents to the respiratory tract. Crit Rev Ther Drug Carrier Syst 6:273–313

Gray RD, McCullagh BN, McCray PB (2015) NETs and CF lung disease: current status and future prospects. Antibiotics 4:62–75

Green JD (1994) Pharmaco-toxicological expert report Pulmozyme rhDNase Genentech, Inc. Hum Exp Toxicol 13:S1–S42

Gueroult M, Picot D, Abi-Ghanem J, Hartmann B, Baaden M (2010) How cations can assist DNase I in DNA binding and hydrolysis. PLoS Comput Biol 6:e1001000

Guggino WB, Stanton BA (2006) New insights into cystic fibrosis: molecular switches that regulate CFTR. Nat Rev Mol Cell Biol 7:426–436

Gupta S, Kaplan MJ (2016) The role of neutrophils and NETosis in autoimmune and renal diseases. Nat Rev Nephrol 12:402–413

Hakkim A, Fürnrohr BG, Amann K, Laube B, Abed UA, Brinkmann V, Herrmann M, Voll RE, Zychlinsky A

(2010) Impairment of neutrophil extracellular trap degradation is associated with lupus nephritis. Proc Natl Acad Sci USA 107:9813–9818

Hawes MC, Wen F, Elquza E (2015) Extracellular DNA: a bridge to cancer. Cancer Res 75:4260–4264

Hendriks T, de Hoog M, Lequin MH, Devos AS, Merkus PJ (2005) DNase and atelectasis in non-cystic fibrosis pediatric patients. Crit Care 9:R351–R356

Hitchcock SE, Carisson L, Lindberg U (1976) Depolymeri zation of F-actin by deoxyribonuclease I. Cell 7:531–542

Honda M, Kubes P (2018) Neutrophils and neutrophil extracellular traps in the liver and gastrointestinal system. Nat Rev Gastroenterol Hepatol 15:206–221

Horton NC (2008) DNA nucleases. In: Rice PA, Correll CC (eds) Protein-nucleic acid interactions: structural biology. Royal Society of Chemistry Publishing, Cambridge, pp 333–363

Hubbard RC, McElvaney NG, Birrer P, Shak S, Robinson WW, Jolley C, Wu M, Chernick MS, Crystal RG (1992) A preliminary study of aerosolized recombinant human deoxyribonuclease I in the treatment of cystic fibrosis. N Engl J Med 326:812–815

Jiménez-Alcázar M, Kim N, Fuchs TA (2017a) Circulating extracellular DNA: cause or consequence of thrombosis? Semin Thromb Hemost 243:553–561

Jiménez-Alcázar M, Rangaswamy C, Panda R, Bitterling J, Simsek YJ, Long AT, Bilyy R, Krenn V, Renné C, Renné T, Kluge S, Panzer U, Mizuta R, Mannherz HG, Kitamura D, Herrmann M, Napirei M, Fuchs TA (2017b) Host DNases prevent vascular occlusion by neutrophil extracellular traps. Science 358: 1202–1206

Jorch SK, Kubes P (2017) An emerging role for neutrophil extracellular traps in noninfectious disease. Nat Med 23:279–287

Jubin V, Ranque S, Le bel NS, Sarles J, Dubus J-C (2010) Risk factors for *Aspergillus* colonization and allergic bronchopulmonary aspergillosis in children with cystic fibrosis. Pediatr Pulmonol 45:764–771

Kabsch W, Mannherz HG, Suck D, Pai EF, Holmes KC (1990) Atomic structure of the actin: DNase I complex. Nature 347:37–44

Kaplan JB, LoVetri K, Cardona ST, Madhyastha S, Sadovskaya I, Jabbouri S, Izano EA (2012) Recombinant human DNase I decreases biofilm and increases antimicrobial susceptibility in Staphylococci. J Antibiot (Tokyo) 65:73–77

Kerem B, Rommens JM, Buchanan JA, Markiewicz D, Cox TK, Chakravarti A, Buchwald M, Tsui LC (1989) Identification of the cystic fibrosis gene: genetic analysis. Science 245:1073–1080

Keyel PA (2017) Dnases in health and disease. Dev Biol 429:1–11

King M, Dasgupta B, Tomkiewicz RP, Brown NE (1997) Rheology of cystic fibrosis sputum after in vitro treatment with hypertonic saline alone and in combination with recombinant human deoxyribonuclease I. Am J Respir Crit Care Med 156:173–177

Kominato Y, Ueki M, Iida R, Kawai Y, Nakajima T, Makita C, Itoi M, Tajima Y, Kishi K, Yasuda T (2006) Characterization of human deoxyribonuclease I gene (DNASE1) promoters reveals the utilization of two transcription-starting exons and the involvement of Sp1 in its transcriptional regulation. FEBS J 273:3094–3105

Konstan MW, Ratjen F (2012) Effect of dornase alfa on inflammation and lung function: potential role in the early treatment of cystic fibrosis. J Cyst Fibros 11:78–83

Konstan MW, Byard PJ, Hoppel CL, Davis PB (1995) Effect of high-dose ibuprofen in patients with cystic fibrosis. N Engl J Med 332:848–854

Konstan MW, Schluchter MD, Xue W, Davis PB (2007) Clinical use of Ibuprofen is associated with slower FEV_1 decline in children with cystic fibrosis. Am J Respir Crit Care Med 176:1084–1089

Konstan MW, VanDevanter DR, Rasouliyan L, Pasta DJ, Yegin A, Morgan WJ, Wagener JS (2010) Trends in the use of routine therapies in cystic fibrosis: 1995–2005. Pediatr Pulmonol 45:1167–1172

Konstan MW, Wagener JS, Pasta DJ, Millar SJ, Jacobs JR, Yegin A, Morgan WJ (2011) Clinical use of dornase alfa is associated with a slower rate of FEV_1 decline in cystic fibrosis. Pediatr Pulmonol 46:545–553

Lachmann PJ (2003) Lupus and desoxyribonuclease. Lupus 12:202–206

Laskowski M Sr (1971) Deoxyribonuclease I. In: Boyer PD (ed) The enzymes, vol 4, 3rd edn. Academic, New York, pp 289–311

Laube BL, Auci RM, Shields DE, Christiansen DH, Lucas MK, Fuchs HJ, Rosenstein BJ (1996) Effect of rhDNase on airflow obstruction and mucociliary clearance in cystic fibrosis. Am J Respir Crit Care Med 153:752–760

Law SM, Gray RD (2017) Neutrophil extracellular traps and the dysfunctional innate immune response of cystic fibrosis lung disease: a review. J Inflamm 14:29

Lazarides E, Lindberg U (1974) Actin is the naturally occurring inhibitor of deoxyribonuclease I. Proc Natl Acad Sci USA 71:4742–4746

Lazarus RA (2002) Human deoxyribonucleases. In: Creighton TE (ed) Wiley encyclopedia of molecular medicine. Wiley, New York, pp 1025–1028

Lieberman J (1962) Enzymatic dissolution of pulmonary secretions. An in vitro study of sputum from patients with cystic fibrosis of pancreas. Am J Dis Child 104:342–348

Lieberman J (1968) Dornase aerosol effect on sputum viscosity in cases of cystic fibrosis. JAMA 205:312–313

Lood C, Blanco LP, Purmalek MM, Carmona-Rivera C, De Ravin SS, Smith CK, Malech HL, Ledbetter JA, Elkon KB, Kaplan MJ (2016) Neutrophil extracellular traps enriched in oxidized mitochondrial DNA are interferogenic and contribute to lupus-like disease. Nat Med 22:146–153

MacKinnon R, Wheeler KI, Sokol J (2011) Endotracheal DNase for atelectasis in ventilated neonates. J Perinatol 31:799–801

Mainz JG, Schiller I, Ritschel C, Mentzel H-J, Riethmuller J, Koitschev A, Schneider G, Beck JF, Wiedemann B (2011) Sinonasal inhalation of dornase alfa in CF: a double-blind placebo-controlled cross-over pilot trial. Auris Nasus Larynx 38:220–227

Mainz JG, Schien C, Schiller I, Schädlich K, Koitschev A, Koitschev C, Riethmüller J, Graepler-Mainka U, Wiedemann B, Beck JF (2014) Sinonasal inhalation of dornase alfa administered by vibrating aerosol to cystic fibrosis patients: a double-blind placebo-controlled cross-over trial. J Cyst Fibros 13:461–470

Martinod K, Wagner DD (2014) Thrombosis: tangled up in NETs. Blood 123(18):2768–2776

Matthews LW, Specter S, Lemm J, Potter JL (1963) The overall chemical composition of pulmonary secretions from patients with cystic fibrosis, bronchiectasis and laryngectomy. Am Rev Respir Dis 88:119–204

McCoy K, Hamilton S, Johnson C (1996) Effects of 12-week administration of dornase alfa in patients with advanced cystic fibrosis lung disease. Chest 110:889–895

Merza M, Hartman H, Rahman M, Hwaiz R, Zhang E, Renström E, Luo L, Mörgelin M, Regner S, Thorlacius H (2015) Neutrophil extracellular traps induce trypsin activation, inflammation, and tissue damage in mice with severe acute pancreatitis. Gastroenterology 149:1920–1931

Mittal BB, Wang E, Sejpal S, Agulnik M, Mittal A, Harris K (2013) Effect of recombinant human deoxyribonuclease on oropharyngeal secretions in patients with head-and-neck cancers treated with radiochemotherapy. Int J Radiat Oncol Biol Phys 87:282–289

Mohler M, Cook J, Lewis D, Moore J, Sinicropi D, Championsmith A, Ferraiolo B, Mordenti J (1993) Altered pharmacokinetics of recombinant human deoxyribonuclease in rats due to the presence of a binding protein. Drug Metab Dispos 21:71–75

Mol CD, Izumi T, Mitra S, Tainer JA (2000) DNA-bound structures and mutants reveal abasic DNA binding by APE1 and DNA repair coordination. Nature 403:451–456

Moore S (1981) Pancreatic DNase. In: Boyer PD (ed) The enzymes, vol 14, 3rd edn. Academic, New York, pp 281–296

Morgan WJ, Butler SM, Johnson CA, Colin AA, FitzSimmons SC, Geller DE, Konstan MW, Light MJ, Rabin HR, Regelmann WE, Schidlow DV, Stokes DC, Wohl ME, Kaplowitz H, Wyatt MM, Stryker S (1999) Epidemiologic study of cystic fibrosis: design and implementation of a prospective, multicenter, observational study of patients with cystic fibrosis in the U.S. and Canada. Pediatr Pulmonol 28:231–241

ten Berge M, Brinkhorst G, Kroon AA, de Jongste JC (1999) DNase treatment in primary ciliary dyskinesia—assessment by nocturnal pulse oximetry. Pediatr Pulmonol 27:59–61

Nasr SZ, Strouse PJ, Soskolne E, Maxvold NJ, Garver KA, Rubin BK, Moler FW (2001) Efficacy of recombinant human deoxyribonuclease I in the hospital management of respiratory syncytial virus bronchiolitis. Chest 120:203–208

O'Donnell AE, Barker AF, Ilowite JS, Fick RB (1998) Treatment of idiopathic bronchiectasis with aerosolized recombinant human DNase I. rhDNase Study Group. Chest 113:1329–1334

Pan CQ, Lazarus RA (1997) Engineering hyperactive variants of human deoxyribonuclease I by altering its functional mechanism. Biochemistry 36:6624–6632

Pan CQ, Lazarus RA (1999) Ca^{2+}-dependent activity of human DNase I and its hyperactive variants. Protein Sci 8:1780–1788

Pan CQ, Ulmer JS, Herzka A, Lazarus RA (1998a) Mutational analysis of human DNase I at the DNA binding interface: implications for DNA recognition, catalysis, and metal ion dependence. Protein Sci 7:628–636

Pan CQ, Dodge TH, Baker DL, Prince WS, Sinicropi DV, Lazarus RA (1998b) Improved potency of hyperactive and actin-resistant human DNase I variants for treatment of cystic fibrosis and systemic lupus erythematosus. J Biol Chem 273:18374–18381

Pan CQ, Sinicropi DV, Lazarus RA (2001) Engineered properties and assays for human DNase I mutants. Methods Mol Biol 160:309–321

Park J, Wysocki RW, Amoozgar Z, Maiorino L, Fein MR, Jorns J, Schott AF, Kinugasa-Katayama Y, Lee Y, Won NH, Nakasone ES, Hearn SA, Küttner V, Qiu J, Almeida AS, Perurena N, Kessenbrock K, Goldberg MS, Egeblad M (2016) Cancer cells induce metastasis-supporting neutrophil extracellular DNA traps. Sci Transl Med 8:361ra138

Parsiegla G, Noguere C, Santell L, Lazarus RA, Bourne Y (2012) The structure of human DNase I bound to magnesium and phosphate ions points to a catalytic mechanism common to members of the DNase I-like superfamily. Biochemistry 51:10250–10258

Paul K, Rietschel E, Ballmann M, Griese M, Worlitzsch D, Shute J, Chen C, Schink T, Döring G, van Koningsbruggen S, Wahn U, Ratjen F (2004) Effect of treatment with dornase alpha on airway inflammation in patients with cystic fibrosis. Am J Respir Crit Care Med 169:719–725

Piccolo F, Popowicz N, Wong D, Lee YC (2015) Intrapleural tissue plasminogen activator and deoxyribonuclease therapy for pleural infection. J Thorac Dis 7:999–1008

Potter JL, Specter S, Matthews LW, Lemm J (1969) Studies on pulmonary secretions. 3. The nucleic acids in whole pulmonary secretions from patients with cystic fibrosis bronchiectasis and laryngectomy. Am Rev Respir Dis 99:909–915

Prince WS, Baker DL, Dodge AH, Ahmed AE, Chestnut RW, Sinicropi DV (1998) Pharmacodynamics of recombinant human DNase I in serum. Clin Exp Immunol 113:289–296

Puterman AS, Weinberg EG (1997) rhDNase in acute asthma. Pediatr Pulmonol 23:316–317

Quan JM, Tiddens HA, Sy JP, McKenzie SG, Montgomery MD, Robinson PJ, Wohl ME, Konstan MW (2001) A two-year randomized, placebo-controlled trial of dornase alfa in young patients with cystic fibrosis with mild lung function abnormalities. J Pediatr 139:813–820

Rahman NM, Maskell NA, West A, Teoh R, Arnold A, Mackinlay C, Peckham D, Davies CW, Ali N, Kinnear W, Bentley A, Kahan BC, Wrightson JM, Davies HE, Hooper CE, Lee YC, Hedley EL, Crosthwaite N, Choo L, Helm EJ, Gleeson FV, Nunn AJ, Davies RJ (2011) Intrapleural use of tissue plasminogen activator and DNase in pleural infection. N Engl J Med 365:518–526

Ramphal R, Lhermitte M, Filliat M, Roussel P (1988) The binding of anti-pseudomonal antibiotics to macromolecules from cystic fibrosis sputum. J Antimicrob Chemother 22:483–490

Ramsey BW, Astley SJ, Aitken ML, Burke W, Colin AA, Dorkin HL, Eisenberg JD, Gibson RL, Harwood IR, Schidlow DV, Wilmott RW, Wohl ME, Meyerson LJ, Shak S, Fuchs H, Smith AL (1993) Efficacy and safety of short-term administration of aerosolized recombinant human deoxyribonuclease in patients with cystic fibrosis. Am Rev Respir Dis 148:145–151

Ramsey BW, Pepe MS, Quan JM, Otto KL, Montgomery AB, Williams-Warren J, Vasiljev KM, Borowitz D, Bowman CM, Marshall BC, Marshall S, Smith AL (1999) Intermittent administration of inhaled tobramycin in patients with cystic fibrosis. N Engl J Med 340:23–30

Ramsey BW, Davies J, NG ME, Tullis E, Bell SC, Dřevínek P, Griese M, EF MK, Wainwright CE, Konstan MW, Moss R, Ratjen F, Sermet-Gaudelus I, Rowe SM, Dong Q, Rodriguez S, Yen K, Ordoñez C, Elborn JS, VX08-770-102 Study Group (2011) A CFTR potentiator in patients with cystic fibrosis and the G551D mutation. New Engl J Med 365:1663–1672

Raskin P (1968) Bronchospasm after inhalation of pancreatic dornase. Am Rev Respir Dis 98:697–698

Raynor EM, Butler A, Guill M, Bent JP 3rd (2000) Nasally inhaled dornase alfa in the postoperative management of chronic sinusitis due to cystic fibrosis. Arch Otolaryngol Head Neck Surg 126:581–583

Ren CL, Pasta DJ, Rasouliyan L, Wagener JS, Konstan MW, Morgan WJ (2008) Relationship between inhaled corticosteroid therapy and rate of lung function decline in children with cystic fibrosis. J Pediatr 153:746–751

Riethmueller J, Borth-Bruhns T, Kumpf M, Vonthein R, Wiskirchen J, Stern M, Hofbeck M, Baden W (2006) Recombinant human deoxyribonuclease shortens ventilation time in young, mechanically ventilated children. Pediatr Pulmonol 41:61–66

Riordan JR, Rommens JM, Kerem B, Alon N, Rozmahel R, Grzelczak Z, Zielenski J, Lok S, Plavsic N, Chou JL, Drumm ML, Iannuzzi MC, Collins FS, Tsui LC (1989) Identification of the cystic fibrosis gene: cloning and characterization of complementary DNA. Science 245:1066–1073

Robinson M, Hemming AL, Moriarty C, Eberl S, Bye PT (2000) Effect of a short course of rhDNase on cough and mucociliary clearance in patients with cystic fibrosis. Pediatr Pulmonol 30:16–24

Rozov T, de Oliveira VZ, Santana MA, Adde FV, Mendes RH, Paschoal IA, Reis FJC, Higa LYS, de Castro Toledo AC Jr, Pahl M (2010) Dornase alfa improves the health-related quality of life among Brazilian patients with cystic fibrosis—a one-year prospective study. Pediatr Pulmonol 45:874–882

Saiman L, Mayer-Hamblett N, Campbell P, Marshall BC (2005) Heterogeneity of treatment response to azithromycin in patients with cystic fibrosis. Am J Respir Crit Care Med 172:1008–1012

Sanders NN, Franckx H, De Boeck K, Haustraete J, De Smedt SC, Demeester J (2006) Role of magnesium in the failure of rhDNase therapy in patients with cystic fibrosis. Thorax 61:962–968

Sawicki GS, Signorovitch JE, Zhang J, Latremouille-Viau D, von Wartburg M, Wu EQ, Shi L (2012) Reduced mortality in cystic fibrosis patients treated with tobramycin inhalation solution. Pediatr Pulmonol 47:44–52

Sawicki GS, Chou W, Raimundo K, Trzaskoma B, Konstan MW (2015) Randomized trial of efficacy and safety of dornase alfa delivered by eRapid nebulizer in cystic fibrosis patients. J Cyst Fibros 14:777–783

Scala M, Hoy D, Bautista M, Palafoutas JJ, Abubakar K (2017) Pilot study of dornase alfa (Pulmozyme) therapy for acquired ventilator-associated infection in preterm infants. Pediatr Pulmonol 52:787–791

Scherer T, Geller DE, Owyang L, Tservistas M, Keller M, Boden N, Kesser KC, Shire SJ (2011) A technical feasibility study of dornase alfa delivery with eFlow vibrating membrane nebulizers: aerosol characteristics and physicochemical stability. J Pharm Sci 100:98–109

Shah PI, Bush A, Canny GJ, Colin AA, Fuchs HJ, Geddes DM, Johnson CA, Light MC, Scott SF, Tullis DE, De Vault A, Wohl ME, Hodson ME (1995) Recombinant human DNase I in cystic fibrosis patients with severe pulmonary disease: a short-term, double-blind study followed by six months open-label treatment. Eur Respir J 8:954–958

Shak S (1995) Aerosolized recombinant human DNase I for the treatment of cystic fibrosis. Chest 107:65S–70S

Shak S, Capon DJ, Hellmiss R, Marsters SA, Baker CL (1990) Recombinant human DNase I reduces the viscosity of cystic fibrosis sputum. Proc Natl Acad Sci USA 87:9188–9192

Shiokawa D, Tanuma S (2001) Characterization of human DNase I family endonucleases and activation of DNase gamma during apoptosis. Biochemistry 40:143–152

Shire SJ (1996) Stability characterization and formulation development of recombinant human deoxyribonuclease I [Pulmozyme, (dornase alfa)]. In: Pearlman R, Wang YJ (eds) Pharmaceutical biotechnology: formulation, characterization and stability of protein drugs, vol 9. Plenum Press, New York, pp 393–426

Silverman RA, Foley F, Dalipi R, Kline M, Lesser M (2012) The use of rhDNAse in severely ill, non-intubated adult asthmatics refractory to bronchodilators: a pilot study. Respir Med 106:1096–1102

Simpson G, Roomes D, Reeves B (2003) Successful treatment of empyema thoracis with human recombinant deoxyribonuclease. Thorax 58:365–366

Sinicropi DV, Lazarus RA (2001) Assays for human DNase I activity in biological matrices. Methods Mol Biol 160:325–333

Sinicropi DV, Prince WS, Lofgren JA, Williams M, Lucas M, DeVault A (1994a) Sputum pharmacodynamics and pharmacokinetics of recombinant human DNase I in cystic fibrosis. Am J Respir Crit Care Med 149:A671

Sinicropi D, Baker DL, Prince WS, Shiffer K, Shak S (1994b) Colorimetric determination of DNase I activity with a DNA-methyl green substrate. Anal Biochem 222:351–358

Suck D (1994) DNA recognition by DNase I. J Mol Recognit 7:65–70

Suri R (2005) The use of human deoxyribonuclease (rhDNase) in the management of cystic fibrosis. BioDrugs 19:135–144

Thornton RB, Wiertsema SP, Kirkham LS, Rigby PJ, Vijayasekaran S, Coates HL, Richmond PC (2013) Neutrophil extracellular traps and bacterial biofilms in middle ear effusion of children with recurrent acute otitis media—a potential treatment target. PLoS One 8:e53837

Ulmer JS, Herzka A, Toy KJ, Baker DL, Dodge AH, Sinicropi D, Shak S, Lazarus RA (1996) Engineering actin-resistant human DNase I for treatment of cystic fibrosis. Proc Natl Acad Sci USA 93:8225–8229

VanDevanter DR, Craib ML, Pasta DJ, Millar SJ, Morgan WJ, Konstan MW (2018) Cystic fibrosis clinical characteristics asssoiciated with dornase alfa treatment regimen change. Pediatr Pulmonol 53:43–49

Vasconcellos CA, Allen PG, Wohl ME, Drazen JM, Janmey PA, Stossel TP (1994) Reduction in viscosity of cystic fibrosis sputum in vitro by gelsolin. Science 263:969–971

Wagener JS, Kupfer O (2012) Dornase alfa (pulmozyme). Curr Opin Pulm Med 18:609–614

Wagener JS, Rock MJ, McCubbin MM, Hamilton SD, Johnson CA, Ahrens RC (1998) Aerosol delivery and safety of recombinant human deoxyribonuclease in young children with cystic fibrosis: a bronchoscopic study. J Pediatr 133:486–491

Wang H, Morita M, Yang X, Suzuki T, Yang W, Wang J, Ito K, Wang Q, Zhao C, Bartlam M, Yamamoto T, Rao Z (2010) Crystal structure of the human CNOT6L nuclease domain reveals strict poly(A) substrate specificity. EMBO J 29:2566–2576

Widlak P, Garrard WT (2005) Discovery, regulation, and action of the major apoptotic nucleases DFF40/CAD and endonuclease G. J Cell Biochem 94:1078–1087

Wills PJ, Wodehouse T, Corkery K, Mallon K, Wilson R, Cole PJ (1996) Short-term recombinant human DNase in bronchiectasis. Effect on clinical state and in vitro sputum transportability. Am J Respir Crit Care Med 154:413–417

Wilmott RW, Amin RS, Colin AA, DeVault A, Dozor AJ, Eigen H, Johnson C, Lester LA, McCoy K, McKean LP, Moss R, Nash ML, Jue CP, Regelmann W, Stokes DC, Fuchs HJ (1996) Aerosolized recombinant human DNase in hospitalized cystic fibrosis patients with acute pulmonary exacerbations. Am J Respir Crit Care Med 153:1914–1917

Wolf E, Frenz J, Suck D (1995) Structure of human pancreatic DNase I at 2.2 Å resolution. Protein Eng 8:79

Wong SL, Demers M, Martinod K, Gallant M, Wang Y, Goldfine AB, Kahn CR, Wagner DD (2015) Diabetes primes neutrophils to undergo NETosis, which impairs wound healing. Nat Med 21:815–819

Yang W (2011) Nucleases: diversity of structure, function and mechanism. Q Rev Biophys 44:1–93

Zahm JM, Girod de Bentzmann S, Deneuville E, Perrot-Minnot C, Dabadie A, Pennaforte F, Roussey M, Shak S, Puchelle E (1995) Dose-dependent in vitro effect of recombinant human DNase on rheological and transport properties of cystic fibrosis respiratory mucus. Eur Respir J 8:381–386

23 Monoclonal Antibodies in Cancer

Jürgen Barth

INTRODUCTION

More than 60 years ago the first chemotherapeutic drugs were used to support surgery and/or radiation therapy against cancer. In the following decades, chemotherapy developed to a mainstay of therapy rather than being supporting in character. In the last two decades monoclonal antibodies (MABs) have faced a growing interest as antitumor therapeutics. In November 1997, Rituximab was the first-in-class therapeutic MAB approved by the FDA. In June 1998 followed the approval in the European Union. At that time, even the manufacturer believed the approval as monotherapy for relapsed/refractory, CD20 positive, low-grade or follicular B-cell Non-Hodgkin's lymphoma would be a niche indication. The following rapid development of many different MABs in multiple different cancer indications shows how incorrect this assessment was. Nowadays, a large number of MABs has been approved for use in numerous cancer indications with many more in different stages of clinical development.

CLASSIFICATION OF MONOCLONAL ANTIBODIES

Structure, functionality, classes and possible modifications of MABs and their mode of action are described in Chap. 8. MABs can be roughly divided into unconjugated antibodies and conjugated antibodies. The latter ones can be subdivided into toxin coupled antibodies—so called chemoimmunoconjugates or antibody drug conjugates (ADC)—and radionuclide coupled antibodies, the radio immune conjugates (RIC). These "naked", uncoupled toxins given alone would be too toxic for the patient. The antibody works as a tugboat, tugging the toxin to accumulate selectively nearby or in the tumor. A RIC can be considered "inner radiation therapy".

PHARMACOLOGICAL TARGETS OF ONCOLOGIC ANTIBODIES

MABs can be directed against surface structures of malignant cells. These structures comprise receptors or proteins, such as the epidermal growth factor receptor (EGFR) or the cluster of differentiation (CD) antigens. Besides that, some MABs intercept soluble (growth) factors in the blood and peripheral tissue fluids, which could lead to a tumor survival benefit. One example in oncology is the vascular endothelial growth factor (VEGF), which is intercepted by bevacizumab or aflibercept ("*VEGF-Trap*"). The most recent and rapidly growing class of MABs are immune agonistic antibodies, currently directed against the cytotoxic T-lymphocyte antigen 4 (CTLA4), the programmed cell death receptor1 (PD 1) or against its ligand (PD-L1). The main difference in the mode of action compared to all the other classes of MABs and even chemotherapeutics is that not the tumor itself is attacked, but the immune system of the patient is held "under fire" to re-recognize the tumor. Table 23.1 gives an overview over the present MABs with an oncology indication, ordered by the target structure.

All mentioned targets can also be found on non-malignant tissues, which explains the observed toxicity. At present time, none of the approved MABs is directed against a tumor specific molecular driver, as they are known for instance in Philadelphia chromosome positive CML (the fusion protein BCR/Abl), in anaplastic lymphoma kinase (Alk) positive non-small cell lung cancer (NSCLC), in EGFR mutated NSCLC (mutated EGFR), or in the FLT3-positive AML. Her2 (=ErbB2), for example, can also be found in normal tissues, but in Her2 positive breast cancers it is overexpressed.

J. Barth (✉)
Justus-Liebig-Universität, Medizinische Klinik IV, Universitätsklinik, Giessen, Germany
e-mail: juergen.barth@innere.med.uni-giessen.de

D. J. A. Crommelin et al. (eds.), *Pharmaceutical Biotechnology*, https://doi.org/10.1007/978-3-030-00710-2_23

Anti-CD-antibodies	
Obinutuzumab	Anti-CD-20 (B-lymphocytes)
Ofatumumab	Anti-CD-20 (B-lymphocytes)
Rituximab	Anti-CD-20 (B-lymphocytes)
I^{131}-Tositumumab-Tiuxetan	Anti-CD-20 (B-lymphocytes) + radionuclide
Y^{90}-Ibritumumab-Tiuxetan	Anti-CD-20 (B-lymphocytes) + radionuclide
Inotuzumab Ozogamicin	Anti-CD22 + toxin
Blinatumumab	Anti-CD3/-CD19 (T- & B-cells)
Brentuximab Vedotin	Anti-CD30 + toxin (HD, sALCL)
Gemtuzumab Ozogamicin	Anti-CD33 + toxin (myeloid cells)
Daratumumab	Anti-CD38 (myeloma cells)
Elotuzumab	Anti-SLAMF7 (=anti-CD319; myeloma cells)
Alemtuzumab	Anti-CD-52 (lymphocytes)
Anti EGFR-antibodies	
Cetuximab	Anti-EGFR (ErbB1)
Necitumumab	Anti-EGFR (ErbB1)
Panitumumab	Anti-EGFR (ErbB1)
Pertuzumab	Anti-HER2/neu (ErbB2) / -HER3
Trastuzumab	Anti-HER2/neu (ErbB2)
(Ado-)Trastuzumab Emtansin (T-DM1)	Anti-HER2/neu (ErbB2) + toxin
Anti angiogenic antibodies	
Bevacizumab	Anti-VEGF („ligand capture“)
(Zif-)Aflibercept	Anti-VEGF („VEGF-Trap“)
Ramucirumab	Anti-VEGF-R2
Immune agonistic antibodies	
Ipilimumab	Anti-CTLA4 (T-cells)
Nivolumab	Anti-PD-1 (T-cells)
Pembrolizumab	Anti-PD-1 (T-cells)
Atezolizumab	Anti-PD-L1 (expressed on tumor tissue)
Avelumab	Anti-PD-L1 (expressed on tumor tissue)
Durvalumab	Anti-PD-L1 (expressed on tumor tissue)
Other antibodies	
Catumaxomab	Anti-EpCAM
Denosumab	Anti-RANKL
Dinutuxumab	Anti-GD2
Olaratumab	Anti-PDGFRα

Table 23.1 ■ Therapeutic MABs clustered by their targets

PHARMACOKINETICS OF MABS: GENERAL REMARKS

Unlike small, defined molecules, the pharmacokinetic properties of MABs differ markedly. Distribution into tissue is slow (internalization) because of the molecular size of MABs. Volumes of distribution are generally low. Metabolism is similar to catabolic degradation of endogenous and dietetic peptides and proteins. The half-life is usually relatively long, which allows for long dosing intervals during maintenance therapy. Rituximab, for instance, is given every 2 months in the first line setting and every 3 months in the relapsed or refractory situation. Possible factors influencing the pharmacokinetics include the amount of the target antigen, which corresponds to the total tumor mass, immune reactions to the antibody (anti-drug antibodies) and patient demographics such as gender or age (see section on rituximab). Population pharmacokinetic analyses have been applied in assessing covariates in the disposition of MABs. Both linear and nonlinear elimination have been reported for MABs, which is probably caused by target mediated disposition (overview Keizer et al. 2010). If a tumor responds to a MAB therapy, the amount of the remaining target antigen diminishes and the half-life can be prolonged. However, MAB dosing is based on different pharmacokinetic models, leading to approved dosing strategies of body surface area-based (rituximab), body weight-based (trastuzumab, pertuzumab) or flat dosing (atezolizumab, obinutuzumab).

ANTI-CD ANTIBODIES

The cluster of differentiation (also known as cluster of designation or classification determinant and often abbreviated as CD) denotes groups of immune phenotyping surface properties for the identification and investigation of cell surface molecules providing targets on cells in order to classify these cells according to their biochemical or functional characteristics. CD molecules are membrane bound proteins, often glycosylated, in part cell specific. In terms of physiology, CD molecules can act in numerous ways, often acting as receptors important to cell functioning and/or survival. Others have enzymatic activity. A signaling cascade is usually initiated or modulated, altering the behavior of the cell. Additionally to the mechanisms of ADCC and CDC (Chap. 8), MABs can alter or even block signal transduction pathways, leading to cell death via apoptosis (overview Ludwig et al. 2003).

Anti CD20 Antibodies

In the 1980s, CD20 was identified as a B-cell marker by Stashenko et al. (1980). CD20 is expressed on early pre-B cells, it remains through B-cell development, and is then lost from plasma cells (Tedder and Engel 1994). It is not found on hematopoietic stem cells. Therefore, anti CD20 antibodies are also designated as anti-lymphocytic antibodies. The antigen is neither shed nor internalized. CD20 is expressed on the majority of B-cell lymphomas (Stashenko et al. 1980; Tedder and Engel 1994; Nadler et al. 1981). It is a nonglycosylated member of the membrane-spanning 4-A (MS4A) family (Ishibashi et al. 2001). The antigen consists of three hydrophobic regions forming a tetraspan transmembrane molecule with a single extracellular loop and intracellular N- and C-terminal regions (Tedder et al. 1988). CD20 has been shown to be present on the cell surface as a homo-multimer, in tetramer complexes (Polyak and Deans 2002; Polyak et al. 2008). Despite decades of research, no natural ligand for CD20 could be detected (Cragg et al. 2005). However, subsequent data revealed that CD20 is resident in lipid raft domains of the plasma membrane where it probably functions as a store-operated calcium (SOC) channel following ligation of the B cell receptor (BCR) with the antigen, implying that it plays a role in regulating cytoplasmic calcium levels after antigen engagement (Bubien et al. 1993; Kanzaki et al. 1995; Li et al. 2003).

Pharmacology

Anti-CD20 antibodies can be classified into type I and type II antibodies with different pharmacodynamics (Cragg and Glennie 2004). Type I (rituximab-like) MABs induce CD20 to redistribute into large detergent resistant microdomains (lipid rafts), whereas type II (tositumomab-like) MABs do not (Deans et al. 1998). These lipid microenvironments on the cell surface—known as lipid rafts—also take part in the process of signal transduction. Lipid rafts containing a given set of proteins can change their size and composition in response to intra- or extracellular stimuli. This favors specific protein–protein interactions, resulting in the activation of signaling cascades. For details see Simons and Toomre (2000). Rituximab and ofatumumab are type I, whereas obinutuzumab is the first glyco-engineered type II MAB. Type I antibodies display a remarkable ability to activate complement and elicit complement-dependent cytotoxicity (CDC, Chap. 8). This is a result of enhanced recruitment of the complement factor C1q. This ability, however, appears to be directly linked to their (CD20 bound) translocation into lipid rafts, which cluster the antibody Fc regions thus enabling improved C1q binding (Cragg et al. 2003). Type II MABs do not show these characteristics: They do not change CD20 distribution after binding; no concomitant clustering is observed and they are relatively ineffective in CDC. Interestingly, they evoke far more homotypic adhesion and direct killing of target cells in a caspase independent manner (Chan et al. 2003; Ivanov et al. 2008). In summary, type I MABs have to cross-link the homo-tetrameric CD20 antigen for a pharmacodynamic effect. In diseases like CLL, with a lower density of CD20 antigens compared with other B-cell lymphomas, the tetramers have to be bridged with more than one molecule of rituximab. That is the explanation why rituximab in CLL is given at a higher dose of 500 mg/m^2 in subsequent cycles after the usual starting dose of 375 mg/m^2. For illustration see Fig. 23.1.

Type II MABs bind within a CD20 tetramer, without lipid raft redistribution. They induce a "closed conformation" (Beers et al. 2010; Niederfellner et al. 2011) (Fig. 23.2). The antigens don't have to be bridged. The

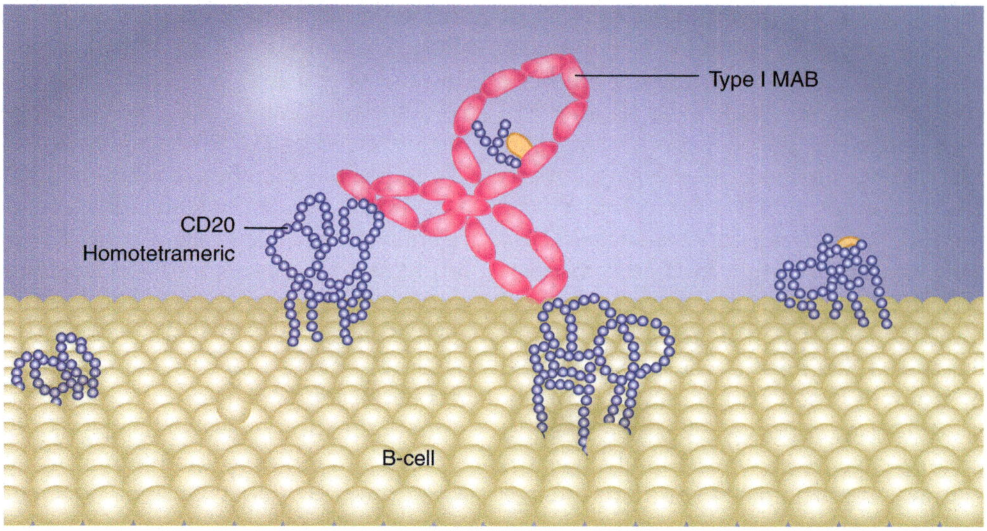

Figure 23.1 ■ Anti-CD20 MABs can be divided into two distinct subtypes, termed type I and II. Type I MABs induce CD20 to redistribute into large detergent resistant microdomains (rafts) whereas type II MABs do not. This differential ability of anti-CD20 mAbs to redistribute CD20 in the cell membrane impacts on many of the binding properties and effector functions that control the therapeutic success of anti-CD20 mAbs. Type I and II MABs have the ability to evoke different effects: type I MABs engage ADCC and cause CD20 modulation but do not elicit direct cell death, whereas type II MABs mediate direct cell death and engage ADCC, but do not promote CD20 modulation (Beers et al. 2010). In diseases with a low CD20 density, more than one rituximab molecule has to bridge the CD20 antigens

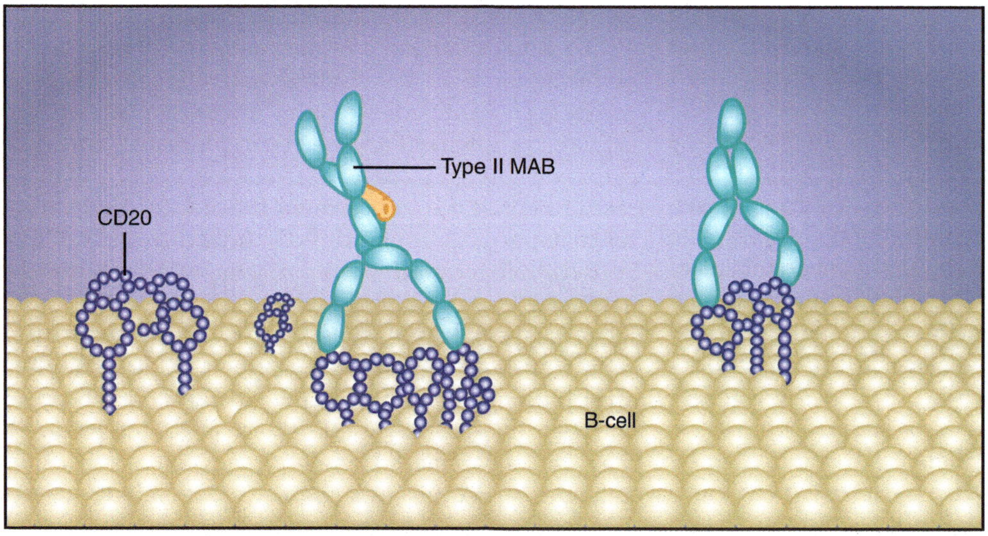

Figure 23.2 ■ Typ II MAB (Tositumomab like) bind within a CD20 tetramer, and the antigens don't have to be bridged. No redistribution into lipid rafts occurs (Beers et al. 2010; Niederfellner et al. 2011)

type II MAB-induced cell death is dependent on homotypic adhesion, requires cholesterol, and is energy-dependent, involving the relocalization of mitochondria to the vicinity of the cell–ell contact (Beers et al. 2010).

The pharmacodynamic mechanism of action and the resulting effects of rituximab are illustrated in Fig. 23.3 (from Stolz and Schuler 2009).

Rituximab

Rituximab is used as a monotherapy as well as in combinations with chemotherapy. It has become a mainstay in the treatment of B-cell malignancies such as aggressive and indolent non-Hodgkin's lymphomas (NHLs) and chronic lymphocytic leukemia (CLL), as well as other B-cell triggered diseases. It is also widely utilized in an off label fashion for numerous clinical conditions like immune thrombocytopenia (ITP). Histology subtype has been described as the main tumor parameter that influences rituximab efficacy. In an early trial, when rituximab was given for four doses as monotherapy, small lymphocytic lymphoma histology negatively influenced the objective response rate compared with other low-grade lymphomas (McLaughlin et al. 1998). Several studies have

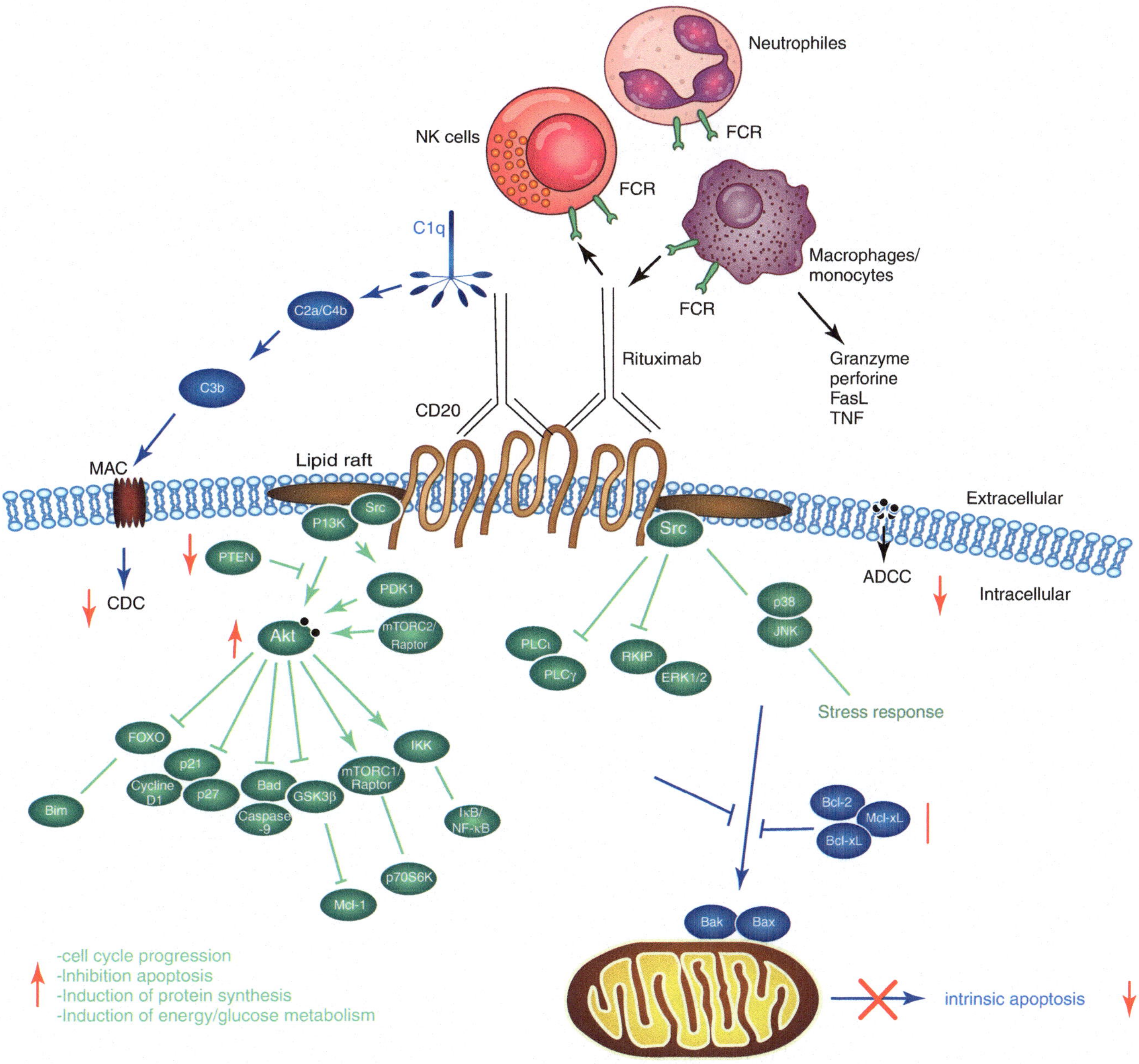

Figure 23.3 ■ Overview of rituximab-inducible indirect (ADCC und CDC) effector mechanisms and intracellular, CD20 triggered signal transduction cascades after CD20 cross linking (Stolz and Schuler 2009)

described a low objective response rate in patients with CLL treated with the standard dose of 375 mg/m² rituximab monotherapy used in other NHL (Huhn et al. 2001; Nguyen et al. 1999; O'Brien et al. 2001). As mentioned above, the level of CD20 expression (density) may differ depending on tumor histology (Manches et al. 2003). This was initially used to explain the variation in rituximab efficacy among different histological subtypes. Despite conflicting in vitro data, the dosing in CLL was adjusted to 500 mg/m² for subsequent doses after an initial dosing of the well-known 375 mg/m² finally. The reduced dose for the first infusion is necessary because of an usually high tumor load in need for therapy in CLL blast crisis. Responding to rituximab therapy bears a high risk of tumor lysis and cytokine release syndrome as well as other infusion related reactions (IRR); see also under 'safety'. For induction therapy as well as for maintenance therapy (used in follicular lymphoma—FL) a minimum serum concentration has to be achieved for tumor response (Berinstein et al. 1998; Gordan et al. 2005).

Responses to therapeutic MABs have also been reported to correlate with specific polymorphisms in the Fcγ receptor (FcγR), especially when ADCC is a major part in the mechanism of action (Mellor et al. 2013). These polymorphisms are associated with differential affinity of the receptors to MABs. At present, these functional FcγR polymorphisms are not suitable to be used as pharmacogenetic biomarkers that could be used to better target the use of MABs in cancer patients. The available studies do not describe a consistent effect of FcγR genotype on the clinical anti-tumor activity of therapeutic IgG1 MABs. Inconsistencies observed in studies are likely related to differences in tumor type, the cytotoxic agents used in combination, the clinical settings, like metastatic vs. adjuvant situation, the clinical benefit parameters measured, the therapeutic antibody used, as well as the magnitude and even the direction of the effect. However, even patients with an "unfavorable" FcγR genotype do benefit from an antibody containing regimen (overview Mellor et al. 2013).

To minimize IRR, the infusion rate is increased slowly from the initial infusion rate of 50 mg/h every 30 min by doubling the subsequent infusion rate if no reactions occur up to 400 mg/h. Shortly before approval of rituximab biosimilars, a fixed dose, subcutaneous (s.c.) formulation was launched in the EU. Rituximab is concentrated up to 120 mg/mL in recombinant hyaluronidase, a penetration enhancer ("spreading factor"). The dose for follicular lymphoma is 1400 mg (12 mL), for CLL 1600 mg (16 mL). The first dose has still to be given by the i.v. route due to tolerability concerns. The subsequent s.c. doses can be given over 6 min—an substantial advantage from the patient's point of view.

As shown by the SABRINA study, the pharmacokinetic profile of s.c. rituximab was non-inferior to i.v. rituximab. I.v. and s.c. rituximab had similar efficacy and safety profiles, and no new safety concerns were noted. S.c. administration does not compromise the anti-lymphoma activity of rituximab when given with chemotherapy.

Rituximab Safety

From today's point of view, dose finding and scheduling of rituximab administration, the first approved therapeutic anti-cancer antibody, were more empirical than rational or biologic target based. As no dose-limiting toxicity or clear dose–response relationship was found during a phase I study with single doses of 10, 50, 100, 250 or 500 mg/m^2 (Maloney et al. 1994), the 375 mg/m^2 dose level with a 4 weekly dosing scheme was chosen for phase II studies (McLaughlin et al. 1998; Maloney et al. 1997) without an apparent reasoning. A dose escalation trial was conducted in CLL and even at 2250 mg/m^2 (monotherapy) the maximum tolerated dose was not reached (O'Brien et al. 2001). Rituximab has significant activity in patients with CLL at the higher dose levels. However, the dose-response-curve is not steep. Myelosuppression and infections are uncommon.

Rituximab is generally well tolerated, in patients with both malignant and non-malignant disease, including children (Quartier et al. 2001) and even pregnant women (Herold et al. 2001). Severe adverse events are rare but possible. The most common adverse events are infusion-/foreign protein-related and occur most frequently during or shortly after the first infusion. However, extremely rare, hypersensitivity reactions can occur even after years of maintenance therapy, leading to permanent discontinuation of its use. This syndrome consists of chills, fever, headache, rhinitis, pruritus, vasodilation, asthenia and angioedema. A cytokine release syndrome is possible. Less often reported are hypotension, rash, bronchospasm, pain at tumor sites and rash or severe skin toxicity inclusive Stevens-Johnson-Syndrome and Toxic Epidermal Necrolysis (=Lyell-Syndrome). Routine premedication consists of corticosteroids, if they are not already a component of the chemotherapy- or antiemetic scheme. The same drug classes are used for intervention in case of hypersensitivity reactions (HSR) despite correct premedication.

Rituximab induces a rapid depletion of CD20$^+$ B-cells in the peripheral blood. B-cells remain at low levels for at least 2–6 months with recovery to pretreatment values occurs within 12 months (Maloney et al. 1997). Other hematological toxicities comprise temporary reduction of platelets or neutrophils, and occasionally reduced immunoglobulin levels, which also can be caused by the underlying disease and its bone marrow involvement. Despite the fact that the drug is generally well tolerated, a small number of patients experience unexpected and severe toxicities. It is speculated, that these patients have a rituximab serum level dramatically above the average. However, so far, this could not be proven in clinical routine.

Also, gender and age seem to influence rituximab kinetics and clinical outcome. The German High-Grade Non-Hodgkin Lymphoma Study Group (DSHNHL) first detected in elderly women with diffuse large B cell lymphoma (DLBCL) a slower elimination of rituximab compared with men, which translated in a better outcome for these women (Pfreundschuh et al. 2014). Consequently, the DSHNHL conducted a phase II trial increasing the number of rituximab infusions to achieve high rituximab levels early during treatment. In this DENSE-R-CHOP-14 trial, 100 elderly patients with aggressive CD20$^+$ B-cell lymphoma received 6 cycles of biweekly CHOP-14 combined with 12 x rituximab

(375 mg/m^2) on days 0, 1, 4, 8, 15, 22, 29, 43, 57, 71, 85, and 99. (CHOP-14 treatment regimen: **C**yclophosphamide 600 mg/m^2 day 1; doxorubicin (=**H**ydroxydaunorubicin) 50 mg/m^2 day 1; Vincristine (**O**ncovin®) 1.4 mg/m^2 max. 2 mg day 1; Predniso(lo)ne 100 mg day 1–5 every 14 days).

This intensification of rituximab administration achieved higher rituximab serum levels and resulted in higher complete remission and event-free survival rates in elderly patients with poor-prognosis DLBCL (Pfreundschuh et al. 2007). The negative impact of male gender in DLBCL was confirmed by a meta-analysis (Yildirim et al. 2015). While body weight contributes to a faster elimination in males according to (Muller et al. 2012), others found a significant longer five-year OS in a high BMI group (>22.55 kg/m^2) when compared to that of the low BMI group (Weiss et al. 2017).

With the increasing use of Rituximab, a growing number of rare adverse effects have been recognized. Late-onset neutropenia (LON) is, according to the National Cancer Institute Common Toxicity Criteria defined as grade III–IV neutropenia, in which absolute neutrophil count is less than 1.0 × 10^3/L, occurring 4 weeks after the last rituximab administration. LON has been reported in 5–27% of rituximab-treated lymphoma patients. Similar figures apply for autoimmune patients but those appear to have more infections during the neutropenic period (Tesfa et al. 2011; Tesfa and Palmblad 2011).

The mechanisms of LON after rituximab treatment still has not been elucidated. One hypothesis is, that LON may result from hematopoietic lineage competition due to an excessive B-cell recovery in the bone marrow by promotion of B-cell lymphopoiesis over granulopoiesis (Anolik et al. 2003). Others see a correlation between a high-affinity *FCGR3 158 V* allele and LON in lymphoma patients (Weng et al. 2010). A clinically relevant question is if it is safe to re-treat patients with rituximab who previously developed LON. Recurrence of LON episodes upon re-exposed patients has been reported. Nevertheless, a close clinical follow-up or complete blood count monitoring is considered adequate in most LON cases (Tesfa and Palmblad 2011).

Following Rituximab administration, reactivation of hepatitis B, in some cases resulting in fulminant hepatitis, hepatic failure, and death, has been reported. This led to testing of active replicating hepatitis as well as to screening of all patients for HBV infection by measuring HBsAg and anti-HBc before initiating treatment with rituximab as a therapeutic precondition. Monitoring and/or reactivation of antiviral prophylaxis should be considered, and is advised by the FDA's Full Prescribing Information (FPI) and the European Medicines Agency's Summary of Product Characteristics (SmPC). HBV reactivation can occur up to 24 months following completion of rituximab therapy.

The immune suppressing antibody ± chemotherapy can lead to reactivation of latent JC polyoma virus, leading to potentially fatal Progressive Multifocal Leukoencephalopathy (PML). Patients presenting with onset of neurologic manifestations should consult a neurologist with this suspected diagnosis. For natalizumab, an anti-alpha4-integrin antibody used against multiple sclerosis, that induced PML in some patients, removal of the drug via plasma exchange was an important part of the therapy, as it reconstituted the immune system. In a case report, the first successful removal of rituximab with plasma exchange therapy (rituximab apheresis) and accompanying complement-dependent cytotoxicity test (CDC) assay for monitoring, has been described. Neurologic symptoms of the patient improved within the first 2 weeks (Burchardt et al. 2012).

Ofatumumab

Ofatumumab is a type I, human immunoglobulin (Ig) G1k antibody. Ofatumumab binds with greater avidity than rituximab to another epitope of CD20, which encompasses the small extracellular loop (residues 74–80) and the N-terminal region of the second large extracellular loop (Fig. 23.4). Several crystal structure based analyses of the Fab fragment of the antibody suggests that ofatumumab can bind closer and tighter to the cell membrane than rituximab, leading to more effective CDC. Induction of CDC appears to be greater than with rituximab and occurs even at a lower density of CD20 on the cell surface (Cheson 2010). After binding to CD20 on malignant B cells, ofatumumab induces clustering of CD20 into lipid rafts, similar to other type I antibodies as described above. In contrast to rituximab, ofatumumab does not induce apoptosis of B-cell lines (Cheson 2010).

Initially licensed for double refractory CLL, namely those resistant or refractory to fludarabine and alemtuzumab, ofatumumab can be used in previously untreated as well as relapsed patients after conventional chemotherapy. As already mentioned, CLL in need for therapy (blast crisis) bears a risk of rapid cell breakdown in the sense of a tumor lysis syndrome. Therefore a reduced initial flat dose of 300 mg is given. The subsequent flat dose is 1000 mg or 2000 mg, depending on the clinical situation (details see FPI and SmPC).

Ofatumumab Safety

Qualitatively the toxicity profile of ofatumumab is similar to that of rituximab. This includes HBV reactivation and the potential for PML. No additional toxicity or safety signals have been observed so far.

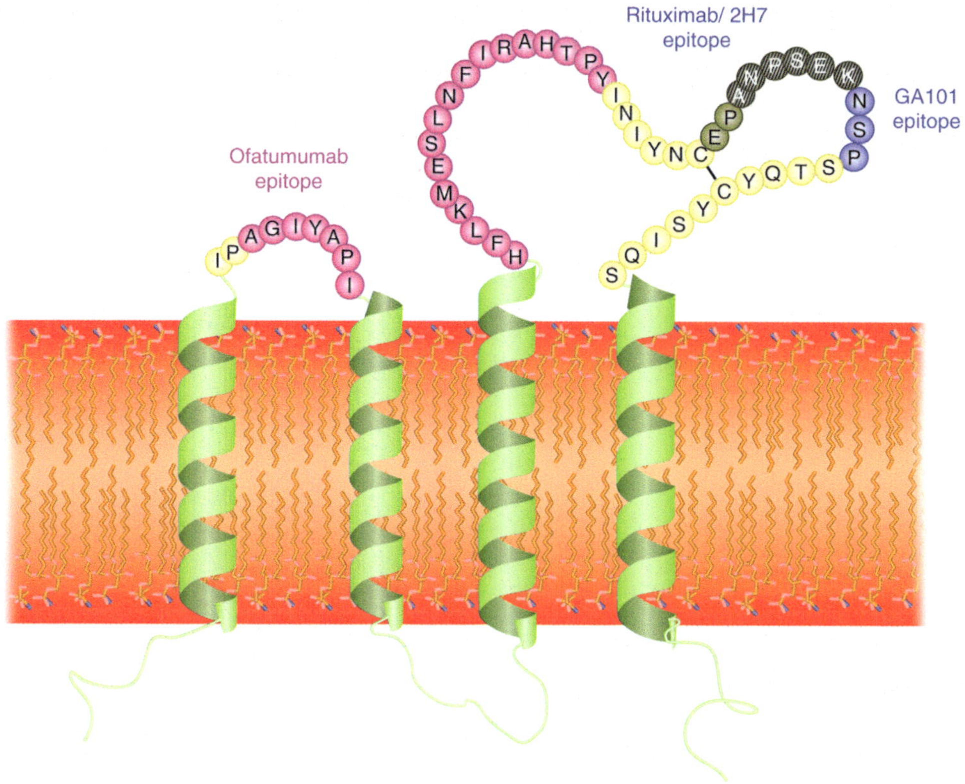

Figure 23.4 ■ Distinct CD20 binding epitopes of rituximab, ofatumumab and obinutuzumab (designated as GA101). Ofatumumab binds to the so called "small loop" (from Klein et al. 2013)

Obinutuzumab

Obinutuzumab is the first glycoengineered, type II humanized anti-CD20 MAB. It is post-translational defucosylated, resulting in the absence of a fucose sugar residue from IgG oligosaccharides in the Fc region of the MAB molecule (Tobinai et al. 2017). Obinotuzumab binds within the CD20 tetramer, as depicted in Fig. 23.2. CDC, probably, does not contribute to the overall activity of obinutuzumab. The limited capacity of obinutuzumab to fix complement via its Fc portion may further enhance its capability to bind to FcγRIII and mediate ADCC (summarized in Tobinai et al. 2017). Obinutuzumab was significantly more effective than rituximab in depleting B cells in whole blood samples from healthy donors (n = 10) and from an individual with CLL (Mossner et al. 2010). In CLL, the dosing of obinutuzumab is 100 mg on day 1, followed by 900 mg on day 2 in cycle 1. If tolerated and no IRR occur, the second part of the split dose can be given on day 1. In subsequent cycles there is no dose splitting on day 1. As mentioned before, starting therapy of CLL may lead to the tumor lysis syndrome. Therefore, the split dose is a safety measure and not necessary in other diseases, e.g. indolent NHL. According to the FPI and SmPC no dose splitting is advised for follicular lymphoma.

In contrast to rituximab, obinutuzumab is ramped up in cycle 1 with a flat dose of 1000 mg on days 1, 8 and 15. Consequently, patients in head-to-head comparisons of obinutuzumab with rituximab received 3000 mg obinutuzumab in cycle 1, whereas rituximab patients received 375 mg/m^2. This was often seen as a dosing imbalance. However, the manufacturer did not study a second experimental arm with the same flat dose for rituximab, which would have been considered a real head-to-head study. Different dosing regimens were tested for obinutuzumab. For achieving the desired serum concentration, 1600 mg on days 1 and 8 in cycle 1, followed by 800 mg on day 1 in subsequent cycles was determined. 1600 mg might need very long infusion times due to possible IRR, especially in CLL. Results in the GAUGUIN study (Morschhauser et al. 2013) and pharmacokinetic modeling showed that obinutuzumab 1000 mg per cycle with additional 1000 mg doses on days 8 and 15 of cycle 1 can achieve exposures similar to the 1600/800 mg regimen. This simplified flat-dose 1000 mg schedule was adopted for subsequent phase II and III investigations (Cartron et al. 2016).

Obinutuzumab Safety

The safety profile of obinutuzumab is similar to the other anti-CD20 antibodies rituximab and ofatumumab.

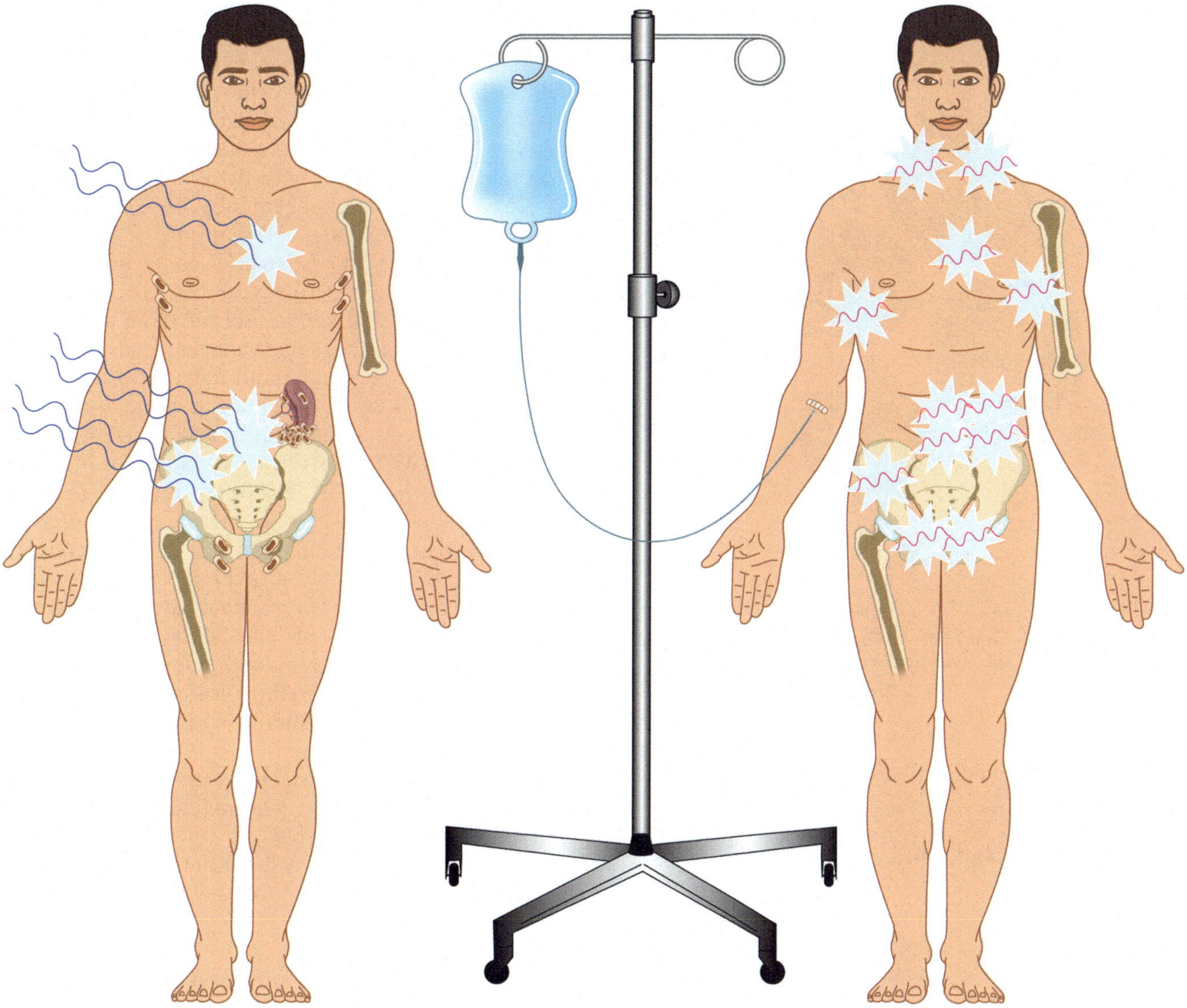

Figure 23.5 ■ Comparison of conventional radiotherapy (left) with an external radiation source. Radiation from inside (right) by RICs

Y^{90} Ibritumumab and I^{131} Tositumumab Tiuxetan

Y^{90} Ibritumumab and *I^{131} Tositumumab Tiuxetan* are murine RICs. Yttrium-90 is a beta-emitter; Iodine-131 is a beta-emitter and an emitter of gamma radiation. Their activity is mainly achieved through their radioisotopes rather than their intrinsic antibody activity (Fig. 23.5). The radiation can penetrate through several cell layers, which is termed "cross fire" or "bystander" effect (Fig. 23.6). Adjacent cells, not marked by the antibody are also effected. Although active, these antibodies never gained a broad acceptance in the medical community. As of February 2014, the production of tositumomab and I^{131} tositumomab has been discontinued by the manufacturer and is no longer available (National Cancer Institute 2014), Y^{90} ibritumumab tiuxetan is still approved in the EU, but rarely used.

■ Other Anti CD Antibodies: Unconjugated

Alemtuzumab

Alemtuzumab was another anti-lymphocytic antibody, directed against the CD52 antigen. The CD52 antigen is mainly found on mature B- and T lymphocytes, but can also be found on monocytes/macrophages, NK cells, eosinophils and epithelial cells of the male reproductive tract. Alemtuzumab was used for the treatment of double refractory B-CLL (refractory to an alkylator plus fludarabine). This hematological approval was retracted in 2012 to

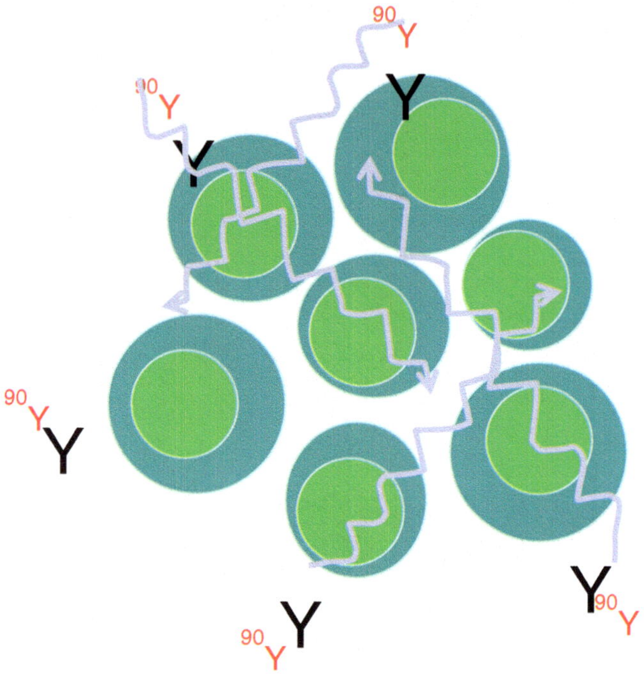

Figure 23.6 ■ "Cross fire" or "bystander" effect of radiation, penetrating more cell layers than marked by the antibody

favor the development as an immunosuppressant against multiple sclerosis, for which it is currently approved.

■ Anti Myeloma Antibodies

Elotuzumab

Elotuzumab is an immunostimulatory monoclonal antibody that recognizes SLAMF7 (Signaling Lymphocyte Activation Molecule Family Member 7; CD319), a glycoprotein highly expressed on myeloma and natural killer cells but not on normal tissues (Hsi et al. 2008). Elotuzumab causes myeloma cell death via a dual mechanism of action (Collins et al. 2013) (Fig. 23.7).

1. *Direct activation:* Binding to SLAMF7 directly activates natural killer cells (Collins et al. 2013), but not myeloma cells (Guo et al. 2015).
2. *Tagging for recognition:* Elotuzumab activates natural killer cells via CD16, enabling selective killing of myeloma cells via antibody-dependent cellular cytotoxicity (ADCC) with minimal effects on normal tissue (Collins et al. 2013).

Elotuzumab is not active as a monotherapy (Radhakrishnan et al. 2017), so it is combined with an immune modulating drug, usually lenalidomide, and dexamethasone. This combination lowers the killing threshold for myeloma cells. Further combinations, for example with proteasome inhibitors, are currently being tested.

Daratumumab

Daratumumab is directed against the CD38 antigen, found on T cells (precursors, activated), B cells (precursors, activated), myeloid cells (monocytes, macrophages, dendritic cells), NK cells, erythrocytes and platelets. CD38 has multiple functions. It acts as a receptor in close contact with the B cell receptor complex and CXCR4. In engagement with CD31 or hyaluronic acid, it activates NF-kappaB, ZAP-70, and ERK1/2 pathways. It also works as an ectoenzyme. CD38 interacts with NAD^+ and $NADP^+$, which are converted to cADPR, ADPR, and NAADP, all intracellular Ca^{2+} mobilizing agents (Malavasi et al. 2011).

Because of marked quantitative differences in expression levels of CD38 between normal cells and leukemic cells, combined with its role in cell signaling, suggests that CD38 is an attractive target for immunotherapy treatment of multiple myeloma (MM) (Malavasi et al. 2008). It is highly and uniformly expressed on myeloma cells (Lin et al. 2004; Santonocito et al. 2004), whereas only a relatively low expression was detected on normal lymphoid and myeloid cells and in some tissues of non-hematopoietic origin (Deaglio et al. 2001). In summary, daratumumab binding to CD38 elicits a signaling cascade and immune effector function engagement, leading to (de Weers et al. 2011)

- Complement-dependent cytotoxicity (CDC)
- Antibody-dependent cell-mediated cytotoxicity (ADCC)
- Antibody-dependent cell-mediated phagocytosis (ADCP), a rather new/unknown mode of action (Overdijk et al. 2015)
- Induction of apoptosis
- Modulation of cellular enzymatic activities associated with calcium mobilization and signaling
- Combination of these activities leads to elimination of plasma cells from bone marrow in MM patients

Daratumumab also kills myeloid-derived suppressor cells—Tregs or negatively regulating T cells. A graphical overview of Daratumumab's mode of action is presented in Fig. 23.8.

Daratumumab and Elotuzumb Safety

Both antibodies need an intensive premedication. Despite correct pre-treatment with antipyretics, antihistamines and multiple doses of oral and i.v corticosteroids, IRR occur during daratumumab and elotuzumab administration, which makes a close patient-monitoring mandatory. Especially for daratumumab, IRR can occur hours after completing the infusion. A suddenly stuffy nose, cough, throat irritation, allergic rhinitis, hoarseness during the infusion can be regarded as early signs of an upcoming IRR. Due to necessary infusion interrup-

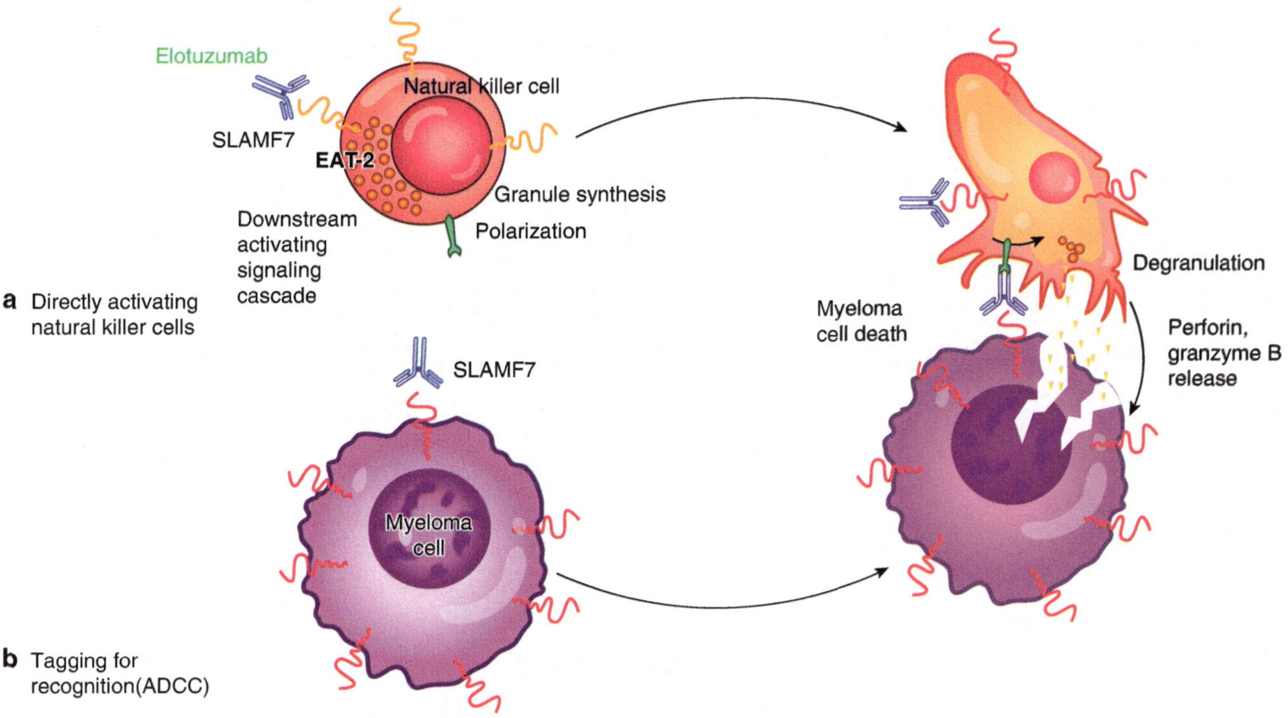

Figure 23.7 ■ Dual mechanism of action of elotuzumab (Collins et al. 2013)

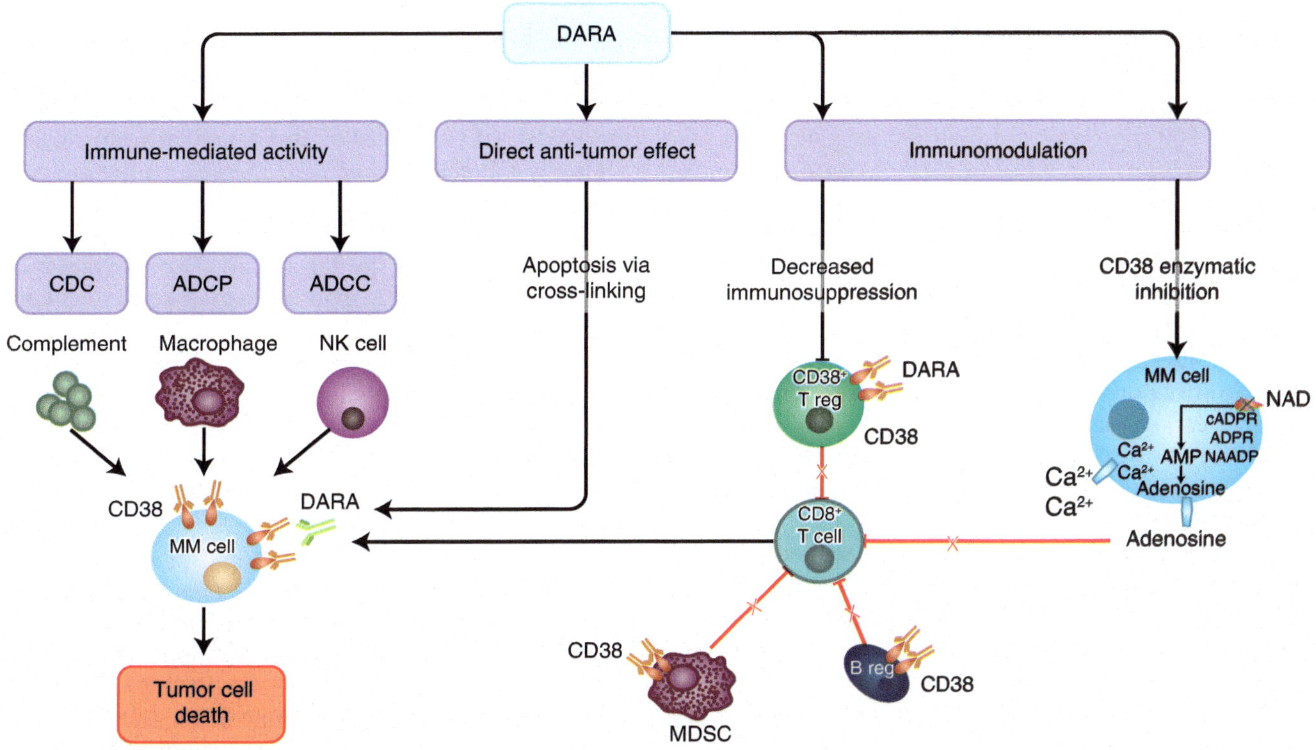

Figure 23.8 ■ Modes of action of daratumumab (de Weers et al. 2011; Overdijk et al. 2015). Antibody mediated phagocytosis is a rather new pharmacodynamic process. Details see text

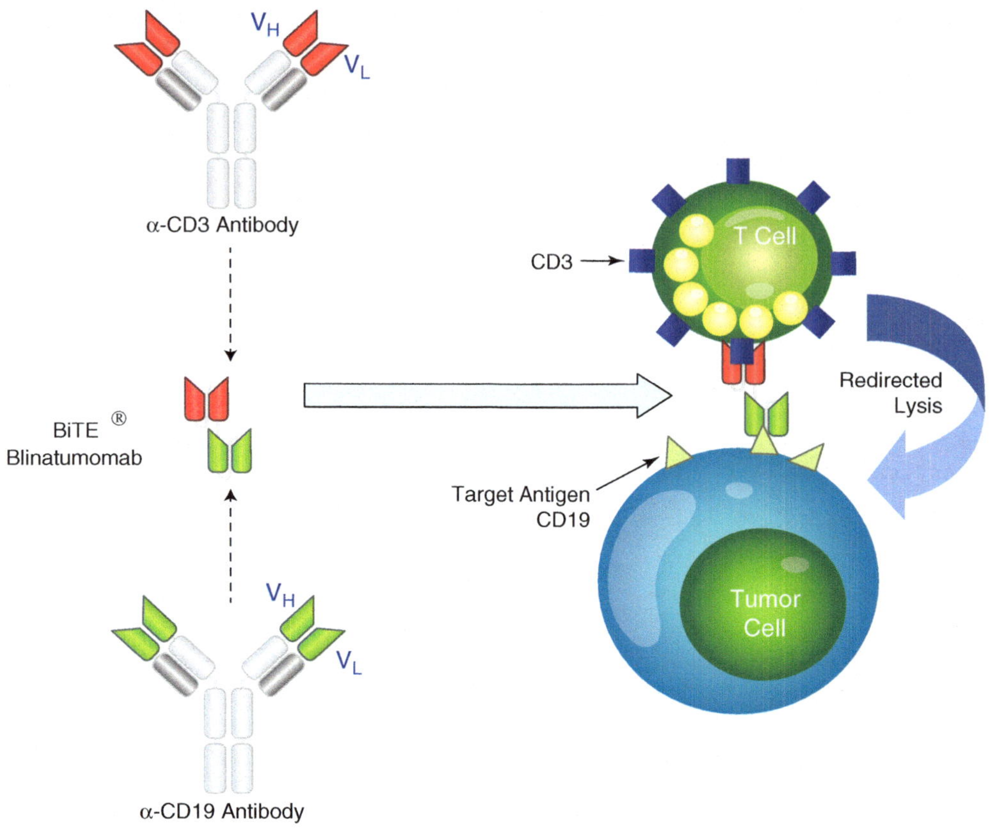

Figure 23.9 ■ Two fused scFv of anti CD3/antiCD19 antibodies result in the blinatumumab construct. One arm of blinatumomab binds to CD3, the other binds to CD19. This engages unstimulated T cells, which destroys the $CD19^+$ cells

tions caused by these IRR, a s. c. formulation as described for rituximab may resolve the problem. Dissolved in recombinant hyaluronidase, the fixed dose of 1800 mg daratumumab (90 mL) achieves the same trough level on day 1 of cycle 3, compared to the i.v. dosage form.

Because CD38 is also expressed on erythrocytes, the indirect Coombs test used prior to blood transfusions is false positive, up to 6 months after the last infusion of daratumumab. Blood typing at baseline is therefore highly recommended before the first daratumumab infusion. Meanwhile, daratumumab in blood samples can be destroyed by incubation with dithiothreitol (DTT) prior to the blood compatibility test. DTT cracks the structure stabilizing disulfide bridges of the antibody.

Both, elotuzumab and daratumumab also interfere with serum protein electrophoresis or immune fixation assays, leading to false positive results in patients with IgGκ myeloma protein, making the assessment of the initial response difficult.

■ Bispecific Antibodies

Blinatumumab

Blinatumumab is a first-in-class bispecific antibody, directed against CD3 on T cells and CD19 on B cells. It is also designated as a BiTE, a Bispecific T cell Enhancer. This antibody construct is made of two single chain variable fragments (scFv) of anti CD3/CD19, enabling a patient's T cells to recognize malignant B cells (Fig. 23.9). CD3 is part of the T cell receptor. CD19, originally a B cell marker, is expressed on the majority of B cell malignancies in normal to high levels. By linking these two cell types, T cells are activated to exert cytotoxic activity on the target cell. The usual clinical use is the Philadelphia chromosome negative B (precursor) ALL.

Blinatumumab has a molecular weight of 54.1 kDa, approximately one-third of the size of a traditional monoclonal antibody (Wu et al. 2015). It is eliminated rather quickly by the kidneys with a half-life of 1.2 h. Therefore, blinatumumab has to be continuously infused over 1 month.

Blinatumomab Safety

Blinatumumab can cause cytokine release as well as fulminant neurological toxicities even with fatal outcome. Some of them were caused by prescription, calculation or handling errors. When changing the infusion lines, for instance, the used lines must not be flushed. This would result in an erroneous bolus application with severe toxicities or death. To avoid all this and to make blinatumumab therapy safer, the manufacturer developed risk minimization information brochures for physicians, other health care professionals and patients. The preparation protocol is rather complicated and a high-precision infusion pump is necessary.

Other Anti CD Antibodies: Toxin Conjugated

Antibody drug conjugates (ADC) are chemically linked combinations of MABs and small molecule drugs with anti-tumor activity. As mentioned above, the unconjugated drug alone is too toxic for the patient. Therefore, common features of toxin-coupled antibodies are:

- The ADC has to be stable in circulation in vivo
- The antigen has to be predominantly tumor specific
- After binding to the tumor antigen, the ADC has to be internalized
- When internalized, the ADC has to be degradable inside the cell to release the lethal cargo.

The linker between the MAB and toxin can be distinguished into enzymatically cleavable linkers, such as the dipeptide linker used in brentuximab vedotin, or enzymatically uncleavable linkers, such as the thioether linker in ado-trastuzumab emtansine (trastuzumab emtansine in the EU, syn. TDM1). The linker itself contributes to the properties of the ADC including PK and ADME (overview Han and Zhao 2014).

Gemtuzumab Ozogamicin

Gemtuzumab Ozogamicin (GO) is an anti-CD33 MAB, coupled with a cytotoxic enediyne -antibiotic N-acetyl derivate from *Micromonospora echinospora* ssp. *Calichenensis*, termed calicheamicin γ_1^I (gamma-one-iodine, Fig. 23.10).

The calicheamicin cleaves double stranded DNA via a radical mechanism. Like bleomycin, it belongs to the so-called *free radical-based-DNA-cleaving-natural-products*. Calicheamicin binds with sequence specificity to TCCT-, TCTC- and TTT in the minor grove of the DNA (minor groove binding agent).

Gemtuzumab ozogamicin originally received accelerated approval in May 2000 as a stand-alone treatment for older patients with CD33-positive AML who had experienced a relapse. It was voluntarily withdrawn from the market after subsequent confirmatory trials failed to verify clinical benefit and demonstrated safety concerns, including a high number of early deaths. Gemtuzumab ozogamicin was re-approved in September 2017 with a modified dosing regimen. This approval includes a lower recommended dose, a different schedule in combination with chemotherapy or on its own, and a new patient population (FDA 2017).

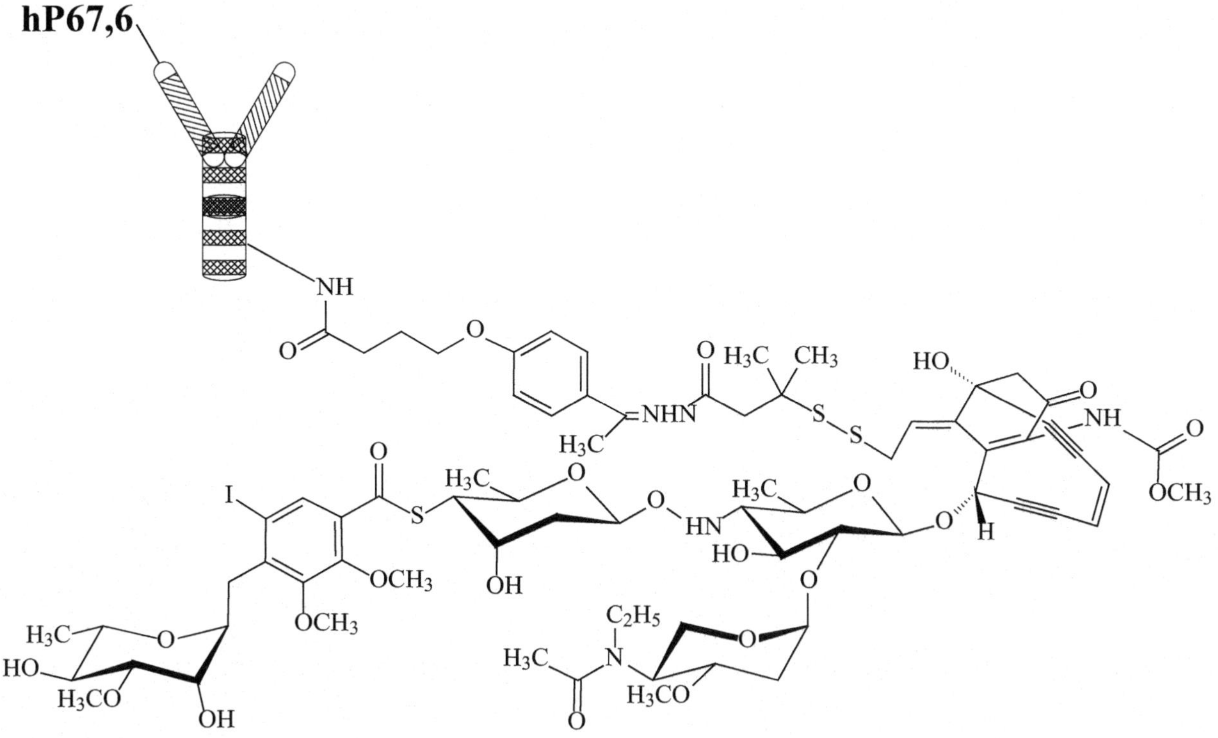

Figure 23.10 ■ The complex chemical structure of N-acetyl-calicheamicin γ_1^I coupled to an anti CD33 MAB (symbolized in the upper left; © J. Barth)

Gemtuzumab Ozogamicin Safety

Worrisome adverse events are end organ damages such as veno-occlusive disease or the sinusoidal obstruction syndrome, which can lead to fatalities. Other, in part severe, treatment-emergent adverse events are hemorrhage, mucositis, nausea, vomiting, constipation, headache, increased liver enzymes (AST and ALT), rash, fever and infection.

Inotuzumab Ozogamicin

Inotuzumab Ozogamicin carries the same toxin as gemtuzumab in gemtuzumab ozogamicin, but the MAB component of the ADC is directed against the CD22 antigen on (precursor) B-ALL cells. Safety and treatment emergent adverse events are similar to those of gemtuzumab ozogamicin.

Brentuximab Vedotin

Brentuximab Vedotin is directed against the CD30 antigen, expressed on classical Hodgkin's Lymphoma Reed-Sternberg and anaplastic large cell lymphoma cells and, in part, mycosis fungoides. It is expressed in embryonal carcinomas, but not in seminomas and is thus a useful marker in distinguishing between these germ cell tumors. The toxin in this ADC is monomethyl auristatin E (MMAE), a dolastatin 10 derivate, derived from peptides occurring in marine shell-less mollusk *Dolabella auricularia* (Blunt-end Sea Hare) (Fig. 23.11). MMAE is a synthetic drug with a comparable mechanism of action as the taxanes. It inhibits cell division by blocking the polymerization of tubulin. MMAE is 100–1000 times more potent than doxorubicin.

Brentuximab Vedotin Safety

The drug has a myelotoxic potential with possible grade 3/4 neutropenia, thrombocytopenia and anemia. Neutropenia can result in severe infections and/or opportunistic infections. In the presence of severe renal or hepatic impairment, a higher frequency of ≥grade 3 toxicities and deaths was observed. Besides severe but rare dermatologic reactions including Stevens-Johnson-Syndrome and Toxic Epidermal Necrolysis, a cumulative, peripheral sensory neurotoxicity, has been observed. This may require a delay, change in dose, or discontinuation of treatment.

Brentuximab and ado Trastuzumab (see below) each carry a toxin that, in case of extravasation, could cause skin necrosis like the vinca alkaloids. As mentioned, the antibodies are conjugated with a cleavable or an uncleavable linker to the toxin. Whether cleavable linkers will be lysed in the extravasation area is unclear at the current time. ADCs with an uncleavable liker will be degraded like proteins and after that, the toxin is released. If and how this may happen to a clinically relevant degree in an extravasation area is also unclear at the current time. Limited clinical experience so far suggests that extravasated ADCs may only cause slight skin reactions.

ANTI GROWTH FACTOR RECEPTOR ANTIBODIES: ANTI-EGFR

■ Anti-EGFR-Strategies

The cell membranous receptors of the epidermal growth factor family consist of four related, functionally different members with tyrosine kinase activity, the homologues EGFR1 to EGFR4 (also called HER1 to HER4 or ErbB1 to ErbB4). The inactive monomers homo- (HER1 with HER1) or hetero-dimerize (HER1 with HER2, or -3, or -4) after external ligand binding. Conformational change leads to auto phosphorylation and subsequent signal transduction for diverse cellular functions including proliferation, cell survival—comprising inhibition of apoptosis-, adhesion, and DNA damage repair. In tumors, this pro survival signal transduction is activated permanently, without binding of a physiological, external ligand such as trans-

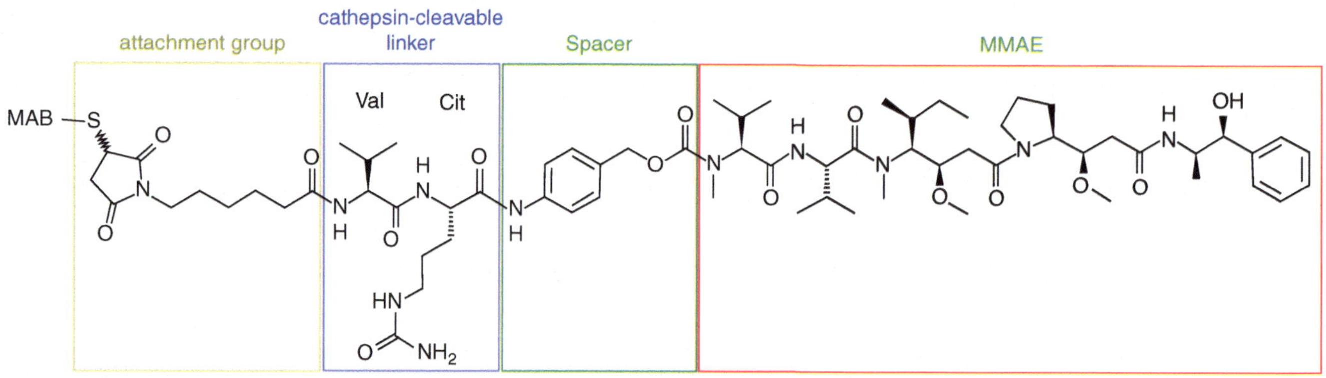

Figure 23.11 ■ MMAE and the attached MAB-linker-conjugate. Via a spacer (para-aminobenzylcarbamate), MMAE is attached to a cathepsin cleavable amino acid linker, followed by an attachment group, consisting of maleimide and caproic acid

forming growth factor-alpha (TGFA), heparin-binding EGF-like growth factor (HBEGF), betacellulin (BTC), amphiregulin (AREG), epiregulin (EREG), epigen (EPGN) and neuregulins (Rubin and Yarden 2001; Schneider and Wolf 2009; Singh et al. 2016). Diseases with malignancy associated overexpression of EGFR1 (HER1) are, for example, colorectal carcinomas (CRC), NSCLC, pancreas carcinomas and squamous cell cancers of the head and neck. Her2 is overexpressed by certain breast and gastric cancers. Over-expression is also known to occur in ovarian, (English et al. 2013; Teplinsky and Muggia 2014; Tuefferd et al. 2007) stomach, and aggressive forms of uterine cancer, such as uterine serous endometrial carcinoma (Buza et al. 2014; Santin et al. 2008). HER2 is over-expressed in 30% of salivary duct carcinomas (Chiosea et al. 2015), however, without any therapeutic consequences up to now. Overexpression has to be demonstrated by immunohistochemistry (IHC) or fluorescent in-situ hybridization (FISH) as a prerequisite for the use of anti-EGFR MABs.

Cetuximab

Cetuximab is a chimeric IgG1 antibody composed of the Fv region of a murine anti-EGFR antibody with human IgG heavy and kappa light chain constant regions. It binds to the extracellular domain of EGFR1 with an affinity five to tenfold greater than endogenous ligands, resulting in inhibition of EGFR signaling. Moreover, it also exerts the cytotoxic immune effector mechanisms described in Chap. 8. It is indicated in the treatment of metastatic colorectal cancer as mono- and combination therapy. Cetuximab also binds to a number of EGFR antigen negative tissues, therefore a saturating loading dose of 400 mg/m^2 has to be given as a first dose and again, if the weekly interval is exceeded. The weekly follow-up dose is 250 mg/m^2. Many commonly used chemotherapy regimens for CRC, including irinotecan monotherapy or in combination with infusional fluorouracil, like FolFOx or FolFIri, are administered every 2 weeks (FolFIri treatment regimen (=**Fol**inic acid, **F**luorouracil, **Iri**notecan): irinotecan 180 mg/m^2 day 1; calcium folinate 400 mg/m^2 day 1; fluorouracil (5-FU) 400 mg/m^2 day 1 undiluted bolus injection over 5 min; fluorouracil (5-FU) 2400 mg/m^2 day 1–2 as 48 h as prolonged infusion; FolFOx treatment regimen (=**Fol**inic acid, **F**luorouracil, **Ox**aliplatin): oxaliplatin 100 mg/m^2 day 1; calciumfolinate 400 mg/m^2 day 1; fluorouracil (5-FU) 400 mg/m^2 day 1 undiluted bolus injection over 5 min; fluorouracil (5-FU) 2400 mg/m^2 day 1–2 as 48 h as prolonged infusion).

The ability to synchronize the administration of cetuximab and concomitant chemotherapy is more convenient for the patients. Dosing of 500 mg/m^2 every 2 weeks exhibited predictable pharmacokinetics, which were similar to those of the approved weekly dosing regimen. No differences between the weekly and 2-weekly regimen on pharmacodynamics were observed. Efficacy and safety were also similar (Tabernero et al. 2008). Cetuximab is also used in the treatment of certain squamous cell cancers of the head and neck in combination with radiation or in combination with a platin-based chemotherapy.

Panitumumab

Panitumumab is the fully human version of an anti-EGFR1 MAB and shares the same target as cetuximab with slightly different binding affinity and specificity. In contrast to cetuximab, no loading dose is necessary—it is continuously dosed with 6 mg/kg q2w.

Both antibodies are only effective in pan RAS mutation negative tumors (wild type). K- and N-RAS proteins are G proteins (GTPases) downstream of EGFR and components of EGFR signaling, propagating EGFR signaling events. Activating mutations result in constitutive activation without necessity of ligand binding to the EGFR (Fig. 23.12). In other words: an anti EGFR antibody therapy for patients with activating RAS mutations has no therapeutic benefit, but exposes the patient to the risk of anti-EGFR MAB related toxicity.

Pan RAS tissue testing is mandatory according to clinical guidelines (Van Cutsem et al. 2014) before initiating a cetuximab or panitumumab therapy. The benefit of adding cetuximab to RAS wild type was shown by the pooled analysis of the OPUS and CRYSTAL studies (Bokemeyer et al. 2012).

Approximately up to 10% of CRC tumors also carry a BRAF mutation. RAS mutations and BRAF mutations are usually mutually exclusive (De Roock et al. 2010), so double testing is not necessary. A BRAF mutation is a strong negative prognostic biomarker and patients with a BRAF mutant CRC have a very poor prognosis (Van Cutsem et al. 2011). However, patients with a KRAS wild type but a BRAF mutation benefit from a cetuximab containing chemotherapy (Van Cutsem et al. 2011). Side matters—location of the CRC: it has been observed for years that patients with right sided colorectal cancer had worse outcomes than those with left-sided disease (Brule et al. 2015). Meanwhile, right and left sided tumors are regarded as molecular distinct (Tejpar et al. 2016). This translates into therapeutic consequences. Whereas treatment of patients with right sided tumors should be started with an antiangiogenic component (bevacizumab), patients with left sided tumors benefit from an anti-EGFR treatment (Venook et al. 2016) (Fig. 23.13).

Necitumumab

Necitumumab is an anti-EGFR recombinant human monoclonal antibody of the IgG1κisotype, currently

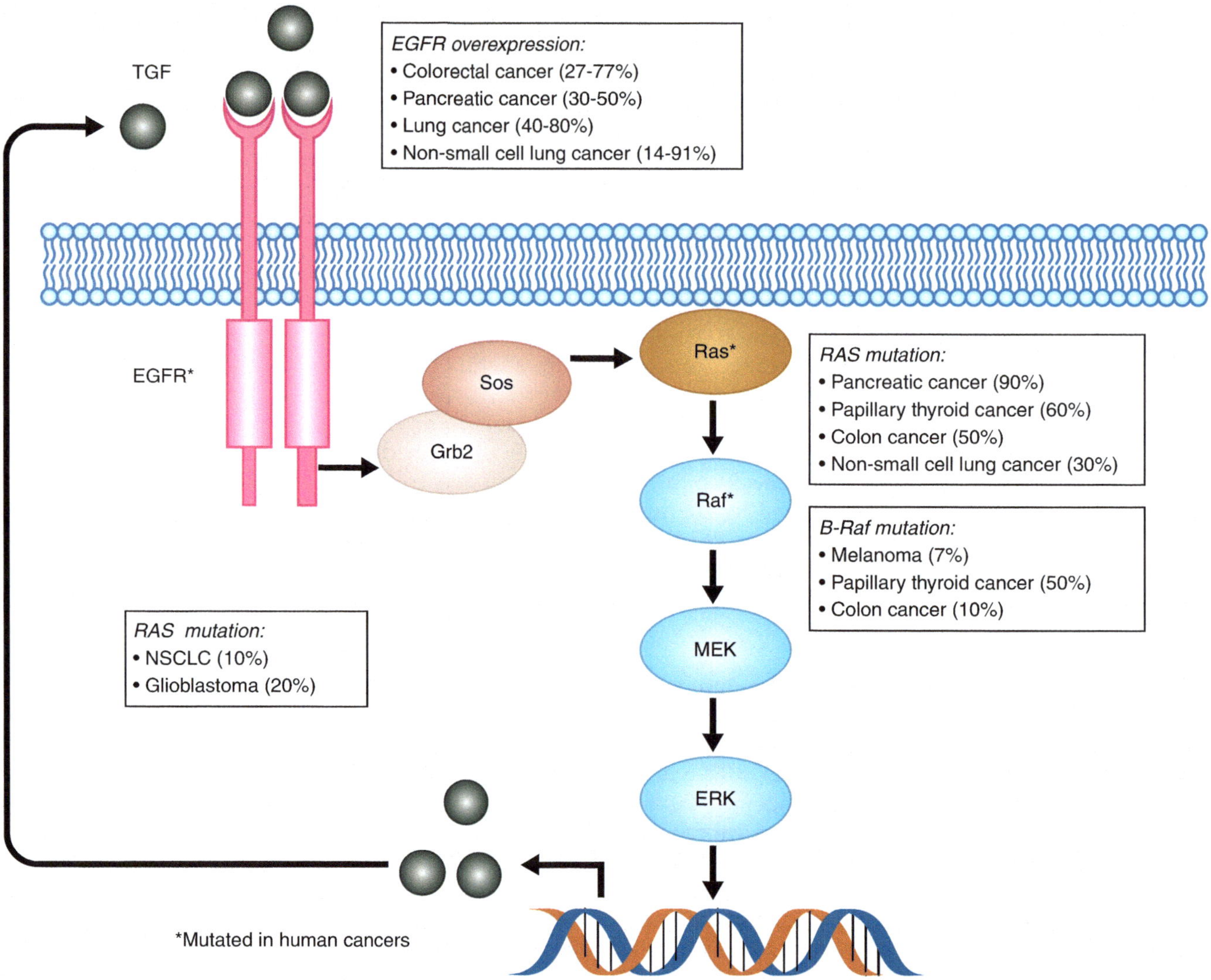

Figure 23.12 ■ Mutated RAS carcinomas are resistant to anti EGFR antibodies due to constitutively activated downstream signaling and thus growth promotion

used against NSCLC in combination with cisplatin (75–80 mg/m^2 on day 1) and gemcitabine 1200–1250 mg/m^2 on days 1 and 8). It was approved with a statistically significant difference in median overall survival (OS) of 1.6 months, compared to cisplatin and gemcitabine without antibody (11.5 vs 9.9 months). There is a fixed dosing for necitumumab of 800 mg q3w.

Anti-EGFR MAB Safety

Common anti EGFR therapy associated adverse events include acneiform rash, diarrhea, hypomagnesemia, hypocalcemia, and infusion reactions. Most common are papulopustular rash of the upper trunk and face skin (60–90%), dry and itchy skin (12–16%), and resulting microbial infections (38–70%), conditioned by open pustules as portal of entry for germs. Less frequently, pruritus, hair modifications, and paronychial inflammation occur (Holcmann and Sibilia 2015). By now, the mechanisms underlying skin disorders induced by EGFR inhibitors are well understood (Holcmann and Sibilia 2015). Alterations in chemokine and cytokine production in keratinocytes may result in attraction of inflammatory cells. Disturbed keratinocyte differentiation impairs proper formation of tight junctions and physiological barrier function. The barrier defect and reduced expression of antimicrobial peptides result in bacterial infections. Prophylactic—rather than reactive—management of skin reactions for all patients receiving EGFR inhibitors is recommended. Appropriate prophylaxis can effectively reduce the severity of skin reactions and also a stigmatization as a cancer patients, discernible by their skin eruptions. Skin care has the potential to directly benefit patients and their quality of life. Several recommendations and

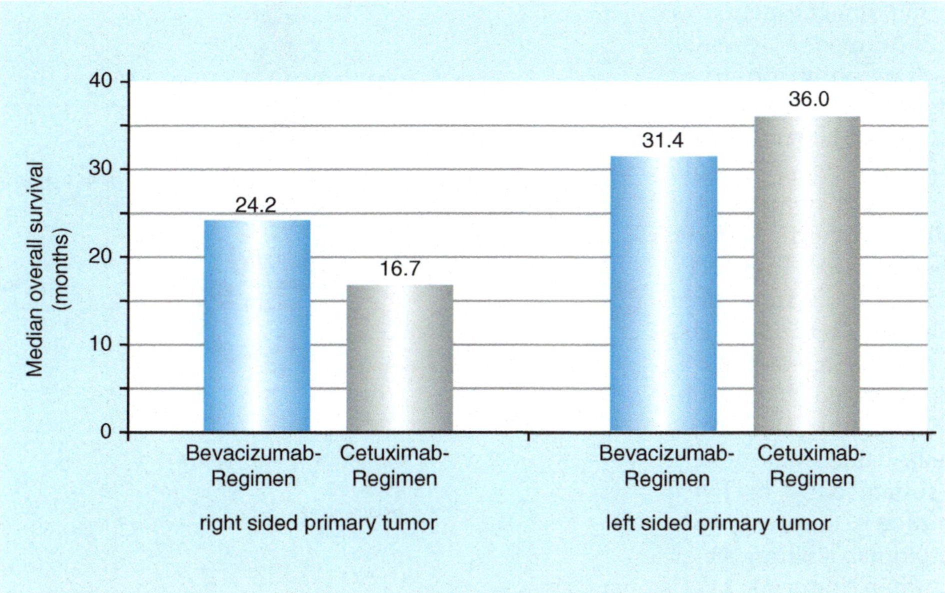

KRAS-WT (n = 1025)	Median overall survival with a right sided tumor	Median overall survival with a left sided tumor	HR (95%-CI)	p-value
Bevacizumab/ Chemotherapy	24.2	31.4	1.32 (1.05; 1.65)	p = 0.01
Cetuximab/ Chemotherapy	16.7	36.0	1.87 (1.48; 2.32)	p < 0.0001

Figure 23.13 ■ Median survival dependent on the tumor location and first-line regimen in colorectal cancer (CRC (based on Venook et al. 2016)). KRAS-WT = KRAS wild type, not mutated. HR hazard ratio

guidelines have been published (assorted samples: Gutzmer et al. 2011; Hofheinz et al. 2016; Lacouture et al. 2011; Potthoff et al. 2011). Skin changes during therapy proceed in three phases. Skin care has to be adapted to these phases

- Phase I: acneiform skin changes
- Phase II: desiccation phase
- Phase III: dry, sensitive skin

During phase III, the skin is very sensitive to sun light. An unnecessary sun exposure should be avoided, long sleeved outer clothing be worn, and the use of sun blockers should be considered. Furthermore, micro traumatization should be avoided. That is:

- No mechanical manipulation of alleged spots
- No hot hair drying
- No use of curlers, especially no tight wrapped curlers
- No long and hot showering or bathing
- No vigorous rubbing with towels (hard to comply in case of additional, tantalizing itching)
- No occlusion for instance with rubber gloves
- No too tight footwear
- Shaving, electric or blade shaving, always causes (unavoidable) micro traumatization.

Skin cracking that is hardly healing and possibly painful can be sealed with instant glue (like cyanoacrylate glue). This can keep these lesions from worsening or becoming infected. Superglue is also supposed to have some local anesthetic properties (Lacouture et al. 2011).

Electrolyte disturbances (Ca^{2+}, Mg^{2+}) were initially "simply reported" in the SmPC/FPI. However, especially Mg^{2+} loss occurs frequently. The EGFR is also found in the distal part of the collecting duct and other parts of the kidneys, but with a rather high expression in the ascending part of Henle's loop and in the distal convoluted tubule, where active re-absorption of magnesium ions takes place (~70%).The EGFR regulates the protein TRPM6 (=transient receptor potential cation channel, under family M member 6) (Schlingmann et al. 2007). By blocking this pump with anti EGFR antibodies, magnesium losses develop (Izzedine et al. 2010) (Patients with a *loss-of-function* germline mutation in the TRPM6-gene suffer from severe, congenital hypomagnesemia). The elimination half-life of cetuximab is approximately 3–7 days. Assuming that the half-life is 3 days and 5 half-lives are necessary to quantitatively eliminate a drug to have no residual pharmacodynamic activity, then one can be assume that the EGFR dependent magnesium pump is more or less permanently inhibited during the weekly dosing schedules. The same applies for panitumumab with its two-weekly schedule and a half-life of 7.5 days.

As a consequence, cumulative hypomagnesaemia of grade 3/4 can develop. This is termed *Magnesium Wasting Syndrome* (MWS). The (randomly) observed frequency of MWS ranges between 27% (Fakih et al. 2006) to 36% (Schrag et al. 2005), although in a prospective cohort study 97% of the patients were affected (Tejpar et al. 2007). Besides the known symptoms of magnesium loss such as excitability and cardiac effects, a severe fatigue syndrome can be observed. To detect a MWS early, magnesium levels have to be monitored from baseline (as comparative value), because a loss can occur up to 8 weeks after completing therapy. A hypomagnesemia grade 1/2 can be treated by oral substitution. A grade 3/4 hypomagnesemia has to be treated by parenteral substitution. Fakih et al. recommend 6–10 g (!) magnesium sulfate daily or twice weekly (Fakih 2008). This magnitude of necessary substitution was confirmed for cetuximab (Schrag et al. 2005) as well as for panitumumab induced MWS (Cheng et al. 2009). Such an amount of magnesium sulfate has to be given as a protracted infusion, because of a quick compensatory elimination from short infusions by the kidneys. Ambulatory pumps such as those for infusional 5-FU can be used. In contrast to anti-EGFR MABs, no magnesium deficiency—not to mention MWS—has been reported with the use of small molecular inhibitors EGFR tyrosine kinase inhibitors such as erlotinib or gefitinib, except in context with diarrhea. Altundag et al. (2005) argue that the presence of magnesium stearate as a tableting ingredients compensates the drug induced deficiency. However, regarding the doses needed for supplementation, this seems rather unlikely. During a phase I study with erlotinib combined with the multikinase inhibitor sorafenib, phosphate deficiencies were observed (Izzedine et al. 2010). MWS seems to be a class effect of anti EGFR MABs. Detected relatively late after approval of cetuximab and panitumumab, a frequency for hypomagnesemia of 83% is stated in the FPI/SmPC of necitumumab. Meanwhile, electrolyte monitoring (potassium, calcium, magnesium) is recommended to prevent cardiopulmonary arrest.

Hypersensitivity risk by tick bite: an unexpected connection with cetuximab's structure. As with other MABs, hypersensitivity prophylaxis by premedication with an antihistamine is recommended. European product specifications also recommend the use of a corticosteroid premedication. However, severe anaphylaxis during the first exposure to cetuximab has been observed. These reactions to cetuximab developed rapidly and symptoms often peaked during or within 20 min following the first infusion of the antibody and occasionally proved fatal. Many of the affected patients also reported to be intolerant to mammalian (red) meat such as beef and pork. These first events were associated with a specific geographical region: a group of southern US states. The highest occurrence of these hypersensitivity reactions was observed in Virginia, North Carolina, Tennessee, Arkansas, Oklahoma, and Missouri (Chung et al. 2008). Subsequently, it has become clear that the syndrome of delayed anaphylaxis to red meat is also most common in these same states (Commins et al. 2009). The similarity between the region for reactions to cetuximab and the maximum incidence of Rocky Mountain spotted fever suggested that tick bites might be relevant to these reactions.

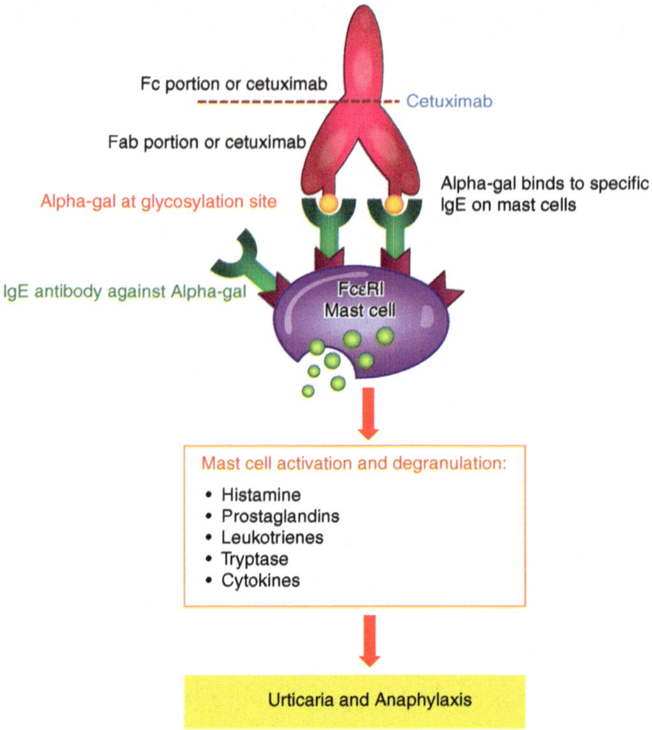

Figure 23.14 ■ Infusion reactions with cetuximab are linked to the presence of IgE antibodies directed against the alpha-gal component of the Fab fragment of the cetuximab heavy chain

Subsequently, it could be shown that tick bites can induce an immunological reaction against the oligosaccharide galactose-alpha-1,3-galactose (alpha-gal), most likely through components in the tick saliva. Alpha-gal is naturally not present in humans. Immunocompetent individuals may form antibodies to alpha-gal, that makes alpha-gal an immunogenic carbohydrate. The alpha-gal oligosacharide is also present at a glycosylation site (Asn88) on the Fab region of the heavy chain of cetuximab, a chimeric IgG1 with murine components. Each cetuximab molecule contains two alpha-gal epitopes that can cross-link the high affinity receptor for IgE on mast cells leading to mast cell activation and release of hypersensitivity mediators (Saleh et al. 2012) (Fig. 23.14). IgE binding to alpha-gal was later linked to allergic reactions to red meat in America and Europe.

Despite the development of an ELISA test for anti-cetuximab IgE for the identification of patients with high risk (Mariotte et al. 2011), no recommendations for pre-therapeutic testing exist up to now. The phenomenon, however, is mentioned in the SmPC. For further reading consult (Chung et al. 2008; Commins et al. 2009; Saleh et al. 2012; Berg et al. 2014; Commins et al. 2011; Steinke et al. 2015).

Anti Growth Factor Receptor Antibodies Anti-EGFR2 (=Anti HER2/NEU)

Trastuzumab

Trastuzumab is mainly indicated for HER2/*neu* overexpressing breast cancers in different clinical situations, as monotherapy as well as in combination therapy. It is also approved for HER2/*neu* overexpressing gastric cancers in combination with chemotherapy. Overexpression has to be verified by IHC or FISH testing. Dosing depends on the interval. For the weekly regimen, a 4 mg/kg loading dose is necessary, followed by 2 mg/kg weekly. The loading dose for the 3 weekly interval is 8 mg/kg followed by 6 mg/kg. Like rituximab, a fixed dose preparation of s. c. trastuzumab is available (in Europe). 600 mg are given q3w over 2–5 min in the thigh. No loading dose is necessary. However, this time-saving procedure compared to i.v. infusions is counteracted by the EMA's demand to supervise the patients for 6 h (!) after the first and for 2 h after subsequent injections.

Pertuzumab

Pertuzumab is another anti HER2 antibody. Trastuzumab binds to the HER2 subdomain IV and disrupts ligand-*in*dependent HER2 signaling (Fig. 23.15). Pertuzumab binds to subdomain II and blocks ligand-dependent HER2 heterodimerization with HER1, HER3, and HER4. Therefore, pertuzumab has been classified as the first HDI = HER2 dimerization inhibitor. The combination of pertuzumab and trastuzumab significantly augmented anti-tumor activity in HER2-overexpressing xenograft models, which was the rationale for the development of this double antibody based anti-Her2 strategy. Improved anticancer activity was proven in patients treated with pertuzumab in combination with trastuzumab compared to either drug alone (Baselga et al. 2012; Cortes et al. 2012).

Pertuzumab is given as a combination therapy with trastuzumab on a 3 weekly basis (with docetaxel). The initial loading dose is 840 mg followed by 240 mg q3w (Trastuzumab: 8 mg/kg loading dose followed by 6 mg/kg q3W).

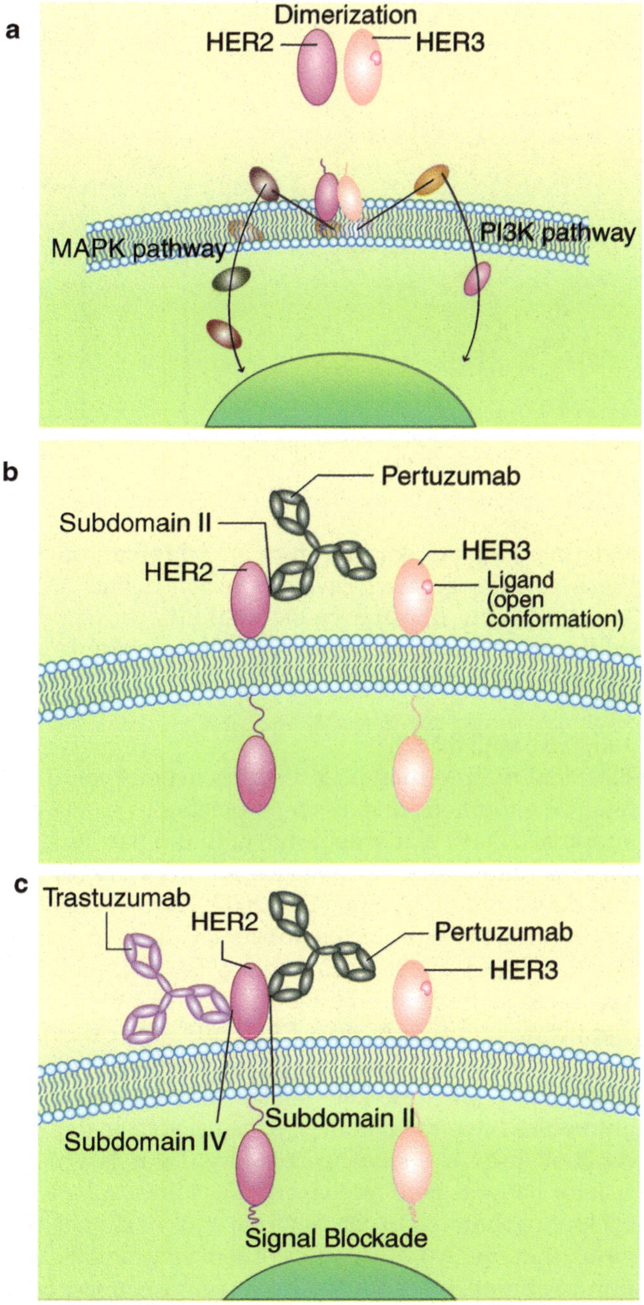

Figure 23.15 (**a**) HER2/3 heterodimerization with subsequently the strongest mitogenic signaling and activation of two key pathways that regulate cell survival and growth (**b**) Pertuzumab binds to subdomain II and blocks ligand-dependent HER2 heterodimerization with HER1, HER3, and HER4. (**c**) Trastuzumab binds to subdomain IV and disrupts ligand-independent HER2 signaling. Trastuzumab in combination with pertuzumab provide a more comprehensive blockade of HER2-driven signaling pathways

Ado-Trastuzumab-/Trastuzumab Emtanside

Ado-Trastuzumab-/Trastuzumab Emtanside (TDM-1) is the third anti-HER2 antibody, an ADC coupled with a toxin. This mertansinoide is a 19 unit lactam of the

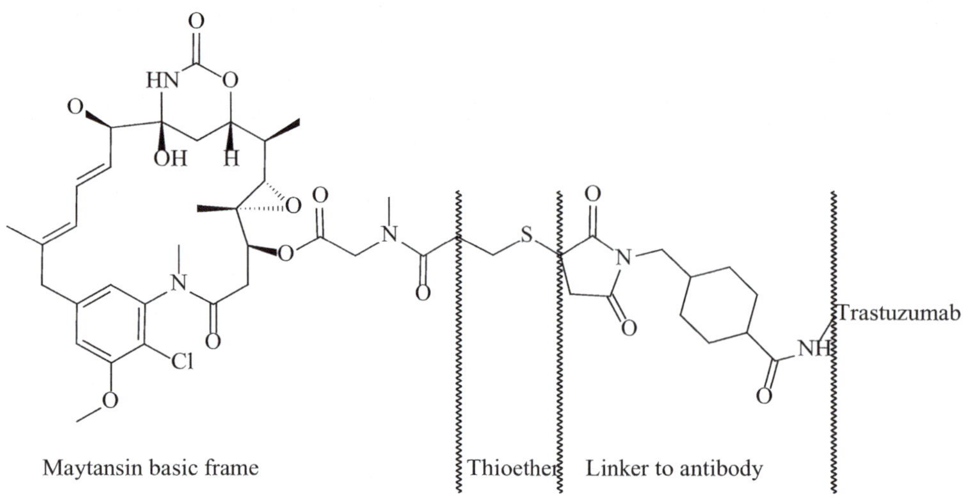

Figure 23.16 ■ The antibody-toxin-construct in TDM-1

ansamycine type, derived from an Ethiopian bush of the *Maytenus* genus (*Maytenus serrata*) (Fig. 23.16). The toxin acts like the vinca alkaloids as a mitosis inhibitor. Dosing is based on body weight with 3.6 mg/kg q3w.

Anti-HER2 MAB Safety

The Her2 receptor has essential roles in embryonal and fetal development and tissue protection, i.e. via anti apoptosis. Particularly neuronal and non-neuronal tissues, including cardiac myocytes, require Her2 for normal development (Negro et al. 2004; Zhao et al. 1998). By blocking these protective functions, the corresponding toxicity, namely cardiotoxicity, is observed. This applies to all three anti-HER2 MABs. All of them carry a warning message in their FPI/SmPC for cardiomyopathy and/or the development of a reduced left ventricular ejection function. That means all anti-HER2 antibodies have the potential to cause ventricular dysfunction and congestive heart failure. There is a higher risk for patients who receive anthracyclines, taxanes or cyclophosphamide in combination and/or during previous therapy. An evaluation of left ventricular function in all patients prior to and during treatment with these MABs is mandatory. Post approval surveys revealed a potential for lung toxicity, including interstitial lung disease. Some (rare) cases developed respiratory distress syndrome, including some with fatal outcome. Exacerbation of chemotherapy-induced neutropenia can occur with trastuzumab, and can also occur when combining pertuzumab and trastuzumab. For TDM-1, hepatotoxicity, has been reported, predominantly as asymptomatic elevations of transaminases, and neurotoxicity. This is most probably attributable to MMAE. The most common adverse reaction are infusion reactions (usually mild to moderate), which rarely require discontinuation of therapy. A routine prophylaxis with antihistamines, antipyretics and/or corticosteroids is not recommended. Skin toxicity like rash, pruritus and dry skin is described. However an intense prophylaxis therapy as required for the anti-EGFR MABs- is apparently not necessary.

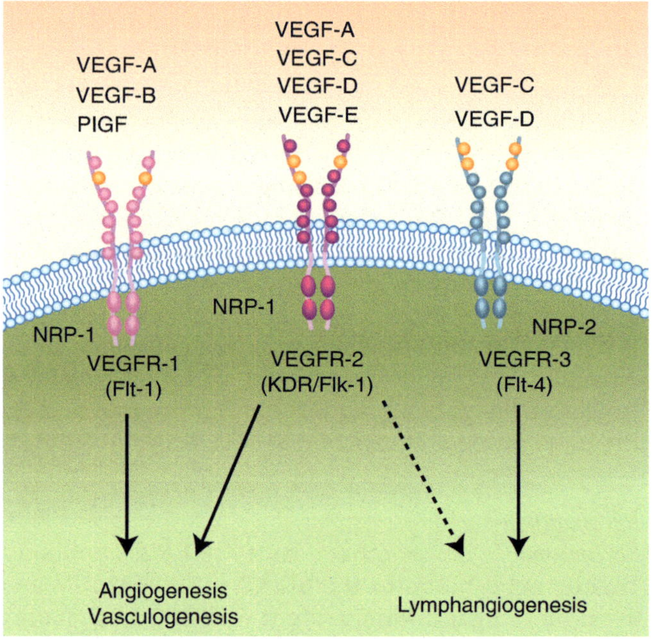

Figure 23.17 ■ VEGF-family and their corresponding receptors. PlGF was discovered in human placenta and shares a 50% homology to VEGF-A. *VEGF* vascular endothelial growth factor, *PlGF* placenta growth factor, *VEGF-R* vascular endothelial growth factor receptor, *NRP* neuropilin

ANTI-ANGIOGENIC ANTIBODIES

A small (undetectable) tumor is nourished by passive diffusion. When it has reached dimensions of 1 to 2 mm across, diffusion is not sufficient any longer. This leads to evolutionary pressure for the tumor and, in the sense of gain-of-function, it can secrete autocrine pro angiogenic growth factors such as VEGF (Vascular Endothelial Growth Factor). The angiogenic switch has been turned on. The subsequent formation of new blood vessels from pre-existing vessels (angiogenesis) is crucial for tumor development, growth and metastasis (Ohta et al. 1996). VEGF, with its different subtypes (VEGF-A–E), is a secretory, proangiogenic cytokine and one of the major regulators of the process of neovascularization (Ohta et al. 1996). An important regulating process in angiogenesis is the interaction of the VEGF subtypes with their receptors. Fig. 23.17 shows the members of the VEGF family with their receptors and the resulting effects.

Anti-angiogenic therapy leads to:

- Regression of existing microvasculature, known as antivascularisation
- Normalization of the surviving vasculature offering optimal chemotherapy delivery within the tumor, thus enhancing antitumor properties
- Antiangiogenic effect leading to the inhibition of new vessel growth, offering improved response rates and tumor death with the potential of improving patient relevant outcomes (progression free survival—PFS, time to progression—TTP, overall survival—OS).

Up to now, there are two principles of anti-angiogenic therapy.

1. Intercepting the soluble growth factors in the peripheral blood before they can interact with their receptors (bevacizumab, aflibercept)
2. Blocking the receptor a) by a MAB (ramucirumab) from the extracellular space, b) by a small molecule kinase inhibitor from the intracellular space (examples: axitinib, cabozantinib, nintedanib, pazopanib, regorafenib, sorafenib, sunitinib—not further discussed here).

■ Bevacizumab

Bevacizumab is directed against VEGF-A and its isoforms. VEGF is intercepted in the peripheral blood and tumor microenvironment, and thus neutralized before it can exert proangiogenic effects. Bevacizumab is used against several solid tumors like CRC (initial approval), NSCLC, breast- and renal cancer. Dosing depends on the schedule interval and the underlying disease. 5–10 mg/kg q2w or 7.5–15 mg/kg q3w are given.

■ Ziv-aflibercept

Ziv-aflibercept/Aflibercept (in EU) is a recombinant fusion protein consisting of the VEGF binding extracellular domain of human VEGF-receptors 1 and 2, fused to the Fc-part of human IgG1. It binds to all VEGF-A isoforms with a 100-fold higher affinity than bevacizumab. It also binds to VEGF-C and -D and to PlGF. It is designated as VEGF trap. The clinical use in oncology is restricted to CRC in combination with FolFIri at a dose of 4 mg/kg q2w. A non-oncologic indication of aflibercept (of note the INN) is the treatment of patients with neovascular (wet) age-related macular degeneration by ophthalmic intravitreal injection.

■ Ramucirumab

Ramucirumab is a recombinant human IgG1 monoclonal antibody that specifically binds to vascular endothelial growth factor receptor 2. Its clinical use comprises NSCLC, gastric, and colorectal cancer as single agent (gastric or gastro-esophageal junction adenocarcinomas) or in combination with selected chemotherapy regimens. The dosage for gastric cancer/CRC is 8 mg/kg qw2, whereas for NSCLC it is 10 mg/kg q3w.

Anti-Angiogenic MAB Safety

Initially it was assumed that VEGF-targeted therapies would be toxicity free. However, clinical trials and experience revealed a number of adverse events associated with anti-angiogenic agents, MABS as well as small kinase inhibitors, which can be summarized as a class effect (Chen and Cleck 2009; Hutson et al. 2008). These treatment-emergent adverse events comprise:

- Hypertension
- Impaired wound healing
- Haemorrhage, including severe courses
- Proteinuria
- Nephrotic syndrome or thrombotic microangiopathy
- Gastrointestinal perforation
- Fistula formation
- Arterial thromboembolic events
- Grade 4 venous thromboembolic events (including pulmonary embolism)
- Posterior reversible encephalopathy syndrome (PRES), also known as reversible posterior leukoencephalopathy syndrome (RPLS), colloquially referred to as "cortical blindness".

Pre-therapeutic hypertension has to be adjusted and monitored through therapy. Sometimes, "aggressive" interventions for blood pressure control have to be undertaken or therapy has to be discontinued. Blood pressure is mainly driven by the VEGF-R2, e.g. by NO and prostacyclin I_2 release from endothelial cells. By blocking VEGF-R2 and intercepting its ligands, the synthesis of vasodilators is suppressed, which in turn increases the peripheral resistance and in consequence the blood pressure (Verheul and Pinedo 2007). Elevated peripheral vascular resistance can also contribute to a reduced left ventricular ejection function and thus be the cause for (congestive) heart insufficiency.

Wound healing depends on neoangiogenesis. Therefore, it is easy to understand that wound healing is impaired by anti-angiogenic therapy. The mentioned MABs may be used at the earliest 4 weeks after surgery and after complete wound healing. They also have to be interrupted for 4 weeks before a planned surgery. Gastrointestinal perforations, especially along surgical sutures, have occurred.

PRES or RPLS is a rare (<1%) but severe side effect of anti-angiogenic or blood pressure elevating drugs (examples of the latter: proteasome inhibitors). RPLS is a brain-capillary leak syndrome related to hypertension, fluid retention, and the cytotoxic effects of immunosuppressive agents on the vascular endothelium. It seems that severe hypertensive encephalopathy leads to RPLS and vasogenic edema of the posterior cerebral white matter, induced by endothelial dysfunction and a disrupted blood–brain barrier (Verheul and Pinedo 2007; Widakowich et al. 2007). This rare syndrome regained attention after the approval of bevacizumab, but for most of the anti-angiogenic kinase inhibitors this side effect has been described, as well as for proteasome inhibitors such as carfilzomib, which also elevates blood pressure. Patients who experience a RPLS must never be exposed again to the causative drug.

IMMUNE ONCOLOGY

■ Immune Agonistic Antibodies

In principle, the human immune system can prevent tumorigenesis. Tumor cells, however, have the capability to escape the immune system (Vesely et al. 2011). (Re-) activating the immune system to eliminate cancer cells to produce clinically relevant responses has been a long-standing "dream of mankind". T cells have an important role to play in fighting cancers. To avoid collateral damage of host tissues and organs, T cell action is balanced by inhibitory signals and molecules—the so-called immune checkpoints. They are critical for maintaining

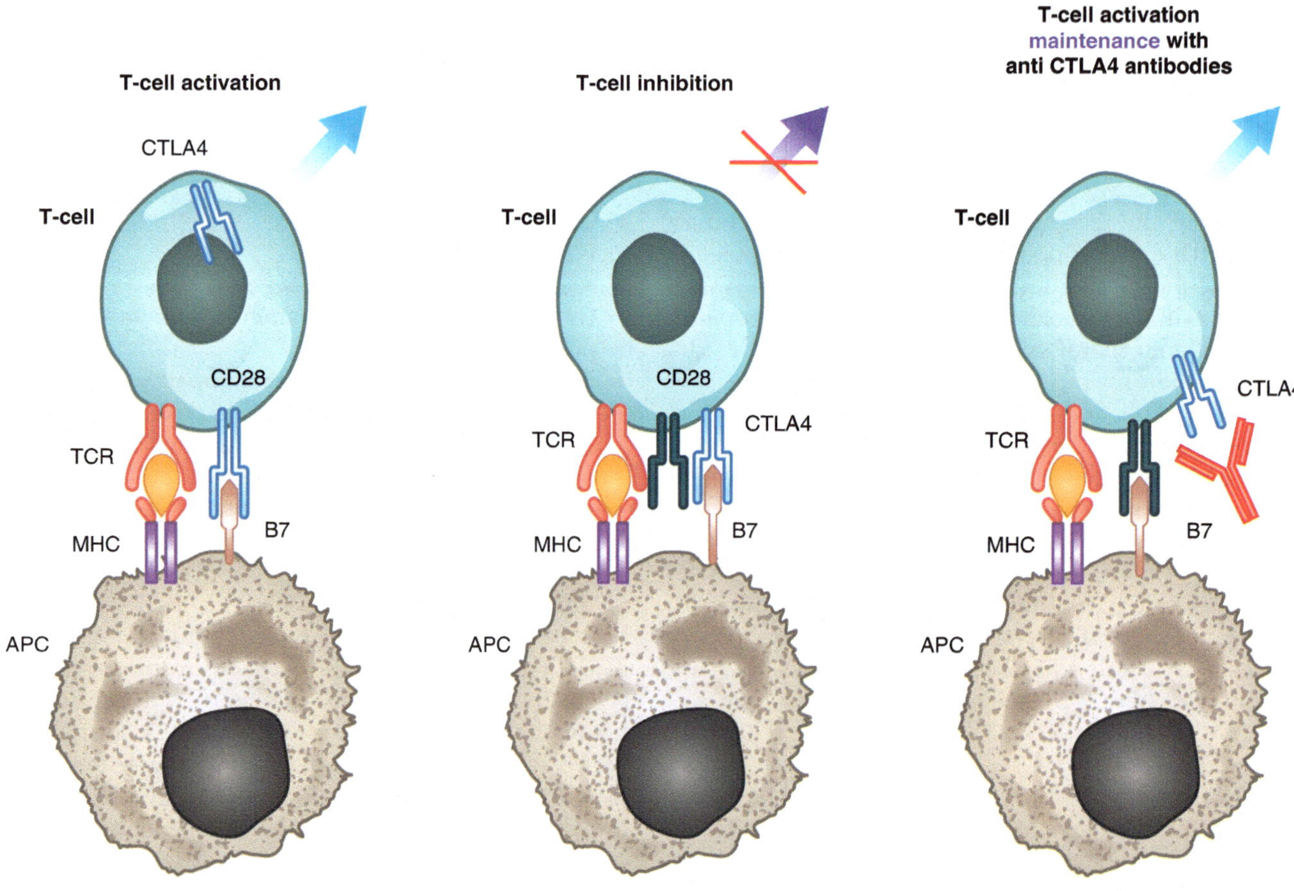

Figure 23.18 ■ Simplified mechanism of action of anti CTLA4 antibodies. *Left:* T cell activation by antigen presenting to the T cell receptor with the co-stimulatory signal B7 to CD28. *Middle:* Under physiological conditions, the activated T cells are downregulated after 48–72 h by the displacement of costimulatory CD28 with CTLA4. The B7-CTLA4-axis slows down the T cells up to complete inhibition and maintains self-tolerance in the periphery. *Right:* By blocking CTLA4 with MABs, the T cell remains activated, attacking tumor tissues. (*APC* antigen presenting cell, *CTLA4* cytotoxic T-lymphocyte antigen 4, *MHC* major histocompatibility complex, *TCR* T cell receptor)

self-tolerance on the one hand and modulating the duration and amplitude of immune responses on the other.

Normally, after T-cell activation, CTLA4 (Cytotoxic T-Lymphocyte Antigen 4; CD152), is upregulated on the plasma membrane. Its functions is to downregulate T-cell activity through a variety of mechanisms, including preventing co-stimulation by outcompeting CD28 for its ligand, B7, and also by inducing T-cell cycle arrest. Through these mechanisms and others, CTLA-4 has an essential role in maintaining normal immunologic homeostasis. CTLA4 downmodulates the amplitude of T cell activation. Blockade of CTLA4 by MABs such as ipilimumab keeps T cells stimulated (Fig. 23.18).

In contrast to CTLA4, which primarily regulates the amplitude of the early stages of T cell activation, the major role of PD1 is to limit the T cell activity in peripheral tissues. Despite its name—programmed cell death protein-1—PD1 does not induce cell death directly. When engaged with one of its ligands, PD-L1 or PD-L2, PD1 inhibits kinases that are involved in T cell activation. In summary, this pathway is a "stop signal" for T cells. Tumors use these inhibitory pathways to evade an immune attack through overexpression of PD-L1. As a result, this blocks the generation of an immune response to the tumor (cf. Figs. 23.19 and 23.20).

Long-term exposure to antigens in the presence of inflammatory cytokines induces a distinct phenotype in T cells, characterized by loss of effector functions, sustained expression of inhibitory receptors, poor proliferative capacity and decreased cyto-

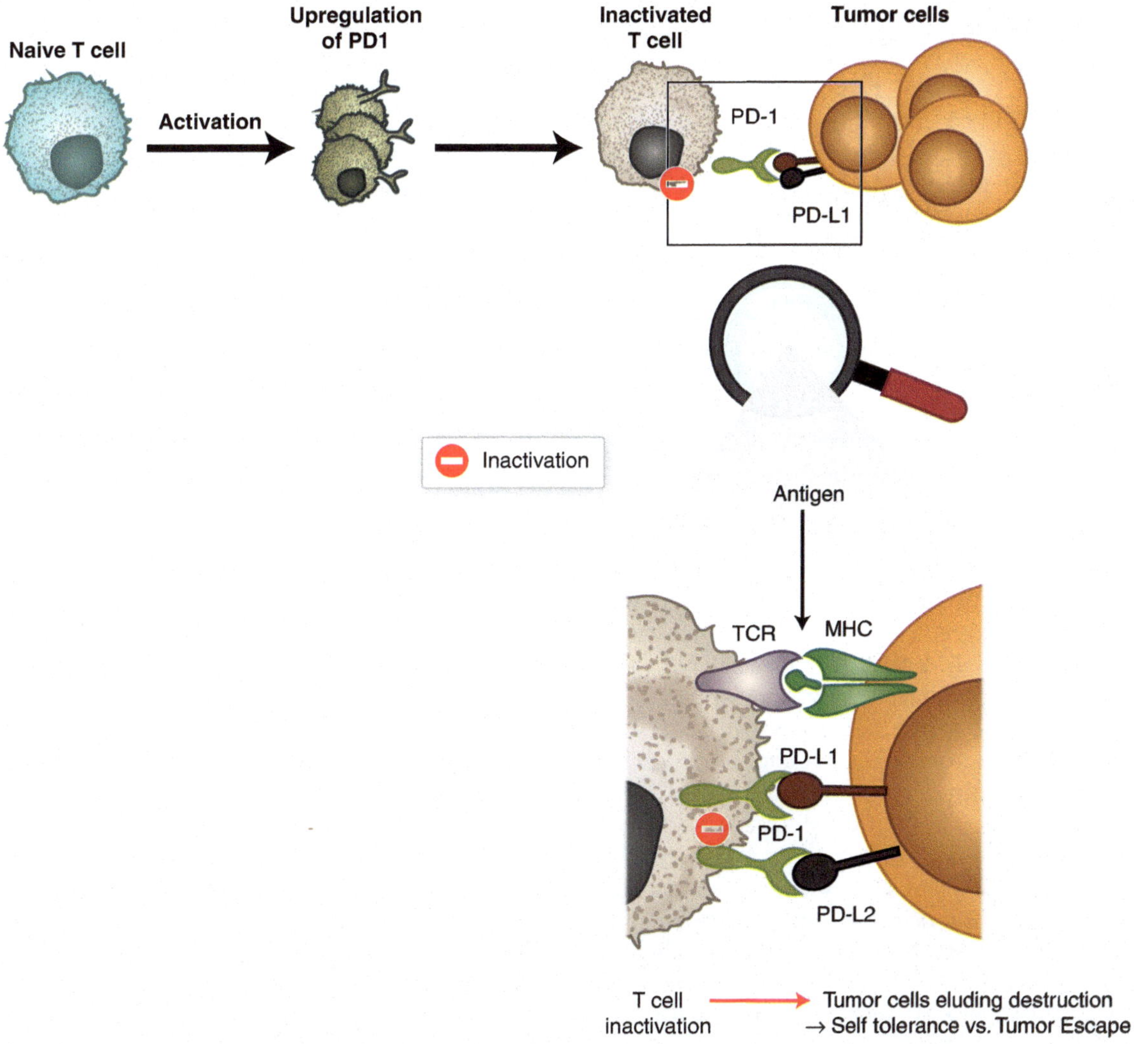

Figure 23.19 ■ Naive T cells are activated by the presentation of tumor antigens. During this priming phase, PD-1 is upregulated as a physiological reaction to protect unaffected host tissue. The corresponding ligand, PD-L1, expressed on tumor cells, downregulates T cells, pretending to be "friendly", healthy tissue. The magnifier shows the details of the T cell receptor (TCR) interaction with tumor antigen presenting Major Histocompatibility Complex (MHC). Inactivating programmed cell death receptor 1 (PD-1) is stimulated by the corresponding ligands (PD-L1/2), resulting in T cell exhaustion. (*MHC* major histocompatibility complex, *PD-1* programmed cell death receptor1, *PD-L1/2* PD1/2-ligand, *TCR* T cell receptor)

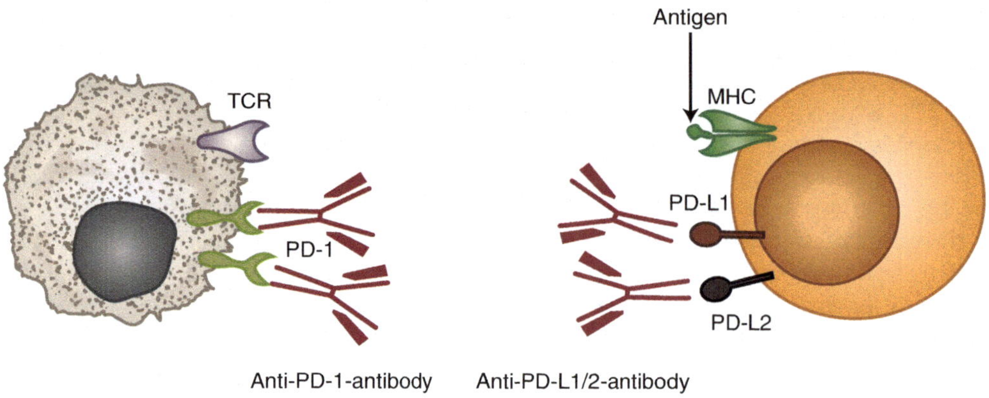

Figure 23.20 ■ Anti PD-1 and/or anti PD-L antibodies prevent the inactivation of immune competent T cells

toxic functions. This progressive loss of T-cell effector functions is commonly seen during chronic viral infections and in cancer. It is termed "T-cell exhaustion". T cells detect the tumor, accumulate in the tumor microenvironment, however, are silenced by inhibitory molecules expressed on the tumor surface such as PD-L1/2. PD-1/PD-L1 inhibitors pharmacologically prevent the PD-1/PD-L1 interaction, thus facilitating a positive immune response to kill the tumor. For further immune oncology (IO) information, the reader is referred to Alsaab et al. (2017), Ferris (2013), Intlekofer and Thompson (2013), Li et al. (2016), Pardoll (2012), Rotte et al. (2018), Suzuki et al. (2016)).

Immune oncology MABs do not show a clear dose-response relationship. They are either dosed by body weight or with a fixed dose. For the future it may be possible that antibodies currently dosed by body weight may be switched to fixed dosing.

Due to their mechanism of action, infiltrating the tumor tissue followed by tumor cell killing, an initial increase of tumor lesions was observed. From the formal point of view, these patients were RECIST progressive (RECIST = Response Evaluation Criteria In Solid Tumors). However, it would have been a mistake to stop treatment too early, as biopsies confirmed inflammatory cell infiltrates with an apparent enlargement of the tumor. This phenomenon is termed pseudoprogression or "tumor flare" (short overview Chiou and Burotto 2015). Thus, to ascertain a clinical benefit, it can take 12 weeks or more after the first infusion and may include the emergence of (temporary) new lesions. To avoid misclassification according WHO in immune oncology, immune-related response criteria (irRC) were developed in 2009 (Wolchok et al. 2009).

■ Anti CTLA4 Antibodies

Ipilimumab

Ipilimumab is the first anti CTLA4, recombinant human monoclonal antibody. It is used as monotherapy for the treatment of melanoma in different clinical situations. 3 mg/kg q3w for 4 doses are used for unresectable or metastatic melanoma. In a certain adjuvant setting (cutaneous melanoma with pathologic involvement of regional lymph nodes of more than 1 mm that have undergone complete resection, including total lymphadenectomy), 10 mg/kg q3w for 4 doses followed by 10 mg/kg q12w up to 3 years are recommended. Fig. 23.18 illustrates the simplified mechanism of action.

■ Anti PD1- and Anti PD-L1 Antibodies

While development of new anti PD1/anti PD-L1 antibodies is rapidly progressing and will likely provide new agents, the following MABs were on the market at the time of the creation of this manuscript (Table 23.2):

The anti PD1/anti PD-L1 antibodies are used against different solid tumors. Depending on the underlying disease and the clinical situation (first-line treatment or relapsed tumor), PD-L1 testing is sometimes mandatory. The relevance and usefulness of PD-L1 as a predicting biomarker is still under debate. Fig. 23.19 illustrates the pathological mechanisms, Fig. 23.20 the pharmacodynamic intervention with MABs.

Immune Oncology MAB Safety: Playing with Fire?

Due to their mechanism of action, immune checkpoint inhibitors in the form of MABs against CTLA-4, PD-1, and PD-L1, have a unique spectrum of toxicity that differs from the typical adverse events seen with chemotherapeutic agents. By inhibiting checkpoint molecules, the immune system is activated or even over-activated or, from the viewpoint of the normal tissue, deregulated (non-recognizing "self"). These new kind of autoimmune-like symptoms are based on the loss of self-tolerance and termed immune-related adverse events (irAEs). For CTLA-4–blocking antibodies, toxicities seem to be dose related, because the rate of grade 3 to 4 drug-related serious irAEs increased from 5% to 18% when the dose was increased from 3 to 10 mg/kg whereas it was 0% at a dose of 0.3 mg/kg. In contrast, the toxicities related to PD-1 blockade are similar at doses ranging from 0.3 to 10 mg/kg, exemplary observed with nivolumab. The observed toxicities depend on

- The patient population/the underlying disease
- The dose (especially for CTLA-4 antibodies)
- The schedule

That means, the same dose or schedule in different diseases might result in different toxicity profiles. Combinational checkpoint blockade can result in an increase of grade 3/4 treatment emergent adverse events (TEAE) up to 53% (Wolchok et al. 2013). The toxicity pattern is based on induced autoimmunity and comprises:

- Skin irAEs, including Stevens-Johnson-Syndrome and Toxic Epidermal Necrolysis (both rare)
- Gastrointestinal irAEs—autoimmune colitis
- Autoimmune hepatitis
- Autoimmune pancreatitis
- Autoimmune thyroiditis
- Autoimmune hypophysitis
- Neurological irAEs
- Autoimmune pneumonitis
- Ocular irAE (rare), like autoimmune uveitis and autoimmune episcleritis

In December 2016 the Federal Institute for Drugs and Medical Devices, Germany, informed the medical professional circles about suspected cases of pancytopenia/agranulocytosis. Onset was between 12 and 274 days after start of therapy. Three instances were fatal. Another rare irAE was myocarditis (9 cases), with two of them having an additional myositis and rhabdomyolysis. Four cases had a fatal outcome. In

Anti PD-1 antibodies	Anti PD-L1 antibodies
Nivolumab	Durvalumab
Pembrolizumab	Atezolizumab
	Avelumab

Table 23.2 ■ Approved anti PD-1 and anti PD-L1 antibodies, effective April 2018

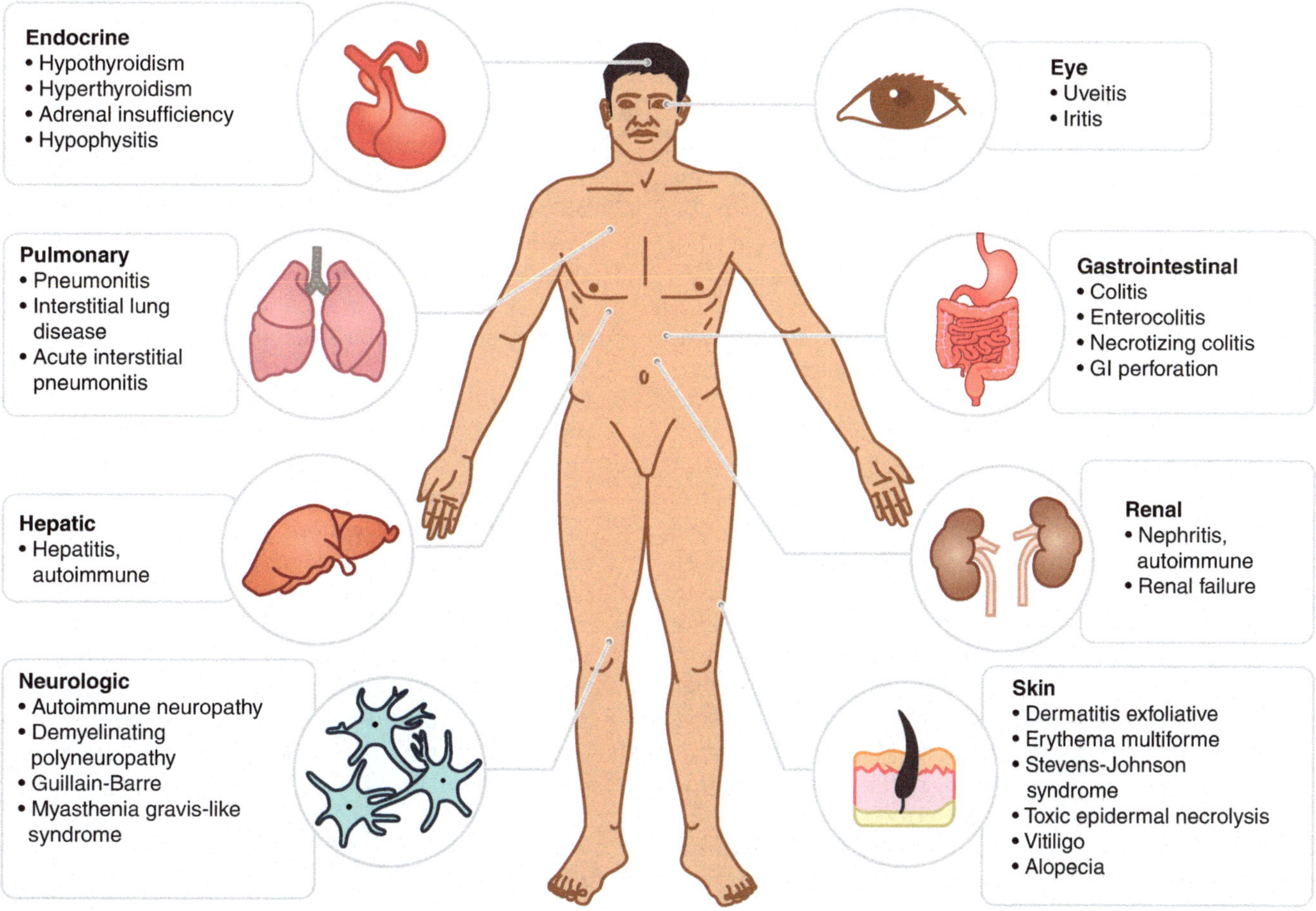

Figure 23.21 ■ Affected tissues organs and symptoms by autoimmune related adverse reactions. Listing is not intended to be exhaustive

principle, every tissue and organ can be affected (Fig. 23.21).

Toxicity/iRAE Management

Physicians and pharmacists should know about and be able to recognize irAE as such and the recommended interventions (Davies and Duffield 2017; Haanen et al. 2015; Weber et al. 2012; Weber et al. 2015).

In severe diarrhea with associated signs of colitis, the usual counter-measures (fluid + electrolytes ⇨ loperamide ⇨ budesonide) are insufficient. Intravenous or oral steroid therapy has to be initiated. For patients in whom intravenous steroids followed by high-dose oral steroid therapy does not lead to initial resolution of symptoms within 48–72 h, treatment with infliximab at 5 mg/kg can be used as an "emergency brake". Once relief of symptoms is achieved with infliximab, it should be discontinued. A prolonged steroid taper over 45–60 days should be instituted. There may be a waxing and waning of the GI adverse effects. As steroids are tapered, there can be a recrudescence of symptoms, mandating a retapering of steroids starting at a higher dose, a more prolonged taper, and the (re-) use of infliximab. Prophylactic use of budesonide cannot be recommended, based on a phase II study (Wolchok et al. 2010).

Autoimmune hepatitis is likewise treated with (high dose) corticosteroids. If serum transaminase levels do not decrease within 48 h after initiation of systemic steroids, oral mycophenolate mofetil 500 mg q12h should be considered. Infliximab has to be avoided, because of its potential own hepatotoxicity. As described above, resurgence of symptoms and steroid tapering is necessary.

Difficult in diagnosis can be the auto hypophysitis with symptoms of headache, nausea, vertigo, behavior change, visual disturbances such as diplopia, and weakness. In this context new occurrence of brain metastases have to be excluded. Baseline measurement of pituitary, thyroid, adrenal, and gonadal status, i.e. serum morning cortisol, adrenocorticotropic hormone [ACTH], free triiodothyronine [T3], free thyroxine [T4], thyroid-stimulating hormone [TSH], testosterone in males and follicle-stimulating hormone, luteinizing hormone, and prolactin in females is recommended.

Immune-related pancreatitis generally manifests as an asymptomatic increase of amylase and lipase. Some patients experience more or less unspecific symptoms like fevers, malaise, nausea and vomiting and/or abdominal pain. As described for other irAEs, a steroid taper is indicated, but often this has minimal *immediate* effects. The symptoms of an autoimmune pancreatitis resolve slowly.

The irAEs caused by checkpoint blockade exhibit a characteristic pattern in the timing of their occurrence, shown in Fig. 23.22 (Weber et al. 2012).

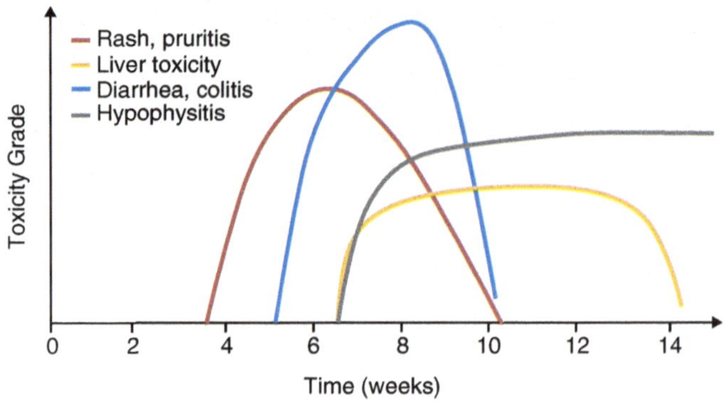

Figure 23.22 ■ irAEs exhibit a characteristic pattern in the timing of their occurrence. The frequency is not considered (from Weber et al. 2012)

After 2–3 weeks of initiation of a checkpoint blocker therapy, skin-related irAEs can be expected. Gastrointestinal side effects emerge after approximately 5–6 weeks. Hepatic irAEs occur after 6–7 weeks, and endocrinological irAEs (autoimmune hypothyroiditis or hypophysitis) after an average of 9 weeks. Long-term effects of immune oncology therapy are currently still largely unknown.

SELF ASSESSMENT QUESTIONS

■ Questions

1. Against what kind of molecular targets can MABs be directed? Give examples
2. By which factors can the pharmacokinetics of MABs be influenced?
3. What stands ADC for?
4. Why is Rituximab in CLL dosed with 375 mg/m^2 initially but escalated to 500 mg/m^{2}in subsequent cycles?
5. Describe the differences in clinical effects between type I and type II anti-lymphoma antibodies.
6. How many subtypes of the epidermal growth factor receptors exist and how are they designated?
7. Which diagnostic actions are mandatory before using anti-EGFR/anti-Her2 antibodies?
8. Does it make therapeutically a difference if a colorectal carcinoma is right sided or left sided?
9. What is the main difference in the mechanism of action between 'classical' antibody treatment of cancers and immune agonistic antibodies?
10. Describe the toxicity profile of checkpoint inhibitors.

■ Answers

1. MABs can be directed against
   - Surface antigens like CD antigens (CD20, CD30)
   - Receptors (EGFR)
   - Growth factors (VEGF)

- Activating immune checkpoints on T cells (PD1)
- Suppressing immune checkpoints on tumor cells (PD-L1)

2. Tumor burden which corresponds to the amount of target antigen.
   - Neutralizing anti-MAB-antibodies
   - Gender
   - Age
3. ADC is the abbreviation for antibody drug conjugate, where an antibody is chemically linked to a toxin with anti-tumor activity. The toxins are too toxic to be given in unconjugated form.
4. In CLL the CD20 antigen density is lower than in other CD20 positive lymphomas. The reduced dose for the first infusion is necessary because of a usually high tumor load in need for therapy in CLL blast crisis. Responding to rituximab therapy bears a high risk of tumor lysis and cytokine release syndrome as well as other infusion related reactions.
5. Type I antibodies cause predominant CDC, type II antibodies ADCC
6. 4 subtypes, EGFR 1–4 or ErbB 1–4 or Her 1–4
7. Verification of EGFR or Her2 overexpression, in case of Her2 with IHC or FISH. Pan-RAS wild type testing for cetuximab and panitumumab.
8. Depending on the localization, these tumors are regarded as biologically different. Patients with a right sided tumor benefit from an antiangiogenic drug containing first line therapy, whereas left sided tumors benefit from an anti EGFR strategy if they are not RAS mutated.
9. The so-called check point inhibiting antibodies do not attack the tumor itself, they restore their immunogenicity and/or (re-)activate immune competent cells.
10. The toxicity pattern consists of loss of self-olerance, resulting in autoimmune reactions (immune related adverse events) such as
    - Skin irAEs, including Stevens-Johnson-Syndrom and Toxic Epidermal Necrolysis (both rare)
    - Gastrointestinal irAEs—auto immune colitis
    - Autoimmune hepatitis
    - Autoimmune pancreatitis
    - Autoimmune thyreodits
    - Autoimmune hypophysitis
    - Neurological irAEs
    - Autoimmune pneumonitis
    - Ocular irAE (rare), such as autoimmune uveitis and autoimmune episcleritis

REFERENCES

Alsaab HO et al (2017) PD-1 and PD-L1 checkpoint signaling inhibition for Cancer immunotherapy: mechanism, combinations, and clinical outcome. Front Pharmacol 8:561

Altundag K et al (2005) Re: cetuximab therapy and symptomatic hypomagnesemia. J Natl Cancer Inst 97(23):1791–1792

Anolik JH et al (2003) The relationship of FcgammaRIIIa genotype to degree of B cell depletion by rituximab in the treatment of systemic lupus erythematosus. Arthritis Rheum 48(2):455–459

Baselga J et al (2012) Pertuzumab plus trastuzumab plus docetaxel for metastatic breast cancer. N Engl J Med 366(2):109–119

Beers SA et al (2010) CD20 as a target for therapeutic type I and II monoclonal antibodies. Semin Hematol 47(2):107–114

Berg EA, Platts-Mills TA, Commins SP (2014) Drug allergens and food--the cetuximab and galactose-alpha-1,3-galactose story. Ann Allergy Asthma Immunol 112(2):97–101

Berinstein NL et al (1998) Association of serum rituximab (IDEC-C2B8) concentration and anti-tumor response in the treatment of recurrent low-grade or follicular non-Hodgkin's lymphoma. Ann Oncol 9(9):995–1001

Bokemeyer C et al (2012) Addition of cetuximab to chemotherapy as first-line treatment for KRAS wild-type metastatic colorectal cancer: pooled analysis of the CRYSTAL and OPUS randomised clinical trials. Eur J Cancer 48(10):1466–1475

Brule SY et al (2015) Location of colon cancer (right-sided versus left-sided) as a prognostic factor and a predictor of benefit from cetuximab in NCIC CO.17. Eur J Cancer 51(11):1405–1414

Bubien JK et al (1993) Transfection of the CD20 cell surface molecule into ectopic cell types generates a Ca2+ conductance found constitutively in B lymphocytes. J Cell Biol 121(5):1121–1132

Burchardt A, Wienzek-Lischka S, Schoelz C, Hackstein H, Rummel M (2012) Plasma exchange (PE) therapy (rituximab apheresis) for rituximab (R) induced progressive multifocal Leukoencephalopathy (PML) in hematologic disorders. Onkologie:133

Buza N, Roque DM, Santin AD (2014) HER2/neu in endometrial Cancer: a promising therapeutic target with diagnostic challenges. Arch Pathol Lab Med 138(3):343–350

Cartron G et al (2016) Rationale for optimal obinutuzumab/GA101 dosing regimen in B-cell non-Hodgkin lymphoma. Haematologica 101(2):226–234

Chan HT et al (2003) CD20-induced lymphoma cell death is independent of both caspases and its redistribution into triton X-100 insoluble membrane rafts. Cancer Res 63(17):5480–5489

Chen HX, Cleck JN (2009) Adverse effects of anticancer agents that target the VEGF pathway. Nat Rev Clin Oncol 6(8):465–477

Cheng H, Gammon D, Dutton TM, Piperdi B (2009) Panitumumab-related Hypomagnesemiain patients with colorectal Cancer. Hosp Pharm 44:234–238

Cheson BD (2010) Ofatumumab, a novel anti-CD20 monoclonal antibody for the treatment of B-cell malignancies. J Clin Oncol 28(21):3525–3530

Chiosea SI et al (2015) Molecular characterization of apocrine salivary duct carcinoma. Am J Surg Pathol 39(6):744–752

Chiou VL, Burotto M (2015) Pseudoprogression and immune-related response in solid tumors. J Clin Oncol 33(31):3541–3543

Chung CH et al (2008) Cetuximab-induced anaphylaxis and IgE specific for galactose-alpha-1,3-galactose. N Engl J Med 358(11):1109–1117

Collins SM et al (2013) Elotuzumab directly enhances NK cell cytotoxicity against myeloma via CS1 ligation: evidence for augmented NK cell function complementing ADCC. Cancer Immunol Immunother 62(12):1841–1849

Commins SP et al (2009) Delayed anaphylaxis, angioedema, or urticaria after consumption of red meat in patients with IgE antibodies specific for galactose-alpha-1,3-galactose. J Allergy Clin Immunol 123(2):426–433

Commins SP et al (2011) The relevance of tick bites to the production of IgE antibodies to the mammalian oligosaccharide galactose-alpha-1,3-galactose. J Allergy Clin Immunol 127(5):1286–1293. e6

Cortes J et al (2012) Pertuzumab monotherapy after trastuzumab-based treatment and subsequent reintroduction of trastuzumab: activity and tolerability in patients with advanced human epidermal growth factor receptor 2-positive breast cancer. J Clin Oncol 30(14):1594–1600

Cragg MS, Glennie MJ (2004) Antibody specificity controls in vivo effector mechanisms of anti-CD20 reagents. Blood 103(7):2738–2743

Cragg MS et al (2003) Complement-mediated lysis by anti-CD20 mAb correlates with segregation into lipid rafts. Blood 101(3):1045–1052

Cragg MS et al (2005) The biology of CD20 and its potential as a target for mAb therapy. Curr Dir Autoimmun 8:140–174

Davies M, Duffield EA (2017) Safety of checkpoint inhibitors for cancer treatment: strategies for patient monitoring and management of immune-mediated adverse events. Immunotargets Ther 6:51–71

De Roock W et al (2010) Effects of KRAS, BRAF, NRAS, and PIK3CA mutations on the efficacy of cetuximab plus chemotherapy in chemotherapy-refractory metastatic colorectal cancer: a retrospective consortium analysis. Lancet Oncol 11(8):753–762

de Weers M et al (2011) Daratumumab, a novel therapeutic human CD38 monoclonal antibody, induces killing of multiple myeloma and other hematological tumors. J Immunol 186(3):1840–1848

Deaglio S, Mehta K, Malavasi F (2001) Human CD38: a (r) evolutionary story of enzymes and receptors. Leuk Res 25(1):1–12

Deans JP et al (1998) Rapid redistribution of CD20 to a low density detergent-insoluble membrane compartment. J Biol Chem 273(1):344–348

English DP, Roque DM, Santin AD (2013) HER2 expression beyond breast cancer: therapeutic implications for gynecologic malignancies. Mol Diagn Ther 17(2):85–99

Fakih M (2008) Management of anti-EGFR-targeting monoclonal antibody-induced hypomagnesemia. Oncology (Williston Park) 22(1):74–76

Fakih MG, Wilding G, Lombardo J (2006) Cetuximab-induced hypomagnesemia in patients with colorectal cancer. Clin Colorectal Cancer 6(2):152–156

FDA (2017) FDA approves mylotarg for treatment of acute myeloid leukemia. https://www.fda.gov/NewsEvents/Newsroom/PressAnnouncements/ucm574507.htm

Ferris R (2013) PD-1 targeting in cancer immunotherapy. Cancer 119(23):E1–E3

Gordan LN et al (2005) Phase II trial of individualized rituximab dosing for patients with CD20-positive lymphoproliferative disorders. J Clin Oncol 23(6):1096–1102

Guo H et al (2015) Immune cell inhibition by SLAMF7 is mediated by a mechanism requiring src kinases, CD45, and SHIP-1 that is defective in multiple myeloma cells. Mol Cell Biol 35(1):41–51

Gutzmer R et al (2011) Management of cutaneous side effects of EGFR inhibitors: recommendations from a German expert panel for the primary treating physician. J Dtsch Dermatol Ges 9(3):195–203

Haanen JB, Thienen H, Blank CU (2015) Toxicity patterns with immunomodulating antibodies and their combinations. Semin Oncol 42(3):423–428

Han TH, Zhao B (2014) Absorption, distribution, metabolism, and excretion considerations for the development of antibody-drug conjugates. Drug Metab Dispos 42(11):1914–1920

Herold M, Schnohr S, Bittrich H (2001) Efficacy and safety of a combined rituximab chemotherapy during pregnancy. J Clin Oncol 19(14):3439

Hofheinz RD et al (2016) Recommendations for the prophylactic management of skin reactions induced by epidermal growth factor receptor inhibitors in patients with solid tumors. Oncologist 21(12):1483–1491

Holcmann M, Sibilia M (2015) Mechanisms underlying skin disorders induced by EGFR inhibitors. Mol Cell Oncol 2(4):e1004969

Hsi ED et al (2008) CS1, a potential new therapeutic antibody target for the treatment of multiple myeloma. Clin Cancer Res 14(9):2775–2784

Huhn D et al (2001) Rituximab therapy of patients with B-cell chronic lymphocytic leukemia. Blood 98(5):1326–1331

Hutson TE et al (2008) Targeted therapies for metastatic renal cell carcinoma: an overview of toxicity and dosing strategies. Oncologist 13(10):1084–1096

Intlekofer AM, Thompson CB (2013) At the bench: preclinical rationale for CTLA-4 and PD-1 blockade as cancer immunotherapy. J Leukoc Biol 94(1):25–39

Ishibashi K et al (2001) Identification of a new multigene four-transmembrane family (MS4A) related to CD20, HTm4 and beta subunit of the high-affinity IgE receptor. Gene 264(1):87–93

Ivanov A et al (2008) Radiation therapy with tositumomab (B1) anti-CD20 monoclonal antibody initiates extracellular signal-regulated kinase/mitogen-activated protein kinase-dependent cell death that overcomes resistance to apoptosis. Clin Cancer Res 14(15):4925–4934

Izzedine H et al (2010) Electrolyte disorders related to EGFR-targeting drugs. Crit Rev Oncol Hematol 73(3):213–219

Kanzaki M et al (1995) Expression of calcium-permeable cation channel CD20 accelerates progression through the G1 phase in Balb/c 3T3 cells. J Biol Chem 270(22):13099–13104

Keizer RJ et al (2010) Clinical pharmacokinetics of therapeutic monoclonal antibodies. Clin Pharmacokinet 49(8):493–507

Klein C et al (2013) Epitope interactions of monoclonal antibodies targeting CD20 and their relationship to functional properties. MAbs 5(1):22–33

Lacouture ME et al (2011) Clinical practice guidelines for the prevention and treatment of EGFR inhibitor-associated dermatologic toxicities. Support Care Cancer 19(8):1079–1095

Li H et al (2003) Store-operated cation entry mediated by CD20 in membrane rafts. J Biol Chem 278(43):42427–42434

Li Y et al (2016) A mini-review for Cancer immunotherapy: molecular understanding of PD-1/PD-L1 pathway & translational blockade of immune checkpoints. Int J Mol Sci 17(7):E1151

Lin P et al (2004) Flow cytometric immunophenotypic analysis of 306 cases of multiple myeloma. Am J Clin Pathol 121(4):482–488

Ludwig DL et al (2003) Monoclonal antibody therapeutics and apoptosis. Oncogene 22(56):9097–9106

Malavasi F et al (2008) Evolution and function of the ADP ribosyl cyclase/CD38 gene family in physiology and pathology. Physiol Rev 88(3):841–886

Malavasi F et al (2011) CD38 and chronic lymphocytic leukemia: a decade later. Blood 118(13):3470–3478

Maloney DG et al (1994) Phase I clinical trial using escalating single-dose infusion of chimeric anti-CD20 monoclonal antibody (IDEC-C2B8) in patients with recurrent B-cell lymphoma. Blood 84(8):2457–2466

Maloney DG et al (1997) IDEC-C2B8 (rituximab) anti-CD20 monoclonal antibody therapy in patients with relapsed low-grade non-Hodgkin's lymphoma. Blood 90(6):2188–2195

Manches O et al (2003) In vitro mechanisms of action of rituximab on primary non-Hodgkin lymphomas. Blood 101(3):949–954

Mariotte D et al (2011) Anti-cetuximab IgE ELISA for identification of patients at a high risk of cetuximab-induced anaphylaxis. MAbs 3(4):396–401

McLaughlin P et al (1998) Rituximab chimeric anti-CD20 monoclonal antibody therapy for relapsed indolent lymphoma: half of patients respond to a four-dose treatment program. J Clin Oncol 16(8):2825–2833

Mellor JD et al (2013) A critical review of the role of Fc gamma receptor polymorphisms in the response to monoclonal antibodies in cancer. J Hematol Oncol 6:1

Morschhauser FA et al (2013) Obinutuzumab (GA101) monotherapy in relapsed/refractory diffuse large b-cell lymphoma or mantle-cell lymphoma: results from the phase II GAUGUIN study. J Clin Oncol 31(23):2912–2919

Mossner E et al (2010) Increasing the efficacy of CD20 antibody therapy through the engineering of a new type II anti-CD20 antibody with enhanced direct and immune effector cell-mediated B-cell cytotoxicity. Blood 115(22):4393–4402

Muller C et al (2012) The role of sex and weight on rituximab clearance and serum elimination half-life in elderly patients with DLBCL. Blood 119(14):3276–3284

Nadler LM et al (1981) A unique cell surface antigen identifying lymphoid malignancies of B cell origin. J Clin Invest 67(1):134–140

National Cancer Institute 2014 FDA approval for tositumomab and iodine I 131 tositumomab. Internet: https://www.cancer.gov/about-cancer/treatment/drugs/fda-tositumomab-I131iodine-tositumomab

Negro A, Brar BK, Lee KF (2004) Essential roles of Her2/erbB2 in cardiac development and function. Recent Prog Horm Res 59:1–12

Nguyen DT et al (1999) IDEC-C2B8 anti-CD20 (rituximab) immunotherapy in patients with low-grade non-Hodgkin's lymphoma and lymphoproliferative disorders: evaluation of response on 48 patients. Eur J Haematol 62(2):76–82

Niederfellner G et al (2011) Epitope characterization and crystal structure of GA101 provide insights into the molecular basis for type I/II distinction of CD20 antibodies. Blood 118(2):358–367

O'Brien SM et al (2001) Rituximab dose-escalation trial in chronic lymphocytic leukemia. J Clin Oncol 19(8):2165–2170

Ohta Y et al (1996) Significance of vascular endothelial growth factor messenger RNA expression in primary lung cancer. Clin Cancer Res 2(8):1411–1416

Overdijk MB et al (2015) Antibody-mediated phagocytosis contributes to the anti-tumor activity of the therapeutic antibody daratumumab in lymphoma and multiple myeloma. MAbs 7(2):311–321

Pardoll DM (2012) The blockade of immune checkpoints in cancer immunotherapy. Nat Rev Cancer 12(4):252–264

Pfreundschuh M, Zeynalova S, Poeschel V, Haenel M, Schmitz N, Hensel M, Reiser M, Loeffler M, Schubert J (2007) Dose-dense rituximab improves outcome of elderly patients with poor-prognosis diffuse large B-cell lymphoma (DLBCL): results of the DENSE-R-CHOP-14 trial of the German high-grade non-Hodgkin lymphoma study group (DSHNHL). Blood 110(11):789

Pfreundschuh M et al (2014) Suboptimal dosing of rituximab in male and female patients with DLBCL. Blood 123(5):640–646

Polyak MJ, Deans JP (2002) Alanine-170 and proline-172 are critical determinants for extracellular CD20 epitopes; heterogeneity in the fine specificity of CD20 monoclonal antibodies is defined by additional requirements imposed by both amino acid sequence and quaternary structure. Blood 99(9):3256–3262

Polyak MJ et al (2008) CD20 homo-oligomers physically associate with the B cell antigen receptor. Dissociation upon receptor engagement and recruitment of phosphopro-

teins and calmodulin-binding proteins. J Biol Chem 283(27):18545–18552
Potthoff K et al (2011) Interdisciplinary management of EGFR-inhibitor-induced skin reactions: a German expert opinion. Ann Oncol 22(3):524–535
Quartier P et al (2001) Treatment of childhood autoimmune haemolytic anaemia with rituximab. Lancet 358(9292):1511–1513
Radhakrishnan SV et al (2017) Elotuzumab as a novel anti-myeloma immunotherapy. Hum Vaccin Immunother 13(8):1751–1757
Rotte A, Jin JY, Lemaire V (2018) Mechanistic overview of immune checkpoints to support the rational design of their combinations in cancer immunotherapy. Ann Oncol 29(1):71–83
Rubin I, Yarden Y (2001) The basic biology of HER2. Ann Oncol 12(Suppl 1):S3–S8
Saleh H et al (2012) Anaphylactic reactions to oligosaccharides in red meat: a syndrome in evolution. Clin Mol Allergy 10(1):5
Santin AD et al (2008) Trastuzumab treatment in patients with advanced or recurrent endometrial carcinoma overexpressing HER2/neu. Int J Gynaecol Obstet 102(2):128–131
Santonocito AM et al (2004) Flow cytometric detection of aneuploid CD38(++) plasmacells and CD19(+) B-lymphocytes in bone marrow, peripheral blood and PBSC harvest in multiple myeloma patients. Leuk Res 28(5):469–477
Schlingmann KP et al (2007) TRPM6 and TRPM7—gatekeepers of human magnesium metabolism. Biochim Biophys Acta 1772(8):813–821
Schneider MR, Wolf E (2009) The epidermal growth factor receptor ligands at a glance. J Cell Physiol 218(3):460–466
Schrag D et al (2005) Cetuximab therapy and symptomatic hypomagnesemia. J Natl Cancer Inst 97(16):1221–1224
Simons K, Toomre D (2000) Lipid rafts and signal transduction. Nat Rev Mol Cell Biol 1(1):31–39
Singh B, Carpenter G, Coffey RJ 2016 EGF receptor ligands: recent advances. F1000Res 5. https://doi.org/10.12688/f1000research.9025.1
Stashenko P et al (1980) Characterization of a human B lymphocyte-specific antigen. J Immunol 125(4):1678–1685
Steinke JW, Platts-Mills TA, Commins SP (2015) The alpha-gal story: lessons learned from connecting the dots. J Allergy Clin Immunol 135(3):589–596
Stolz C, Schuler M (2009) Molecular mechanisms of resistance to rituximab and pharmacologic strategies for its circumvention. Leuk Lymphoma 50(6):873–885
Suzuki S et al (2016) Current status of immunotherapy. Jpn J Clin Oncol 46(3):191–203
Tabernero J, Pfeiffer P, Cervantes A (2008) Administration of cetuximab every 2 weeks in the treatment of metastatic colorectal cancer: an effective, more convenient alternative to weekly administration? Oncologist 13(2):113–119
Tedder TF, Engel P (1994) CD20: a regulator of cell-cycle progression of B lymphocytes. Immunol Today 15(9):450–454
Tedder TF et al (1988) Isolation and structure of a cDNA encoding the B1 (CD20) cell-surface antigen of human B lymphocytes. Proc Natl Acad Sci U S A 85(1):208–212
Tejpar S et al (2007) Magnesium wasting associated with epidermal-growth-factor receptor-targeting antibodies in colorectal cancer: a prospective study. Lancet Oncol 8(5):387–394
Tejpar S, et al. 2016 Prognostic and predictive relevance of primary tumor location in patients with RAS wild-type metastatic colorectal Cancer: retrospective analyses of the CRYSTAL and FIRE-3 trials. JAMA Oncol. https://doi.org/10.1001/jamaoncol.2016.3797
Teplinsky E, Muggia F (2014) Targeting HER2 in ovarian and uterine cancers: challenges and future directions. Gynecol Oncol 135(2):364–370
Tesfa D, Palmblad J (2011) Late-onset neutropenia following rituximab therapy: incidence, clinical features and possible mechanisms. Expert Rev Hematol 4(6):619–625
Tesfa D et al (2011) Late-onset neutropenia following rituximab therapy in rheumatic diseases: association with B lymphocyte depletion and infections. Arthritis Rheum 63(8):2209–2214
Tobinai K et al (2017) A review of Obinutuzumab (GA101), a novel type II anti-CD20 monoclonal antibody, for the treatment of patients with B-cell malignancies. Adv Ther 34(2):324–356
Tuefferd M et al (2007) HER2 status in ovarian carcinomas: a multicenter GINECO study of 320 patients. PLoS One 2(11):e1138
Van Cutsem E et al (2011) Cetuximab plus irinotecan, fluorouracil, and leucovorin as first-line treatment for metastatic colorectal cancer: updated analysis of overall survival according to tumor KRAS and BRAF mutation status. J Clin Oncol 29(15):2011–2019
Van Cutsem E et al (2014) Metastatic colorectal cancer: ESMO clinical practice guidelines for diagnosis, treatment and follow-up. Ann Oncol 25 Suppl 3:iii1-9
Venook A, Niedzwiecki D, Innocenti F, Fruth B, Greene B, O'Neil BH, Shaw JE, Atkins JN, Horvath LE, Polite BN, Meyerhardt JA, O'Reilly EM, Goldberg RM, Hochster HS, Blanke CD, Schilsky RL, Mayer RJ, Bertagnolli MM, Lenz H-J (2016) Impact of primary (1°) tumor location on overall survival (OS) and progression-free survival (PFS) in patients (pts) with metastatic colorectal cancer (mCRC): analysis of CALGB/SWOG 80405 (Alliance). J Clin Oncol 34:3504
Verheul HM, Pinedo HM (2007) Possible molecular mechanisms involved in the toxicity of angiogenesis inhibition. Nat Rev Cancer 7(6):475–485
Vesely MD et al (2011) Natural innate and adaptive immunity to cancer. Annu Rev Immunol 29:235–271
Weber JS, Kahler KC, Hauschild A (2012) Management of immune-related adverse events and kinetics of response with ipilimumab. J Clin Oncol 30(21):2691–2697

Weber JS et al (2015) Toxicities of immunotherapy for the practitioner. J Clin Oncol 33(18):2092–2099
Weiss L et al (2017) Influence of body mass index on survival in indolent and mantle cell lymphomas: analysis of the StiL NHL1 trial. Ann Hematol 96(7):1155–1162
Weng WK et al (2010) Immunoglobulin G Fc receptor FcgammaRIIIa 158 V/F polymorphism correlates with rituximab-induced neutropenia after autologous transplantation in patients with non-Hodgkin's lymphoma. J Clin Oncol 28(2):279–284
Widakowich C et al (2007) Review: side effects of approved molecular targeted therapies in solid cancers. Oncologist 12(12):1443–1455
Wolchok JD et al (2009) Guidelines for the evaluation of immune therapy activity in solid tumors: immune-related response criteria. Clin Cancer Res 15(23):7412–7420
Wolchok JD et al (2010) Ipilimumab monotherapy in patients with pretreated advanced melanoma: a randomised, double-blind, multicentre, phase 2, dose-ranging study. Lancet Oncol 11(2):155–164
Wolchok JD et al (2013) Nivolumab plus ipilimumab in advanced melanoma. N Engl J Med 369(2):122–133
Wu J et al (2015) Blinatumomab: a bispecific T cell engager (BiTE) antibody against CD19/CD3 for refractory acute lymphoid leukemia. J Hematol Oncol 8:104
Yildirim M et al (2015) The role of gender in patients with diffuse large B cell lymphoma treated with rituximab-containing regimens: a meta-analysis. Arch Med Sci 11(4):708–714
Zhao YY et al (1998) Neuregulins promote survival and growth of cardiac myocytes. Persistence of ErbB2 and ErbB4 expression in neonatal and adult ventricular myocytes. J Biol Chem 273(17):10261–10269

24 Hematopoietic Growth Factors

Juan Jose Pérez-Ruixo

INTRODUCTION

Hematopoiesis is an intricate, well-regulated, and homeostatic multistep process that allows immature precursor cells in the bone marrow to proliferate, differentiate, mature, and become functional blood cells that transport oxygen and carbon dioxide; contribute to host immunity; and facilitate blood clotting. In the early 1900s, scientists recognized the presence of circulating factors that regulate hematopoiesis. It took approximately 50 years to develop in vitro cell culture systems in order to definitively prove that the growth and survival of early blood cells require the presence of specific circulating factors, called hematopoietic growth factors (HGF). The presence of many HGF with different targets at extremely small amounts in blood, bone marrow, and urine confounded the search for a single HGF with a specific activity. Scientific progress was slow until it became possible to purify sufficient quantities to evaluate the characteristics and biologic potential of the isolated materials. The introduction of recombinant DNA technology triggered a flurry of studies and an information explosion, which confirmed hematopoiesis is mediated by a series of HGF that acts individually and in various combinations involving complex feedback mechanisms. Today, many HGF have been isolated; some have been studied extensively, and a few have been manufactured for clinical use.

Different mature blood cells have been identified, each derived from primitive hematopoietic stem cells in the bone marrow. The most primitive pool of pluripotent stem cells comprises approximately 0.1% of the nucleated cells of the bone marrow, and 5% of these cells may be actively cycling at a given time. The stem cell pool maintains itself, seemingly without extensive depletion, by asymmetrical cell division. When a stem cell divides, one daughter cell remains in the stem cell pool and the other becomes a committed colony-forming unit (CFU). The CFU proliferates at a greater rate than the other stem cells and are more limited in self-renewal than pluripotent hematopoietic stem cells. Proliferation and differentiation are regulated by different mechanisms that necessarily involve HGF, which eventually convert the dividing cells into a population of terminally differentiated functional cells committed to the myeloid or the lymphoid pathway. Functional hematopoietic-derived blood cells from the myeloid pathway are red blood cells (erythrocytes), granulocytes (neutrophils, eosinophils, and basophils), monocytes and macrophages, tissue mast cells, and platelets (thrombocytes). Cells committed to the lymphoid pathway give rise to B- or T-lymphocytes and plasma cells.

Most HGF are glycosylated single-chain polypeptides encoded by a specific gene. Production of a recombinant HGF protein is accomplished by first identifying and isolating the particular HGF gene coding region, inserting the HGF DNA into a plasmid, and then expressing the recombinant growth factor protein in a biologic system (e.g., bacteria, yeast, or mammalian cells). The carbohydrate content of HGF varies by the particular protein and production method, which affects not only the molecular weight of the glycoprotein, but potentially the specific biologic activity and the circulating half-life as well. For these reasons why the recombinant copies of HGF proteins cannot be exactly identical to the original HGF protein, however, they might become biosimilars of the original HGF protein. An extensive review of the characteristics of the biosimilar products has been recentaly published (Schellekens et al. 2016). In addition, a summary of the HGF and their activities is provided in Table 24.1.

This chapter focus on reviewing the molecular structure, mechanism of action, pharmacokinetics and pharmacodynamics, clinical indications, and adverse events of HGF proteins stimulating erythropoiesis, granulopoiesis and thrombopoiesis. The common phar-

J. J. Pérez-Ruixo (✉)
Department of Clinical Pharmacology, Janssen Research & Development, Beerse, Belgium
e-mail: jjperezr@its.jnj.com

D. J. A. Crommelin et al. (eds.), *Pharmaceutical Biotechnology*, https://doi.org/10.1007/978-3-030-00710-2_24

Factor	Molecular weight (kDa)	Target cells	Actions
Erythropoietin (EPO)	34–39	Erythroid progenitors	Increase red blood cell counts
Granulocyte colony-stimulating factor (G-CSF)	18	Granulocyte progenitors and mature neutrophils	Increase neutrophil counts
Granulocyte-macrophage colony-stimulating factor (GM-CSF)	14–35	Granulocyte-macrophage progenitors and eosinophil progenitors	Increase neutrophil, eosinophil, and monocyte counts
Stem cell factor (SCF)	18	Granulocyte-erythroid progenitors, lymphoid progenitors, and natural killer cells	Increase pluripotent stem cells and progenitor cells for all other cell types
Thrombopoietin (TPO)	35	Stem cells, megakaryocytes, and erythroid progenitors	Increase platelet counts

Table 24.1 ■ Hematopoietic growth factors and their activities

macokinetic and pharmacodynamic features across the HGF are presented in detail for erythropoietin-stimulating agents (ESA), and then briefly discussed for other HGF. In this context, the existence of flip-flop pharmacokinetics justifying efficiency of the subcutaneous administration relative to the intravenous administration, as well as the concentration-dependent disposition mediated by its binding to the target receptor and the time-dependent pharmacokinetics, consequence of its pharmacodynamic action extending the receptor pool over time, are common features of the recombinant proteins targeting the receptors for erythropoietin, G-CSF and thrombopoietin.

ERYTHROPOIESIS-STIMULATING AGENTS

Erythropoietin (EPO) is a 30.4 kDa glycoprotein hormone secreted by the kidneys in response to tissue hypoxia, which stimulates red blood cell (RBC) production. EPO requires glycosylation to regulate erythrocyte production by activating the EPO receptor (EPOR) and stimulating the proliferation and differentiation of erythrocytic progenitors in the bone marrow, which leads to reticulocytosis, erythrocytosis and the increase of hemoglobin concentration in the blood. The gene that encodes EPO is located on chromosome 7. The cloning of the *EPO* gene in the early 1980s allowed for the development of recombinant erythropoietins and analogs (erythropoiesis-stimulating agents [ESAs]), offering an alternative to transfusion as a method of raising hemoglobin levels that has been successfully used for over 25 years to treat anemia in millions of anemic patients.

Epoetin alfa (Epogen®), the first commercial form of recombinant human erythropoietin (rHuEPO) marketed in the USA, EU, Japan, and China, and epoetin beta (Recormon®, NeoRecormon®), marketed outside of the USA, are both expressed in Chinese hamster ovary cells. Both have the same 165 amino acid sequence, which is identical to human EPO, and contain two disulfide bonds and three N-linked and one O-linked sialic acid-containing carbohydrate chains (Halstenson et al. 1991) and lead to the same biological effects as endogenous EPO (Egrie et al. 1986). No important differences in clinical efficacy are apparent between epoetin alfa and beta (Jelkmann 2000). Darbepoetin alfa (Aranesp®) is a hyperglycosylated erythropoietin analog with five amino acid changes and two additional N-linked carbohydrate chains, which has the same mechanism of action as EPO (Elliott et al. 2004a). However, darbepoetin alfa has a threefold increased serum half-life (Macdougall et al. 1999; Elliott et al. 2003; Sinclair and Elliott 2005) and increased in vivo potency (Egrie et al. 2003), allowing for more convenient modes of administration, including extended dosing intervals (Vansteenkiste et al. 2002; Nissenson et al. 2002) up to monthly dosing as described in the US label. It is marketed globally and is indicated to treat the anemia of patients with chronic kidney disease and chemotherapy-induced anemia in cancer patients.

A large methoxy polyethylene glycol (PEG) polymer chain was integrated into the epoetin beta molecule via amide bonds between either the N-terminal amino group or the ε-amino group of lysine by means of a succinimidyl butanoic acid linker (Macdougall 2005). The resulting pegylated epoetin beta molecule has been marketed as Mircera® to treat the anemia of patients with chronic kidney disease (CKD), but its clinical development as treatment for chemotherapy-induced anemia was stopped (Gascon et al. 2010). The pegylated epoetin beta stimulates erythropoiesis by binding to EPOR; however, the EPOR binding affinity is reduced (Jarsch et al. 2008). This biologic disadvantage is counterbalanced with an extended half-life in humans, which allows for extended dosing intervals in CKD patients (Chanu et al. 2010), similar to the dosing interval of darbepoetin.

Five rHuEPO biosimilars manufactured by two companies have been approved in the EU. Abseamed®, Binocrit® and Epoetin alfa HEXAL® all produced by Rentschler Biotechnologie GmbH, but marketed by three different companies, are epoetin alfa biosimilars of the reference product Eprex®. Comparable safety and efficacy between these three biosimilars and Eprex® was demonstrated in randomized controlled trials in hemodialysis patients with renal anemia. Although the EMA regulatory guidelines for rHuEPO biosimilars recommend that comparable efficacy and safety are demonstrated with two randomized trials in the nephrology setting, these biosimilars were approved based on a single nephrology trial. Two additional biosimilar versions of Eprex®, Retacrit® and Silapo® are manufactured by Norbitec GmbH, under the international nonproprietary name (INN) of epoetin zeta. The comparability of epoetin zeta to Eprex® was demonstrated in two randomized clinical trials, a correction phase study and a maintenance phase study, involving hemodialysis patients with renal anemia. In the correction phase study, the comparability between epoetin zeta and Eprex® over the evaluation period was demonstrated for mean hemoglobin levels, but not for mean dose. Similar results were reported in the maintenance phase study, suggesting a possible difference in the bioactivity of epoetin zeta and Eprex®. Data from studies in cancer patients receiving chemotherapy and treated with epoetin alfa biosimilars and epoetin zeta were also submitted for approval, but these studies were not adequately powered to demonstrate therapeutic equivalence to the reference product in this patient population. However, epoetin alfa biosimilars and epoetin zeta were approved in EU for indications in renal anemia, chemotherapy-induced anemia and for pre-donation of blood prior to surgery for autologous transfusion (Schellekens and Moors 2010). Retacrit® was approved in May 2018 in the US for the treatment of anemia caused by chronic kidney disease, chemotherapy or use of zidovudine in patients with HIV infection.

Regulation of Erythropoietin

The primary site of EPO synthesis in adults is the peritubular cells of the kidney (Jelkmann 2000; Jelkmann 1992). The liver is a secondary site of EPO production, with synthesis occurring in both hepatocytes and fibroblastoid interstitial cells (Spivak 1998). No preformed stores of EPO exist, and serum EPO concentrations are maintained at a constant concentration by homeostatic turnover, which consists of the basal production and elimination of the hormone (Fisher 2003). Within a healthy individual, the serum EPO concentration tends to be controlled tightly; however, large interindividual variability is evident from the normal range, 5–35 IU/L (Fisher 2003). Maintenance of normal serum concentrations of endogenous EPO requires the synthesis of about 2–3 IU/kg/day, or approx. 1000–1500 IU/week for a 70-kg man. Sex differences and regular-to-moderate athletic training do not appear to affect endogenous EPO serum concentrations. The blood flow in the kidney has a circadian rhythm in normal individuals; therefore, the endogenous production of EPO has diurnal variations with the highest levels in the evening and at night (Wide et al. 1989).

The overexpression of EPO occurs in a number of adaptive and pathologic conditions. In response to acute hypoxic stress, such as severe blood loss or severe anemia, EPO production rate can increase 100- to 1000-fold. Numerous studies have shown an exponential increase in serum EPO, with increasing degrees of anemia, although the maximal bone marrow response to such stimulation is only a four to sixfold increase in RBC production rate (Jelkmann 2000). Overproduction of EPO with accompanying erythrocytosis may be an adaptive response to conditions that produce chronic tissue hypoxia, such as living at high altitude, chronic respiratory diseases, cyanotic heart disease, sleep apnea, smoking, localized renal hypoxia, radiotherapy, or hemoglobinopathies with increased oxygen affinity. Paraneoplastic production of EPO from some tumors and cysts can also result in high serum concentrations of EPO. Following bone marrow ablation, aplastic anemia, or anemia in patients with hypoplastic marrows, serum EPO levels are disproportionately increased relative to slightly decreased hemoglobin levels. Conversely, individuals with hyperactive marrow owing to hemolytic anemia had disproportionately low serum EPO levels and rapid EPO serum disappearance.

In chronic kidney disease, up to 60% of patients have hemoglobin concentrations below 11 g/dL before beginning dialysis (Jungers et al. 2002). Multiple mechanisms contribute to the low hemoglobin levels (Fisher 2003), but the most important is the inability of the diseased kidneys to produce an appropriate EPO response for the given degree of anemia or an inability to meet the increased RBC demands of uremic patients (Adamson and Eschbach 1990). In addition, the uremic state itself appears to blunt the bone marrow response to EPO (Fisher 2003). It is of interest that serum EPO concentrations in chronically anemic dialysis patients increase to some extent in response to acute hypoxic stress (from either acute bleeding or systemic hypoxemia), suggesting that kidney failure does not result in a complete inability to produce EPO (Kato et al. 1994).

In cancer patients, anemia is of multifactorial etiology (Fisher 2003), and there are three distinct types of anemia: cancer-related anemia (nontreatment related), anemia related to myelosuppressive chemotherapy, and anemia related to other causes such as bleeding, nutritional deficiency, or iron deficiency, among others. As with other anemias of chronic disease, including those associated with chronic infection and inflammatory disorders, the anemia of cancer is characterized by a decreased production of endogenous EPO (Miller et al. 1990), cytokine-induced suppression of bone marrow function, disordered iron absorption and metabolism (Bron et al. 2001), and decreased erythrocyte survival. In the anemia related to chemotherapy treatment, the amount of endogenous EPO transiently increases up to sixfold within the 48 h after the administration of chemotherapy and returns to baseline within a week (Glaspy et al. 2005). After myeloablative chemotherapy, severe thrombocytopenia and bleeding might contribute to a significant loss of RBC. Finally, the anemias associated with infant prematurity, pregnancy, allogeneic bone marrow transplantation, and HIV infection are often characterized by inappropriately low EPO concentrations (Spivak 1998).

Pharmacokinetics

Absorption

After subcutaneous (s.c.) dosing of rHuEPO, its absorption is slow, leading to peak serum concentrations at 5–30 h and a longer terminal half-life (24–79 h) than that obtained after intravenous (i.v.) administration (McMahon et al. 1990). These results indicate the presence of flip-flop pharmacokinetics, where the rate of absorption is slower than the rate of elimination. Thus, the absorption process is the rate limiting process for its disposition, and the observed terminal half-life after s.c. dosing reflects the absorption rate rather than elimination rate.

Following s.c. administration, protein therapeutics, including the marketed recombinant HGF proteins, typically enter into the systemic circulation via the blood capillaries or the lymphatic system (Porter and Charman 2000; McLennan et al. 2006). The lymphatic system is considered to be the primary route of absorption from the s.c. injection site for protein therapeutics greater than 16 kD due to the restricted vascular access afforded by the continuous endothelial layer of blood capillaries (Supersaxo et al. 1990). In both healthy subjects and cancer patients, the fraction of dose absorbed via the lymphatics is about 80–90% and increases at doses higher than 300 IU/kg (Olsson-Gisleskog et al. 2007; Ait-Oudhia et al. 2011; Krzyzanski et al. 2005; Ramakrishnan et al. 2004). The s.c. absorption rates of rHuEPO vary according to the administration site, with a more rapid and extensive absorption when injected into the thigh compared with the abdomen or arm (Jensen et al. 1994). This relatively small difference is most likely reflecting regional differences in blood and lymph flow, and not considered to be clinically relevant as the pharmacodynamic profile (i.e., reticulocytes time course) did not evidence any difference across the site of administration. Small differences in the absorption due to the administration site has been also observed for other HGF, such as G-CSF and romiplostim, but they are of limited clinical relevance.

The s.c. absorption of darbepoetin alfa in humans is also slow, with peak concentrations reached at 34–58 h post-dose, followed by a generally monophasic decline. Similarly to rHuEPO, darbepoetin alfa also displays flip-flop pharmacokinetics, with a longer terminal half-life after s.c. dosing than after i.v. dosing (Agoram et al. 2007). The mean terminal half-life of darbepoetin alfa, 73 h, is associated with large variability between patients, consistent with the variability observed for other ESAs (Glaspy et al. 2005). The mean absorption time of darbepoetin alpha is 56 h, substantially longer than the mean absorption time reported for rHuEPO (Olsson-Gisleskog et al. 2007).

The reported 20–30% reduction in the darbepoetin alfa absorption rate per decade of age (Agoram et al. 2007) is consistent with the estimated effect of age on the rHuEPO absorption rate in healthy subjects (Olsson-Gisleskog et al. 2007) and cancer patients (Ait-Oudhia et al. 2011) and reflects the longer terminal half-life and the larger exposure to both drugs in older patients. It has been hypothesized (Agoram et al. 2007) that the age-dependent reduction in lymphatic flow rate could be the physiological reason behind this relationship, as it has also been reported for monoclonal antibodies administered by s.c. route (Sutjandra et al. 2011; Kakkar et al. 2011). The data available also suggest that the pharmacokinetic profile of rHuEPO and darbepoetin alfa after s.c. administration is similar in adults and children; however, s.c. absorption in children may be more rapid than in adults for both drugs (Heatherington 2003).

Bioavailability

Initial bioavailability estimates for rHuEPO after s.c. administration range from about 15 to 40% and are similar for epoetin alfa and beta (Deicher and Horl 2004). When the pharmacokinetics of s.c. rHuEPO and darbepoetin alfa were studied over a wider dose range in healthy volunteers and the rHuEPO nonlinear clearance was accounted for, exposure was found to increase more than proportional with dose (Olsson-Gisleskog et al. 2007; Agoram et al. 2007; Cheung et al. 1998, 2001). The s.c. bioavailability of darbepoetin alfa increases from 57 to 69% when the 200 μg dose is increased up to 400 μg, while the s.c. bioavailability of rHuEPO increases from 54 to 65% when the 40 kIU dose is increased up to 80 kIU. The apparent increase in s.c. bioavailability with dose of ESA might indicate saturable pre-systemic processes. Nevertheless, despite the apparent low bioavailability, s.c. administration of ESA has been reported to produce equivalent or better efficacy relative to i.v. administration, although there is a wide range of inter-patient variability (Kaufman et al. 1998). The flip-flop kinetics, together with the increase in absolute bioavailabitlity following s.c. dosing, results in a substantial increase in the efficiency of the ESA s.c. administration relative to i.v. administration. This phenomenon has been also reported for the G-CSF agonists (filgrastim, lenograstim and pegfilgrastim) as well as the c-Mpl agonist (romiplostim).

Distribution

During i.v. infusion, serum rHuEPO and darbepoetin alfa concentrations rise rapidly and then decline in a bi-exponential manner (Olsson-Gisleskog et al. 2007; Doshi et al. 2010). The peak serum rHuEPO and darbepoetin alfa concentrations correlate linearly with dose. A rHuEPO dose of 50 IU/kg produces concentrations of about 1000 mIU/mL 15 min after the end of the infusion, while a darbepoetin alfa dose of 0.75 μg/kg generates serum concentrations of about 10–20 ng/mL after the end of the infusion (Doshi et al. 2010). As expected from its large molecular weight, the volume of distribution of rHuEPO is similar to the plasma volume (40–60 mL/kg), suggesting confinement of rHuEPO within the plasma circulation (McMahon et al. 1990; Olsson-Gisleskog et al. 2007). The data available also suggest that the volume of distribution, normalized by body weight, in adults and children is similar after i.v. administration of rHuEPO and darbepoetin alfa. These results are also consistent with the findings observed for the G-CSF agonists (filgrastim, lenograstim and pegfilgrastim) as well as the c-Mpl agonist (romiplostim).

Elimination

Despite the long clinical experience with ESAs, the mechanism(s) of their clearance have not been fully elucidated, and there is a paucity of information regarding which organ(s) and tissue(s) are important in the metabolism of these drugs. Two ESA clearance pathways have been suggested to explain ESA elimination: (1) a capacity-limited clearance pathway utilizing EPO receptor-mediated endocytosis by erythroid progenitor cells and (2) a EPOR-independent linear clearance reflecting other mechanism(s). In vivo studies demonstrate that the kidney, liver, and lymph exert a negligible effect on in vivo EPOR-independent clearance. Clearly our understanding of the nature of the EPOR-independent clearance pathways is incomplete. However, it is important to recognize that renal excretion and hepatic metabolism of ESAs plays a minor role in their elimination and altered renal or hepatic function does not warrant dose adjustments. Notably, the presence of two clearance pathways also determines the elimination of the G-CSF agonists (filgrastim and lenograstim) as well as the c-Mpl agonist (romiplostim).

An investigation of the trafficking and degradation of rHuEPO by EPOR-expressing cells (BsF3) in cell culture found that rHuEPO was subjected to EPO receptor-mediated endocytosis followed by degradation in lysosomes (Gross and Lodish 2006). The rHuEPO receptor-binding, dissociation, and trafficking properties affected the relative rate of rHuEPO cellular uptake and intracellular degradation (Walrafen et al. 2005). About 57% of surface-bound rHuEPO was internalized ($k_{in} = 0.06\ min^{-1}$) and, after internalization, 60% of the ligand was recycled intact to the cell surface, while 40% was degraded. In spite of the in vitro results suggesting the role of EPOR on ESA clearance, the in vivo evidence is indirect and mostly arises from chemotherapy studies in patients treated with rHuEPO and darbepoetin alfa (Chapel et al. 2001). Chemotherapy-based approaches may also affect EPOR-independent clearance mechanisms, due to destruction of macrophages or neutrophils. The reduction in the number of these cells may explain, or at least contribute to, the decrease in ESA clearance observed after chemotherapy treatment.

Studies investigating the pharmacokinetics of rHuEPO analogs with different EPOR binding activity, suggested that EPOR-independent pathway plays a major role in the ESA clearance since decreasing the number of receptors with chemotherapy or, blocking the EPOR pathway with analogs without binding activity, were unable to completely shut down the elimination of rHuEPO. In addition, since pegylation has been shown to mainly affect the EPOR-independent clearance pathway, EPOR-mediated clearance may not be the dominant route of ESA elimination (Agoram et al. 2009).

It has been shown that carbohydrate side chains of EPO are necessary for persistence and in vivo biologic activity of the molecule, but not for in vitro receptor binding or stimulation of proliferation. Indeed rHuEPO molecules with increased sialic acid content have less affinity for the EPOR (Sinclair and Elliott 2005; Elliott et al. 2004b). Darbepoetin alfa is a hyperglycosylated analog of rHuEPO, with three to fivefold lower affinity for the EPOR compared to rHuEPO (Gross and Lodish 2006; Elliott et al. 2004b), but has three to fourfold longer serum half-life and greater in vivo activity than rHuEPO (Egrie et al. 2003). Surface-bound darbepoetin alfa was internalized at the same rate than rHuEPO, and after internalization, 60% of each ligand was re-secreted intact and 40% degraded (Gross and Lodish 2006). While in vitro experiments suggested that relative to rHuEPO, darbepoetin may have reduced clearance in vivo because of reduced EPOR-mediated endocytosis and degradation, darbepoetin alfa has other biophysical characteristics, such as increased molecular size and decreased isoelectric point, suggesting that the reduced clearance might be better explained by other mechanisms. In this context, studies investigating the pharmacokinetics of rHuEPO analogs with different EPOR binding activity suggest that hyperglycosylation mainly impacts the EPOR-independent clearance pathway, which also supports the hypothesis that EPOR-mediated clearance may not play a dominant role in ESA elimination (Agoram et al. 2009).

A population pharmacokinetic meta-analysis of rHuEPO in 533 healthy subjects enrolled in 16 clinical studies, where a wide range of i.v. and s.c. rHuEPO doses were administered, has helped in quantifying the two separate elimination pathways and understanding the influence of demographic characteristics and other covariates on the pharmacokinetic parameters of rHuEPO (Olsson-Gisleskog et al. 2007). At low concentrations, including the endogenous EPO concentrations observed at baseline or in ESA-untreated states, the nonlinear clearance operates at full capacity, giving a total clearance of about 0.9 L/h. As concentrations increase, the nonlinearity of pharmacokinetics becomes more important and, at the concentration of 394 IU/L, the clearance is 0.6 L/h. When the concentration are above 3546 IU/L, the nonlinear clearance of rHuEPO was fully (>90%) saturated and the total clearance decreased to almost one third, being mainly represented by the linear component. At concentrations higher than 3546 IU/L, rHuEPO pharmacokinetics is approximately linear. The concentration-dependent clearance appears to be independent of the type of rHuEPO (epoetin alfa vs. epoetin beta) or population (healthy subjects or patients with chronic renal failure).

A further indication of the possible involvement of EPOR binding in the disposition of rHuEPO can be found when investigating the rHuEPO pharmacokinetics after multiple dosing. A rHuEPO time-dependent clearance, with a 10–30% increase after several weeks of treatments with no subsequent changes (McMahon et al. 1990; Cheung et al. 1998; Yan et al. 2012) has been attributed to the limited number of EPOR located on the finite, but expandable, number of bone marrow erythroid progenitors. The pharmacodynamic action of rHuEPO increases BFU-E and CFU-E cell expansion and, consequently, the number of EPOR, which in turn results in an increase in rHuEPO clearance, a decrease in the apparent volume of distribution and a reduction in terminal half-life. The term pharmacodynamic-mediated drug disposition (PDMDD) has been coined to describe these types of TMDD models where pharmacodynamics affects the size of the target pool and influences the drug clearance, as has been described for ESAs. Consequently, the pharmacokinetics of rHuEPO is considered nonlinear because it is concentration dependent and nonstationary (time-dependent) (Yan et al. 2012).

The rHuEPO pharmacokinetic models for healthy subjects can be applied to patients with anemia due to renal insufficiency; however, it may have limited predictive value when applied to patients receiving chemotherapy. The consequences of the chemotherapy effect on the pharmacokinetics of rHuEPO in oncology patients are derived from the reduced number of EPOR available to clear rHuEPO in progenitor cells and the reduction of non-EPOR-mediated clearance (Olsson-Gisleskog et al. 2007). In cancer patients treated with chemotherapy, a correlation between the decline in the absolute reticulocyte count and the decrease in the clearance of rHuEPO over time has been observed (Ait-Oudhia et al. 2011). As a consequence, the rHuEPO elimination process becomes slower than the absorption process, and the flip-flop phenomenon observed in healthy subjects disappears when rHuEPO is given s.c. to cancer patients receiving chemotherapy (Olsson-Gisleskog et al. 2007; Ait-Oudhia et al. 2011). Furthermore, this phenomenon has clinical implications with respect to the synchronicity of ESA and chemotherapy administration, suggesting asynchronous dosing might be superior (Glaspy et al. 2005).

Pharmacodynamics

After rHuEPO is administered, it binds to the EPOR on the surface of the BFU-E, CFU-E, and proerythroblast and activates the signal transduction pathways. CFU-E cells have the highest EPOR density (1000 receptors per cell) and are the most sensitive to EPO. Experimental data suggest that approximately only 5–10% of EPOR must be continuously occupied with rHuEPO in order to prevent apoptosis and stimulate proliferation and differentiation of erythroid precursors. Then, CFU-Es will differentiate into normoblasts (including proerythroblast, basophilic erythroblast, polychromatophilic erythroblast, and orthochromatic erythroblast) and, upon normoblast denucleation, reticulocytes will be formed and reside in the bone marrow for 1 day before they are released into the bloodstream, where they circulate for about 1 day before maturing to erythrocytes. In healthy adults, the RBC life span is about 120 days and shows a relatively narrow distribution. The RBC life span is similar in cancer patients but markedly reduced in patients with chronic kidney disease, 60–65 days in dialysis patients and 82 days in nondialysis patients, with a moderate interindividual variability (Uehlinger et al. 1992; Chanu et al. 2010).

Previous studies have demonstrated that highly glycosylated rHuEPO has increased in vivo biological activity and serum half-life, but decreased receptor binding affinity (Egrie and Browne 2001). Given these relationships, a comparison of clearance among different ESAs has to be interpreted in conjunction with EPOR binding affinity and/or in vivo activity. Darbepoetin alfa stimulates erythropoiesis by the same mechanisms as those previously discussed for endogenous EPO and rHuEPO. In vitro, the affinity of darbepoetin alfa for the EPOR is one third to one fifth of the rHuEPO affinity (Gross and Lodish 2006); however, the increase in mean residence time of darbepoetin alfa results in a prolonged period above an erythropoietic threshold that more than compensates for the reduced receptor affinity, yielding an increased in vivo activity (Elliott et al. 2003; Egrie et al. 2003; Krzyzanski et al 2005).

Different mechanisms have been proposed to explain the pharmacodynamic tolerance of the rHuEPO effect. Besides the increase in rHuEPO clearance over time due to the increase in the number of EPOR, an oxygen-mediated feedback mechanism, erythroid precursor pool depletion, and iron-restricted erythropoiesis have been also proposed as tolerance mechanisms (Krzyzanski et al. 2005; Ramakrishnan et al. 2004). The oxygen feedback mechanism is regulated through an oxygen-sensing system: a high hemoglobin level leads to an increased oxygen level and eventually inhibits the production of endogenous EPO. Erythroid progenitor cells are EPO dependent; they cannot survive without EPO. On the other hand, extensive rHuEPO treatment results in anemia due to depletion of the erythroid precursor pool (Piron et al. 2001). This anemia is not due to low endogenous EPO levels but rather exhaustion of erythroid progenitors (Krzyzanski et al. 2005; Perez-Ruixo et al. 2009). Furthermore, iron-restricted erythropoiesis occurs in the presence of absolute iron deficiency, functional iron deficiency, and/or iron sequestration. Absolute iron deficiency is a common nutritional deficiency in women's health, pediatrics, and the elderly. Functional iron deficiency occurs in patients with significant EPO-mediated erythropoiesis or therapy with ESAs, even when storage iron is present. Iron sequestration, mediated by hepcidin, is an underappreciated but common cause of iron-restricted erythropoiesis in patients with chronic inflammatory disease. It has been shown that iron supplementation improves the hematopoietic response of ESAs used for chemotherapy-induced anemia. In multiple-dosing regimens, even though the endogenous EPO production might be suppressed, the total concentration of EPO is still high, and tolerance may occur due to precursor pool depletion and/or iron-restricted erythropoiesis. However, the oxygen feedback mechanism might be present, especially at the end of dosing intervals in regimens that extend longer than four rHuEPO half-lives.

■ Indications for Cancer Patients and Potential Adverse Events

Unless otherwise indicated, the information pertaining to ESA indications in cancer patients provided in this section is derived from the product prescribing information package inserts as well as the National Comprehensive Cancer Network for cancer- and chemotherapy-induced anemia. ESAs are indicated for the treatment of anemia due to the effects of concomitantly administered chemotherapy for a duration of ≥2 months in patients with metastatic, nonmyeloid malignancies. However, ESA treatment is not indicated for patients receiving hormonal agents, biologics, or radiotherapy, unless they are receiving concomitant myelosuppressive chemotherapy. Notably, ESA therapy should not be used to treat anemia associated with malignancy or anemia of cancer in patients with either solid or nonmyeloid hematological malignancies who are not receiving concurrent chemotherapy (Rizzo et al. 2008). Furthermore, ESA treatment is not indicated for patients receiving myelosuppressive therapy when the anticipated outcome is cure, due to the absence of studies that adequately characterize the impact of ESA therapy on progression-free and overall survival. ESA therapy is also not indicated for the treatment of anemia in cancer patients due to other factors such as absolute or functional iron deficiency, folate deficiencies, hemolysis, or gastrointestinal bleeding. ESA use in cancer patients has not been demonstrated in controlled clinical trials to improve symptoms of anemia, quality of life, fatigue, or patient well-being.

Depending on the clinical situation and the severity of anemia, red blood cell transfusion could be an alternative option to ESA therapy (Rizzo et al. 2008). Otherwise, a s.c. rHuEPO dose of 150 IU/kg three times in a week (TIW) or 40 kIU weekly (QW) is recommended to increase hemoglobin and decrease transfusions in patients with chemotherapy-associated anemia when the hemoglobin concentration is approaching, or has fallen below, 10 g/dL. Alternatively, s.c. rHuEPO dose of 80 kIU biweekly (Q2W) or 120 kIU every 3 weeks (Q3W) can be used as initial dosing because these two dosage schedules have not been found to have any differences in efficacy with respect to the approved TIW and QW dosing schedules. The dose of ESA therapy should be titrated for each patient to achieve and maintain the lowest hemoglobin level sufficient to avoid the need for blood transfusion. Therefore, the TIW s.c. dose of rHuEPO should be increased to 300 IU/kg if no reduction in transfusion requirements or rise in hemoglobin after 8 weeks of treatment has been observed. Similarly, the QW dose should increase to 60 kIU if no increase in hemoglobin by at least 1 g/dL after 4 weeks of treatment is observed. In addition, if hemoglobin exceeds 11 g/dL, but not 12 g/dL, the dose should be reduced by 25%. However, if hemoglobin exceeds 12 g/dL, therapy should be held until hemoglobin falls below 11 g/dL and then restarted at a 25% dose reduction. The pediatric dosing guidance is based on an initial i.v. dose of 600 IU/kg QW (maximum 40 kIU). If there is no increase in hemoglobin by at least 1 g/dL after 4 weeks of treatment (in the absence of RBC transfusion), the rHuEPO dose should be increased to 900 IU/kg (maximum 60 kIU) in order to maintain the lowest hemoglobin level sufficient to avoid RBC transfusion.

The recommended initial s.c. dose of darbepoetin alfa is 2.25 μg/kg QW or 500 μg once every 3 weeks (Q3W). The initial darbepoetin alfa s.c. dose of 2.25 μg/kg QW should be increased to 4.5 μg/kg QW if hemoglobin increase is less than 1 g/dL after 6 weeks of treatment. In addition, if hemoglobin increases by more than 1 g/dL in any 2-week period or when the hemoglobin reaches a level needed to avoid transfusion, the dose should be reduced by 40%. If hemoglobin exceeds a level needed to avoid transfusion, therapy should be held until hemoglobin approaches a level where transfusions may be required then restarted at a 40% dose reduction. A s.c. darbepoetin alfa dose of 100 μg QW, 200 μg Q2W, or 300 μg Q3W can be used as alternative initial dosing since differences in efficacy have not been found. If needed, these initial dose levels should be increased to 150–200 μg QW, 300 μg Q2W, or 500 μg Q3W, respectively. At this time the safety and efficacy of darbepoetin alfa in children receiving chemotherapy has not been established.

Although no specific serum rHuEPO level has been established which predicts which patients would be unlikely to respond to epoetin alfa therapy, treatment is not recommended for patients with grossly elevated serum rHuEPO levels (e.g., greater than 200 mUnits/mL). The hemoglobin should be monitored on a weekly basis in patients receiving ESA therapy until hemoglobin becomes stable and then at regular intervals thereafter.

Patients with multiple myeloma, especially those with renal failure, may benefit from adjunctive ESA therapy to treat anemia. Endogenous EPO levels should be monitored in order to assist in planning ESA therapy. No high-quality, published studies support the exclusive use of epoetin or darbepoetin in anemic myeloma, non-Hodgkin's lymphoma, or chronic lymphocytic leukemia in the absence of chemotherapy. Treatment with chemotherapy and/or corticosteroids should be initiated first. If a rise in hemoglobin does not result, treatment with epoetin or darbepoetin may begin in patients with particular caution exercised with chemotherapeutic agents and disease states where the risk of thromboembolism is increased. Blood transfusion is also an option (Rizzo et al. 2008). The current standard of care for symptomatic anemia in patients with myelodysplastic syndrome (MDS) is supportive care with RBC transfusion. Patients with serum EPO levels less than or equal to 500 IU/L, normal cytogenetics, and less than 15% marrow-ringed sideroblasts may respond to relatively high doses of rHuEPO (40–60 kIU s.c.TIW) or darbepoetin alfa (150–300 μg QW s.c.). Evidence supports the use of epoetin or darbepoetin in patients with anemia associated with low-risk myelodysplasia (Rizzo et al. 2008). Supportive care with RBC transfusion is the standard of care for symptomatic anemia in patients with hematologic malignancies (non-Hodgkin's lymphoma, chronic lymphocytic leukemia). There is insufficient data to recommend ESA therapy for patients responding to treatment with good prognosis and persistent transfusion-dependent anemia.

Iron supplementation improves the hematopoietic response of ESAs used for chemotherapy-induced anemia. A recent meta-analysis of randomized, controlled trials, comparing parenteral or oral iron and no iron, when added to ESAs in anemic cancer patients, evidenced that overall parenteral iron reduces the risk of transfusions by 23% and increases the chance of hematopoietic response by 29% when compared with ESAs alone. On the contrary, oral iron does not increase hematopoietic response or transfusion rate. The significance of these results is that the proportion of nonresponders to ESAs treated with parenteral iron will have strongly improved quality of life and cost ameliorated (Petrelli et al. 2012).

Several studies have reported a possible decreased survival rate in cancer patients receiving ESA for correction of anemia. Analyses of eight randomized studies in patients with cancer found a decrease in overall survival and/or locoregional disease control associated with ESA therapy for correction of anemia with an off-label target hemoglobin level greater than 12 g/dL. These results were confirmed in three recent meta-analyses (Bennett et al. 2008; Bohlius et al. 2009; Tonelli et al. 2009) and refuted in other two meta-analyses (Ludwig et al. 2009; Glaspy et al. 2010). There are also observational data and data from randomized studies that show no increase in mortality with ESA use according to prescribing label specifically in patients receiving chemotherapy. In addition, an increased risk for thromboembolic events has been reported with ESA therapy in cancer patients. Besides the intrinsic risk associated with the malignancy itself, the chemotherapy, and other concomitant factors, results from several meta-analyses established a significant association between the increased risk for thrombotic events and ESA use, with relative risk point estimates ranging from 1.48 to 1.69 (Bennett et al. 2008; Tonelli et al. 2009; Ludwig et al. 2009; Glaspy et al. 2010). The increased risk for mortality and thrombotic events in cancer patients receiving ESA therapy is specified in the black box warning included in the FDA label. Seizures and antibody-associated pure red cell aplasia (PRCA) have occurred in chronic renal failure patients receiving ESA therapy. While it is unclear whether cancer patients receiving ESA therapy are at risk of seizures and/or PRCA, ESA treatments should be closely monitored.

MYELOID HEMATOPOIETIC GROWTH FACTORS

■ Granulocyte Colony-Stimulating Factor (G-CSF)

The chemical properties of the myeloid hematopoietic growth factors, G-CSF and granulocyte-macrophage colony-stimulating factor (GM-CSF), have been characterized (Table 24.2) and extensively reviewed (Armitage 1998). The gene that encodes G-CSF is located on chromosome 17; the mature G-CSF polypeptide has 174 amino acids and is produced in monocytes, fibroblasts, endothelial cells, and bone marrow stromal cells. Filgrastim, a non-glycosylated r-metHuG-CSF, is marketed by several companies under various trade names throughout the world, and several filgrastim biosimilars have also been approved. Lenograstim, a glycosylated rHuG-CSF, is not marketed in the United States but is marketed in other countries under several trade names. Pegfilgrastim, a sustained-duration form of filgrastim to which a 20 kDa polyethylene glycol molecule is covalently bound to the N-terminal methionine residue, is marketed as Neulasta® in the European Union, the United States, and other countries, and several pegfilgrastim biosimilars are in development. Although not all indications are approved in every country, filgrastim, lenograstim, and pegfilgrastim are indicated for the prevention and treatment of chemotherapy-induced febrile neutropenia in cancer patients receiving chemotherapy, mobilization of stem cells for transplantation in oncology patients, and support of induction/consolidation chemotherapy for AML and hematopoiesis after bone marrow transplantation, among others (Aapro et al. 2011).

Filgrastim is primarily eliminated by glomerular filtration in the kidney and binding to the G-CSF receptor on the cell surface of neutrophils and neutrophil precursors, with subsequent internalization of the growth factor-receptor complexes via endocytosis and degradation inside the cells. Pegylation of filgrastim renders renal clearance insignificant, and neutrophil-mediated clearance becomes the predominant elimination pathway. After subcutaneous administration, both filgrastim and pegfilgrastim exhibits flip-flop phenomenon, justifying efficiency of the s.c. administration relative to the i.v. dosing, as well as nonlinear and nonstationary pharmacokinetics due to pharmacodynamic-mediated drug disposition. These findings were quantitatively characterized in a recent population pharmacokinetic and pharmacodynamic meta-analysis using data from 10 phase I-III clinical studies, conducted in 110 healthy adults, and 618 adult and 52 paediatric patients on chemotherapy, following administration of a wide range of i.v. and s.c. doses of filgrastim or pegfilgrastim (Melhem et al. 2018).

	G-CSF	GM-CSF
Nonproprietary name	Filgrastim, lenograstim, and pegfilgrastim	Molgramostim and sargramostim
Chromosome location	17	4
Amino acids	174[a]	127 or 128[b]
Glycosylation	*O*-linked (lenograstim)	*N*-linked (sargramostim)
Pegylation	Pegfilgrastim	None
Source of gene	Bladder carcinoma cell line (filgrastim, pegfilgrastim) and squamous carcinoma cell line (lenograstim)	Human monocyte cell line (molgramostim) and mouse T-lymphoma cell line (sargramostim)
Expression system	*E. coli* (bacteria): filgrastim and pegfilgrastim	*E. coli* (bacteria): molgramostim
	Chinese hamster ovary cell line (mammalian): lenograstim	*Saccharomyces cerevisiae* (yeast): sargramostim

[a]Native G-CSF has two forms, one with 177, which is less active than the other form with 174 amino acids; filgrastim has an N-terminal methionine

[b]Molgramostim has 128 amino acids; sargramostim 127

Table 24.2 ■ Characteristics of the marketed myeloid growth factors, rhG-CSF, and rhGM-CSF

Filgrastim and pegfilgrastim increases the proliferation and differentiation of neutrophils from committed progenitor cells, induces maturation, and enhances the survival and function of mature neutrophils, resulting in dose-dependent increases in neutrophils counts. Although similar dissociation constant for filgrastim and pegfilgrastim were found *in vitro*, a four-fold increase in the pegfilgrastim dissociation constant, relative to that from filgrastim, have been observed in human, which suggest pegfilgrastim had lower affinity for the G-CSF receptor than filgrastim. However, the longer half-life of pegfilgrastim, relative to filgrastim, counter balance the lower receptor affinity to the point that, in humans, the net stimulatory effects of pegfilgrastim were significantly greater than those of filgrastim. Actually, during chemotherapy-induced neutropenia, the clearance of pegfilgrastim is significantly reduced, and the concentration of pegfilgrastim is sustained until the onset of neutrophil recovery. Data from a pivotal study confirmed that a once-per-chemotherapy-cycle injection of pegfilgrastim at 6 mg was as safe and effective as 11 daily injections of filgrastim at 5 μg/kg in reducing neutropenia and its complications in patients with breast cancer receiving four cycles of doxorubicin/docetaxel chemotherapy (Green et al. 2003). Because of the highly efficient regulation of pegfilgrastim clearance via neutrophils and neutrophil precursors, a single fixed dose of pegfilgrastim can be given once per chemotherapy cycle in conjunction with a variety of myelosuppressive chemotherapy regimens (Yang and Kido 2011). Extensive clinical reviews on the myeloid growth factors have been published elsewhere (Keating 2011; Crawford et al. 2009).

Granulocyte-Macrophage Colony-Stimulating Factor (GM-CSF) and Stem Cell Factor (SCF)

The granulocyte-macrophage colony-stimulating factor (GM-CSF) is a polypeptide of 128 amino acids encoded by a gene located on chromosome 4, secreted by macrophages, T cells, mast cells, NK cells, endothelial cells, and fibroblasts. Molgramostim (marketed in the EU) and sargramostim (marketed in the USA) are two versions of rHuGM-CSF rarely used today. rHuGM-CSF is indicated for neutropenia associated with bone marrow transplantation and antiviral therapy for AIDS-related cytomegalovirus. rHuGM-CSF is also indicated for failed bone marrow transplantation or delayed engraftment and for use in mobilization and after transplantation of autologous PBPCs.

Similarly to G-CSF and GM-CSF, stem cell factor (SCF), encoded on chromosome 12, is a membrane-bound polypeptide of 248 amino acids that proteolytically release a soluble SCF containing 165 amino acids. SCF is an early-acting hematopoietic growth factor that stimulates the proliferation of primitive hematopoietic and non-hematopoietic cells. In vitro, SCF alone has minimal colony-stimulating activity on hematopoietic progenitor cells; however, it synergistically increases colony-forming or stimulatory activity of other HGF. Unlike most hematopoietic growth factors, SCF circulates in relatively high concentrations in normal human plasma. Ancestim® is a non-glycosylated version of the soluble r-metHuSCF marketed in Canada, Australia, and New Zealand and is rarely used in combination with G-CSF to increase the mobilization of peripheral blood progenitor cells (PBPC) for harvesting and support of autologous transplantation after myeloablative chemotherapy in patients with cancer. Comprehensive reviews of r-metHuSCF have been published (Langley 2004).

Megakaryocyte Hematopoietic Growth Factors

Megakaryocytopoiesis is a continuous developmental process of platelet production regulated by a complex network of HGF. In this process, hematopoietic stem cells undergo proliferation, differentiation, and maturation, generating megakaryocytes and platelets. Platelet production is controlled by signaling through the hematopoietic c-Mpl receptor. The ligand for this receptor, thrombopoietin (TPO) is the primary regulator of megakaryocyte development and subsequent platelet formation. TPO is a HGF encoded on chromosome 3 and produced in the liver and bone marrow stroma. Depending on the source, the mature polypeptide has between 305 and 355 amino acids, which may undergo cleavage to a smaller polypeptide that retains biologic activity. Upon binding to the c-Mpl receptor, TPO triggers several cellular signal transduction processes, which involve the FOLLOWING pathways: JAK-STAT and TYK2 tyrosine kinase, mitogen-activated protein kinase (MAPK), phosphatidylinositol 3-kinase (PI3K), and nuclear factor kappa B (NF-κB).

Early recombinant forms of TPO, rHu-TPO and the pegylated megakaryocyte growth and development factor (Peg-MGDF), showed promising results in clinical trials. However, later studies failed to meet their clinical endpoints, because the recombinant proteins generated antibodies that cross-reacted with c-Mpl ligands and resulted in paradoxical thrombocytopenia (Li et al. 2001). Further clinical development of these molecules was therefore suspended. An extensive compilation of the biology of rHu-TPO and Peg-MGDF has been published elsewhere (Kuter et al. 1997).

Romiplostim (Nplate®), previously known as AMG 531, is a novel biological thrombopoiesis-stimulating agent that was developed to overcome the problem of cross-reacting autoantibodies by use of a peptide sequence with no homology to endogenous TPO to activate the c-Mpl receptor. Structurally, romiplostim is a 59 kDa fusion protein that consists of two identical subunits, each containing a human IgG_1 Fc domain covalently linked at the C-terminus to a peptide consisting of two c-Mpl binding domains. The four copies of the TPO mimetic peptide stimulate megakaryocytopoiesis by binding the TPO receptor, yet because they bear no sequence homology with TPO, there is a reduced potential for the generation of anti-TPO antibodies. In vitro, romiplostim competes with TPO for binding to the c-Mpl receptor on normal platelets and Mpl-transfected cells (BaF3-Mpl cells). Upon binding to the c-Mpl receptor, romiplostim activates the Janus kinase/signal transducers and activators of transcription (JAK-STAT) and other pathways in the same way as endogenous TPO (Broudy and Lin 2004). When cocultured with murine bone marrow cells, romiplostim promotes the growth of CFU-megakaryocytes and promotes the proliferation as well as the maturation of megakaryocytes. During preclinical development, romiplostim led to robust dose-dependent platelet responses in mice, rats, rabbits, and monkeys. The pharmacokinetics and pharmacodynamics of romiplostim in animals, healthy subjects, and patients with immune thrombocytopenia purpura (ITP) have been extensively investigated during clinical development (Wang et al. 2010, 2011; Yan and Krzyzanski 2013; Perez-Ruixo et al. 2012). Similar to erythropoietin stimulating agents and G-CSF analogs, romiplostim exhibits flip-flop phenomenon after s.c. administration, justifying efficiency of the s.c. route relative to the i.v. dosing, as well as nonlinear and nonstationary pharmacokinetics due to pharmacodynamic-mediated drug disposition (Wang et al. 2010). Similar to rHu-EPO, clinical data suggest that approximately only 20–30% of c-Mpl receptors must be occupied with thrombopoietin receptor agonist in order to have 50% of the maximal effect in stimulating the proliferation and differentiation of precursors cells (Wang et al. 2010, Samtani et al. 2009).

Currently, romiplostim has been approved in the USA and the EU and is indicated for the treatment of thrombocytopenia in patients with chronic immune thrombocytopenia (ITP) who have had an insufficient response to corticosteroids, immunoglobulins, or splenectomy (Bussel et al. 2006). An extensive review of the use of romiplostim in ITP patients has been published (Keating 2012). At this time, romiplostim or other protein-based c-Mpl ligands are not approved for clinical use in cancer patients; however, clinical trial data in oncology patients have been recently reported (Kantarjian et al. 2010a, b).

SELF-ASSESSMENT QUESTIONS

Questions

1. What do hematopoietic factors do?
2. What are the major lineages or types of mature blood cells?
3. In general, describe chemically the hematopoietic growth factors.
4. How do hematopoietic growth factors function?
5. What are the in vivo actions of rhG-CSF and rhGM-CSF in patients with advanced cancer?
6. What is the physiologic role of EPO?
7. What are the currently commercially available hematopoietic growth factors?
8. What are the indications for rhG-CSF?
9. What are the indications for rhEPO?
10. What is the indication for romiplostim?
11. What are the relevant and common pharmacokinetic and pharmacodynamic properties of the HGF?

Answers

1. Hematopoietic growth factors regulate both hematopoiesis and the functional activity of blood cells (including proliferation, differentiation, and maturation). Some hematopoietic growth factors mobilize progenitor cells to move from the bone marrow to the peripheral blood.
2. The myeloid pathway gives rise to red blood cells (erythrocytes), platelets, monocytes/macrophages, and granulocytes (neutrophils, eosinophils, and basophils). The lymphoid pathway gives rise to lymphocytes.
3. They are glycoproteins, which can be distinguished by their amino acid sequence and glycosylation (carbohydrate linkages). Hematopoietic growth factors have folding patterns that are dictated by physical interactions and covalent cysteine-cysteine disulfide bridges. Correct folding is necessary for biologic activity. Most hematopoietic growth factors are single-chain polypeptides weighing approximately 14–35 kDa. The carbohydrate content varies depending on the growth factor and production method, which in turn affects the molecular weight but not necessarily the biologic activity.
4. HGF act by binding to specific cell surface receptors. The resultant complex sends a signal to the cell to express genes, which in turn induce cellular proliferation, differentiation, or activation. A hematopoietic growth factor may also act indirectly if the cell expresses a gene that causes the production of a different hematopoietic growth factor or another cytokine, which in turn binds to and stimulates a different cell.
5. Both HGF cause a transient leucopenia that is followed by a dose-dependent increase in the number of circulating mature and immature neutrophils. Both HGF enhance the in vitro function of neutrophils obtained from treated patients. rhGM-CSF, but not rhG-CSF, also increases the number of circulating monocytes/macrophages and eosinophils, as well as in vitro monocyte cytotoxicity and cytokine production.
6. EPO maintains a normal red blood cell count by causing committed erythroid progenitor cells to proliferate and differentiate into normoblasts.

EPO also shifts marrow reticulocytes into circulation.

7. Besides the biosimilars, five HGF are commercially available, rhG-CSF (filgrastim, lenograstim, pegfilgrastim), rhGM-CSF (molgramostim and sargramostim), rhEPO (epoetin alfa, epoetin beta, darbepoetin alfa), rhSCF (ancestim), and rhIL-11 (oprelvekin).
8. Approval for marketing varies by country and not all countries have all labeled uses. rhG-CSF is indicated for neutropenia associated with myelosuppressive cancer chemotherapy, bone marrow transplantation, and severe chronic neutropenia; rhG-CSF is also indicated to mobilize peripheral blood progenitor cells (PBPC) for PBPC transplantation; and rhG-CSF is indicated for the reversal of clinically significant neutropenia and subsequent maintenance or adequate neutrophil counts in patients with HIV infection during treatment with antiviral and/or other myelosuppressive medications.
9. rhEPO is indicated to treat anemia associated with chronic renal failure, zidovudine-induced anemia in HIV-infected patients, and chemotherapy-induced anemia. rhEPO is also indicated to reduce allogeneic blood transfusions and hasten erythroid recovery in surgery patients.
10. Romiplostim is indicated for the treatment of thrombocytopenia in patients with chronic immune thrombocytopenia (ITP) who have had an insufficient response to corticosteroids, immunoglobulins, or splenectomy.
11. There are two main characteristics that are common to erythropoietin stimulating agents, G-CSF analogs and thrombopoietin receptor agonist. The first one is the presence of the flip-flop pharmacokinetics that justifies the efficiency of the s.c. administration relative to the i.v. dosing. The second is the nonlinear (concentration-dependent) and nonstationary pharmacokinetics due to pharmacodynamic-mediated drug disposition, which justify the dose approved since they achieve the level of receptor coverage needed to achieve clinically relevant endpoints.

Acknowledgements Parts of this chapter are updated versions of previously published portions of several other chapters and/or review manuscripts, that include:

1. Heatherington AC (2003) Clinical pharmacokinetic properties of rHuEPO: a review. In: Molineux G, Foote MA, Elliott S (eds) Erythropoietins and erythropoiesis: molecular, cellular, preclinical, and clinical biology. Birkhauser, Basel, pp 87–112
2. Elliot S, Heatherington AC, Foote MA (2004) Erythropoietic factors: clinical pharmacology and pharmacokinetics. In: Morstyn G, Foote MA, and Lieschke GJ (eds) Hematopoietic growths factors in oncology. Humana Press, Totowa, pp 97–123
3. Foote AN (2008) Hematopoietic growth factors. In: Crommelin DJA, Sindelar RD, Meibohm B (eds) Pharmaceutical biotechnology. Fundamentals and applications, 3rd edn. Informa Healthcare USA, New York, pp 225–242
4. Doshi S, Perez-Ruixo JJ, Jang GR, Chow A, Elliot S (2008) Pharmacocinétique de les agents stimulant l'érythropoïèse. In: Rossert J, Casadevall N, Gisselbrecht C (eds) Les agents stimulant l'érythropoïèse. Paris, France
5. Doshi S, Perez-Ruixo JJ, Jang GR, Chow AT (2009) Pharmacokinetics of erythropoiesis-stimulating agents. In: Molineux G, Foote MA, Elliott S (eds) Erythropoietins and erythropoiesis: molecular, cellular, preclinical, and clinical biology. 2nd edn. Birkhäuser Verlag AG, Basel, pp 195–224.
6. Doshi S, Krzyzanski W, Yue S, Elliott S, Chow A, Pérez-Ruixo JJ. Clinical pharmacokinetics and pharmacodynamics of erythropoiesis-stimulating agents. Clin Pharmacokinet. 2013 Dec;52(12):1063-83.

REFERENCES

Aapro MS, Bohlius J, Cameron DA et al (2011) 2010 update of EORTC guidelines for the use of granulocyte-colony stimulating factor to reduce the incidence of chemotherapy-induced febrile neutropenia in adult patients with lymphoproliferative disorders and solid tumours. Eur J Cancer 47:8–32

Adamson JW, Eschbach JW (1990) Treatment of the anemia of chronic renal failure with recombinant human erythropoietin. Annu Rev Med 41:349–360

Agoram B, Sutjandra L, Sullivan JT (2007) Population pharmacokinetics of darbepoetin alfa in healthy subjects. Br J Clin Pharmacol 63:41–52

Agoram B, Aoki K, Doshi S et al (2009) Investigation of the effects of altered receptor binding activity on the clearance of erythropoiesis-stimulating proteins: nonerythropoietin receptor-mediated pathways may play a major role. J Pharm Sci 98:2198–2211

Ait-Oudhia S, Vermeulen A, Krzyzanski W (2011) Non-linear mixed effect modeling of the time-variant disposition of erythropoietin in anemic cancer patients. Biopharm Drug Dispos 32:1–15

Armitage JO (1998) Emerging applications of recombinant human granulocyte colony-stimulating factor. Blood 92:4491–4508

Bennett CL, Silver SM, Djulbegovic B et al (2008) Venous thromboembolism and mortality associated with recombinant erythropoietin and darbepoetin administration for the treatment of cancer-associated anemia. JAMA 299:914–924

Bohlius J, Schmidlin K, Brillant C et al (2009) Recombinant human erythropoiesis-stimulating agents and mortality in patients with cancer: a meta-analysis of randomised trials. Lancet 373:1532–1542

Bron D, Meuleman N, Mascaux C (2001) Biological basis of anemia. Semin Oncol 28:1–6

Broudy VC, Lin NL (2004) AMG531 stimulates megakaryopoiesis in vitro by binding to Mpl. Cytokine 25:52–60

Bussel JB, Kuter DJ, George JN et al (2006) AMG 531, a thrombopoiesis-stimulating protein, for chronic ITP. N Engl J Med 355:1672–1681

Chanu P, Gieschke R, Charoin JE, Pannier A, Reigner B (2010) Population pharmacokinetic – pharmacodynamic model for a C.E.R.A. in both ESA-naive and ESA-treated chronic kidney disease patients with renal anemia. J Clin Pharmacol 50:507–520

Chapel S, Veng-Pedersen P, Hohl RJ, Schmidt RL, McGuire EM, Widness JA (2001) Changes in erythropoietin pharmacokinetics following busulfan-induced bone marrow ablation in sheep: evidence for bone marrow as a major erythropoietin elimination pathway. J Pharmacol Exp Ther 298:820–824

Cheung WK, Goon BL, Guilfoyle MC, Wacholtz MC (1998) Pharmacokinetics and pharmacodynamics of recombinant human erythropoietin after single and multiple subcutaneous doses to healthy subjects. Clin Pharmacol Ther 64:412–423

Cheung WK, Minton N, Gunawardena K (2001) Pharmacokinetics and pharmacodynamics of epoetin alfa once weekly and three times weekly. Eur J Clin Pharmacol 57:411–418

Crawford J, Armitage J, Balducci L et al (2009) Myeloid growth factors. J Natl Compr Cancer Netw 7:64–83

Deicher R, Horl WH (2004) Differentiating factors between erythropoiesis-stimulating agents: a guide to selection for anemia of chronic kidney disease. Drugs 64:499–509

Doshi S, Chow A, Pérez Ruixo JJ (2010) Exposure-response modeling of darbepoetin alfa in anemic patients with chronic kidney disease not receiving dialysis. J Clin Pharmacol 50(9 Suppl):75S–90S

Egrie JC, Browne JK (2001) Development and characterization of novel erythropoiesis stimulating protein (NESP). Br J Cancer 84(Suppl 1):3–10

Egrie JC, Strickland TW, Lane J et al (1986) Characterization and biological effects of recombinant human erythropoietin. Immunobiology 72:213–224

Egrie JC, Dwyer E, Browne JK, Hitz A, Lykos MA (2003) Darbepoetin alfa has a longer circulating half-life and greater in vivo potency than recombinant human erythropoietin. Exp Hematol 31:290–299

Elliott S, Lorenzini T, Asher S et al (2003) Enhancement of therapeutic protein in vivo activities through glycoengineering. Nat Biotechnol 21:414–421

Elliott S, Heatherington AC, Foote MA (2004a) Erythropoietic factors. In: Morstyn G, Foote MA, Lieschke GJ (eds) Hematopoietic growth factors in oncology: basic science and clinical therapeutics. Humana Press Inc, Totowa, pp 97–123

Elliott S, Egrie J, Browne J et al (2004b) Control of rHuEPO biological activity: the role of carbohydrate. Exp Hematol 32:1146–1155

Fisher JW (2003) Erythropoietin: physiology and pharmacology update. Exp Biol Med 228:1–14

Gascon P, Pirker R, Del Mastro L, Durrwell L (2010) Effects of CERA (continuous erythropoietin receptor activator) in patients with advanced non-small-cell lung cancer (NSCLC) receiving chemotherapy: results of a phase II study. Ann Oncol 21:2029–2039

Glaspy J, Henry D, Patel R et al (2005) The effects of chemotherapy on endogenous erythropoietin levels and the pharmacokinetics and erythropoietic response of darbepoetin alfa: a randomised clinical trial of synchronous versus asynchronous dosing of darbepoetin alfa. Eur J Cancer 41:1140–1149

Glaspy J, Crawford J, Vansteenkiste J et al (2010) Erythropoiesis stimulating agents in oncology: a study-level meta-analysis of survival and other safety outcomes. Br J Cancer 102:301–315

Green MD, Koelbl H, Baselga J et al (2003) A randomized double-blind multicenter phase III study of fixed-dose single-administration pegfilgrastim versus daily filgrastim in patients receiving myelosuppressive chemotherapy. Ann Oncol 14:29–35

Gross AW, Lodish HF (2006) Cellular trafficking and degradation of erythropoietin and novel erythropoiesis stimulating protein (NESP). J Biol Chem 281:2024–2032

Halstenson CE, Macres M, Katz SA et al (1991) Comparative pharmacokinetics and pharmacodynamics of epoetin alfa and epoetin beta. Clin Pharmacol Ther 50:702–712

Heatherington AC (2003) Clinical pharmacokinetic properties of rHuEPO: a review. In: Molineux G, Foote MA, Elliott S (eds) Erythropoietins and erythropoiesis: molecular, cellular, preclinical, and clinical biology. Birkhauser, Basel, pp 87–112

Jarsch M, Brandt M, Lanzendörfer M, Haselbeck A (2008) Comparative erythropoietin receptor binding kinetics of C.E.R.A. and epoetin-beta determined by surface plasmon resonance and competition binding assay. Pharmacology 81:63–69

Jelkmann W (1992) Erythropoietin: structure, control of production, and function. Physiol Rev 72:449–489

Jelkmann W (2000) Use of recombinant human erythropoietin as an antianemic and performance enhancing drug. Curr Pharm Biotechnol 1:11–31

Jensen JD, Jensen LW, Madsen JK (1994) The pharmacokinetics of recombinant human erythropoietin after subcutaneous injection at different sites. Eur J Clin Pharmacol 46:333–337

Jungers PY, Robino C, Choukroun G, Nguyen-Khoa T, Massy ZA, Jungers P (2002) Incidence of anaemia, and use of Epoetin therapy in pre-dialysis patients: a prospective study in 403 patients. Nephrol Dial Transplant 17:1621–1627

Kakkar T, Sung C, Gibiansky L et al (2011) Population PK and IgE pharmacodynamic analysis of a fully human monoclonal antibody against IL4 receptor. Pharm Res 28:2530–2542

Kantarjian H, Fenaux P, Sekeres MA et al (2010a) Safety and efficacy of romiplostim in patients with lower-risk myelodysplastic syndrome and thrombocytopenia. J Clin Oncol 28:437–444

Kantarjian HM, Giles FJ, Greenberg PL et al (2010b) Phase 2 study of romiplostim in patients with low- or intermediate-risk myelodysplastic syndrome receiving azacitidine therapy. Blood 116:3163–3170

Kato A, Hishida A, Kumagai H, Furuya R, Nakajima T, Honda N (1994) Erythropoietin production in patients with chronic renal failure. Ren Fail 16:645–651

Kaufman JS, Reda DJ, Fye CL et al (1998) Subcutaneous compared with intravenous epoetin in patients receiving hemodialysis. Department of Veterans Affairs Cooperative Study Group on erythropoietin in hemodialysis patients. N Engl J Med 339:578–583

Keating GM (2011) Lenograstim: a review of its use in chemotherapy-induced neutropenia, for acceleration of neutrophil recovery following haematopoietic stem cell transplantation and in peripheral blood stem cell mobilization. Drugs 71:679–707

Keating GM (2012) Romiplostim. Drugs 72:415–435

Krzyzanski W, Jusko WJ, Wacholtz MC, Minton N, Cheung WK (2005) Pharmacokinetic and pharmacodynamic modeling of recombinant human erythropoietin after multiple subcutaneous doses in healthy subjects. Eur J Pharm Sci 26:295–306

Kuter DJ, Hunt P, Sheridan W, Zucker-Franklin D (eds) (1997) Thrombopoiesis and thrombopoeitin. Humana Press Inc, Totowa, p 412

Langley KE (2004) Stem cell factor and its receptor, c-Kit. In: Morstyn G, Foote MA, Lieschke GJ (eds) Hematopoietic growth factors in oncology. Humana Press Inc, Totowa, pp 153–184

Li J, Yang C, Xia Y et al (2001) Thrombocytopenia caused by the development of antibodies to thrombopoietin. Blood 98:3241–3248

Ludwig H, Crawford J, Osterborg A et al (2009) Pooled analysis of individual patient-level data from all randomized, double-blind, placebo controlled trials of darbepoetin alfa in the treatment of patients with chemotherapy-induced anemia. J Clin Oncol 27:2838–2847

Macdougall IC (2005) CERA (continuous erythropoietin receptor activator): a new erythropoiesis-stimulating agent for the treatment of anemia. Curr Hematol Rep 4:436–440

Macdougall IC, Gray SJ, Elston O et al (1999) Pharmacokinetics of novel erythropoiesis stimulating protein compared with epoetin alfa in dialysis patients. J Am Soc Nephrol 10:2392–2395

McLennan DN, Porter CJ, Edwards GA, Heatherington AC, Martin SW, Charman SA (2006) The absorption of darbepoetin alfa occurs predominantly via the lymphatics following subcutaneous administration to sheep. Pharm Res 23:2060–2066

McMahon FG, Vargas R, Ryan M et al (1990) Pharmacokinetics and effects of recombinant human erythropoietin after intravenous and subcutaneous injections in healthy volunteers. Blood 76:1718–1722

Melhem M, Delor I, Pérez-Ruixo JJ et al (2018) Pharmacokinetic-pharmacodynamic modelling of neutrophil response to G-CSF in healthy subjects and patients with chemotherapy-induced neutropenia. Br J Clin Pharmacol 84:911–925

Miller CB, Jones RJ, Piantadosi S, Abeloff MD, Spivak JL (1990) Decreased erythropoietin response in patients with the anemia of cancer. N Engl J Med 322:1689–1692

Nissenson AR, Swan SK, Lindberg JS et al (2002) Randomized, controlled trial of darbepoetin alfa for the treatment of anemia in hemodialysis patients. Am J Kidney Dis 40:110–118

Olsson-Gisleskog P, Jacqmin P, Perez-Ruixo JJ (2007) Population pharmacokinetics meta-analysis of recombinant human erythropoietin in healthy subjects. Clin Pharmacokinet 46:159–173

Perez-Ruixo JJ, Krzyzanski W, Bouman-Thio E et al (2009) Pharmacokinetics and pharmacodynamics of the erythropoietin mimetibody construct CNTO 528 in healthy subjects. Clin Pharmacokinet 48:601–613

Perez-Ruixo JJ, Green B, Doshi S, Wang YM, Mould DR (2012) Romiplostim dose-response in patients with immune thrombocytopenia. J Clin Pharmacol 52:1540–1551

Petrelli F, Borgonovo K, Cabiddu M, Lonati V, Barni S (2012) Addition of iron to erythropoiesis-stimulating agents in cancer patients: a meta-analysis of randomized trials. J Cancer Res Clin Oncol 138:179–187

Piron M, Loo M, Gothot A, Tassin F, Fillet G, Beguin Y (2001) Cessation of intensive treatment with recombinant human erythropoietin is followed by secondary anemia. Blood 97:442–448

Porter CJ, Charman SA (2000) Lymphatic transport of proteins after subcutaneous administration. J Pharm Sci 89:297–310

Ramakrishnan R, Cheung WK, Wacholtz MC, Minton N, Jusko WJ (2004) Pharmacokinetic and pharmacodynamic modeling of recombinant human erythropoietin after single and multiple doses in healthy volunteers. J Clin Pharmacol 44:991–1002

Rizzo JD, Somerfield MR, Hagerty KL et al (2008) Use of epoetin and darbepoetin in patients with cancer: 2007 American Society of Clinical Oncology/American Society of Hematology clinical practice guideline update. J Clin Oncol 26:132–149

Samtani MN, Perez-Ruixo JJ, Brown KH et al (2009) Pharmacokinetic and pharmacodynamic modeling of pegylated thrombopoietin mimetic peptide (PEG-TPOm) after single intravenous dose administration in healthy subjects. J Clin Pharmacol 49:336–350

Schellekens H, Moors E (2010) Clinical comparability and European biosimilar regulations. Nat Biotechnol 28:28–31

Schellekens H, Smolen JS, Dicato M, Rifkin RM (2016) Safety and efficacy of biosimilars in oncology. Lancet Oncol 17:e502–e509

Sinclair AM, Elliott S (2005) Glycoengineering: the effect of glycosylation on the properties of therapeutic proteins. J Pharm Sci 94:1626–1635

Spivak JL (1998) The biology and clinical applications of recombinant erythropoietin. Semin Oncol 25(3 suppl 7):7–11

Supersaxo A, Hein WR, Steffen H (1990) Effect of molecular weight on the lymphatic absorption of water-soluble compounds following subcutaneous administration. Pharm Res 7:167–169

Sutjandra L, Rodriguez RD, Doshi S et al (2011) Population pharmacokinetic meta-analysis of denosumab in healthy subjects and postmenopausal women with osteopenia or osteoporosis. Clin Pharmacokinet 50:793–807

Tonelli M, Hemmelgarn B, Reiman T et al (2009) Benefits and harms of erythropoiesis-stimulating agents for anemia related to cancer: a meta-analysis. CMAJ 180:E62–E71

Uehlinger DE, Goth FA, Sheiner LB (1992) A pharmacodynamic model of erythropoietin therapy for uremic anemia. Clin Pharmacol Ther 51:76–89

Vansteenkiste J, Pirker R, Massuti B et al (2002) Double-blind, placebo-controlled, randomized phase III trial of darbepoetin alfa in lung cancer patients receiving chemotherapy. J Natl Cancer Inst 94:1211–1220

Walrafen P, Verdier F, Kadri Z, Chrétien S, Lacombe C, Mayeux P (2005) Both proteasomes and lysosomes degrade the activated erythropoietin receptor. Blood 105:600–608

Wang YM, Krzyzanski W, Doshi S, Xiao JJ, Pérez-Ruixo JJ, Chow AT (2010) Pharmacodynamics-mediated drug disposition (PDMDD) and precursor pool lifespan model for single dose of romiplostim in healthy subjects. AAPS J 12:729–740

Wang YM, Sloey B, Wong T, Khandelwal P, Melara R, Sun YN (2011) Investigation of the pharmacokinetics of romiplostim in rodents with a focus on the clearance mechanism. Pharm Res 28:1931–1938

Wide L, Bengtsson C, Birgegard G (1989) Circadian rhythm of erythropoietin in human serum. Br J Haematol 72:85–90

Yan X, Lowe PJ, Fink M, Berghout A, Balser S, Krzyzanski W (2012) Population pharmacokinetic and pharmacodynamic model-based comparability assessment of a recombinant human epoetin alfa and the biosimilar HX575. J Clin Pharmacol 52:1624–1644

Yan X, Krzyzanski W (2013) Quantitative assessment of minimal effective concentration of erythropoiesis-stimulating agents. CPT Pharmacometrics Syst Pharmacol 2:e62. https://doi.org/10.1038/psp.2013.39

Yang BB, Kido A (2011) Pharmacokinetics and pharmacodynamics of pegfilgrastim. Clin Pharmacokinet 50:295–306

25

Monoclonal Antibodies in Solid Organ Transplantation

Nicole A. Pilch, Holly B. Meadows, and Rita R. Alloway

INTRODUCTION

Administration of targeted immunosuppression, in the form of genetically engineered antibodies, is commonplace in solid organ transplantation. Polyclonal antibodies, such as rabbit antithymocyte globulin, offer global immunosuppression by targeting several cell surface antigens on B and T lymphocytes. However, secondary to their broad therapeutic targets, they are associated with infection, infusion-related reactions, inter-batch variability, and posttransplant malignancies. Nevertheless, polyclonal antibodies are still commonly administered for induction and treatment of allograft rejection and offer an important role in current solid organ transplantation, which is beyond the scope of this chapter.

In an attempt to target solid organ transplant immunosuppression, monoclonal antibodies directed against key steps in specific immunologic pathways were introduced. The first agent, muromonab-CD3 (OKT3), was initially introduced in the early 1980s for the treatment of allograft rejection (Morris 2004). The use of monoclonal antibodies has evolved and expanded over the past two decades and today monoclonal antibodies are routinely included as part of the overall immunosuppression regimen. Both the innate and adaptive immune systems have multiple components and signal transduction pathways aimed at protecting the host from a foreign body, such as transplanted tissue. The ultimate goal of posttransplant immunosuppression is tolerance, a state in which the host immune system recognizes the foreign tissue but does not react to it. This goal has yet to be achieved under modern immunosuppression secondary to immune system redundancy as well as the toxicity of currently available agents. Therefore, monoclonal antibodies are used to provide targeted, immediate immunomodulation aimed at attenuating the overall immune response. Specifically, monoclonal antibodies have been used to (1) decrease the inherent immunoreactivity of the potential transplant recipient prior to engraftment, (2) induce global immunosuppression at the time of transplantation allowing for modified introduction of other immunosuppressive agents (calcineurin inhibitors or corticosteroids), (3) spare exposure to maintenance immunosuppressive agents, and (4) treat acute allograft rejection. Monoclonal antibody selection, as well as dose, is based on patient-specific factors, such as indication for transplantation, type of organ being transplanted, and the long-term immunosuppression objective. To understand the approach that the transplant clinician uses to determine which agent to administer and when, it is necessary to briefly describe how immunoreactivity can be predicted and review the immunological basis for the use and development of monoclonal antibodies in solid organ transplantation.

IMMUNOLOGIC TARGETS: RATIONAL DEVELOPMENT/ USE OF MONOCLONAL ANTIBODIES IN ORGAN TRANSPLANT

The rational use of monoclonal antibodies in transplantation is focused on the prevention of host immune recognition of donor tissue. There are two ways in which allograft tissue can be immediately impaired secondary to the host immune response: complement-dependent antibody-mediated cell lysis (antibody-mediated rejection) and T-cell-mediated parenchymal

N. A. Pilch (✉)
Department of Pharmacy Practice and Outcomes Sciences, Medical University of South Carolina, Charleston, SC, USA
e-mail: weimert@musc.edu

H. B. Meadows
Department of Pharmacy, Medical University of South Carolina, Charleston, SC, USA

R. R. Alloway
Division of Nephrology, Department of Internal Medicine, University of Cincinnati, Cincinnati, OH, USA

D. J. A. Crommelin et al. (eds.), *Pharmaceutical Biotechnology*, https://doi.org/10.1007/978-3-030-00710-2_25

Monoclonal antibody	Molecular weight	Animal epitope	Molecular target	Target cells	Use
Alemtuzumab (Campath-1H®)	150 kDa	Murine/human	CD52	Peripheral blood lymphocytes, natural killer cells, monocytes, macrophages, thymocytes	Induction Antibody-mediated rejection
Daclizumab (Zenapax®)	14.4 kDa	Murine/human	CD25 alpha subunit	IL2-dependent T-lymphocyte activation	Induction
Basiliximab (Simulect®)	14.4 kDa	Murine/human	CD25 alpha subunit	IL2-dependent T-lymphocyte activation	Induction
Muromonab-OKT3 (Orthoclone-OKT3®)	75 kDa	Murine	CD3	T lymphocytes (CD2, CD4, CD8)	Treatment of polyclonal antibody-resistant cellular-mediated rejection
Rituximab (Rituxan®)	145 kDa	Murine/human	CD20	B lymphocytes	Desensitization Antibody-mediated rejection Focal segmental glomerulosclerosis
Belatacept (Nulojix®)	90 kDa	Humanized	CD80 and CD86	T lymphocytes	Maintenance immunosuppression
Eculizumab (Soliris®)	148 kDa	Murine/human	C5	Block formation of membrane attack complex	Desensitization Antibody-mediated rejection Hemolytic uremic syndrome
Tocilizumab (Actenra®)	148 kDa	Murine/human	IL-6 receptor	Blocks proinflammatory effects of IL-6	Desensitization

Table 25.1 ■ Use of monoclonal antibodies in solid organ transplantation

destruction leading to localized allograft inflammation and arteritis (cellular-mediated rejection) (Halloran 2004). Pre-transplant screening for antibodies against donor tissues has significantly reduced the incidence and severity of antibody-mediated rejection. However, as will be discussed, preferential destruction of cells that produce these antibodies using monoclonal technology, such as rituximab, prior to transplant has become an option for recipients with preformed alloantibodies. As such recently the use of monoclonal antibodies to target B-cells has become a focus of transplant clinicians as a way to overcome traditional immunologic barriers pre and post-transplant. Despite this, prevention and treatment of cellular-mediated rejection, has traditionally been the main focus of maintenance immunosuppression and the rationale for use of monoclonal antibodies in the posttransplant period. Cellular-mediated rejection is characterized by initial recognition of donor tissue by T cells. This leads to a complex signal transduction pathway traditionally described as three signals (Halloran 2004):

- Signal 1: Donor antigens are presented to T cells leading to activation, characterized by T-cell proliferation.
- Signal 2: CD80 and CD86 complex with CD28 on the T-cell surface activating signal transduction pathways (calcineurin, mitogen-activated protein kinase, protein kinase C, nuclear factor kappa B) which leads to further T-cell activation, cytokine release, and expression of the interleukin-2 (IL2) receptor (CD25).
- Signal 3: IL-2 and other growth factors cause the activation of the cell cycle and T-cell proliferation (Halloran 2004).

Monoclonal antibodies have been developed against various targets within this pathway to prevent propagation and lymphocyte proliferation providing profound immunosuppression (Table 25.1). Monoclonal antibodies that were originally developed for treatment of various malignancies have also been employed as immunosuppressant agents in solid organ recipients. Use of these agents must be balanced with maintenance immunosuppression to minimize the patient's risk of infection or malignancy from over-immunosuppression. Table 25.2 describes common adverse effects associated with maintenance immunosuppressant medications. Tables 25.3 and 25.4 summarizes recent trends regarding the use of monoclonal antibodies for induction immunosuppression in solid organ transplantation. A plethora of factors influence the trends towards more frequent induction therapy use with T-cell depleting agents all focused on increasing accessibility to transplantation and improving long-term outcomes.

■ Monoclonal Antibodies Administered Pre-transplant

Immunologic barriers to solid organ transplantation are common. Improved management of end-stage organ disease has increased the number of potential

	Hypertension	Hyperlipidemia	Hyperglycemia	Hematologic	Renal dysfunction	Dermatologic
Corticosteroids	+	++	++	–	–	++
Cyclosporine	+++	+++	++	+	+++	++
Tacrolimus	+++	+++	+++	+++	+++	++
Mycophenolate mofetil[a]	–	–	–	+++		–
Sirolimus	++	+++	–	+++	+	+++
Everolimus	++	+++	–	+++	+	+++
Belatacept	–	–	–	–	–	–

Incidence based on manufacturer package insert clinical trial approval reports, + < 1%, ++ 1–10%, +++ > 10%
[a]Adverse effects reported for mycophenolate mofetil (CellCept®) are based on clinical trials using this agent in combination with cyclosporine or tacrolimus and corticosteroids, values modified to account for concurrent agents

Table 25.2 ■ Complications of current maintenance immunosuppressants

Immunosuppression trends from 1994 to 2004					
Organ	Who receive induction (%)	Alemtuzumab (%)	Basiliximab (%)	Daclizumab (%)	Muromonab (%)
Kidney	72	7	20	10	0
Pancreas	80	43	15	5	0
Heart	47	0	10	15	4
Lung	50	3	23	15	0
Liver	11	2	6	5	0
Intestine	50	19	0	9	0

Based on reported immunosuppression trends from 1994 to 2004, with data Adapted from Meier-Kriesche et al. (2006)

Table 25.3 ■ Current trends of monoclonal antibody induction use in solid organ transplantation

Organ	Who receive induction (%)	T-cell depleting[a] (%)	Basiliximab (%)	None (%)
Liver	38	18	20	62
Kidney	95	75	20	5
Pancreas	92.4	84.8	7.6	7.6
Heart	52.2	22.2	30	47.8
Lung	76	15	61	24
Intestine	69.1	52.9	16.2	30.9

Based on estimates from OPTN/SRTR 2016 Annual Reports for Kidney, Pancreas, Heart, Lung, Liver and Intestine (Hart et al. 2017; Kandaswamy et al. 2017; Colvin et al. 2017; Valapour et al. 2017; Kim et al. 2017; Smith et al. 2017)
[a]Includes poly and monoclonal T cell depleting

Table 25.4 ■ Adult induction immunosuppression trends based on scientific registry of transplant recipients 2016 annual report

organ recipients and produced a significant shortage of organs available for transplant in comparison to the growing demand. Therefore, clinicians have sought to transplant across previously contraindicated immunologic barriers. In addition, more patients are surviving through their first transplant and are now waiting for a subsequent transplant. Monoclonal antibodies are now being employed prior to transplant to desensitize the recipient's immune system. Desensitization is a strategy where immunosuppression is administered prior to transplant to prevent hyperacute or early rejection in patients who are known to have circulating antibodies against other human antigens. This strategy is generally reserved for patients who are "highly sensitized" during their evaluation for transplant. As the long-term significance of these sensitizing events is better understood, varying degrees of "desensitization" therapy are initiated based upon varying levels of sensitization. The long-term impact of this empirical therapy is yet to be defined. Specifically, as a patient develops end-stage organ disease, their medical and immunologic profiles are characterized. Blood samples from these potential recipients are screened for the presence of antibodies against the major histocompatibility complexes (MHC) on the surface of other human cells, specifically human leukocyte antigens (HLA). Potential recipients who have received blood products, previous organ transplants, or have a history of pregnancy are at higher risk for the development of antibodies against HLA. In addition, all humans have preformed IgG and IgM antibodies against the major blood group antigens (A, B, AB, and A1) (Reid and Olsson 2005). These antibodies will recognize donor tissue and quickly destroy (hyperacute rejection) the implanted organ if the tissue contains previously recognized HLA within minutes to hours following transplant. Therefore, it is necessary to evaluate the presence of preformed circulating antibodies against HLA in the potential organ recipients. Some centers will implement desensitization, which incorporates monoclonal antibodies prior to transplant to diminish the production of antibodies against a new organ, allowing for transplant across this immunologic barrier.

Monoclonal Antibodies Administered at the Time of Transplant

Current maintenance immunosuppression is aimed at various targets within the immune system to halt its signal transduction pathway. Available agents, although effective, are associated with significant patient and allograft adverse effects, which are correlated with long-term exposure (Table 25.2). The leading cause of death in noncardiac transplant recipients is a cardiovascular event. These cardiovascular events have been linked to long-term corticosteroid exposure. In addition, chronic administration of calcineurin inhibitors (cyclosporine and tacrolimus) is also associated with acute and chronic kidney dysfunction leading to hemodialysis or need for a kidney transplant. Monoclonal antibodies given at the time of transplant (induction) have been used to decrease the need for corticosteroids and allow for the delay or a reduction in the amount of calcineurin inhibitor used. Determination of the solid organ transplant recipient's immunologic risk at the time of transplant is necessary to determine which monoclonal antibody to use in order to minimize the risk of early acute rejection and graft loss. Recipients are stratified based on several donor, allograft, and recipient variables to determine their immunologic risk. Patients at high risk for acute rejection or those in which maintenance immunosuppression is going to be minimized should receive a polyclonal or monoclonal antibody that provides cellular apoptosis, for example, alemtuzumab or rabbit antithymocyte globulin. Recipients at low risk for acute rejection may receive a monoclonal antibody which provides immunomodulation without lymphocyte depletion, such as basiliximab.

Several important pharmacokinetic parameters must be considered when these agents are administered to the various organ transplant recipients. The volume of distribution, biological half-life, and total body clearance can differ significantly from a kidney transplant recipient to a heart transplant recipient. Clinicians must consider when to administer monoclonal antibodies in different transplant populations to maximize efficacy and minimize toxicity. For example, heart and liver transplant recipients tend to lose large volumes of blood around the time of transplant; therefore, intraoperative administration may not be the optimal time to administer a monoclonal antibody since a large portion may be lost during surgery. Monoclonal antibodies are also removed by plasma exchange procedures, such as plasmapheresis, which may be performed during the perioperative period in solid organ transplant recipients (Nojima et al. 2005).

Monoclonal Antibodies Administered Following Transplant

Monoclonal antibodies given following transplantation are used to treat allograft rejection and more recently as maintenance immunosuppressants. Administration of these agents is mainly reserved for severe allograft rejection in which the immunologic insult must be controlled quickly. Under normal homeostatic conditions the humoral immune system provides immediate control of infectious pathogens through secretion of antibodies. Cell-mediated immunity, in addition to fighting infections, provides surveillance against the production of mutant cells capable of oncogenesis. Interruption of either of these immune systems through the use of monoclonal antibodies places these patients at significant risk for infection and malignancy. Careful post-administration assessment of infection and posttransplant malignancy is commonplace. While those monoclonal antibodies employed as maintenance immunosuppressants have been developed to decrease the toxicity of long-term exposure to traditional agents such as calcineurin inhibitors, which can lead to chronic kidney damage in all organ transplant recipients, the use of these monoclonal antibodies is not without their own risks.

SPECIFIC AGENTS USED IN SOLID ORGAN TRANSPLANT

Muromonab

Muromonab was the first monoclonal antibody used in solid organ transplantation. Muromonab is a murine monoclonal antibody directed against human CD3 receptor, which is situated on the T-cell antigen receptor of mature T cells, inducing apoptosis of the target cell (Wilde and Goa 1996). Cells which display the

CD3 receptor include CD2-, CD4-, and CD8-positive lymphocytes (Ortho Biotech 2004). Other investigators suggest that muromonab may also induce CD3 complex shedding, lymphocyte adhesion molecule expression causing peripheral endothelial adhesion, and cell-mediated cytolysis (Wilde and Goa 1996; Ortho Biotech 2004; Buysmann et al. 1996; Magnussen et al. 1994; Wong et al. 1990). Muromonab is approved for the treatment of kidney allograft rejection and steroid-resistant rejection in heart transplant recipients (Ortho biotech 2004). Muromonab was initially employed as an induction agent for kidney transplant recipients, in conjunction with cyclosporine, azathioprine, and corticosteroids. When compared to patients who received no muromonab induction, the rate of acute rejection was lower and the time to first acute rejection was substantially greater (Wilde and Goa 1996). Liver recipients with renal dysfunction at the time of transplant who received muromonab induction were also able to run their posttransplant cyclosporine levels lower without an increased incidence of acute rejection (Wilde and Goa 1996). Therefore, administration of OKT3 enabled preservation of renal function in the setting of reduced calcineurin inhibitor exposure when compared to those who did not receive muromonab (Wilde and Goa 1996). The use of OKT3 as an induction agent is nearly extinct with the introduction of newer agents that have more favorable side effect profiles.

Today, muromonab is of historical value as it is no longer being manufactured. Although prior to its withdrawal from the market, it was reserved for treatment of refractory rejection. Muromonab is extremely effective at halting most corticosteroid as well as polyclonal antibody-resistant rejections. These rejections are treated with 5 mg of muromonab given daily for 7–14 days (Ortho Biotech 2004). The dose and duration of therapy is often dependent on clinical or biopsy resolution of rejection or may be correlated with circulating CD3 cell concentrations in the serum.

Most patients who are exposed to OKT3 will develop human anti-mouse antibodies (HAMA) following initial exposure. These IgG antibodies may lead to decreased efficacy of subsequent treatment courses, but premedication with corticosteroids or antiproliferative agents during initial therapy may reduce their development (Wilde and Goa 1996). Following administration, in vitro data indicates that a serum concentration of 1000 μg/L is required to inhibit cytotoxic T-cell function (Wilde and Goa 1996). In vivo concentrations near the in vivo threshold immediately (1 h) following administration but diminish significantly by 24 h (Wilde and Goa 1996). Steady-state concentrations of 900 ng/mL can be achieved after three doses, with a plasma elimination half-life of 18 h when used for treatment of rejection and 36 h when used for induction (Wilde and Goa 1996; Ortho Biotech 2004).

Muromonab administration is associated with significant acute and chronic adverse effects. Immediately following administration, patients will experience a characteristic OKT3 cytokine release syndrome. The etiology of this syndrome is characterized by the pharmacodynamic interaction the OKT3 molecule has at the CD3 receptor. Muromonab will stimulate the target cell following its interaction with the CD3 receptor prior to inducing cell death. Consequently, CD3 cell stimulation leads to cytokine production and release, which is compounded by acute cellular apoptosis leading to cell lysis and release of the intracellular contents. The cytokine release syndrome associated with muromonab manifests as high fever, chills, rigors, diarrhea, capillary leak, and in some cases aseptic meningitis (Wilde and Goa 1996). Capillary leak has been correlated with increased tumor necrosis factor release leading to an initial increase in cardiac output secondary to decreased peripheral vascular resistance, followed by a reduction in right heart filling pressures which leads to a decrease in stroke volume (Wilde and Goa 1996). Sequelae of this cytokine release syndrome can occur immediately, within 30–60 min, and last up to 48 h following administration (Wilde and Goa 1996; Ortho Biotech 2004). This syndrome appears to be the most severe following the initial dose when the highest inoculum of cells is present in the patient's serum or when preformed antibodies against the mouse epitope exist. Subsequent doses appear to be better tolerated, though cytokine release syndrome has been reported after five doses, typically when the dose has been increased or the CD3-positive cell population has rebounded from previous dose baseline (Wilde and Goa 1996). Pretreatment against the effects of this cytokine release is necessary to minimize the host response. Specifically, corticosteroids to prevent cellular response to cytokines, nonsteroidal anti-inflammatory agents to prevent sequelae of the arachidonic acid cascade, acetaminophen to halt the effects of centrally acting prostaglandins, and diphenhydramine to attenuate the recipient's response to histamine.

In addition to immediate adverse effects, the potency of muromonab has been associated with a high incidence of posttransplant lymphoproliferative disease and viral infections. For all patients, the 10-year cumulative incidence of posttransplant lymphoproliferative disease is 1.6% (Opelz and Dohler 2004). Review of large transplant databases revealed that deceased donor kidney transplant recipients who received muromonab for induction or treatment had a cumulative incidence of posttransplant lymphoproliferative disease that was three times higher than those who did not received muromonab or other T-cell depleting induction (Opelz and Dohler 2004). This observation may be multifactorial. It is well known that posttransplant lymphoproliferative disease may be induced secondary to Epstein-Barr viral B-cell malignant transformation. Muromonab's potent inhibition of T lymphocytes over a sustained period of time diminishes the immune system's normal surveillance and destruction of malignant cell lines, consequently leading to unopposed transformed B-cell proliferation and subsequent posttransplant lymphoma (Opelz and Dohler 2004).

Early use and development of muromonab in solid organ transplantation was beneficial for the novel development and use of newer monoclonal agents. The immunodepleting potency of muromonab, combined with the significant risk for malignancy, has made its use obsolete in the setting of modern transplantation. However, this agent still serves as a template for treatment of severe allograft rejection and the use of monoclonal antibodies posttransplant.

Interleukin-2 Receptor Antagonists

Interleukin-2 antagonists were the next monoclonal antibodies to be used and were specifically developed for use in solid organ transplantation. As previously mentioned, monoclonal antibody use and development in solid organ transplantation is rational. The IL-2 receptor was targeted for several reasons. Interleukin-2, the ligand for the IL-2 receptor, is a highly conserved protein, with only a single gene locus on chromosome 4 (Church 2003). Animal IL-2 knockout models have decreased lymphocyte function at 2–4 weeks of age and early mortality at 6–9 weeks of age (Chen et al. 2002). These models also display significantly diminished myelopoiesis leading to severe anemia and global bone marrow failure (Chen et al. 2002). This observation confirms the significant role that IL-2 and the IL-2 receptor complex play in immunity. The function and biological effect of IL-2 binding to the IL-2 receptor was first reported by Robb and colleagues in 1981 (Robb et al. 1981). This in vitro study evaluated murine lymphocytes and found that the IL-2 receptor is only present on activated cells (CD4+ and CD8+) (Church 2003). Uchiyama et al. (1981) reported one of the first monoclonal antibodies developed against activated human T cells. This compound displayed in vitro preferential activity against activated T cells, including terminally mature T cells, but did not exhibit activity against B cells or monocytes (Uchiyama et al. 1981). Later it was determined that this antibody actually bound to the alpha subunit of the activated T-cell receptor, CD25 (Church 2003). The actual T-cell receptor is made up of three subunits, alpha, beta, and gamma. When the beta and gamma subunits combine, they can only be stimulated by high concentrations of IL-2; however, in conjunction with the alpha subunit, the receptor shows high affinity for IL-2 and can be stimulated at very low concentrations. The expression of IL-2 and the IL-2 receptor alpha region is highly regulated at the DNA transcription level and is induced following T-cell activation (Shibuya et al. 1990). The alpha subunit is continuously expressed during allograft rejection, T-cell-mediated autoimmune diseases, and malignancies (Church 2003). The beta and gamma subunits, however, have constitutive expression, resulting in low levels of expression in resting T lymphocytes (Vincenti et al. 1997, 1998). There is no constitutive expression of IL-2 or the alpha receptor subunit (Shibuya et al. 1990; Noguchi et al. 1993). Both, the beta and gamma subunits, have similar molecular structures and are members of the cytokine receptor superfamily, but are structurally dissimilar to the alpha subunit (Noguchi et al. 1993). Therefore, the alpha subunit (CD25) became a rational target for monoclonal development since it is only expressed on activated T cells. Blockade of the CD25 receptor was to halt the activity of IL-2, thereby decreasing proliferation and clonal expansion of T cells when activated by foreign donor antigens.

Daclizumab

In 1997, daclizumab became the first anti-CD25 monoclonal antibody approved for use in the prevention of allograft rejection in kidney transplant recipients, when combined with cyclosporine and corticosteroids. Daclizumab was the first "humanized" monoclonal antibody approved in the United States for human administration (Tsurushita et al. 2005). The daclizumab molecule is a humanized IgG1 adapted from a mouse antibody against the alpha portion of the IL-2 receptor (Uchiyama et al. 1981). Daclizumab was developed as an alternative to the initial mouse antibody developed against the IL-2 receptor. The mouse antibody led to the development of human anti-mouse antibodies (HAMA) and inability to administer subsequent doses. Although daclizumab bound with one-third the affinity for the T-cell receptor site when compared to the original mouse molecule, it was still able to exhibit a high-binding capacity ($Ka = 3 \times 10^9\ M^{-1}$) (Tsurushita et al. 2005; Queen et al. 1988). A daclizumab serum concentration of 1 μg/mL is required for 50% inhibition of antigen-induced T-cell proliferation (Junghans et al. 1990). Early, phase I clinical trials in kidney transplant recipients, who received corticosteroids in combination with cyclosporine and azathioprine, used five doses of daclizumab (Vincenti et al. 1997). Pharmacokinetic studies revealed a mean serum half-life of 11.4 days, a steady-state volume of distribution of 5 l, and displayed weight-dependent elimination. There was no change in the number of circulating CD3-positive cells following administration. Five doses of 1 mg per kg body weight given every other week were required to produce the serum concentrations needed to achieve 90% inhibition of T-cell proliferation for 12 weeks. One patient did develop neutralizing antibodies against the daclizumab molecule after receiving weekly doses for 2 weeks. Saturation of the IL-2 receptor did not change. Intravenous doses were well tolerated with no infusion-related reactions. No infection or malignancies were reported up to 1 year following daclizumab administration. The authors concluded that daclizumab stayed within the intravascular space and doses should be based on patient weight at the time of transplant (Vincenti et al. 1997). Subsequent premarketing clinical trials confirmed these results and dosing schematic and were able to show that daclizumab administration reduced the incidence of acute rejection by 13% in low-risk kidney transplant recipients (Vincenti et al. 1998). Following daclizumab's approval, several trials have been conducted using various dosing regimens and immunosuppression combinations within various solid organ recipients. Secondary to low utilization in solid organ transplant, however, its manufacturing for transplant has recently been halted. The drug, however, has been repurposed under the name of Zinbryta® with indications for treatment of relapsing forms of multiple sclerosis.

Basiliximab

Basiliximab was developed as a more potent anti-IL-2 receptor antagonist when compared to daclizumab and may have several logistical advantages. Basiliximab, in combination with cyclosporine and corticosteroids, was approved for the prevention of acute allograft rejection in renal transplant recipients in May of 1998. Basiliximab is a murine/human (chimeric) monoclonal antibody directed against the alpha subunit of the IL-2 receptor on the surface of activated T lymphocytes. The antibody is produced from genetically engineered mouse myeloma cells. The variable region of the purified monoclonal antibody is comprised of murine hypervariable region, RFT5, which selectively binds to the IL-2 receptor alpha region. The constant region is made up of human IgG1 and kappa light chains (Novartis Pharmaceuticals 2005). Since the variable region is the only portion with a nonhuman epitope, there appears to be low antigenicity and increased circulating half-life associated with its administration (Amlot et al. 1995). Following administration, basiliximab rapidly binds to the alpha region of the IL-2 receptor and serves as a competitive antagonist against IL-2. The estimated receptor binding affinity (Ka) is 1×10^{10} M^{-1}, which is three times more potent than daclizumab (Novartis Pharmaceuticals 2005). Complete inhibition of the CD25 receptor occurs after the serum concentration of basiliximab exceeds 0.2 μg/mL and inhibition correlated with increasing dose (Novartis Pharmaceuticals 2005; Kovarik et al. 1996). Initial dose finding studies of basiliximab were similar to daclizumab. Basiliximab, combined with cyclosporine and corticosteroids, was administered to adult kidney transplant recipients for the prevention of acute cellular rejection.

Kovarik et al. (1997) performed a multicenter, open-label pharmacodynamic analysis evaluating basiliximab dose escalation in adult patients undergoing primary renal transplantation. Patients received a total of 40 or 60 mg of basiliximab in combination with cyclosporine, corticosteroids, and azathioprine. Thirty-two patients were evaluated and were primarily young (34 ± 12 years), Caucasian (29/32) males (23/32). Basiliximab infusions were well tolerated without changes in blood pressure, temperature, or hypersensitivity reactions. Thirty patients underwent pharmacokinetic evaluation. Basiliximab blood concentrations showed biphasic elimination with an average terminal half-life of 6.5 days. Significant intra- and interpatient variability in observed volume of distribution and drug clearance was observed. This could not be corrected through body weight adjustment. Gender did not appear to influence the pharmacokinetic parameters of basiliximab; however, this cohort contained only a small number of female recipients that may have limited the detection of a difference.

Results also indicated that the use of basiliximab with a combination of cyclosporine, corticosteroids, and azathioprine may be an inadequate immunosuppression regimen to prevent acute rejection, especially if cyclosporine initiation is delayed posttransplant. A total of 22 patients had an acute rejection episode, 16 patients in the 40 mg groups and six in the 60 mg group. These rejections appeared within the first 2 weeks following transplantation with a mean time to rejection of 11 days. The study was designed for cyclosporine to begin on day ten posttransplant. Also, three patients experienced graft loss, two of which were immunologically mediated. There was no difference in the basiliximab serum concentration in the patients who experienced rejection versus those who did not. The authors concluded that increased cyclosporine concentrations, which would inhibit IL-2 production, within the first few days posttransplant may increase the efficacy of basiliximab when used for induction (Kovarik et al. 1996).

The clinical efficacy of basiliximab has been confirmed in several prospective post-marketing trials. Currently, the recommended basiliximab dosing regimen is a total dose of 40 mg, with 20 mg administered

2 h prior to transplanted organ reperfusion and a subsequent 20 mg dose on postoperative day 4.

IL-2 receptor antagonists are currently used in all solid organ transplant populations for induction (Tables 25.3 and 25.4), but are only approved for use in kidney transplant recipients. Administration does not reduce the total number of circulating lymphocytes or the number of T lymphocytes expressing other markers of activations, such as CD26, CD38, CD54, CD69, or HLA-DR (Chapman and Keating 2003). Consequently, it is necessary that additional immunosuppressive agents, such a calcineurin inhibitors and antiproliferative agents, be administered as soon as possible to decrease the risk of early acute rejection.

The advantage of IL-2 receptor antagonists is that they confer a decreased risk of infusion-related reactions, posttransplant infection, and malignancy when compared to immunodepleting agents. The use of these agents has increased since the introduction of more potent maintenance immunosuppressant agents, although their preference for induction has fluctuated over the years depending on organ transplant type (Tables 25.3 and 25.4). Although these agents have been evaluated in organ recipients who are at high risk for acute rejection, they are mainly reserved for patients who are at low to moderate risk. Also, these agents are still being evaluated for use in immunosuppression protocols which withdraw or avoid corticosteroids or calcineurin inhibitors.

There may be an increased risk of anti-idiotypic IgE anaphylactic reaction in patients who receive repeat courses of IL-2 receptor antagonists. Two published case reports describe patients who had been previously exposed to an IL-2 receptor antagonist and upon subsequent exposure developed dyspnea, chest tightness, rash, and angioedema. However, in one case where basiliximab was the offending agent, daclizumab was successfully administered following a negative skin test. Therefore, caution may be warranted in patients who receive a dose of an IL-2 antagonist without concomitant corticosteroids following previous exposure in the past 6 months when circulating antibodies are expected to be present.

Alemtuzumab

Alemtuzumab is a recombinant DNA-derived, humanized, rat IgG1k monoclonal antibody targeting the 21–28 kDa cell surface protein glycoprotein CD52, which is produced in a Chinese hamster ovary cell suspension (Genzyme Corporation 2009; Kneuchtle et al. 2004). Initially, the first anti-CD52 antibodies were developed from rat hybrid antibodies that were produced to lyse lymphocytes in the presence of complement (Morris and Russell 2006). Campath-1 M was the first agent developed. This molecule was a rat IgM antibody which produced little biological effect. In contrast, the rat IgG (Campath-1G) produced profound lymphopenia (Morris and Russell 2006). In order to prevent the formation of antibodies against the rat IgG, the molecule was humanized and called alemtuzumab or Campath-1H (Morris and Russell 2006). The biologic effects of alemtuzumab are the same as Campath-1G and include complement-mediated cell lysis, antibody-mediated cytotoxicity, and target cell apoptosis (Magliocca and Knechtle 2006). The CD52 receptors account for 5% of lymphocyte surface antigens (Morris and Russell 2006). Cells which express the CD52 antigen include T and B lymphocytes, natural killer cells, monocytes, macrophages, and dendritic cells (Genzyme Corporation 2009; Bloom et al. 2006). However, plasma cells and memory type cells appear to be unaffected by alemtuzumab (Magliocca and Knechtle 2006). Following administration, a marked decrease in circulating lymphocytes is observed. Use in the hematology population indicates that this effect is dose dependent (see Chap. 23). However, single doses of 30 mg or two doses of 20 mg are currently used in the solid organ transplant population.

The plasma elimination half-life after single doses is reported to be around 12 days, and the molecule may be removed by posttransplant plasmapheresis (Magliocca and Knechtle 2006). The biological activity of alemtuzumab, however, may last up to several months. One in vivo study of kidney transplant recipients aimed to observe the recovery and function of lymphocytes following administration of 40 mg of alemtuzumab (Bloom et al. 2006). Authors reported a 2-log reduction in peripheral lymphocytes following administration. Absolute lymphocyte counts at 12 months remained markedly depleted, falling below 50% of their original baseline. Monocytes and B lymphocytes were the first cell lines to recover at 3–12 months post-administration. T lymphocytes returned to 50% of their baseline value by 36 months.

Until recently, alemtuzumab was primarily FDA approved for the treatment of B-cell chronic lymphocytic leukemia. The first report of alemtuzumab use in solid organ transplantation appeared in 1991. Friend et al. (1991) published a case series on the use of alemtuzumab to reverse acute rejection in renal transplant recipients. Shortly thereafter, Calne et al. (1999) issued the first report of alemtuzumab use as an induction agent. The authors reported the results of 31 consecutive renal transplant recipients. Patients received two 20 mg doses of alemtuzumab; the first dose was given in the operating room and the second dose was given on postoperative day 1. Patients were initiated on low-dose cyclosporine monotherapy 72 h after transplant, with a target trough range of 75–125 ng/mL. Six patients experienced corticosteroid responsive rejection (20%). Three of these were maintained on corticosteroids and azathioprine following rejection, while the other three remained on cyclosporine monotherapy. Allografts remained functional in 94% (29/31) of patients at 15–28 months posttransplant (Calne et al. 1999).

The largest multicenter randomized controlled trial assessing alemtuzumab induction in low- and high-risk renal transplant recipients showed that biopsy-confirmed acute rejection was reduced in low-risk patients receiving alemtuzumab when compared to basiliximab after 3 years of follow-up. In high-risk renal transplant patients, alemtuzumab and Thymoglobulin® appeared to have similar efficacy. However, patients who received alemtuzumab had increased rates of late rejections (between 12 and 36 months) when compared to conventional therapies (8% versus 3%, $p = 0.03$). All patients were withdrawn from steroids by postoperative day 5. Adverse effects were similar with more leukopenia observed in the alemtuzumab group (54%) compared to basiliximab (29%), and more serious adverse effects related to malignancy were seen with alemtuzumab (5%) when compared to a composite of all basiliximab- and Thymoglobulin®-treated patients (1%). However, overall adverse events related to malignancy were similar between treatment groups (Hanaway et al. 2011).

Currently, the most data on the use of alemtuzumab in solid organ transplantation are with kidney transplant recipients and literature suggests that it is used in 13% of all kidney transplants (Serrano et al. 2015). However, alemtuzumab is currently being used for induction and for treatment of rejection in other organs as well (Morris and Russell 2006). In the most recent review of immunosuppression trends in the United States, alemtuzumab use markedly increased from 2001 to 2004 and has been lumped in with other T-cell depleting induction in most recent reports, with use primarily limited to induction of immunosuppression (see Tables 25.3 and 25.4).

In 2004, alemtuzumab was the predominant agent used for induction in both pancreas and intestinal transplant recipients (Meier-Kriesche et al. 2006). Use in liver transplant has been limited but has appeared in a couple of published trials. Specific findings from these trials indicate that patients without hepatitis C were able to tolerate lower levels of calcineurin inhibitors which corresponded to lower serum creatinine levels at 1-year posttransplant (Tzakis et al. 2004). In contrast, administration of alemtuzumab positively correlated with early recurrence of hepatitis C viral replication (Marcos et al. 2004).

Alemtuzumab in heart transplantation has been rarely reported in the literature with only 2% of heart transplant patients receiving alemtuzumab for induction in 2004 (Meier-Kriesche et al. 2006). Teuteberg and colleagues recently published a retrospective study on 1-year outcomes on the use of alemtuzumab for induction in cardiac transplantation at a single center. Freedom from rejection was higher in the alemtuzumab group (versus no induction); however, survival at 1 year was similar between groups with more adverse effects in the alemtuzumab group (Teuteberg et al. 2010). Despite this recent publication, there remains a paucity of data in the cardiac transplant population regarding alemtuzumab for induction immunosuppression, which has resulted in limited use in this population. The use of alemtuzumab in lung transplant is also under investigation with some initial analysis of registry data suggesting that it may be beneficial in preventing bronchiolitis obliterans syndrome, a form of chronic rejection, when used for induction and as a rescue (Furuya et al. 2016, Ensor et al. 2017).

A retrospective review of 5-year outcomes on the use of alemtuzumab induction in lung transplant recipients at a single center showed an improvement in patient and graft survival with alemtuzumab compared to no induction or daclizumab induction and higher rates of freedom from cellular rejection than no induction or Thymoglobulin® or daclizumab induction (Shyu et al. 2011). The results of the previous study are consistent with another retrospective study that showed decreased rejection rates with alemtuzumab induction in comparison to Thymoglobulin® and daclizumab in lung transplant patients (McCurry et al. 2005). In 2004, 3% of lung transplant recipients received alemtuzumab for induction (Meier-Kriesche et al. 2006); however, this number may be increasing as more data emerges regarding alemtuzumab use in the lung transplant population.

Alemtuzumab induction has allowed for early withdrawal of corticosteroids in several clinical trials, thereby decreasing long-term steroid exposure. This may lead to improved clinical outcomes since the use of steroids has been correlated with an increased incidence of cardiovascular disease, endocrine, and metabolic side effects. However, the long-term benefit of steroid withdrawal after alemtuzumab induction requires further study. Several trials have also shown success with using low-dose calcineurin inhibitors with alemtuzumab induction. However, early trials in which calcineurin inhibitor avoidance was initiated, the rate of early acute antibody-mediated rejection was 17% compared to 10% under traditional immunosuppression which included calcineurin inhibitors (Magliocca and Knechtle 2006).

The infusion of alemtuzumab is well tolerated. In general, induction doses are administered immediately preceding reperfusion of the transplanted allograft.

Pretreatment with corticosteroids, diphenhydramine, and acetaminophen is generally advised to prevent sequelae from cellular apoptosis. However, cytokine release associated with alemtuzumab is insignificant in comparison to other agents (Morris and Russell 2006).

Until recently, there were few published experiences detailing long-term outcomes in patients who received alemtuzumab induction (Magliocca and Knechtle 2006). Initially clinicians were concerned that the profound lymphodepletion that was observed following administration would lead to a significant increase in the number of severe infections. Therefore, lymphocyte response to donor antigens following alemtuzumab administration was also evaluated in vitro (Bloom et al. 2006). Lymphocytes from patients treated with alemtuzumab were able to respond to donor antigens and cytokines. However, a small subset of patients were hyporesponsive, which is similar to the control patients observed in this study (Bloom et al. 2006). In addition, several reports detailing the use of alemtuzumab thus far suggest that both infection and malignancy rates are minimal when compared to other agents used for the same indication (Morris and Russell 2006; Magliocca and Knechtle 2006). These findings are confirmed with the prospective 3-year data published by Hanaway et al. in kidney transplant recipients as well as the retrospective 5-year data published by Shyu et al. in lung transplant recipients (Hanaway et al. 2011; Shyu et al. 2011). Recent analysis of kidney registry data also indicate that long-term outcomes with alemtuzumab induction are similar to that of Thymoglobulin® induction (Serrano et al. 2015).

At present, a concern associated with alemtuzumab administration is an increased incidence of autoimmune diseases. The exact incidence and etiology of autoimmune diseases following alemtuzumab administration in solid organ transplant is currently unknown, although the most well-designed trial with 3-year follow-up to date did not report autoimmune diseases developing in kidney transplant recipients receiving alemtuzumab for induction (Hanaway et al. 2011). Initial reports of autoimmune diseases associated with alemtuzumab administration came from the multiple sclerosis population. A single center observed the development of Grave's disease in 9 out of 27 patients who received alemtuzumab (Coles et al. 1999). Thyroid function in all patients was normal prior to alemtuzumab and the mean time to development of autoimmune hyperthyroidism was 19 months (range 9–31 months) (Coles et al. 1999). Autoimmune hyperthyroidism was first reported in a kidney transplant recipient who received alemtuzumab induction 4 years earlier (Kirk et al. 2006). Watson et al. (2005) published a 5-year experience with alemtuzumab induction, in which they reported a 6% (2/33) incidence of autoimmune disease development following administration. One patient developed hyperthyroidism in the early posttransplant period, and one patient developed hemolytic anemia, which was refractory to corticosteroids. With the increased use of alemtuzumab in solid organ transplantation, it is important to continually assess the risk of autoimmune disease development in this population.

Alemtuzumab became such a popular option in solid organ transplant and for other non-transplant indications that the pharmaceutical company removed it from the market in 2012. (Enderby and Keller 2015) Similar to other medications mentioned the drug has been repurposed as a medication to treat multiple sclerosis under the name Lemtrada®. Transplant centers were able to obtain alemtuzumab for transplantation since then but under scrutinized conditions and limited qualities associated with a distribution program (Serrano et al. 2015).

■ Rituximab

Rituximab is a chimeric murine/human IgG1 monoclonal antibody directed at the CD20 cell surface protein (Tobinai 2003). Rituximab is currently FDA approved for the CD20-positive forms of non-Hodgkin's lymphoma and chronic lymphocytic leukemia (CLL) and Wegener granulomatosis, microscopic polyangiitis, and refractory rheumatoid arthritis (see Chaps. 23 and 26) (Genentech 2011). The CD20 antigen is a 35-kDa phosphoprotein expressed on B cells, from pre-B cells to mature B cells. This protein is not expressed on hematopoietic stem cells, plasma cells, T lymphocytes, or other tissues (Tobinai 2003). The CD20 protein is a calcium channel and is responsible for B-cell proliferation and differentiation (Tobinai 2003). Early monoclonal antibodies developed against CD20 revealed that antibody binding did not result in modulation of activity or shedding of the surface protein, making the development of a humanized anti-CD20 antibody rational (Tobinai 2003). Rituximab was originally developed to treat B-cell lymphomas, as the vast majority of malignant B cells express the CD20 receptor. Following continuously infused, high doses of engineered anti-CD20 monoclonal antibodies clearance of CD20-positive cells occurred within 4 h of administration (Press et al. 1987). Circulating B-cell clearance was immediate; however, lymph node and bone marrow B-cell clearance were dose dependent.

Rituximab was initially used in solid organ transplant recipients to treat posttransplant lymphoproliferative disorder (PTLD). PTLD is a malignancy that develops following exposure to high levels of T-cell depleting immunosuppression (see section "Immunologic Targets: Rational Development/Use of Monoclonal Antibodies in Organ Transplant"). Under normal physiologic conditions, both the humoral and cellular immune systems work in concert to fight infection. In addition, cytotoxic T lymphocytes survey the body for malignant cells. Current immunosuppression and induction therapy are focused on decreasing communication and proliferation of T lymphocytes, which may lead to unopposed B-cell proliferation. The most significant risk factors for the development of PTLD are the use of potent T-cell depleting therapies as well as an Epstein-Barr virus (EBV) negative recipient serostatus. Approximately 60–70% of PTLD cases are associated with EBV. Certain B cells that are infected with EBV or other viruses may go into unopposed cellular differentiation leading to PTLD (Evens et al. 2010).

This disorder was first reported in five living donor renal transplant recipients in 1969 with four of the five patients dying from their disease. The fifth patient survived following radiation and reduction in immunosuppression (Penn et al. 1969). The incidence of posttransplant malignancy, specifically PTLD, increased as the number of solid organ transplants increased. Specific agents linked to the development of PTLD included OKT3 and rabbit antithymocyte globulin (Swinnen et al. 1990; Evens et al. 2010). The initial treatment for PTLD is a reduction in maintenance immunosuppression, to allow T-cell surveillance to resume and aid in the destruction of malignancy causing cells. However, pharmacotherapeutic agents have been used successfully in patients who fail to respond to decreased immunosuppression. Rituximab is the most studied medication for the treatment of PTLD and can be considered in patients with CD20-positive tumors. Rituximab was initially used in the 1990s to target B-cell-specific forms of PTLD that did not involve the central nervous system (Faye et al. 1998; Cook et al. 1999; Davis and Moss 2004). The molecular size of rituximab generally precludes its use for central nervous system tumors with <5% of rituximab penetrating the blood brain barrier, although some recent reports have shown success with rituximab for the treatment of CNS PTLD (Patrick et al. 2011; Kordelas et al. 2008; Jagadeesh et al. 2012). Administration of rituximab in patients with peripheral lymphomas resulted in clearance of malignant B cells for up to 12 months (Davis and Moss 2004). Currently, rituximab is reserved for patients with CD20-positive PTLD who fail to respond to reduction in maintenance immunosuppression. Rituximab can be used alone or in combination with chemotherapy in patients with severe or refractory PTLD.

Rituximab has also been employed as a desensitizing agent (see section "Monoclonal Antibodies Administered Pre-transplant") prior to solid organ transplant. Doses of 375 mg per m^2 administered prior to transplant enabled transplantation across ABO incompatible blood types and transplantation of highly sensitized patients. Often rituximab is given in combination with other immunosuppressants to halt the production of new B lymphocytes and prevent the formation of new plasma cells. Desensitization protocols involve administration of pooled immunoglobulin followed by plasmapheresis to remove donor-specific antibody complexes. Rituximab is administered following the course of plasmapheresis for two reasons: (1) rituximab is removed by plasmapheresis and (2) rituximab only targets B lymphocytes, not the plasma cells currently secreting antibody. Therefore, timing of administration is crucial to the success of the desensitization protocol (Pescovitz 2006). Several protocols with various outcomes exist. One example is a recent study by Vo and colleagues where they evaluated intravenous immunoglobulin with and without rituximab for desensitization in a double-blind placebo controlled trial. This trial was halted early secondary to serious adverse events in the placebo arm however did suggest some benefit of rituximab based regimens in preventing rebound of antibodies (Vo et al. 2014).

Following transplant, rituximab is also used for the treatment of acute, refractory antibody-mediated rejection. Antibody-mediated rejection is characterized by host recognition of donor antigens followed by T-cell proliferation and antigen presentation to B cells. B cells then undergo clonal expansion and differentiation into mature plasma cells, which secrete anti-donor antibody. This immune process may occur before or after transplantation. Often the presence of antibodies against donor tissue is discovered prior to transplant, during final crossmatch, thus preventing hyperacute rejection. In some cases, low levels of antibody or memory B cells exist which can facilitate antibody-mediated rejection within the first several weeks following transplant. Rituximab, therefore, is used to induce apoptosis of the B cells producing or capable of producing antibodies against the allograft. Unfortunately, the CD20 receptor is absent on mature plasma cells; therefore, rituximab can only stop new B cells from forming. Plasmapheresis is necessary to remove antibodies produced by secreting plasma cells. It is important to remember that rituximab may be removed by plasmapheresis and timing of administration is necessary to ensure optimal drug exposure. The optimal number of doses and length of therapy necessary to suppress antibody-mediated rejection is unknown (Pescovitz 2006; Stegall and Gloor 2010).

In 2005 and 2006, rituximab was shown to improve the clinical course of renal transplant patients with recurrent focal segmental glomerulosclerosis (FSGS) in patients who were receiving rituximab for the treatment of PTLD (Nozu et al. 2005; Pescovitz et al. 2006). A subsequent study described seven pediatric patients who had a relapse of proteinuria after transplantation and who failed to respond to initial plasmapheresis. After failure of plasmapheresis, patients received rituximab for treatment of refractory FSGS. Three patients had complete resolution of proteinuria; urine protein decreased by 70% in one patient and by 50% in one patient. One patient failed to respond to therapy and one patient was unable to tolerate the rituximab infusion. This study confirmed that rituximab is a possible treatment option for recurrent FSGS (Strologo et al. 2009). Additional studies are needed to further delineate the role of rituximab in the treatment of recurrent FSGS.

Eculizumab

Eculizumab is a recombinant-humanized IgG2/4 monoclonal antibody with murine complementarity-determining regions grafted onto the framework of the human antibody on the light- and heavy-chain variable regions. Eculizumab binds with specificity and with high affinity to C5, a complement protein. By binding to C5, eculizumab prevents cleavage of C5 to C5a and C5b, which prevents the formation of the membrane attack complex. Currently, eculizumab is approved for use in the treatment of paroxysmal nocturnal hemoglobinuria and atypical hemolytic uremic syndrome (Alexion Pharmaceuticals 2011; McKeage 2011).

Because antibody-mediated rejection (AMR) is associated with complement activation evidenced by $C4d^+$ staining on biopsy, the use of eculizumab for the prevention and treatment of AMR holds promise (Stegall and Gloor 2010). The first case describing the use of eculizumab for the treatment of severe AMR was published in 2009. The patient was a highly sensitized kidney transplant recipient who received desensitization therapy before and after transplant. However, he became anuric with a biopsy that was positive for AMR approximately 8 days after transplant. After clinical failure of plasmapheresis and intravenous immunoglobulin, eculizumab was initiated. Intravenous immunoglobulin was also given in order to decrease donor-specific antibodies, and rituximab was given in order to prevent B-cell proliferation. Donor-specific antibodies did not decrease initially; however, C5d-9 staining was reduced on biopsy, and AMR was completely resolved on follow-up biopsies (Locke et al. 2009).

The use of eculizumab for the prevention of AMR has also been reported. In one study, patients with a positive crossmatch to their living kidney donor received plasmapheresis and eculizumab preoperatively and were compared to a historical control who received only plasmapheresis pre- and postoperatively. The treatment group also received eculizumab post-transplant for at least 4 weeks. Treatment continued in patients who did not have a decrease in donor-specific antibody. The incidence of AMR at 3 months was 7% in the eculizumab group compared to 41% in the historical control group (Stegall and Gloor 2010).

Recent evidence has proven that complement activation is involved in the development of hemolytic uremic syndrome. There have been a few case reports that show that eculizumab can improve the outcomes of patients who develop hemolytic uremic syndrome after renal transplant (Van den Hoogen and Hilbrands 2011). More recently a case series detailing use post-transplant in patients either prophylactically, with known hemolytic uremic syndrome, or who developed hemolytic uremic syndrome indicated good response without a significant increase in opportunistic infections (de Andrade et al. 2017).

There is limited data, mainly case reports and series, on the use of eculizumab in solid organ transplantation at this time. However, it is likely that its role in the prevention and treatment of AMR, hemolytic uremic syndrome after transplantation, and other possible indications will be more clearly defined by the next decade.

Tocilizumab

Tocilizumab is a humanized monoclonal antibody directed at the IL-6 receptor and is approved in the United States to treat various forms of arthritis. Tocilizumab is a novel mAb therapy that competitively inhibits the binding of IL-6 to its receptor. Inhibiting the entire receptor complex prevents IL-6 signal transduction to inflammatory mediators that summon B and T cells. IL-6 signaling can be inhibited by suppressors of cytokine signaling, such as antibodies directed against IL-6R. In order to signal, IL-6 and its receptors form a four-part complex at the cell surface that comprises IL-6, an IL-6R, and two gp130 proteins. The signal is then transduced through several members of the Janus-activated kinase-signal transducer and activator of transcription (JAK-STAT) pathway. The signal ultimately leads to the transcription of genes with IL-6 response elements. The most commonly known members of the JAK-STAT pathway are the acute-phase proteins, which are a collection of macromolecules that flood the circulation during certain inflammatory disorders (Sebba 2008).

As attempts to reduce HLA antibodies levels in sensitized transplant recipients have not been universally effective, many drugs with favorable mechanisms of action have been tested in desensitization. Since IL-6 is a pleiotropic cytokine that has powerful stimulatory effects on B cells and plasma cells and its function is responsible for normal antibody production, it is reasonable to evaluate its efficacy for desensitization. In November 2016, the first published experience with tocilizumab in patients undergoing desensitization awaiting kidney transplant was reported. Tocilizumab was added to a common intravenous immunoglobulin (IVIG) based desensitization protocol and resulted in decrease in the mean time to transplant and outcomes free of biopsy proven antibody mediated rejection. These early results encourage further studies with tocilizumab and other agents developed outside of transplant indications which possess a novel approach to reducing antibody production (Vo et al. 2015).

Belatacept

In an effort to achieve the "immunotolerant" state posttransplant, research has been focused in the area of co-stimulation blockade. Simplistically, when a T cell is exposed to an antigen particle expressed on an antigen presenting cell through the T-cell receptor, additional co-stimulation is required for full activation of the T cell (Wekerle and Grinyo 2012). If co-stimulation is blocked, then the T cell becomes unresponsive and in essence tolerant. CD28 is expressed on human T cells and is upregulated on activated T cells, while its ligands, on the surface of the antigen presenting cell, are CD80 and CD86 (Wekerle and Grinyo 2012). Cytotoxic T-lymphocyte antigen-4 (CTLA-4) was identified as a compound that would bind the same ligands as CD28 but to a much higher affinity (Wekerle and Grinyo 2012). A modification of CTLA-4, giving it higher binding affinity for CD80/86, was fused with a mutated (no longer able to fix complement) human IgG1, yielding belatacept (Wekerle and Grinyo 2012). Therefore, belatacept binds to CD80 and CD86 with high affinity, blocking their interaction with CD28 on T cells. An artifact of belatacept is that it also blocks intrinsic CTLA-4, which normally acts as an inhibitory ligand on the surface of activated T cells, responsible for limiting the proliferation of the immune response (Wekerle and Grinyo 2012). Blockade of CTLA-4 could prevent tolerance from being achieved when administered posttransplant; however, phase II trials indicate that the synthesis of CD4+ CD25+ regulatory T cells is not interrupted following belatacept exposure (Gupta and Womer 2010). Belatacept is an intravenous infusion, dosed based on actual body weight, and is unaffected by renal or hepatic function, which is administered frequently during the first 1–3 months posttransplant then monthly thereafter (Martin et al. 2011).

Belatacept has been mainly studied and demonstrated efficacy in kidney transplant recipients in combination with basiliximab induction and mycophenolate mofetil/prednisone maintenance immunosuppression. Belatacept has been touted as calcineurin inhibitor sparing and therefore more renal protective posttransplant. Recently the 3-year results of the BENEFIT study were published detailing the safety and efficacy of belatacept versus cyclosporine in combination with mycophenolate mofetil and prednisone (Vincenti et al. 2012). The BENEFIT trial evaluated 663 kidney transplant recipients who received low intensity (0–3 months; 10 mg/kg on days 1 and 5, 10 mg/kg on weeks 2, 4, 8, 12, 3–36 months 5 mg/kg every 4 weeks; $n = 226$), moderate intensity (0–6 months) 10 mg/kg on days 1 and 5, 10 mg/kg on weeks 2, 4, 6, 8, 10, 12, 16, 20, and 24; 7–36 months 5 mg/kg ($n = 219$) belatacept or cyclosporine ($n = 221$) in combination with mycophenolate mofetil and prednisone. Graft survival at 3 years was 92% in the low- and moderate-intensity groups and 89% in the cyclosporine group. A total of 6 patients died, 2 in each group, and 9 patients lost their graft (4 in the low intensity, 3 in the moderate intensity, and 2 in the cyclosporine group). Calculated glomerular filtration rate was 66 ± 27 mL/min/1.73 m^2 in the low intensity, 65 ± 26 mL/min/1.73 m^2 in the moderate intensity, and 44 ± 24 mL/min/1.73 m^2 in the cyclosporine group, $p < 0.0001$. Acute rejection mainly occurred in the first-year posttransplant with a cumulative rate of 17% in the low intensity and 24% in the moderate intensity versus 10% in the cyclosporine group. There were no new rejectins in the belatacept treatments arms between years 2–3. Donor specific antibody production was reduced by 50% in the belatacept treated patients. PTLD occurred in five patients who received belatacept versus one patient in the cyclosporine group (Vincenti et al. 2012). In 2016, 7 years after transplantation of this same cohort, patient and graft survival and the mean eGFR were significantly higher with belatacept than with cyclosporine. A 43% reduction in the risk of death or graft loss was observed as compared with the cyclosporine regimen with equal contributions from the lower rates of death and graft loss. The mean estimated glomerular filtration rate increased over the 7-year period with belatacept, but declined with the cyclosporine regimen. (Vincenti et al. 2016) Similar results were found at 3 and 7 years in extended criteria kidney transplant recipients (Pestana et al. 2012, Durrbach et al. 2016). When more intensive belatacept dosing was used in combination with mycophenolate mofetil ($n = 33$) or sirolimus ($n = 26$) versus tacrolimus with mycophenolate mofetil ($n = 30$) following rabbit antithymocyte globulin and early corticosteroid withdrawal (4 days), acute rejection rates were low (12% belatacept-mycophenolate, 4% belatacept-sirolimus, and 3% in the tacrolimus-mycophenolate). Graft survival was 100% at 1 year in the tacrolimus group versus 91% in the belatacept-mycophenolate group and 92% in the belatacept-sirolimus group; however, graft function was roughly 8 mL/min/1.73 m^2 higher in the belatacept groups. However, less than 80% of patients in the belatacept groups remained steroid-free at 12 months versus 93% in the tacrolimus group (Ferguson et al. 2011). Patients 6–36 months post-kidney transplant were also enrolled in a conversion trial in which they were randomized to continue their current immunosuppression or be converted to belatacept to evaluate if an improvement in renal function could be obtained following discontinuation of a calcineurin inhibitor (Rostaing et al. 2011). An average improvement in glomerular filtration rate was noted in the belatacept group (7 mL/min versus 2.1 mL/min, $p = 0.0058$) at

12 months following conversion. Six patients did develop acute rejection following their conversion to belatacept, but these rejections did not result in graft loss (Rostaing et al. 2011).

Evidence for the use of belatacept is currently lacking in nonrenal transplant recipients and high immunologic risk and non-Caucasian organ recipients. Additionally, patients who are EBV positive are at high risk of developing posttransplant lymphoproliferative disease in the central nervous system. This observation warranted a black box warning to be issued in the belatacept package insert detailing that the use of belatacept is contraindicated in patients who are EBV negative (Bristol Myers Squibb Company 2011). As a result of this warning, a risk evaluation and mitigation strategy (REMS) for belatacept was originally approved by the Food and Drug Administration (FDA) on June 15, 2011. On May 9, 2017, the FDA determined that a REMS is no longer required for belatacept and has eliminated the REMS requirement citing current labeling is adequate to address the serious and significant public health concerns to ensure the benefits of the drug outweigh the risks.

OTHER MONOCLONAL ANTIBODIES USED IN TRANSPLANT RECIPIENTS

Monoclonal antibodies to treat other comorbid conditions is commonplace in prospective transplant candidates. The use of these antibodies post-transplant becomes a discussion and the therapeutic impact on overall immunosuppression is unknown. Careful consideration of each monoclonal antibody used in combination with transplant immunosuppression is needed. The patient and clinical team need to weigh the risks and benefits of continuing the monoclonal antibody and potentially see if symptoms resolve for conditions previously treated with maintenance immunosuppression. If monoclonal antibodies used for non-transplant indications after transplant are needed the team should consider timing based on immunosuppression given at the time of transplantation, and if additional monitoring for opportunistic infections and malignancies is needed.

CONCLUSION

Currently, there are several challenges remaining in solid organ transplantation. These challenges may be grouped as follows. One challenge is optimizing patient-specific immunosuppression based on risk factors for acute rejection. Monoclonal antibodies provide targeted immunosuppression that when used in conjunction with specific maintenance immunosuppressants may allow more specific therapy. Another challenge is preventing over-immunosuppression, which may lead to infection and malignancy. Although monoclonal antibodies provide targeted therapy, the toxicity and potency must be balanced with over-immunosuppression. Consideration of the mechanism of action of both the monoclonal antibody and maintenance immunosuppression must be evaluated to ensure that appropriate antimicrobial prophylaxis and malignancy screening tools are utilized to minimize the patient's risk. Finally, increasing patient and graft survival through reducing the incidence of adverse effects associated with long-term exposure to maintenance immunosuppression, such as cardiovascular events or kidney dysfunction, is necessary. Monoclonal, along with polyclonal antibodies, may allow for withdrawal or minimization of specific maintenance immunosuppressants that lead to the increased incidence of these long-term adverse effects. Oftentimes the use of specific monoclonal antibodies in institutional protocols is driven by cost or changing availability (Table 25.5) with careful consideration of the goals of therapy.

Monoclonal antibody	Dose[a]	US cost per course (AWP)[b]
Alemtuzumab	30 mg × 1	$[c]
Basiliximab	20 mg × 2	$5605
Rituximab	375 mg/m² weekly × 4 doses	$20,682
Belatacept	10 mg/kg days 1 and 5	$42,090 for the first year
	10 mg/kg after 2 and 4 weeks	$28,798 subsequent years
	10 mg/kg after 8 and 12 weeks	
	5 mg/kg after 16 weeks and every 4 weeks thereafter	
Eculizumab	1200 mg × 1[d]	$74,880
Tocilizumab	600 mg × 1 then	$23,860
	600 mg weekly × 3 8 mg/kg on Day 15, then monthly for 6 months[e]	

[a]Based on 70 kg dosing weight, rounded to nearest vial size
[b]Actual wholesale price (AWP) Adapted from Red Book; Thomson Reuters (2012)
[c]Only available through specialized distribution program
[d]Dosing is based on Stegall et al. (2011) study. Adequate dose for transplantation has not yet been established
[e]Dosing is based on Vo et al. (2015) study. Adequate dose for desensitization has not yet been established

Table 25.5 ■ Per dose cost comparison estimates between monoclonal antibodies currently used in solid organ transplantation

SELF-ASSESSMENT QUESTIONS

Questions

1. Monoclonal antibodies are used for several reasons in solid organ transplantation. What benefit do they provide over polyclonal antibodies?
2. The rational development and use of monoclonal antibodies in solid organ transplantation is focused on the prevention of host recognition of donor tissue (rejection). What are the two ways in which the host immune system recognizes donor tissue and may cause tissue damage?
3. What are the molecular targets for monoclonal antibodies currently used in solid organ transplantation?
4. Monoclonal antibodies are used at various times in solid organ transplantation. Describe the reasons why a monoclonal antibody would be administered before transplant, at the time of transplant, or following transplant?
5. There are several important pharmacokinetic parameters that must be considered when administering monoclonal antibodies to solid organ transplant recipients. What are these pharmacokinetic parameters?
6. Muromonab has a characteristic infusion-related reaction. Why does this reaction occur and how can it be attenuated?
7. Daclizumab and basiliximab are two monoclonal antibodies directed against the alpha subunit of the interleukin-2 receptor. What is the difference between these two antibodies?
8. There are several benefits, as well as several risks associated with the use of monoclonal antibodies in solid organ transplantation. What are these benefits and risks?

Answers

1. Monoclonal antibodies provide targeted immunosuppression. The advantage monoclonal antibodies offer over polyclonal antibodies is that the receptor target is known. Polyclonal antibody development involves the introduction of human lymphocytes into an animal host immune system. The animal will then develop polyclonal antibodies directed against human lymphocyte cell surface targets. As a consequence, inter-batch variability and potency may vary. Although significant outcome data exists with the use of polyclonal antibodies, monoclonal antibodies have a known target allowing for in vivo and in vitro pharmacokinetic and pharmacodynamic data to aid incorporation into novel immunosuppression regimens.
2. The two ways in which the host immune system recognizes donor tissue: Complement-dependent antibody-mediated rejection occurs when the host (recipient) develops or has preformed antibodies against the donor tissue. Preformed antibodies will aggregate to the implanted tissue and initiate the complement cascade, which facilitates cell lysis. The majority of these antibodies are usually directed against the major histocompatibility complexes (MHC) located on the surface of the donor tissue. An absolute contraindication to transplantation is the presence of preformed antibodies against MHC complex I, which is located on the surface of all nucleated cells. The second way in which the host immune system attacks donor tissue is through T-cell-mediated rejection. This occurs when the donor tissue is recognized as foreign by host antigen presenting cells. Antigen presenting cells present donor tissue antigens to the T cells which stimulates T-cell proliferation and graft infiltration leading to inflammation and arteritis.
3. Alemtuzumab (Campath-1H®) targets the CD52 receptor, located on peripheral blood lymphocytes, natural killer cells, monocytes, macrophages, and thymocytes.
   - Daclizumab (Zenapax®) targets the CD25 alpha subunit of the IL-2 receptor, located on activated T lymphocytes.
   - Basiliximab (Simulect®) targets the CD25 alpha subunit of the IL-2 receptor, located on activated T lymphocytes.
   - Muromonab-OKT3 (Orthoclone-OKT3®) targets the CD3 receptor located on CD2-, CD4-, and CD8-positive lymphocytes.
   - Rituximab (Rituxan®) targets the CD20 receptor located on B lymphocytes.
   - Eculizumab (Soliris®) targets C5 in the complement pathway.
   - Tocilizumab targets the IL-6 receptor.
4. The administration of monoclonal antibodies prior to transplant is called desensitization. This strategy is reserved for "highly sensitized" patients, meaning they have high titers of circulating antibodies against donor-specific antigens. Monoclonal antibodies that target cells which produce these antibodies are employed, in conjunction with plasmapheresis and pooled human immune globulins. Removal of these antibodies may facilitate successful transplantation across this immunologic barrier.
   - Monoclonal antibodies administered at the time of transplant are called induction. Induction is provided at the time of transplant to decrease the ability of the host immune system to respond to implantation of foreign tissue. In addition, monoclonal antibodies which provide profound T-cell depletion given at the time of transplant may facilitate the need for certain maintenance immunosuppressants.

- Following transplantation, monoclonal antibodies may be used to treat cell-mediated or antibody-mediated rejection. Cell and antibody infiltrates found in biopsy specimens in correlation with the clinical status of the patient will dictate the type, dose, and duration of the monoclonal antibody chosen.

5. The volume of distribution, biological half-life, and total-body clearance can differ significantly between solid organ transplant recipients. Careful consideration of these pharmacokinetic parameters must be employed to maximize the efficacy and minimize the toxicity associated with administration of these agents. For example, weight-based dosing in obese patients must be carefully considered, and biological markers of efficacy should be evaluated to determine the appropriate dose and dosing schedule. In addition, monoclonal antibodies are also removed by plasma exchange procedures, such as plasmapheresis, which may be performed during the perioperative period. Therefore, it would be prudent to administer the monoclonal antibody following the plasma exchange prescription to avoid removal of the drug and avoid a possible decrease in efficacy.
6. Muromonab's infusion-related reaction occurs because when the molecule binds to the CD3 receptor. It actually activates the cell prior to inducing apoptosis. T-cell activation leads to increased production of inflammatory cytokines and when the cell undergoes apoptosis these cytokines are released causing a "cytokine release syndrome." This cytokine release syndrome is characterized by fever, chills, rigors, diarrhea, and potentially capillary leak leading to pulmonary edema. Often times this reaction is the worst when the largest number of cells are present, namely, the first dose. However, this reaction can occur after several days of dosing. This reaction can be attenuated by administration of corticosteroids, histamine blockers, and cyclooxygenase antagonists. Pharmacotherapy aimed at reducing the production or the interaction of cytokines with their receptors may decrease the severity of the cytokine release syndrome.
7. *Structure activity relationship*: Daclizumab has a binding capacity of $3 \times 10^9\ M^{-1}$ versus basiliximab which has a binding capacity of $1 \times 10^{10}\ M^{-1}$. Therefore, basiliximab is three times more potent than daclizumab. *Dosing*: Daclizumab is dosed based on weight, while basiliximab is given as a 20 mg dose. The dosing schedule varies based on the type of solid organ transplanted as well as concomitant immunosuppression given. These agents, however, are only approved for prevention of acute rejection in kidney transplant recipients.
8. Benefits include targeted immunosuppression, no batch variability, and low antigenicity in humanized products. The risks associated with any type of immunosuppression include an increased risk for infection, as well as malignancy. Patients who receive monoclonal antibodies which specifically target a cell line, such as muromonab, are associated with a significantly increased risk of posttransplant lymphoproliferative disease. Appropriate antimicrobial prophylaxis and vigilant screening for posttransplant malignancy may allow for safe and effective use of these monoclonal antibodies in solid organ transplantation.

REFERENCES

Alexion Pharmaceuticals: Eculizumab (Soliris) Package Insert. Alexion Pharmaceuticals, Cheshire. Last updated: 2011

Amlot PL, Rawlings E, Fernando ON, Griffin PJ, Heinrich G, Schreier MH, Castaigne JP, Moore R, Sweny P (1995) Prolonged action of a chimeric interleukin-2 receptor (CD25) monoclonal antibody used in cadaveric renal transplantation. Transplantation 60:748–756

Bloom DD, Hu H, Fechner JH, Knechtle SJ (2006) T-lymphocyte alloresponses of Campath-1H treated kidney transplant patients. Transplantation 81:81–87

Bristol Myers Squibb Company: Belatacept (Nulojix) Package Insert. Bristol Myers Squibb, Princeton. Last updated: June 2011

Buysmann S, Bemelman FJ, Schellekens PT, van Kooyk Y, Figdor CG, ten Berge IJ (1996) Activation and increased expression of adhesion molecules on peripheral blood lymphocytes is a mechanism for the immediate lymphocytopenia after administration of OKT3. Blood 87:404–411

Calne R, Moffatt SD, Friend PJ, Jamieson NV, Bradley JA, Hale G, Firth J, Bradley J, Smith KG, Waldmann H (1999) Campath IH allows low-dose cyclosporine monotherapy in 31 cadaveric renal allograft recipients. Transplantation 68:1613–1616

Chapman TM, Keating GM (2003) Basiliximab: a review of its use as induction therapy in renal transplantation. Drugs 63:2803–2835

Chen J, Astle CM, Harrison DE (2002) Hematopoietic stem cell functional failure in interleukin-2-deficient mice. J Hematother Stem Cell Res 11:905–912

Church AC (2003) Clinical advances in therapies targeting the interleukin-2 receptor. QJM 96:91–102

Coles AJ, Wing M, Smith S, Coraddu F, Greer S, Taylor C, Weetman A, Hale G, Chatterjee VK, Waldmann H, Compston A (1999) Pulsed monoclonal antibody treatment and autoimmune thyroid disease in multiple sclerosis. Lancet 354:1691–1695

Colvin M, Smith JM, Hadley N, Skeans MA, Carrico R, Uccellini K, Lehman R, Robinson A, Israni AK, Snyder

JJ, Kasiske BL (2017) OPTN/SRTR 2016 annual report: heart. Am J Transplant 18:291–362

Cook RC, Connors JM, Gascoyne RD, Fradet G, Levy RD (1999) Treatment of post-transplant lymphoproliferative disease with rituximab monoclonal antibody after lung transplantation. Lancet 354:1698–1699

Davis JE, Moss DJ (2004) Treatment options for post-transplant lymphoproliferative disorder and other Epstein-Barr virus-associated malignancies. Tissue Antigens 63:285–292

de Andrade LGM, Contti MM, Nga HS, Bravin AM, Takase HM, Viero RM, da Silva TN, Chagas KN, Palma LMP (2017) Long-term outcomes of the Atypical Hemolytic Uremic Syndrome after kidney transplantation treated with eculizumab as first choice. PLoS One 12:e0188155

Durrbach A, Pestana JM, Florman S, Del Carmen Rial M, Rostaing L, Kuypers D, Matas A, Wekerle T, Polinsky M, Meier-Kriesche HU, Munier S, Grinyó JM (2016) Long-term outcomes in belatacept- versus cyclosporine-treated recipients of extended criteriadonor kidneys: final results from BENEFIT-EXT, a phase III randomized study. Am J Transplant 16:3192–3201

Enderby C, Keller CA (2015) An overview of immunosuppression in solid organ transplantation. Am J Managed Care 21:s12–s23

Ensor CR, Rihtarchik LC, Morrell MR, Hayanga JW, Lichvar AB, Pilewski JM, Wisniewski S, Johnson BA, D'Cunha J, Zeevi A, McDyer JF (2017) Rescue alemtuzumab for refractory acute cellular rejection and bronchiolitis obliterans syndrome after lung transplantation. Clin Transpl 31:e12899

Evens AM, Roy R, Sterrenberg D, Moll MZ, Chadburn A, Gordon LI (2010) Post-transplantation lymphoproliferative disorders: diagnosis, prognosis, and current approaches to therapy. Curr Oncol Rep 12:383–394

Faye A, Van Den Abeele T, Peuchmaur M, Mathieu-Boue A, Vilmer E (1998) Anti-CD20 monoclonal antibody for post-transplant lymphoproliferative disorders. Lancet 352:1285

Ferguson R, Grinyo J, Vincenti F, Kaufman DB, Woodle ES, Marder BA, Citterio F, Marks WH, Agarwal M, Wu D, Dong Y, Garg P (2011) Immunosuppression with belatacept-based, corticosteroid-avoiding regimens in de novo kidney transplant recipients. Am J Transplant 11:66–76

Friend PJ, Waldmann H, Hale G, Cobbold S, Rebello P, Thiru S, Jamieson NV, Johnston PS, Calne RY (1991) Reversal of allograft rejection using the monoclonal antibody, Campath-1G. Transplant Proc 23:2253–2254

Furuya Y, Jayarajan SN, Taghavi S, Cordova FC, Patel N, Shiose A, Leotta E, Criner GJ, Guy TS, Wheatley GH, Kaiser LR, Toyoda Y (2016) The impact of Alemtuzumab and Basiliximab induction on patient survival and time to bronchiolitis obliterans syndrome in double lung transplantation recipients. Am J Transplant 16:2334–2341

Genentech: Rituximab (Rituxan) Package Insert. Genentech, Inc, San Francisco. Last updated: 2011

Genzyme Corporation: Alemtuzumab (Campath) Package Insert. Genzyme Corporation, Cambridge. Last updated: 2009

Gupta G, Womer KL (2010) Profile of belatacept and its potential role in prevention of graft rejection following renal transplantation. Drug Des Devel Ther 4:375–382

Halloran PF (2004) Immunosuppressive drugs for kidney transplantation. N Engl J Med 351:2715–2729

Hanaway MJ, Woodle ES, Mulgaonkar S, Peddi VR, Kaufman DB, First MR, Croy R, Holman J (2011) Alemtuzumab induction in renal transplantation. N Engl J Med 364:1909–1919

Hart A, Smith JM, Skeans MA, Gustafson SK, Wilk AR, Robinson A, Wainright JL, Haynes CR, Snyder JJ, Kasiske BL, Israni AK (2017) OPTN/SRTR 2016 annual report: kidney. Am J Transplant 18:18–113

Jagadeesh D, Woda BA, Draper J, Evens AM (2012) Post transplant lymphoproliferative disorders: risk, classification, and therapeutic recommendations. Curr Treat Options in Oncol 13(1):122–136

Junghans RP, Waldmann TA, Landolfi NF, Avdalovic NM, Schneider WP, Queen C (1990) Anti-Tac-H, a humanized antibody to the interleukin 2 receptor with new features for immunotherapy in malignant and immune disorders. Cancer Res 50:1495–1502

Kandaswamy R, Stock PG, Gustafson SK, Skeans MA, Curry MA, Prentice MA, Fox A, Israni AK, Snyder JJ, Kasiske BL (2017) OPTN/SRTR 2016 annual report: pancreas. Am J Transplant 18:114–171

Kim WR, Lake JR, Smith JM, Schladt DP, Skeans MA, Harper AM, Wainright JL, Snyder JJ, Israni AK, Kasiske BL (2017) OPTN/SRTR 2016 annual report: liver. Am J Transplant 18:172–253

Kirk AD, Hale DA, Swanson SJ, Mannon RB (2006) Autoimmune thyroid disease after renal transplantation using depletional induction with alemtuzumab. Am J Transplant 6:1084–1085

Kneuchtle SJ, Fernandez LA, Pirsch JD et al (2004) Campath-1H in renal transplantation: the University of Wisconsin experience. Surgery 136:754–760

Kordelas L, Trenschel R, Koldehoff M, Elmaagacli A, Beelan DW (2008) Successful treatment of EBV PTLD with CNS lymphomas with the monoclonal anti-CD20 antibody rituximab. Onkologie 31:691–693

Kovarik JM, Rawlings E, Sweny P, Fernando O, Moore R, Griffin PJ, Fauchald P, Albrechtsen D, Sodal G, Nordal K, Amlot PL (1996) Pharmacokinetics and immunodynamics of chimeric IL-2 receptor monoclonal antibody SDZ CHI 621 in renal allograft recipients. Transpl Int 9:S32–S33

Kovarik J, Wolf P, Cisterne JM, Mourad G, Lebranchu Y, Lang P, Bourbigot B, Cantarovich D, Girault D, Gerbeau C, Schmidt AG, Soulillou JP (1997) Disposition of basiliximab, an interleukin-2 receptor antibody, in recipients of mismatched cadaver renal allografts. Transplantation 64:1701–1705

Locke JE, Magro CM, Singer AL, Segev DL, Haas M, Hillel AT, King KE, Kraus E, Lees LM, Melancon JK, Stewart

ZA, Warren DS, Zachary AA, Montgomery RA (2009) The use of antibody to complement protein C5 for salvage treatment of severe antibody-mediated rejection. Am J Transplant 9:231–235

Magliocca JF, Knechtle SJ (2006) The evolving role of alemtuzumab (Campath-1H) for immunosuppressive therapy in organ transplantation. Transpl Int 19:705–714

Magnussen K, Klug B, Moller B (1994) CD3 antigen modulation in T-lymphocytes during OKT3 treatment. Transplant Proc 26:1731

Marcos A, Eghtesad B, Fung JJ, Fontes P, Patel K, Devera M, Marsh W, Gayowski T, Demetris AJ, Gray EA, Flynn B, Zeevi A, Murase N, Starzl TE (2004) Use of alemtuzumab and tacrolimus monotherapy for cadaveric liver transplantation: with particular reference to hepatitis C virus. Transplantation 78:966–971

Martin ST, Tichy EM, Gabardi S (2011) Belatacept: a novel biologic for maintenance immunosuppression after renal transplantation. Pharmacotherapy 31:394–407

McCurry KR, Iacono A, Zeevi A, Yousem S, Girnita A, Husain S, Zaldonis D, Johnson B, Hattler BG, Starzl TE (2005) Early outcomes in human lung transplantation with Thymoglobulin or Campath-1H for recipient pretreatment followed by posttransplant tacrolimus near-monotherapy. J Thorac Cardiovasc Surg 130:528–537

McKeage K (2011) Eculizumab: a review of its use in paroxysmal nocturnal haemoglobinuria. Drugs 71:2327–2345

Meier-Kriesche HU, Li S, Gruessner RWG, Fung JJ, Bustami RT, Barr ML, Leichtman AB (2006) Immunosuppression: evolution in practice and trends, 1994–2004. Am J Transplant 6:1111–1131

Morris PJ (2004) Transplantation–a medical miracle of the 20th century. N Engl J Med 351:2678–2680

Morris PJ, Russell NK (2006) Alemtuzumab (Campath-1H): a systematic review in organ transplantation. Transplantation 81:1361–1367

Noguchi M, Adelstein S, Cao X, Leonard WJ (1993) Characterization of the human interleukin-2 receptor gamma gene. J Biol Chem 268:13601–13608

Nojima M, Yoshimoto T, Nakao A, Itahana R, Kyo M, Hashimoto M, Shima H (2005) Sequential blood level monitoring of basiliximab during multisession plasmapheresis in a kidney transplant recipient. Transplant Proc 37:875–878

Novartis Pharmaceuticals: Basiliximab (Simulect) Package Insert. Novartis Pharmaceuticals Corporation, East Hanover. Last updated: 2005

Nozu K, Iijima K, Fujisawa M, Nakagawa A, Yoshikawa N, Matsuo M (2005) Rituximab treatment for posttransplant lymphoproliferative disorder (PTLD) induces complete remission of recurrent nephritic syndrome. Pediatr Nephrol 20:1660–1663

Opelz G, Dohler B (2004) Lymphomas after solid organ transplantation: a collaborative transplant study report. Am J Transplant 4:222–230

Ortho Biotech: Muromonab (Orthoclone) Package Insert. Ortho Biotech, Raritan. Last updated: 2004

Patrick A, Wee A, Hedderman A, Wilson D, Weiss J, Govani M (2011) High-dose intravenous rituximab for multifocal, monomorphic primary central nervous system posttransplant lymphoproliferative disorder. J Neuro-Oncol 103:739–743

Penn I, Hammond W, Brettschneider L, Starzl TE (1969) Malignant lymphomas in transplantation patients. Transplant Proc 1:106–112

Pescovitz MD (2006) Rituximab, an anti-CD20 monoclonal antibody: history and mechanism of action. Am J Transplant 6:859–866

Pescovitz MD, Book BK, Sidner RA (2006) Resolution of recurrent focal segmental glomerulosclerosis proteinuria after rituximab treatment. N Engl J Med 354:1961–1963

Pestana JOM, Grinyo JM, Vanrenterghen Y, Becker T, Campistol JM, Florman S, Garcia VD, Kamar N, Lang P, Manfro RC, Massari P, Rial MD, Schnitzler MA, Vitko S, Duan T, Block A, Harler MB, Durrbach A (2012) Three year outcomes from BENEFIT-EXT: a phase III study of belatacept versus cyclosporine in recipients of extended criteria donor kidneys. Am J Transplant 12(3):630–639

Press OW, Appelbaum F, Ledbetter JA, Martin PJ, Zarling J, Kidd P, Thomas ED (1987) Monoclonal antibody 1F5 (anti-CD20) serotherapy of human B cell lymphomas. Blood 69:584–591

Queen C, Schneider WP, Selick HE, Payne PW, Landolfi NF, Duncan JF, Avdalovic NM, Levitt M, Junghans RP, Waldmann TA (1988) A humanized antibody that binds to the interleukin 2 receptor. Proc Natl Acad Sci U S A 86:10029–10033

Reid ME, Olsson ML (2005) Human blood group antigens and antibodies. In: Hoffman R, Benz EJ (eds) Hematology: basic principles and practice, 4th edn. Churchill Livingstone, Philadelphia, pp 2370–2374

Robb RJ, Munck A, Smith KA (1981) T cell growth factor receptors: quantitation, specific and biological relevance. J Exp Med 154:1455–1474

Rostaing L, Massari P, Garcia VD, Mancilla-Urrea E, Nainan G, del Carmen RM, Steinberg S, Vincenti F, Shi R, Di Russo G, Thomas D, Grinyo J (2011) Switching from calcineurin inhibitor based regimens to a belatacept based regimen in renal transplant recipients: a randomized phase II study. Clin J Am Soc Nephrol 6:430–439

Sebba A (2008) Tocilizumab: the first interleukin-6-receptor inhibitor. Am J Health Syst Pharm 65:1413–1418

Serrano OK, Friedmann P, Ahsanuddin S, Millan C, Ben-Yaacov A, Kayler LK (2015) Outcomes associated with steroid avoidance and Alemtuzumab among kidney transplant recipients. Clin J Am Soc Nephrol 10:2030–2038

Shibuya H, Yoneyama M, Nakamura Y, Harada H, Hatakeyama M, Minamoto S, Kno T, Doi T, White R, Taniguchi T (1990) The human interleukin-2 receptor beta-chain gene: genomic organization, promoter analysis and chromosomal assignment. Nucleic Acids Res 18:3697–3703

Shyu S, Dew MA, Pilewski JM, Dabbs AJD, Zaldonis DB, Studer SM, Crespo MM, Toyoda Y, Bermudez CA, McCurry KR (2011) Five-year outcomes with alemtuzumab induction after lung transplantation. J Heart Lung Transplant 30:743–754

Smith JM, Weaver T, Skeans MA, Horslen SP, Harper AM, Snyder JJ, Israni AK, Kasiske BL (2017) OPTN/SRTR 2016 annual report: intesting. Am J Transplant 18:254–290

Stegall MD, Gloor JM (2010) Deciphering antibody-mediated rejection: new insights into mechanisms and treatment. Curr Opin Organ Transplant 15:8–10

Stegall MD, Diwan T, Raghavaiah S, Cornell LD, Burns J, Dean PG, Cosio FG, Gandhi MJ, Kremers W, Gloor JM (2011) Terminal complement inhibition decreases antibody-mediated rejection in sensitized renal transplant recipients. Am J Transplant 11:245–2413

Strologo LD, Guzzo I, Laurenzi C, Vivarelli M, Parodi A, Barbano G, Camilla R, Scozzola F, Amore A, Ginevri F, Murer L (2009) Use of rituximab in focal glomerulosclerosis relapses after renal transplantation. Transplantation 88:417–420

Swinnen LJ, Costanzo-Nordin MR, Fisher SG, O'Sullivan EJ, Johnson MR, Heroux AL, Dizikes GJ, Pifarre R, Fisher RI (1990) Increased incidence of lymphoproliferative disorder after immunosuppression with the monoclonal antibody OKT3 in cardiac-transplant recipients. N Engl J Med 323:1723–1728

Teuteberg JJ, Shullo MA, Zomak R, Toyoda Y, McNamara DM, Bermudex C, Kormos RL, McCurry KR (2010) Alemtuzumab induction prior to cardiac transplantation with lower intensity maintenance immunosuppression: one-year outcomes. Am J Transplant 10:382–388

Tobinai K (2003) Rituximab and other emerging antibodies as molecular target-based therapy of lymphoma. Int J Clin Oncol 8:212–223

Tsurushita N, Hinton PR, Kumar S (2005) Design of humanized antibodies: from anti-Tac to Zenapax. Methods 36:69–83

Tzakis AG, Tryphonopoulos P, Kato T, Nishida S, Levi DM, Madariaga JR, Gaynor JJ, De Faria W, Regev A, Esquenazi V, Weppler D, Ruiz P, Miller J (2004) Preliminary experience with alemtuzumab (Campath-1H) and low-dose tacrolimus immunosuppression in adult liver transplantation. Transplantation 77:1209–1214

Uchiyama T, Border S, Waldmann TA (1981) A monoclonal antibody (anti-Tac) reactive with activated and functionally mature human T cells. J Immunol 126:1393–1397

Valapour M, Lehr CJ, Skeans MA, Smith JM, Carrico R, Uccellini K, Lehman R, Robinson A, Israni AK, Snyder JJ, Kasiske BL (2017) OPTN/SRTR 2016 annual report: lung. Am J Transplant 18:363–433

Van den Hoogen MWF, Hilbrands LB (2011) Use of monoclonal antibodies in renal transplantation. Immunotherapy 3:871–880

Vincenti F, Lantz M, Birnbaum J, Garovoy M, Mould D, Hakimi J, Nieforth K, Light S (1997) A phase I trial of humanized anti-interleukin 2 receptor antibody in renal transplantation. Transplantation 63:33–38

Vincenti F, Kirkman R, Light S, Bumgardner G, Pescovitz M, Halloran P, Neylan J, Wilkinson A, Ekberg H, Gaston R, Backman L, Burdick J (1998) Interleukin-2-receptor blockade with daclizumab to prevent acute rejection in renal transplantation. Daclizumab Triple Therapy Study Group. N Engl J Med 338:161–165

Vincenti F, Larsen CP, Alberu J, Bresnahan B, Garcia VD, Kothari J, Lang P, Urrea EM, Massari P, Mondragon-Ramirez G, Reyes-Acevedo R, Rice K, Rostaing L, Steinberg S, Xing J, Agarwal M, Harler MB, Charpentier B (2012) Three-year outcomes from BENEFIT, a randomized, active-controlled, parallel-group study in adult kidney transplant recipients. Am J Transplant 12:210–217

Vincenti F, Rostaing L, Grinyo J, Rice K, Steinberg S, Gaite L, Moal MC, Mondragon-Ramirez GA, Kothari J, Polinsky MS, Meier-Kriesche HU, Munier S, Larsen CP (2016) Belatacept and long-term outcomes in kidney transplantation. N Engl J Med 374:333–343

Vo AA, Choi J, Cisneros K, Reinsmoen N, Haas M, Ge S, Toyoda M, Kahwaji J, Peng A, Villicana R, Jordan SC (2014) Benefits of rituximab combined with intravenous immunoglobulin for desensitization in kidney transplant recipients. Transplantation 98:312–319

Vo AA, Choi J, Kim I, Louie S, Cisneros K, Kahwaji J, Toyoda M, Ge S, Haas M, Puliyanda D, Reinsmoen N, Peng A, Villicana R, Jordan SC (2015) A phase I/II trial of the interleukin-6 receptor-specific humanized monoclonal (tocilizumab) + intravenous immunoglobulin in difficult to desensitize patients. Transplantation 99:2356–2363

Watson CJ, Bradley JA, Friend PJ, Firth J, Taylor CJ, Bradley JR, Smith KG, Thiru S, Jamieson NV, Hale G, Waldmann H, Calne R (2005) Alemtuzumab (CAMPATH 1H) induction therapy in cadaveric kidney transplantation—efficacy and safety at five years. Am J Transplant 5:1347–1533

Wekerle T, Grinyo JM (2012) Belatacept: from rational design to clinical application. Transpl Int 25:139–150

Wilde MI, Goa KL (1996) Muromonab CD3: a reappraisal of its pharmacology and use of prophylaxis of solid organ transplant rejection. Drugs 51:865–894

Wong JT, Eylath AA, Ghobrial I, Colvin RB (1990) The mechanism of anti-CD3 monoclonal antibodies. Mediation of cytolysis by inter-T cell bridging. Transplantation 50:683–689

26 Antibody-Based Biotherapeutics in Inflammatory Diseases

Honghui Zhou, Yan Xu, and Amarnath Sharma

INTRODUCTION

Inflammatory diseases encompass a broad and diverse spectrum of serious chronic disorders, many of which have significant need for safe and effective pharmacotherapies. The conventional drugs used to treat immune-mediated inflammatory diseases include nonsteroidal anti-inflammatory drugs (NSAIDs), corticosteroids, sulfasalazine, 5-aminosalicylates, methotrexate, azathioprine, and 6-mercaptopurine which have exhibited limited efficacy with significant side effects. The initial rationale and promise of antibody-based biotherapeutics, such as monoclonal antibodies (mAbs), was focused on oncology and organ transplantation (Ehrlich 1891; Gura 2002). Over the last two decades, there has been significant success in developing a number of antibody-based biotherapeutics as a very effective and relatively safe treatment for several inflammatory diseases, and this area of research and development is rapidly expanding. Five of the top-selling mAbs are for the treatment of chronic inflammatory conditions.

Antibody-based biotherapeutics are a subclass of protein therapeutics. These are large molecular weight glycoproteins designed and produced through recombinant DNA technology and require production in eukaryotic cells using bioreactor technology. These modalities have provided many efficacious therapeutic options for patients and are providing significant insights into the underlying complex pathological pathways of these disorders, which, in turn, are identifying new targets for treatment of these diseases. A significant translational insight derived from the clinical development programs of antibody-based pharmacotherapy is the dysregulation of common proinflammatory mediators, such as tumor necrosis factor alpha (TNFα), across diverse rheumatologic, dermatologic, and gastroenterological pathologies. In addition, the observation of patient subsets that are refractory to a particular therapy indicates that dysregulation of different mediators (targets) may be the primary driver of the underlying disease and require a different treatment. Antibody-based biotherapeutics embody structural, biochemical, and pharmacologic properties distinct from other biologic or chemically synthesized molecular drugs. In general, they exhibit relatively long half-lives (~2–3 weeks) at therapeutic doses, and have high affinity and target specificity with minimum off-target effects, which usually translate into potent and sustained pharmacodynamic (PD) effects.

Currently approved antibody-based therapies for autoimmune/inflammatory disorders include chimeric, humanized, human mAbs and fusion proteins. The mechanism of action of these agents includes either neutralizing a soluble ligand(s) such as cytokines or binding to receptors to block signaling through ligands, or acting as direct agonist or antagonist. The examples of neutralizing soluble ligands include TNFα (infliximab, golimumab, adalimumab, etanercept, certolizumab), interleukin (IL)-12/IL-23 (ustekinumab), IL-23 (guselkumab), IL-17A (secukinumab and ixekizumab), IL-5 (mepolizumab and reslizumab), IL-1β (canakinumab, rilonacept) and soluble immunoglobulin E (IgE, omalizumab). The examples of binding to receptors include IL-4 receptor (dupilumab), IL-5 receptor (benralizumab), IL-6 receptor (tocilizumab, sarilumab) and IL-17 receptor A (brodalumab). The examples of direct agonist or anti-agonist include anti-CD80/CD86 agents to inhibit lymphocyte activation (abatacept, belimumab), CD20 directed cytolytic agents (rituximab and ocrelizumab) and anti-integrin agents to inhibit lymphocyte migration (natalizumab and vedolizumab). Table 26.1 summarizes the 25 antibody-based biotherapeutics that are currently approved and

Updated from Chapter 20 in the fourth Edition authors Zhou, Xu, Mascelli and Davis.

H. Zhou (✉) · Y. Xu · A. Sharma
Clinical Pharmacology and Pharmacometrics, Janssen Research and Development, Spring House, PA, USA
e-mail: hzhou2@its.jnj.com

D. J. A. Crommelin et al. (eds.), *Pharmaceutical Biotechnology*, https://doi.org/10.1007/978-3-030-00710-2_26

Part A: Indication, mechanism of action, recommended dose regimen and pharmaceuticals considerations					
Product	**Target**	**Indication[a]**	**Mechanism of action**	**Recommended dose regimen[a]**	**Pharmaceutical considerations[a]**
Anti-TNFα					
Adalimumab (Humira®)	TNFα	RA, PsA, AS, pJIA, PsO, CD, pediatric CD, UC, HS and UV	Adalimumab binds specifically to TNFα and blocks its interaction with the p55 and p75 cell surface TNF receptors. Adalimumab also lyses surface TNF expressing cells *in vitro* in the presence of complement. Adalimumab does not bind or inactivate lymphotoxin (TNF-β)	Adalimumab should be administered as SC injection *RA, PsA, and AS*: The recommended dose of adalimumab is 40 mg SC q2w *pJIA (2 years and older):* The recommended dose of adalimumab is SC q2w at a dose level of 10, 20 and 40 mg for pediatric patients weighting 10 to <15 kg, 15 to <30 kg and ≥30 kg, respectively *PsO and UV*: The recommended dose of adalimumab is 80 mg initial SC dose followed by 40 mg SC q2w *CD and UC*: The recommended dose of adalimumab is 160 mg initial dose, 80 mg dose 2 weeks later, followed by 40 mg SC q2w *Pediatric CD (6 years and older)*: The recommended dose for pediatric patients weighing 17 to <40 kg is 80 mg initial dose, 40 mg dose 2 weeks later, followed by 20 mg SC q2w. Pediatric patients weighing ≥40 kg should be administered following the adult dose regimen *HS*: The recommended dose is 160 mg initial dose, 80 mg dose 2 weeks later, followed by 40 mg SC qw	Adalimumab is a human IgG1 mAb with an apparent MW of ~ 148 kDa Adalimumab is supplied as a preservative-free, sterile solution and is provided as single-use pens (80 mg/0.8 mL, 40 mg/0.8 mL, 40 mg/0.4 mL), prefilled syringes (80 mg/0.8 mL, 40 mg/0.8 mL, 40 mg/0.4 mL, 20 mg/0.4 mL, 20 mg/0.2 mL, 10 mg/0.2 mL, 10 mg/0.1 mL) and a single-use institutional use vial (40 mg/0.8 mL) Keep refrigerated at 2 °C–8 °C. Store in original carton until time of use. Do not freeze. If needed, may be stored at room temperature up to a maximum of 25 °C for a period of up to 14 days, with protection from light
Certolizumab pegol (Cimzia®)	TNFα	RA, PsA, AS and CD	Certolizumab pegol binds to human TNFα and selectively neutralizes TNFα (but not TNFβ) TNFα is a key pro-inflammatory cytokine with a central role in inflammatory processes	Certolizumab pegol should be administered as SC injection *RA and PsA*: The recommended dose of certolizumab pegol is 400 mg SC initially and at weeks 2 and 4, followed by 200 mg SC q2w. For maintenance dosing, 400 mg SC q4w can also be considered *AS*: The recommended dose of certolizumab pegol is 400 mg SC initially and at weeks 2 and 4, followed 200 mg SC q2w or 400 mg SC q4w *CD*: The recommended dose of certolizumab pegol is 400 mg SC initially and at weeks 2 and 4. For patients achieving clinical response, the recommended maintenance dose regimen is 400 mg SC q4w	Certolizumab pegol is a humanized antibody Fab' fragment, conjugated to an approximately 40-kDa PEG. The MW of certolizumab pegol is ~ 91 kDa Certolizumab pegol is a clear to opalescent solution that is colorless to pale yellow and essentially free from particulates. Certolizumab pegol is supplied as either 200 mg sterile, white, lyophilized powder for reconstitution in a single use vial or as a 200 mg/mL sterile solution in a single-use prefilled syringe Keep refrigerated at 2 °C–8 °C. Store in original carton until time of use. Protect from light. Do not freeze

Table 26.1 ■ Antibody-based biotherapeutics in immune-mediated inflammatory diseases

Etanercept (Enbrel®)	TNFα	RA, PsA, AS, pJIA and PsO	Etanercept is a dimeric soluble form of the p75 TNF receptor that can bind TNF molecules. Etanercept inhibits binding of TNF-α and TNF-β to cell surface TNF receptors, rendering TNF biologically inactive	Etanercept should be administered as SC injection *RA, PsA, and AS*: The recommended dose of etanercept is 50 mg SC qw with or without methotrexate *Adult PsO*: The recommended dose of etanercept is 50 mg twice weekly for 3 months, followed by 50 mg SC qw *pJIA (2 years and older) and pediatric PsO (4 years and older):* The recommended dose of etanercept is 0.8 mg/kg SC qw, with a maximum of 50 mg per week	Etanercept is a dimeric fusion protein with an apparent MW of ~ 150 kDa Etanercept is supplied as clear and colorless, sterile, preservative-free solution in single-dose prefilled syringes (50 mg/mL and 25 mg/mL) and a single-dose prefilled SureClick autoinjector (50 mg/mL). Etanercept is also supplied in a multiple-dose vial (25 mg/vial) as a sterile, white, preservative-free, lyophilized powder for reconstitution prior to injection Keep refrigerated at 2 °C–8 °C. Store in original carton until time of use. Protect from light. Do not freeze or shake. For convenience, storage of individual syringes or autoinjectors at room temperature (20 °C–25 °C) for a maximum single period of 14 days is permissible, with protection from light and sources of heat
Golimumab (Simponi®, Simponi Aria®)	TNFα	RA, PsA, AS, and UC nr-AxSpA and pJIA (EU only, SmPC)	Golimumab binds to both the soluble and transmembrane bioactive forms of human TNFα. This interaction prevents the binding of TNFα to its receptors, thereby inhibiting the biological activity of TNFα	Golimumab may be administered as IV infusion and SC injection *IV infusion for RA, PsA, and AS*: The recommended dose of golimumab is 2 mg/kg IV infusion over 30 mins at weeks 0 and 4, then 2 mg/kg IV q8w thereafter *SC injection for RA, PsA, AS and nr-AxSpA*: The recommended dose of golimumab is 50 mg SC monthly. Consider 100 mg SC monthly if no adequate clinical response after 3 or 4 doses *SC injection for UC*: The recommended dose of golimumab is 200 mg SC at week 0, followed by 100 mg SC at week 2 and then 100 mg SC q4w SC injection for pJIA (≥40 kg): The recommended dose of golimumab is 50 mg SC q4w	Golimumab is a human IgG1κ mAb with an apparent MW of ~ 150–151 kDa For IV use, golimumab used is supplied as a preservative-free, colorless to light yellow solution in a single-dose vial (50 mg/vial) For SC use, golimumab is supplied as a preservative-free, clear to slightly opalescent, colorless to light yellow solution in single-dose prefilled syringes (50 mg/0.5 mL and 100 mg/1 mL) and single-dose prefilled SmartJet® autoinjectors (50 mg/0.5 mL and 100 mg/1 mL) Keep refrigerated at 2 °C–8 °C. Store in original carton until time of use. Protect from light. Do not freeze or shake

Table 26.1 ■ (continued)

Part A: Indication, mechanism of action, recommended dose regimen and pharmaceuticals considerations

Product	Target	Indication[a]	Mechanism of action	Recommended dose regimen[a]	Pharmaceutical considerations[a]
Infliximab (Remicade®)	TNFα	RA, PsA, AS, PsO, CD, UC, pediatric CD, pediatric UC	Infliximab neutralizes the biological activity of TNFα by binding to the soluble and transmembrane forms of TNFα and inhibits binding of TNFα with its receptors. Infliximab does not neutralize TNFβ	Infliximab should be administered as IV infusion *RA*: The recommended dose of infliximab is 3 mg/kg at 0, 2, and 6 weeks, followed by 3 mg/kg q8w thereafter. Some patients may benefit from increasing the dose up to 10 mg/kg or treating as often as q4w *PsA and PsO*: The recommended dose of infliximab is 5 mg/kg at 0, 2, and 6 weeks, followed by 5 mg/kg q8w thereafter *AS*: The recommended dose of infliximab is 5 mg/kg at 0, 2, and 6 weeks, followed by 5 mg/kg q6w thereafter *CD and UC*: The recommended dose of infliximab is 5 mg/kg at 0, 2, and 6 weeks, followed by 5 mg/kg q8w thereafter. Some CD patients who initially respond to treatment may benefit from increasing the dose to 10 mg/kg if they later lose their response *Pediatric CD and UC (6 years of age and older)*: The recommended dose of infliximab is 5 mg/kg at 0, 2, and 6 weeks, followed by 5 mg/kg q8w thereafter	Infliximab is a chimeric IgG1κ mAb with an apparent MW of ~ 149.1 kDa Infliximab is supplied as sterile, preservative free, white, lyophilized powder in a single-dose vial for reconstitution prior to IV infusion. Each vial contains 100 mg of infliximab for final reconstitution volume of 10 mL Keep refrigerated at 2 °C–8 °C. Store in original carton until time of use. Protect from light. Unopened infliximab vials may also be stored at temperatures up to a maximum of 30 °C for a single period of up to 6 months but not exceeding the original expiration date. Any unused portion of the infusion solution should not be stored for reuse
Anti-IL-1β					
Canakinumab (Ilaris®)	IL-1β	CAPS and sJIA	Canakinumab binds to human IL-1β and neutralizes its activity by blocking its interaction with IL-1 receptors, but it does not bind IL-1α or IL-1 receptor antagonist	Canakinumab may be administered as IV infusion and SC injection depending on the age and body weight categories *CAPS (4 years and older)*: The recommended dose of canakinumab is 150 mg SC q8w for patients weighing >40 kg and 2 mg/kg SC q8w for patients weighing ≥15 kg and ≤ 40 kg. For children 15–40 kg with an inadequate response, the dose can be increased to 3 mg/kg SC q8w *sJIA (2 years and older)*: The recommended dose of canakinumab is 4 mg/kg (with maximum of 300 mg) SC q4w for pediatric patients weighing ≥7.5 kg	Canakinumab is a human IgG1κ mAb with an apparent MW of ~ 145 kDa For IV use, canakinumab is supplied as white, preservative-free, lyophilized powder in a single-dose vial (150 mg/vial) for reconstitution and dilution prior to IV infusion For SC use, canakinumab is supplied as a sterile, preservative-free, clear to opalescent, colorless to slightly pale-yellow solution in a single-dose glass vial (150 mg/mL) Keep refrigerated at 2 °C–8 °C. Store in original carton until time of use. Protect from light. Do not freeze

Rilonacept (Arcalyst®)	IL-1β	CAPS	Rilonacept blocks IL-1β signaling by acting as a soluble decoy receptor that binds IL-1β and prevents its interaction with cell surface receptors. Rilonacept also binds IL-1α and IL-1 receptor antagonist with reduced affinity	Rilonacept should be administered as SC injection *Adult CAPS*: The recommended dose of rilonacept is 320 mg SC as a loading dose, followed by a maintenance dose regime of 160 mg SC qw *Pediatric CAPS (12 years of age and older)*: The recommended dose of rilonacept is 4.4 mg/kg (up to 320 mg) SC as a loading dose, followed by a maintenance dose regime of 2.2 mg/kg (up to 160 mg) SC qw	Rilonacept is a dimeric fusion protein with an apparent MW of ~ 147 kDa Rilonacept is supplied as sterile, preservative-free, white to off-white, lyophilized powder in a single-use vial. After reconstitution, each vial contains 80 mg/mL rilonacept and a volume of up to 2 mL can be withdrawn. The resulting solution is viscous, clear, colorless to pale yellow, and essentially free from particulates Keep refrigerated at 2 °C–8 °C. Protect the vials from light by storing in the original package until time of use. After reconstitution, rilonacept may be kept at room temperature, should be kept from light, and should be used within 3 h of reconstitution
Anti-IL-5					
Mepolizumab (Nucala®)	IL-5	Asthma, EGPA	Mepolizumab binds to IL-5, inhibiting the bioactivity of IL-5 by blocking its binding to the alpha chain of the IL-5 receptor complex expressed on the eosinophil cell surface IL-5 is the major cytokine responsible for the growth and differentiation, recruitment, activation, and survival of eosinophils, which plays a role in the pathogenesis of asthma and EGPA	Mepolizumab should be administered as SC injection *PsO*: The recommended dose of mepolizumab is 300 mg administrated as three separate 100-mg SC injections q4w *EGPA*: The recommended dose of mepolizumab is 300 mg administrated as three separate 100-mg SC injections q4w	Mepolizumab is a humanized IgG1 mAb with an apparent MW of ~ 149 kDa Mepolizumab is supplied as sterile, clear, white to off-white, preservative-free, lyophilized powder in cartons of a single-dose glass vial and a flip-off seal for reconstitution and SC injection (100 mg/vial) Keep refrigerated below 25 °C. Store in the original package to protect from light
Reslizumab (Cinqair®)	IL-5	Asthma	Reslizumab binds to IL-5, inhibiting the bioactivity of IL-5 by blocking its binding to the α chain of the IL-5 receptor complex expressed on the eosinophil cell surface IL-5 is the major cytokine responsible for the growth and differentiation, recruitment, activation, and survival of eosinophils, which plays a role in the pathogenesis of asthma	Reslizumab should be administered as IV infusion *Asthma*: The recommended dose of reslizumab is 3 mg/kg q4w by IV infusion over 20–50 mins	Reslizumab is a human IgG4κ mAb with an apparent MW of ~ 147 kDa Reslizumab is a sterile, preservative-free, clear to slightly hazy/opalescent, colorless to slightly yellow solution and supplied in a single-use vial (100 mg/10 mL) Keep refrigerated at 2 °C–8 °C. Do not freeze or shake. Protect the vials from light by storing in the original package until time of use
Anti-IL-17A					
Ixekizumab (Taltz®)	IL-17A	PsA, PsO	Ixekizumab selectively binds with IL-17A and inhibits its interaction with the IL-17 receptor IL-17A is a naturally occurring cytokine that is involved in normal inflammatory and immune responses. Ixekizumab inhibits the release of proinflammatory cytokines and chemokines	Ixekizumab should be administered as SC injection *PsO*: The recommended dose of ixekizumab is 160 mg SC at week 0, followed by 80 mg SC at weeks 2, 4, 6, 8, 10, and 12, then 80 mg SC q4w thereafter *PsA*: The recommended dose of ixekizumab is 160 mg SC at week 0, followed by 80 mg SC q4w thereafter. For PsA patients with coexistent moderate-to-severe PsO, the dose regimen for PsO can be used	Ixekizumab is a human IgG4 mAb with an apparent MW of ~ 146.2 kDa Ixekizumab is supplied as a sterile, preservative free, clear, colorless to light yellow solution in a single-dose prefilled syringe or single-dose prefilled autoinjector (80 mg/mL) Keep refrigerated at 2 °C–8 °C. Store in original carton until time of use. Protect from light. Do not freeze or shake. Discard any unused portion

Table 26.1 ■ (continued)

Part A: Indication, mechanism of action, recommended dose regimen and pharmaceuticals considerations

Product	Target	Indication[a]	Mechanism of action	Recommended dose regimen[a]	Pharmaceutical considerations[a]
Secukinumab (Cosentyx®)	IL-17A	PsA, AS and PsO	Secukinumab binds to IL-17A and inhibits its interaction with the IL-17 receptor IL-17A is a naturally occurring cytokine that is involved in normal inflammatory and immune responses. Secukinumab inhibits the release of proinflammatory cytokines and chemokines	Secukinumab should be administered as SC injection *PsO*: The recommended dose of secukinumab is 300 mg SC at weeks 0, 1, 2, 3, and 4 followed by 300 mg SC q4w. For some patients, a dose of 150 mg may be acceptable *PsA*: For PsA patients with coexistent moderate to severe PsO, use the secukinumab dose for PsO. For other PsA patients, the recommended dose of secukinumab is 150 mg SC q4w with or without of a loading dosage (i.e., 150 mg SC at weeks 0, 1, 2, 3, and 4). If a patient continues to have active PsA, consider a dosage of 300 mg *AS:* The recommended dose of secukinumab is 150 mg SC q4w with or without of a loading dosage (i.e., 150 mg SC at weeks 0, 1, 2, 3, and 4)	Secukinumab is a human IgG1κ mAb with an apparent MW of ~ 151 kDa Secukinumab is supplied in a single-dose Sensoready pen or prefilled syringe as a sterile, preservative-free, clear to slightly opalescent, colorless to slightly yellow solution (150 mg/1.14 mL). Secukinumab is also supplied as sterile, preservative free, white to slightly yellow, lyophilized powder in a single-use vial (150 mg /vial) for reconstitution and injection Keep refrigerated at 2 °C–8 °C. Protect from light by storing in the original package until time of use. Do not freeze or shake
Anti-IL12/IL-23					
Ustekinumab (Stelara®)	IL12/IL23	PsO, PsA, CD and adolescent PsO	Ustekinumab binds to the p40 protein subunit used by both the IL-12 and IL-23 cytokines IL-12 and IL-23 are naturally occurring cytokines that are involved in inflammatory and immune responses, such as natural killer cell activation and CD4+ T-cell differentiation and activation. IL-12 and IL-23 have been implicated as important contributors to chronic inflammations	Ustekinumab may be used as IV infusion and as SC injection *PsO*: The recommended dose of ustekinumab is 45 mg SC initially and 4 weeks later, followed by 45 mg SC q12w for patients weighing ≤100 kg; the recommended dose for patients weighing >100 kg is 90 mg SC initially and 4 weeks later, followed by 90 mg SC q12w *PsO adolescent (12 years of age and older):* The recommended dose of ustekinumab is SC weight-based-dosing (0.75 mg/kg, 45 mg and 90 mg for weight range of <60 kg, 60–100 kg and ≥100 kg, respectively) at the initial dose, 4 weeks later, then q12w thereafter *PsA*: The recommended dose of ustekinumab is 45 mg SC initially and 4 weeks later, followed by 45 mg SC q12w. For patients with co-existent moderate-to-severe PsO weighing >100 kg, consider a dosage of 90 mg *CD*: The recommended induction dose of ustekinumab is a singe IV infusion using weight-based-dosing (~ 6.g/kg, i.e., 260 mg, 390 mg, and 520 mg for weight range of ≤55 kg, 55–85 kg and >85 kg, respectively). The recommended maintenance dose of ustekinumab is 90 mg SC 8 weeks after the initial IV dose, then q8w thereafter	Ustekinumab is a human IgG1κ mAb with an apparent MW of ~ 148.1–149.7 kDa Ustekinumab is a sterile, preservative-free, colorless to light yellow solution and may contain a few small translucent or white particles For IV use, ustekinumab is supplied as a single-dose glass vial with a coated stopper (130 mg/26 mL) For SC use, ustekinumab is supplied in single-dose prefilled syringes (45 mg/0.5 mL and 90 mg/ 1 mL) or a single-dose vial with a coated stopper (45 mg/0.5 mL) Keep refrigerated at 2 °C–8 °C. Store vials upright. Do not freeze or shake. Keep the product in the original carton to protect from light until the time of use

Anti-IL-23					
Guselkumab (Tremfya®)	IL-23	PsO	Guselkumab selectively binds to the p19 subunit of IL-23 and inhibits its interaction with the IL-23 receptor IL-23 is a naturally occurring cytokine that is involved in normal inflammatory and immune responses. Guselkumab inhibits the release of proinflammatory cytokines and chemokines	Guselkumab should be administered as SC injection *PsO*: The recommended dose of guselkumab is 100 mg SC at weeks 0 and 4, followed by 100 mg SC q8w thereafter	Guselkumab is a human IgG1λ mAb with an apparent MW of ~ 143.6 kDa Guselkumab is supplied as a sterile, preservative free, clear, colorless to light yellow solution that may contain small translucent particles in a single-dose prefilled syringe (100 mg/mL) Keep refrigerated at 2 °C–8 °C. Store in original carton until time of use. Protect from light. Do not freeze or shake
Anti-IL-4 receptor					
Dupilumab (Dupixent®)	IL-4 receptor subunit α	AD	Dupilumab inhibits IL-4 and IL-13 signaling by binding to the IL-4 receptor subunit α shared by the IL-4 and IL-13 receptor complexes Blocking IL-4 receptor subunit α with dupilumab inhibits IL-4 and IL-13 cytokine-induced responses, including the release of proinflammatory cytokines, chemokines and IgE	Dupilumab should be administered as SC injection *AD*: The recommended dose of dupilumab is 600 mg (two 300 mg injections) SC initially, followed by 300 mg SC q2w	Dupilumab is a human IgG4 mAb with an apparent MW of ~ 147 kDa Dupilumab is supplied as a sterile, preservative-free, clear to slightly opalescent, colorless to pale yellow solution in a single-use prefilled syringe with or without needle shield (300 mg/2 mL) Keep refrigerated at 2 °C–8 °C. Store in original carton until time of use. Protect from light. Do not freeze or shake. Do not expose to heat. If necessary, pre-filled syringes may be kept at room temperature up to 25 °C for a maximum of 14 days
Anti-IL-5 receptor					
Benralizumab (Fasenra®)	IL-5 receptor	Asthma	Benralizumab binds to the α subunit of the human IL-5 receptor, which expressed on the surface of eosinophils and basophils The absence of fucose in the Fc domain of benralizumab facilitates binding to FcγRIII receptors on immune effectors cells, such as natural killer cells, leading to apoptosis of eosinophils and basophils through antibody-dependent cell-mediated cytotoxicity (ADCC)	Benralizumab should be administered as SC injection *Asthma*: The recommended dose of benralizumab is 30 mg SC at weeks 0, 4 and 8, followed by 30 mg q8w	Benralizumab is a humanized afucosylate IgG1κ mAb with an apparent MW of 150 kDa Benralizumab is supplied in a single-dose prefilled syringe (30 mg/1 mL) with needle safety guard as few translucent or white to off-white particles may be present in the solution and may contain a few translucent or white to off-white particles Keep refrigerated at 2 °C–8 °C. Store in original carton to protect from light. Do not freeze or shake. Prior to administration, warm benralizumab by leaving carton at room temperature for about 30 mins. Administer benralizumab within 24 h

Table 26.1 ■ (continued)

Part A: Indication, mechanism of action, recommended dose regimen and pharmaceuticals considerations

Product	Target	Indication[a]	Mechanism of action	Recommended dose regimen[a]	Pharmaceutical considerations[a]
Anti-IL-6 receptor					
Sarilumab (Kevzara®)	IL-6 receptor	RA	Sarilumab binds to both soluble and membrane-bound IL-6 receptors, and has been shown to inhibit IL-6-mediated signaling through these receptors IL-6 is a pleiotropic pro-inflammatory cytokine produced by a variety of cell types including T-and B-cells, lymphocytes, monocytes, and fibroblasts. IL-6 is also produced by synovial and endothelial cells leading to local production of IL-6 in joints affected by inflammatory processes	Sarilumab should be administered as SC injection *RA*: The recommended dose of sarilumab is 200 mg SC q2w	Sarilumab is a human IgG1 mAb with an apparent MW of ~ 150 kDa Sarilumab is supplied as a sterile, colorless to pale yellow, preservative-free solution in single-dose pre-filled syringes (150 mg/1.14 mL or 200 mg/1.14 mL) Keep refrigerated at 2 °C–8 °C. Protect from light by storing in the original package until time of use. Do not freeze or shake. If needed, sarilumab may be stored at room temperature up to 25 °C up to 14 days in the outer carton. Do not store above 25 °C. After removal from the refrigerator, use sarilumab within 14 days or discard

Table 26.1 ■ (continued)

Tocilizumab (Actemra®)	IL-6 receptor	RA, pJIA, sJIA, GCA, and CRS	Tocilizumab binds to both soluble and membrane-bound IL-6 receptors, and has been shown to inhibit IL-6-mediated signaling through these receptors IL-6 is a pleiotropic pro-inflammatory cytokine produced by a variety of cell types including T-and B-cells, lymphocytes, monocytes, and fibroblasts. IL-6 is also produced by synovial and endothelial cells leading to local production of IL-6 in joints affected by inflammatory processes	Tocilizumab may be used as IV infusion and SC injection *RA*: for IV use, the recommended starting dose of tocilizumab is 4 mg/kg IV q4w, followed by an increase to 8 mg/kg IV q4w based on clinical response For SC use, the recommended dose of tocilizumab is 162 mg SC q2w, followed by an increase to qw based on clinical response for patients <100 kg; the recommended dose for patients ≥100 kg is 162 mg SC qw *pJIA (2 years of age and older)*: The recommended dose of tocilizumab is 10 mg/kg or 8 mg/kg IV q4w for patients weighing <30 kg or ≥30 kg, respectively, alone or in combination with methotrexate *sJIA (2 years of age and older)*: The recommended dose is 12 mg/kg or 8 mg/kg IV q2w for patients weighing <30 kg or ≥30 kg, respectively, alone or in combination with methotrexate *GCA*: The recommended dose is 162 mg SC qw, in combination with a tapering course of glucocorticoids. Dose regimen of 162 mg SC q2w in combination with a tapering course of glucocorticoids may be prescribed based on clinical considerations. Tocilizumab can be used alone following discontinuation of glucocorticoids *CRS (2 years of age and older)*: The recommended dose of tocilizumab is 12 mg/kg or 8 mg/kg IV for patients weighing <30 kg or ≥ 30 kg, respectively, alone or in combination with corticosteroids. If no clinical improvement after the first dose, up to three additional doses of tocilizumab may be administered. The interval between consecutive doses should be at least 8 h. Doses exceeding 800 mg per infusion are not recommended	Tocilizumab is a human IgG1κ mAb with an apparent MW of ~ 151 kDa For IV use, tocilizumab is supplied as a sterile, preservative-free, clear, colorless to pale yellow liquid in single-use vials at a concentration of 20 mg/mL (80 mg/4 mL, 200 mg/10 mL, and 400 mg/20 mL) for further dilution prior to IV infusion For SC use, tocilizumab is supplied as a sterile, preservative-free, clear, colorless to slightly yellowish solution and is provided in a single-dose prefilled syringe (162 mg/0.9 mL) Keep refrigerated at 2 °C–8 °C. Do not freeze. Protect from light by storing in the original package until time of use, and keep syringes dry

Part A: Indication, mechanism of action, recommended dose regimen and pharmaceuticals considerations

Product	Target	Indication[a]	Mechanism of action	Recommended dose regimen[a]	Pharmaceutical considerations[a]
Anti-IL-17 receptor A					
Brodalumab (Siliq®)	IL-17 receptor A	PsO	Brodalumab selectively binds to human IL-17 receptor A and inhibits its interactions with cytokines IL-17A, IL-17F, IL-17C, IL-17A/F heterodimer and IL-25 IL-17 receptor A is a protein expressed on the cell surface and is a required component of receptor complexes utilized by multiple IL-17 family cytokines. Blocking IL17 receptor A inhibits IL-17 cytokine-induced responses including the release of pro-inflammatory cytokines and chemokines	Brodalumab should be administered as SC injection *PsO*: The recommended dose of brodalumab is 210 mg SC at weeks 0, 1 and 2 followed by 210 mg q2w	Brodalumab is a human IgG2κ mAb with an apparent MW of ~ 144 kDa Brodalumab is supplied in a single-dose prefilled syringe (210 mg/1.5 mL) as a clear to slightly opalescent, colorless to slightly yellow solution and may contain a few translucent to white, amorphous particles Keep refrigerated at 2 °C–8 °C. Store in original carton until time of use. Do not freeze or shake. Protect from light. If needed, may be stored at room temperature up to a maximum of 25 °C for a single period of up to 14 days, with protection from light and source of heat
Anti-IgE					
Omalizumab (Xolair®)	IgE	Asthma and CIU	Omalizumab binds to IgE and lowers free IgE levels. Subsequently, IgE receptors (FcεRI) on cells down-regulate, such as mast cells and basophils Reduction in surface-bound IgE on FcεRI-bearing cells limits the degree of release of mediators of the allergic response	Omalizumab should be administered as SC injection *Asthma (6 years of age and older)*: The recommended dose of omalizumab is 75–375 mg SC q2w or q4w, with dose and dosing frequency determined by pretreatment serum IgE levels and body weight *CIU (12 years of age and older)*: The recommended dose of omalizumab is 150 or 300 mg SC q4w	Omalizumab is a humanized IgG1κ mAb with an apparent MW of ~ 149 kDa Omalizumab is supplied as sterile, preservative free, clear, white to off-white, lyophilized powder in a single-dose vial (150 mg/vial) for reconstitution and SC injection Keep refrigerated below 25 °C. Protect from light. Use the solution within 8 h following reconstitution when stored in the vial at 2–8 °C, or within 4 h of reconstitution when stored at room temperature
Anti-integrin					
Natalizumab (Tysabri®)	Integrin	CD and MS	Natalizumab binds to the α4-subunit of α4β1 and α4β7 integrins expressed on the surface of all leukocytes except neutrophils, and inhibits the α4-mediated adhesion of leukocytes to their counter-receptor(s)	Natalizumab should be administered as IV infusion *CD and MS*: The recommended dose of natalizumab is 300 mg q4w by IV infusion over 1 h	Natalizumab is a human IgG4κ mAb with an apparent MW of ~ 149 kDa Natalizumab is supplied as a colorless and clear to slightly opalescent solution for dilution prior to IV infusion and is provided in a sterile, single-use vial free of preservatives (300 mg/15 mL) Keep refrigerated at 2 °C–8 °C. Protect from light. Do not freeze or shake. If not used immediately, store the diluted Natalizumab solution for infusion at 2 °C–8 °C. Natalizumab solution for infusion must be administered within 8 h of preparation

Vedolizumab (Entyvio®)	Integrin	CD and UC	Vedolizumab binds to the α4β7 integrin and blocks the interaction of α4β7 integrin with MAdCAM-1 and inhibits the migration of memory T-lymphocytes across the endothelium into inflamed gastrointestinal parenchymal tissue. Vedolizumab does not bind to or inhibit function of the α4β1 and αEβ7 integrins and does not antagonize the interaction of α4 integrins with VCAM-1	Vedolizumab should be administered as IV infusion *CD and UC*: The recommended dose of vedolizumab is 300 mg at 0, 2, and 6 weeks by IV infusion over approximately 30 mins, then q8w thereafter	Vedolizumab is a humanized IgG1 mAb with an apparent MW of ~ 147 kDa Vedolizumab is supplied as sterile, preservative free, white to off-white, lyophilized cake in a single-use vial (300 mg/vial) for reconstitution and dilution prior to IV infusion Keep refrigerated at 2 °C–8 °C. Retain in original package to protect from light. Administer infusion solution within 4 h of reconstitution and dilution
Anti-CD80/CD86 Lymphocyte Activation Inhibitor					
Abatacept (Orencia®)	CTLA-4	RA, PsA, and pJIA	Abatacept is a selective costimulation modulator that inhibits T lymphocyte activation by binding to CD80 and CD86, thereby blocking interaction with CD28. This interaction provides a costimulatory signal necessary for full activation of T lymphocytes	Abatacept may be administered as IV infusion and SC injection *IV infusion for RA and PsA*: The recommended dose of abatacept is weight based dosing (~ 10 mg/kg, i.e., 500, 750, and 1000 mg for patients weighing <60 kg, 60–100 kg, and >100 kg, respectively) administered as IV infusion at weeks 0, 2, and 4 and q4w thereafter *SC injection for RA*: The recommended dose of abatacept is 125 mg SC qw with or without an initial IV loading dose (according to body weight categories described above) *SC injection for PsA*: The recommended dose of abatacept is 125 mg SC qw (without the need of an IV loading dose) *IV infusion for pJIA (6 years and older)*: The recommended dose for pediatrics weighing <75 kg is 10 mg/kg at weeks 0, 2, and 4 and q4w by IV infusion. Pediatric patients weighing ≥75 kg should be administered following the IV dose regimen for adult RA (not to exceed 1000 mg/injection) *SC injection for pJIA (2 years and older)*: The recommended dose is SC qw at a body-weight-tired dosing of 50, 87.5 and 125 mg for pJIA patients weighing 10 to <25 kg, 25 to <50 kg and ≥50 kg, respectively	Abatacept is a soluble fusion protein with an apparent MW of ~ 92 kDa For IV use, abatacept is supplied as sterile, white, preservative-free, lyophilized powder in a single-use vial (250 mg/vial) for reconstitution and dilution prior to IV infusion For SC use, abatacept is supplied as a sterile, preservative-free, clear to slightly opalescent, colorless to pale-yellow solution and is provided in single-dose prefilled syringes (50 mg/0.4 mL, 87.5 mg/0.7 mL, and 125 mg/mL), or in a single-dose prefilled ClickJect autoinjector (125 mg/mL) Keep refrigerated at 2 °C–8 °C. Do not freeze. Store in original carton until time of use. Protect from light

Table 26.1 ■ (continued)

Part A: Indication, mechanism of action, recommended dose regimen and pharmaceuticals considerations

Product	Target	Indication[a]	Mechanism of action	Recommended dose regimen[a]	Pharmaceutical considerations[a]
Belimumab (Benlysta®)	BLyS	SLE	Belimumab is a BLyS-specific inhibitor that blocks the binding of soluble BLyS, a B-cell survival factor, to its receptors on B cells. Belimumab does not bind B cells directly, but by binding BLyS Belimumab inhibits the survival of B cells, including autoreactive B cells, and reduces the differentiation of B cells into immunoglobulin-producing plasma cells	Belimumab may be administered as IV infusion and SC injection *IV infusion for SLE*: The recommended dose of belimumab is 10 mg/kg q2w for the first three doses, followed by 10 mg/kg q4w thereafter *SC injection for SLE*: The recommended dose of belimumab is 200 mg qw	Belimumab is a human IgG1λ mAb with an apparent MW of ~ 147 kDa For IV use, belimumab is supplied as a sterile, white to off-white, preservative-free, lyophilized powder in single-dose vials (120 mg/vial or 400 mg/vial) for reconstitution and dilution prior to IV infusion For SC use, belimumab is supplied in a single-dose prefilled syringe or autoinjector as a sterile, preservative-free, clear to opalescent, colorless to pale-yellow solution (200 mg/mL) Keep refrigerated at 2 °C–8 °C. Store in original carton until time of use. Protect from light. Do not freeze or shake. May be stored outside of the refrigerator up to 30 °C for up to 12 h in the original container
Anti-CD-20 cytolytic agent					
Ocrelizumab (Ocrevus®)	CD20	MS	Ocrelizumab directed against CD20-expressing B-cells CD20 is a cell surface antigen present on pre-B and mature B lymphocytes. Following cell surface binding to B lymphocytes, ocrelizumab results in antibody-dependent cell-mediated cytotoxicity (ADCC) and complement-mediated lysis	Ocrelizumab should be administered as IV infusion *MS*: The recommended dose of ocrelizumab is 300 mg IV infusion initially, followed 2 weeks by a second 300 mg IV infusion, and then 600 mg IV infusion every 6 months Pre-medicate with methylprednisolone (or an equivalent corticosteroid) and an antihistamine (e.g., diphenhydramine) prior to each infusion. Monitor patients closely during and for at least 1 h after infusion	Ocrelizumab is a glycosylated human IgG1 mAb with an apparent MW of ~ 149 kDa Ocrelizumab is supplied as preservative-free, sterile, clear or slightly opalescent, and colorless to pale brown solution supplied as a carton containing one 300 mg/10 mL (30 mg/mL) single-dose vial Keep refrigerated at 2 °C–8 °C in the outer carton to protect from light. Do not freeze or shake
Rituximab (Rituxan®)	CD20	RA	Rituximab targets the CD20 antigen expressed on the surface of pre-B and mature B-lymphocytes. Upon binding to CD20, rituximab mediates B-cell lysis	Rituximab should be administered as IV infusion *RA*: The recommended dose of rituximab in combination with methotrexate is two 1000 mg IV infusions separated by 2 weeks (one course) every 24 weeks or based on clinical evaluation, but no more frequent than every 16 weeks. Methylprednisolone 100 mg IV or equivalent glucocorticoid is recommended 30 mins prior to each infusion	Rituximab is a chimeric IgG1κ mAb with an apparent MW of ~ 145 kDa Rituximab is supplied a sterile, clear, colorless, preservative-free liquid concentrate for IV infusion at a concentration of 10 mg/mL in either 100 mg/10 mL or 500 mg/50 mL single-use vials Keep refrigerated at 2 °C–8 °C. Protect from direct sunlight. Do not freeze or shake

Part B: Pharmacokinetics and pharmacokinetics/pharmacodynamics

Product	Target	Indication	Pharmacokinetics	Pharmacokinetics/Pharmacodynamics	Reference[a]
Anti-TNFα					
Adalimumab (Humira®)	TNFα	RA, PsA, AS, pJIA, PsO, CD, pediatric CD, UC, HS and UV	Adalimumab exhibits linear pharmacokinetics with mean terminal half-life being about 2 weeks. The systemic clearance of adalimumab was approximately 12 mL/h. The mean bioavailability of SC adalimumab was 64% In patients with RA, the mean steady-state trough concentrations were about 5 and 8–9 μg/mL without and with concomitant methotrexate, respectively, following 40 mg q2w SC dosing. Methotrexate reduced adalimumab apparent clearance after single and multiple dosing by 29% and 44%, respectively, in patients with RA. Adalimumab concentrations in the synovial fluid from five rheumatoid arthritis patients ranged from 31–96% of those in serum In patients with PsA treated with 40 mg adalimumab SC q2w, the mean steady-state trough concentrations were slightly higher (6–10 μg/mL and 8.5–12 μg/mL, without and with methotrexate, respectively) compared to the concentrations in RA patients treated with the same dose	In patients with RA, relationships between adalimumab concentration and the time course in the reduction of DAS28-ESR score and the serum CRP level were characterized using a direct P/PD model and an indirect response PK/PD model respectively, following E_{max} relationship. The estimated EC_{50} was 11 and 3.6 μg/mL, respectively In patients with RA and PsA, analysis of the adalimumab trough concentration- effect relationship for reduction in DAS28 score suggested that steady-state trough concentration in a range of 5–8 μg/mL was sufficient to reach adequate clinical response In patients with PsO, analysis of the adalimumab trough concentration- effect relationship for improvement in PASI score adalimumab suggested that steady-state trough concentration in a range of 3.5–7 μg/mL was sufficient to reach adequate clinical response	Ternant et al. (2015) (RA) Vogelzang et al. (2014) (PsA), (2015) (RA) Menting et al. (2015) (PsO) Hoseyni et al. (2018) (CD/UC) EMA/CHMP/364731/2015 (2015b) (HS) EMA/501143/2016 (2016a) (UV) EMA/CHMP/829007/2017 (2017d) (pJIA) EMA/56352/2013 (2013a) (Pediatric CD) EMA/CHMP/177541/2015 (2015a) (Pediatric PsO)

Table 26.1 ■ (continued)

Part B: Pharmacokinetics and pharmacokinetics/pharmacodynamics

Product	Target	Indication	Pharmacokinetics	Pharmacokinetics/Pharmacodynamics	Reference[a]
			In patients with AS, the pharmacokinetics of adalimumab were similar to those in patients with RA In patients with CD/UC, the adalimumab loading dose of 160 mg SC at week 0 followed by 80 mg SC at week 2 achieved mean serum trough concentrations of approximately 12 μg/mL at week 2 and week 4. Mean steady-state trough concentrations of 7–8 μg/mL were observed after receiving an adalimumab maintenance dose of 40 mg SC q2w In patients with PsO, the mean steady-state trough concentration was approximately 5–6 μg/mL during adalimumab 40 mg SC q2w monotherapy treatment In patients with HS, the adalimumab loading dose of 160 mg SC at week 0 followed by 80 mg SC at week 2 achieved mean serum adalimumab trough concentrations of 7–8 μg/mL at week 2 and week 4. The mean steady-state trough concentrations were 7–11 μg/mL during adalimumab 40 mg SC qw treatment In patients with UV, the mean steady-state trough concentration was 8–10 μg/mL during adalimumab 40 mg SC q2w treatment In pJIA patients 4–17 years of age, the mean steady-state trough serum adalimumab concentrations for patients weighing <30 kg who received 20 mg adalimumab SC q2w as monotherapy or with concomitant methotrexate were 6.8 μg/mL and 10.9 μg/mL, respectively. The mean steady-state trough concentrations for patients weighing ≥30 kg who received 40 mg SC q2w as monotherapy or with concomitant methotrexate were 6.6 μg/mL and 8.1 μg/mL, respectively. In pJIA patients weighing <15 kg, the mean steady-state trough concentrations following SC adalimumab of 24 mg/m^2 (maximum 20 mg) q2w as monotherapy or with concomitant methotrexate were 6.0 μg/mL and 7.9 μg/mL, respectively	In patients with CD and UC, several reports suggested that higher adalimumab trough concentrations were associated with higher proportions of patients achieving the desired clinical efficacy endpoints, including clinical remission, mucosal healing and CRP remission In patients with HS, Hidradenitis Suppurativa Clinical Response (HiSCR) responders had higher adalimumab trough concentrations compared to non-responders. In HiSCR responders, higher adalimumab concentrations were associated with less probability of loss of response In patients with UV, patients with treatment failure had lower adalimumab exposure compared to those without treatment failure. The estimated EC_{50} for inhibition of treatment failure event was 6.4–9.7 μg/mL In pediatric patients with CD, relationship between adalimumab concentration and the clinical remission rate over time was characterized by two types of PK/PD models, namely the indirect response model and the Markov chain model. Clear E-R relationship was established and the Markov chain model estimated EC_{50} was 3.4 μg/mL In pediatric patients with pJIA and PsO, relationships between adalimumab exposure and the probability of achieving pediatric ACR response (PedACR30/PedACR50) and the PASI75 response, respectively, were characterized by non-linear logistic regression models. Clear E-R relationships were shown in these two pediatric populations, with higher adalimumab concentration associated with higher probability of achieving the clinical endpoints In patients with RA, significant E-R relationship for effectiveness (ACR20/50/70 responses over time) was shown using a continuous-time Markov model. Increased certolizumab pegol exposure resulted in an increased probability of attaining higher level of ACR20/50/70 responses, with majority of the clinical effect being attained at the exposure associated with the recommended 200 mg q2w label maintenance dose. Additionally, change from baseline in DAS28(CRP) (ΔDAS) increased with certolizumab concentration, where certolizumab concentration threshold ≥24 μg/mL was associated with ΔDAS ≥2 at weeks 12 and 24	

Certolizumab pegol (Cimzia®)	TNFα	RA, PsA, AS and CD	In pediatric patients with CD weighing ≥40 kg, the mean serum concentrations were 15.7 μg/mL at week 4 following SC doses of 160 mg at week 0 and 80 mg at week 2, and the mean steady-state trough concentrations during maintenance therapy were 10.5 μg/mL following 40 mg SC q2w. In pediatric patients with CD weighing <40 kg, the mean serum concentrations were 10.6 μg/mL at week 4 following SC doses of 80 mg at week 0 and 40 mg at week 2, and the mean steady-state trough concentrations during maintenance therapy were 6.9 μg/mL following 20 mg SC q2w Certolizumab pegol exhibits linear pharmacokinetics with mean terminal half-life being about 14 days. The systemic clearance ranged from 9.21 to 14.38 mL/h in healthy subjects. The mean bioavailability of SC certolizumab pegol was 80%. Apparent clearance following SC injections were estimated to be 17 mL/h and 21 mL/h in CD and RA populations, respectively	In patients with CD, certolizumab pegol concentrations at weeks 2, 4, and 6 were higher in patients with clinical response, remission, CRP ≤ 5 mg/L and fecal calprotectin ≤250 μg/g at week 6 than without. Certolizumab concentrations of at least 36.1 μg/mL at week 6 and at least 14.8 μg/mL at week 12 were associated with the desired outcomes at weeks 6 and 26 respectively	Lacroix et al. (2014) (RA) Wolbink et al. (2016) (RA) Vande Casteele et al. (2018) (CD)
Etanercept (Enbrel®)	TNFα	RA, PsA, AS, pJIA and PsO	Etanercept exhibits linear pharmacokinetics with mean terminal half-life being 102 h. The mean clearance was 160 mL/h In patients with RA and PsO, the mean steady-state trough concentrations were 1.2 and 1.5 μg/mL, respectively, following 50 mg SC qw dosing In patients with pJIA, the mean serum concentrations were 2.1 μg/mL following 0.4 mg/kg SC twice weekly (maximum of 50 mg per week) dosing In pediatric PsO patients, the mean steady-state trough concentrations were 1.6–2.1 μg/mL following 0.8 mg/kg (maximum of 50 mg) SC qw dosing	In patients with RA, relationships between predicted etanercept cumulative AUC and the ACR20/50/70 responses rates and the reduction in DAS28 score over time were characterized by a logistic regression model and a direct inhibitory E_{max} model, respectively, with respect to time. Clear E-R relationships were established In patients with PsO, significant E-R relationship for effectiveness (probability of achieving PASI75 over time) was shown using time series logistic regression models with cumulative etanercept dose, predicted cumulative etanercept AUC and predicted etanercept trough before each PASI75 assessment as the exposure variables. Cumulative AUC was determined to be the most adequate exposure predictor	Lee et al. (2003) (RA) Hsu and Huang (2014) (RA) Hutmacher et al. (2007) (PsO)

Table 26.1 ■ (continued)

Part B: Pharmacokinetics and pharmacokinetics/pharmacodynamics

Product	Target	Indication	Pharmacokinetics	Pharmacokinetics/Pharmacodynamics	Reference[a]
Golimumab (Simponi®, Simponi Aria®)	TNFα	RA, PsA, AS, and UC nr-AxSpA and pJIA (EU only, SmPC)	Golimumab exhibits linear pharmacokinetics with mean terminal half-life being about 2 weeks. The mean systemic clearance was estimated to be 7.6 mL/day/kg in patients with RA. The mean bioavailability of SC golimumab was 53% Following IV administration of 2 mg/kg golimumab at weeks 0, 4 and q8w thereafter, the mean steady-state serum trough concentrations in patients with active RA, PsA and AS were 0.4, 0.7 and 0.8 μg/mL respectively Following SC administration of 50 mg golimumab q4w with concomitant methotrexate, the mean steady-state trough concentrations in patients with active RA, PsA and AS were 0.4–0.6, 0.5 and 0.8 μg/mL respectively. Concomitant use of methotrexate reduced the apparent clearance of golimumab by approximately 52, 36 and 21% in patients with RA, PsA and AS respectively Treatment of patients with UC with 100 mg golimumab SC q4w during maintenance resulted in a mean steady-state trough concentration of approximately 1.8 μg/mL	In patients with RA, the relationship between golimumab concentration and the time course of ACRN (a continuous measure of clinical improvement derived from ACR20 response criteria) score following golimumab 50 or 100 mg q4w was characterized using an indirect response PK/PD model. E_{max} relationship was attempted but EC_{50} cannot be reliably estimated; golimumab 50 and 100 mg doses likely results in a range of exposures located in the upper domain of a saturating E-R response curve In patients with pJIA, the relationship between golimumab concentration and the time course of log-transformed Juvenile Arthritis Disease Activity Score (JADAS) score was characterized using an indirect response PK/PD model following E_{max} relationship. Clear E-R relationship was established and the estimated EC_{50} was 0.412 μg/ml In patients with UC, higher serum golimumab concentrations were associated with higher efficacy response rates (including clinical response, clinical remission and mucosal healing) during induction and maintenance. Golimumab concentrations of 2.5 μg/ml (induction at week 6) and 1.4 μg/ml (maintenance steady-state trough) are estimated to be the concentration targets for attainment of optimal clinical outcomes	Hu et al. (2011) (RA) EMA/CHMP/404217/2016 (2016b) (pJIA) Adedokun et al. (2017) (UC)

Infliximab (Remicade®)	TNFα	RA, PsA, AS, PsO, CD, UC, pediatric CD, pediatric UC	Infliximab exhibits linear pharmacokinetics with median terminal half-life being 7.7–9.5 days Following IV infusions of a maintenance dose of 3–10 mg/kg q8w, median steady-state serum infliximab concentrations ranged approximately 0.5–6 μg/mL. Development of antibodies to infliximab increased infliximab clearance and lead to lower infliximab concentration Infliximab pharmacokinetic characteristics were similar in pediatric (aged 6–17 years) and adult patients with CD or UC following infliximab 5 mg/kg IV dosing	In patients with RA, higher infliximab serum pre-infusion concentrations at week 54 were associated with increased magnitude of ACR response (assessed by ACRN, a continuous measure of clinical improvement derived from ACR20 response criteria), greater reduction from baseline in CRP, and less progression of radiographic joint damage at week 54, as shown by the graphical exploratory analysis and/or the regression modeling analysis In patients with PsO, the maintenance of clinical response was related to the achievement of stable infliximab serum concentrations. Patients who maintained their PASI improvement had median pre-infusion serum infliximab concentrations above 1 μg/mL during maintenance therapy, while patients who lost response had median pre-infusion serum infliximab concentrations less than 1 μg/mL In patients with luminal CD, higher infliximab serum pre-infusion concentrations at week 14 were associated with greater reduction from baseline in CDAI (CD activity index) and higher clinical remission rate at week 14. In patients with fistulizing CD, higher infliximab serum pre-infusion concentrations at week 30 were associated with a higher probability of complete fistula response at week 30 In patients with UC, higher serum infliximab concentrations were associated with higher efficacy response rates (including clinical response, clinical remission and mucosal healing) during induction and maintenance. Infliximab concentrations of 41 μg/ml (induction at week 8) and 3.7 μg/ml (maintenance steady-state trough) are estimated to be the concentration targets for attainment of optimal clinical outcomes In pediatric patients with UC (6–17 years of age), a positive E-R relationship was identified between infliximab serum concentration and clinical effect following induction therapy by a logistic regression analysis (similar to adults). In addition, maintaining trough serum infliximab concentrations above detectable levels may be associated with maintenance of clinical response	St. Clair et al. (2002) (RA) Reich et al. (2005) (PsO) Fasanmade et al. (2002) (CD) Fasanmade et al. (2003) (CD) Adedokun et al. (2014) (UC) Adedokun et al. (2013) (Pediatric UC)

Table 26.1 (continued)

Part B: Pharmacokinetics and pharmacokinetics/pharmacodynamics

Product	Target	Indication	Pharmacokinetics	Pharmacokinetics/Pharmacodynamics	Reference[a]
Anti-IL-1β					
Canakinumab (Ilaris®)	IL-1β	CAPS and sJIA	Canakinumab exhibits linear pharmacokinetics with mean terminal half-life being 26 days. The mean bioavailability of SC canakinumab was 66%. Clearance of canakinumab varied according to body weight and was estimated to be 0.174 L/day in a CAPS patient weighing 70 kg and 0.11 L/day in a sJIA patient weighing 33 kg Pharmacokinetic properties of canakinumab are similar in CAPS and sJIA pediatric populations. In patients less than 2 years of age, the exposure of canakinumab were comparable to older age groups with a same weight-based-dose	In patients with CAPS, a mechanistic PK-biomarker-symptom model was developed to characterize the relationship between canakinumab concentration and the time course in the suppression of peripheral IL-1β, and IL-1β was linked further to the probability of flare and the changes in serum CRP, serum amyloid A and absolute neutrophil count over time. It indicated that CAPS is entirely mediated by IL-1β and that canakinumab treatment can restore physiological IL-1β production In patients with sJIA, the relationships between canakinumab concentration and the time course of peripheral IL-1β was characterized by a dynamic drug-ligand binding and turnover PK/PD model. The relationship between canakinumab exposure and sJIA flare reduction was characterized using a discrete hazard model. These modeling analyses supported the dose selection of canakinumab in patients with sJIA	Lachmann et al. (2009) (CAPS) Sun et al. (2016) (sJIA) Xiong et al. (2013) (sJIA)
Rilonacept (Arcalyst®)	IL-1β	CAPS	Following weekly SC doses of 160 mg in patients with CAPS, serum rilonacept concentration appeared to reach steady state by week 6 with average trough levels being approximately 24 μg/mL	In patients with CAPS, there was no apparent relationship between dose (or rilonacept concentrations at the respective time points) and either IL-1ß complex levels or total IL-1 receptor antagonist levels in blood in the Phase III study. The rilonacept concentrations were high compared to the affinity to the cytokines; therefore, cytokines were likely almost completely bound at any time and dose	EMEA/541561/2009 (2009) (CAPS)

Anti-IL-5					
Mepolizumab (Nucala®)	IL-5	Asthma, EGPA	Mepolizumab exhibited linear pharmacokinetics in patients with asthma, with mean terminal half-life being 16–22 days. Apparent clearance was estimated to be 0.28 L/day for a 70-kg individual. The bioavailability of SC mepolizumab was approximately 80% The pharmacokinetic properties of mepolizumab observed in patients with EGPA were similar to the pharmacokinetic properties displayed in patients with severe asthma	In patients with asthma, the relationship between mepolizumab concentration and the percentage change from baseline in blood eosinophils over time was described by an indirect response PK/PD model following E_{max} relationship. The estimated maximal decrease in eosinophil count was 85% from baseline and the estimated EC_{50} was 0.45 µg/mL	Smith et al. (2011)
Reslizumab (Cinqair®)	IL-5	Asthma	Reslizumab exhibits linear pharmacokinetics with a terminal half-life being about 24 days. The systemic clearance was approximately 7 mL/h. Peak serum concentrations were typically observed at the end of the infusion and serum concentrations generally declined from peak in a biphasic manner	In patients with asthma, clear E-R relationship between reslizumab exposure and the inhibition of peripheral blood eosinophil response over time was shown using an indirect response PK/PD model. Significant E-R relationships for improvement of lung function (forced expiratory volume in 1 s [FEV1]) and Asthma Control Questionnaire (ACR) score were also shown using the direct sigmoid E_{max} models. These analyses supported the proposed dose regimen for registration	US FDA Advisory Committee Briefing Document (BLA#761033) (2015a) (Asthma)
Anti-IL-17A					
Ixekizumab (Taltz®)	IL-17A	PsA, PsO	Ixekizumab exhibits linear pharmacokinetics in patients with PsO, with mean terminal half-life being 13 days. Apparent clearance was 0.39 L/day. The bioavailability of SC ixekizumab ranged from 60 to 81%. Administration of ixekizumab via SC injection in the thigh achieved a higher bioavailability relative to that achieved using other injection sites including the arm and abdomen Following SC administration of 160 mg ixekizumab at week 0 and 80 mg q2w thereafter, steady-state concentrations were achieved at week 8 in patients with PsO, with a mean trough level of 9.3 µg/mL. After switching from 80 mg q2w to 80 mg q4w dose regimen, steady-state concentrations were achieved 10 weeks later, with a mean trough level of 3.5 µg/mL The pharmacokinetic properties of ixekizumab observed in PsA patients were similar to the pharmacokinetic properties displayed in PsO patients	In patients with PsO, the relationship between ixekizumab concentration and Static Physicians Global Assessment (SPGA) response over time was characterized using an indirect response PK/PD model following E_{max} relationship. Clear E-R relationship was established and the modeling results supported the proposed dose regimen for registration	Choi et al. (2016)

Table 26.1 ■ (continued)

Part B: Pharmacokinetics and pharmacokinetics/pharmacodynamics

Product	Target	Indication	Pharmacokinetics	Pharmacokinetics/Pharmacodynamics	Reference[a]
Secukinumab (Cosentyx®)	IL-17A	PsA, AS and PsO	Secukinumab exhibited linear pharmacokinetics in patients with PsO, with mean terminal half-life being 22–31 days. Apparent clearance ranged from 0.14 to 0.22 L/day in patients with PsO. The bioavailability of SC secukinumab ranged from 55 to 77% The mean steady-state trough concentrations in PsO patients following 150 mg and 300 mg SC q4w dosing were 16.7 and 34.4 μg/mL, respectively Secukinumab concentrations in interstitial fluid in lesional and non-lesional skin of PsO patients ranged from 27% to 40% of those in serum at 1 and 2 weeks after a single SC dose of secukinumab 300 mg The pharmacokinetic properties of secukinumab observed in patients with PsA and AS were similar to the pharmacokinetic properties observed in patients with PsO	In patients with PsO, significant E-R relationship was shown between the observed secukinumab serum concentrations at week 12 and the PASI75 and IGA 0/1 at week 12, using logistic regression and/or graphical quartile analyses In patients with PsA, clear E-R relationships were observed at week 12 efficacy parameters of ACR, PASI, DAS28-CRP and HAQ-DI (Health Assessment Questionnaire Disability Index) by graphical exploratory analysis, with a trend of increased response with higher secukinumab trough concentration. E-R curves of endpoints reflecting the arthritic components of the disease (ACR20/50/70, DAS) appeared to plateau at trough levels higher than 20 μg/ml (20 μg/ml corresponds to the typical steady-state trough concentrations achieved following 150 mg SC q4w dosing) In patients with AS, clear E-R relationships were observed at week 16 efficacy parameters of ASAS (Assessment of SpondyloArthritis international Society response criterion), BASDAI (Bath Ankylosing Spondylitis Disease Activity Index), and SF36- PCS (short form 36—Physical Component Summary) by graphical exploratory analysis, with a trend of increased response with higher secukinumab trough concentration. The E-R curves appeared to plateau at trough levels higher than 25 μg/ml, which was approximate the mean trough concentrations following 150 mg SC q4w dosing	FDA Clinical Pharmacology Review (BLA#125504) (2015b) (RA) EMA/CHMP/665427/2015 (2015d) (PsA) EMA/CHMP/665405/2015 (2015c) (AS)

Anti-IL12/IL-23					
Ustekinumab (Stelara®)	IL12/IL23	PsO, PsA, CD and adolescent PsO	Ustekinumab exhibits linear pharmacokinetics In patients with PsO, the mean systemic clearance ranged from 1.90 to 2.22 mL/day/kg, with mean terminal half-life being 14.9–45.6 days. Following SC administration of 45 or 90 mg q12w, the mean steady-state trough concentrations were 0.31 and 0.64 μg/mL, respectively In patients with PsA, PK profiles were in general consistent with what were observed in patients with PsO In patients with CD, clearance was estimated to be 0.19 L/day with a median terminal half-life being approximately 19 days. Following the recommended IV induction dose (260 mg, 390 mg, and 520 mg for weight range of ≤55 kg, 55–85 kg and > 85 kg, respectively), mean peak serum ustekinumab concentration was 125.2 μg/mL. Mean steady-state trough concentration was 2.51 μg/mL following a maintenance dose of 90 mg SC q8w	In patients with PsO, relationship between ustekinumab exposure and the reduction of PASI score over time was characterized by an indirect response PK/PD model following an E_{max} relationship. The estimated median EC_{50} in partial responders (achieved 50% or more but less than 75% improvement in PASI score) was approximately 30-fold higher than that in responders (achieving 75% improvement in PASI score) In patients with PsA, the proportion of patients who achieved ACR20, ACR50, and PASI75 responses at week 24 was higher in patients with quantifiable serum ustekinumab concentrations at week 16 when compared with patients with serum ustekinumab concentrations below limit of quantitation (BLQ) at week 16 In patients with CD, relationship between ustekinumab concentration and the reduction of CDAI score over time were characterized by an indirect response PK/PD model following an E_{max} relationship with an autocorrelation residual error. Clear E-R relationship were established and the estimated EC_{50} was 6.37 μg/mL	Zhou et al. (2010) (PsO) EMA/CHMP/431551/2013 (2013b) (PsA) Hu et al. (2017a) (CD)
Anti-IL-23					
Guselkumab (Tremfya®)	IL-23	PsO	Guselkumab exhibited linear pharmacokinetics in patients with PsO, with mean terminal half-life being 15–18 days. Apparent clearance was approximately 0.516 L/day. The bioavailability of SC guselkumab was 49% in healthy subjects Following SC administration of 100 mg guselkumab at weeks 0 and 4, and q8w thereafter in PsO patients, mean steady-state serum guselkumab trough concentration was approximately 1.2 μg/mL	In patients with PsO, the relationship between guselkumab concentration and the time course of PASI75/90/100 responses rates and the Physician's Global Assessment (PGA) score was characterized using a joint indirect response PK/PD model following E_{max} relationship. Clear E-R relationship was established and the estimated EC_{50} was 0.0663 μg/ml	Hu et al. (2017b) (PsO)

Table 26.1 ■ (continued)

Part B: Pharmacokinetics and pharmacokinetics/pharmacodynamics

Product	Target	Indication	Pharmacokinetics	Pharmacokinetics/Pharmacodynamics	Reference[a]
Tocilizumab (Actemra®)	IL-6 receptor	RA, pJIA, sJIA, GCA, and CRS	Tocilizumab exhibits target-mediated nonlinear pharmacokinetics. Clearance of tocilizumab decreased with increased doses. The terminal half-life of tocilizumab is concentration-dependent, up to 13 and 5 days at steady state for 162 mg SC qw and 162 mg SC q2w, respectively, in patients with RA. The bioavailability of SC tocilizumab was 80% In adult patients with RA, following 4 mg/kg IV q4w, the model-predicted mean steady state peak and trough concentrations were 88.3 and 1.49 μg/mL, respectively. Following 162 mg SC q2w, the estimated mean steady-state peak and trough concentrations were 12.3 and 5.6 μg/mL, respectively In patients with GCA, following 162 mg SC qw, the estimated mean steady-state peak and trough concentrations were 73 and 68.1 μg/mL, respectively In patients with pJIA, the estimated mean steady-state peak and trough concentrations were 182 and 7.49 μg/mL, respectively, and 175 and 2.35 μg/mL, respectively, following 8 mg/kg IV q4w (patients weighing ≥30 kg) and 10 mg/kg IV q4w (patients weighing <30 kg), respectively In patients with sJIA, the estimated mean steady-state peak and trough concentrations were 245 and 57.5 μg/mL, respectively, at the recommended dose regimen (8 and 12 mg/kg SC q2w for patients ≥30 kg and <30 kg respectively)	In patients with RA, relationship between tocilizumab exposure and the improvement in DAS28-ESR (erythrocyte sedimentation rate) score over time following tocilizumab IV administration were characterized using an indirect response PK/PD model following E_{max} relationship, with the estimated EC_{50} being 3.7 μg/mL. Following tocilizumab SC administration, clinical response (probability of achieving ACR20/50/70 responses) increased with increasing tocilizumab trough concentration as indicated by quartile analysis and/or logistic regression analysis In patients with sJIA, dosing regimens of 8 mg/kg in patients weighing ≥30 kg and 12 mg/kg in sJIA patients weighing <30 kg achieved uniform exposure across the entire bodyweight range, which were associated comparable changes in markers related to inflammation (CRP and ESR); markers related to tocilizumab mechanism of action (IL-6 and soluble IL-6 receptor); and efficacy results (JIAACR30 at week 12 with absence of fever). There was no apparent correlation between the tocilizumab exposure and the PD/efficacy end points, suggesting that adalimumab exposures associated with the doses studied in Phase III studies were at the plateau of the E-R curve In patients with pJIA following the recommended dose regimen, analysis by tocilizumab exposure (AUC) quartiles showed that the proportion of patients who achieved JIAACR50 and JIAACR70 responses at week 16 was slightly lower with lower exposure (quartile 1) than the upper three quartiles. There was no apparent correlation between the tocilizumab exposure and the other PD/efficacy end points, such as change from baseline in the 27-joint Juvenile Arthritis Disease Activity Score [JADAS-27], IL-6 and soluble IL-6 receptor. These data suggest the adalimumab exposures associated with the doses studied in Phase III were at the plateau of the E-R curve	Levi et al. (2013) (RA) Abdallah et al. (2017) (RA) Zhang et al. (2013) (sJIA) Zhang et al. (2017) (pJIA) Gibiansky et al. (2017) (GCA)

Anti-IL-4 receptor					
Dupilumab (Dupixent®)	IL-4 receptor subunit α	AD	Dupilumab exhibits nonlinear target-mediated pharmacokinetics with exposures increasing in a greater than dose-proportional manner. The systemic exposure increased by 30-fold when the dose increased eightfold following a single dose of dupilumab from 75 mg to 600 mg. The bioavailability of SC dupilumab was 64% Steady state was achieved by week 16 following 600 mg SC initially and 300 mg SC q2w thereafter, and the mean steady-state trough concentrations ranged from 73.3 to 79.9 μg/mL	In patients with AD, quartile analysis by dupilumab trough concentration at week 16 and predicted cumulative AUC from week 0 to week 16 showed clear E-R relationships for the efficacy endpoints including percent change from baseline eczema area and severity index (EASI) score, proportion of patients achieving IGA 0/1 and percent change from baseline for peak NRS (pruritus Numerical Rating Scale) Based on an E_{max} model linking dupilumab trough concentration and EASI score at week 16, EC_{50} was estimated to be 30 μg/mL	EMA/512262/2017 (2017b) (AD)
Anti-IL-5 receptor					
Benralizumab (Fasenra®)	IL-5 receptor	Asthma	Benralizumab exhibits linear pharmacokinetics n patients with asthma over a SC dose range of 20–200 mg, with mean terminal half-life being 15 days. The mean bioavailability of SC benralizumab was 58%. Typical systemic clearance of benralizumab was estimated to be 0.29 L/day for a subject weighing 70 kg	In patients with asthma (and heathy subjects), blood eosinophil count data following benralizumab treatment was characterized by a semi-mechanistic PK/PD model. Depletion of blood eosinophil counts was depicted by a hematopoietic transit model in which benralizumab induced depletion of eosinophils in each age compartment. Modeling results supported selection of dose regimen for future studies in patients with asthma	Wang et al. (2017) (Asthma)
Anti-IL-6 receptor					
Sarilumab (Kevzara®)	IL-6 receptor	RA	Sarilumab exhibits target-mediated nonlinear pharmacokinetics. The half-life of sarilumab is concentration-dependent, up to 8 and 10 days at steady state following 150 and 200 mg SC q2w dose regimens, respectively, in patients with RA. Steady state exposure over the dosing interval measured by area under curve (AUC) increased twofold with an increase in dose from 150 to 200 mg q2w Following 200 mg SC q2w, the estimated mean steady-state AUC, C_{min} and C_{max} of sarilumab were 395 mg·day/L, 16.5 mg/L, and 35.6 mg/L, respectively	In patients with RA, relationships between sarilumab exposure and DAS28-CRP score and the absolute neutrophil count over time were characterized using two separate indirect response PK/PD models following E_{max} relationships. Model estimated potency (EC_{50}) were 2.32 and 10.3 μg/mL, respectively	Ma et al. (2016a, b) (RA)

Table 26.1 ■ (continued)

Part B: Pharmacokinetics and pharmacokinetics/pharmacodynamics

Product	Target	Indication	Pharmacokinetics	Pharmacokinetics/Pharmacodynamics	Reference[a]
Anti-IL-17 receptor A					
Brodalumab (Siliq®)	IL-17 receptor A	PsO	Brodalumab exhibits non-linear pharmacokinetics with exposures increased greater than dose-proportionally over the dose range of 140 mg SC to 350 mg SC in PsO patients. The clearance of brodalumab increased with decreasing doses due to nonlinear elimination. The mean apparent total clearance was 3.0 L/day following a single brodalumab SC dose of 210 mg. Bioavailability of SC brodalumab was 55% Steady-state was achieved by week 4 following 210 mg SC q2w, and the mean peak concentration and AUC over the two-week dosing interval were 20.6 μg/mL and 227 μg·day/mL, respectively	In patients with GCA, a Cox proportional hazards modeling analysis was conducted for time-to-first-flare (TFF). Risk for flare decreased with increasing tocilizumab exposure following an E_{max} relationship. Patients receiving tocilizumab 162 mg SC q2w compared to qw were at higher risk for shorter TFF In patients with PsO, relationship between brodalumab concentration and the time course of PASI score was characterized by an indirect response PK/PD model following E_{max} relationship. Clear E-R relationship was established and the estimated EC_{50} was 0.637 μg/mL	Salinger et al. (2014) (PsO)
Anti-IgE					
Omalizumab (Xolair®)	IgE	Asthma and CIU	Omalizumab exhibits target-mediated nonlinear pharmacokinetics (linear at doses greater than 0.5 mg/kg). The mean bioavailability of SC omalizumab was 62% In patients with asthma, the mean apparent clearance of omalizumab was estimated to be 2.4 mL/kg/day with a mean terminal half-life being 26 days In patients with CIU, the mean apparent clearance of omalizumab was estimated to be 240 mL/day with a mean terminal half-life being 24 days	In patients with asthma, relationship between omalizumab concentration and blood IgE level (total and free) over time was characterized by a dynamic drug-ligand binding and turnover model. Model predicted free IgE concentrations correlated well with clinical signs and symptoms, allowing a target concentration of 14 ng/mL, at the midpoint of 4-week clinical observation periods, to be set for the determination of dose regimen in asthma patients In patients with CIU, relationship between omalizumab concentration and blood IgE level over time was characterized by a target-mediated population PK/PD model incorporating omalizumab-IgE binding and turnover. Modeling results supported the flat dosing regimen for omalizumab in CIU patients	Hochhaus et al. (2003); Lowe et al. (2009) (Asthma) Zheng et al. (2014) (CIU)

Anti-integrin					
Natalizumab (Tysabri®)	Integrin	CD and MS	In patients with CD, the mean systemic clearance of natalizumab was 22 mL/h with mean half-life being 10 days. The mean steady-state trough concentration was 10 μg/mL following 300 mg IV infusion q4w dosing In patients with MS, the mean systemic clearance of natalizumab was 16 mL/h with mean half-life being 11 days. The mean steady-state trough concentrations ranged from 23 to 29 μg/mL following 300 mg IV infusion q4w dosing	In patients with CD, the probability of clinical response at week 6 was found to correlate with natalizumab cumulative AUC from week 0 to week 6 in a dose ranging study. However, an inverse U-shaped dose- and exposure-response relationship was found with the highest dose group of 6 mg/kg q4w having lower response rate compared to the lower dose of 3 mg/kg q4w; the reason was not identified In patients with MS, the relationship between predicted natalizumab concentration and α4 integrin saturation over time was described by a direct PK/PD model following sigmodal E_{max} relationship. The estimated EC_{50} was 2.51 μg/mL with a hill factor of 1.35. Using log-linear models with natalizumab average concentration during dosing interval as the exposure variable, significant E-R relationship for effectiveness was shown for gadolinium-enhancing lesion count data and annualized relapse rate (ARR) over time	US FDA Clinical Pharmacology Review (BLA# 125104/33) (2008) (CD) Muralidharan et al. (2017a, b) (MS)
Vedolizumab (Entyvio®)	Integrin	CD and UC	Vedolizumab exhibits nonlinear pharmacokinetics. Clearance depends on both linear and nonlinear pathways; the nonlinear clearance decreases with increasing concentrations. Linear clearance was estimated to be 0.157 L/day and the terminal half-life was approximately 25 days at 300 mg IV dosage In adult patients with CD and UC, the vedolizumab induction dose of 300 mg IV at weeks 0 and 2 achieved mean serum trough concentration of approximately 26–27 μg/mL at week 6. Mean steady-state trough concentration of 11–13 μg/mL were observed after receiving an a vedolizumab maintenance dose of 300 mg IV q8w	In patients with CD and UC, relationship between vedolizumab concentration and the time course in the percentage of peripheral MAdCAM-1 (mucosal addressin cell adhesion molecule-1) binding by lymphocytes expressing high levels of α4β7 integrin was characterized by a direct effect PK/PD model with sigmoid E_{max} relationship. Model estimated EC_{50} was 0.093 μg/mL with a hill factor of 0.801. Significant E-R relationships were also shown for remission at week 6 after induction therapy using logistic regression with predicted cumulative average concentration through week 6 as the exposure variable, and the E-R relationship was steeper for UC than CD	Rosario et al. (2015, 2017)

Table 26.1 ■ (continued)

Part B: Pharmacokinetics and pharmacokinetics/pharmacodynamics

Product	Target	Indication	Pharmacokinetics	Pharmacokinetics/Pharmacodynamics	Reference[a]
Anti-CD80/CD86 lymphocyte activation inhibitor					
Abatacept (Orencia®)	CTLA-4	RA, PsA, and pJIA	Abatacept exhibits linear pharmacokinetics in adult RA patients with mean terminal half-life being 13.1–14.3 days. The mean systemic clearance was 0.22 mL/h/kg. The bioavailability of SC abatacept was 78.6%. Following IV infusions of 10 mg/kg q4w, the mean steady-state peak and trough concentrations were 295 and 24 μg/mL, respectively. Following SC injections of 125 mg weekly, the mean steady-state peak and trough concentrations were 48.1 and 32.5 μg/mL, respectively In patients with PsA, the geometric mean steady-state trough concentration was 24.3 μg/mL at 10 mg/kg IV dosing. Following 125 mg SC weekly dosing, the geometric mean of steady-state trough concentration was 25.6 μg/mL. Relative to the RA patients with the same body weight, abatacept clearance in PsA patients was approximately 8% lower In pJIA patients 6–17 years of age, the mean systemic clearance was estimated to be 0.4 mL/h/kg. Following IV infusions of 10 mg/kg q4w, the mean steady-state peak and trough concentrations were 217 and 11.9 μg/mL, respectively In pJIA patients 2–17 years of age, following SC weekly injections at the recommended body-weight–tiered dosing, the mean steady-state trough concentrations were 44.4, 46.6 and 38.5 μg/mL in patients weighing 10 to <25 kg, 25 to <50 kg, and ≥50 kg, respectively	In patients with RA, relationship between abatacept exposure and the time course in the suppression of serum IL-6 was characterized by an indirect-response PK/PD model following E_{max} relationship. Clear E-R relationship was established and the estimated EC_{50} was 11.3 μg/mL. Significant relationship between abatacept trough concentration and the probability of achieving ACR20 over time was also shown using time-series generalized estimating equations. Steady-state trough concentration over 10 μg/mL was suggested to be the target exposure for near-maximal efficacy In patients with PsA, relationships between abatacept exposure and the clinical endpoints (ACR20, ACR50, ACR70, PASI50, PASI75) on Day 169 were described by logistic regression models using steady-state trough, average and maximum concentration as the exposure variables. Steady state trough concentration was identified as the best exposure predictor for efficacy where patients with higher trough concentrations were associated with higher probability of achieving the binary efficacy endpoints. Significant E-R relationships between abatacept exposure and the DAS28-CRP score over time was also shown using an inhibitory E_{max} model with respect to time In pediatric patients with pJIA, a proportional odds model with a log linear function of steady-state abatacept trough concentration adequately described the E–R relationship for JIAACR responses (JIAACR30/50/70/100) at month 4. Steady state trough concentration threshold of 10 μg/mL provided a near-maximal efficacy response	Roy et al. (2017) (RA) Hasegawa et al. (2011) (RA) Li et al. (2017) (pJIA) EMA/455579/2017 (2017a) (PsA)

Belimumab (Benlysta®)	BLyS	SLE	The model predicted systemic clearance of belimumab was 215 mL/day with a terminal half-life being19.4 days. The peak concentration of belimumab was estimated to be 313 μg/mL following 10 mg/kg belimumab by IV infusion at 2-week intervals for the first 3 doses and at 4-week intervals thereafter Model predicted SC bioavailability of belimumab was 74%. Following SC belimumab dosing of 200 mg qw, the peak and trough concentration were estimated to be 108 and 97 μg/mL, respectively	In patients with SLE, belimumab 200 mg SC qw plus standard of care significantly improved the SLE responder index (SRI). However, at this dose, no apparent relationship was identified between belimumab average steady-state concentration and the SRI response at week 52 by the logistic regression analysis. Belimumab 200-mg dose likely results in a range of exposures located in the upper domain of a saturating E-R response curve	Struemper et al. (2017) (SLE)
Anti-CD-20 cytolytic agent					
Ocrelizumab (Ocrevus®)	CD20	MS	Ocrelizumab exhibits nonlinear pharmacokinetics with time-dependent clearance (linear at doses between 400 mg and 2000 mg). Constant clearance was estimated at 0.17 L/day, and initial time-dependent clearance at 0.05 L/day, which declined with a half-life of 33 weeks. The terminal elimination half-life was 26 days In patients with relapsing forms of MS, the maximum concentration was 212 μg/mL at a maintenance dose of 600 mg IV infusion every 6 months In patients with primary progressive MS, the mean maximum concentration was 141 μg/mL at a maintenance dose of two 300 mg infusions separated by 14 days every 6 months	In patients with primary progressive (PPMS) and relapsing forms (RMS) of MS, relationships between ocrelizumab exposure and the clinical efficacy endpoints were evaluated using ocrelizumab cumulative average concentration over treatment period as the main exposure metric. Although all ocrelizumab groups showed a benefit compared with control (hazard ratio < 1), there was no apparent E-R relationship for the primary endpoint of 12-week annualized relapse rate (ARR) in RMS patients. However, both RMS and PPMS patients showed a trend for greater risk reduction for 12-week clinical disability progression (CDP) with higher exposure of ocrelizumab	EMA/790835/2017 (2017c) (MS)
Rituximab (Rituxan®)	CD20	RA	The estimated clearance of rituximab was 0.335 L/day in patients with RA with mean terminal half-life being 18.0 days Following administration of two 1000 mg rituximab IV infusions separated by 2 weeks in patients with RA, the mean concentrations after the first infusion and second infusion were 318 and 381 μg/mL, respectively	There are no published reports describing E-R relationships of rituximab in patients with RA. However, significant relationships between rituximab exposure (AUC and trough concentration) and therapeutic effect had been shown in patients with B non-Hodgkin lymphoma (B-NHL) and chronic lymphocytic leukemia (CLL)	Golay et al. (2013) (review)

ACR20/50/70 20%,50% and 70% improvement in American College of Rheumatology (ACR) Criteria, *AS* ankylosing spondylitis, *AD* atopic dermatitis, *BLyS* B-lymphocyte stimulator, *CAPS* cryopyrin-associated periodic syndromes, *CD* Crohn's disease, *CD2* T-lymphocyte antigen CD2, *CD20/80/86* B-lymphocyte antigen CD20, CD80, CD86, *CIU* chronic idiopathic urticaria, *CRP* C-reactive protein, *CRS* cytokine release syndrome, *CTLA-4* cytotoxic T-lymphocyte-associated antigen 4, *DAS28-CRP* 28-joints disease activity score (DAS) using C-reactive protein, EC_{50} concentration to achieve half the maximal drug effect, E_{max} maximal drug effect, *E-R* exposure-response, *GCA* giant cell arteritis, *HS* hidradenitis suppurativa, *IGA0/1* investigator's global assessment (IGA) score of 1 or 1 and an improvement of 2 points or more compared to baseline, *IgE* immunoglobulin E, *IL* interleukin, *IV* intravenous, *JIAACR30/50/70/100* 30%, 50%, 70%, 100% improvement in the juvenile idiopathic arthritis ACR response criterion, *KD* kilodalton, *mAb* monoclonal antibody, *MAdCAM-1* mucosal addressin cell adhesion molecule-1, *MW* molecular weight, *MS* multiple sclerosis, *NLR-3* nucleotide-binding domain, leucine rich family (NLR), pyrin domain containing 3, nr-*Axial SpA* non-radiographic axial spondyloarthritis, *PASI50/75/90* 50%,75% and 90% improvement in Psoriasis Area and Severity Index (PASI) score from baseline, *pJIA* polyarticular juvenile idiopathic arthritis, *PK/PD* pharmacokinetics/pharmacodynamics, *PsA* psoriatic arthritis, *PsO* plaque psoriasis, *q12w* every 12 weeks, *q2w* every 2 weeks, *q4w* every 4 weeks, *q8w* every 8 weeks, *qw* every week, *RA* rheumatoid arthritis, *SC* subcutaneous, *SLE* systemic lupus erythematosus, *sJIA* systemic juvenile idiopathic arthritis, *TNFα* tumor necrosis factor alpha, *UC* ulcerative colitis, *UV* uveitis, *VCAM-1* vascular cell adhesion molecule-1

[a]From US prescription information (USPI), unless otherwise indicated

on market for the treatment of immune-mediated inflammatory diseases (as of February 2018).

One challenge in the long-term treatment with antibody-based biotherapeutics of immune-mediated disorders is to avoid the side effects due to the potent and sustained suppression of the immune system. The expectation for these newer therapies is that they can be used earlier in the course of disease to not only maintain control over episodic disease flares but also prevent the less reversible organ damage posed by long-term uncontrolled chronic inflammation or even reversal of disease such as joint damage caused by rheumatoid arthritis (Taylor et al. 2004).

The primary focus of this chapter is on describing the pharmacologic properties of approved biologic therapies for major classes of inflammatory diseases, such as arthritides, systemic lupus erythematosus (SLE), psoriasis, inflammatory bowel disease (IBD), asthma, and a few other less common inflammatory disorders (including atopic dermatitis [AD], chronic idiopathic urticaria [CIU], cryopyrin-associated periodic syndrome [CAPS], cytokine release syndrome [CRS], eosinophilic granulomatosis with polyangiitis [EGPA], giant-cell arteritis [GCA], hidradenitis suppurativa [HS], multiple sclerosis [MS], and uveitis [UV]). Within each of these disease category, biologic agents will be introduced according to their mechanisms of action, and listed alphabetically when having a same mechanism of action. Notably information described in this chapter is based on the original 'innovator' products.

ARTHRITIDES

Arthritides are a class of chronic autoimmune inflammatory conditions of unknown etiology, characterized by pain and stiffness of the affected joints and tissue (Davis and Mease 2008; McInnes and Schett 2011). Arthritides consist of a variety of clinical diseases, such as rheumatoid arthritis (RA), psoriatic arthritis (PsA), and ankylosing spondylitis (AS), involving skeletal joints. Juvenile idiopathic arthritis (JIA) is a chronic inflammatory arthropathy with an age of onset of <16 years, including polyarticular JIA (pJIA), and systemic JIA (sJIA). Although these arthritic diseases may have different clinical manifestations, they are considered to have a similar underlying etiology. RA is the most common of the autoimmune arthritides, affecting at least 1% of the general population in the United States. If not properly treated, the chronic inflammation can result in progressive and irreversible joint destruction. Although early intervention with corticosteroids and conventional non-biologic disease-modifying antirheumatic drugs (DMARDs) has been proven to attenuate inflammation, these therapies are not very effective in slowing down the progression of joint damage in large subsets of patients. In addition, these conventional therapies often have significant off-target side effects (O'Dell 2004).

Several biologic agents have been approved for patients with RA, PsA, AS, or JIA (Table 26.1). These therapeutic proteins provide valuable treatment options for patients, particularly for those who experience significant side effects and/or have inadequate clinical efficacy with conventional DMARDs. These biotherapeutics significantly improve the signs and symptoms of the disease, effectively inhibit (and sometimes even reverse) the progression of joint damage, and greatly improve physical functions and quality of life. Anti-TNFα agents (adalimumab, certolizumab, etanercept, golimumab and infliximab) are considered the gold standard biologic therapy for RA; however, the availability of biologic agents with different mechanisms of action such as anti-IL-6 receptor agents (sarilumab and tocilizumab) provides alternative options when patients do not achieve adequate response to anti-TNFα agents. Other non-TNFα targeting biologic agents demonstrating effectivness for the treatment of arthritides including agents neutralizing soluble cytokines such as IL-1β (canakinumab), IL-17A (ixekizumab and secukinumab) and IL-12/IL-23 (ustekinumab), and acting as direct agonist or anti-agonist to inhibit T-cell activation (abatacept) or depletion of B lymphocytes (rituximab). Compared to conventional DMARDs, the most attractive attribute of antibody-based therapeutic proteins is their binding to the target with high specificity, consequently producing greater efficacy and fewer off-target adverse effects. In addition, antibody-based therapeutic proteins usually have long half-lives (up to 2–3 weeks), which allow for infrequent dosing which is desirable for the patients with chronic diseases.

■ Anti-TNFα Agents

TNFα is a naturally occurring cytokine that is involved in normal inflammatory and immune responses. Elevated levels of TNFα are found in the synovial fluid of patients with RA, JIA, PsA, and AS and play an important role in both the pathologic inflammation and the joint destruction that are hallmarks of these diseases.

The approved anti-TNFα agents such as etanercept, infliximab, adalimumab, golimumab, and certolizumab pegol, are presently one of the most successful classes of therapeutic proteins with many approved clinical indications. Etanercept, a dimeric fusion protein consisting of the p75 human TNFα receptor linked to the Fc portion of human IgG1, was the first anti-TNFα biologic agent approved for an arthritide indication. Infliximab is a chimeric IgG1 mAb containing

~ 25% mouse sequence and ~ 75% human sequence. Certolizumab pegol is a Fab antibody fragment linked to polyethylene glycol that enhances solubility and prolongs elimination half-life. Adalimumab and golimumab are two human IgG1 mAbs, which were created using phage display libraries and the expression of human immunoglobulin genes by transgenic mice, respectively. Human antibodies were developed to minimize immunogenicity; however, patients treated with either adalimumab or golimumab still develop antidrug antibodies. Future efforts are still required to generate therapeutic mAbs that not only have the human sequence as the primary structure, but also have secondary and tertiary structures like natural human immunoglobulins. Although no head-to-head comparative trials are currently available, these anti-TNFα agents appear to have similar efficacy for the treatment of adult RA patients alone or as an add-on to methotrexate (Salliot et al. 2011). These anti-TNFα agents have different elimination half-lives and offer a variety of dosing options. Infliximab is administered intravenously, while the other three anti-TNFα agents can be administered subcutaneously. Golimumab can also be administrated either intravenously or subcutaneously. Etanercept has the shortest half-life (~ 4 days) and needs to be dosed once or twice a week. Infliximab is administered intravenously every 4–8 weeks, while adalimumab, certolizumab, and golimumab are administered subcutaneously every 2 weeks, every 2–4 weeks, or monthly, respectively (Tracey et al. 2008).

Although these antibody-based drugs offer targeted therapy with high specificity, there are adverse effects associated with them that need to be closely monitored (Bongartz et al. 2006; Brown et al. 2002; Ellerin et al. 2003). Certain adverse events such as infections are the result of inhibition of the protective functions of the targeted cytokines and related immune cells. Serious infections due to bacterial, mycobacterial, invasive fungal, viral, protozoal, or other opportunistic pathogens have been reported in patients with RA, PsA, AS, or JIA who received TNFα blockers and other immunosuppressant therapeutic proteins. Patients should be closely monitored for the development of signs and symptoms of infection during and after treatment with these therapeutic proteins, including the development of tuberculosis in patients who tested negative for latent tuberculosis infection prior to the initiation of therapy. Malignancy, albeit rare, has been another important concern when using these immunosuppressant therapeutic proteins. In controlled clinical trials of TNFα blockers, more cases of lymphoma and leukemia have been observed among patients receiving anti-TNFα treatment compared to patients in the control groups; however, there are confounders when assessing the risk of malignancy associated with the use of these therapeutic proteins in patients with chronic inflammatory diseases. Patients with chronic inflammatory diseases, particularly patients with highly active disease and/or chronic exposure to immunosuppressant therapies, may be at higher risk (up to several folds) than the general population for the development of lymphoma and leukemia, even in the absence of TNF-blocking therapy (Smedby et al. 2008). Other notable adverse events associated with these complex proteins include demyelinating disorders, liver enzyme elevation, autoimmune diseases (such as lupus), immunogenicity (formation of antibodies to the therapeutic protein), infusion/injection site reactions, and other hypersensitivity reactions. Overall, a large number of clinical trials have demonstrated that the benefits outweigh the risks for anti-TNF biologic agents in patients with various arthritides.

Adalimumab

Adalimumab (Humira®) is a recombinant human IgG1 mAb, which was created using phage display technology resulting in a human antibody. Adalimumab binds specifically to TNF-α and blocks its interaction with the p55 and p75 cell surface TNF receptors. Adalimumab does not bind or inactivate lymphotoxin (Humira®, US prescribing information 2017).

The efficacy and safety of adalimumab have been assessed in various adult RA populations (DMARD [including methotrexate]-inadequate responders and methotrexate-naïve patients), polyarticular JIA, PsA, and AS. In a randomized, double-blind, controlled Phase III study in patients with active RA despite methotrexate therapy, 6-month treatment with subcutaneous adalimumab in combination with methotrexate at the recommended dose regimen (40 mg every 2 weeks) resulted in 63, 39, and 21% of RA patients achieving ACR20, ACR50, and ACR70 (20, 50 and 70% improvement in the American College of Rheumatology response criterion), respectively, while the control group (methotrexate plus placebo) had only 30, 10, and 3% of patients with ACR20, ACR50, and ACR70 responses, respectively.

Serious infection and malignancy Black-Box warnings were placed on the adalimumab label (Humira®, US prescribing information 2017), similar to the labels of other TNF antagonists. Patients treated with adalimumab are at increased risk for developing serious infections involving various organ systems and sites that may lead to hospitalization or death. Adalimumab should not be started during an active infection. If an infection develops, monitor carefully, and stop adalimumab if infection becomes serious. Lymphoma and other malignancies, some fatal, have been reported in children and adolescent patients treated with TNF blockers including adalimumab.

Risks and benefits of TNF-blocker treatment including adalimumab should be considered prior to initiating therapy in patients with a known malignancy other than a successfully treated non-melanoma skin cancer (NMSC) or when continuing a TNF blocker in patients who develop a malignancy.

The concomitant use of a TNF blocker and abatacept (lymphocyte activation inhibitor) or anakinra (IL-1 receptor antagonist) was associated with a higher risk of serious infections in patients with RA. Therefore, the concomitant use of adalimumab and these biologic products is not recommended in the treatment of patients with RA (Humira®, US prescribing information 2017).

For the treatment of arthritides, adalimumab is indicated for the treatment of adult patients with moderately to severely active RA, active PsA, or active AS. Adalimumab is also indicated for reducing signs and symptoms in pediatric patients 2 years of age and older with moderately to severely active polyarticular JIA (Humira®, US prescribing information 2017).

Certolizumab Pegol

Certolizumab pegol (Cimzia®) is a recombinant, humanized antibody Fab fragment that is conjugated to an approximately 40 kDa polyethylene glycol. Certolizumab pegol binds to human TNFα with high affinity and selectively neutralizes TNFα activity, but does not neutralize lymphotoxin (Cimzia®, US prescribing information 2016).

The efficacy and safety of certolizumab pegol have been assessed in adult RA patients who had active disease despite methotrexate therapy or who had failed at least one conventional DMARD other than methotrexate. Assessments in adult patients with active PsA and active AS have also been conducted. In a randomized, double-blind, controlled Phase III study in patients with active RA despite methotrexate therapy, 6-month treatment with subcutaneous certolizumab pegol at the recommended dose regimen (400 mg initially and at weeks 2 and 4, following by 200 mg every 2 weeks) in combination with methotrexate resulted in 59, 37, and 21% of RA patients achieving ACR20, ACR50, and ACR70, respectively, while the control group (methotrexate plus placebo) had only 14, 8, and 3% of patients with ACR20, ACR50, and ACR70 response, respectively.

Serious infection and malignancy Black-Box warnings were placed on the certolizumab pegol label (Cimzia®, US prescribing information 2016), similar to the labels of other TNF antagonists.

Of the arthritides, certolizumab pegol is indicated for the treatment of adult patients with moderately to severely active RA, active PsA and active AS. Certolizumab pegol is not indicated for use in pediatric patients (Cimzia®, US prescribing information 2016).

Etanercept

Etanercept (Enbrel®) is the first anti-TNF biologic agent approved for arthritide indication. Etanercept is a dimeric fusion protein consisting of the extracellular ligand-binding portion of the human 75 kDa (p75) TNF receptor linked to the Fc portion of human IgG1. Etanercept inhibits binding of TNF-α and TNF-β (lymphotoxin alpha) to cell surface TNF receptors, rendering TNF biologically inactive (Enbrel®, US prescribing information 2016).

The efficacy and safety of etanercept have been assessed in various adult RA populations (DMARD [including methotrexate]-inadequate responders and methotrexate-naïve patients), active polyarticular JIA, active PsA, and active AS. In a randomized, double-blind, controlled Phase III study in patients with active RA despite methotrexate therapy, 6-month treatment with subcutaneous etanercept in combination with methotrexate at the recommended dose regimen (50 mg weekly) resulted in 71, 39, and 15% of RA patients achieving ACR20, ACR50, and ACR70, respectively, while the control group (methotrexate plus placebo) had only 27, 3, and 0% of patients exhibiting ACR20, ACR50, and ACR70 responses, respectively.

Serious infection and malignancy Black-Box warnings were placed on the etanercept label (Enbrel®, US prescribing information 2016), similar to the labels of other TNF antagonists.

Use of etanercept with anakinra (IL-1 receptor antagonist) or abatacept (T-lymphocyte activation inhibitor) is not recommended. Concurrent administration of etanercept with anakinra or abatacept resulted in increased incidences of serious adverse events, including infections, and did not demonstrate increased clinical benefit. In a 24-week study in patients with active RA on background methotrexate, the ACR50 response rate was 31% for patients treated with the combination of anakinra and etanercept and 41% for patients treated with etanercept alone, indicating no added clinical benefit of the combination over etanercept alone. A higher rate of serious infections was observed in RA patients with concurrent anakinra and etanercept therapy (7%) than in patients treated with etanercept alone (0%). Therefore, use of anakinra in combination with TNF blocking agents is not recommended (Enbrel®, US prescribing information 2016). In controlled clinical trials in patients with active RA, patients receiving concomitant intravenous abatacept and etanercept therapy experienced more infections (63%) and serious infections (4.4%) compared to patients treated with only etanercept (43% and 0.8%, respectively). In addition, these trials failed to demonstrate an enhancement of efficacy with concomitant administration of abatacept with etanercept (Orencia®, US prescribing information 2017). As a result, abatacept should not be given concomitantly with TNF antagonists.

For the treatment of arthritides, etanercept is indicated for the treatment of adult patients with moderately to severely active RA, active PsA, or active AS. Etanercept is also indicated for reducing signs and symptoms of polyarticular JIA in pediatric patients 2 years of age and older (Enbrel®, US prescribing information 2016).

Golimumab

Golimumab (Simponi®[subcutaneous], Simponi Aria®[intravenous]) is a human IgG1κ mAb which was created using genetically engineered mice immunized with human TNF. Golimumab binds to both the soluble and transmembrane bioactive forms of human TNFα and therefore inhibits the biologic activity of TNFα. There is no evidence of golimumab binding to other TNF superfamily ligands; golimumab does not bind or neutralize human lymphotoxin. Golimumab does not lyse human monocytes expressing transmembrane TNF in the presence of complement or effector cells (Simponi®, US prescribing information 2017a; Simponi Aria®, US prescribing information 2017).

The efficacy and safety of golimumab have been assessed in various adult RA populations (methotrexate-inadequate responders, methotrexate-naïve patients, and patients with previous use of other anti-TNFα agents), active PsA, active AS and pediatric patients with active polyarticular JIA. In a randomized, double-blind, controlled Phase III study in patients with active RA despite methotrexate therapy, six-month treatment with subcutaneous golimumab in combination with methotrexate at the recommended dose regimen (50 mg every 4 weeks) resulted in 60, 37, and 20% of RA patients achieving ACR20, ACR50, and ACR70, respectively, while the control group (methotrexate plus placebo) had only 28, 14, and 5% of patients exhibiting ACR20, ACR50, and ACR70 responses, respectively. Recently, another Phase III study demonstrated similar efficacy and safety for treating adult RA patients with intravenous golimumab with a longer dosing interval (every 8 weeks) as an alternative to the previously established subcutaneous route of administration (every 4 weeks).

Serious infection and malignancy Black-Box warnings were placed on the golimumab label, similar to the labels of other TNF antagonists. The concomitant use of golimumab with biologics approved to treat RA, PsA, or AS is not recommended because of the possibility of an increased risk of infection (Simponi®, US prescribing information, 2017a; Simponi Aria®, US prescribing information 2017).

Within arthritides, golimumab is indicated for the treatment of adult patients with moderately to severely active RA, active PsA, or active AS (Simponi®, US prescribing information, 2017a; Simponi Aria®, US prescribing information 2017). Golimumab is also indicated for the treatment of adult patients with nonradiographic axial spondyloarthritis (nr-AxSpA), and children with polyarticular JIA with a body weight of at least 40 kg, who have responded inadequately to previous therapy with methotrexate (Simponi®, SmPC 2017b).

Infliximab

Infliximab (Remicade®) is a chimeric IgG1κ mAb that is composed of human constant and murine variable regions. Infliximab neutralizes the biologic activity of TNFα by binding with high affinity to the soluble and transmembrane forms of TNFα and inhibits binding of TNFα with its receptors. Infliximab does not neutralize TNFβ (lymphotoxin-α) (Remicade®, US prescribing information 2017).

The efficacy and safety of infliximab have been assessed in various adult RA populations (methotrexate-inadequate responders and methotrexate-naïve patients), active PsA, and active AS. In a randomized, double-blind, controlled Phase III study in patients with active RA despite methotrexate therapy, 30-week treatment with intravenous infliximab (3 mg/kg at 0, 2, and 6 weeks, following by 3 mg/kg every 8 weeks thereafter) in combination with methotrexate resulted in 50, 27, and 8% of RA patients achieving ACR20, ACR50, and ACR70, respectively, while the control group (methotrexate plus placebo) had only 20, 5, and 0% of patients exhibiting ACR20, ACR50, and ACR70 responses, respectively.

Serious infection and malignancy Black-Box warnings were placed on the infliximab label (Remicade®, US prescribing information 2017), similar to the labels of other TNF antagonists.

There is insufficient information regarding the concomitant use of infliximab with other biological therapeutics used to treat the same conditions as infliximab. The concomitant use of infliximab with these biologics is not recommended because of the possibility of an increased risk of infection. An increased risk of serious infections has been seen in clinical RA trials of other TNF blockers used in combination with anakinra or abatacept, with no added benefit (described earlier in this chapter); therefore, use of infliximab with abatacept or anakinra is not recommended. The use of tocilizumab (IL-6 receptor antagonist) in combination with TNF antagonists, including infliximab, should also be avoided because of the possibility of increased immunosuppression and increased risk of infection (Remicade®, US prescribing information 2017).

Within arthritides, infliximab is indicated for reducing signs and symptoms, inhibiting the progression of structural damage, and improving physical function in patients with moderately to severe active RA. Infliximab is also indicated for reducing signs and symptoms in patients with active AS and in patients with active PsA, inhibiting the progression of structural damage, and improving physical function in patients with PsA (Remicade®, US prescribing information 2017).

■ Anti-IL-1β Biologic Agent

As of February 2018, canakinumab (Ilaris®) is the only anti-IL-β biologic agent approved for arthritides related disorders, i.e., systemic JIA (sJIA). Systemic JIA (sJIA) is a severe autoinflammatory disease, driven by innate immunity by means of proinflammatory cytokines such as IL-1β.

Canakinumab

Canakinumab (Ilaris®) is a recombinant human IgG1κ anti-IL-1β mAb. Canakinumab binds to human IL-1β and neutralizes its activity by blocking its interaction with IL-1 receptors, but it does not bind IL-1α or IL-1 receptor antagonist (IL-1Ra) (Ilaris®, US prescribing information 2016).

The efficacy and safety of canakinumab have been assessed in two Phase III studies (Study 1 and Study 2) in sJIA patients aged 2 to less than 20 years. Study 1 was a randomized, double-blind, placebo-controlled, single-dose 4-week study in sJIA patients who were randomized to receive a single subcutaneous dose of 4 mg/kg canakinumab or placebo. At Day 29, 81, 79 and 67% of sJIA patients who received a single subcutaneous dose of 4 mg/kg canakinumab achieved PEDACR30, PEDACR50, and PEDACR70 responses (30, 50 and 70% improvement in an adapted Pediatric American College of Rheumatology response criterion), respectively, while the control group had only 10, 5, and 2% of patients with PEDACR30, PEDACR50, and PEDACR70 responses, respectively. Study 2 was a two-part study to assess the flare prevention by canakinumab in patients with active sJIA, with an open-label, single-arm active treatment period (Part I) followed by a randomized, double-blind, placebo-controlled, event-driven withdrawal design (Part II). The probability of experiencing a flare (defined by worsening of greater than or equal to 30% in at least 3 of the 6 core Pediatric ACR response variables combined with improvement of greater than or equal to 30% in no more than 1 of the 6 variables, or reappearance of fever not due to infection for at least 2 consecutive days) over time in Part II was statistically lower for the canakinumab group than for the placebo group. This corresponded to a 64% relative reduction in the risk of flare for patients in the canakinumab group as compared to those in the placebo group.

An increased incidence of serious infections and an increased risk of neutropenia have been associated with administration of another IL-1 blocker in combination with TNF inhibitors (anakinra in combination with etanercept) in another patient population (adult RA). Use of canakinumab with TNF inhibitors may also result in similar toxicities and is not recommended because this may increase the risk of serious infections (Ilaris®, US prescribing information 2016).

Of the arthritides, canakinumab is indicated for the treatment of active systemic JIA in patients aged 2 years and older (Ilaris®, US prescribing information 2016).

■ Anti IL-17A Agent

Two anti-IL-17A biologic agents have been approved for arthritides related disorders, ixekizumab (Taltz®) and secukinumab (Cosentyx®). Ixekizumab is a humanized IgG4 mAb while secukinumab (Cosentyx®) is a human IgG1κ mAb. Each of these two agents selectively binds with the IL-17A cytokine and inhibits its interaction with the IL-17 receptor. IL-17A is a naturally occurring cytokine that is involved in normal inflammatory and immune responses. Ixekizumab or secukinumab inhibits the release of proinflammatory cytokines and chemokines.

Ixekizumab

Ixekizumab (Taltz®) is a humanized anti-IL17A IgG4 mAb produced by recombinant DNA technology in a recombinant mammalian cell line (Taltz®, US prescribing information 2017).

The efficacy and safety of ixekizumab have been assessed in two randomized, double-blind, controlled Phase III studies in patients with active PsA despite NSAIDs, corticosteroid or non-biologic conventional DMARD therapy. In the randomized, double-blind, controlled Phase III study in biologic-naive PsA patients (43% patients with concomitant methotrexate use), 6-month treatment with subcutaneous ixekizumab at the recommended dose regimen (160 mg at week 0, followed by 80 mg every 4 weeks thereafter) resulted in 58, 40, and 23% of RA patients achieving ACR20, ACR50, and ACR70, respectively, while the control group had only 30, 15, and 6% of patients with ACR20, ACR50, and ACR70 responses, respectively. In the other Phase III study in anti-TNFα experienced PsA patients, greater responses compared to placebo were seen regardless of prior anti-TNF exposure.

Of the arthritides, ixekizumab is indicative for the treatment of adult patients with moderately to severely active PsA (Taltz®, US prescribing information 2017).

Secukinumab

Secukinumab (Cosentyx®) is a recombinant human anti-IL-17A IgG1/κ mAb expressed in a recombinant Chinese Hamster Ovary cell line (Cosentyx®, US prescribing information 2017).

The efficacy and safety of secukinumab have been assessed in adult patients with active PsA and active AS. In a randomized, double-blind, controlled Phase III study in patients with active PsA despite NSAIDs, corticosteroid or DMARD therapy, 6-month treatment with subcutaneous secukinumab at the recommended dose regimen (150 mg every 4 weeks) resulted in 51, 35, and 21% of RA patients (55% of these patients had concomitant methotrexate use) achieving ACR20, ACR50, and ACR70, respectively, while the control group had only 15, 7, and 1% of patients with ACR20, ACR50, and ACR70 responses, respectively.

Of the arthritides, secukinumab is indicated for the treatment of adult patients with active PsA and active AS (Cosentyx®, US prescribing information 2017).

■ Anti-IL-12/IL-23 Agent

As of February 2018, ustekinumab (Stelara®) is the only anti-IL-12/IL-23 biologic agent approved for arthritides related disorders, i.e., PsA. IL-12 and IL-23 are naturally occurring cytokines that are involved in inflammatory and immune responses, such as natural killer cell activation and CD4+ T-cell differentiation and activation.

Ustekinumab

Ustekinumab (Stelara®) is a human IgG1κ mAb that binds with high affinity and specificity to the p40 protein subunit used by both the IL-12 and IL-23 cytokines. In *in vitro* models, ustekinumab was shown to disrupt IL-12- and IL-23-mediated signaling and cytokine cascades by disrupting the interaction of these cytokines with a shared cell surface receptor chain, IL-12β1 (Stelara®, US prescribing information 2017).

The safety and efficacy of ustekinumab have been assessed in adult patients with active PsA (≥5 swollen joints and ≥ 5 tender joints) despite NSAIDs or DMARD therapy. In a randomized, double-blind, controlled Phase III studies in TNF blocker naïve PsA patients (approximately 50% of patients continued on stable doses of methotrexate), 6-month treatment in patients received subcutaneous ustekinumab treatment at the recommend dose regimen (45 mg at weeks 0 and 4 followed by every 12 weeks thereafter) resulted in 42, 25, 12 and 57% of PsA patients achieving ACR20, ACR50, ACR70, and PASI75 (at least a 75% reduction in PASI [Psoriasis Activity and Severity Index] score from baseline) respectively, while the control group (placebo) had only 23, 9, 2, and 11% of patients with ACR20, ACR20, ACR50, ACR70, and PASI75 respectively.

Of the arthritides, ustekinumab is indicated for the treatment of adult patients with active PsA, alone or in combination with methotrexate (Stelara®, US prescribing information 2017).

■ Anti-IL-6 Receptor Agent

Two anti-IL-6 receptor biologic agents have been approved for arthritides related disorders, sarilumab (Kevzara®) and tocilizumab (Actemra®). Sarilumab is a human IgG1 mAb while tocilizumab is a humanized IgG1κ mAb. Each of these two agents selectively binds to both soluble and membrane-bound IL-6 receptors (sIL-6R and mIL-6R), and has been shown to inhibit IL-6-mediated signaling through these receptors. IL-6 is a pleiotropic pro-inflammatory cytokine produced by a variety of cell types including T- and B-cells, lymphocytes, monocytes and fibroblasts. IL-6 has been shown to be involved in diverse physiological processes such as T-cell activation, induction of immunoglobulin secretion, initiation of hepatic acute phase protein synthesis, and stimulation of hematopoietic precursor cell proliferation and differentiation. IL-6 is also produced by synovial and endothelial cells leading to local production of IL-6 in joints affected by inflammatory processes such as RA (Actemra®, US prescribing information 2017).

Sarilumab

Sarilumab (Kevzara®) is a human recombinant anti-IL-6 receptor mAb of the IgG1 subclass, which is produced by recombinant DNA technology in Chinese Hamster Ovary cell suspension culture (Kevzara®, US prescribing information 2017).

The efficacy and safety of sarilumab have been assessed in patients with moderately to severely active RA who had inadequate clinical response to methotrexate and who had an inadequate clinical response or were intolerant to one or more TNFα antagonists. In a randomized, double-blind, controlled Phase III study in RA patients with inadequate clinical response to methotrexate, 6-month treatment with subcutaneous sarilumab at the recommended dose regimen (200 mg every 2 weeks) with concomitant methotrexate use resulted in 66, 46, and 25% of RA patients achieving ACR20, ACR50, and ACR70, respectively, while the control group had only 33, 17, and 7% of patients with ACR20, ACR50, and ACR70 responses, respectively.

Serious infection Black-Box warning was placed on the sarilumab label (Kevzara®, US prescribing information 2017). Serious infections leading to hospitalization or death including bacterial, viral, invasive fungal, and other opportunistic infections have occurred in patients receiving sarilumab. In the 52-week placebo-controlled population, the rate of serious infections in the 200 mg and 150 mg sarilumab with concomitant DMARD group was 4.3 and 3.0 events per 100 patient-years, respectively, compared to 3.1 events per 100 patient-years in the placebo plus DMARD group. In the long-term safety population, the overall rate of serious infections was consistent with rates in the controlled periods of the studies. The most frequently observed serious infections included pneumonia and cellulitis. Cases of opportunistic infections have been reported. Therefore, signs and symptoms of infection should be closely monitored during treatment with sarilumab. Sarilumab use should be avoided during an active infection.

Sarilumab was approved for the treatment of adult patients with moderately to severely active RA who have had an inadequate response or intolerance to one or more DMARDs (Kevzara®, US prescribing information 2017).

Tocilizumab

Tocilizumab (Actemra®), a recombinant humanized anti-IL-6 receptor mAb of IgG 1κ, was the first drug approved in this class (Actemra®, US prescribing information 2017).

The efficacy and safety of tocilizumab have been assessed in various adult RA populations (DMARD [including methotrexate]-inadequate responders, and methotrexate-naïve patients, and patients with an inadequate clinical response or intolerant to one or more TNF antagonist therapies), and pediatrics with polyarticular JIA and systemic JIA. In a randomized, double-blind, controlled Phase III study in RA patients, treatment with intravenous tocilizumab (4 or 8 mg/kg) in combination with methotrexate resulted in 51–56%, 25–32%, and 11–13% of RA patients achieving ACR20, ACR50, and ACR70, respectively, at week 24, while the control group (methotrexate plus placebo) had only 27, 10, and 2% of patients exhibiting ACR20, ACR50, and ACR70 responses, respectively. Recently, another Phase III study demonstrated similar efficacy and safety for treating RA patients using a subcutaneous route of administration as an alternative to the previously established intravenous route of administration.

Serious infection Black-Box warning was placed on the tocilizumab label (Actemra®, US prescribing information 2017). Serious infections leading to hospitalization or death including tuberculosis (TB), bacterial, viral, invasive fungal, and other opportunistic infections have occurred in patients receiving tocilizumab. In the 24-week, controlled clinical studies, the rate of serious infections in the tocilizumab intravenously administrated 8 mg/kg monotherapy group was 3.6 per 100 patient-years compared to 1.5 per 100 patient-years in the methotrexate group. The rate of serious infections in the 8 mg/kg intravenously administrated tocilizumab plus DMARD group was 5.3 events per 100 patient-years, respectively, compared to 3.9 events per 100 patient-years in the placebo plus DMARD group. Therefore, tocilizumab should not be administered during an active infection, including localized infections. If a serious infection develops, interrupt tocilizumab until the infection is controlled.

Of the arthritides, tocilizumab is indicated as a second-line biologic therapy for the treatment of adult patients with moderately to severely active RA who have had an inadequate response to one or more TNF antagonist therapies. It is also indicated for the treatment of pediatric patients 2 years of age and older with active polyarticular JIA and systemic JIA (Actemra®, US prescribing information 2017).

■ Anti-CD80/CD86 Agent to Inhibit Lymphocyte Activation

Abatacept

Abatacept (Orencia®) is a soluble fusion protein that consists of the extracellular domain of human cytotoxic T-lymphocyte-associated antigen 4 (CTLA-4) linked to the Fc portion of human IgG1. Abatacept inhibits T-lymphocyte activation by binding to CD80 and CD86 on antigen presenting cells (APC), thereby blocking interaction with CD28 on T-cells which is required for their activation (Orencia®, US prescribing information 2017). Activated T lymphocytes are implicated in the pathogenesis of RA.

The efficacy and safety of abatacept have been assessed in various adult RA populations (DMARD [including methotrexate]-inadequate responders, anti-TNFα-inadequate responders, and methotrexate-naïve patients), active polyarticular JIA and active PsA. In a randomized, double-blind, controlled Phase III study in patients with active RA despite methotrexate therapy, 6-month treatment with intravenous abatacept in combination with methotrexate at the recommended dose regimen (500, 750, and 1000 mg for patients weighing <60 kg, 60–100 kg, and > 100 kg, respectively) resulted in 68, 40, and 20% of RA patients achieving ACR20, ACR50, and ACR70, respectively, while the control group (methotrexate plus placebo) had only 40, 17, and 7% of patients achieving ACR20, ACR50, and ACR70 responses, respectively. Recently, another Phase III study demonstrated similar efficacy and safety for treating RA patients using a subcutaneous route of administration as an alternative to the previously established intravenous route of administration.

As described earlier in this chapter, abatacept should not be given concomitantly with TNF antagonists due to an increased risk of serious adverse events, including infections, whereas no clear signal in clinical benefit when compared to anti-TNF therapy alone.

Abatacept is indicated for the treatment of adult patients with moderately to severely active RA and

PsA. It is also indicated for reducing signs and symptoms in pediatric patients 2 years of age and older with moderately to severely active polyarticular JIA (Orencia®, US prescribing information 2017).

Anti-CD20 Cytolytic Agent

Rituximab

Rituximab (Rituxan®) is a genetically engineered chimeric murine/human IgG1κ mAb that binds specifically to the antigen CD20 on pre-B and mature B lymphocytes. In the pathogenesis of RA, B cells may be involved in the autoimmune/inflammatory process through production of rheumatoid factor (RF) and other autoantibodies, antigen presentation, T-cell activation, and/or proinflammatory cytokine production. Rituximab binds to the CD20 antigen on B lymphocytes, and the Fc domain recruits immune effector functions to mediate B-cell lysis, resulting in B-cell depletion of circulating and tissue-based B cells (Rituxan®, US prescribing information 2016).

The efficacy and safety of rituximab have been assessed in adult patients with moderately to severely active RA who had a prior inadequate response to at least one anti-TNFα agent. In a randomized, double-blind, controlled Phase III study in RA patients, treatment with one course of intravenous rituximab (2 doses of 1000 mg rituximab separated by 2 weeks) in combination with methotrexate resulted in 51, 27, and 12% of RA patients achieving ACR20, ACR50, and ACR70, respectively, at week 24, while the control group (methotrexate plus placebo) had only 18, 5, and 1% of patients exhibiting ACR20, ACR50, and ACR70 responses, respectively.

Black-Box warnings of fatal infusion reactions, severe mucocutaneous reactions, hepatitis B virus (HBV) reactivation and progressive multifocal leukoencephalopathy (PML) were placed on the rituximab label (Rituxan®, US prescribing information 2016). Rituximab can cause severe, including fatal, infusion reactions. Severe reactions typically occurred during the first infusion with time to onset of 30–120 min. Therefore, rituximab should only be administered by a healthcare professional with appropriate medical support to manage severe infusion reactions that can be fatal if they occur. The incidence of serious infections was 2% in the rituximab-treated patients with RA and 1% in the placebo group in the pre-marketing trials. Mucocutaneous reactions, some with fatal outcome, can occur in patients treated with rituximab. These reactions include paraneoplastic pemphigus, Stevens-Johnson syndrome, lichenoid dermatitis, vesiculobullous dermatitis, and toxic epidermal necrolysis. The onset of these reactions has been variable and includes reports with onset on the first day of rituximab exposure. HBV reactivation, in some cases resulting in fulminant hepatitis, hepatic failure and death, can occur in patients treated with drugs classified as CD20-directed cytolytic antibodies, including rituximab. John Cunningham virus infection resulting in PML and death can occur in rituximab treated patients with autoimmune diseases. Most cases of PML were diagnosed within 12 months of their last infusion of rituximab. Rituximab should be discontinued in patients who experienced/developed these reactions, and rituximab is not recommended for use in patients with severe, active infections.

Within arthritides, rituximab is indicated as a second-line biologic therapy for the treatment of adult patients with moderately to severely active RA who have had an inadequate response to one or more TNF antagonist therapies. The estimated median terminal half-life of rituximab is 18 days in RA patients; however, the pharmacodynamic effect on B cells lasts much longer than the drug presence. B-cell recovery begins at approximately 6 months, and median B-cell levels return to normal by 12 months following completion of treatment with rituximab. Consequently, treatment courses of rituximab should be administered every 24 weeks or based on clinical evaluation, but no more frequent than every 16 weeks (Rituxan®, US prescribing information 2016).

SYSTEMIC LUPUS ERYTHEMATOSUS

Systemic lupus erythematosus (SLE) is an autoimmune disease characterized by the involvement of multiple organ systems, a clinical pattern of unpredictable exacerbations and remissions, and the presence of autoantibodies. The immunopathogenic characteristic of this disease is polyclonal B-cell activation that leads to hyperglobulinemia, autoantibody production, and immune complex formation, which in turn leads to inflammation and damage that can affect multiple organ systems. Generalized SLE symptoms may include fever, fatigue, rash, oral ulceration, hair loss, and arthralgias. US prevalence estimates for various types of lupus, including SLE, vary greatly, with estimates as high as 100 per 100,000 persons affected. Approximately 80–90% of patients with SLE are women.

The primary causes of SLE remain unclear. Current therapies tend to be generally immunosuppressive, often providing suboptimal control over disease manifestation and long-term outcomes due to ineffectiveness or side effects. These SLE therapies have targeted nonspecific sites for inflammatory reduction (e.g., NSAIDs and antimalarials) and immune system suppression (e.g., corticosteroids, azathioprine, cyclophosphamide, methotrexate and mycophenolate). Belimumab (Benlysta®), a B-lymphocyte stimulator (BLyS) neutralizing agent, is currently the only approved biologic therapy for SLE.

Anti- BLyS Agent

Belimumab

Belimumab (Benlysta®) is a human IgG1λ mAb specific for B-lymphocyte stimulator (BLyS) produced by recombinant DNA technology in a murine cell (NS0) expression system. Belimumab blocks the binding of soluble BLyS, a B-cell survival factor, to its receptors on B cells. Belimumab does not bind B cells directly, but by binding BLyS, it inhibits the survival of B cells, including autoreactive B cells, and reduces the differentiation of B cells into immunoglobulin-producing plasma cells (Benlysta®, US prescribing information 2017).

The safety and effectiveness of belimumab were evaluated in four randomized, double-blind, placebo-controlled studies in patients with SLE according to criteria from the American College of Rheumatology, with intravenous belimumab administration in Trials 1–3 and subcutaneous belimumab administration in Trial 4. Patients were on a stable SLE standard of care treatment regimen comprising any of the following (alone or in combination): corticosteroids, antimalarials, NSAIDs, and immunosuppressives.

The first Phase III study (Trial 1) evaluated intravenous doses of 1, 4, and 10 mg/kg belimumab plus standard of care compared to placebo plus standard of care over 52 weeks in patients with SLE. The co-primary endpoints were percent changes in SELENA-SLEDAI score (a sum of all marked SLE-related descriptors) at week 24 and time to flare over 52 weeks. Exploratory analysis of this study identified a subgroup of patients (72%), who were autoantibody positive, in whom belimumab appeared to offer benefit. The results of this study informed the design of the next two Phase III studies (Trial 2 and Trial 3) and led to the selection of a target population and indication that was limited to autoantibody-positive SLE patients. Trial 2 and Trial 3 were both randomized, double-blind, placebo-controlled trials in patients with SLE. The studies were similar in design except Trial 2 had a 52-week duration and Trial 3 had a 76-week duration. Both studies compared intravenous belimumab 1 and 10 mg/kg plus standard of care to placebo plus standard of care. Eligible patients had active SLE disease, defined as a SELENA-SLEDAI score ≥ 6, and positive autoantibody test results at screening. The primary efficacy determination was based on a composite endpoint (SLE Responder Index or SRI) response at week 52 compared to baseline. The proportion of SLE patients achieving a SRI response in Trial 2 and Trial 3 was significantly higher in the belimumab 10 mg/kg group than in the placebo group (odds ratio of 1.5–1.8 after 52 weeks of treatment). Trial 4 is another randomized, double-blind, placebo-controlled Phase III study in autoantibody-positive SLE patients, who received subcutaneous administrated belimumab (200 mg weekly dosing plus standard of care) or placebo plus standard of care. Statistically significant efficacy was achieved in the subcutaneous belimumab group versus the placebo group, with odds ratio of 1.7 after 52 weeks of treatment.

In Phase III trials, reports suggest that overall rates for adverse events, infections, treatment discontinuations due to adverse events, and fatalities were not significantly different between the belimumab- and the placebo-treated patients; however, serious and severe infusion-related reactions were reported more often in belimumab-treated patients.

Belimumab is indicated for the treatment of adult patients with active autoantibody-positive SLE who are receiving standard therapy (Benlysta®, US prescribing information 2017).

PSORIASIS

Psoriasis is the most common chronic, immune-mediated skin disorder, affecting approximately 2% of the world's population (Nestle et al. 2009). Thickened epidermal layers resulting from excessive keratinocyte cell proliferation characterize psoriasis. The majority of sufferers are afflicted with psoriasis for most of their lives. Symptoms typically present between the ages of 15 and 35, with the majority of individuals diagnosed before the age of 40. Plaque psoriasis is the most common form, affecting approximately 85–90% of individuals with the condition. The disease manifests as raised, well-demarcated, erythematous, and frequently pruritic and painful plaques with silvery scales (Christophers 2001; Griffiths and Barker 2007). Approximately 25% of individuals with psoriasis develop moderate to severe disease with widely disseminated lesions. In clinical development and in managing patient care, the Psoriasis Activity and Severity Index (PASI) is commonly used as an instrument to measure and evaluate patient care and treatment effects of anti-psoriasis therapies (Feldman and Krueger 2005).

Prior to the availability of biologic agents in psoriasis, multiple therapeutic options existed for the treatment of the disease; however, a significant unmet need remained for a safe, highly effective, convenient systemic therapy for patients with moderate to severe forms of the disease (Papp et al. 2011). Psoralen plus ultraviolet A light therapy, while effective, is inconvenient and is associated with an increased risk of skin malignancies and photodamage. Significant safety concerns and organ toxicity are associated with chronic administration of conventional systemic agents such as methotrexate, cyclosporine, and acitretin, thus limiting their use in long-term psoriasis management.

Three anti-TNFα biologic agents are approved for use in psoriasis: etanercept, adalimumab, and infliximab. Two anti-IL-17A mAbs are approved for treatment of psoriasis, ixekizumab and secukinumab. Other approved biologic agents for the treatment of psoriasis include ustekinumab (anti-IL-12/IL-23), guselkumab (anti-IL23) and brodalumab (anti-IL-17 receptor A) (Table 26.1). Efalizumab (Raptiva®) is a humanized IgG1 mAb directed against CD11 and inhibits leukocyte function. Efalizumab was approved in 2003 for the treatment of moderate to severe psoriasis but was voluntarily withdrawn in 2009 due to reports of PML, an opportunistic viral infection of the brain that usually leads to death or severe disability. Alefacept (Amevive®), is a CD2-directed human leukocyte function antigen-3 (LFA-3)/Fc fusion protein. It interferes with lymphocyte activation via CD2 and causes a reduction in subsets of CD2+ T lymphocytes and circulating total CD4+ and CD8+ T-lymphocyte counts. Alefacept was approved in 2003 for the treatment of moderate to severe psoriasis; however, because of the availability of better tolerated and more effective biologics for psoriasis, alefacept was withdrawn from use by its sponsor in 2011.

Anti-TNFα Agents

TNFα antagonists (adalimumab, etanercept, and infliximab) block the binding of TNFα to its receptor, interrupting the subsequent signaling and inflammatory pathways driven by TNFα. This activity suppresses inflammation and the increased activation of T cells that are characteristics of psoriasis (Humira®, US prescribing information 2017; Enbrel®, US prescribing information 2016; Remicade®, US prescribing information 2017).

An evidence-based comparison from clinical trials of three TNFα antagonists (adalimumab, etanercept, and infliximab) has indicated better efficacy of infliximab and adalimumab than etanercept in treating psoriasis (Langley 2012).

A meta-analysis comparing three TNFα antagonists and traditional systemic therapy (e.g., cyclosporine) used in the treatment of moderate to severe psoriasis demonstrated high efficacy and tolerability of TNFα antagonists (Langley 2012). Due to the mode of action, there is a concern that patients receiving TNFα antagonists may become more susceptible to infection; however, a meta-analysis of trial data for these TNFα antagonists showed that serious infection rates were not much higher than those in placebo-treated patients.

Another meta-analysis was completed from 20 trials employing anti-psoriatic biologics. Based on an indirect comparison and a placebo PASI50 (50% improvement in PASI score from baseline) response of 13%, infliximab had the highest predicted mean probability of response of 93, 80, and 54% for PASI50, PASI75, and PASI90 (50%, 75% and 90% improvement in PASI score from baseline), respectively, followed by ustekinumab 90 mg at 90, 74, and 46%, respectively, and then ustekinumab 45 mg, adalimumab, etanercept, and efalizumab (Reich et al. 2012).

A more recent network meta-analysis (Gomez-Garcia et al. 2017) based on 27 randomized controlled trials was conducted to assess the short-term efficacy and safety of biologic therapies for psoriasis. From the available evidence (direct and indirect comparison) collected from six biologics (infliximab, adalimumab, etanercept, secukinumab and ustekinumab), infliximab and secukinumab were shown to be the most effective short-term treatments (as ranked by PASI75 and PASI90 responses), but were the biologics most likely to produce at least one adverse event or an infectious adverse event, respectively. Ustekinumab demonstrated the best efficacy–safety profile among the six biologics (it had the third most efficacious treatment effect, and was the only agent that did not show increased risk of adverse events compared with placebo). These results are consistent with results from another recent meta-analysis (Jabbar-Lopez et al. 2017) where ustekinumab was shown to fall into the category of high efficacy and tolerability for the treatment of (together with adalimumab and secukinumab).

Adalimumab, etanercept, and infliximab have been indicative for the treatment of plaque psoriasis in adult patients. In addition, etanercept is approved for pediatric plaque psoriasis (age 4 years and older) based on the beneficial clinical evidence from a randomized, double-blind, placebo-controlled study in children 4–17 years of age with moderate to severe plaque psoriasis.

Anti IL-17A Agents

Two anti-IL-17A biologic agents have been approved for psoriasis, ixekizumab (Taltz®) and secukinumab (Cosentyx®).

Ixekizumab

An overview of ixekizumab, a humanized anti-IL-17A mAb, has been provided earlier in this chapter (Taltz®, US prescribing information 2017). In addition to the use of this antibody for the treatment of PsA, ixekizumab has also been evaluated in patients with moderate to severe plaque psoriasis. Elevated levels of IL-17A are found in psoriatic plaques. Treatment with IL-17A antagonists may reduce epidermal neutrophils and IL-17A levels in psoriatic plaques.

The safety and effectiveness of ixekizumab have been evaluated in three randomized, double-blind, placebo-controlled Phase III trials (Trials 1, 2, and 3) in patients with moderate to severe psoriasis. In the two active comparator trials (Trials 2 and 3), patients who randomized to the etanercept arm received subcutaneous etanercept 50 mg twice weekly. Three-month treatment with subcutaneous ixekizumab at the recommended dose regimen (160 mg at week 0, followed by 80 mg at weeks 2, 4, 6, 8 10, and 12, then 80 mg every 4 weeks thereafter) resulted in 87–90%, 68–71%, and 35–40% of psoriatic patients achieving PASI75, PASI90, and PASI100, respectively, while the etanercept group had 41%, 18% and 4% of patients achieving PASI75, PASI90 and PASI100, respectively; and the placebo control group had only 2–7%, 1–3% and 0–1% of patients exhibiting PASI75, PASI90 and PASI100 responses, respectively. Among clinical responders at week 12, the percentage of patients who maintained this response (i.e., static Physician Global Assessment [sPGA] score 0 or 1) at week 60 (48 weeks following re-randomization) in Trials 1 and 2 was higher for patients treated with ixekizumab (75%) compared to those treated with placebo (7%).

Ixekizumab is indicated for the treatment of adults with moderate to severe plaque psoriasis who are candidates for systemic therapy or phototherapy (Taltz®, US prescribing information 2017).

Secukinumab

An overview of secukinumab has been provided earlier in this chapter (Cosentyx®, US prescribing information 2017). In addition to the use of this human anti-IL17A mAb for the treatment of PsA and AS, secukinumab has also been evaluated in patients with plaque psoriasis.

Four randomized, double-blind, placebo-controlled Phase III trials (Trials 1, 2, 3, and 4) have been conducted for secukinumab in patients with moderate to severe psoriasis. In the active comparator trial (Trial 2), patients who randomized to the etanercept arm received subcutaneous etanercept 50 mg twice weekly. Three-month treatment with secukinumab of 300 mg subcutaneously administrated at weeks 0, 1, 2, 3 and 4, and every 4 weeks thereafter resulted in 75–87% of psoriasis patients achieving PASI75, while the etanercept group had 44% of patients achieving PASI75; and the placebo control group had only 0–5% of patients exhibiting PASI75 response (Langley et al. 2014). With continued treatment over 52 weeks, PASI75 responders maintained their responses in 81–84% patients treated with secukinumab (300 mg every 4 weeks).

A head-to-head randomized controlled trial was conducted comparing the efficacy and safety between secukinumab and ustekinumab in patients with moderate to severe psoriasis (Blauvelt et al. 2017). Secukinumab was administered 300 mg subcutaneously at baseline and at weeks 1, 2, and 3, and then every 4 weeks from week 4 onward. Ustekinumab was dosed subcutaneously at 45 mg in patients ≤100 kg and at 90 mg in those >100 kg, and given at baseline, at week 4, and then every 12 weeks. Secukinumab has demonstrated superior efficacy to ustekinumab at weeks 4 and 16 in patients with plaque psoriasis. This superior efficacy is sustained over 52 weeks in the proportion of patients achieving PASI90 (76% vs. 61%) and PASI100 (46% vs. 36%). In addition, patients received secukinumab had greater improvement in health-related quality of life and comparable safety.

Secukinumab is indicated for the treatment of adults with moderate-to-severe plaque psoriasis who are candidates for systemic therapy or phototherapy (Cosentyx®, US prescribing information 2017).

■ Anti-IL-12/IL-23 Agents

Ustekinumab

An overview of ustekinumab has been provided earlier in this chapter (Stelara®, US prescribing information 2017). In addition to its use for the treatment of PsA, the efficacy and safety of ustekinumab have been assessed in adult and adolescent patients (12 years or older) with moderate to severe psoriasis.

The safety and efficacy of ustekinumab in treatment of psoriasis were assessed in two Phase III trials (PHOENIX 1 and PHOENIX 2). The results from these two trials demonstrated that ustekinumab was effective in ameliorating psoriatic plaques, pruritus, and nail psoriasis (Leonardi et al. 2008; Papp et al. 2008). Within 12 weeks of initiating subcutaneous ustekinumab treatment (45 or 90 mg/kg at weeks 0 and 4), more than two-thirds of patients exhibited ≥75% reduction in PASI (PASI75 response). Maximum efficacy was achieved at approximately 24 weeks after initiation of therapy, with approximately 75% of ustekinumab-treated patients achieving a PASI75 response. Clinical response to ustekinumab was associated with serum ustekinumab concentrations that were somewhat correlated with patient body weight. While efficacy of the 45 and 90 mg doses of ustekinumab was similar in patients weighing ≤100 kg, the 90-mg dose was more effective than the 45-mg dose in patients weighing >100 kg, who represented approximately one-third of the combined PHOENIX 1 and PHOENIX 2 population. Thus, to optimize efficacy in all patients while minimizing unnecessary drug exposure, fixed dose administration of ustekinumab based on body weight is indicated, i.e., for patients weighing >100 kg, the recommended dose is 90 mg initially and 4 weeks later, followed by 90 mg every 12 weeks; for patients weighing ≤100 kg, the recommended dose is 45 mg initially and 4 weeks later, followed by 45 mg every 12 weeks.

Results of the Phase III psoriasis clinical trials indicated that ustekinumab was generally well tolerated. Rates and types of adverse events, serious adverse events, adverse events leading to treatment discontinuation, and laboratory abnormalities were generally comparable among patients receiving subcutaneously administration of placebo, ustekinumab 45 or 90 mg during the 12-week placebo-controlled phases of PHOENIX 1 and PHOENIX 2. Dose–response relationships for safety events were not apparent. Rates of serious infections and malignancies in PHOENIX 1 and PHOENIX 2 were low and comparable across treatment groups during the placebo-controlled phases, no apparent increase in the frequency of these adverse events was observed through 18 months of treatment, and no mycobacterial or salmonella infections were reported (Leonardi et al. 2008; Papp et al. 2008).

A head-to-head controlled trial was conducted comparing the efficacy and safety of a TNFα antagonist, etanercept, and ustekinumab in patients with moderate to severe psoriasis (Griffiths et al. 2010). Ustekinumab was administered subcutaneously at either 45 or 90 mg at weeks 0 and 4, and etanercept was administered subcutaneously 50 mg twice weekly for 12 weeks. There was at least 75% improvement in the PASI (PASI75) at week 12 in 67.5% of patients who received 45 mg of ustekinumab and 73.8% of patients who received 90 mg of ustekinumab, as compared to 56.8% of those who received etanercept ($p = 0.01$ and $p < 0.001$, respectively). The efficacy of ustekinumab at 45 or 90 mg was superior to that of etanercept over a 12-week period while the safety profiles were similar.

Ustekinumab is indicated for the treatment of adult patients with moderate-to-severe plaque psoriasis who are candidates for systemic therapy or phototherapy. Ustekinumab is also indicative for adolescent patients (12 years or older) with moderate to severe plaque psoriasis (Stelara®, US prescribing information 2017).

Anti-IL-23 Agents

As of February 2018, guselkumab (Tremfya®) is the only anti-IL-23 biologic agent approved for psoriasis. IL-23 pathway is suggested contributing to the chronic inflammation underlying the pathophysiology of psoriasis. Guselkumab, by neutralizing IL-23, inhibits the release of proinflammatory cytokines and chemokines.

Guselkumab

Guselkumab (Tremfya®) is a human IgG1λ mAb, which is produced in a mammalian cell line using recombinant DNA technology. It selectively binds to the p19 subunit of IL-23 and inhibits its interaction with the IL-23 receptor (Tremfya®, US prescribing information 2017).

The safety and efficacy of guselkumab have been evaluated in three multicenter, randomized, double-blind Phase III trials (VOYAGE 1, VOYAGE 2 and NAVIGATE) in patients with moderate to severe plaque psoriasis. In VOYAGE 1 and VOYAGE 2, patients were randomized to either guselkumab (100 mg SC at weeks 0 and 4 and every 8 weeks thereafter), placebo or U.S. licensed adalimumab (80 mg SC at week 0 and 40 mg at week 1, followed by 40 mg every other week thereafter). Sixteen-weeks treatment with subcutaneous guselkumab resulted in 70–73% of psoriasis patients achieving PASI90, while the placebo control group had only 2–3% patients exhibiting PASI90 response. An analysis based on clinical data from all the North America sites (i.e., U.S. and Canada) demonstrated superiority of guselkumab to U.S. licensed adalimumab. The PASI90 response rates at weeks 16, 24 and 48 were 64–73%, 71–80% and 73% respectively, for guselkumab; and 41–42%, 44–51% and 46% respectively, for adalimumab. NAVIGATE evaluated the efficacy of guselkumab in patients who had not achieved an adequate response at week 16 after initial treatment with ustekinumab (dosed 45 mg or 90 mg according to the subject's baseline weight [≤ and > 100 kg respectively] at week 0 and week 4). These patients were randomized to either continue with ustekinumab treatment every 12 weeks or switch to guselkumab. Twelve-weeks after randomization, a greater proportion of patients on guselkumab treatment compared to ustekinumab (31% vs. 14%) achieved an Investigator's Global Assessment (IGA) score of 0 or 1 with a ≥ 2 grade improvement.

Results of the Phase III moderate to severe plaque psoriasis clinical trials indicated that guselkumab was generally well tolerated at the recommended dose regimen. Rates and types of adverse events, serious adverse events, adverse events leading to treatment discontinuation, and laboratory abnormalities were generally comparable among patients receiving placebo and guselkumab during the 16-week placebo-controlled periods of the pooled clinical trials (VOYAGE 1 and VOYAGE 2). Infections occurred in 23% of the guselkumab group compared to 21% of the placebo group. The most common (≥ 1%) infections were upper respiratory infections, gastroenteritis, tinea infections, and herpes simplex infections; all cases were mild to moderate in severity and did not lead to discontinuation of guselkumab. Through week 48, no new adverse reactions were identified with guselkumab use and the frequency of the adverse reactions was similar to the safety profile observed during the first 16 weeks of treatment.

Guselkumab is indicated for the treatment of adult patients with moderate-to-severe plaque psoriasis who are candidates for systemic therapy or phototherapy (Tremfya®, US prescribing information 2017).

Anti-IL-17 Receptor A Agents

As of February 2018, brodalumab (Siliq®) is the only anti-IL-17 receptor A (IL-17RA) biologic agent approved for psoriasis. IL-17RA is a protein expressed on the cell surface and is a required component of receptor complexes utilized by multiple IL-17 family cytokines. Blocking IL-17RA inhibits IL-17 cytokine-induced responses including the release of pro-inflammatory cytokines and chemokines.

Brodalumab

Brodalumab (Siliq®) is a human IgG2κ mAb expressed in a Chinese Hamster Ovary cell line. It selectively binds to human IL-17 receptor A (IL-17RA) and inhibits its interactions with cytokines IL-17A, IL-17F, IL-17C, IL-17A/F heterodimer and IL-25. (Siliq®, US prescribing information 2017).

The safety and effectiveness of brodalumab have been evaluated in three multicenter, randomized, double-blind, controlled Phase III trials (Trials 1, 2, and 3) in patients with moderate to severe plaque psoriasis. In these trials, patients were randomized to placebo or subcutaneous brodalumab treatment of 210 mg at weeks 0, 1, and 2, followed by 210 mg every 2 weeks thereafter. In the two active comparator trials (Trials 2 and 3), patients randomized to the subcutaneous ustekinumab group received a 45-mg dose if their weight was ≤100 kg and a 90-mg dose if their weight was >100 kg at weeks 0, 4, and 16, followed by the same dose every 12 weeks. Treatment with brodalumab resulted in 83–86% and 37–42% of psoriatic patients achieving PASI75 and PASI100, respectively, at week 12, while the ustekinumab group had 69–70% and 19–22% of patients achieving PASI75 and PASI100, respectively; and the placebo control group had only 3–8% and 0–1% of patients exhibiting PASI75 and PASI100 responses, respectively. Maintenance of the treatment effect of brodalumab was demonstrated. Among PASI100 responders at week 12, 72% of the patients who continued on brodalumab 210 mg every 2 weeks maintained the response at week 52.

Suicidal ideation and behavior Black-Box warnings were placed on the brodalumab label (Siliq®, US prescribing information 2017). Suicidal ideation and behavior, including four completed suicides, occurred in patients treated with brodalumab in the psoriasis pre-marketing trials. There were no completed suicides in the 12-week placebo-controlled portion of the trials. A causal association between treatment with brodalumab and increased risk of suicidal ideation and behavior has not been established. Because of the observed suicidal ideation and behavior in subjects treated with brodalumab, in the United States, brodalumab is only available through a restricted program under REMS (Risk Evaluation and Mitigation Strategy). Prescribers should weigh the potential risks and benefits before using brodalumab in patients with a history of depression or suicidality. Patients with new or worsening suicidal thoughts and behavior should be referred to a mental health professional, as appropriate.

Brodalumab is indicated for the treatment of moderate to severe plaque psoriasis in adult patients who are candidates for systemic therapy or phototherapy and have failed to respond or have lost response to other systemic therapies (Siliq®, US prescribing information 2017).

INFLAMMATORY BOWEL DISEASE

Inflammatory bowel disease (IBD) refers to a group of chronic inflammatory diseases of the gastrointestinal tract that mainly comprise two well-defined clinical entities, Crohn's disease (CD) and ulcerative colitis (UC). A study in 2012 (Molodecky et al. 2012) found that prevalence of UC in North America between 1980 and 2008 was 198.1–298.5 cases per 100,000 persons and prevalence of CD was 135.7–318.5 cases/100,000 persons. CD and UC are two idiopathic IBD. They have some similarities and unique differences (Baumgart and Sandborn 2007).

CD is a relapsing, transmural inflammatory disease of the gastrointestinal mucosa that can affect the entire gastrointestinal tract from the mouth to the anus, while UC is a relapsing, nontransmural inflammatory disease that is restricted to the colon. CD may involve all layers of the intestine, and there can be normal healthy bowel between patches of diseased bowel, while UC does not affect all layers of the bowel but only affects the top layers of the colon in an even and continuous distribution. In CD, pain is commonly experienced in the lower right abdomen, while in UC, in the lower left part of the abdomen. In CD, colon wall may be thickened and may have a rocky appearance, while in UC the colon wall is thinner and shows continuous inflammation. In clinical practice, disease activity of CD is typically described as mild to moderate (ambulatory patients able to tolerate oral alimentation without manifestations of dehydration, toxicity, abdominal tenderness, painful mass, obstruction, or > 10% weight loss), moderate to severe disease (failure to respond to treatment for mild disease, more prominent symptoms of fever, weight loss, abdominal pain or tenderness, intermittent nausea and vomiting without obstruction, or significant anemia), and severe to fulminant disease (persisting symptoms on corticosteroids, high fevers, persistent vomiting, evidence of intestinal obstruction, rebound tenderness, cachexia, or evidence of an abscess). While disease activity of UC is typically described as mild (up to four bloody stools daily and no systemic toxicity), moderate (four to six blood stools daily and minimal toxicity), or severe (more than six stools daily and signs of toxicity, such as fever, tachycardia, anemia, and raised erythrocyte sedimentation rate), patients with fulminant UC usually have more than ten bloody stools daily, continuous bleeding, anemia requiring blood transfusion, abdominal tenderness, and colonic dilation on plain abdominal radiographs (Baumgart and Sandborn 2007).

Conventional pharmacologic treatments for IBD include aminosalicylates, corticosteroids, immunomodulators (azathioprine, 6-mecaptopurine, methotrexate, cyclosporine), and antibiotics (metronidazole, ciprofloxacin, clarithromycin). The aim of traditional therapy is to induce and maintain remission in patients. Treatment guidelines generally recommend initiating treatment with first-line agents such as sulfasalazine and systemic corticosteroids, followed by immunomodulators. These conventional pharmacologic therapies are often effective in patients with IBD, particularly in those with mildly to moderately active disease; however, a significant proportion of patients have severely active disease that is often refractory to these conventional therapies. Furthermore, these small molecule drugs have limitations in the treatment of IBD. Corticosteroids have many side effects and are not suitable for long-term maintenance therapy. Corticosteroids are also ineffective for healing bowel ulcerations (Modigliani et al. 1990). Immunomodulators promote mucosal healing, but the onset of action is slow. The use of anti-TNFα agents can overcome the shortcomings of the conventional treatment options and provide greater improvement for severe or refractory IBD. Anti-TNFα therapy can rapidly improve signs and symptoms (i.e., induce and maintain clinical response and clinical remission), promote mucosal healing, eliminate corticosteroid use, and has the potential to alter the natural history of IBD. Historically, therapeutic proteins have been used as rescue therapy for patients with IBD refractory to conventional therapies. Recently, evidence has emerged that early use of anti-TNFα therapy in patients at high risk may induce a greater response and prevent irreversible damage to the intestine (D'Haens et al. 2008). There are also concerns with respect to increased risks of infections and malignancy associated with the use of anti-TNFα agents in patients with IBD (Hoentjen and van Bodegraven 2009). The timing of initiating therapy with therapeutic proteins and the identification of the subset of patients who can achieve maximal benefit from treatment using therapeutic proteins remain active areas of debate, and further clinical research is required to provide evidence-based guidelines. Anti-integrin and anti-IL-12/IL-23 agents are non-TNF biologic therapies developed recently for the treatment of IBD; they provide alternative in case of treatment failures to conventional drugs (such as glucocorticoids and immunomodulators) and/or anti-TNFα therapies.

There are seven biologic agents approved for the treatment of CD and/or UC; those are four anti-TNFα agents (infliximab, adalimumab, certolizumab pegol and golimumab), one anti-IL-12/IL-23 agent (ustekinumab), and two anti-integrin agents (natalizumab and vedolizumab) (Table 26.1).

■ Anti-TNFα Agents

Four anti-TNFα agents (infliximab, adalimumab, certolizumab pegol and golimumab) have been approved for the treatment of CD and/or UC. Not all anti-TNFα agents have been shown to be effective for IBD. For example, infliximab, the first-in-class anti-TNFα biologic agent approved for treating CD, has been shown to be highly effective in the treatment of CD, but etanercept was shown to be ineffective for this disease. A mechanism postulated to explain the differential effects of infliximab and etanercept for CD was that infliximab could bind membrane-associated TNFα and induce apoptosis of activated T cells and macrophages, but etanercept only binds to soluble TNFα (Van den Brande et al. 2003). However, this theory is questioned by later data showing induction of apoptosis by etanercept and clinical efficacy of certolizumab pegol, a non-apoptotic anti-TNFα agent (Chaudhary et al. 2006; Sandborn et al. 2006). As of February 2018, infliximab is the only antibody-based therapeutic protein approved for pediatric patients with CD or UC. For pediatric patients with CD, adalimumab is also approved as an anti-TNFα biologic therapy.

Adalimumab

An overview of adalimumab, a human anti-TNFα mAb, has been provided earlier in this chapter (Humira®, US prescribing information 2017). In addition to the use of this therapeutic protein for the treatment of arthritides and psoriasis, the efficacy and safety of adalimumab have been assessed in adult and pediatric patients with active CD, and adult patients with active UC.

The efficacy and safety of adalimumab in the treatment of adult CD have been evaluated in patients with moderately to severely active CD (Crohn's Disease Activity Index [CDAI] $\geq$ 220 and $\leq$ 450) in three randomized, double-blind, controlled Phase III studies (CD-1I, CD-II and CD-III). In a Phase III Study (CD-I) in CD patients who were naïve to TNF blocker, treatment with subcutaneous adalimumab at the recommended induction dose regimen (160 and 80 mg at weeks 0 and 2, respectively) resulted in 58 and 36% of patients achieving clinical response (defined as a decrease in CDAI of at least 70 points) and clinical remission (defined as CDAI <150), respectively, at week 4, while the control group (placebo) had 34 and 12% of patients with clinical response and clinical remission, respectively. A greater percentage of the patients treated with adalimumab also achieved induction of clinical response and remission versus placebo at week 4 in CD patients who had lost response to or were intolerant to infliximab in another Phase III trial (CD-II). The adalimumab group had 52 and 21% of patients who were in clinical response and clinical remission, respectively, at week 4, while the placebo group had 34 and 7% of patients in clinical response and clinical remission, respectively. In the third Phase III trial (CD-III), maintenance of clinical remission was evaluated. Among clinical responders at week 4, further maintenance treatment with 40 mg adalimumab administrated subcutaneously every other week demonstrated greater efficacy than the placebo maintenance group. The adalimumab maintenance group had 43 and 36% of patients who were in clinical response and clinical remission, respectively, at week 56, while the placebo maintenance group had 18 and 12% of patients in clinical response and clinical remission, respectively.

Two randomized, double-blind, placebo-controlled Phase III studies (UC-I and UC-II) have been conducted for adalimumab in patients with moderately to severely active UC (Mayo score 6–12 on a 12-point scale, with an endoscopy subscore of 2–3 on a scale of 0–3) despite concurrent or prior treatment with immunosuppressants such as corticosteroids, azathioprine, or 6-mercaptopurine. All patients in Study UC-I were TNF blocker naïve and 40% patients enrolled in Study UC-II had previously used another TNF-blocker. In both UC-I and UC-II studies, a greater percentage of the patients treated with subcutaneous adalimumab at the recommended subcutaneous dose regimen (160 and 80 mg at weeks 0 and 2, respectively) compared to patients treated with placebo (16.5–18.5% vs. ~ 9%) achieved induction of clinical remission (defined as Mayo score ≤ 2 with no individual subscores >1). In Study UC-II, a greater percentage of the patients treated with maintenance adalimumab of 40 mg every other week compared to patients treated with placebo (8.5% vs. 4.1%) achieved sustained clinical remission (defined as clinical remission at both weeks 8 and 52). The subgroup of patients with prior TNF-blocker use in Study UC-II achieved induction of clinical remission at 9% in the adalimumab group versus 7% in the placebo group, and sustained clinical remission at 5% in the adalimumab group versus 1% in the placebo group.

In addition to adult CD and UC, safety and efficacy of adalimumab for pediatric patients 6 years of age or older with CD have also been established. Use of adalimumab in this age group is supported by evidence from adult CD trials with additional data in pediatric CD patients (6–17 years of age) from a randomized, double-blind Phase III study.

Among IBD indications, adalimumab is indicated for treatment of CD by reducing signs and symptoms and inducing and maintaining clinical remission in adult patients with moderately to severely active CD who have had an inadequate response to conventional therapy, and by reducing signs and symptoms and inducing clinical remission in these patients if they have also lost response to or are intolerant to infliximab. Adalimumab is also indicated for treatment of UC by inducing and sustaining clinical remission in adult patients with moderately to severely active ulcerative colitis who have had an inadequate response to immunosuppressants such as corticosteroids, azathioprine or 6-mercaptopurine. Adalimumab is also indicated for treatment of pediatric CD in patients 6 years of age and older who have had an inadequate response to corticosteroids or immunomodulators (Humira®, US prescribing information 2017).

Certolizumab Pegol

An overview of certolizumab pegol, a TNF blocker, has been provided earlier in this chapter (Cimzia®, US prescribing information 2016). In addition to its use for the treatment of RA and PsA, the efficacy and safety of certolizumab pegol have also been assessed in adult patients with moderately to severely active CD.

In a randomized, double-blind, controlled Phase III study in patients with active CD (CDAI ≥220 and ≤ 450), treatment with subcutaneous certolizumab pegol at the recommended induction dose regimen (400 mg at weeks 0, 2, and 4) resulted in 35 and 22% of patients achieving clinical response (defined as a decrease in CDAI ≥100) and clinical remission (defined as CDAI ≤150), respectively, at week 6, while the control group (placebo) had 27 and 17% of patients with clinical response and clinical remission, respectively. Among clinical responders at week 6, further maintenance treatment with 400 mg certolizumab pegol administrated subcutaneously every 4 weeks demonstrated greater efficacy than the placebo maintenance group. The certolizumab pegol maintenance group had 63 and 48% of patients who were in clinical response and clinical remission, respectively, at week 26, while the placebo maintenance group had 36 and 29% of patients in clinical response and clinical remission, respectively.

Among IBD indications, Certolizumab pegol is indicated for reducing signs and symptoms of CD and maintaining clinical response in adult patients with moderately to severely active disease who have had an inadequate response to conventional therapy (Cimzia®, US prescribing information 2016).

Golimumab

An overview of golimumab, an anti-TNFα human mAb, has been provided earlier in this chapter (Simponi®, US prescribing information, 2017a; Simponi Aria®, US prescribing information 2017). In addition to its use for the treatment of RA, PsA and AS, the efficacy and safety of golimumab have been assessed in adult patients with moderately to severely active UC.

In a randomized, double-blind, controlled Phase III study in patients with active UC (Mayo score of 6–12), treatment with subcutaneous golimumab at the recommended induction dose regimen (200 mg at week 0, followed by 100 mg at week 2) resulted in 51 and 18% of patients achieving clinical response (defined as a decrease from baseline in the Mayo score of ≥30% and ≥ 3 points, accompanied by a decrease in the rectal bleeding subscore of ≥1 or a rectal bleeding subscore of 0 or 1) and clinical remission (defined as defined as a Mayo score ≤ 2 points, with no individual subscore >1; improvement of endoscopic appearance of the mucosa was defined as a Mayo endoscopy subscore of 0 [normal or inactive disease] or 1 [erythema, decreased vascular pattern, mild friability]), respectively, at week 6, while the control group (placebo) had 30 and 6% of patients with clinical response and clinical remission, respectively. Among clinical responders at week 6, further maintenance treatment with 100 mg subcutaneous golimumab every 4 weeks demonstrated greater efficacy than the placebo maintenance group. The golimumab maintenance group had 50 and 28% of patients who were in clinical response at week 54 and clinical remission at both week 30 and week 54, respectively, while the placebo maintenance group had 31 and 16% of patients in clinical response and clinical remission, respectively.

Among IBD indications, golimumab is indicated for adult patients with moderately to severely active UC with an inadequate response or intolerant to prior treatment or requiring continuous steroid therapy who have had an inadequate response to conventional therapy, for inducing and maintaining clinical response, improving endoscopic appearance of the mucosa during induction, inducing clinical remission, and achieving and sustaining clinical remission in induction responders (Simponi®, US prescribing information 2017a).

Infliximab

An overview of infliximab, an anti-TNFα chimeric mAb, has been provided earlier in this chapter (Remicade®, US prescribing information 2017). In addition to its use for the treatment of arthritides and psoriasis, the efficacy and safety of infliximab have also been assessed in adult and pediatric patients with moderately to severely active CD or UC.

In a randomized, double-blind, controlled Phase III study in patients with moderately to severely active CD (CDAI ≥220 and ≤ 400), treatment with an initial intravenous dose of 5 mg/kg infliximab at week 0 resulted in 57% of patients achieving clinical response (defined as a decrease in CDAI ≥70) at week 2. All patients who received 5 mg/kg infliximab at week 0 were then randomized to placebo or infliximab maintenance groups (5 or 10 mg/kg at weeks 2 and 6, followed by every 8 weeks). Maintenance treatment with infliximab demonstrated greater efficacy than placebo maintenance treatment. The 5 and 10 mg/kg infliximab maintenance groups had 25 and 34% of patients who were in clinical remission and discontinued corticosteroid use, respectively, at week 54, while the placebo maintenance group had 11% of patients in clinical remission with corticosteroid discontinuation.

In another randomized, double-blind, controlled Phase III study in patients with moderately to severely active UC (Mayo score of 6–12, Endoscopy subscore ≥2), patients were randomized at week 0 to receive either placebo or infliximab at weeks 0, 2, and 6 and every 8 weeks thereafter. At week 8, a greater proportion of patients in the 5 mg/kg infliximab treatment group were in clinical response (defined as a decrease in Mayo score by ≥30% and ≥ 3 points;) and clinical remission (defined as a Mayo score ≤ 2 points with no individual subscore >1) compared to the placebo treatment group (69% vs. 37% for clinical response; 39% vs. 15% for clinical remission). The clinical efficacy was maintained over time. At week 54, the 5 mg/kg infliximab maintenance group had 45 and 35% of patients who were in clinical response and clinical remission, respectively, while the placebo maintenance group had 20 and 17% of patients in clinical response and clinical remission, respectively.

For both CD and UC, maintenance therapy with infliximab every 8 weeks significantly reduced disease-related hospitalizations and surgeries. A reduction in corticosteroid use and improvements in quality of life were observed. In addition, the safety and efficacy of infliximab for pediatric patients 6 years of age or older with CD or UC have also been established.

Among IBD indications, infliximab is indicated for treatment of CD by reducing signs and symptoms and inducing and maintaining clinical remission in adult patients with moderately to severely active disease who have had an inadequate response to conventional therapy and by reducing the number of draining enterocutaneous and rectovaginal fistulas and maintaining fistula closure in adult patients with fistulizing disease. Infliximab is also indicated for treatment of UC by reducing signs and symptoms, inducing and maintaining clinical remission and mucosal healing, and eliminating corticosteroid use in adult patients with moderately to severely active disease who have had an inadequate response to conventional therapy. Additionally, infliximab is indicated for treatment of pediatric patients 6 years of age or older with CD or UC who have had an inadequate response to conventional therapy (Remicade®, US prescribing information 2017).

Anti-IL-12/IL-23 Agents

Ustekinumab

An overview of ustekinumab, a human anti-IL-12/IL-23 mAb, has been provided earlier in this chapter (Stelara®, US prescribing information 2017). In addition to its use for the treatment of PsA and psoriasis, the safety and efficacy of ustekinumab, an IL-12/IL-23 inhibitor, in treatment of CD has been recently established (Stelara®, US prescribing information 2017). IL-12 and IL-23 have been implicated as important contributors to the chronic inflammation that is a hallmark of CD and UC.

The efficacy and safety of ustekinumab have been assessed in three randomized, double-blind, placebo-controlled Phase III studies in adult patients with moderately to severely active CD (CDAI ≥220 and ≤ 450). These were two 8-week intravenous induction studies (CD-1 and CD-2) followed by a 44-week subcutaneous randomized withdrawal maintenance study (CD-3) representing 52 weeks of therapy. In both induction studies (CD-1 and CD-2), patients were randomized to receive a single intravenous administration of ustekinumab at either approximately 6 mg/kg (recommended induction dose), placebo, or 130 mg (a lower dose than recommended). Patients who had failed or were intolerant to prior treatment with a TNF blocker were enrolled for Study CD-1, while patients who had never received a TNF blocker or previously received but had not failed a TNF blocker were enrolled for Study CD-2. Concomitant stable dosages of aminosalicylates, corticosteroids, and immunomodulators were allowed in both studies. In Study CD-1, the ustekinumab group had 34 and 21% of patients who were in clinical response (defined as reduction in CDAI score by at least 100 points) at week 6 and clinical remission (defined as CDAI score < 150) at week 8, respectively, while the placebo group had 21 and 7% of patients in clinical response at week 6 and clinical remission at week 8, respectively. In Study CD-2, the ustekinumab group had 56 and 40% of patients who were in clinical response at week 6 and clinical remission at week 8, respectively, while the placebo group had 29 and 20% of patients in clinical response at week 6 and clinical remission at week 8, respectively. The maintenance study (CD-3) evaluated patients who achieved clinical response at week 8 of induction in studies CD-1 or CD-2. At week 44 of the maintenance treatment (i.e., week 52 from the initiation of induction therapy), 47% of patients received 90 mg subcutaneous ustekinumab every 8 weeks maintenance treatment demonstrated corticosteroid-free and in clinical remission, compared to 30% of patients in the placebo group.

Among IBD indications, ustekinumab is indicated for treatment of adult patients with moderately to severely active CD who have failed or were intolerant to treatment with immunomodulators or corticosteroids, but never failed a TNF blocker or who failed or were intolerant to treatment with one or more TNF blockers (Stelara®, US prescribing information 2017).

Anti-integrin Agent

Natalizumab and vedolizumab are both anti-integrin agents approved for treatment of CD (vedolizumab is also indicated for the treatment of UC). Natalizumab has a more restricted use with a requirement for patient registration due to its potential risk of PML. It has been hypothesized that preventing α4β1/α4β7 integrin binding to vascular cell adhesion molecule-1 (VCAM-1) may result in decreased immune surveillance within the central nervous system (CNS), in turn increasing the risk of developing PML. Unlike natalizumab, vedolizumab specifically targets α4β7 and does not inhibit binding at VCAM-1 (Soler et al. 2009). Overall, vedolizumab seems to be safe with respect to the risk of PML but continuous and careful monitoring of patients is needed to explore its full safety profile.

Natalizumab

Natalizumab (Tysabri®) is a recombinant humanized IgG4κ mAb that is produced in murine myeloma cells. Natalizumab binds to the α4-subunit of α4β1 and α4β7 integrins expressed on the surface of all leukocytes, and inhibits the α4-mediated adhesion of leukocytes to their counter-receptor(s). Disruption of these molecular interactions prevents transmigration of leukocytes across the endothelium into inflamed parenchymal tissue (Tysabri®, US prescribing information 2017).

The efficacy and safety of natalizumab have been assessed in adult patients with moderately to severely active CD (CDAI ≥220 and ≤450). In a randomized, double-blind, controlled Phase III study in patients with active CD, treatment with intravenous natalizumab at the recommended induction dose regimen (300 mg every 4 weeks) resulted in 56% of patients achieving clinical response (defined as a decrease in CDAI ≥70 from baseline) at week 10, while the control group (placebo) had 49% of patients achieving clinical response ($p = 0.067$). Among clinical responders at both weeks 10 and 12, maintenance treatment with 300 mg natalizumab every 4 weeks demonstrated greater efficacy than that observed in the placebo maintenance group. The natalizumab maintenance group had 54 and 40% of patients who were in clinical response and clinical remission (defined as CDAI score < 150) at month 15, respectively, while the placebo maintenance group had 20 and 15% of patients in clinical response and clinical remission, respectively.

Natalizumab was first approved in November 2004 and was suspended soon after (February 2005) because of the occurrence of three cases of PML, an opportunistic viral infection of the brain that usually leads to death or severe disability. Two of the three PML cases were reported in multiple sclerosis patients (another indication of natalizumab) and one in a patient with CD. In June 2006, the US FDA and European Medicine Agency (EMA) granted approval for the reintroduction of natalizumab under a specific risk management plan designed to redefine the safety profile of natalizumab (with Black-Box Warning in label) (Gold et al. 2007).

Among IBD indications, natalizumab is indicated for the induction and maintenance of clinical response and remission in adult patients with moderately to severely active CD with evidence of inflammation who have had an inadequate response to, or are unable to tolerate, conventional CD therapies and TNF-α inhibitors. Natalizumab should not be used in combination with immunosuppressants or inhibitors of TNFα in CD (Tysabri®, US prescribing information 2017).

■ Vedolizumab

Vedolizumab (Entyvio®) is a humanized IgG1 mAb produced in Chinese hamster ovary cells. Vedolizumab specifically binds to the α4β7 integrin and blocks the interaction of α4β7 integrin with mucosal addressin cell adhesion molecule-1 (MAdCAM-1) and inhibits the migration of memory T-lymphocytes across the endothelium into inflamed gastrointestinal parenchymal tissue. Vedolizumab does not bind to or inhibit function of the α4β1 and αEβ7 integrins and does not antagonize the interaction of α4 integrins with VCAM-1. The interaction of the α4β7 integrin with MAdCAM-1 has been implicated as an important contributor to the chronic inflammation that is a hallmark of CD and UC. (Entyvio®, US prescribing information 2014).

The efficacy and safety of vedolizumab have been assessed in three randomized, double-blind, placebo-controlled Phase III studies (Trials CD-1, CD-II and CD-III) in adult patients with moderately to severely active CD (CDAI ≥220 and ≤450). Trials CD-I and CD-II both assessed induction regimens. A higher number of patients who had an inadequate response, loss of response, or intolerance to one or more TNF blockers were enrolled in CD-II when compared to CD-II (76% vs. 46%). Concomitant stable dosages of aminosalicylates, corticosteroids, and immunomodulators were allowed in both CD-1 and CD-II. In Study CD-I, a statistically significantly higher proportion of patients treated with vedolizumab at the recommended dose regimen (300 mg intravenous infusion at weeks 0 and 2) achieved clinical remission (defined as CDAI ≤150) as compared to placebo at week 6 (15% vs. 7%, $p = 0.041$). In Study CD-II, among patients who had an inadequate response, loss of response, or intolerance to one or more TNF blockers, no statistical significant difference was shown in the proportion of patients achieving clinical remission between the 300 mg vedolizumab group and the placebo group at week 6 (15% vs. 12%). Study CD-III evaluated the maintenance regimen. Among clinical responders ((≥70 decrease in CDAI score from baseline) at week 6, 39% of patients who received maintenance treatment with 300 mg vedolizumab intravenous infusion every 8 weeks demonstrated clinical remission (defined as the proportion of patients in this subgroup that discontinued corticosteroids by week 52 and were in clinical remission at week 52), compared to 22% of patients in the placebo group.

The efficacy and safety of vedolizumab have also been assessed in two randomized, double-blind, placebo-controlled Phase III studies (Trials UC-1 and UC-II) in adult patients with moderately to severely active UC (Mayo score of 6–12 with endoscopy subscore of 2 or 3). UC-I assessed the induction therapy and UC-II assessed the maintenance therapy. Concomitant stable dosages of aminosalicylates, corticosteroids, and immunomodulators were allowed in both studies. Six-weeks treatment with vedolizumab (300 mg intravenous infusion at week 0 and week 2) compared to placebo resulted in a greater proportion of patients achieved clinical response at week 6 (47% vs. 26%, defined as reduction in complete Mayo score of ≥3 points and ≥30% from baseline with an accompanying decrease in rectal bleeding subscore of ≥1 point or absolute rectal bleeding subscore of ≤1 point), clinical remission at week 6 (17% vs. 5%, defined as complete Mayo score of ≤2 points and no individual subscore >1 point), and improvement of endoscopic appearance of the mucosa at week 6 (41% vs. 25%, defined as Mayo endoscopy subscore of 0 [normal or inactive disease] or 1 [erythema, decreased vascular pattern, mild friability]). Among clinical responders at week 6, 42% of patients who received maintenance treatment with 300 mg vedolizumab intravenous infusion every 8 weeks demonstrated clinical remission at week 52, compared to 16% of patients in the placebo group.

Among IBD indications, vedolizumab is indicated for treatment of adult patients with moderately to severely active CD and UC who have had an inadequate response with, lost response to, or were intolerant to a TNF blocker or immunomodulator; or had an inadequate response with, were intolerant to, or demonstrated dependence on corticosteroids (Entyvio®, US prescribing information 2014).

ASTHMA

Asthma is a complex chronic inflammatory syndrome of the airways and is characterized by variable symptoms of cough, breathlessness, and wheezing. These episodes may be punctuated by periods of more severe and sustained deterioration in control of symptoms, termed exacerbations, which can result in potentially life-threatening bronchospasm. Asthma affects almost 20 million individuals in the USA, six million of which are children. Pharmacotherapeutic management of the disease has progressed but is suboptimal for a subset of moderately to severely affected patients. Treatment with inhaled corticosteroids and short- and long-acting β-adrenoceptor agonists is considered the standard of care and is generally effective at attenuating symptoms, particularly in mild to moderate asthma; however, these therapeutic modalities do not necessarily address the underlying pathology of the disease. A subset of patients with moderate to severe asthma remain symptomatic despite treatment with corticosteroids, suggesting persistent inflammation of the airways.

The limitations of existing asthma therapies justify continued research into novel interventions, particularly those that modify disease processes. To that aim, a number of therapeutic proteins targeting cytokines linked to the underlying pathology of the disease have been developed, and four biologic agents have been approved for use in asthma, including omalizumab (Xolair®), a humanized mAb against IgE; mepolizumab (Nucala®) and reslizumab (Cinqair®), two humanized mAbs against IL-5; and benralizumab (Fasenra®), a humanized mAb against IL-5 receptor.

■ Anti-IgE Agent

Omalizumab

Omalizumab (Xolair®) is a recombinant human IgG1κ mAb that selectively binds IgE and inhibits the binding of IgE to the high-affinity IgE receptor (FcεRI) on the surface of mast cells and basophils. IgE plays a central role in increasing allergen uptake by dendritic cells, activated mast cells, and basophils. Reduction in surface-bound IgE on FcεRI-bearing cells limits the degree of the allergic response. Omalizumab also reduces the number of FcεRI receptors on basophils in atopic patients. Omalizumab is a first-in-class selective IgE inhibitor approved for use by patients with allergic asthma inadequately controlled by inhaled corticosteroids (Xolair®, US prescribing information 2016).

The safety and efficacy of omalizumab in treatment of asthma have been evaluated in in three randomized, double-blind, placebo-controlled, multicenter trials in patients 12–76 years old, with moderate to severe persistent asthma for at least 1 year, and a positive skin test reaction to a perennial. Omalizumab dosing was based on body weight and baseline serum total IgE concentration. All patients were required to have a baseline IgE between 30 and 700 IU/mL and body weight not more than 150 kg. Patients were treated according to a dosing table to administer at least 0.016 mg/kg/IU (IgE/mL) of omalizumab or a matching volume of placebo over each 4-week period. The maximum omalizumab dose per 4 weeks was 750 mg. Two of the Phase III trials (Trials 1 and 2) were conducted in patients with concomitant controller medications of inhaled corticosteroids (ICS) and short acting β2-agonists. Both trials included a run-in period followed by randomization to omalizumab or placebo. Patients received omalizumab for 16 weeks with an unchanged corticosteroid dose unless an acute exacerbation necessitated an increase. Patients then entered a 12-weeks ICS reduction phase during which ICS dose reduction was attempted in a step-wise manner. Omalizumab efficacy was based primarily on the reduction of asthma exacerbations, which were defined as a worsening of asthma that required treatment with systemic corticosteroids or a doubling of baseline-inhaled corticosteroid dose. In Trial 1 and Trial 2, the number of exacerbations per patient was reduced in patients treated with omalizumab compared with placebo in both the 12-weeks steroid free period (asthma exacerbation frequencies of 0, 1 and ≥2 per patient in 86–87%, 11–12% and 1–2% of patients receiving omalizumab, and in 70–77%, 17–25% and 5–7% of patients receiving placebo) and the 16-week steroid reduction period (asthma exacerbation frequencies of 0, 1 and ≥2 per patient in 79–84%, 14–19% and 1–2% of patients receiving omalizumab, and in 68–70%, 26–28%, 3–4% of patients receiving placebo). Trial 3 had a similar design to that of Trials 1 and 2, but long-acting β2-agonists were allowed. In Trial 3, the number of exacerbations in patients treated with omalizumab was similar to that in placebo-treated patients. The absence of an observed treatment effect in Trial 3 may be related to differences in the patient population compared with Asthma Trials 1 and 2, study sample size (lower in Trial 3), or other factors.

The safety and efficacy of omalizumab in treatment of asthma have also been evaluated in children 6 to <12 years of age with moderate to severe asthma who had a positive skin test or *in vitro* reactivity to a perennial aeroallergen. Omalizumab-treated children had a statistically significant reduction in the rate of asthma exacerbations versus the placebo group.

An anaphylaxis Black-Box warning was placed on the omalizumab (Xolair®) label based on clinical evidence. Anaphylaxis has been reported to occur after administration of omalizumab in pre-marketing clinical trials and in post-marketing spontaneous reports. In pre-marketing clinical trials in patients with asthma, anaphylaxis was reported in 3 of 3507 (0.1%) patients. In post-marketing spontaneous reports, the frequency of anaphylaxis attributed to omalizumab use was at least 0.2% of patients based on an estimated exposure of about 57,300 patients from June 2003 through December 2006. Anaphylaxis has occurred after the first dose of omalizumab but also has occurred beyond 1 year after beginning treatment. Therefore, omalizumab should be available only in a healthcare setting by healthcare providers prepared to manage anaphylaxis that can be life-threatening (Xolair®, US prescribing information 2016).

Omalizumab is indicated for moderate to severe persistent asthma in patients 6 years of age and older with a positive skin test or *in vitro* reactivity to a perennial aeroallergen and symptoms that are inadequately controlled with inhaled corticosteroids. (Xolair®, US prescribing information 2016).

Anti-IL-5 Agents

Two anti-IL-5 biologic agents have been approved for asthma, mepolizumab (Nucala®) and reslizumab (Cinqair®). Mepolizumab is a humanized Ig1κ mAb while reslizumab is a humanized IgG4κ mAb. IL-5 is the major cytokine responsible for the growth and differentiation, recruitment, activation, and survival of eosinophils. Mepolizumab or reslizumab binds to IL-5, inhibiting the bioactivity of IL-5 by blocking its binding to the α chain of the IL-5 receptor complex expressed on the eosinophil cell surface. Mepolizumab or reslizumab, by inhibiting IL-5 signaling, reduces the production and survival of eosinophils; however, their mechanism of action in asthma has not been definitively established (Nucala®, US prescribing information 2017; Cinqair®, US prescribing information 2016).

Mepolizumab

Mepolizumab (Nucala®) is a humanized IgG1κ mAb against IL-5, which is produced by recombinant DNA technology in Chinese hamster ovary cells (Nucala®, US prescribing information 2017).

The safety and efficacy of mepolizumab as add-on treatment of severe asthma have been evaluated in patients aged 12 years and older who had asthma despite regular use of high-dose inhaled corticosteroid (ICS) plus additional controller(s), or use of daily oral corticosteroids (OCS) in addition to regular use of high-dose ICS plus additional controller(s). These patients had markers of eosinophilic airway inflammation and continued their background asthma therapy throughout the duration of the trials. In a 32-week double-blind, randomized, placebo- controlled Phase III trial, patients receiving add-on mepolizumab treatment at the recommended dose regimen (100 mg administrated subcutaneously every 4 weeks) in combination with background therapy, compared with placebo (plus background therapy), experienced significantly fewer (52% reduction) exacerbations (defined as worsening of asthma requiring use of oral/systemic corticosteroids and/or hospitalization and/or emergency department visits). Additionally, compared with placebo (plus background therapy), there were fewer exacerbations requiring hospitalization and/or emergency department visits and exacerbations requiring only in-patient hospitalization with mepolizumab add-on treatment. In a 24-week OCS-reduction trial, effect of mepolizumab on reducing the use of maintenance OCS was evaluated. Compared with placebo (plus background therapy), add-on mepolizumab at the recommended dose regimen for 24 weeks resulted in greater reductions in daily maintenance OCS dose, while maintaining asthma control. Twenty-three per cent (23%) patients in the add-on mepolizumab treatment group versus 11% in the placebo group (plus background therapy) had a 90–100% reduction in their OCS dose. Thirty-six per cent (36%) patients in the add-on mepolizumab group versus 56% in the placebo group (plus background therapy) were classified as having no improvement for OCS dose (i.e., no change or any increase or lack of asthma control or withdrawal of treatment). Additionally, 54% of patients receiving add-on mepolizumab treatment achieved at least half reduction in the daily prednisone dose compared with 33% of subjects who received placebo (plus background therapy).

In the Phase III trials for asthma, total 28 adolescents aged 12–17 years with severe asthma were enrolled. These adolescent patients showed a reduction in the rate of exacerbations that trended in favor of mepolizumab. The adverse event profiles in adolescents was generally comparable to the overall population in the Phase III studies.

Mepolizumab is indicated for add-on maintenance treatment of patients with severe asthma aged 12 years and older, and with an eosinophilic phenotype.

Reslizumab

Reslizumab (Cinqair®) is a humanized IL-5 antagonist IgG4κ mAb produced by recombinant DNA technology in murine myeloma non-secreting 0 (NS0) cells (Cinqair®, US prescribing information 2016).

The safety and efficacy of reslizumab as add-on treatment of asthma have been evaluated in adult and adolescent patients aged 12 years and older who had at least one asthma exacerbation requiring systemic corticosteroid use over the past 12 months. Most patients had markers of eosinophilic airway inflammation and all patients continued their background asthma therapy throughout the duration of the trials. While patients aged 12–17 years were included in these trials, reslizumab is not approved for use in this age group. The safety and effectiveness of reslizumab in pediatric patients (aged 17 years and younger) have not been established.

In two 52-week double-blind, randomized, placebo-controlled Phase III trials, patients receiving add-on reslizumab treatment at the recommended dose regimen (3 mg/kg administrated intravenously every 4 weeks), compared with placebo (with background therapy), had significantly reduction (50–59% reduction) in the rate of all asthma exacerbations (defined as worsening of asthma requiring use of systemic corticosteroids or twofold increase in the use of ICS for 3 or more days, and/or asthma-related emergency treatment including visit to their healthcare professional for nebulizer treatment or other urgent treatment to prevent worsening of asthma symptoms, or a visit to the emergency room or hospitalization). Exacerbations requiring the use of a systemic corticosteroid such as OCS as well as exacerbations resulting in hospitalization or an emergency room visit were also reduced with add-on reslizumab treatment. In two other 16-week double-blind, randomized, placebo-controlled Phase III trials, add-on reslizumab treatment at the recommended dose regimen resulted in improvements in lung function (as assessed by FEV1 [forced expiratory volume in 1 s]) 4 weeks following the first dose of reslizumab and maintained through week 52.

An anaphylaxis Black-Box warning was placed on the reslizumab (Cinqair®, US prescribing information 2016) label. Anaphylaxis occurred with reslizumab infusion in 0.3% of patients in placebo-controlled Phase III studies. Patients should be observed for an appropriate period of time after reslizumab infusion; healthcare professionals should be prepared to manage anaphylaxis that can be life-threatening.

Reslizumab is indicated for add-on maintenance treatment of patients with severe asthma aged 18 years and older, and with an eosinophilic phenotype. (Cinqair®, US prescribing information 2016).

■ Anti-IL-5 Receptor Agent

In addition to directly neutralizing the IL-5 cytokine, blockage of IL-5 receptor has also been explored as an alternative mechanism of action to target the IL-5 pathway for the treatment of asthma, such as benralizumab.

Benralizumab

Benralizumab (Fasenra®) is a humanized afucosylated IL-5 receptor antagonist IgG1κ mAb produced by recombinant DNA technology in Chinese hamster ovary cells. The IL-5 receptor is expressed on the surface of eosinophils and basophils, Inflammation is an important component in the pathogenesis of asthma. Multiple cell types (e.g., mast cells, eosinophils, neutrophils, macrophages, lymphocytes) and mediators (e.g., histamine, eicosanoids, leukotrienes, cytokines) are involved in inflammation. Benralizumab, by binding to the α chain of IL-5 receptor, reduces eosinophils through antibody-dependent cell-mediated cytotoxicity (ADCC); however, its mechanism of action in asthma has not been definitively established (Fasenra®, US prescribing information 2017).

The safety and efficacy of benralizumab have been evaluated in patients aged 12 years and older who had at least two asthma exacerbation requiring systemic corticosteroid use over the past 12 months. Most patients had markers of eosinophilic airway inflammation and all patients continued their background asthma therapy throughout the duration of the trials. In a 48-week double-blind, randomized, placebo-controlled Phase III trial, patients receiving add-on benralizumab treatment at the recommended dose regimen (30 mg administrated subcutaneously at weeks 0, 4 and 8, followed by every 8 weeks), compared with placebo (plus background therapy of high dose ICS), had significant reduction (35% vs. 51%) in the rate of all asthma exacerbations (defined as a worsening of asthma requiring use of oral/systemic corticosteroids for at least 3 days, and/or emergency department visits requiring use of oral/systemic corticosteroids and/or hospitalization). Exacerbations requiring hospitalization or an emergency room visit and exacerbations requiring hospitalization were also reduced with add-on benralizumab treatment. Compared to placebo (plus background therapy), add-on benralizumab treatment at the recommended dose regimen also provided consistent improvements over time in the mean change from baseline in lung function, s assessed by FEV1.

Benralizumab is indicated for add-on maintenance treatment of patients with severe asthma aged 12 years and older, and with an eosinophilic phenotype. (Fasenra®, US prescribing information 2017).

ATOPIC DERMATITIS

Atopic dermatitis (AD) is a common chronic pruritic inflammatory skin disease with the prevalence rates worldwide up to 2–5% for adults and up to 10–20% for children. It is the most common form of eczema and is characterized by rashes on the skin that can include symptoms such as intense, persistent itching and skin dryness, cracking, redness, crusting, and oozing. The pathogenesis of AD is multifactorial and is not completely understood. The abnormalities in the skin of AD patients include an activation of the immune system (especially the type 2 T helper [Th2]-pathway) without an adequate stimulus, epithelial barrier dysfunction (often associated with a mutation of filaggrin gene), and an imbalance in the skin microbiota composition. Treatment of patients suffering from mild or moderate AD includes the use of emollients and topical glucocorticoids or topical calcineurin inhibitors. Patients with chronic and severe AD where topical therapy is usually insufficient require the use of systemic immunosuppressive drugs, which is often limited due to toxicity and severe adverse effects. There is an immense unmet need for new therapy concepts for moderate to severe AD, which impacts the quality of life of patients and has become a global health problem.

With a better understanding of the pathophysiology of the disease, multiple new therapeutic proteins have been developed for the treatment of AD (Boguniewicz 2017). These biologic agents exhibit several novel mechanisms of action including anti-IL-31 (nemolizumab) (Ruzicka et al. 2017), anti-IL-12/IL-23 (ustekinumab) (Saeki et al. 2017; Khattri et al. 2017), anti-IL-4 receptor α (dupilumab) (Kraft and Worm 2017), and anti-IL-13 (tralokinumab [NCT02347176, NCT03160885, ClinicalTrials.gov, accessed 22Jan2018] and lebrikizumab [NCT02340234, NCT02465606, ClinicalTrials.gov, accessed 22Jan2018]). One of these agents, dupilumab (Dupixent®) was recently approved by the FDA and EMA for the treatment of adults with inadequately controlled moderate to severe AD. Dupilumab is the first biologic medicine approved for AD.

■ Dupilumab

Dupilumab (Dupixent®) is a human mAb of the IgG4 subclass, which is produced by recombinant DNA technology in Chinese Hamster Ovary cell suspension culture. Dupilumab inhibits IL-4 and IL-13 signaling by specifically binding to the IL-4 receptor α (IL-4Rα) subunit shared by the IL-4 and IL-13 receptor complexes. Blocking IL-4Rα with dupilumab inhibits IL-4 and IL-13 cytokine-induced responses, including the release of proinflammatory cytokines, chemokines and IgE (Dupixent®, US prescribing information 2017).

The efficacy and safety of dupilumab have been evaluated in three randomized, double-blind, controlled Phase III trials in adult patients with moderate to severe AD who were not adequately controlled by topical medication(s). Disease severity was defined by an Investigator's Global Assessment (IGA) score ≥ 3 in the overall assessment of AD lesions on a severity scale of 0–4, and an Eczema Area and Severity Index (EASI) score ≥ 16 on a scale of 0–72. In the two dupilumab monotherapy Phase III trials, 12-week treatment with subcutaneous dupilumab at the recommended dose regimen (600 mg initially followed by 300 mg every 2 weeks) resulted in 36–38% and 44–51% of AD patients achieving IGA 0/1 (IGA 'clear' or 'almost clear' with a reduction of ≥2 points on a 0–4 IGA scale) and EASI 75 (improvement of at least 75% in EASI score from baseline) responses, respectively, while the control group had only 9–10% and 12–15% of patients with IGA 0/1 and EASI 75 responses, respectively. Clinical efficacy was also shown in the concomitant Phase III trial, where 12-week treatment with dupilumab at the recommended subcutaneous dose regimen (600 mg initially followed by 300 mg every 2 weeks) in combination with topical corticosteroids resulted in 39 and 69% of AD patients achieving IGA 0/1 and EASI 75 responses, respectively, while the control group (placebo plus topical corticosteroids) had only 12 and 23% of patients with IGA 0/1 and EASI 75 responses, respectively.

Dupilumab is indicated for the treatment of adult patients with moderate-to-severe atopic dermatitis (AD) whose disease is not adequately controlled with topical prescription therapies or when those therapies are not advisable. Dupilumab can be used with or without topical corticosteroids (Dupixent®, US prescribing information 2017).

CHRONIC IDIOPATHIC URTICARIA

Chronic idiopathic urticaria (CIU) is a common autoimmune skin condition characterized by spontaneously recurring hives, occurring either intermittently or continuously for 6 weeks or longer (Vestergaard and Deleuran 2015). A significant association of CIU is a deeper localized swelling called angioedema, which is observed in about one-third of patients. This leads to remarkable psychosocial morbidity with a negative impact on overall quality of life. CIU occurs largely in young women between 20 and 40 years of age. The exact prevalence of CIU is difficult to determine. A recently published article indicated a point prevalence of at least 0.5% in the general population for CIU (Maurer et al. 2011). Conventional treatment for CIU prescribes a stepwise approach with non-sedating non-impairing antihistamines as first-line agents followed by increasing to four times the licensed doses as second-line treatment. However, close to half of CIU patients do not achieve adequate symptom relief with antihistamines alone. Third-line treatments include cyclosporine, which is associated with toxicity and requires frequent monitoring.

An autoimmune mechanism is thought to mediate the disease process in up to 50% of patients with CIU. Autoantibody to the α chain of the high affinity IgE receptor and/or intrinsic IgE immune modulation may play an important role. Toward this, omalizumab, a humanized anti-IgE antibody, is developed as an alternative treatment option for patients with CIU. Omalizumab (Xolair®) is the first and only biologic agent currently approved for the treatment of CIU. Rituximab, a humanized anti-CD-20 mAb, has been reported in a few cases to be effective in the treatment of CIU; whereas other case did not show any effect (Mallipeddi and Grattan 2007). Antibodies against TNFα have also been used in the treatment of CIU but with variable success and only in small numbers of patients (Cooke et al. 2015).

Omalizumab

An overview of omalizumab, a humanized anti-IgE mAb, has been provided earlier in this chapter (Xolair®, US prescribing information 2016). In addition to asthma, the efficacy and safety of omalizumab have been evaluated in patients with CIU. The mechanism of action has been described earlier as an antibody targeting IgE; however, the specific mechanism by which omalizumab results in an improvement of CIU symptoms has not been fully defined.

Two randomized, placebo-controlled, multiple-dose clinical trials have been conducted for omalizumab in adult and adolescent patients 12 years of age and older with CIU. Disease severity was measured by a weekly urticaria activity score (UAS7, range 0–42), which is a composite of the weekly itch severity score (range 0–21) and the weekly hive count score (range 0–21). In both trials, patients who received subcutaneous omalizumab 150 mg or 300 mg every 4 weeks in addition to their baseline antihistamine therapy had greater decreases from baseline in itch severity scores and hive count scores than patients receiving placebo (plus background therapy) at week 12. In one trial, the change from baseline to week 12 were −3.63, −6.66, −9.40 for placebo, omalizumab 150 mg and 300 mg, respectively, in itch severity score, and were −4.37, −7.78, −11.35 for placebo, omalizumab 150 mg and 300 mg, respectively, in hive count score. Similar results were shown in the other trial.

In addition to asthma, omalizumab is also indicated for chronic idiopathic urticaria in adults and adolescents 12 years of age and older who remain symptomatic despite antihistamine treatment. (Xolair®, US prescribing information 2016).

CRYOPYRIN-ASSOCIATED PERIODIC SYNDROMES

Cryopyrin-associated periodic syndrome (CAPS) comprises three genetic autoinflammatory disorders including familial cold autoinflammatory syndrome (FCAS), Muckle-Wells syndrome (MWS), and neonatal-onset, multisystem, inflammatory disorder (NOMID) (Kubota and Koike 2010). These three phenotypically distinct disorders are recognized as a clinical continuum of the same disease in an increasing order of severity since all three disorders are associated with mutations in the NACHT, LRR and PYD domains-containing protein 3 (NLRP3) gene that encodes the cryopyrin protein. NLRP3 mutations result in overactivation of caspase-1, the enzyme that cleaves precursors of IL-1β, IL-18, and IL-33 into active cytokine forms. CAPS is rare with a prevalence of one in about one million people, however many cases of this disease are believed to be undiagnosed.

Therapeutic treatments of CAPS include nonsteroidal anti-inflammatory drugs, colchicine, immunosuppressants, corticosteroids, and the recent addition of anti-IL-1β biologic therapy (Kubota and Koike 2010). Anti-IL-1β therapy is very effective for the treatment of CAPS since it exerts pharmacologic action directly against the underlying cause of the disease. Clinical evidence suggests that use of anti-IL-1β agents can achieve rapid and complete control of both clinical manifestations and laboratory parameters.

Anti-IL-1β Agents

Currently, there are two long-acting anti-IL-1β therapeutic proteins (canakinumab [Ilaris®] and rilonacept [Arcalyst®]) that have been approved for the treatment of CAPS, although a short-acting IL-1 receptor antagonist, anakinra, is also effective for this disease (Hawkins and Lachmann 2003). Excessive production of IL-1β is the central pathophysiology of CAPS. Both canakinumab and rilonacept were generally well tolerated in the Phase III trials with infections being a commonly reported adverse event due to the immunosuppressant effect of anti-IL-1β therapy.

Canakinumab

An overview of canakinumab, a human anti-IL-1β mAb, has been provided earlier in this chapter (Ilaris®, US prescribing information 2016). In addition to the use of this therapeutic protein for the treatment of sJIA, canakinumab has also been evaluated in patients with CAPS. Canakinumab binds to human IL-1β and neutralizes its activity.

The efficacy and safety of canakinumab for the treatment of CAPS has been assessed in a double-blind, placebo-controlled, randomized withdrawal trial in in patients 9–74 years of age with the MWS phenotype of CAPS. This study consisted of three parts. Part 1 was an 8-week open-label, single-dose period where all patients received canakinumab. Patients who achieved a complete clinical response and did not relapse by week 8 were randomized to receive either placebo or canakinumab every 8 weeks for 24 weeks in Part 2 of the study. Patients who completed Part 2 or experienced a disease flare entered Part 3, a 16-week open-label active treatment phase. Throughout the trial, patients weighing more than 40 kg received subcutaneous canakinumab 150 mg and patients weighing 15–40 kg received canakinumab 2 mg/kg. In Part 1, a complete clinical response was observed in 71% of patients 1 week following initiation of treatment and in 97% of patients by week 8. In the randomized withdrawal period, a total of 81% of the patients randomized to placebo flared compared to none (0%) of the patients randomized to canakinumab treatment. In a second trial, patients 4–74 years of age with both MWS and FCAS phenotypes of CAPS were treated in an open-label manner. Treatment with canakinumab resulted in clinically significant improvement of signs and symptoms in majority of patients within 1 week.

Among inflammatory diseases, in addition to sJIA, canakinumab is also indicated for the treatment of CAPS, including FCAS and MWS, in adults and children 4 years of age and older (Ilaris®, US prescribing information 2016).

Rilonacept

Rilonacept (Arcalyst®) is a dimeric fusion protein consisting of the ligand-binding domains of the extracellular portions of the human IL-1 receptor component (IL-1RI) and IL-1 receptor accessory protein (IL-1RAcP) linked in-line to the Fc portion of human IgG1. Rilonacept blocks IL-1β signaling by acting as a soluble decoy receptor that binds IL-1β and prevents its interaction with cell surface receptors. Rilonacept also binds IL-1α and IL-1 receptor antagonist (IL-1RA) with reduced affinity (Arcalyst®, US prescribing information 2016).

The safety and efficacy of rilonacept for the treatment of CAPS have been assessed in a randomized, double-blind, placebo-controlled Phase III trial in patients with FCAS and MWS phenotypes of CAPS. After 6 weeks of treatment, a higher proportion of adult patients in the rilonacept group at the recommended subcutaneous dose regimen (320 mg initially followed by 160 mg every week onward) experienced improvement from baseline in a composite CAPS disease score by at least 30% (96% vs. 29% of patients), by at least 50% (87% vs. 8%), and by at least 75% (70% vs. 0%) compared to the placebo group. Six pediatric patients (12–17 years of age) were enrolled directly into the open-label extension phase of this study and improvements in symptoms were shown in these patients following rilonacept treatment.

Taking rilonacept with TNF inhibitors is not recommended because this may increase the risk of serious infections. An increased incidence of serious infections has been associated with administration of an IL-1 blocker in combination with TNF inhibitors. IL-1 blockade may interfere with the immune response to infections. Serious, life-threatening infections have been reported in patients taking rilonacept. In an open-label extension study, one patient developed bacterial meningitis and died (Arcalyst®, US prescribing information 2016).

Rilonacept is indicated for the treatment of CAPS, including FCAS and MWS, in adults and children 12 years of age and older (Arcalyst®, US prescribing information 2016).

CAR-T CELL-INDUCED CYTOKINE RELEASE SYNDROME

T lymphocytes can be genetically modified to target tumors through the expression of a chimeric antigen receptor (CAR). Most notably, CAR T cells have demonstrated clinical efficacy in hematologic malignancies with more modest responses when targeting solid tumors. However, CAR T cells also have the capacity to elicit expected and unexpected toxicities, including neurologic toxicity, "on target/off tumor" recognition, anaphylaxis, and the life-threating cytokine release syndrome (CRS) (Bonifant et al. 2016).

■ Tocilizumab

An overview of tocilizumab, a human anti-IL-6 receptor mAb, has been provided earlier in this chapter (Actemra®, US prescribing information 2017). In addition to use of this therapeutic protein for the treatment of RA, pJIA and sJIA (and giant-cell arteritis as described later in this chapter), tocilizumab is also indicated for treatment of CAR T cell-induced severe or life-threatening CRS in adults and pediatric patients 2 years of age and older (Actemra®, US prescribing information 2017).

The efficacy of tocilizumab for the treatment of CRS have been assessed in a retrospective analysis of pooled outcome data from clinical trials of CAR T-cell therapies for hematological malignancies. Evaluable patients had been treated with intravenous tocilizumab 8 mg/kg (12 mg/kg for patients <30 kg) with or without additional high-dose corticosteroids for severe or life-threatening CRS; only the first episode of CRS was included in the analysis. The study population included 24 male and 21 female subjects of median age 12 years (range, 3–23 years). The median time from start of CRS to first dose of tocilizumab was 4 days (range, 0–18 days). Resolution of CRS was defined as lack of fever and off vasopressors for at least 24 h. Patients were considered responders if CRS resolved within 14 days of the first dose of tocilizumab, no more than two doses of tocilizumab were needed, and no drugs other than tocilizumab and corticosteroids were used for treatment. Thirty-one patients (69%) achieved a response. Achievement of resolution of CRS within 14 days was confirmed in a second study using an independent cohort that included 15 subjects (range: 9–75 years old) with CAR T cell-induced CRS.

EOSINOPHILIC GRANULOMATOSIS POLYANGIITIS

Eosinophilic granulomatosis with polyangiitis (EGPA) is a rare disease characterized by disseminated necrotizing vasculitis with extravascular granulomas occurring exclusively among patients with asthma and tissue eosinophilia (Greco et al. 2015). EGPA usually manifests between 7 and 74 years of age, with a mean age at onset of 38–54 years. The estimated incidence is approximately 0.11–2.66 new cases per one million people per year, with an overall prevalence of 10.7–14 per one million adults. Although still considered an idiopathic condition, EGPA is generally considered a Th2-mediated disease. Recent evidence also points to B cells and the humoral response as further contributors to EGPA's pathogenesis. EGPA patients without poor-prognosis factors are usually treated with glucocorticoids alone, whereas those with a worse prognosis are recommended glucocorticoids and immunosuppressants. Recently, biologic agents such as mepolizumab (anti-IL-5 antibody) are considered promising therapeutic alternatives for EGPA.

■ Mepolizumab

An overview of mepolizumab, a humanized anti-IL-5 mAb, has been provided earlier in this chapter (Nucala®, US prescribing information 2017). In addition to the use of this therapeutic protein for the treatment of asthma, mepolizumab has also been evaluated in patients with EGPA. Eosinophils and their mediators are considered to be critical effectors to EGPA. Mepolizumab, by inhibiting IL-5 signaling, reduces the production and survival of eosinophils; however, its mechanism of action in EGPA has not been definitively established (Nucala®, US prescribing information 2017).

In a randomized, placebo-controlled, multicenter study, patients with EGPA received 300 mg mepolizumab or placebo administered subcutaneously once every 4 weeks while continuing their stable OCS therapy. A greater percentage of the patients receiving 300 mg mepolizumab treatment achieved remission versus placebo within the first 24 weeks and remained in remission for the remainder of the 52-week treatment period (19% vs. 1%).

In addition to severe asthma, mepolizumab is indicated for the treatment of adult patients with EGPA (Nucala®, US prescribing information 2017).

GIANT CELL ARTERITIS

Giant-cell arteritis (GCA) is an inflammatory vasculopathy that typically occurs in medium and large arteries with well-developed wall layers and adventitial vasa vasorum (Pradeep and Smith 2018). It is the most common systemic vasculitis in the elderly with an estimated incidence of 27 cases in 100,000 people in those over 50 years old with peak incidence at 70–80 years of age. GCA is a medical emergency which, if left untreated, can result in vision loss. Current standard of care is prompt initiation of glucocorticoid treatment when there is a suspicion of GCA. In most patients with GCA, administration of glucocorticoids can improve signs and symptoms; however, glucocorticoid-related morbidity is a common treatment challenge. When glucocorticoids are tapered, disease flares may occur frequently (an average of one to two episodes per person-year). Recent findings suggested a fundamental failure of T regulatory cell function as a main contributor to GCA's pathogenesis. This represents an opportunity for novel therapeutic medicines as possible glucocorticoid-sparing agents, such as abatacept (a lymphocyte activation inhibitor by targeting CTLA-4) (Langford et al. 2017) and tocilizumab (an IL-6 receptor antagonist). In 2017, tocilizumab (Actemra®) was approved for GCA by US FDA (and EMA). This is the first FDA-approved therapy specific to the disorder.

■ Tocilizumab

An overview of tocilizumab, a human anti-IL-6 receptor mAb, has been provided earlier in this chapter (Actemra®, US prescribing information 2017). In addition to use of this therapeutic protein for the treatment of RA, pJIA, sJIA, and CRS, tocilizumab is also indicative for the treatment of GCA in adult patients (Actemra®, US prescribing information 2017).

In a randomized, double-blind, placebo-controlled Phase III study in patients with active GCA, treatment with subcutaneous tocilizumab 162 mg weekly and 162 mg every other week (in combination with 26 weeks prednisone taper) resulted in 56 and 53% of GCA patients, respectively, achieving sustained remission (defined as absence of GCA signs and symptoms from week 12 through week 52, along with normalization of erythrocyte sedimentation rate [ESR], normalization of C-reactive protein [CRP], and adherence to the prednisone taper regime), while the control groups (placebo with 26- or 52-week prednisone taper) had only 14–18% of patients with sustained remission.

HIDRADENITIS SUPPURATIVA

Hidradenitis suppurativa (HS) is a chronic, inflammatory, recurrent, debilitating skin disease of the hair follicle that usually presents with painful, deep-seated, inflamed lesions in the apocrine gland-bearing areas of the body, most commonly the axillae, inguinal and anogenital regions. The prevalence of HS is approximately 1–4% in general population, with an onset after puberty and before age of 40, peaking in the second and third decades of life. HS has the highest impact on patients' quality of life among the overall dermatological diseases, and is associated with multiple comorbidities, including obesity, metabolic syndrome, inflammatory bowel disease, and spondyloarthropathy. The general approach to HS includes non-medical interventions, topical and systemic medications, and surgery. Until now, surgery remains the first-line therapy for HS patients with extensive disease. However, even with extensive surgical intervention HS often recurs. This led to the recent interest in the use of adjunctive biologic therapy in the management of HS (Shanmugam et al. 2017).

The role of immune system in the pathophysiology of HS is being increasingly recognized and several therapeutic proteins are under investigation. The TNF antagonists of infliximab and adalimumab are considered to be efficacious in the treatment of moderate to severe HS, as demonstrated in case series, retrospective studies and randomized controlled trials (Shanmugam et al. 2017). Some benefits of ustekinumab, an anti-IL12/IL-23 mAb, in HS have been indicated in case reports and a prospective open-label study (Blok et al. 2016). Use of IL-1 receptor antagonist (such as anakinra) in HS had mixed results with some studies showing lack of efficacy, but a recent randomized controlled trial (Tzanetakou et al. 2016) have shown efficacy. IL-17 antagonist therapy is also being investigated in the clinic such as bimekizumab (NCT03248531, ClinicalTrials.gov, accessed 22Jan2018) and secukinumab (NCT02421172, ClinicalTrials.gov, accessed 22Jan2018). Recently, adalimumab (Humira®) was approved by US FDA (and EMA) for the treatment of moderate to severe HS. This is the first biologic medicine approved for HS.

■ Adalimumab

An overview of adalimumab, a human anti-TNFα mAb, has been provided earlier in this chapter (Humira®, US prescribing information 2017). In addition to arthritides, psoriasis, CD and UC (and uveitis as described later in this chapter), adalimumab is also indicated for the treatment of moderate to severe HS in adult patients (Humira®, US prescribing information 2017). Elevated levels of TNFα, an inflammatory cytokine, are seen in blood and skin lesions of patients with HS.

The safety and efficacy of adalimumab for the treatment of HS have been assessed in two randomized, double-blind, placebo-controlled Phase III studies in adult patients with moderate to severe HS with Hurley Stage II or III disease and with at least three abscesses or inflammatory nodules. Hurley staging system is a three-stage classification system developed for assessing extent and severity of HS, with Stage 0 being no active HS and Stages I-III associated with increased severity. All patients used topical antiseptic wash daily in these two studies. Concomitant oral antibiotic use was allowed in Study HS-II but not Study HS-I. Hidradenitis Suppurativa Clinical Response (HiSCR) was used to assess the treatment effect, which was defined as at least a 50% reduction in total abscess and inflammatory nodule count with no increase in abscess count and no increase in draining fistula count relative to baseline. Twelve-week treatment with subcutaneous adalimumab at the recommended dose regimen (160 mg initial dose, 80 mg 2 weeks later, followed by 40 mg weekly dosing thereafter) resulted in 42 and 59% of HS patients achieving HiSCR in Study HS-I and Study HS-II, respectively, while the control group had only 26 and 28% of patients with HiSCR response in Study HS-I and Study HS-II, respectively.

MULTIPLE SCLEROSIS

Multiple sclerosis (MS) is a chronic demyelinating disease of the CNS. The main pathological findings in MS are inflammation, demyelination, and axonal degeneration. Inflammation and demyelination are responsible for the acute symptoms of the disease, and axonal degeneration is the underlining cause of the progressive disability associated with MS. Although the etiology of MS remains undetermined, it is considered to be an autoimmune disorder. Blood autoreactive T and B lymphocytes, once activated against myelin constituents, migrate across the blood–brain barrier and initiate inflammatory and demyelinating processes within the CNS leading to MS lesions. Currently, two therapeutic proteins have been approved for the treatment of MS, including an $\alpha4\beta1/\alpha4\beta7$ integrin antagonist, natalizumab (Tysabri®), and a CD20-directed cytolytic agent, ocrelizumab (Ocrevus®).

■ Anti-integrin Agents

Natalizumab

An overview of natalizumab, a $\alpha4\beta1/\alpha4\beta7$ integrin antagonist, has been provided earlier in this chapter (Tysabri®, US prescribing information 2017). In addition to the use of this therapeutic protein for the treatment of

CD, natalizumab (Tysabri®) was the first mAb developed for the treatment of MS. The mechanism of action has been described earlier as an antibody targeting integrins; however, the specific mechanism(s) by which natalizumab exerts its effects in MS has not been fully defined (Tysabri®, US prescribing information 2017).

The safety and efficacy of natalizumab in treatment of MS have been evaluated in two randomized, double-blind, placebo-controlled, multicenter Phase III studies in patients with relapsing forms of MS who had not received any interferon (IFN)-β or glatiramer acetate (Study MS1) (Polman et al. 2006) or patients who had experienced relapses despite INF-β-1a treatment (Study MS2) (Rudick et al. 2006). In Study MS1, 2-years treatment with intravenous natalizumab monotherapy at the recommended intravenous dose regimen (300 mg every 4 weeks), when compared to the placebo treatment, lowered the proportion of patients with increased disability (17% vs. 29%) and the annualized relapse rate (68% reduction). Natalizumab also suppressed the formation of new gadolinium enhancing lesions and reduced the mean number of active lesions based on MRI assessment. In Study MS2, natalizumab or placebo was evaluated in combination with IFN-β-1a. The clinical and MRI-associated efficacies associated with natalizumab treatment were similar to those observed in Study MS1. However, Study MS2 ended 1 month earlier than planned because of the occurrence of PML in two patients receiving natalizumab plus IFN-β-1a.

PML is a demyelinating infectious disease of the CNS caused by reactivation of the John Cunningham virus (JCV). PML may be fatal or result in severe disability. Risk factors for the development of PML include duration of therapy, prior use of immunosuppressants, and presence of anti-JCV antibodies. These factors should be considered in the context of expected benefit when initiating and continuing treatment with natalizumab (Tysabri®, US prescribing information 2017). As of July 2001, 145 cases of PML have been reported among 88,100 patients treated with natalizumab worldwide in the post-marketing setting (Laffaldano et al. 2011).

In addition to CD, natalizumab is also indicated as monotherapy for the treatment of patients with relapsing forms of multiple sclerosis (MS). It is generally recommended for patients who have had an inadequate response to, or are unable to tolerate, an alternate MS therapy. Because of the risk of PML, in the United States, natalizumab is available only through a restricted program under REMS called the TOUCH® Prescribing Program. Natalizumab must be given as monotherapy, and any prior immunomodulator or immunosuppressive therapy must be discontinued prior to use (Tysabri®, US prescribing information 2017).

■ Anti-CD20 Cytolytic Agent

Ocrelizumab

Ocrelizumab (Ocrevus®) is a humanized CD20-directed cytolytic IgG1 antibody. The precise mechanism by which ocrelizumab exerts its therapeutic effects in MS is unknown, but is presumed to involve binding to CD20, a cell surface antigen present on pre-B and mature B lymphocytes. Following cell surface binding to B lymphocytes, ocrelizumab results in antibody-dependent cellular cytolysis (ADCC) and complement-mediated lysis (Ocrevus®, US prescribing information 2017).

The safety and efficacy of ocrelizumab have been evaluated in patients with relapsing or primary progressive forms of MS. In two double-blind, randomized, active comparator-controlled Phase III trials, treatment of ocrelizumab at the recommended dose regimen (initial treatment of two 300 mg IV infusions administered 2 weeks apart, and subsequent doses administered as a single 600 mg IV infusion every 24 weeks) in patients with relapsing forms of MS resulted in significantly lower annualized relapse rate compared with placebo (46–47% reduction, $p < 0.0001$), as well as the proportion of patients with confirmed disability progression (40% reduction, $p = 0.0006$). In a double-blind, randomized, placebo-controlled Phase III trial, treatment of ocrelizumab at the recommended dose regimen in patients with primary progressive form of MS resulted in significantly lower proportion of patients with confirmed disability progression (24% reduction, $p = 0.0321$).

Ocrelizumab is indicated for the treatment of patients with relapsing or primary progressive forms of MS (Ocrevus®, US prescribing information 2017).

UVEITIS

Uveitis (UV) is a term that describes a heterogeneous collection of diseases including infections, systemic immune-mediated diseases like sarcoidosis, and immune-mediated syndromes confined to the eye like sympathetic ophthalmia. Uveitis is rare with a prevalence of 115.3 cases per 100,000 people; however, it can damage vital eye tissue, leading to permanent vision loss. Most uveitis is anterior in location, which generally permits successful therapy with topical medication alone. Challenge in the treatment of uveitis relates to patients who have inflammation involving the posterior segment, either primarily in the vitreous (intermediate uveitis), the choroid or retina (posterior uveitis), or involving the entire eye (panuveitis). These patients can have refractory uveitis where systemic corticosteroids or other immunosuppressive therapy are required. Weighting of the risk of blindness and the complications related to these drugs need to be carefully planned (Lin et al. 2014).

Uveitis is considered an immune-mediated disease. A recent literature review suggests that anti-TNFα agents, such as infliximab, adalimumab and golimumab, are reasonably effective for controlling ocular inflammation and sparing patients corticosteroid treatment in non-infectious refractory uveitis (Borrás-Blasco et al. 2015). Adalimumab (Humira®) is currently the first and only FDA-approved non-corticosteroid therapy for uveitis, though other anti-TNFα agents are also being used 'off-label'.

Adalimumab

An overview of adalimumab, a human anti-TNFα mAb, has been provided earlier in this chapter (Humira®, US prescribing information 2017). In addition to arthritides, psoriasis, CD, UC and HS, adalimumab is also indicated for the treatment of moderate to severe uveitis (UV) in adult patients (Humira®, US prescribing information 2017).

The safety and efficacy of adalimumab in treatment of uveitis have been assessed in two randomized, double-masked, placebo-controlled Phase III studies (UV I and UV II) in adult patients with non-infectious intermediate, posterior and panuveitis despite corticosteroids therapy. The primary efficacy endpoint was 'time to treatment failure'. Treatment failure was a multi-component outcome defined as the development of new inflammatory chorioretinal and/or inflammatory retinal vascular lesions, an increase in anterior chamber cell grade or vitreous haze grade or a decrease in best corrected visual acuity. Statistically significant reductions in the time to treatment failure were demonstrated in patients treated with subcutaneous adalimumab at the recommended dose regimen (80 mg initial dose followed by 40 mg every 2 weeks) versus patients receiving placebo, with hazard ratio of 0.50 (95% CI: 0.36–0.70) and 0.57 (95% CI: 0.39–0.84) in Study UV I and Study UV II, respectively.

CONCLUSION

The Introduction of more than 20 antibody-based biotherapeutics in the last decades has fundamentally changed the treatment paradigm in immune-mediated inflammatory diseases such as RA, IBD, and psoriasis. Though these "targeted biotherapies" are expensive compared to traditional "small molecular" therapies such as methotrexate, they have provided effective treatment alternatives with highly specific targeted novel mechanisms of action. Some of these biotherapeutics can not only provide relief of symptoms but also offer an opportunity to modify or even reverse the course of these diseases, as has been demonstrated in RA. Notably, despite the remarkable clinical improvement in the treatment of inflammatory diseases using antibody-based biotherapeutics, there is still unmet medical need in achieving 'permanent cure' for these complex multifactorial disorders. Inflammatory diseases such as RA and IBD are not the products of dysfunction in isolated individual entities or linear pathways; they arise from perturbations in complex dynamic networks that shift from patterns representing normal function to others that give rise to disease. Therefore, treatment of the disease is unlikely to be resolved using a one-size-fits-all approach by targeting a single target. It is important to understand how individual biological components interact for a given patient, which could then be used to guide personalization of therapies and the segmentation or stratification of treatment populations. With the further advance in protein engineering technology and better understanding of the etiology and disease progression of immune-mediated inflammatory diseases, equipped with more predictive and diagnostic biomarkers, it is reasonable to anticipate that more effective and safe "targeted biotherapeutics" tailored to the individual patients' needs will be added to the therapeutic armory to successfully treat inflammatory diseases.

SELF-ASSESSMENT QUESTIONS

Questions

1. Are targeted biologic therapies for autoimmune diseases only to be used once drugs like corticosteroids and methotrexate have had an adequate trial of use and have failed to control the patient's symptoms?
2. What is the primary clinical concern with the immunogenicity of biologic therapies?
3. What is the most likely explanation for why a patient who receives a dose of omalizumab might have an increase in their total serum IgE level for many weeks after the first dose?
4. Why do some cell subsets in the peripheral blood increase after dosing with natalizumab?
5. If a trial reports an ACR70 of 20% on active drug, what does that mean?
6. What does PASI 75 mean?
7. Given that there are currently five anti-TNFα biotherapeutic agents on the market, how would you compare and contrast them?
8. What are the key differences in the indication for use of rituximab vs. abatacept in RA?
9. What is the mechanism of action for guselkumab in treating plaque psoriasis?

Answers

1. Though the standard of care in diseases like RA is still to start with older DMARDs like methotrexate, the decision of when to start or switch therapies is complex and impacted by individual issues linked to clinical response like tolerance/adherence to a particular therapeutic regimen, severity and course of disease and its progression, and concomitant medications and medical issues. It is likely that the standard of care will continue to change and incorporate earlier use of biologic therapies that can modify the disease course with fewer generalized side effects.
2. If a biologic therapy is highly immunogenic, there is a concern that an increasing number of patients exposed to the drug, particularly upon repeated exposure after a hiatus, because their antidrug antibodies could sometimes neutralize the majority of the drug and they would not likely get the full dose or effect. Though less likely there are also rare examples of antidrug antibodies resulting in an autoimmune or allergic-type reaction.
3. Therapeutic monoclonal antibodies that target soluble molecules like IgE form complexes. Though immune complexes are typically cleared from the blood more quickly than monomeric IgG, soluble target molecules typically have a shorter serum half-life than IgG. So an assay detecting the soluble target (in this case IgE) that can detect target even when it is bound to the drug (which is typically an longer-lived IgG) will show more target present in the serum post-dosing as compared to baseline. This is called a carrier effect. Assuming the drug neutralized the bound target, the test detecting the target can be misleading, because the target, though present, is effectively inactive.
4. Natalizumab is a monoclonal antibody that blocks lymphocyte movement between the blood and tissues ("trafficking"); when this movement is effectively blocked in one direction (from the blood into the tissues), an apparent increase in the peripheral lymphocyte population will be evident on assessment by flow cytometry (or perhaps even on a CBC with differential) post-dosing.
5. An ACR70 of 20% means the 20% of the patients had a 70% improvement in their RA disease.
6. The PASI score stands for Psoriasis Area and Severity Index. This tool allows researchers and dermatologists to put an objective number on what would otherwise be a very subjective idea: how bad is a person's psoriasis. The PASI evaluates the degree of erythema, thickness, and scaling of psoriatic plaques and estimates the extent of involvement of each of these components in four separate body areas (head, trunk, upper, and lower extremities).
   - If in a clinical study a certain proportion of patients experienced a 75% reduction in their PASI scores, it is reported as a percentage of people achieving "PASI 75."
7. Although the five anti-TNFα biologics have broadly similar efficacy and safety profiles in RA, there are significant differences in the five anti-TNFα agents particularly with respect to dosing characteristics and also in the details of the approved indications for use.
   - Infliximab is the first approved anti-TNFα agent given intravenously, has the longest dosing interval, and is the first FDA-approved anti-TNFα agent for IBD indication. All the other anti-TNFα agents are administered by subcutaneous administration. It is a chimeric monoclonal antibody that neutralizes TNF-α and has approvals in the most indications (including rheumatoid arthritis, psoriatic arthritis, ankylosing spondylitis, adult and pediatric ulcerative colitis, adult and pediatric Crohn's disease, and psoriasis).
   - Etanercept is a dimeric soluble fusion protein and has approvals for use in several indications (rheumatoid arthritis, polyarticular juvenile rheumatoid arthritis, psoriatic arthritis, ankylosing spondylitis, and psoriasis). It is used as weekly injection.
   - Adalimumab is a human monoclonal antibody that neutralizes TNF-α and has FDA approvals for use in patients with rheumatoid arthritis, psoriatic arthritis, ankylosing spondylitis, psoriasis, Crohn's disease, Pediatric Crohn's disease, ulcerative colitis, hidradenitis suppurative, and uveitis. It is used at a frequency of every week or every other week.
   - Golimumab is a human monoclonal antibody that neutralizes TNF-α and has FDA approvals for use in patients with rheumatoid arthritis, psoriatic arthritis, and ankylosing spondylitis, and ulcerative colitis via subcutaneous route of administration. It is used at a frequency of every month. It can also be given via intravenous route of administration with a frequency of every 8 weeks for the treatment of rheumatoid arthritis.
   - Certolizumab pegol is a recombinant, humanized antibody Fab fragment, with specificity for human tumor necrosis factor alpha (TNFα), conjugated to an approximately 40-kDa polyethylene glycol (PEG2MAL40K). It has been approved by FDA for the treatment of rheumatoid arthritis and Crohn's disease.
8. Rituximab in combination with methotrexate is indicated for the treatment of adult patients with moderate to severe rheumatoid arthritis who have had an inadequate response to one or more TNF antagonist therapies. Abatacept is indicated for use as monotherapy or in combination with DMARDS

in patients with moderate to severe active rheumatoid arthritis who have had an inadequate response to DMARDs or TNF antagonists.

9. IL-23 is a naturally occurring cytokine that is involved in inflammatory and immune responses, such as natural killer cell (NK) activation and CD4+ T-cell differentiation and activation. Guselkumab, a human IgG1λ monoclonal antibody that binds with high affinity and specificity to the p19 protein subunit used by IL-23, can prevent human IL-23 from binding to the IL-23 (IL-12Rβ1/23R) receptor complexes on the surface of NK and T cells.

REFERENCES

Abdallah H, Hsu JC, Lu P et al (2017) Pharmacokinetic and pharmacodynamic analysis of subcutaneous tocilizumab in patients with rheumatoid arthritis from 2 randomized, controlled trials: SUMMACTA and BREVACTA. J Clin Pharmacol 57:459–468

Actemra (tocilizumab) (2017) US prescribing information. Genentech Inc., South San Francisco

Adedokun OJ, Xu Z, Padgett L et al (2013) Pharmacokinetics of infliximab in children with moderate-to-severe ulcerative colitis: results from a randomized, multicenter, open-label, phase 3 study. Inflamm Bowel Dis 19:2753–2762

Adedokun OJ, Sandborn WJ, Feagan BG et al (2014) Association between serum concentration of infliximab and efficacy in adult patients with ulcerative colitis. Gastroenterology 147:1296–1307.e5

Adedokun OJ, Xu Z, Marano CW et al (2017) Pharmacokinetics and exposure-response relationship of golimumab in patients with moderately-to-severely active ulcerative colitis: results from phase 2/3 PURSUIT induction and maintenance studies. J Crohns Colitis 11:35–46

Arcalyst (rilonacept) (2016) US prescribing information. Regeneron Pharmaceuticals Inc., Tarrytown

Baumgart DC, Sandborn WJ (2007) Inflammatory bowel disease: clinical aspects and established and evolving therapies. Lancet 369:1641–1657

Benlysta (Belimumab) (2017) US prescribing information. Human Genome Sciences, Inc., (a subsidiary of GlaxoSmithKline), Rockville

Blauvelt A, Reich K, Tsai TF et al (2017) Secukinumab is superior to ustekinumab in clearing skin of subjects with moderate-to-severe plaque psoriasis up to 1 year: Results from the CLEAR study. J Am Acad Dermatol 76:60–69. e9

Blok JL, Li K, Brodmerkel C, Horvátovich P, Jonkman MF, Horváth B (2016) Ustekinumab in hidradenitis suppurativa: clinical results and a search for potential biomarkers in serum. Br J Dermatol 174:839–846

Boguniewicz M (2017) Biologic therapy for atopic dermatitis: moving beyond the practice parameter and guidelines. J Allergy Clin Immunol Pract 5:1477–1487

Bongartz T, Sutton AJ, Sweeting MJ et al (2006) Anti-TNF antibody therapy in rheumatoid arthritis and the risk of serious infections and malignancies: systematic review and meta-analysis of rare harmful effects in randomized controlled trials. JAMA 295:2275–2285

Bonifant CL, Jackson HJ, Brentjens RJ, Curran KJ (2016) Toxicity and management in CAR T-cell therapy. Mol Ther Oncolytics 3:16011

Borrás-Blasco J, Casterá DE, Cortes X, Abad FJ, Rosique-Robles JD, Mallench LG (2015) Effectiveness of infliximab, adalimumab and golimumab for non-infectious refractory uveitis in adults. Int J Clin Pharmacol Ther 53:377–390

Brown SL, Greene MH, Gershon SK et al (2002) Tumor necrosis factor antagonist therapy and lymphoma development: twenty-six cases reported to the Food and Drug Administration. Arthritis Rheum 46:3151–3158

Chaudhary R, Butler M, Playford RJ, Ghosh S (2006) Anti-TNF antibody induced stimulated T lymphocyte apoptosis depends on the concentration of the antibody and etanercept induces apoptosis at rates equivalent to infliximab and adalimumab at 10 micrograms per ml concentration. Gastroenterology 130(Suppl 2). [Abstract A696]

Choi SL, Jackson K, Chigutsa E et al (2016) A longitudinal PKPD model describing the static Physician Global Assessment (sPGA) response to ixekizumab in patients with moderate to severe plaque psoriasis. J Pharmacokinet Pharmacodyn 43:S37. [Abstract M-57]

Christophers E (2001) Psoriasis—epidemiology and clinical spectrum. Clin Exp Dermatol 26:314–320

Cimzia (certolizumab pegol) (2016) US prescribing information. UCB Inc, Smyrna

Cinqair (reslizumab) (2016) US prescribing information. Teva Pharmaceutical Industries Ltd., Frazer

Cooke A, Bulkhi A, Casale T (2015) Role of biologics in intractable urticaria. Biologics 9:25–33

Cosentyx (secukinumab) (2017) US prescribing information. Novartis Pharmaceuticals Corporation, East Hanover

Davis JC, Mease PJ (2008) Insights into the pathology and treatment of spondyloarthritis: from the bench to the clinic. Semin Arthritis Rheum 38:83–100

D'Haens G, Baert F, van Assche G et al (2008) Early combined immunosuppression or conventional management in patients with newly diagnosed Crohn's disease: an open randomised trial. Lancet 371:660–667

Dupixent (dupilumab) (2017) US prescribing information. Sanofi-aventis U.S. LLC/ and Regeneron Pharmaceuticals, Inc., Bridgewater

Ehrlich P (1891) Experimentelle untersuchungen über immunität. I. Ueber Ricin. Dtsch Med Wochenschr 17:976–979

Ellerin T, Rubin RH, Weinblatt ME (2003) Infections and anti-tumor necrosis factor alpha therapy. Arthritis Rheum 48:3013–3022

Enbrel (etanercept) (2016) US prescribing information. Immunex Corporation, Thousand Oaks

Entyvio (vedolizumab) (2014) US prescribing information. Takeda Pharmaceuticals, Deerfield

European Medicines Agency (2009) EMEA/541561/2009-Assessment report (Arcalyst®). http://www.ema.europa.eu/docs/en_GB/document_library/EPAR_-_Public_assessment_report/human/001047/WC500026509.pdf. Accessed 06 Feb 2018

European Medicines Agency (2013a) EMA/56352/2013-Assessment report (Humira®). http://www.ema.europa.eu/docs/en_GB/document_library/EPAR_-_Assessment_Report_-_Variation/human/000481/WC500138422.pdf. Accessed 06 Feb 2018

European Medicines Agency (2013b) EMA/CHMP/431551/2013- Assessment report (Stelara®). http://www.ema.europa.eu/docs/en_GB/document_library/EPAR_-_Assessment_Report_-_Variation/human/000958/WC500150607.pdf. Accessed 06 Feb 2018

European Medicines Agency (2015a) EMA/CHMP/177541/2015- Extension of indication variation assessment report (Humira®). http://www.ema.europa.eu/docs/en_GB/document_library/EPAR_-_Assessment_Report_-_Variation/human/000481/WC500186769.pdf. Accessed 06 Feb 2018

European Medicines Agency (2015b) EMA/CHMP/364731/2015- Assessment report (Humira®). http://www.ema.europa.eu/docs/en_GB/document_library/EPAR_-_Assessment_Report_-_Variation/human/000481/WC500195564.pdf. Accessed 06 Feb 2018

European Medicines Agency (2015c) EMA/CHMP/665405/2015 - Assessment report (Cosentyx®). http://www.ema.europa.eu/docs/en_GB/document_library/EPAR_-_Assessment_Report_-_Variation/human/003729/WC500199574.pdf. Accessed 06 Feb 2018

European Medicines Agency (2015d) EMA/CHMP/665427/2015- Assessment report (Cosentyx®). http://www.ema.europa.eu/docs/en_GB/document_library/EPAR_-_Assessment_Report_-_Variation/human/003729/WC500199573.pdf. Accessed 06 Feb 2018

European Medicines Agency (2016a) EMA/501143/2016-Extension of indication variation assessment report (Humira®). http://www.ema.europa.eu/docs/en_GB/document_library/EPAR_-_Assessment_Report_-_Variation/human/000481/WC500211228.pdf. Accessed 06 Feb 2018

European Medicines Agency (2016b) EMA/CHMP/404217/2016- Assessment report (Simponi®). http://www.ema.europa.eu/docs/en_GB/document_library/EPAR_-_Assessment_Report_-_Variation/human/000992/WC500211888.pdf. Accessed 06 Feb 2018

European Medicines Agency (2017a) EMA/455579/2017-Assessment report (Orencia®). http://www.ema.europa.eu/docs/en_GB/document_library/EPAR_-_Assessment_Report_-_Variation/human/000701/WC500233148.pdf. Accessed 06 Feb 2018

European Medicines Agency (2017b) EMA/512262/2017-Assessment report (Dupixent®). http://www.ema.europa.eu/docs/en_GB/document_library/EPAR_-_Public_assessment_report/human/004390/WC500236509.pdf. Accessed 06 Feb 2018

European Medicines Agency (2017c) EMA/790835/2017-Assessment report (Ocrevusi®). http://www.ema.europa.eu/docs/en_GB/document_library/EPAR_-_Public_assessment_report/human/004043/WC500241126.pdf. Accessed 06 Feb 2018

European Medicines Agency (2017d) EMA/CHMP/829007/2017- Assessment report (Humira®). http://www.ema.europa.eu/docs/en_GB/document_library/EPAR_-_Assessment_Report_-_Variation/human/000481/WC500240431.pdf. Accessed 06 Feb 2018

Fasanmade A, Oison A, Bag W, Pendley C, Davis H, Mayer L (2002) Relationship between Infliximab Pharmacokinetics and Improvement in Crohn's disease. Gastroenterology 122(Suppl 4):A617–A618. [Abstract W1364]

Fasanmade AA, Marsters P, Munsanje E, Graham MA, Davis HM, Van Deventer S (2003) Infliximab pharmacokinetics and improvement in fistulizing Crohn's disease. Gastroenterology 124(Suppl 1):A61. [Abstract 470]

Fasenra (benralizumab) (2017) US prescribing information. AstraZeneca Pharmaceuticals LP, Wilmington

Feldman SR, Krueger GG (2005) Psoriasis assessment tools in clinical trials. Ann Rheum Dis 64(Suppl 2):ii65–ii68

Gibiansky L, Gibiansky E, Frey N et al (2017) Population pharmacokinetic and exposure-efficacy/safety analyses for selection of optimal dose regimen of tocilizumab in patients with giant cell arteritis (GCA). J Pharmacokinet Pharmacodyn 44:S131. [Abstract W-076]

Golay J, Semenzato G, Rambaldi A et al (2013) Lessons for the clinic from rituximab pharmacokinetics and pharmacodynamics. MAbs 5:826–837

Gold R, Jawad A, Miller DH et al (2007) Expert opinion: guidelines for the use of natalizumab in multiple sclerosis patients previously treated with immunomodulating therapies. J Neuroimmunol 187:156–158

Gomez-Garcia F, Epstein D, Isla-Tejera B et al (2017) Short-term efficacy and safety of new biological agents targeting the interleukin-23-T helper 17 pathway for moderate-to-severe plaque psoriasis: a systematic review and network meta-analysis. Br J Dermatol 176:594–603

Greco A, Rizzo MI, De Virgilio A et al (2015) Churg-Strauss syndrome. Autoimmun Rev 14:341–348

Griffiths CE, Barker JN (2007) Pathogenesis and clinical features of psoriasis. Lancet 370:263–271

Griffiths CE, Strober BE, van de Kerkhof P et al (2010) Comparison of ustekinumab and etanercept for moderate-to-severe psoriasis. N Engl J Med 362:118–128

Gura T (2002) Therapeutic antibodies: magic bullets hit the target. Nature 417:584–586

Hasegawa M, Imai Y, Hiraoka M, Ito K, Roy A (2011) Model-based determination of abatacept exposure in support of the recommended dose for Japanese rheumatoid arthritis patients. J Pharmacokinet Pharmacodyn 38:803–832

Hawkins PN, Lachmann HJ (2003) Interleukin-1-receptor antagonist in the Muckle–Wells syndrome. N Engl J Med 348:2583–2584

Hochhaus G, Brookman L, Fox H et al (2003) Pharmacodynamics of omalizumab: implications for optimised dosing strategies and clinical efficacy in the treatment of allergic asthma. Curr Med Res Opin 19:491–498

Hoentjen F, van Bodegraven AA (2009) Safety of anti-tumor necrosis factor therapy in inflammatory bowel disease. World J Gastroenterol 15:2067–2073

Hoseyni HG, Xu Y, Zhou H (2018) Therapeutic drug monitoring (TDM) of biologics for inflammatory bowel disease – an answer to optimized treatment? J Clin Pharmacol 58(7):864–876

Hsu LF, Huang JD (2014) Evaluation of etanercept dose reduction in patients with rheumatoid arthritis using pharmacokinetic/pharmacodynamic modeling and simulation. Int J Clin Pharmacol Ther 52:776–786

Hu C, Xu Z, Zhang Y, Rahman MU, Davis HM, Zhou H (2011) Population approach for exposure-response modeling of golimumab in patients with rheumatoid arthritis. J Clin Pharmacol 51:639–648

Hu C, Adedokun OJ, Chen Y et al (2017a) Challenges in longitudinal exposure-response modeling of data from complex study designs: a case study of modeling CDAI score for ustekinumab in patients with Crohn's disease. J Pharmacokinet Pharmacodyn 44:425–436

Hu C, Randazzo B, Sharma A, Zhou H (2017b) Improvement in latent variable indirect response modeling of multiple categorical clinical endpoints: application to modeling of guselkumab treatment effects in psoriatic patients. J Pharmacokinet Pharmacodyn 44:437–448

Humira (adalimumab) (2017) US prescribing information. AbbVie Inc, North Chicago

Hutmacher MM, Nestorov I, Ludden T, Zitnik R, Banfield C (2007) Modeling the exposure-response relationship of etanercept in the treatment of patients with chronic moderate to severe plaque psoriasis. J Clin Pharmacol 47:238–248

Ilaris (canakinumab) (2016) US prescribing information. Novartis Pharmaceuticals Corporation, East Hanover

Jabbar-Lopez ZK, Yiu ZZN, Ward V et al (2017) Quantitative evaluation of biologic therapy options for psoriasis: a systematic review and network meta-analysis. J Investig Dermatol 137:1646–1654

Kevzara (sarilumab) (2017) US prescribing information. Sanofi-aventis U.S. LLC/Regeneron Pharmaceuticals, Inc., Bridgewater

Khattri S, Brunner PM, Garcet S et al (2017) Efficacy and safety of ustekinumab treatment in adults with moderate-to-severe atopic dermatitis. Exp Dermatol 26:28–35

Kraft M, Worm M (2017) Dupilumab in the treatment of moderate-to-severe atopic dermatitis. Expert Rev Clin Immunol 13:301–310

Kubota T, Koike R (2010) Cryopyrin-associated periodic syndromes: background and therapeutics. Mod Rheumatol 20:213–221

Lachmann HJ, Lowe P, Felix SD et al (2009) In vivo regulation of interleukin 1beta in patients with cryopyrin-associated periodic syndromes. J Exp Med 206:1029–1036

Lacroix BD, Karlsson MO, Friberg LE (2014) Simultaneous exposure-response modeling of ACR20, ACR50, and ACR70 improvement scores in rheumatoid arthritis patients treated with certolizumab pegol. CPT Pharmacometrics Syst Pharmacol. 3:e143

Laffaldano P, Lucchese G, Trojano M (2011) Treating multiple sclerosis with natalizumab. Expert Rev Neurother 11:1683–1692

Langford CA, Cuthbertson D, Ytterberg SR et al (2017) A randomized, double-blind trial of abatacept (CTLA-4Ig) for the treatment of Giant cell arteritis. Arthritis Rheumatol 69:837–845

Langley RG (2012) Effective and sustainable biologic treatment of psoriasis: what can we learn from new clinical data? J Eur Acad Dermatol Venereol 26(Suppl 2):21–29

Langley RG, Elewski BE, Lebwohl M et al (2014) Secukinumab in plaque psoriasis--results of two phase 3 trials. N Engl J Med 371:326–338

Lee H, Kimko HC, Rogge M, Wang D, Nestorov I, Peck CC (2003) Population pharmacokinetic and pharmacodynamic modeling of etanercept using logistic regression analysis. Clin Pharmacol Ther 73:348–365

Leonardi CL, Kimball AB, Papp KA et al (2008) Efficacy and safety of ustekinumab, a human interleukin-12/23 monoclonal antibody, in patients with psoriasis: 76-week results from a randomised, double-blind, placebo-controlled trial (PHOENIX 1). Lancet 371:1665–1674

Levi M, Grange S, Frey N (2013) Exposure-response relationship of tocilizumab, an anti-IL-6 receptor monoclonal antibody, in a large population of patients with rheumatoid arthritis. J Clin Pharmacol 53:151–159

Li X, Passarell JA, Lin K, Roy A, Murthy B, Girgis IG (2017) Population pharmacokinetics and exposure–response analyses for abatacept in juvenile idiopathic arthritis. J Pharmacokinet Pharmacodyn 44:S127–S128. [Abstract W-069]

Lin P, Suhler EB, Rosenbaum JT (2014) The future of uveitis treatment. Ophthalmology 121:365–376

Lowe PJ, Tannenbaum S, Gautier A, Jimenez P (2009) Relationship between omalizumab pharmacokinetics, IgE pharmacodynamics and symptoms in patients with severe persistent allergic (IgE-mediated) asthma. Br J Clin Pharmacol 68:61–76

Ma L, Xu C, Su Y, Paccaly A, Kanamaluru V (2016a) Population pharmacokinetics and pharmacodynamics of the effect of sarilumab on DAS28-CRP in patients with rheumatoid arthritis. J Pharmacokinet Pharmacodyn 43:S106. [Abstract W-46]

Ma L, Xu C, Su Y, Paccaly A, Kanamaluru V (2016b) Population pharmacokinetics and pharmacodynamics of the effect of sarilumab on absolute neutrophil counts in patients with rheumatoid arthritis. J Pharmacokinet Pharmacodyn 43:S106–S107. [Abstract W-47]

Mallipeddi R, Grattan C (2007) Lack of response of severe steroid-dependent chronic urticaria to rituximab. Clin Exp Dermatol 32:333–334

Maurer M, Weller K, Bindslev-Jensen C et al (2011) Unmet clinical needs in chronic spontaneous urticaria. A GA2LEN task force report. Allergy 66:317–330

McInnes IB, Schett G (2011) The pathogenesis of rheumatoid arthritis. N Engl J Med 365:2205–2219

Menting SP, Coussens E, Pouw MF et al (2015) Developing a therapeutic range of adalimumab serum concentrations in management of psoriasis: a step toward personalized treatment. JAMA Dermatol. 151:616–622
Modigliani R, Mary JY, Simon JF et al (1990) Clinical, biological, and endoscopic picture of attacks of Crohn's disease: evolution on prednisolone. Gastroenterology 98:811–818
Molodecky NA, Soon IS, Rabi DM et al (2012) Increasing incidence and prevalence of the inflammatory bowel diseases with time, based on systematic review. Gastroenterology 142:46–54. e42
Muralidharan KK, Kuesters G, Plavina T et al (2017a) Population pharmacokinetics and target engagement of natalizumab in patients with multiple sclerosis. J Clin Pharmacol 57:1017–1030
Muralidharan KK, Steiner D, Amarante D et al (2017b) Exposure-disease response analysis of natalizumab in subjects with multiple sclerosis. J Pharmacokinet Pharmacodyn 44:263–275
Nestle FO, Kaplan DH, Barker J (2009) Psoriasis. N Engl J Med 361:496–509
Nucala (mepolizumab) (2017) US prescribing information. GlaxoSmithKline LLC, Philadelphia
O'Dell JR (2004) Therapeutic strategies for rheumatoid arthritis. N Engl J Med 350:2591–2602
Orencia (abatacept) (2017) US prescribing information. Bristol-Myers Squibb Company, Princeton
Ocrevus (ocrelizumab) (2017) US prescribing information. Genentech, Inc. A Member of the Roche Group, South San Francisco
Papp KA, Langley RG, Lebwohl M et al (2008) Efficacy and safety of ustekinumab, a human interleukin-12/23 monoclonal antibody, in patients with psoriasis: 52-week results from a randomised, double-blind, placebo-controlled trial (PHOENIX 2). Lancet 371:1675–1684
Papp K, Gulliver W, Lynde C et al (2011) Canadian guidelines for the management of plaque psoriasis. J Cutan Med Surg 15:210–219
Polman CH, O'Connor PW, Havrdova E et al (2006) A randomized, placebo-controlled trial of natalizumab for relapsing multiple sclerosis. N Engl J Med 354:899–910
Pradeep S, Smith JH (2018) Giant cell arteritis: practical pearls and updates. Curr Pain Headache Rep 22:2
Reich K, Nestle FO, Papp K et al (2005) Infliximab induction and maintenance therapy for moderate-to-severe psoriasis: a phase III, multicentre, double-blind trial. Lancet 366:367–374
Reich K, Burden AD, Eaton JN, Hawkins NS (2012) Efficacy of biologics in the treatment of moderate to severe psoriasis: a network meta-analysis of randomized controlled trials. Br J Dermatol 166:179–188
Remicade (infliximab) (2017) US prescribing information. Janssen Biotech Inc, Horsham
Rituxan (rituximab) (2016) US prescribing information. Genentech Inc., South San Francisco
Rosario M, Dirks NL, Gastonguay MR et al (2015) Population pharmacokinetics-pharmacodynamics of vedolizumab in patients with ulcerative colitis and Crohn's disease. Aliment Pharmacol Ther 42:188–202
Rosario M, French JL, Dirks NL et al (2017) Exposure-efficacy relationships for vedolizumab induction therapy inp with ulcerative colitis or Crohn's disease. J Crohns Colitis 11:921–929
Roy A, Mould DR, Wang XF, Tay L, Raymond R, Pfister M (2017) Modeling and simulation of abatacept exposure and interleukin-6 response in support of recommended doses for rheumatoid arthritis. J Clin Pharmacol 47:1408–1420
Rudick RA, Stuart WH, Calabresi PA et al (2006) Natalizumab plus interferon-β-1a for relapsing multiple sclerosis. N Engl J Med 354:911–923
Ruzicka T, Hanifin JM, Furue M et al (2017) Anti-interleukin-31 receptor A antibody for atopic dermatitis. N Engl J Med 376:826–835
Saeki H, Kabashima K, Tokura Y et al (2017) Efficacy and safety of ustekinumab in Japanese patients with severe atopic dermatitis: a randomised, double-blind, placebo-controlled, phase II Study. Br J Dermatol 177:419–427
Salinger DH, Endres CJ, Gibbs MA (2014) Exposure-response model of brodalumab in psoriasis: modeling of continuous PASI response predicts categorical PASI 75 and PASI 100 endpoints. J Pharmacokinet Pharmacodyn 41:S52–S53. [Abstract T-030]
Salliot C, Finckh A, Katchamart W et al (2011) Indirect comparisons of the efficacy of biological antirheumatic agents in rheumatoid arthritis in patients with an inadequate response to conventional disease-modifying antirheumatic drugs or to an anti-tumour necrosis factor agent: a meta-analysis. Ann Rheum Dis 70:266–271
Sandborn WJ, Feagan BG, Stoinov S et al (2006) Certolizumab pegol administered subcutaneously is effective and well tolerated in patients with active Crohn's disease: results from a 26-week, placebo-controlled phase III study (PRECiSE 1). Gastroenterology 130:A-107
Shanmugam VK, Zaman NM, McNish S, Hant FN (2017) Review of current immunologic therapies for hidradenitis suppurativa. Int J Rheumatol 2017:8018192. https://doi.org/10.1155/2017/8018192
Siliq (brodalumab) (2017) US prescribing information. Valeant Pharmaceuticals North America LLC, Bridgewater
Simponi (golimumab) (2017a) US prescribing information. Janssen Biotech Inc, Horsham
Simponi (golimumab) (2017b) European Union summary of product characteristics (SmPC). Janssen Biologics B.V, Leiden
Simponi Aria (golimumab) (2017) US prescribing information. Janssen Biotech Inc, Horsham
Smedby KE, Askling J, Mariette X et al (2008) Autoimmune and inflammatory disorders and risk of malignant lymphomas–an update. J Intern Med 264:514–527
Smith DA, Minthorn EA, Beerahee M (2011) Pharmacokinetics and pharmacodynamics of mepolizumab, an anti-interleukin-5 monoclonal antibody. Clin Pharmacokinet 50:215–227
Soler D, Chapman T, Yang LL, Wyant T, Egan R, Fedyk ER (2009) The binding specificity and selective antagonism of vedolizumab, an anti-alpha4beta7 integrin therapeutic antibody in development for inflammatory bowel diseases. J Pharmacol Exp Ther 330:864–875
St Clair EW, Wagner CL, Fasanmade AA et al (2002) The relationship of serum infliximab concentrations to clini-

cal improvement in rheumatoid arthritis: results from ATTRACT, a multicenter, randomized, double-blind, placebo-controlled trial. Arthritis Rheum 46:1451–1459

Stelara (ustekinumab) (2017) US prescribing information. Janssen Biotech Inc, Horsham

Struemper H, Thapar M, Roth D (2018) Population pharmacokinetic and pharmacodynamic analysis of belimumab administered subcutaneously in healthy volunteers and patients with systemic lupus erythematosus. Clin Pharmacokinet 57(6):717–728.

Sun H, Van LM, Floch D et al (2016) Pharmacokinetics and pharmacodynamics of canakinumab in patients with systemic juvenile idiopathic arthritis. J Clin Pharmacol 56:1516–1527

Taltz (ixekizumab) (2017) US prescribing information. Eli Lilly and Company, Indianapolis

Taylor PC, Steuer A, Gruber J et al (2004) Comparison of ultrasonographic assessment of synovitis and joint vascularity radiographic evaluation in a randomized, placebo-controlled study of infliximab therapy in early rheumatoid arthritis. Arthritis Rheum 50:1107–1116

Ternant D, Ducourau E, Fuzibet P et al (2015) Pharmacokinetics and concentration-effect relationship of adalimumab in rheumatoid arthritis. Br J Clin Pharmacol 79:286–297

Tracey D, Klareskog L, Sasso EH et al (2008) Tumor necrosis factor antagonist mechanisms of action: a comprehensive review. Pharmacol Ther 117:244–279

Tremfya (guselkumab) (2017) US prescribing information. Janssen Biotech Inc, Horsham

Tysabri® (natalizumab) (2017) US prescribing information. Biogen Idec Inc, Cambridge

Tzanetakou V, Kanni T, Giatrakou S et al (2016) Safety and efficacy of anakinra in severe hidradenitis suppurativa: a randomized clinical trial. JAMA Dermatol 152:52–59

US Food and Drug Administration (2008) 125104Orig1s0033 [BLA#125104/33]- Clinical pharmacology/biopharmaceutics review (Tysabri®). https://www.accessdata.fda.gov/drugsatfda_docs/bla/2008/125104Orig1s0033.pdf. Accessed 06 Feb 2018

US Food and Drug Administration (2015a) Advisory Committee Briefing Document (BLA#761033, Reslizumab). https://www.fdanews.com/ext/resources/files/12-15/12-07-15-Teva-reslizumab.pdf?1517272698. Accessed 06 Feb 2018

US Food and Drug Administration (2015b) Clinical pharmacology/ Biopharmaceutics Review (Cosentyx®)-125504Orig1s000 (BLA#125504). https://www.accessdata.fda.gov/drugsatfda_docs/nda/2015/125504Orig1s000ClinPharmR.pdf. Accessed 06 Feb 2018

Van den Brande JM, Braat H, van den Brink GR et al (2003) Infliximab but not etanercept induces apoptosis in lamina propria T-lymphocytes from patients with Crohn's disease. Gastroenterology 124:1774–1785

Vande Casteele N, Feagan BG, Vermeire S et al (2018) Exposure-response relationship of certolizumab pegol induction and maintenance therapy in patients with Crohn's disease. Aliment Pharmacol Ther 47:229–237

Vestergaard C, Deleuran M (2015) Chronic spontaneous urticaria: latest developments in aetiology, diagnosis and therapy. Ther Adv Chronic Dis 6:304–313

Vogelzang EH, Kneepkens EL, Nurmohamed MT et al (2014) Anti-adalimumab antibodies and adalimumab concentrations in psoriatic arthritis; an association with disease activity at 28 and 52 weeks of follow-up. Ann Rheum Dis 73:2178–2182

Vogelzang EH, Pouw MF, Nurmohamed M et al (2015) Adalimumab trough concentrations in patients with rheumatoid arthritis and psoriatic arthritis treated with concomitant disease-modifying antirheumatic drugs. Ann Rheum Dis. 74:474–475

Wang B, Yan L, Yao Z, Roskos LK (2017) Population pharmacokinetics and pharmacodynamics of benralizumab in healthy volunteers and patients with asthma. CPT Pharmacometrics Syst Pharmacol 6:249–257

Wolbink G, Goupille P, Sandborn W et al (2016) Association between plasma certolizumab pegol concentration and improvement in disease activity in rheumatoid arthritis and Crohn's disease. Arthritis Rheumatol 68(Suppl 10). [Abstract 596]

Xiong Y, Wang W, Ebling W et al (2013) Exposure-response modeling of canakinumab in the avoidance of flares in children with systemic juvenile idiopathic arthritis. Pediatr Rheumatol 11(Suppl 2):P181. [Abstract]

Xolair (omalizumab) (2016) US prescribing information. Genentech Inc., South San Francisco

Zhang X, Morcos PN, Saito T, Terao K (2013) Clinical pharmacology of tocilizumab for the treatment of systemic juvenile idiopathic arthritis. Expert Rev Clin Pharmacol 6:123–137

Zhang X, Chen YC, Terao K (2017) Clinical pharmacology of tocilizumab for the treatment of polyarticular-course juvenile idiopathic arthritis. Expert Rev Clin Pharmacol 10:471–482

Zheng Y, Le K, Wada R et al (2014) Population PK-PD and exposure–response modeling and simulation to support dose recommendation of Xolair in chronic idiopathic urticaria/chronic spontaneous urticaria. J Pharmacokinet Pharmacodyn 41:S32. [Abstract M-059]

Zhou H, Hu C, Zhu Y et al (2010) Population-based exposure-efficacy modeling of ustekinumab in patients with moderate to severe plaque psoriasis. J Clin Pharmacol 50:257–267

SUGGESTED READINGS

Lagassé HA, Alexaki A, Simhadri VL, Katagiri NH, Jankowski W, Sauna ZE, Kimchi-Sarfaty C (2017) Recent advances in therapeutic protein drug development. F1000Res 6:113. https://doi.org/10.12688/f1000research.9970.1. eCollection2017

Murphy K, Weaver C (2016) Janeway's Immunology. 9th edn. Garland Science. ISBN: 978-0815345053

Zhou H, Theil F-P (eds) (2015) ADME and Translational Pharmacokinetics/Pharmacodynamics of Therapeutic Proteins. John Wiley and Sons, Inc., Hoboken. ISBN: 978-1-118-89864-2

Zhou H, Mould D (eds) (2019) Quantitative pharmacology and individualized therapy strategies in development of therapeutic proteins for immune-mediated inflammatory diseases. Wiley, Hoboken. ISBN: 978-1119289197

27 Interferons and Interleukins

Jean-Charles Ryff and Sidney Pestka[†]

INTRODUCTION

PHARMACOTHERAPY INFORMATION

Further information on the applied pharmacotherapy with interferons and interleukins can be found in the following frequently used textbooks:

Applied Therapeutics: The Clinical Use of Drugs (Koda-Kimble, MA, et al., Eds.), 10th edition, Lippincott Williams & Wilkins, Baltimore 2013.

Pharmacotherapy: A Pathophysiologic Approach (DiPiro, JT, et al., Eds.), 9th edition, McGraw-Hill, New York 2014.

Textbook of Therapeutics: Drug and Disease Management (Helms, RA, et al., Eds.), 8th edition, Lippincott Williams & Wilkins, Baltimore 2006: Chapters 9, 33, 46, 49, 65, 93, 103.

In 1957 Alick Isaacs and Jean Lindenmann described a substance which was produced by virus-infected cell cultures and "interfered" with infection by other viruses; it was called interferon. Over the following decades it was realized that "interferon" comprises a family of related proteins with several additional properties. Starting in the 1960s various "factors" produced primarily by white blood cell (WBC) as well as otherv-cell supernatants were described which acted in various ways on other WBCs or somatic cells. They were usually given a descriptive name either associated with their cell of origin or their activity on other cells resulting in a myriad of names. The application of molecular biological techniques allowed us to determine that some cytokines had multiple activities and that different cytokines had similar overlapping activities. A classification system based on genetic structure and protein characterization is being used. The interactive networks and cascades of cytokines, interferons (IFN), interleukins (IL), growth factors (GF), chemokines (CK), their receptors (r or R) and signaling pathways are highly complex and will be further explored in this chapter.

Cytokine is a term coined in 1974 by Stanley Cohen in an attempt to develop a more systematic approach to

[†]Deceased

J.-C. Ryff (Retired) (✉)
Biotechnology Research and Innovation Network, Basel, Switzerland

S. Pestka[†]
PBL Interferon Source, Piscataway, NJ, USA

D. J. A. Crommelin et al. (eds.), *Pharmaceutical Biotechnology*, https://doi.org/10.1007/978-3-030-00710-2_27

the numerous regulatory proteins secreted by hematopoietic and non-hematopoietic cells. Cytokines play a critical role in modulating the innate and adaptive immune systems. They are multifunctional peptides that are now known to be produced by normal and neoplastic cells, as well as by cells of the immune system. These local messengers and signaling molecules are involved in the development of the immune system, cell growth and differentiation, repair mechanisms and the inflammatory cascade. Traditionally, interleukins can be classified as T-helper cells type 1 (Th1; pro-inflammatory), e.g. IL-2, IL-12, IL-18, IFNγ, or T-helper cells type 2 (Th2; anti-inflammatory) stimulating, e.g. IL-4, IL-10, IL-13, TGF-β. More recently a third category T-helper cells 17 (Th17) have been described which are associated with autoimmunity. A review of the Th1/Th2 and Th17 concept is provided by Steinman (2007).

(a) *Interferons*: proteins produced by eukaryotic cells in response to viral infections, tumors and other biological inducers. They promote an antiviral state in other, neighboring cells and also help to regulate the immune response. They exhibit a variety of activities and represent a wide family of proteins.
(b) *Interleukins*: a group of cytokines mainly secreted by leukocytes and primarily affecting growth and differentiation of hematopoietic and immune cells. They are also produced by other normal and malignant cells and are of central importance in the regulation of hematopoiesis, immunity, inflammation, tissue remodeling, and embryonic development.

"Thus, all interleukins are cytokines however not all cytokines are interleukins"

(c) *Growth factors*: proteins that activate cellular proliferation and/or differentiation. Many growth factors stimulate cellular division in numerous different cell types; others are specific to a particular cell type. They also promote proliferation of connective tissue, glial and smooth muscle cells, enhance normal wound healing and promote proliferation and differentiation of erythrocytes (erythropoietin). Hematopoietic growth factors are reviewed in Chap. 24. Some ILs have a function overlap with growth factors, e.g. IL-2, IL-3, IL-11 (see Table 27.1).
(d) *Chemokines*: (*chemo*tactic cyto*kines*) a large family of structurally related low molecular weight proteins with potent leukocyte activation and/or chemotactic activity. "CXC" (or α) and "C-C" (or β) chemokine subsets are based on presence or absence of an amino acid between the first two of four conserved cysteines. A third subset, "C", has only two cysteines and to date only one member, IL-16, has been identified. The fourth subgroup, the C-X3-C chemokine has three amino acid residues between the first two cysteines.
(e) *Others*, such as tumor necrosis factors (TNF) lymphotoxin alpha (LT)-α] and -β and transforming growth factor (TGF)-α and -β.

All cytokines including interferons and interleukins act by binding to specific transmembrane receptors. In general, these receptors have two main components: a low affinity ligand-binding domain that ensures ligand specificity and a high affinity effector domain activating target gene promoters via an intracellular signaling pathway. Because cytokines can bind to their receptors only where these are expressed on the cell membrane, a functional tissue or cell specificity is ensured.

Cytokine signaling is tightly controlled within the cell through the action of multiple different negative regulators. Members of the suppressors of cytokine signaling (SOCS) family specifically interfere with cytokine signaling by several different mechanisms including direct binding and inhibition of Janus activated kinase (JAK) proteins, competition with janus activated signal transducer and activator of transcription (STAT) for binding sites on the cytokine receptor (see below), and activation of proteosomal degradation of signaling components.

Their action is described as:

- *autocrine*, if the cytokine acts on the cell that secretes it,
- *paracrine*, if the action is restricted to the immediate vicinity of a cytokine's secretion, or
- *endocrine*, if the cytokine diffuses or is otherwise transported to distant regions of the body to affect different tissues.

They can act on many targets, can act in concert, or can antagonize one another:

- *synergy*—action together to induce a different response than either can induce alone
- *antagonism*—cytokines can counteract one another
- *pleiotropy*—action in a similar way on more than one "target" cell
- *redundancy*—more than one cytokine triggers identical or similar responses in a given "target" cell
- *pathway activation*—triggered sequential induction or "cascade"

INTERFERONS: NOMENCLATURE AND FUNCTIONS

Interferons are a family of naturally occurring proteins and glycoproteins with molecular weights of 16,776 to 22,093 Da produced and secreted by cells in

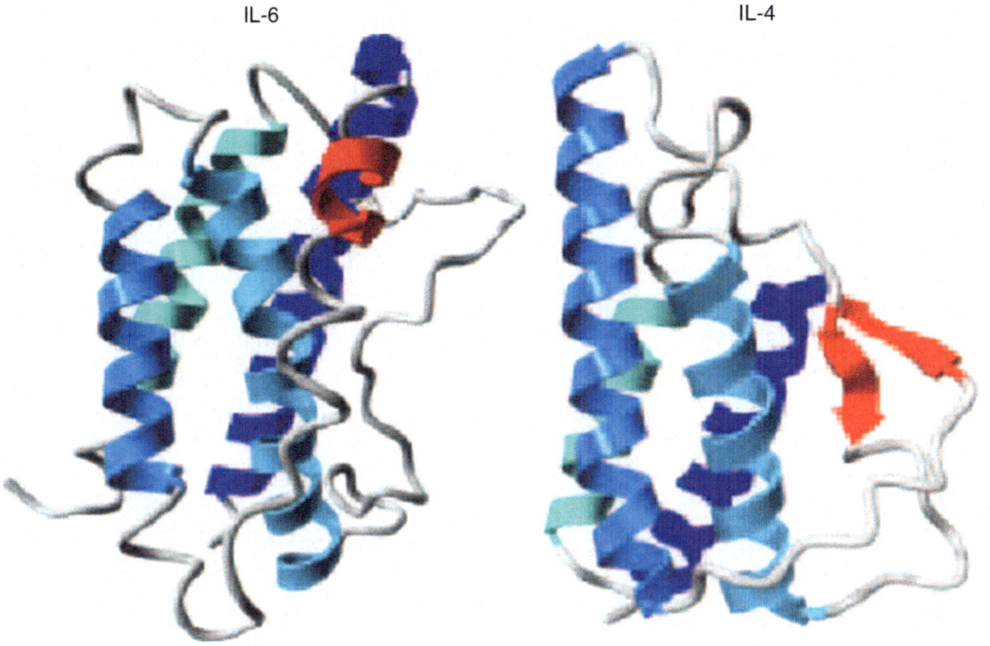

Figure 27.1 ■ Class-1 helical cytokines. Class-1 helical cytokines fold into a bundle of four tightly packed α-helices. On the basis of their helix length, class-I helical cytokines are characterized as (**a**) long chain, such as IL-6, or (**b**) short chain, such as IL-4. From: Journal of Endocrinology (2006) 189, 1–25, with permission

response to viral infections and to synthetic or biological inducers. By interacting with their specific heterodimeric receptors on the surface of cells, the interferons initiate a broad and varied array of signals that induce cellular antiviral states, modulate inflammatory responses, inhibit or stimulate cell growth, produce or inhibit apoptosis, and modulate many components of the immune system. Structurally, they are part of the helical cytokine family (Fig. 27.1). During the past 30 years, major research efforts have been undertaken to understand the signaling mechanisms through which these cytokines induce their effects. Figure 27.2 as a generic example, illustrates the JAK-STAT (Janus activated kinase, originally "just another kinase"—signal transducer and activator of transcription), the best characterized IFN signaling pathway. However, coordination and cooperation of multiple distinct signaling cascades, including the mitogen-activated protein kinase p38 cascade and the phosphatidylinositol 3-kinase cascade, are required for the generation of responses to interferons (Platanias 2005). For a review of the IFN signaling pathways see Journal of Interferon and Cytokine Research 2005; 25: 731–811, Special Issue: The Neoclassical Pathways of Interferon Signaling. Many of the symptoms of acute viral infections are the consequence of the high systemic IFNα response induced by the infecting viruses particularly during the viremic phase.

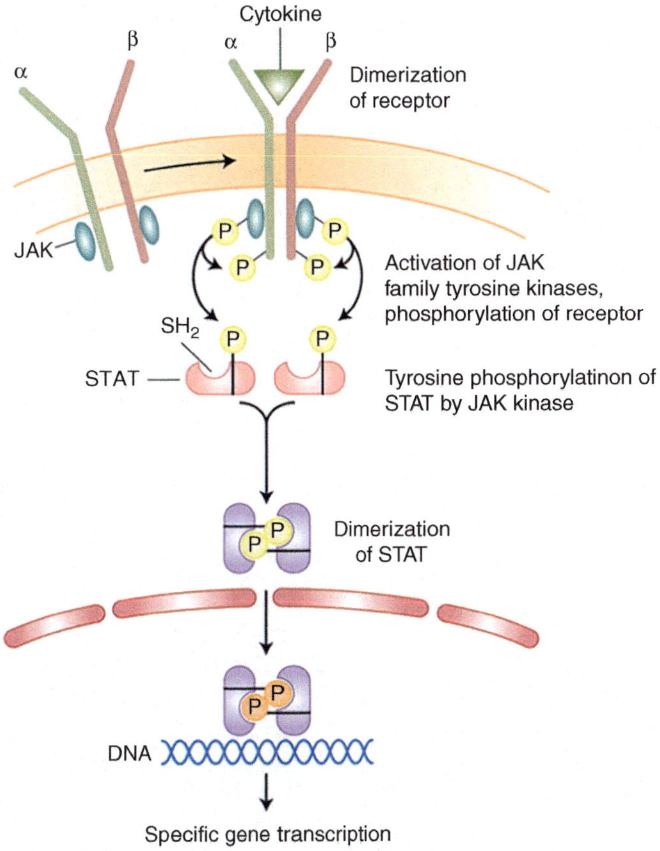

Figure 27.2 ■ Generic JAK-STAT signaling pathway mediated by most cytokine receptors

Human type I interferons comprise 13 different IFNα isoforms or subtypes with varying specificities, e.g. affinities to different cell types, and downstream activities. Although there are 13 human IFNα proteins, two of them (IFNα1 and IFNα13) are identical proteins so that the total number of type I IFNs often is listed as 12 (Pestka 1981a, 1981b, 1986). There is also one subtype each for IFNβ (beta), IFNε (epsilon), IFNκ (kappa) and IFNω (omega). Their ability to establish an "antiviral state" is the distinctive fundamental property of type I IFNs. They are produced by most cells. However, certain types seem to be more selectively expressed, e.g. IFNκ by keratinocytes.

Type II IFN consists of a single representative: IFNγ (gamma) (Pestka 1981a, 1981b, 1986). IFNγ or immune interferon plays an essential role in cell-mediated immune responses. It is produced by NK cells, dendritic cells, cytotoxic T cells, progenitor Th0 cells and Th1 cells. IFNα2, -β and -γ are the most extensively studied to date. All IFNs and IFN-like cytokines have been reviewed in Pestka et al. 2004a.

The names for the human IFNs presently approved by the Human Genome Nomenclature Committee (HGNC) are listed in Table 27.1. For an exhaustive review see Meager 2006.

Symbol	Name	Symbol	Name
IFNα1	Interferon, alpha 1	IFNβ1	Interferon, beta-1, fibroblast
IFNα2	Interferon, alpha 2	IFNε1	Interferon, epsilon-1
IFNα4	Interferon, alpha 4	IFNκ	Interferon, kappa
IFNα5	Interferon, alpha 5	IFNω1	Interferon, omega-1
IFNα6	Interferon, alpha 6	IFNγ	Interferon, gamma
IFNα7	Interferon, alpha 7	There are in addition a number of interferon pseudogenes (Ps) (non-functional and related to interferon genes) mentioned for completion's sake: IFNα22, IFNν (nu) 1, IFN-P 11, 12, 20, 23 and 24, IFNω-P 2, 4, 5, 9, 15, 18 and 19	
IFNα8	Interferon, alpha 8		
IFNα10	Interferon, alpha 10		
IFNα13	Interferon, alpha 13[a]		
IFNα14	Interferon, alpha 14		
IFNα16	Interferon, alpha 16		
IFNα17	Interferon, alpha 17		
IFNα21	Interferon, alpha 21		

P pseudogene
[a]IFNα13 sequence identical to IFNα1

Table 27.1 ■ HGNC approved interferons names (adapted from ExPASy and HGNC)

INTERLEUKINS: NOMENCLATURE AND FUNCTIONS

The first interleukins were identified in the 1970s. Initially it was believed that interleukins were made chiefly by leukocytes to act primarily on other leukocytes. For this reason they were named interleukins, meaning "between leukocytes." It was later realized that they are also produced by and interact with a host of cells not involved in immunity and are involved in many other physiological functions. The role that interleukins play in the body is much greater than was initially understood. They are, however, primarily a collection of immune cell growth, differentiation and maturation factors. Collectively they orchestrate a precise and efficient immune response to toxins and pathogens, including cancer cells, recognized as foreign. As is the case for IFNs, ILs bind to related specific cell surface receptors that activate similar intracellular signaling cascades. Many interleukins, mainly those with pro-inflammatory function, are intrinsically toxic either directly or indirectly, i.e. through induction of toxic gene products. Therefore, the human body has an elaborate system of checks and balances that, under (patho)-physiological conditions, regulates the magnitude and duration of an immune response. ILs are produced upon appropriate stimulation, have a short circulation time. Their production is regulated by positive and negative feedback loops. Furthermore, their effect is mostly localized, and in some cases soluble receptors or neutralizing antibodies limit their dissemination. Specific receptor antagonists can also control their activity.

Table 27.2 lists the ILs for which the protein and gene structure have been characterized. Their names and symbols have been approved by the HGNC.

Under patho-physiological conditions, the sequential concentrations of agonistic and antagonistic interleukins establish a delicate balance in driving pro- and anti-inflammatory phases. This process can be disturbed by various pathogenic agents or mechanisms:

- Infectious agents or toxins
- Allergens
- Malignant tumors
- Genetic variants

These pathogenic agents or mechanisms can result in a self-limited or protracted disequilibrium. Symptoms of disease are the consequence of an adequate immune response at the end of which the steady-state is reestablished. A brisk inflammatory response is the sign of a healthy immune reaction. In some instances, an inadequate response can manifest itself as relapsing remitting progressive disease, e.g. rheumatoid arthritis, asthma, psoriasis, chronic inflammatory

Symbol	Approved name	Previous symbol	Aliases
IL-1A	Interleukin-1, alpha	IL-1	IL-1 alpha, hematopoietin-1, interleukin -1 family member (IL-1F) 1
IL-1B	Interleukin-1, beta		IL-1 beta, IL-1F2, catabolin
IL-1F3	Interleukin-1 family, member 3		IL-1 delta, IL-1 receptor antagonist homolog 1, IL-1-related protein 3
IL-RN	Interleukin 1 receptor antagonist	IL1F3	IL1RA, ICIL-1RA, IRAP, MGC10430
IL-2	Interleukin-2		T-cell growth factor (TCGF) aldesleukin
IL-3	Interleukin-3		Multi-CSF
IL-4	Interleukin-4		BSF1
IL-5	Interleukin-5		TRF, EDF, BCDF 1
IL-6	Interleukin-6	IFNB2	BCSF2, HSF, HGF, CTL differentiation factor, MGI-2
IL-7	Interleukin-7		
IL-8	Interleukin-8		CXCL8 (chemokine), MDNCF, TCCF, NAP1, GCP1, MONAP, emoctakin
IL-9	Interleukin-9		TCGF P40, P40 cytokine
IL-10	Interleukin-10		CSIF, TGIF, IL-10A
IL-11	Interleukin-11		AGIF, oprelvekin
IL-12A	Interleukin-12A	NKSF1	CLMF p35, CLMF1, IL-12 p35
IL-12B	Interleukin-12B	NKSF2	CLMF p40, CLMF2, IL-12 p40
IL-13	Interleukin-13		
IL-15	Interleukin-15		
IL-16	Interleukin-16		LCF, proIL-16
IL-17A	Interleukin-17A	IL-17	CTLA-8
IL-17B	Interleukin-17B		Cytokine Zcyto7, neuronal interleukin-17-related factor, interleukin-20
IL-17C	Interleukin-17C		Cytokine CX2
IL-17D	Interleukin-17D		Interleukin-27
IL-17F	Interleukin-17F		Interleukin-24, cytokine ML-1
IL-18	Interleukin-18	IL-1F4	IFN-gamma-inducing factor, IL-1 gamma, iboctadekin
IL-19	Interleukin-19		Melanoma differentiation-associated protein-like protein, IL-10C
IL-20	Interleukin-20		Zcyto10
IL-21	Interleukin-21		Za11
IL-22	Interleukin-22		Zcyto18, IL-TIF
IL-23A	Interleukin-23A		IL-23 subunit p19, SGRF
IL-24	Interleukin-24		MDA-7, suppression of tumorigenicity 16 protein
IL-25	Interleukin-25	IL-17E	Interleukin-17E
IL-26	Interleukin-26		AK155 protein
IL-27	Interleukin-27	IL-30	IL-27A, p28
IL-28A	Interleukin-28A		IFN lambda-2, Zcyto20
IL-28B	Interleukin-28B		IFN lambda-3, IFN lambda-4 Zcyto22
IL-29	Interleukin-29		IFN lambda-1, Zcyto21
IL-31	Interleukin-31		

Table 27.2 ■ HGNC approved interleukins names (adapted from ExPASy and HGNC)

Symbol	Approved name	Previous symbol	Aliases
IL-32	Interleukin-32		NK cell protein 4, TAIF
IL-33	Interleukin-33	IL-1F11	NF-HEV
IL-34	Interleukin-34		
IL-35	Interleukin-35		
IL-36A	Interleukin-36 alpha	IL-1F6	FIL-1 epsilon
IL-36B	Interleukin-36 beta	IL-1F8	Interleukin-1 eta, interleukin-1 homolog 2
IL-36G	Interleukin-36 gamma	IL-1F9	Interleukin-1 epsilon, interleukin-1 homolog 1, IL-1-related protein 2
IL-36RN	Interleukin 36 receptor antagonist	IL-1F5	FIL1 delta, FIL1D, IL1HY1, IL1RP3, IL1L1, IL-1F5, IL36Ra, MGC29840
IL-37	Interleukin-37	IL-1F7	FIL-1 zeta, IL-1 zeta, IL-1 homolog 4, IL-1-related protein 1
IL-38	Interleukin 38	IL-1F10	Interleukin-1 receptor antagonist-like, FIL-1 theta, IL-1 theta, IL-1 HY2

The symbols IL-14 and IL-30 are no longer used as approved nomenclature

Table 27.2 ■ (continued)

bowel disease, multiple sclerosis, chronic hepatitis, or chronic insulitis leading to diabetes mellitus. All have in common that they need a genetic predisposition and an environmental trigger factor to become active, and are, at best, only partially understood. In many cases these diseases are caused by either insufficient production or overproduction of key interleukins. Thus, in principle, once the diagnosis is made these interleukins can be therapeutically supplemented or suppressed to restore proper balance (Ryff 1996).

Our current knowledge of the interleukins listed in Table 27.2 is briefly summarized below and each referenced article selected expands on the subject. Readers interested in the current knowledge about the protein, DNA, RNA, gene, chromosome location etc. for individual interferons or interleukins are referred to the following databases:

1. www.genatlas.org (with a links to other databases), or
2. http://au.expasy.org/sprot/, or

www.rcsb.org/pdb/ for the 3D models of individual IFNs or ILs. For a better understanding of interleukins and their wide ranging, overlapping, redundant and antagonistic functions we have grouped them into a working classification of various "families" according to gene clustering on chromosomes, gene sequence homologies, secondary and tertiary structure, use of related receptors and also according to their function. This classification should be considered as "work in progress" as it is impossible in many cases to assign a member to a specific "family" or "subfamily". Today structural analysis has become the principal approach for classification; it is therefore likely that these groups will expand as crystallisation data and structural analyses become available (for a recent review see Akdis et al. 2016).

■ Interleukin-1 Family

The IL-1 (Garlanda et al. 2013) family comprises 11 different members: IL-1α, IL-1β, IL-1 receptor antagonist (Ra), IL-18, IL-33, IL-36A, B, C, IL-36Ra, IL-37 and IL-38. All are thought to have arisen from a common ancestral gene that underwent multiple duplications. A tight regulation via receptor antagonists, decoy receptors and signaling inhibitors ensures that amplification of innate immunity does not degenerate into uncontrolled inflammation. All cells of the innate immune system express and/or are affected by IL-1 family members.

Interleukin-1

IL-1 (Towne et al. 2004) is generally used to describe IL-1α and IL-1β both of which have the same biological effects and play a primordial role in the innate and adaptive immune response. Although a prototypical proinflammatory cytokine, it also plays a key role in hematopoiesis, appetite control, and bone metabolism. IL-1 is released as part of the acute phase reaction of hepatocytes. The primary producers of IL-1 are macrophages, B-cells and neutrophils. IL-1α and IL-1β are synthesized as pro-peptides of approximately 30 kDa, and are then cleaved to produce products of 159 and 153 amino acids. Differences in glycosylation are responsible for the variation of reported molecular weights.

Interleukin-1Ra

IL-1Ra (Towne et al. 2004) is a naturally occurring IL-1 receptor antagonist (IL-1Ra), an inhibitor of IL-1. It has limited sequence similarity to either IL-1α or IL-1β, but does have the ability to bind to the IL-1 receptors. Lacking IL-1 activity, it acts as a useful blocker of the receptor. A recombinant IL-1Ra has been investigated for its potential use in sepsis; the clinical trials were inconclusive. Recombinant IL-1Ra has, however, been used successfully for the treatment of rheumatoid arthritis and is marketed under the name of Kineret® (see section "Therapeutic Use of Recombinant Interleukins" below). The interleukin-1 receptor antagonist (IL-1Ra) contributes to tumor survival and progression in multiple cancer entities.

Interleukin-18

IL-18 (Liu et al. 2000) shares unique structural features with the IL-1 family, but it does not have the usual four-helix structure rather an all β-pleated sheet structure. It is produced by activated macrophages such as Kupffer cells of the liver and other resident macrophages from which, after cleavage of its precursor pro-IL-18, the mature protein is released. IL-18 is an early inducer of the Th1 response, co-stimulating with IL-12, the production of IFNγ, TNFα, granulocyte macrophage colony-stimulating factor (GM-CSF) and IL-2. IL-18 is associated with the metabolic syndrome and coronary vascular disease (Trøseid et al. 2010).

Interleukin-33

IL-33 (Schmitz et al. 2005), unlike other members of the IL-1 family which are all pro-inflammatory, has a major role in the development of a Th2 type immune response by inducing IL-5 and IL-13. Human smooth muscle cells as well as epithelial cells forming bronchus and small airways show constitutive expression of IL-33 mRNA; in lung or dermal fibroblasts and keratinocytes IL-33 mRNA is induced after activation with TNFα and IL-1β. Activated dendritic cells and macrophages are the only hematopoietic cells showing low quantities of IL-33 mRNA. In addition, IL-33 and IL-18 are the only known IL-1 family member genes not located on chromosome 2. IL-33 is thought to play a key role in mediating an anaphylactic shock. This effect can be completely neutralized by anti-IL-33 antibodies in an experimental model. Thus IL-33 may be a potential target for the treatment of anaphylactic shock and prevention or treatment of atherosclerosis.

Interleukin-36A, B, and G

IL-36 A, B and G (or α, β, and γ) (Towne et al. 2011) previously classified as interleukin-1 family member (IL-1F) 6, IL-1F8, IL-1F9 respectively.

IL-36A (IL-36 alpha) is a member of the IL-1 family of proteins. Cells reported to express IL-36 alpha include monocytes, B cells, and T cells. Notably, IL-36 alpha is the only novel IL-1 family member expressed on T-cells. It is expressed in the immune system and fetal brain, but not in other tissues tested or in multiple hematopoietic cell lines.

IL-36B (IL-36 beta) is expressed at low levels in tonsils, bone marrow, heart, placenta, lung, testes and colon but not in any hematopoietic cell lines nor in adipose tissue. It is detected at higher levels in psoriatic plaques than in symptomless psoriatic skin or healthy control skin. Increased levels are not detected in inflamed joint tissue. It is induced by proinflammatory cytokines IL-1α, IL-1β and TNF in synovial fibroblasts and by IL-1α and TNF in keratinocytes. It is constitutively expressed in articular chondrocytes. IL-36-B stimulates the production of interleukin-6 and interleukin-8 in synovial fibrobasts, articular chondrocytes and mature adipocytes.

IL-36G (IL-36 gamma), is highly expressed in tissues containing epithelial cells: skin, lung, stomach and esophagus. In the skin it can only be detected in keratinocytes but not in fibroblasts, endothelial cells or melanocytes. TNF and IFNγ up-regulate IL-36G in the keratinocytes of psoriatic skin lesions.

Interleukin-36Ra

IL-36Ra (Towne et al. 2011) acts as an IL-36R antagonist controlling the activity of IL-36. Cells expressing IL-36Ra include monocytes, B cells, dendritic cells/ Langerhans cells, keratinocytes, and gastric fundus parietal and chief cells. IL-36Ra is essential for normal skin maintenance. A variant of interleukin-36Ra shows impaired IL-36R affinity and dysregulated secretion of inflammatory cytokines leading to generalized pustular psoriasis (Marrakchi et al. 2011). Il-36Ra has also been documented to suppress inflammation of the brain by enhancing IL-4 response (Collison et al. 2008).

Interleukin-37

IL-37 (Nold et al. 2010) expressed in human monocytes and epithelial cells is a fundamental inhibitor of innate immunity. The overexpression of IL-37 in cells of monocytic or epithelial origin almost completely abolishes the production of pro-inflammatory cytokines.

Interleukin-38

IL-38 was formerly known and HGNC approved as IL-1F10 (Yuan et al. 2015) or IL-1HY2 and has been shown to be expressed in basal epithelia of in fetal skin, in the spleen and in proliferating B-cells of tonsil. This tissue specific expression pattern and the membership of the IL-1 family suggests a role in establishing a normal immune response and inflammatory pathophysiology.

As an efficient method to generate a relatively large quantity of IL-38 is lacking, its biology is largely unexplored. The association of inflammatory pathologies with IL-38 polymorphisms and structural similarities with IL-1Ra suggested an immune regulatory role.

■ Interleukin-2 Family

Interleukin-2 belongs to a family of cytokines, which also includes IL-4, IL-7, IL-9, IL-15 and IL-21 (Liao et al. 2011). These interleukins all share a common receptor γ chain (γc) and are also known as γc-family cytokines.

Interleukin-2

IL-2 (Malek and Castro 2010) originally described as T-cell growth factor (TCGF) is synthesized and secreted primarily by T-cells. IL-2 stimulates the growth, differentiation and activation of T-cells, B-cells, and NK-cells. The major physiological effect is to promote self-tolerance by suppressing T-cell response in vivo. IL-2 signals through a receptor complex consisting of IL-2 specific IL-2 receptor alpha, IL-2 receptor beta and a common gamma chain, which is shared by all members of this cytokine family. A soluble form of the IL-2R capable of binding IL-2, a truncated version of the α chain without cytoplasmic tail, has been found in human serum (soluble receptor or sR). High levels of IL-2sR have been found in patients with a wide variety of disorders, including chronic hepatitis C, HIV infection, cancer, solid organ transplant rejection, and arthritis. Soluble IL-2R can bind released IL-2 prior to its binding to cells to prevent overflow or over-stimulation. Several other cytokine and adhesion molecule receptors also have circulating forms. This is one manner in which the immunological cascade maintains its checks and balances.

Interleukin-4

IL-4, an anti-inflammatory cytokine (Gilmour and Lavender 2008) is produced by Th2 cells and by mast cells, basophils, and eosinophils and acts as an antagonist to interferon- (IFN) γ. It stimulates B-cell proliferation and activation, induces class switch to IgE and IgG_4 expression by B-cells, as well as class II major histocompatibility complex (MHC) expression. In addition, it induces the differentiation of eosinophils and activity of cytotoxic T-cells. IL-4 regulates the differentiation of helper T-cells to the Th2 type. These T-cells produce the cytokines IL-4, IL-5, IL-9, and IL-13, which can all participate in the allergic response. IL-4 regulates the production of IgE by B-lymphocytes. It also has the ability to stimulate chemokine production and mucus hypersecretion by epithelial cells. Overproduction of IL-4 is associated with allergy and asthma.

Interleukin-7

IL-7 (Fry and Mackall 2002) is an essentially tissue-derived cytokine. Its primary sources are stromal and epithelial cells in various locations including intestinal epithelium, liver and, to a lesser degree, dendritic cells. IL-7 acts primarily on pre-B-cells to stimulate their differentiation. It can also stimulate the development of human T-cells. IL-7 is classified as a type I short chain cytokine of the hematopoietin family which also includes IL-2, IL-3, IL-4, IL-5, GM-CSF, IL-9, IL-13, IL-15, macrophage-colony stimulating factor (M-CSF) and stem cell factor (SCF).

Interleukin-9

IL-9 (Noelle and Nowak 2010) is a Th2 cytokine originally characterized as a factor produced by activated T-cells and able to support the long-term growth of some T-helper clones. IL-9 activities extend to various cell types including mast cells, B-lymphocytes, hematopoietic progenitors, eosinophils, lung epithelial cells, neuronal precursors and T-lymphocytes. Increased IL-9 production has been implicated in major pathologies such as asthma supported by its effects on IgE production, mucus production, mast cell differentiation, eosinophil activation and bronchial hyper-responsiveness. IL-9 stimulates the growth of murine thymic lymphomas and an autocrine loop has been suggested in Hodgkin lymphoma. Finally, IL-9 is required for an efficient immune response against intestinal parasites. IL-9 exerts its effects through a receptor that belongs to the hematopoietic receptor superfamily and consists of two chains, also involved in IL-2, IL-4, IL-7, IL-15 and IL-21 signaling.

Interleukin-15

IL-15 (Waldmann 2015) shares the IL-2βγ receptor complex components IL-2Rβ and IL-2Rγ. However, specificity is conferred by a unique α-chain (IL-15Rα) completing the IL-15Rαβγ heterotrimeric high-affinity receptor complex. While the role of interleukin-2 is in the elimination of self-reactive T cells to prevent autoimmunity, interleukin-15 is dedicated to the prolonged maintenance of memory T-cell responses to invading pathogens. It does not stimulate T regulatory cells (Tregs) formerly suppressor T-cells. Thus, boosting IL-15 activity could enhance innate and specific immunity and fight tumors.

Interleukin-21

IL-21 (Yi et al. 2010) is the most recently discovered member of the IL-2 family of cytokines that utilize the common γ-chain receptor subunit for signal transduction. Structurally, it shows homology to the other interleukins of the IL-2 family. The heterodimeric IL-21R has an IL-21 specific subunit besides the γ-chain. IL-21 expression is restricted primarily to activated $CD4^+$ T-cells. IL-21 expression seems transient and stage specific during T-cell differentiation. It is required for normal humoral immunity and regulates antibody production in cooperation with IL-4. IL-21 also regulates cell-mediated immunity by inducing IFNγ, TNF-α and synthesis of perforin and granzyme B leading to cytolytic activity. It can cooperate with other cytokines to generate potent killer T-cells and thus has anti-tumor activity. Lastly, it also has inhibitory activity by inducing IL-10. Thus, altogether, it is responsible for the coordination of the initiation and cessation of an efficient immune response.

■ Interleukin-10 Family

The IL-10 family (Pestka et al. 2004b) includes, besides IL-10, the interleukines: IL-19, -20, -22, -24, -26, -28A, -28B and -29. They share a classical four-helix bundle, a signature element of all helical cytokines (Fig. 27.1) and all share the IL-10R2 or α chain of their dimeric receptor, while each has its own R1 or α chain.

Interleukin-10

IL-10 (Pestka et al. 2004b) is a major endogenous anti-inflammatory mediator, which acts by profoundly inhibiting the synthesis of proinflammatory molecules such as IFNγ, IL-2, IL-12 and TNFα. Macrophages are the major source of IL-10, a homodimer. Th2 cell subsets, monocytes and several other cells can also synthesize this imterleukin. A number of molecules produced under stress conditions including reactive oxygen species stimulate IL-10 synthesis. Recombinant human IL-10 has been tested in clinical trials in rheumatoid arthritis, inflammatory bowel disease, psoriasis, organ transplantation, and chronic hepatitis C. To date the results are mixed or disappointing. However, they give new insight into the immunobiology of IL-10.

Interleukin-19

IL-19 (Azuma et al. 2010) is a member of the IL-10 family. The induction of IL-19 in human monocytes is down-regulated by IFN-γ and up-regulated by IL-4. IL-19 influences the balance of Th1/Th2 cells in favour of Th2 cells by up-regulating IL-4 and down-regulating IFNγ. IL-19 is essential for the induction and maintenance of endotoxin tolerance and appears to play a key role in innate immunity. IL-19 together with IL-20 with whom it shares the same receptor complex, has been associated with psoriasis and is thought to be involved in regulating inflammatory response in various tissues and be of particular importance for proper skin development and function.

Interleukin-20

IL-20 (Xu 2004) was originally identified from a keratinocyte library, its mRNA isolated from skin and trachea. It is classified as a helical cytokine member of the IL-10 family. Keratinocytes and activated monocytes synthetize IL-20. IL-1β, TGF-α and epidermal growth factor (EGF), factors known to be involved with proliferative and pro-inflammatory signals in the skin, enhance the response to IL-20. It binds to two cell surface receptors: IL-20Rα and IL-20Rβ on keratinocytes and other epithelial cells. IL-20 mediates the hyperproliferation of keratinocytes associated with cutaneous inflammation and has a central role in inflammatory skin diseases such as psoriasis and eczema. It also promotes the expansion of pluripotential hematopoietic progenitor cells indicating a role beyond the response of epithelial cells to inflammation.

Interleukin-22

IL-22 (Kotenko et al. 2001a) also belongs to the family of cytokines structurally related to IL-10. In contrast to IL-10, it has proinflammatory activities: it upregulates the production of acute-phase proteins. The IL-22 receptor is composed of an IL-22-binding chain, IL-22R1 and the IL-10R2 subunit, which is shared with the IL-10R. IL-22 is produced by activated human T-helper cells and mast cells. A soluble IL-22-binding protein, IL22RBP, encoded by a distinct gene, has been identified. This soluble receptor, which has 34% amino acid identity to the extracellular domain of the IL-22R1, binds IL-22 and antagonizes its functional activities (Kotenko et al. 2001b). The skin is also a target for IL-22; high IL-22 expression has been detected in the skin of patients with T-cell-mediated dermatoses. Normal human epidermal keratinocytes express a functional receptor for IL-22 but not for IL-10. IL-22 plays a role in skin inflammatory processes and wound healing.

Interleukin-24

IL-24 (Wang and Liang 2005) is a member of the IL-10 family secreted by activated peripheral blood mononuclear cells and the ligand for two heterodimeric receptors, IL-22R1/IL-20R2 and IL-20R1/IL-20R2. The latter is also a receptor chain for IL-20. Under physiological conditions, the major sources of IL-24 are activated monocytes and Th2 cells, whereas the major IL-24 target tissues, based on the receptor expression pattern, are non-hematopoietic in origin and include skin, lung and reproductive tissues. Structurally and functionally, IL-24 is highly conserved across species. It has shown anti-angiogenic activity and its gene is a tumor suppressor gene (Dent et al. 2010).

Interleukin-26

IL-26 (Donnelly et al. 2010) is part of the IL-10 family and produced by Th17 cells, to some extent in NK cells. It binds to a heterodimeric receptor composed of the IL-20R1 and IL-10R2 chains and is frequently co-expressed with IL17 and IL-22. Targeting epithelial cells that express IL-20R1, IL-26 is likely to play a role in local mechanisms of mucosal and cutaneous immunity. Furthermore, IL-26 appears to play a central role in autoimmune disease.

Interleukin 28A and B and Interleukin 29

Recently, the human genomic sequence for a family of three cytokines, designated IL-28A, IL-28B and IL-29 (Donnelly and Kotenko 2010), that are distantly related to type I IFNs (IFNλ1-3) (Pestka et al. 2004a, b) and the IL-10 family has been described. Like type I IFNs, IL-28 and IL-29 are induced by viral infection and have antiviral activity. However, IL-28 and IL-29 interact with a heterodimeric class II cytokine receptor that consists of the IL-10 receptor II (IL-10R2) and an orphan class 2 receptor chain, designated IL-28R1. This newly described cytokine family may serve as an alternative to type I IFNs in providing resistance to viral infection and antitumor activity.

Interleukin-12 Family

The IL-12 family (Collison et al. 2008) includes IL-12, IL-23, IL-27 and IL-35, consist of mediators of inflammation. Each member is a heterodimeric complex composed of two subunits whose expression is regulated independently (see also IL-23, IL-27 and IL-35 below).

Interleukin-12

IL-12 (Trinchieri 2003) is a 70 kDa heterodimeric proinflammatory cytokine composed of two covalently linked glycosylated chains: p35 and p40. It is mainly produced by activated monocytes, macrophages and dendritic cells DCs), enhances proliferation and cytolytic activity of NK- and T-cells, and stimulates their IFNγ production, towards a Th1 response while it inhibits Th2 cells. Dysregulation of IL-12 production can have a major impact on the modulation of immune and allergic responses. Recombinant IL-12 has several potential therapeutic uses in infectious diseases, allergy, and cancer.

Interleukin-23

IL-23 (Aggarwal et al. 2003) is a heterodimeric cytokine comprising the IL-12 p40 subunit of IL-12 and an IL-23 specific p19 subunit. It is produced by activated dendritic cells and acts on memory CD4+ T-cells. IL-23 induces IL-17 and thus plays an early role in defense against Gram-negative infection. It is also pivotal for establishing and maintaining organ-specific inflammatory autoimmune disease. IL-23 and IL-27 both have potent antitumor activity even against poorly immunogenic tumors using different effector mechanisms.

Interleukin-27

IL-27 (Fabbi et al. 2017) is a pleiotropic two-chain cytokine, composed of EBI3 and IL-27p28 subunits, which is structurally related to both IL-12and IL-6 cytokine families. It acts through a heterodimer receptor consisting of IL-27Rα (WSX1) and gp130 chains. It was initially reported as an immune-enhancing cytokine (Th1-type) acting in concert with IL-12. However, later research outcomes showed that IL-27 displays complex immune-regulatory functions, which may result in either proinflammatory or anti-inflammatory effects. Several pieces of evidence, obtained in preclinical tumor models, indicated that IL-27 has a potent antitumor activity, related not only to the induction of tumor-specific Th1 and cytotoxic T lymphocyte (CTL) responses but also to direct inhibitory effects on tumor cell proliferation, survival, invasiveness, and angiogenic potential. In view of its dual roles, the effects of IL-27 on cancer may also have protumor effects.

Interleukin-35

IL-35 (Collison et al. 2008) is a member of the IL-12 cytokine family, which is linked to the IL-6 cytokine superfamily. The IL-12 family comprises IL-12, IL-23, IL-27 and IL-35. Unlike the other three family members, IL-35 is an anti-inflammatory cytokine produced by regulatory T-cells (T-reg), which are a critical subpopulation of $CD4^+$ T cells essential for maintaining self-tolerance and preventing autoimmunity. IL-35 is a hetero-dimeric protein composed of the IL-12α and IL-27β chains.

Interleukin-17 Family

IL-17 (Iwakura et al. 2011) a homodimeric glycoprotein more recently renamed IL-17A can also form a heterodimer with IL-17F to which it is the most closely related family member. Four additional members IL-17B to IL-17E have been discovered, whereby IL-17E has been renamed IL-25 (see below). IL-17A and IL-17F are predominantly produced upon stimulation of Th17 cells (CD^+ T-helper cells type 17) by IL-23 after induction of differentiation of naive T-cells by IL-6 and TGFβ. IL-17C has a very restricted expression pattern but has been detected in adult prostate and fetal kidney. Aside from their importance in modulating T-cell mediated inflammatory response and effective host defense against pathogen infections, IL-17 s also have a role in the homeostasis of tissues. The IL-17A/F pathway is implicated in the progression of autoimmune diseases such as rheumatoid arthritis, multiple sclerosis, inflammatory bowel disease and psoriasis. Although IL-17A and IL-17F share the highest amino acid sequence homology, they perform distinct functions. IL-17A is involved in the development of autoimmunity, inflammation, and tumors, and also plays important roles in the host defenses against bacterial and fungal infections, whereas IL-17F is mainly involved in mucosal host defense mechanisms. The functions of IL-17B, IL-17C, and IL-17D remain largely elusive. IL-17E (IL-25) is an amplifier of Th2 immune responses.

Interleukin-25

IL-25 (Fort et al. 2001) is a cytokine that shares sequence similarity with IL-17 and was previously called IL-17E. It is produced by Th2-cells, and its biological effects differ markedly from those of the other described IL-17 family members and have been implicated in the promotion of Th2 immunity. IL-25 induces IL-4, -5 and -13 and causes histological changes in the lungs and GI tract, including eosinophilic and mononuclear infiltrates, increased mucus production, and epithelial cell hyperplasia and hypertrophy. IL-25 appears to be a key cytokine for the development of Th2 associated pathologies such as asthma and other allergic reactions, as well as antiparasitic response.

Hematopoietin Family

Because many cytokines are multifunctional and have overlapping activities, several members of the hematopoietin family overlap with other classifications. The hematopoietins (Metcalf 2008) constitute a family of structurally related proteins that includes various interleukins IL-3, IL-4, IL-5, IL-6, IL-9, IL-11 and IL-13, growth factors including G-CSF, GM-CSF, M-CSF and thrombopoietin, erythropoietin, SCF (stem cell factor), SCPF (stem cell proliferation factor) and other proteins identified initially by some biological activities not related to hematopoiesis such as IL-2, IL-12 (see Chap. 24: Haematopoietic Growth Factors).

Interleukin-3

IL-3 (Martinez-Moczygemba and Huston 2003) is produced by activated T cells, monocytes/macrophages and stroma cells. It is a multicolony stimulating, hematopoietic growth factor which stimulates the generation of hematopoietic progenitors of every lineage. Administration of IL-3 produces an increase in erythrocytes, neutrophils, eosinophils, monocytes and platelets. IL-3, however, is not involved in constitutive hematopoiesis but rather in inductive hematopoiesis upon exposure to immunological stress. IL-3 can act synergistically or additively with other hematopoietic growth factors such as GM-CSF, IL-5 and erythropoietin (EPO).

Interleukin-5

IL-5 (Greenfeder et al. 2001) acts as a homodimer originally known as T-cell replacement factor (TRF), eosinophil differentiation factor (EDF) and B-cell growth factor (BCGF) II. It is produced by Th2-helper and mast cells. It acts on the eosinophilic lineage, stimulating eosinophil expansion and chemotaxis and also affects basophils. In humans, IL-5 is a very selective cytokine as only eosinophils and basophils express IL-5 receptors. Interleukin-5 has been associated with the cause of several allergic diseases including allergic rhinitis and asthma and is therefore a target for the treatment of severe asthma.

Interleukin-6

IL-6 (Kamimura et al. 2003) is a proinflammatory cytokine that not only affects the immune system, but also acts in many physiological events in various organs that influence homeostatic processes. It is produced by lymphoid and non-lymphoid cells and was formerly known as interferon-β_2 for its weak antiviral activity. By stimulating hepatocytes to produce "acute phase proteins" it plays a central role in the "acute phase reaction". It is also responsible for the reactive thrombocytosis seen in acute inflammatory processes by stimulating thrombopoietin. Furthermore, IL-6 is associated with insulin resistance in type 2 diabetes mellitus (Kristiansen and Mandrup-Paulsen 2005). Together with IL-11 (below) and IL-27, IL-6 is also a member of the gp130 receptor cytokine family, which also includes other cytokines not classified as interleukins.

Interleukin-11

IL-11 (Du and Williams 1997) initially described as hematopoietic factor with thrombopoietic activity has subsequently been shown to be expressed and active in many other tissues including brain, spinal cord neurons, gut, and testes. IL-11 acts synergistically with other cytokines such as IL-3, -4, -7, -12, -13, SCF and GM-CSF to stimulate various stages and lineages of hematopoiesis. In particular with IL-3 and thrombopoietin (TPO) also termed megakaryocyte growth and development factor (MGDF), it works on various stages of megakaryocytopoiesis and thrombopoiesis. Treatment with IL-11 results in production, differentiation, and maturation of megakaryocytes. IL-11 also has a direct effect on erythroid progenitors and modulates the differentiation and maturation of myeloid progenitor cells. Alveolar and bronchial epithelial cells produce IL-11, which is upregulated by inflammatory cytokines and respiratory syncitial virus (RSV) suggesting that it plays a role in pulmonary inflammation. Moreover, IL-11 is an important regulator of bone metabolism. Evidence indicates that IL-11 together with transforming growth factor (TGF)β, IL-1 and -15 are crucial for successful human implantation and placentation.

■ Interleukin-13

IL-13 (Wills-Karp 2004) is a glycoprotein cloned from activated T-cells. IL-13 was first recognized for its effects on B cells and monocytes, where it upregulated MHC class II expression, promoted IgE class switching and inhibited inflammatory cytokine production. The functions of IL-13 overlap considerably with those of IL-4, especially with regard to changes induced on hematopoietic cells. IL-13 also has several unique effector functions that distinguish it from IL-4. Resistance to most gastrointestinal nematodes is mediated by type-2 cytokine responses, in which IL-13 plays a dominant role. By regulating cell-mediated immunity, IL-13 modulates resistance to intracellular organisms. In the lung, IL-13 is the central mediator of allergic asthma, where it regulates eosinophilic inflammation, mucus secretion, and airway hyperresponsiveness. IL-13 can also inhibit tumor immune-surveillance. Thus, inhibitors of IL-13 might be effective as cancer immunotherapeutics by boosting type-1-associated antitumor defenses. Investigations into the mechanisms that regulate IL-13 production and/or function have shown that IL-4, IL-9, IL-10, IL-12, IL-18, IL-25, IFN-γ, TGF-β, TNF-α, and the IL-4/IL-13 receptor complex are essential for these processes.

■ Others Not (Yet) Assigned to a Family

Interleukin-8

IL-8 (Remick 2005) is a 6–8 kDa CXC chemokine, a potent chemoattractant for neutrophils. It affects the pro-inflammatory effector side, including the stimulation of neutrophil degranulation and the enhancement of neutrophil adherence to endothelial cells. It is produced by monocytes, macrophages, fibroblasts, keratinocytes and endothelial cells. Elevated levels of IL-8 have been found in psoriatic arthritis, synovial fluid and synovium. IL-8 contributes to human cancer progression through its potential functions as a mitogenic, angiogenic, and motogenic factor. Because of the roles that IL-8 plays in favoring tumor progression, several therapeutic strategies are being developed to interfere with its functions (Alfaro et al. 2017).

Interleukin-16

IL-16 (Cruikshank and Little 2008) is a pro-inflammatory cytokine produced by a variety of immune (T-cells, eosinophils, dendritic cells [DCs]) and non-immune (fibroblasts, epithelial and neuronal) cells and induces chemotaxis of not only CD4+ T-cells but also monocyte/macrophages and eosinophils. It is synthesized as a precursor molecule (pro-IL-16), cleaved in the cell cytoplasm and secreted as mature IL-16. It regulates T-cell growth and primes $CD4^{+}$ T cells for IL-2 and IL-15. IL-16 has been shown to play a role in asthma, Crohn's Disease (CD) and systemic lupus erythematosus (SLE). IL-16 also inhibits human (HIV) and simian (SIV) immunodeficiency virus. A neuronal form of IL-16 detected in neurons of the cerebellum and hippocampus has been described.

Interleukin-31

IL-31 (Bilsborough et al. 2006) is a 4-helix bundle cytokine preferentially expressed by activated T-cells with a Th2 bias. Together with IL-4 and IL-13, IL-31 has been implicated in the pathogenesis of atopic dermatitis because they are produced by a subset of T-cells that home to the skin. IL-31 signals through a heterodimeric receptor constitutively expressed by epithelial cells including keratinocytes. IL-31 stimulated keratinocytes induce a whole array of inflammatory chemokines, which also facilitate the recruitment of lymphocytes, monocytes and polymorphonuclear cells to the epidermis.

Interleukin-32

IL-32 (Kim et al. 2005) is a polypeptide, which was described several years ago as natural killer cell transcript 4 (NK4) of activated T-cells and NK-cells and belongs to the pro-inflammatory cytokines. Subsequently it has been detected in higher concentration in patients with sepsis compared to healthy individuals. It was also found to induce the expression of various inflammatory cytokines including TNF-α, IL-6, IL-1β and macrophage inflammatory protein-2 (MIP-2), a chemokine, in different cells via the signal pathway of proinflammatory cytokines. IL-32 is involved in the pathogenesis and progression of inflammatory bowel disease (IBD), gastric inflammation and cancer, rheumatoid arthritis, and chronic obstructive pulmonary disease (COPD). Moreover, it regulates cell growth, metabolism and immune regulation and is therefore involved in the pathology of inflammatory diseases.

Interleukin-34

IL-34 (Lin et al. 2008) forms homodimers and promotes survival and differentiation of monocytes and macrophages. It elicits its activity by binding to the shared (macrophage) colony stimulating factor 1 receptor (CSF-1R). Messenger RNA (mRNA) expression of human IL-34 is found mostly in the spleen but occurs in several other tissues as well: thymus, liver, small intestine, colon, prostate gland, lung, heart, brain, kidney, testes, and ovary. IL 34 also plays an important role in the regulation of osteoclast proliferation and differentiation, and in the regulation of bone resorption (Baud'huin et al. 2010).

THERAPEUTIC USE OF RECOMBINANT INTERFERONS

■ IFNα Therapeutics

Together with recombinant human insulin and growth hormone, recombinant IFNα was one of the first rDNA-derived pharmaceuticals. The drive to produce recombinant interferon and other rDNA-derived pharmaceuticals developed from the need to obtain large amounts of a well defined, purified protein for large-scale therapeutic use (Pestka 1981a, 1981b, 1986). Availability of the necessary basic technologies (see Chaps. 1 and 2) made this possible. Starting in the early 1980s, a number of cytokines produced by recombinant gene technology were developed to become innovative therapeutic modalities called biologicals or biopharmaceuticals. Table 27.3 summarizes the recombinant IFNs approved for therapeutic use.

Interferon alfa-2 (a modified generic name for IFNα2) was developed independently by Hoffmann-LaRoche Ltd. (Interferon alfa-2a; Roferon®A) and Schering Plough Corporation (Interferon alfa-2b; Intron®A). Both were obtained by recombinant DNA technology in *E. coli*, consist of 165 amino acids with an approximate molecular weight of 19 kDa and differ by one amino acid in position 23: Lys for interferon alfa-2a and Arg for interferon alfa-2b (Pestka 1986). For all practical purposes there is no difference between these two products in terms of pharmacological properties or clinical application.

The metabolism of interferon alfa-2a is consistent with that of alfa interferons in general and is therefore used as example. Alfa interferons are totally filtered through the glomeruli and undergo rapid proteolytic degradation during tubular reabsorption (see Chap. 6). Liver metabolism and subsequent biliary excretion are considered minor pathways of elimination for alfa interferons. After intramuscular (IM) and subcutaneous (SC) administrations of 36 million international units (MIU), peak serum concentrations range from 1500 to 2580 picograms/milliliter (pg/mL) (mean 2020 pg/mL) at a mean time to peak of 3.8 h and from 1250 to 2320 pg/mL (mean 1730 pg/mL) at a mean time to peak of

Recombinant Interferons	Company	1st Indication	1st approval
Interferon-α			
IFN-α2a produced in *E.coli;* Roferon A®	Hoffmann–La Roche (Basel, Switzerland)	Hairy cell leukemia	1986 (EU and US)
IFN-α2b produced in *E. coli;* Intron® A; Viraferon®; Alfatronol®	Schering-Plough (Kenilworth NJ, USA)	Hairy cell leukemia	1986 (US and EU)
IFN-αcon1, synthetic type I IFN produced in *E. coli;* Infergen®	Amgen (Thousand Oaks, US), Yamanouchi Europe (Leiderdorp, The Netherlands, EU)	Chronic hepatitis C	2001 (US)
Interferon-β			
IFN-β1a produced in CHO cells; Rebif®	Serono (Geneva, Switzerland)	Relapsing/remitting multiple sclerosis	1998 (EU) 2002 (US)
IFN-β1a produced in CHO cells; Avonex®	Biogen (Cambridge, MA, USA)	Relapsing/remitting multiple sclerosis	1997 (EU), 1996 (US)
IFN-β1b Cys17 Ser substitution; produced in *E. coli*; Betaferon®	Schering AG (Berlin, Germany)	Relapsing/remitting multiple sclerosis	1995 (EU)
IFN-β1b, Cys17 Ser substitution; produced in *E. coli*; Betaseron®	Berlex Labs/Chiron (Richmond/Emeryville, CA, USA)	Relapsing/remitting multiple sclerosis	1993 (US)
Interferon-γ			
Actimmune® (IFN-γ1b; produced in *E. coli*)	Genentech (San Francisco CA, USA), InterMune (Palo Alto, CA, USA)	Chronic granulomatous disease	1990 (US)

Adapted from *Nature Biotechnology* 2006, 24: 769–776

Table 27.3 ■ Interferons approved as biopharmaceuticals approved in the United States and Europe

7.3 h, respectively. The apparent fraction of the dose absorbed after intramuscular injection is >80%. The pharmacokinetics of interferon alfa-2a after single intramuscular doses to patients with disseminated cancer are similar to those found in healthy volunteers. Dose proportional increases in serum concentrations are observed after single doses up to 198 MIU. There are no changes in the distribution or elimination of interferon alfa-2a during twice daily (0.5–36 MIU), once daily (1–54 MIU), or three times weekly (1–136 MIU) dosing regimens up to 28 days of dosing. At the higher doses multiple IM doses of interferon alfa-2a result in an accumulation of two to four times the serum concentrations seen after a single dose.

Roferon®A and Intron®A are approved for the following indications: chronic hepatitis B and C, Kaposi's sarcoma, renal cell carcinoma, malignant melanoma, carcinoid tumor, multiple myeloma, non-Hodgkin lymphoma, hairy cell leukemia, chronic myelogenous leukemia, thrombocytosis associated with chronic myelogenous leukemia and other myeloproliferative disorders. The approved indications vary depending on company and regulatory policies; for detailed information as well as for the recommended dosing the reader is referred to the respective product information current in their countries.

The adverse event profile for these IFNα products is the same; it is generally more or less well tolerated depending on the dose regimen used and subjectively consists primarily of the "influenza-like symptoms" named as such because they mimic the symptoms of early influenza. This, of course, should come as no surprise as these symptoms are caused by peaks of endogenous interferon stimulated by the influenza virus infection. For a detailed reporting of all adverse events, the reader is referred to the product information for each product.

Given the principle that the toxicity of a given medication may be defined by its peak concentration and by the time it is above a toxic threshold concentration and the efficacy by the time the substance is above the minimal therapeutic level, it would be desirable to obtain a therapeutic regimen that minimizes fluctuations in the range below the toxic and above the therapeutic threshold concentration. A constant therapeutic drug concentration would be an ideal goal. The first step towards that goal, as a proof of concept, was to model a long-acting interferon using an insulin pump to inject patients with chronic hepatitis C with interferon α-2a at predetermined rates per hour for 28 days. A similar study was performed in patients with renal cell carcinoma. These studies indicated that interferon α-2a at a constant dose was indeed better tolerated while showing activity when administered by continuous SC infusion (Carreño et al. 1992, Ludwig et al. 1990). The next step therefore was to develop a new longer acting molecule by attaching several polyethylene glycol (PEG) chains to the native interferon molecule (see section "Engineering IFNs and ILs: A Continuing Story - Pegylation", below.)

Pharmaceutical Formulations and Dosing for Interferon alfa Therapeutics

Roferon® A is supplied as pre-filled syringes containing 3 MIU, 4.5 MIU, 6 MIU or 9 MIU in 0.5 mL, or as cartridges containing 18 MIU per mL for SC injection only, or as vials each containing 3 MIU, 6 MIU, 9 MIU or 36 MIU in 1 mL, or multidose injectable solutions containing 9 MIU (each 0.3 mL contains 3 MIU) or 18 MIU of Interferon α-2a (each mL contains 6 MIU) for SC or IM injection. All presentations are human HSA (human serum albumin)-free liquid formulations with 7.21 mg sodium chloride, 0.2 mg polysorbate 80, 10 mg benzyl alcohol (as a preservative), 0.77 mg ammonium acetate and sterile water for injections.

IntronA® is supplied as vials containing 10 MIU, 15 MIU or 50 MIU as lyophilisate and a vial with 1 mL of diluent for reconstitution containing 20 mg glycine, 2.3 mg sodium phosphate dibasic, 0.55 mg sodium phosphate monobasic and 1.0 mg HSA, or as solution vials containing 10 MIU as single dose, 18 MIU or 25 MIU as multidose with 7.5 mg sodium chloride, 1.8 mg sodium phosphate dibasic, 3 mg sodium phosphate monobasic, 0.1 mg edetate disodium, 0.1 mg polysorbate 80, and 1.5 mg m-cresol as a preservative per mL for SC, IM or intralesional injection, or solution in multidose pens containing 6 doses of 3 MIU, 5 MIU or 10 MIU Interferon α-2b per 0.2 mL and excipents as above for SC injection.

Infergen® (interferon alfacon-1) is a synthetic "consensus" interferon consisting of 166 amino acids and not occurring in nature. It was genetically engineered in *E. coli* by Amgen. The amino acid sequence of the product is derived by comparison of the sequences of several natural interferon-α subtypes and assigning the most frequently observed amino acid in each corresponding position. Infergen® is supplied as single-dose, preservative-free vials containing either 9 μg (0.3 mL) or 15 μg (5 mL) of interferon alfacon-1 for SC injection.

■ IFNβ Therapeutics

Three IFNβ-products (Table 27.3) are marketed worldwide for the treatment of multiple sclerosis: the first was Berlex's Betaseron®, marketed by Schering AG as Betaferon® in Europe. It is Interferon β-1b with 165 amino acids and an approximate molecular weight of 18,500 Da, with a cysteine-17-serine substitution. It is produced in *E. coli*, which was then the standard method. It is non-glycosylated, as without further engineering glycosylation is not possible in the *E. coli* system (see Chap. 4). Independently, Biogen and Serono developed a glycosylated IFNβ-1a produced in Chinese hamster ovary cells. Thus, not only is the amino acid sequence of these IFNβs identical to that of natural fibroblast derived human interferon beta, but they are also glycosylated, each containing a single N-linked complex carbohydrate moiety. The two products are marketed as Avonex® and Rebif®, respectively. All three products are indicated for the treatment of multiple sclerosis.

Glycosylating proteins fundamentally alters their pharmacokinetic and pharmacodynamic properties. The non-glycosylated interferon β-1b ($IFN\beta_{ser17}$) has the expected short circulation time: time to peak concentration (C_{max}) between 1 and 8 h with a mean peak serum interferon concentration of 40 IU/mL after a single SC injection of 0.5 mg (16 MIU). Bioavailability is about 50%. Patients receiving single intravenous (IV) doses up to 2.0 mg (64 MIU) show an increase in serum concentrations, which is dose proportional. Mean terminal elimination half-life values ranged from 8.0 min to 4.3 h. Thrice weekly IV dosing for 2 weeks resulted in no accumulation of IFNβ-1b in sera of patients. Pharmacokinetic parameters after single and multiple IV doses were comparable. Following every other day SC administration of 0.25 mg (8 MIU) IFNβ-1b in healthy volunteers, biologic response marker levels (neopterin, β2-microglobulin, myxovirus resistance protein 1 [MxA protein] and IL-10) increased significantly above baseline for 6 to 12 h after the first dose. Biologic response marker levels peaked between 40 and 124 h and remained elevated above baseline throughout the 7-day (168-h) study.

Glycosylated IFNβ-1a such as Rebif®, on the other hand, is slower to reach C_{max}, with a median of 16 h and the serum elimination half-life is 69 ± 37 h (mean ± SD). In healthy volunteers a single SC injection of 60 μg (~18 MIU) of interferon β-1a resulted in a C_{max} of 5.1 ± 1.7 IU/mL. Following every other day SC injections in healthy volunteers, an increase in AUC of approximately 240% was observed, suggesting that accumulation of IFNβ-1a occurs after repeated administration. Biological response markers (e.g. 2′,5′-oligoadenylate synthetase [2,5′ OAS], neopterin and β_2-microglobulin) are induced by IFNβ-1a following a single SC administration of 60 μg. Intracellular 2′,5′-OAS peaked between 12 and 24 h and β_2-microglobulin and neopterin serum concentrations showed a maximum at approximately 24 to 48 h. All three markers remained elevated for up to 4 days. Administration of 22 μg (6 MIU) IFNβ-1a three times per week inhibited mitogen-induced release of pro-inflammatory cytokines (IFNγ, IL-1, IL-6, TNF-α and TNF-β) by peripheral blood mononuclear cells that, on average, was near double that observed with IFNβ-1a administered once per week at either a 22 (6 MIU) or 66 μg (12 MIU) dose.

Pharmaceutical Formulations and Dosing for Interferon Beta Therapeutics

Betaseron®/Betaferon® is formulated as a sterile powder with a 0.54% sodium chloride solution as diluent. Reconstituted it presents as 0.25 mg (8 MIU of antiviral activity) per mL. The recommended dose is 0.25 mg injected SC every other day.

Avonex® is formulated as a lyophilized powder for IM injection. After reconstitution with the supplied diluent (sterile water for injection) each vial contains

30 μg of IFNβ-1a, 15 mg human serum albumin (HSA), 5.8 mg sodium chloride, 5.7 mg dibasic sodium phosphate and 1.2 mg monobasic sodium phosphate in 1.0 mL at a pH of approximately 7.3, or as a prefilled syringe with a sterile solution for IM injection containing 0.5 mL with 30 μg of interferon β-1a, 0.79 mg sodium acetate trihydrate, 0.25 mg glacial acetic acid, 15.8 mg arginine hydrochloride and 0.025 mg polysorbate 20 in water for injection at a pH of approximately 4.8. The recommended dosage is 30 μg injected IM once a week.

Rebif® is supplied in pre-filled 0.5 mL syringes: each 0.5 mL contains either 22 μg (6 MIU) or 44 μg (12 MIU) of IFNβ-1a, 2 or 4 mg HSA, 27.3 mg mannitol, 0.4 mg sodium acetate, and water for injection. The recommended dosage is 22 micrograms (μg) (6 MIU) given 3 times per week by SC injection. This dose is effective in the majority of patients to delay progression of the disease. Patients with a higher degree of disability EDSS (Kurtzke 1983) of 4 or higher may require a dose of 44 μg (12 MIU) 3 times per week.

The adverse event profile for the three IFNβ is similar to IFNα. It is generally reasonably well tolerated and subjectively again consists primarily of the "influenza-like symptoms". For a detailed reporting of all adverse events, the reader is referred to the product information for each biopharmaceutical.

IFNγ Therapeutics

Actimmune® (recombinant interferon γ-1b; immune IFN) is a single-chain polypeptide containing 140 amino acids. It is produced by genetically engineered *E. coli* containing the DNA encoding the human protein. It is a highly purified sterile solution consisting of non-covalent dimers of two identical 16,465 Da monomers. Actimmune® is slowly absorbed; after IM injection of 100 μg/m^2, a C_{max} of 1.5 ng/mL is reached in approximately 4 h, and after SC injection a C_{max} of 0.6 ng/mL is reached in 7 h. The apparent fraction of dose absorbed is >89%. The mean half-life after IV administration was 38 min and after IM and SC dosing with 100 μg/m^2 were 2.9 and 5.9 h, respectively. Multiple-dose SC pharmacokinetics showed no accumulation of Actimmune® after 12 consecutive daily injections of 100 μg/m^2.

Pharmaceutical Formulations and Dosing for Interferon Gamma Therapeutics

Actimmune® is a solution filled in a single-dose vial for SC injection. Each 0.5 mL contains: 100 μg (2 million IU) of IFNγ-1b, formulated in 20 mg mannitol, 0.36 mg sodium succinate, 0.05 mg polysorbate 20 and sterile water for injection. The dosage for the treatment of patients with chronic granulomatous disease or severe, malignant osteopetrosis is 50 μg/m^2 (1 million IU/m^2) for patients with a body surface area greater than 0.5 m^2 and 1.5 mcg/kg/dose for patients with a body surface area equal to or less than 0.5 m^2.

The adverse event profile of IFNγ is similar to IFNα; it is generally well tolerated and subjectively consists primarily of the "influenza-like symptoms". For a detailed reporting of all adverse events, the reader is referred to the Actimmune® product information.

THERAPEUTIC USE OF RECOMBINANT INTERLEUKINS

In general, the approach to the development of interleukins as a therapeutic modality is even more challenging than for IFNs. Most interleukins are embedded in a regulatory network and so far, the therapeutic use of interleukins has been somewhat disappointing. This was largely due to our lack of understanding of the role of these molecules and of the best way to use them; they are less well studied than IFNs. IL-2, for example, was initially developed by oncologists in the days when "go in fast, hit them hard and get out" was the prevalent strategy. Terms such as maximal tolerated dose (which we called minimal poisonous dose) actually defined the dose at which a given drug was in most cases no longer tolerated. Thus, IL-2 got an undeserved bad reputation. Similar thinking nearly killed the development of IFNα for the treatment of chronic viral hepatitis and was ultimately the main reason for discontinuing the development of IL-2 in chronic hepatitis B (Pardo et al. 1997, Artillo et al. 1998) and IL-12 in chronic hepatitis B and C (Zeuzem et al. 1999, Carreño et al. 2000, Pockros et al. 2003). In spite of this progress has been made and our understanding of the complexities of such substances and their antagonists is growing. Interleukins currently approved as biopharmaceuticals worldwide are listed in (Table 27.4).

Recombinant interleukins	Company	1st Indication	1st approval
Proleukin® (aldesleukin; IL-2, lacking N-terminal alanine, C125 S substitution, produced in *E. coli*)	Chiron therapeutics (Emeryville, CA)	RCC (renal-cell carcinoma)	1992 (EU and US)
Neumega® (oprelvekin; IL-11, lacking N-terminal proline produced in *E. coli*.)	Genetics Institute (Cambridge, MA) now Pfizer Inc	Prevention of chemo-therapy induced thrombocytopenia	1997 (US)
Kineret® (anakinra; IL-1 receptor antagonist (produced in *E. coli*)	Amgen (Thousand Oaks, CA)	RA (rheumatoid arthritis)	2001 (US)

Adapted from *Nature Biotechnology* 2006, 24: 769–776

Table 27.4 Interleukins approved as biopharmaceuticals worldwide

Aldesleukin

Proleukin® (aldesleukin), a non-glycosylated human recombinant interleukin-2 product, is a highly purified protein with a molecular weight of approximately 15 kDa. The chemical name is des-alanyl-1, serine-125 human interleukin-2. It is produced by recombinant DNA technology using a genetically engineered *E. coli* containing an analog of the human interleukin-2 gene. The modified human IL-2 gene encodes a modified human IL-2 differing from the native form: the molecule has no N-terminal alanine; the codon for this amino acid was deleted during the genetic engineering procedure; moreover, serine was substituted for cysteine at amino acid position 125. Aldesleukin exists as biologically active, non-covalently bound microaggregates with an average size of 27 recombinant interleukin-2 molecules. The pharmacokinetic profile of aldesleukin is characterized by high plasma concentrations following a short IV infusion, rapid distribution into the extravascular space and elimination from the body by metabolism in the kidneys with little or no bioactive protein excreted in the urine. Studies of aldesleukin administered IV indicate that upon completion of infusion, approximately 30% of the administered dose is detectable in plasma. Observed serum levels are dose proportional. The distribution and elimination half-life after a 5-min IV infusion are 13 and 85 min, respectively. In humans and animals, aldesleukin is cleared from the circulation by both glomerular filtration and peritubular extraction in the kidney. The rapid clearance of aldesleukin has led to dosage schedules characterized by frequent, short infusions. The adverse event profile of IL-2 is similar to that seen for IFNs and many ILs; it is generally reasonably well tolerated and subjectively consists primarily of the "influenza-like symptoms". For a detailed reporting of all adverse events, rarely severe, and pharmacological properties the reader is referred to the product information for Proleukin®.

Pharmaceutical Formulations and Dosing of Aldesleukin

Proleukin® is supplied as a sterile, lyophilized cake in single-use vials intended for IV injection. After reconstitution with 1.2 mL sterile water for injection, each mL contains 18 million IU (1.1 mg) aldesleukin, 50 mg mannitol and 0.18 mg sodium dodecyl sulfate, without preservatives, buffered with approximately 0.17 mg monobasic and 0.89 mg dibasic sodium phosphate to a pH of 7.5. It is indicated for the treatment of adults with metastatic renal cell carcinoma or metastatic melanoma. Each treatment course consists of two 5-day treatment cycles: 600,000 IU/kg (0.037 mg/kg) are administered every 8 h by a 15-min IV infusion for a maximum of 14 doses. Following 9 days of rest, the schedule is repeated for another 14 doses, or a maximum of 28 doses per course, as tolerated.

Oprelvekin

Neumega® (oprelvekin) a non-glycosylated form of IL-11 is produced in *E. coli* by recombinant DNA technology and consists of a 177 amino acid sequence and a molecular mass of approximately 19 kDa. It differs from the 178 amino acid primary sequence of native IL-11 in lacking the amino-terminal proline residue. It is used as a thrombopoietic growth factor that directly stimulates the proliferation of hematopoietic stem cells and megakaryocyte progenitor cells and induces megakaryocyte maturation resulting in increased platelet production. Pharmacokinetics show a rapid clearance from the serum and distribution to highly perfused organs. The kidneys are the primary route of elimination and little intact product can be found in the urine (see Chap. 6). After injection the C_{max} of 17.4 ± 5.4 ng/mL is reached after 3.2 ± 2.4 hrs (T_{max}) with a half-life of 6.9 ± 1.7 hrs. The absolute bioavailability is >80%. There is no accumulation after multiple doses. Patients with severely impaired renal function show a marked decrease in clearance to 40% of that seen in subjects with normal renal function.

Pharmaceutical Formulations and Dosing of Oprelevkin

Neumega® is supplied as single use vials containing 5 mg of oprelvekin (specific activity approximately 8 x 10^6 U/mg) as a sterile lyophilized powder with 23 mg of glycine, 1.6 mg of dibasic sodium phosphate heptahydrate, and 0.55 mg monobasic sodium phosphate monohydrate. When reconstituted with 1 mL of sterile water for injection, the solution has a pH of 7.0. It is indicated for the prevention of severe thrombocytopenia following myelosuppressive chemotherapy. The recommended dose is 50 µg/kg given once daily by SC injection after a chemotherapy cycle in courses of 10 to 21 days. Platelet counts should be monitored to assess the optimal course of therapy. Treatment beyond 21 days is not recommended. Oprelvekin is generally well tolerated. Reported adverse events, mainly as a consequence of fluid retention, include edema, tachycardia/palpitations, dyspnea, and oral moniliasis. For a detailed reporting of all adverse events, rarely severe, the reader is referred to the product information for Neumega®.

Anakinra

Kineret® (anakinra) is a recombinant, non-glycosylated form of the human interleukin-1 receptor antagonist (IL-1Ra) produced using an *E coli* bacterial expression system. It consists of 153 amino acids, has a molecular weight of 17.3 kDa and differs from native human IL-1Ra in that it has a single methionine residue added to its amino terminus. The absolute bioavailability of Kineret® after a 70 mg SC bolus injection is 95%. C_{max} occurs 3 to 7 h after SC administration at clinically relevant doses (1 to 2 mg/kg) and the half-life ranges from 4 to 6 h. There is no accumulation of Kineret® after daily SC doses for up to 24 weeks. The mean plasma clearance with mild and moderate (creatinine clearance 50-80 mL/min and 30-49 mL/min) renal insufficiency was reduced by 16% and 50%, respectively. In severe renal insufficiency and end stage renal disease (creatinine clearance <30 mL/min), mean plasma clearance declined by 70% and 75%, respectively. Less than 2.5% of the administered dose is removed by hemodialysis or continuous peritoneal dialysis. A dose schedule change should be considered for subjects with severe renal insufficiency or end stage renal disease.

Pharmaceutical Formulations and Dosing of Anakirna

Kineret® is supplied in single use prefilled glass syringes with 27-gauge needles as a sterile, clear, preservative-free solution for daily SC administration. Each prefilled glass syringe contains: 0.67 mL (100 mg) of anakinra in a solution (pH 6.5) containing 1.29 mg sodium citrate, 5.48 mg sodium chloride, 0.12 mg disodium EDTA, and 0.70 mg polysorbate 80 in water for injection. It is indicated for the reduction of signs and symptoms and slowing of the progression of structural damage in moderately to severely active rheumatoid arthritis and can be used alone or in combination with disease-modifying anti-rheumatic drugs (DMARD) other than TNF-blocking agents (see Chap. 26). The recommended dose for the treatment of patients with rheumatoid arthritis is 100 mg/day. Patients with severe renal insufficiency or end stage renal disease should receive 100 mg every other day. Anakinra is generally well tolerated; the most common adverse reaction is injection-site reactions, the most serious adverse reactions neutropenia, particularly when used in combination with TNF-blocking agents, and serious infections. For a detailed reporting of all adverse events, rarely severe, the reader is referred to the product information for Kineret®.

Because all therapeutic interleukins or interleukin-antagonists act by correcting an inadequate immune reaction they have been classified as BRMs.

ENGINEERING IFNS AND ILS: A CONTINUING STORY

Pegylation

Since 1977 it has been known that polyethylene glycol (PEG) conjugated proteins are frequently more effective than their native parent molecule. Our understanding of PEG chemistry and how it affects the behavior of a biopharmaceutical has increased with the number of PEGylated proteins developed as therapeutic agents (Table 27.5 gives some examples). PEG is hydrophilic, inert, nontoxic, non-immunogenic and in its most common form either linear or branched terminated with hydroxyl groups that can be activated to couple to the desired target protein. It has been approved for human administration by mouth, injection, and topical application. Its general structure is:

$$HO-(CH_2CH_2O)_n-CH_2CH_2-OH \text{ bifunctional linear PEG (diol)}$$

For polypeptide modification one hydroxyl group is usually inactivated by conversion to monomethoxy or mPEG, which is monofunctional, i.e., only one hydroxyl group is activated during the PEGylation process, thus avoiding the formation of interprotein (oligomerisation) or intraprotein bridges:

$$CH_3O-(CH_2CH_2O)_n-CH_2CH_2-OH \text{ monofunctional linear mPEG}$$

To couple PEG to molecules such as polypeptides, polysaccharides, polynucleotides or small organic molecules it is necessary to chemically activate it. This is done by preparing a PEG derivative with a functional group chosen according to the desired profile for the final product. In addition to the linear PEGs, branched structures have proven useful for peptide and protein modifications:

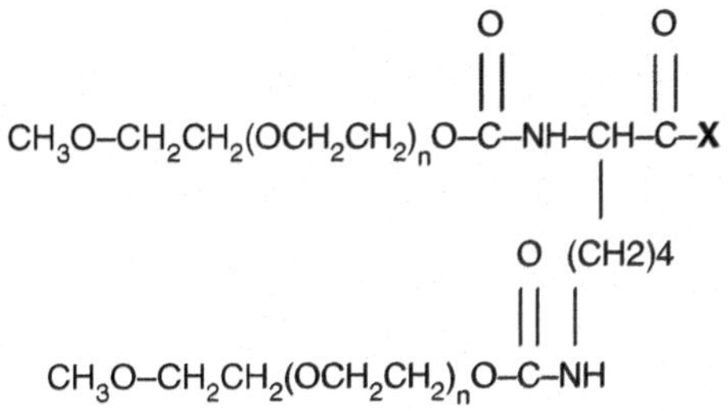

branched PEG

Branched PEG or PEG2 have a number of advantages over linear structures:

- Attached to proteins they'act' much larger than a linear mPEG of the same molecular weight.
- Two PEG chains are added per attachment site, reducing the chance of protein inactivation.
- They are more effective in protecting proteins from proteolysis, reducing antigenicity and immunogenicity.

Depending on the desired use for the PEG-modified molecule different PEGylation strategies can be chosen, for example:

- Multiple shorter chain PEGylation if the biological activity should be preserved.
- A weak PEG-protein bond if a slow release effect is desired.

- A branched chain with high molecular weight and a strong bond if prolonged circulation and receptor saturation is the goal.

Table 27.5 lists the PEGylated interferons approved in the United States and Europe. For a more in-depth review of PEG chemistries and characteristics the interested reader is referred to Roberts et al. 2002 and Bailon et al. 2001.

The development of rhIFNα from the native, unmodified molecule to the PEGylated form with the desired pharmacological profile is an example of how the understanding of PEG chemistry progressed with experience (Zeuzem et al. 2003). Increasing the length of the PEG chain resulted in progressively longer circulating half-life due to protracted resorption and lower clearance, ultimately resulting in a near constant serum concentration over an entire week summarized in Fig. 27.3.

The first PEGylated interferon, IFN alfa-2a, used a linear, 5 kDa mPEG with a weak urethane PEG-IFN alfa-2a link. Clinical trials conducted with this compound were unsuccessful because the blood circulation half-life for the conjugate (Fig. 27.3b) was only slightly improved relative to that of the native protein (Fig. 27.3a) (Wills 1990). Development of the product was therefore halted at Phase II clinical trials (Zeuzem et al. 2003). The second compound was developed by Schering Plough, Kenilworth, NJ in collaboration with Enzon Pharmaceutical Inc., Bridgewater, NJ. It used of a longer (12 kDa), linear PEG with an urethane linkage

PEGylated recombinant interferons	company	1st indication,	1st approval
Pegasys® (PEGylated IFN α-2a produced in *E. coli*)	Hoffman–La Roche (Basel, Switzerland)	Chronic hepatitis B and C	2002 (EU and US)
ViraferonPeg® (PEGylated IFN α-2b produced in *E. coli*)	Schering-Plough (Kenilworth NJ, USA)	Chronic hepatitis C	2000 (EU)
PegIntron® (PEGylated IFN α-2b produced in *E. coli*)	Schering-Plough (Kenilworth NJ, USA)	Chronic hepatitis C	2000 (EU) 2001 (US)

Adapted from *Nature Biotechnology* 2006, 24: 769–776

Table 27.5 ■ PEGylated interferons approved in the United States and Europe

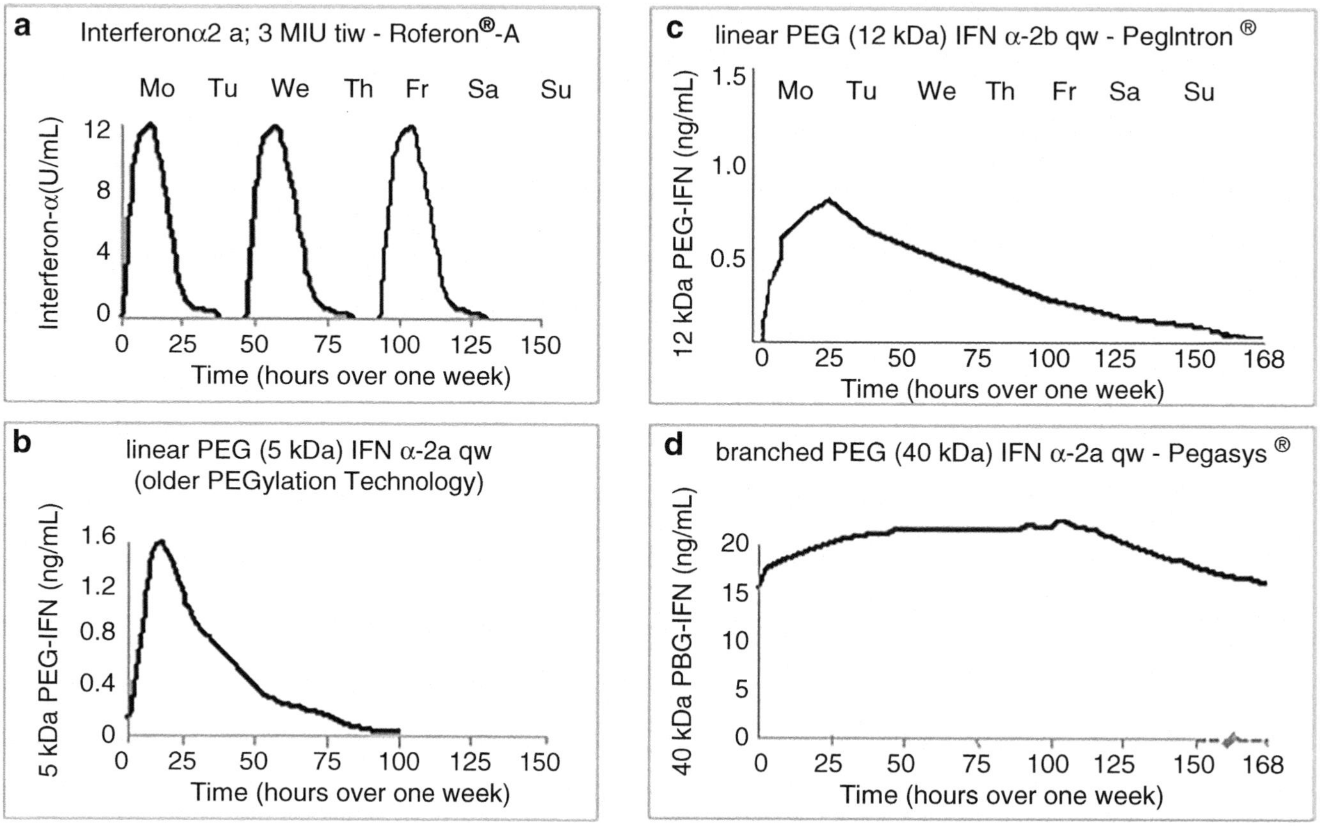

Figure 27.3 ■ Pharmacokinetic Profiles for IFN and PEG-IFN (repeated dosing)

to IFN alfa-2b. The chosen strategy was to combine the advantages of high specific activity with slower serum clearance resulting in PegIntron® (Wang et al. 2002) with markedly improved pharmacological properties allowing once a week administration (Fig. 27.3c) (Glue et al. 2000). PegIntron®, also marketed as Viraferon® in some countries, is approved worldwide for the treatment of chronic hepatitis C.

The development of the third PEGylated interferon, IFN alfa-2a, took a different approach. The strategic goal was to achieve lasting and constant serum concentrations over an entire week. In a collaboration of Roche with Shearwater Polymers in Huntsville, AL, now Nektar; San Carlos, CA, IFNα-2a was linked by a stable amide bond to four different PEG chains of various sizes, structures, and site-attachment numbers. The resulting products were tested for antiviral activity and a variety of pharmacokinetic parameters including half-life, absorption rate, and mean residence time:

- 20-kDa linear mono-PEGIFN alfa-2a,
- 40-kDa linear di-PEGIFN alfa-2a,
- 20-kDa branched mono-PEGIFN alfa-2a
- 40-kDa branched mono-PEGIFN alfa-2a

The 40-kDa, branched PEGylated molecule (later named Pegasys®) exhibited sustained absorption, decreased systemic clearance, and an approximate ten-fold increase in serum half-life over regular interferon. The biological activity was similarly prolonged resulting in an optimal pharmacological profile Fig. 27.3d, (Algranati et al. 1999). It was therefore chosen for further clinical development (Reddy et al. 2002) leading to its approval worldwide for the treatment of chronic hepatitis B and C.

The rapidly growing understanding of the potential of advanced PEGylation chemistry to improve the stability and pharmacological properties of biopharmaceuticals has fostered the development of an increasing number of PEG-biopharmaceuticals. Several of those have proven to offer significant advantages over their native counterparts and found their place in our therapeutic armamentarium. PEG is also used for a variety of other (non-bio) pharmaceutical applications. Table 27.6 lists several examples of different marketed products.

Further Cytokine Engineering

Based on the understanding of the function and limitations of a given therapeutic protein product (TPP) rational protein engineering allows the creation of a new product with improved and expanded activities. Having shown a degree of activity in the treatment of certain cancers, IL-2 is a good example to illustrate this line of thought. Systemic IL-2 (Aldesleukin) treatment has shown significant clinical benefit in a minority of renal cell and melanoma patients, with long term survival in some cases. However, a number of limiting factors have been identified. Its pharmacological properties, short half-life, and its adverse effects, mainly vascular leak syndrome (VLS) with different organ manifestations -a pathophysiological manifestation of acute inflammation- make it difficult to handle. Acute inflammation is a process typical of vascularized tissues whereby interstitial fluid and white blood cells accumulate at the site of injury. Thus, flooding the body with exogenously administered IL-2 can induce a dose dependent "vascular leak

Protein Name	PEGylation	Product name	Reference
IFN α-2a IFN α-2b	Branched, 40 kDa Linear, 12 kDa	Pegasys® PegIntron®	Reddy et al. (2002) Wang et al. (2002)
Interferon β	Linear, 20 kDa	Plegridy® (mPEGIFN β1a)	Biogen PI
Erythropoietin[a]	60 kDa	Mircera® (mPEG epoetinβ)	Schellekens (2006)
G-CSF[a]	Linear, 20 kDa	Neulasta® (pegfilgrastim)	Lyman (2005)
Adenosine deaminase	Linear, 5 kDa	Adagen® (pegademase)	FDA drug label
Arginine deiminase	Linear, 20 kDa	ADI-SS PEG20	Tsai et al. (2017)
Asparaginase	Linear, 5 kDa	Oncaspar®(pegaspargase)	Cao et al. (1990)
rhGH analog[b]	Linear, 5 kDa	Somavert® (pegvisomant)	Ross et al. (2001)
rhFactor VIII[c]	Linear, 40 kDa	Adynovate® (octocog alfa pegol)	Lieuw (2017)
RNA aptamer	40 kDa	Macugen® (pegaptanib)	Ng et al. (2006)

[a]See Chap. 24: hematopoietic growth factors
[b]See Chap. 20: growth hormones
[c]See Chap. 21: recombinant coagulation factors and thrombolytic agents

Table 27.6 ■ Examples of PEGylated (bio)-pharmaceuticals

syndrome" in any vascularized organ. So far, we have been "playing the piano with boxing gloves – now is the time to take off our boxing gloves". What is needed is a possibility to specifically target those cells we wish to impact and only those.

IL-2 has dual properties: one, the ability to expand and activate innate and adaptive effector cells which is the basis of its anticancer activity. Two, to coordinate an immunosuppressive microenvironment by recruiting regulatory T-cells (Tregs) and myeloid derived suppressor cells (MDSCs) as a regulatory mechanism that prevents excessive immune responses and autoimmunity. Unfortunately, the expansion of immune-suppressive Treg cells as well as other immune dysregulation limit or impede IL-2's anticancer activity (Setrerrahmane and Xu 2017).

While PEGylating IL-2 may have resolved the issue of short halflife and ensuing peak toxicity, we are still repeatedly flooding the whole organism with a TPP of known toxicity. With a better understanding of the factors limiting its mechanism of action as well as the structure-function relationship of proteins, rational design and engineering strategies allow adaptation of its beneficial or deleterious (toxic) activity or the creation of new activities.

Reengineering IL-2 by creating a recombinant fusion protein composed of a genetically engineered human monoclonal antibody directed against carcinoembryonic antigen (CEA), i.e. cergutuzumab, linked to an engineered, variant form of interleukin-2 (IL-2v): amunaleukin, with potential immunostimulating and antineoplastic activities (see Chaps. 1, 7, and 9). Upon administration of cergutuzumab amunaleukin (Fig. 27.4), the antibody moiety recognizes and binds to CEA, thereby specifically targeting IL-2v to CEA-expressing tumor tissue. Subsequently, the IL-2v moiety stimulates a local immune response, which activates both natural killer cells and cytotoxic T cells, and eventually leads to tumor cell killing. CEA is a cell surface protein that is expressed on a wide variety of cancer cells. The mutations found in IL-2v inhibit its binding to the IL-2 receptor-alpha (IL-2Rα), which prevents the activation of Treg. However, it can still bind to and induce signaling through the IL-2Rβγ, which allows the preferential expansion of NK cells and CD8-positive T cells. The Fc domain of cergutuzumab has been modified to prevent Fc-gamma binding and downstream cell activation (Klein et al. 2017).

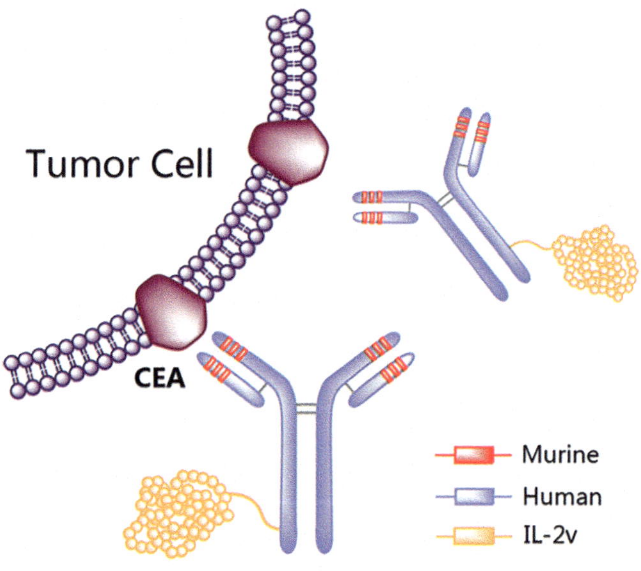

Figure 27.4 Graphic model of the cergutuzumab amunaleukin fusion protein

OUTLOOK AND CONCLUSIONS

There is a very precise and organized order in the intricate function of the immune system to make it work effectively and we are well on our way to map it. But, a lot of hard work still lies ahead. The fundamental approach to cytokine or cytokine antagonist therapy with biopharmaceuticals is to identify diseases caused by insufficient or excessive cytokine production. In the first case, e.g. with certain chronic viral diseases or cancers, appropriate cytokines are used pharmacologically to boost the immune response. Examples include IFNα with antiviral as well as immunomodulatory properties in chronic viral hepatitis, or IL-2 or IL-12 in renal cell cancer and malignant melanoma. For chronic inflammatory or atopic diseases caused by unchecked overproduction of interleukins, two options are available: one can either inhibit the interleukin or its receptor(s), e.g. with human(ized) monoclonal antibodies such as Remicade®, Cinqair®, Nucala®, Sylvant®, Taltz®, Cosentyx®, Humira®, Stelara® or Enbrel® (see Chap. 26) for various indications, or the IL-1R antagonist (Kineret®, see above) in rheumatoid arthritis. Another option would be to downregulate excessively produced interleukin using its antagonistic cytokine, e.g. PEGylated IL-12 in asthma or IL-10 in psoriasis. To date it appears that the first option is more successful than downregulation by anti-inflammatory cytokines, which has so far not resulted in any approved product.

Considering the great potential of cytokines and anti-cytokines, the success stories to-date may appear modest, but they do set the scene. In parallel with the exponential boost of basic knowledge initiated by mastering the tools of biotechnology our understanding of the complex systems we are dealing with has progressed. Diagnostic and therapeutic applications are following closely behind, as well as the capability to monitor the effect of our interventions accurately. As a consequence, an interesting paradigm shift in our approach to many diseases has taken place. Atherosclerosis, psoriasis, insulitis, insulin resistance and asthma as examples for chronic inflammatory diseases in which interleukins and other cytokines play central roles have become therapeutic targets for treatment with biological response modifiers (BRMs). A huge amount of knowledge and experience is available. What is sometimes missing is an integrative view of the many islands of knowledge: "Join the dots to see the greater picture". The tools are there: polymerase chain reaction, genomics, sequencing, cloning, proteomics, microarrays (see Chaps. 1 and 9). Time is an essential factor as we need to learn to recognize potential or established disease in an early stage when intervention is often more effective. Time is, lastly, also a consideration when treating patients, as a beneficial response can require weeks, months, years or a life-time of therapy. There are still issues in need of solutions: how to manage toxicities of mainly the pro-inflammatory cytokines, particularly for their therapeutic use in cancer. Better understanding of the interaction with their receptors, where those receptors are expressed, the dynamics of that expression, and the actions of the cascade their interaction induces. Can we develop a computer model to visualize and help us understand the intricacies of the immune system better? How much can cell and animal models tell us? Can we predict individuals at risk for certain chronic inflammatory diseases or cancer due to allelic variants of interferon-, interleukin- or their receptor-genes? Will gene therapy ultimately displace pharmacological replacement or inhibition of cytokines? Most importantly, can biopharmaceuticals be targeted for better efficacy and less toxicity? New, engineered BRMs with cell specific affinity are a first step in the right direction. They are activated locally when they bind to their receptors and as a consequence can drastically reduce systemic toxicity.

It is no longer visionary to anticipate that proteins will be more extensively engineered in the future. These new "design TPPs" beside showing prolonged half-life, increased target specificity and decreased intrinsic toxicity, will carry neo-sequences not found in nature. The potential risks of immunogenicity will also increase and require immunogenicity risk assessment and mitigation (see also Chap. 7).

SELF-ASSESSMENT QUESTIONS

Questions

Decide whether each of the statements below is true or false. If you believe a statement is false explain why.

1. Interferons are defined:
   (a) by the cell type which produces them,
   (b) by their anti-inflammatory properties,
   (c) by their antiviral activity,
   (d) by their protein structure,
   (e) by their genetic structure.
2. Human interferon alpha:
   (a) is produced selectively by leukocytes
   (b) is a virucidal substance
   (c) triggers antiviral effects in cells expressing appropriate receptors
   (d) acts on the immune system to booster specific antiviral response
   (e) comprises twelve subtypes.
3. Interleukins are characterized by:
   (a) their action on target cells,
   (b) their protein structure,
   (c) their genetic structure,
   (d) pro- or anti-inflammatory effect,
   (e) their cell of origin.
4. The following interleukins are generally considered to be "pro-inflammatory" i.e. induce and/or be part of a Th1 response:
   (a) the IL-1 family, IL-2, -8, -12.
   (b) IL-3.
   (c) IL-4, -5, -9.
   (d) IL-10, -19, -20, -22, -24, -26, -28A, -28B and -29.
   (e) IL-15, -16, -17, -18, -22, -23, and -32.
5. Interleukins are:
   (a) secreted specifically by leukocytes to act on other leukocytes,
   (b) bound to a specific receptor complex to exert their effect,
   (c) a family of proteins which co-regulate the immune response,
   (d) non-toxic products of the body in response to pathogens and other potentially harmful agents,
   (e) long-acting immune modulators.
6. Interferons and interleukins can be toxic, several (patho-) physiological containment mechanisms exist to counteract excessive production:
   (a) soluble receptors,
   (b) binding to cell surface receptors,
   (c) neutralizing antibodies,
   (d) negative feedback mechanisms,
   (e) naturally occurring IL receptor antagonists.
7. The following interferons are used as approved therapy:
   (a) IFNα2,
   (b) IFNβ,
   (c) IFNγ,
   (d) IFNω,
   (e) IFNα8.

   Where appropriate, specify some of the indications they are used for.
8. The following interleukins are approved for therapeutic use:
   (a) IL-1
   (b) IL-2.
   (c) IL-10
   (d) IL-11
   (e) IL-12

Where appropriate, specify some of the indications they are used for.

9. Protein PEGylation:
   (a) prolongs circulation half-life of the PEGylated protein,
   (b) decreases antigenicity of the PEGylated protein,
   (c) protects the protein from proteolysis,
   (d) is difficult due to the toxicity of polyethylene glycol,
   (e) improves the therapeutic efficacy of the PEGylated protein.
10. The following PEGylated IFNs and ILs have been approved for therapeutic use:
    (a) Interferon α2,
    (b) Interferon β,
    (c) Interleukin-1,
    (d) Interleukin-2,
    (e) Interleukin-12.

Answers

1. Interferons are defined:
   a. false. Although IFNα used to be called "leukocyte interferon" and IFNβ "fibroblast interferon" because they were initially produced from buffy coats (leukocytes) infected with Sendai virus and human diploid fibroblasts stimulated with poly(I)-poly(C) or Newcastle disease virus (NDV) respectively, interferons and their Units (IU) are defined by their antiviral activity.
   b. false: while they can act as immune-modulators and on occasion have anti-inflammatory properties (e.g. IFNβ, for the treatment of multiple sclerosis), they will more often induce a Th1 or pro-inflammatory response. IFNγ is one of the classical pro-inflammatory markers.
   c. true.
   d. and e. false. The full protein and genetic sequences of the different interferons and their subtypes were only defined long after the initial crude IFN mixtures had been tested in the clinic initially against viral diseases and subsequently against cancers.

Today however the protein and genetic sequences are necessary to specify an interferon and its purity during the production by biotechnological techniques. Also new interferons or interleukins will be accepted as such by the Human Genome Nomenclature Committee (HGNC) based on their function and a previously unknown genetic sequence.

2. Human interferon alpha:
a. false. Interferon alpha is produced by many cell types, including T-cells and B-cells, macrophages, fibroblasts, endothelial cells and osteoblasts among others.
b. false. By interacting with their specific heterodimeric receptors on the surface of cells, the interferons initiate a broad and varied array of signals that induce antiviral state.
c. true.
d. true.
e. true. See Table 27.2. Each IFNα subtype has a distinct antiviral, antiproliferative, and stimulation of cytotoxic activities of NK and T-cells. To date only one recombinant subtype, IFNα2, has been predominantly used therapeutically.
3. Interleukins are classified according:
a. and e. false. ILs are characterised by their protein and gene structures registered in the HCGN database (and similar centralised databases). Their names and symbols must be approved by the HGNC.
b. true.
c. true.
d. false. While some ILs can be classified as pro- or anti-inflammatory this is not what basically defines them.
4. The following interleukins are generally considered to be "pro-inflammatory" i.e. induce and/or be part of a Th1 response:
a. true.
b. false. IL-3 is a multicolony stimulating, hematopoietic growth factor which stimulates the generation of hematopoietic progenitors of every lineage.
c. false. These three interleukins all play a role in the differentiation and activation of basophils and eosinophils leading to a Th2 response.
d. false. These interleukins are all part of the IL-10 family. However IL-10,-19, and -20 are "anti-inflammatory", IL-22, -24, -26, -28A, -28B and -29 are considered "pro-inflammatory".
e. true.
5. Interleukins are:
a. false. Interleukins are mainly secreted by leukocytes and primarily affecting growth and differentiation of hematopoietic and immune cells. They are also produced by other normal and malignant cells and are of central importance in the regulation of hematopoiesis, immunity, inflammation, tissue remodeling, and embryonic development.
b. true.
c. true.
d. false. Many interleukins, primarily those with pro-inflammatory function, are intrinsically toxic either directly or indirectly, i.e. through induction of toxic gene products.
e. false. Interleukins usually have a short circulation time, and their production is regulated by positive and negative feedback loops.
6. Interferons and interleukins can be toxic, several (patho-) physiological containment mechanisms exist to counteract excessive production.

a. true.
b. false. Binding to cell surface receptor is a physiological process and has negligible effect on "circulating" interferons or interleukins.
c. to e. are true.
7. The following interferons are used as approved therapy.
a. true. IFNα (Roferon® A, IntronA®, Infergen®) are indicated for the treatment of chronic hepatitis B and C, Kaposi's sarcoma, renal cell carcinoma, malignant melanoma, carcinoid tumor, multiple myeloma, non-Hodgkin lymphoma, hairy cell leukemia, chronic myelogenous leukemia, thrombocytosis associated with chronic myelogenous leukemia, and other myeloproliferative disorders.
b. true. IFNβ (Betaseron®, Betaferon®, Avonex®, Rebif®) are indicated for the treatment of multiple sclerosis.
c. true. IFNγ (Actimmune®) is indicated for the treatment of chronic granulomatous disease, severe, malignant osteopetrosis.
d. false. IFNω has only been studied in vitro and in the nude mouse model where it has shown anticancer activity against several tumor cell lines and transplants.
e. false. IFNα8 has only been studied in various cell lines where it has consistently shown the most powerful antiviral effect of the subtypes tested.
8. The following interleukins are approved for therapeutic use:
a. true. An IL-1 analog/antagonist (Kineret®) is indicated for the treatment of rheumatoid arthritis.
b. true. IL-2 (Proleukin®) is indicated for the treatment of adults with metastatic renal cell carcinoma or metastatic melanoma.
c. false. Clinical development IL-10 (Tenovil™) as an anti-inflammatory drug for several indications such as: psoriasis, Crohn's disease, rheumatoid arthritis was discontinued in phase III due to insufficient efficacy to warrant further development.
d. true. IL-11 (Neumega®) is indicated for the prevention of severe thrombocytopenia following myelosuppressive chemotherapy.
e. false. Early clinical trials have been performed in patients with chronic hepatitis C. The programme was, however, discontinued in early phase II due to toxicity.
9. Protein PEGylation:
a. true.
b. true.
c. true.
d. false. PEG is inert, nontoxic, non-immunogenic and in its most common form either linear or branched terminated with hydroxyl groups that can be activated to couple to the desired target protein.
e. true.
10. The following PEGylated IFNs and ILs have been approved for therapeutic use:
a. true: for chronic hepatitis C and B. Limited clinical trials have also been conducted in renal cell carcinoma, malignant melanoma and non-Hodgkin lymphoma.
b. c. d. and e. are false although early clinical trials have been conducted with PEGylated IL-2 in RCC and malignant melanoma and pharmacokinetic studies with PEGylated IFNβ in animal models.

REFERENCES

Aggarwal S, Ghilardi N, Xie M-H et al (2003) Interleukin-23 promotes a distinct CD4 T cell activation state characterised by the production of IL-17. J Biol Chem 278:1910–1914

Akdis M, Aab A, Altunbilakli C et al (2016) Interleukins (from IL-1 to IL-38), interferons, transforming growth factor β, and TNF-α: receptors, functions, and roles in diseases. J Allergy Clin Immunol 138(4):984–1010

Alfaro C, Sanmamed MF, Rodriguez ME et al (2017) Interleukin-8 in cancer pathogenesis, treatment and follow-up. Cancer Treat Rev 60:24–31

Algranati NE, Sy S, Modi M (1999) A branched methoxy 40-kDa polyethylene glycol (PEG) moiety optimizes the pharmacokinetics of peginterferon alpha-2a (PEG-IFN) and may explain its enhanced efficacy in chronic hepatitis C. Hepatology 40:190A

Artillo S, Pastore G, Alberti A et al (1998) Double-blind, randomized controlled trial of interleukin-2 for the treatment of chronic hepatitis B. J Med Virol 54:167–172

AzumaYT,MatsuoY,KuwamuraM,YancopoulosGD,Valenzuela DM,MurphyAJ,NakajimaH,KarowM,TakeuchiT(2010) Interleukin-19 protects mice from innate-mediated colonic inflammation. Inflammatory Bowel Disease 16(6):1017–1028

Baud'huin M, Renault R, Charrier C et al (2010) Interleukin-34 is expressed by giant cell tumours of bone and plays a key role in RANKL-induced osteoclastogenesis. J Pathol 221:77–86

Bilsborough J, Leung DYM, Maurer M et al (2006) IL-31 is associated with cutaneous lymphocyte antigen-positive skin homing T cells in patients with atopic dermatitis. J Allergy Clin Immunol 117:418–425

Cao SG, Zhao QY, Ding ZT et al (1990) Chemical modification of enzyme molecules to improve their characteristics. Ann N Y Acad Sci 613:460–467

Carreño V, Zeuzem S, Hopf U et al (2000) A phase I/II study of recombinant human interleukin-12 in patients with chronic hepatitis B. J Hepatol 32:317–324

Carreño V, Tapia L, Ryff JC et al (1992) Treatment of chronic hepatitis C by continuous subcutaneous infusion of interferon-alpha. J Med Virol 37:215–219

Collison LW, Workman CJ, Kuo TT, Boyd K, Wang Y, Vignali KM, Cross R, Sehy D, Costelloe C, Watson M, Murphy A, McQuillan K, Loscher C, Armstrong ME, Garlanda C, Mantovani A, O'Neill LA, Mills KH, Lynch MA (2008) IL-1F5 mediates anti-inflammatory activity in the brain through induction of IL-4 following interaction with SIGIRR/TIR8. J Neurochem 105(5):1960–1969

Cruikshank WW, Little F (2008) Interleukin-16: the ins and outs of regulating T-cell activation. Crit Rev Immunol 28(6):467–483

Dent P, Yacoub A, Hamed HA et al (2010) The development of MDA-7/IL-24 as a cancer therapeutic. Pharmacol Ther 128(2):375–384

Donnelly RP, Sheikh F, Dickensheets H, Savan R, Young HA, Walter MR (2010) Interleukin-26: an IL-10 related cytokine produced by Th-17 cells. Cytokine Growth Factor Rev 21(5):393–401

Donnelly RP, Kotenko SV (2010) Interferon-lambda: a new addition to an old family. J Interf Cytok Res 30(8):555–564

Du X, Williams DA (1997) Interleukin-11: review of molecular, cell biology, and clinical use. Blood 89:3897–3908

ExPASy. http://au.expasy.org/uniprot/Q9UBH0—(Expert Protein Analysis System) proteomics server of the Swiss Institute of Bioinformatics (SIB)

Fabbi M, Carbotti G, Ferrini S (2017) Dual roles of IL-27 in cancer biology and immunotherapy. Mediators Inflamm. Article ID 3958069, p 14. https://doi.org/10.1155/2017/3958069

Fort MM, Cheung J, Yen D et al (2001) IL-25 induces IL-4, IL-5, and IL-13 and Th2-associated pathologies in vivo. Immunity 15:985–995

Fry TJ, Mackall CL (2002) Interleukin-7: from bench to clinic. Blood 99:3892–3904

Garlanda C, Dinarello CA, Mantovani A (2013) Interleukin-1 family: back to the future. Immunity 39(6):1003–1018

Gilmour J, Lavender P (2008) Control of IL-4 expression in T-helper 1 and 2 cells. Immunology 124:437–444

Glue P, Fang JWS, Rouzier-Panis R et al (2000) Pegylated interferon-α2b: pharmacokinetics, pharmacodynamics, safety, and preliminary efficacy data. Clin Pharm Ther 68:556–567

Greenfeder S, Umland SP, Cuss FM et al (2001) Th2 cytokines and asthma: the role of interleukin-5 in allergic eosinophilic disease. Respir Res 2:71–79

HGNC. www.gene.ucl.ac.uk/nomenclature/—Gene families and grouping—Interferons (IFN)—Interleukins and interleukin receptor genes (IL)

Iwakura Y, Ishigame H, Saijo S, Nakae S (2011) Functional specialization of Interleukin-17 family members. Immunity 34:149–162

Kamimura D, Ishihara K, Hirano T (2003) IL-6 signal transduction and its physiological roles: the signal orchestration model. Rev Physio Biochem Parmacol 149:1–38

Kim S-H, Han S-Y, Azam T et al (2005) Interleukin 32: a cytokine and inducer of TNFα. Immunity 22:131–142

Klein C, Waldhauera I, Nicolinia VG et al (2017) Cergutuzumab amunaleukin (CEA-IL2v), a CEA-targeted IL-2 variant-based immunocytokine for combination cancer immunotherapy: overcoming limitations of aldesleukin and conventional IL-2-based immunocytokines. Oncoimmunology 6(3):15. https://doi.org/10.1080/2162402X.2016.1277306

Kotenko SV, Izotova LS, Mirochnitchenko OV et al (2001a) Identification of the functional IL-TIF (IL-22) receptor complex: the IL-10R2 chain (IL-10Rβ) is a common chain of both IL-10 and IL-TIF (IL-22) receptor complexes. J Biol Chem 276:2725–2732

Kotenko SV, Izotova LS, Mirochnitchenko OV et al (2001b) Identification, cloning and characterization of a novel soluble receptor which binds IL-22, and neutralizes its activity. J Immunol 166:7096–7103

Kristiansen OF, Mandrup-Paulsen T (2005) Interleukin-6 and diabetes: the good, the bad or the indifferent. Diabetes 54(Suppl 2):S114–S124

Kurtzke JF (1983) Rating neurologic impairment in multiple sclerosis: an expanded disability status scale (EDSS). Neurology 33:1444–1452

Liao W, Lin JX, Leonard WJ (2011) IL-2 family cytokines: new insights into the complex roles of IL-2 as a broad regulator of T helper cell differentiation. Curr Opin Immunol 23(5):598–604

Lieuw K (2017) Many factor VIII products available in the treatment of hemophilia A: an embarrassment of riches? J Blood Med 8:67–73

Lin H, Lee E, Hestir K et al (2008) Discovery of a cytokine and its receptor by functional screening of the extracellular proteome. Science 320(5877):807–811

Liu B, Nivick D, Kim SH, Rubinstein M (2000) Production of a biologically active human interleukin 18 requires its prior synthesis as PRO-IL-18. Cytokine 12(10):1519–1525

Ludwig CU, Ludwig-Habemann R, Obrist R et al (1990) Improved tolerance of interferon alpha-2a by continuous subcutaneous infusion. Onkologie 13:117–122

Lyman GH (2005) Pegfilgrastim: a granulocyte colony-stimulating factor with sustained duration of action. Expert Opin Biol Ther 5:1635–1646

Malek TR, Castro I (2010) Interleukin-2 receptor signaling: at the interface between tolerance and immunity. Immunity 33(2):153–165

Marrakchi S, Guigue P, Renshaw BL et al (2011) Interleukin-36–receptor antagonist deficiency and generalized Pustular psoriasis. N Engl J Med 365:620–628

Martinez-Moczygemba M, Huston DP (2003) Biology of common beta receptor-signalling cytokines: IL-3, IL-5 and GM-CSF. J Allergy Clin Immunol 112(4):653–665

Metcalf D (2008) Hematopoietic Cytokines. Blood 111(2):485–491

Ng EWM, Shima DT, Calias P et al (2006) Pegaptanib, a targeted anti-VEGF aptamer for ocular vascular disease. Nat Rev 5:123–132

Noelle RJ, Nowak EC (2010) Cellular source and immune functions of interleukin-9. Nat Rev 10:683–687

Nold MF, Nold-Petry CA, Zepp JA, Palmer BE, Bufler P, Dinarello CA (2010) IL-37 is a fundamental inhibitor of innate immunity. Nat Immunol 11:1014–1022

Pardo M, Castillo I, Oliva H et al (1997) A pilot study of recombinant interleukin-2 for treatment of chronic hepatitis C. Hepatology 26(5):1318–1321

Platanias L (2005) Mechanism of type I- and type II-interferon mediated signaling. Nat Rev Immunol 5:375–386

Pockros P, Patel K, O'Brien CB (2003) A multicenter study of recombinant human interleukin-12 for the treatment of chronic hepatitis C infection in patients with non-responsiveness to previous therapy. Hepatology 37:1368–1374

Reddy KR, Modi WM, Pedder S (2002) Use of peginterferon alfa-2a (40 KD) (Pegasys®) for the treatment of hepatitis C. Adv Drug Deliv Rev 54:571–586

Remick DG (2005) Interleukin-8. Crit Care Med 33(Suppl):S466–S467

Ross RJM, Leung KC, Maamra M et al (2001) Binding and functional studies with the growth hormone receptor antagonist, B2036-PEG (Pegvisomant), reveal effects of pegylation and evidence that it binds to a receptor dimer. J Clin Endocrinol Metab 86:1716–1723

Ryff JC (1996) Both cytokines and their antagonists have a place in clinical medicine. Eur Cytokine Netw 7:437. Abstract 40

Schellekens H (2006) Erythropiesis-stimulating agents—present and future. European Endocrine Review Touch Briefings Publishers, Business Briefing

Schmitz J, Owyang A, Oldham E et al (2005) IL-33, an Interleukin-1-like cytokine that signals via the IL-1 receptor-related protein ST2 and induces T helper type 2-associated cytokines. Immunity 23:479–490

Setrerrahmane S, Xu H (2017) Tumor-related interleukins: old validated targets for new anti-cancer drug development. Mol Cancer 16:153–170

Steinman L (2007) A brief history of TH17, the first major revision in the TH1/TH2 hypothesis of T cell-mediated tissue damage. Nat Med 13(2):139–145

Towne JE, Garka KE, Renshaw BR, Virca GD, Sims JE (2004) Interleukin (IL)-F6m IL-1F8, and IL-1F9 signal through IL-Rrp2 and IL-1RacP to activate the pathway leading to NF-κB and MAPKs. J Biol Chem 279:13677–13688

Towne JE, Blair R, Renshaw BR, Douangpanya J, Lipsky BP, Shen M, Gabel CA, John E, Sims JE (2011) Interleukin-36 (IL-36) ligands require processing for full agonist (IL-36α, IL-36β and IL-36γ) or antagonist (IL-36Ra) activity. J Biol Chem 286:42594–42602

Trinchieri G (2003) Interleukin-12 and the regulation of innate resistance and adaptive immunity – review. Nat Rev Immunol 3:133–146

Trøseid M, Seljeflot I, Amesen H (2010) The role of interleukin-18 in the metabolic syndrome. Cardiovasc Diabetol 9:11–19

Tsai H-J, Jiang SS, Hung W-C et al (2017) A phase II study of arginine Deiminase (ADI-PEG20) in relapsed/refractory or poor-risk acute myeloid leukemia patients. Sci Rep 7:11253. https://doi.org/10.1038/s41598-017-10542-4

Waldmann TA (2015) The shared and contrasting roles of interleukin-2 (IL-2) and interleukin in the life and death of normal and neoplastic lymphocytes: implications for cancer therapy. Cancer Immunol Res 3(3):219–227

Wang M, Liang P (2005) Interleukin-24 and its receptors. Immunology 114:166–170

Wang YS, Youngster S, Grace M, Bausch J, Bordens R, Wyss DF (2002) Structural and biological characterization of pegylated recombinant interferon alpha-2b and its therapeutic implications. Adv Drug Deliv Rev. 54(4):547–570

Wills RJ (1990) Clinical pharmacokinetics of interferons. Clin Pharmacokinet 19:390–399

Wills-Karp M (2004) Interleukin-13 in asthma pathogenesis. Immunol Rev 202:175–190

Xu W (2004) Interleukin-20. Int Immunopharmacol 4:527–633

Yi JS, Cox MA, Zajac AJ (2010) Interleukin-21: A multifunctional Regulator of Immunity to Infections. Microbes Infect 12(14–15):1111–1119

Yuan X, Peng X, Li Y and Li M (2015) Role of IL-38 and its related cytokines in inflammation. Mediators Inflamm. Article ID 807976, p 7. https://doi.org/10.1155/2015/807976

Zeuzem S, Hopf U, Carreño V et al (1999) A phase I/II study of recombinant human interleukin-12 in patients with chronic hepatitis C. Hepatology 29:1280–1286

Zeuzem S, Welsch C, Herrmann E (2003) Pharmacokinetics of Peginterferons. Semin Liver Dis 23(Suppl 1):23–28

SUGGESTED READING[1]

INTERFERONS

Meager A (2006) The interferons: characterization and application. Wiley, Weinheim. ISBN:3-527-31180-7

Pestka S, Krause CD, Walter M (2004a) Interferons, interferon-like cytokines, and their receptors. Immunol Rev 202:8–32

Pestka S (1981a) Interferons. In: Pestka S (ed) Methods in enzymology, vol 78. Academic, New York, p 632

Pestka S (1981b) Interferons. In: Pestka S (ed) Methods in enzymology, vol 79. Academic, New York, p 677

Pestka S (1986) Interferons. In: Pestka S (ed) Methods in enzymology, vol 119. Academic, New York, p 845

Special Issue (2005) The neoclassical pathways of interferon signaling. J Interferon Cytokine Res 25:731–811

INTERLEUKINS

Pestka S, Krause CD, Sarkar C (2004b) IL-10 and related cytokines and receptors. Ann Rev Immunol 22:929–979

Sigal LH (2004) Interleukins of current clinical relevance (part I). J Clin Rheumatol 10:353–359

Sigal LH (2004) Interleukins of current clinical relevance (part II). J Clin Rheumatol 11:34–39

PEGYLATION

Bailon P, Palleroni A, Schaffer CA et al (2001) Rational design of a potent, long-lasting form of interferon: a 40 kDa branched polyethylene glycole conjugated interferon α-2a for the treatment of hepatitis C. Bioconjugate Chem 12:195–202

Roberts MJ, Bentley MD, Harris JM (2002) Chemistry for peptide and protein PEGylation. Adv Drug Deliv Rev 54:459–476

[1] Reviews that summarize the referenced subject in more detail.

Index

D. J. A. Crommelin et al. (eds.), *Pharmaceutical Biotechnology*, https://doi.org/10.1007/978-3-030-00710-2

Printed by Printforce, the Netherlands